Endotherapy in Biliopancreatic Diseases: ERCP Meets EUS

Massimiliano Mutignani • Jörg G. Albert
Carlo Fabbri
Editors

Endotherapy in Biliopancreatic Diseases: ERCP Meets EUS

Two Techniques for One Vision

Springer

Editors
Massimiliano Mutignani
Digestive and Interventional
Endoscopy Unit
Grande Ospedale Metropolitano
Niguarda
Piazza dell'Ospedale Maggiore, Milano
Italy

Jörg G. Albert
Hepatologie und Endokrinologie
Abteilung für Gastroenterologie,
Robert-Bosch-Krankenhaus
Auerbachstraße, Stuttgart
Germany

Carlo Fabbri
Department of Gastroenterology
Azienda USL di Forlì-Cesena
Bologna
Italy

ISBN 978-3-030-42571-5 ISBN 978-3-030-42569-2 (eBook)
https://doi.org/10.1007/978-3-030-42569-2

This Springer imprint is published by the registered company Springer Nature Switzerland AG
The registered company address is: Gewerbestrasse 11, 6330 Cham, Switzerland

To Marilena, Elena and Lucrezia who support me with love in my daily commitment

—Massimiliano Mutignani

Foreword

Biliopancreatic endoscopy described in this collaborative book has very little to do with the one I have learned in the early 1980s. Thanks to the extraordinary improvements in technologies and techniques, and to the marriage of ERCP with therapeutic EUS, biliopancreatic endoscopy has become today the first-line treatment for an impressive number of clinical scenarios involving the liver, the pancreas and the biliopancreatic ductal system.

While ERCP, thanks to the advent and development of non-invasive cross-sectional imaging techniques, has currently become almost exclusively a therapeutic tool, for some decades after its introduction EUS has been mostly used as a diagnostic technique. Only recently, especially thanks to the development of lumen-apposing metal stents, and to the improvement of EUS-guided needles and devices for local tissue ablation, EUS has permanently joined and integrated ERCP in the operative treatment of several biliopancreatic diseases. I believe that this "marriage" has no chances to experience a "divorce" in the next decades, but we are still in the phase where we try to understand *which* technique is better for the particular indication and *when*. By *whom* we already know: more and more the protagonist will be the same physician, trained in both ERCP and therapeutic EUS. We are not yet completely there because training in ERCP and EUS needs at least one additional year (if not two!) after completion of the regular post-graduate training in gastroenterology or surgery, and this is not structured in most countries. The hope is that this issue will be considered and solved in the appropriate way very soon.

The authors of this book have to be commended because they have embraced this modern concept of complementarity between ERCP and EUS providing a comprehensive overview of the current available endoscopic techniques in biliopancreatic diseases, also by entrusting several chapters to very well-known experts in the field.

The last part of the book, which is dedicated to therapeutic algorithms, is an original and extremely useful tool for all those clinicians involved in the management of biliopancreatic diseases.

Finally, I would like to emphasize my personal gratification in seeing Massimiliano Mutignani as leading author of this book: Max has been my first trainee when he was a student and then for many years my principal co-worker. This book certifies the outstanding position he has been able to reach in the world of therapeutic endoscopy.

Guido Costamagna
Digestive Endoscopy Unit
Department of Translational Medicine and Surgery
Fondazione Policlinico Universitario A. Gemelli—IRCCS
Università Cattolica S. Cuore
Rome, Italy

The dedication content has been translated correctly in the updated proof.

Acknowledgement

A special thanks by the editors to Dr. Lorenzo Dioscoridi. Without his perseverance and "self-sacrifice", this book would not be released.

Contents

Part I

ERCP and EUS: Armamentarium and Surroundings

1 ERCP/EUS Room

Rita Conigliaro, Claudio Conti, Giuseppe Grande, and Helga Bertani

1.1 ERCP Room

1.1.1 Introduction

Endoscopic retrograde cholangiopancreatography (ERCP) is still one of the most technically demanding and practically challenger of endoscopic procedure.

Born as a diagnostic investigation, it is now a therapeutic modality and now plays a major role in biliopancreatic diseases.

Many patients requiring ERCP are elderly and fragile, and the surgical therapy could be often risky. Demand for endoscopic therapy today is about 800 per year for 750,000 users; therefore, every large or provincial hospital could be able to provide this service.

The benefits to the patient in terms of efficacy and safety are high, but the converse is also true that poor technique and skill expose the patient to complications and failures and, in turn, becomes more risky than surgery.

Therefore, nowadays, the location and the environment are particularly important because, together with the technology, they must meet the minimum quality standards.

1.2 Some Definitions

Invasive procedure is defined as a procedure that penetrates the protective surfaces of a patient's body (e.g., skin or mucous membranes), is performed in a surgical field, generally requires entry into a body cavity, and may involve insertion of an indwelling foreign body.

Procedures performed through orifices normally colonized with bacteria do not involve an incision of the skin.

Procedure room is defined as a room for the performance of procedures that do not require an aseptic field but may require use of sterile instruments or supplies. Procedure rooms are considered unrestricted areas. Local anesthesia and minimal and moderate sedation may be administered in a procedure room, but anesthetic agents used in procedure rooms must not require special ventilation or scavenging equipment.

1.3 The Room

The ERCP room is equivalent to an operating theater, and the international reference legislation is that of operating theaters.

R. Conigliaro (✉) · G. Grande · H. Bertani
Gastroenterology and Digestive Endoscopy Unit, Civil and University Hospital, Modena, Italy
e-mail: r.conigliaro@ausl.mo.it

C. Conti
Clinical Engineering Institute, Civil and University Hospital, Modena, Italy

M. Mutignani et al. (eds.), *Endotherapy in Biliopancreatic Diseases: ERCP Meets EUS*,
https://doi.org/10.1007/978-3-030-42569-2_1

An operating room (OR) is defined as a room in the surgical suite that meets the requirements of a restricted area and is designated and equipped for performing surgical operations or other invasive procedures that require an aseptic field. Any form of anesthesia may be administered in an OR as long as appropriate anesthesia gas administration devices and exhaust systems are provided [1]. Furthermore, for ERCP, it is not possible to disregard the use of a radiological device; therefore, the operating room where ERCP is performed must be screened for the RX. In ERCP, a hybrid room would be very useful, but a hybrid operating room is an operating room that has permanently installed equipment, like an angiographer, to enable diagnostic imaging before, during, and after surgical procedures: the use of portable imaging technology does not make an OR a hybrid operating room.

1.3.1 Requirements

The following items are requirements that guarantee a regulatory environment and are related to the patient safety [1–5] (Fig. 1.1).

- Procedure rooms may be sized to accommodate the equipment required; the minimum room area recommended for basic endoscopy is 36 m^2. Rooms to accommodate ERCP or video equipment will require a larger space for sterile setup, general anesthesia, and fluoroscopy equipment; a minimum of 42 m^2 is recommended. The minimum square footage for an operating room is determined by combining the square footage of the minimum amount of equipment required, including the endoscopist's table for accessories, the square footage for the minimum number of people required, and a space of approximately 1.22 m

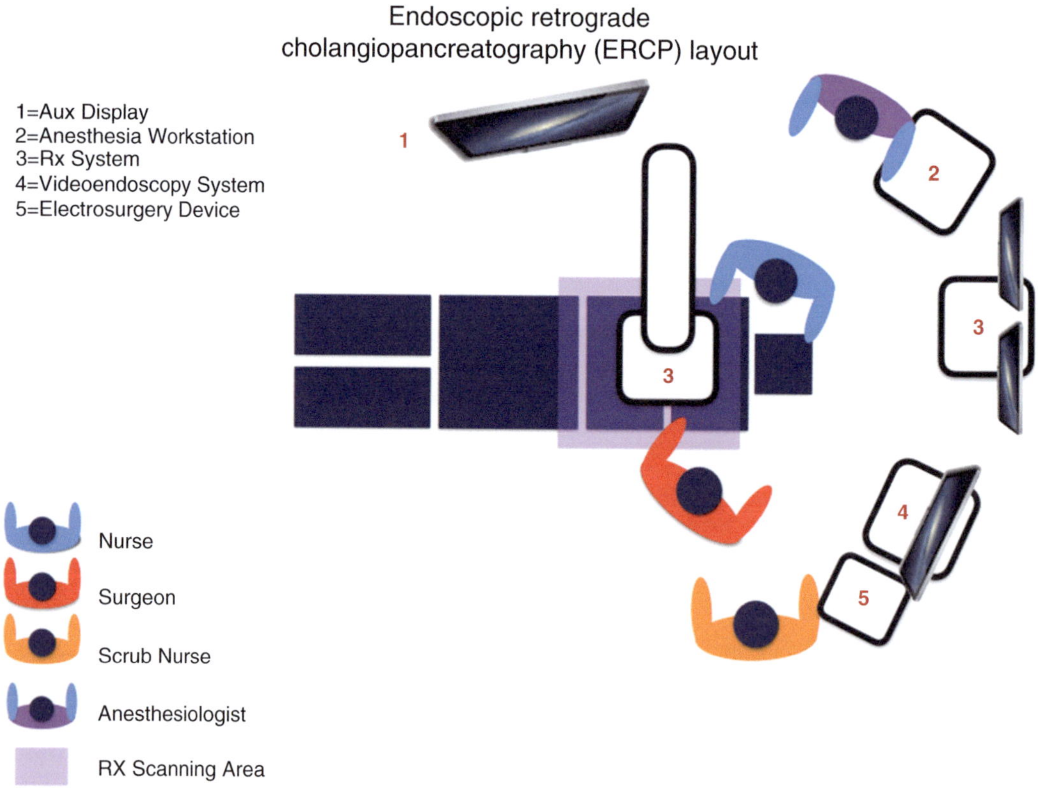

Fig. 1.1 Sample layout of ERCP room

for a minimum safe traffic pathway on all four sides of the operating table [1].

- A reliable and adequate source for oxygen is required. Sources may include in-wall or free-standing oxygen.
- Carbon dioxide (CO_2) must be used instead of room air insufflation of the gastrointestinal lumen. It can be in-wall included.
- A suction source for the equipment and patient must be present either in-wall or portable. For tubing and portable suction, the manufacturer's guidelines must be followed.
- An uninterruptible source of power, supplied either by a generator or battery source is required. The need for a secondary energy source is to allow the procedure to be terminated in the event of a failure of the primary power source. Procedures should not be initiated when the only source of energy is the secondary source.
- The routine monitoring of temperature and humidity within the endoscopic procedure area, although theoretically related to curtail growth of microorganisms and reduce fire hazard, has not yet been associated with safety outcomes in endoscopic units. In the absence of published guidelines on the optimal ranges for these parameters, routine monitoring of temperature and humidity is not currently warranted.
- Puncture-resistant containers for biohazardous materials and sharps should be located so that sharps are not passed over the patient [3].
- Specific room features are required as leaded walls since the flat table fluoroscopy is utilized, with the sign indicating the delivery of X-rays [4, 5] (Figs. 1.2 and 1.3).
- Easy access is required for the movement of trolleys and beds into and out of the room.

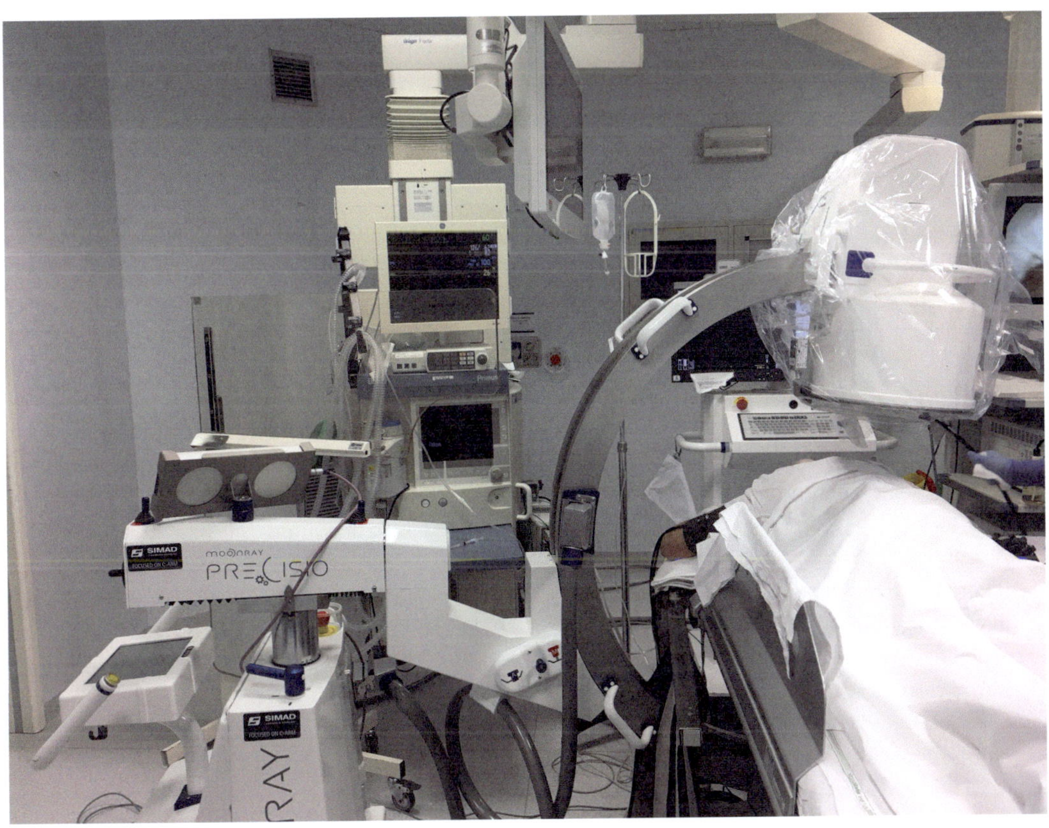

Fig. 1.2 ERCP room with X-ray portable imaging technology

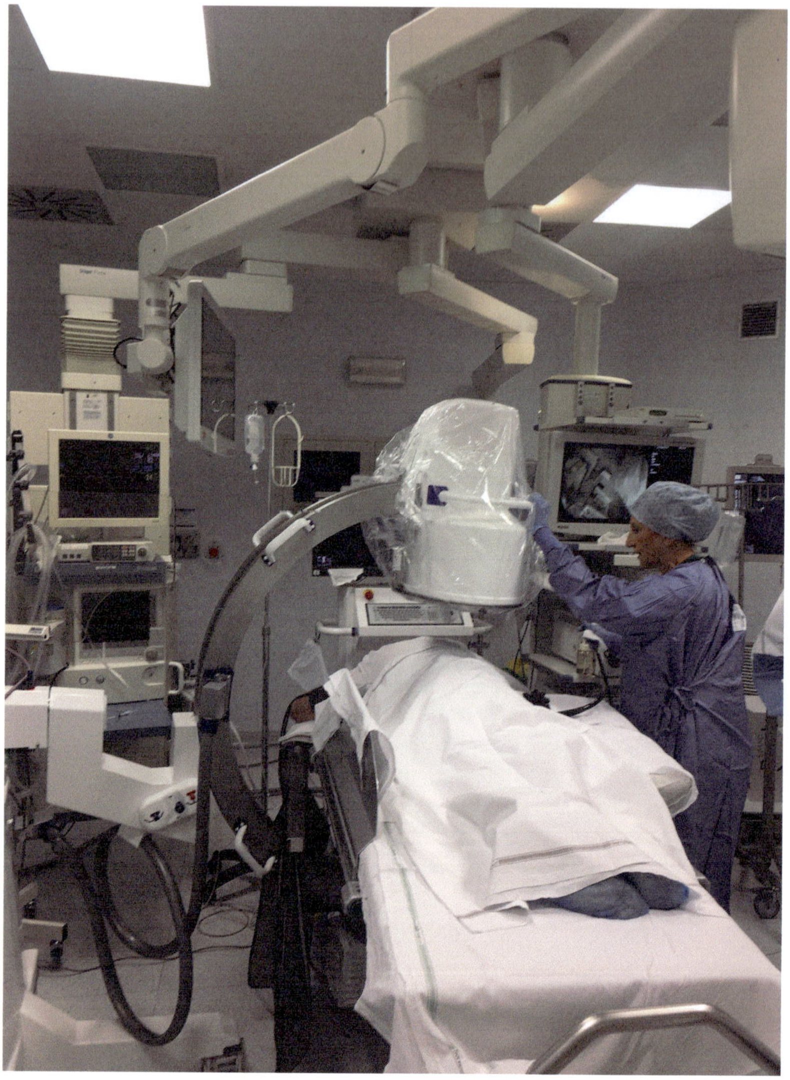

Fig. 1.3 ERCP room with the operator maneuvering portable imaging technology

- Door widths of 1200 mm are recommended for all wheeled traffic. The doors should accommodate this, and they must have the door lock [6].
- A **restricted area** in a surgical suite is a designated space that can only be accessed through a semi-restricted area in order to achieve a high level of asepsis control. Traffic in the restricted area is limited to authorized personnel and patients, and personnel are required to wear surgical attire and cover head and facial hair (Fig. 1.4).

1.3.1.1 Postanesthetic Care Area

A recovery room is required to monitor patients after the endoscopic intervention who have received sedation until the patient is stabilized and to assess for adverse events related to the endoscopic procedure.

In the "postanesthetic care unit," patient care stations are required in both inpatient and outpatient settings and has been defined as 1.5 per OR. If that calculation yields a fraction, the number of patient care stations provided is to be rounded up to the next whole number.

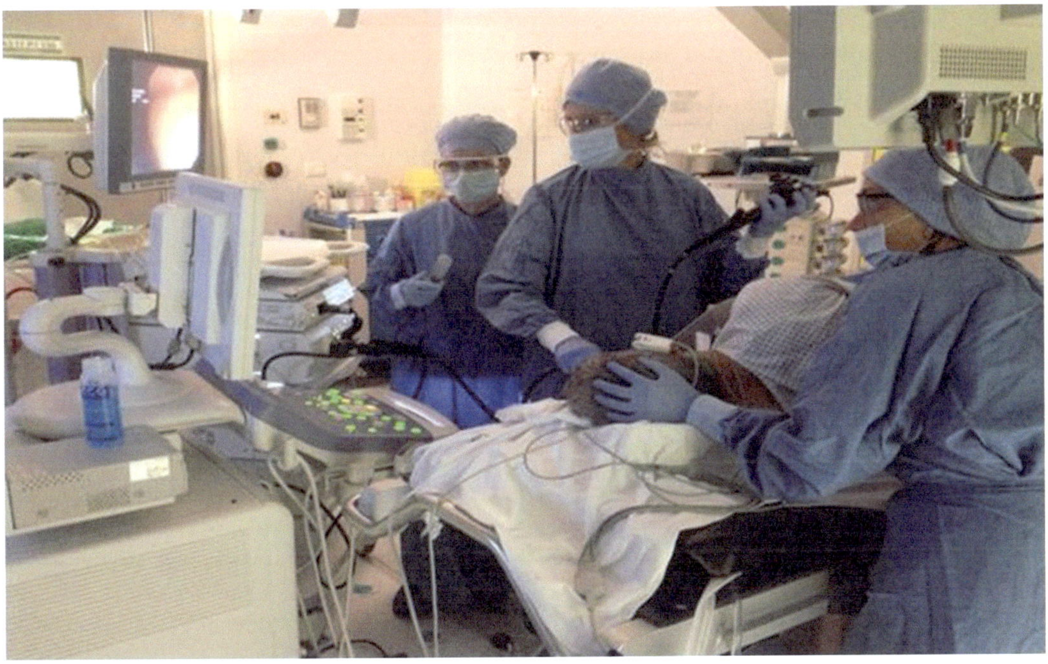

Fig. 1.4 EUS room during interventional procedure

1.3.2 Infection Control

Consideration of infection control is important in the design of the operative unit and for all daily workflow.

Separation of clean and dirty workflows in treatment and cleanup areas and separation of patient care areas and contaminated spaces and equipment is critical to the function of the unit and to prevent cross infection. Procedure/operating rooms will be used for a variety of clients whose infection status may be unknown. Standard precautions must be taken for all clients regardless of their diagnosis or presumed infectious status. Staff hand washing facilities, including disposable paper towels, must be readily available. Specific infection prevention plan must be implemented to prevent the transmission of pathogens in the unit and to provide in case of breach.

The standard practice includes the following:

- Hand hygiene
- Personal protective equipment
- Safe medication administration practices
- Safe handling of potentially contaminated equipment or surfaces in the patient environment.

1.3.3 The Cleaning of the Room

The cleaning of the room should be done at the end of every procedure and not only at the end of the day when the session is finished [6].

1.3.4 Staffing

Complex interventional procedures, such as endoscopic ultrasound (EUS) and ERCP, may require additional staff (registered nurse, RN) for efficiency, but there is no evidence to suggest that this improves safety or patient outcomes [2]. Currently, two RNs are still present during these procedures [6].

1.4 Technical Rules According to European Legislation

ERCP room is a medical suite where medical doctors perform high-complexity endoscopic surgery in full safety and ergonomics.

1.4.1 Technical Plant and Electrical Safety

About plants, the technical reference legislation for this kind of unit is the same as the operating rooms and some in particular [7–10].

According to the legislation, medical rooms are usually classified into three different groups (1-2-3), which are characterized by an increasing level of protection and related plant complexity.

Very briefly (refer to the full-text legislation for more detail), the type 2 rooms (that include endoscopy and ERCP room) are the ones in which patient is exposed to the high electrical shock risks.

Safety systems in group 2 rooms can be described as follows (all of them are present at the same time):

- **Medical Grade Insulation Transformer**: Special power supply systems are able to electrically insulate the facility (with a specific built-in insulation monitoring system). These systems are intended to let doctors safely finish the current procedure even in case of first failure. To achieve this level of protection, all medical devices, which could potentially get in touch to the patient (the patient zone), must be connected to it.
- **Equipotential Grounding**: In order to prevent micro- and macroshock risks, normally, non-current-carrying conductive surfaces must be held rigidly the same potential to prevent the patient from becoming part of an electrical circuit and thus subject to current flow. Accordingly, all branch circuits supplying patient care areas must be provided with an effective ground fault current path. This is accomplished by installing wiring in an impeccably grounded metal race way system or in a cable having a metallic armor or sheath assembly. Room's plant has to be designed to bring the same potential in every point of the ground circuit.
- **Safety Power Supply**: This system is intended to manage power supply continuity in case of central electric supply failure. In this scenario, the hospital have a general UPS, but the activation can take some minutes, which means unacceptable risk for patient under surgery. For high-risk medical suites, specific fast activation of UPS must be foreseen. For specific medical devices present in the room, such as surgical lights or life support, the performance must be at "no break" level.

Modern medical units are becoming increasingly demanding in terms of connectivity toward the "external world." Communication between "in" and "out" of the room must be managed with a specific separation device certified to keep the desired level of electrical insulation. If possible fiber-optic media conversion is highly recommended. Fiber optics is a high-performance material and grants a native electrical insulation (the signal is made by light) without the need of other devices.

1.5 Technological Layout Guidelines

Modern ERCP room project should be managed from a multidisciplinary team and should start from a deep work flow analysis aimed to identify specific organization peculiarity and needs. Internal technical setup and ergonomics should represent the best solution to the various issues arising during the process.

For the internal generic medical supply distribution and device positioning, ceiling pendant technology should be taken in consideration in the first place after a static and structural analysis of the room.

1.5.1 Ceiling Pendant Technology

- **Ceiling pendant** offer many advantages both for their versatility in terms of endowment of technical supplements (medical gas, electrical supply, net and multimedia connection) and for the advanced functions of positioning in the work space and high load capacity. A specific study of the positioning scenarios is recommended to define the exact configuration of the ceiling units (coupling point, outreach). In the event that the room does not multifunction but is dedicated exclusively to endoscopic procedures, it is also advisable to consider the installation systems for video-endoscopy directly on the ceiling unit. This setup brings a benefit to ergonomics deriving from the constant connection with the technical supplies, which are many and different, including the multimedia ones.

The configuration ceiling unit technical appliances must be sufficient in typical use, eliminating the need to connect wall-mounted supplies for the benefit of safety (no cables from the operating theater to the wall). These utilities must however be foreseen but only to manage any faults.

1.5.2 Gases Centralized

- Among the available gases (surely a source for oxygen) in a centralized system, it is advisable to also **include CO_2**, an inert gas indicated for long and complex procedures, eliminating the need for cylinders.

1.5.3 Multimedia Integrated Network

- Given the essentially video-driven nature of the specialty, the room equipment should include a **multimedia integrated network**, designed to connect in a more ergonomic way the different signal sources (video processor, ultrasound, RX) to the various possible destinations (auxiliary room displays, registration system, streaming system). A preliminary analysis is recommended to define first the two sets. This solution allows to minimize "exposed" wiring, decreasing the level of risk.

The multimedia network should include standard input and output connectors appropriately placed on a ceiling unit or—if not possible—on a wall. The recommended connection logic is an "active" matrix type, with the possibility of logical selection of the associations between input and output without having to alter the physical connections. The installation of a ERCP room technical rack is recommended as a point of concentration for the various wiring steps, configuring the net in "star" topology, particularly practical.

1.5.4 Auxiliary Displays

- **It is strongly recommended** to install **auxiliary displays** (at least two screens) installed on a mobile ceiling arm, to be integrated into the aforementioned network. The range of possible movements should be studied to guarantee wide positioning options on the field compared to the main display of the video endoscopy system, so as to allow the whole team the optimal vision while maintaining the ideal posture for the procedure.

1.5.5 Use of Laser Instruments

- If procedures requiring **the use of laser instruments** are foreseen, a selection of specific nonreflective technical interior furnishings is recommended. The external "laser in use" light signaling system and a safety door locking system controlled by the device must also be provided.

1.5.6 Net Connection Point

- The integration of the room with the hospital information system should be considered. For this reason, it is advisable to provide **net connection points inside the room**, connected to a dedicated switch, and at least one workstation strictly with intraoperative application use. The PC must be medical grade, being in the patient area.

It is advisable to deepen needs and predispositions for the following macro ICT functions:

- Computerized system of endoscopic reporting (complete with image acquisition) connected to the hospital information system request manager to send work list
- Connection with PACS for intraoperative consultation and possible radiological image storage of the ERCP
- Streaming/videoconferencing function for interactive teaching

1.6 EUS Room

1.6.1 Introduction

Endoscopic ultrasounds (EUS) are considered one of the most "move on" techniques of the last decades. The change of EUS perspective from a diagnostic to an interventional procedure focused the attention on the room setting and human sources mandatory before starting with an EUS program.

In the 1980s, endoscopic ultrasounds were usually carried out in a standard endoscopic room without dedicated requirements except the skill of operator and EUS equipment. Nowadays, EUS procedures, in tertiary care centers, are usually carried out in dedicated rooms, i.e., as facilities specifically configured for endoscopic ultrasounds, preferably in an endoscopy room (i.e., procedure room) rather than an operating room (OR) except in cases where an interventional procedure is to be carried out (Fig. 1.5).

Starting an EUS program in an endoscopy unit needs some special requirements:

1. Room
2. Equipment
3. Staff (human resources)

The topic of this chapter is the room requirements.

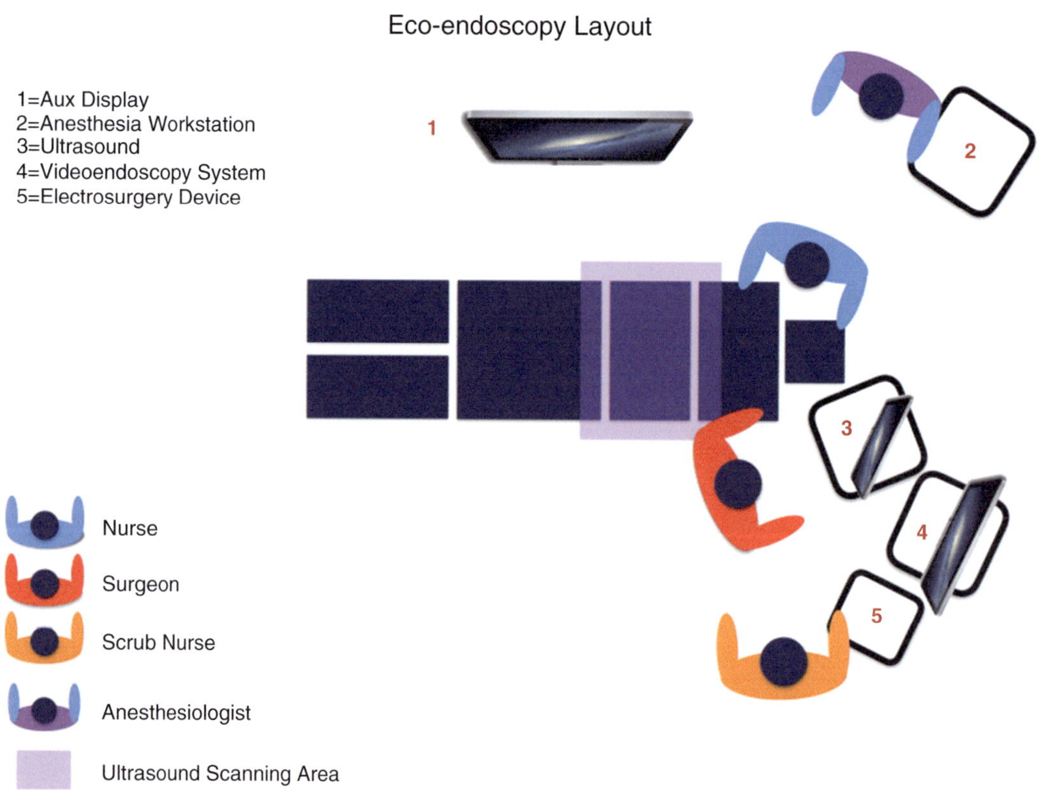

Fig. 1.5 Sample layout of EUS room

1.7 Requirements

There are no published documents on minimal requirement for EUS room or peculiar characteristic different from other endoscopic room; however, operators' personal experience and preferences find a consensus on a list of minimal requirements specific for EUS procedure.

The choice of dedicated EUS room or of "switchable" room depends on the number of procedures that are performed annually, and the above cited requirements should be considered specific for EUS room requirements and consequently added to a standard endoscopic suite.

The diagnostic EUS, including the fine-needle aspiration (FNA) procedure, can be performed in a normal and unpowered endoscopic room, as is the ERCP room.

The interventional EUS instead requires the following:

1.7.1 Room

The size of the interventional EUS room should be able to accommodate all the equipment necessary for this kind of EUS: specific X-ray table, X-ray equipment, one video processor, and one ultrasound machine; recently, some brands of EUS equipment combined together EUS and endoscopy in one source, but both processors should be considered. Combining together all these sources and processors by all means needs a room bigger than a standard endoscopic room and must be like an ERCP room where minimum of 42 m^2 is recommended.

1.7.1.1 Leaded Walls

Interventional EUS procedure is widely diffused and is highly recommended to provide all interventional procedure; even if it is a fluoreless procedure, it is necessary to work in a room fitted for X-ray as a possible salvage procedure.

1.7.2 Equipment Support Tools

- The endoscopy stack accommodates at least two screens, one for EUS room images and one for endoscopic images. Sometimes, during EUS procedures, operators need to change position, and body rotations up to 180° are required; consequently, more than one screen is suggested or positioned on arm able to rotate (see Auxiliary displays above).
- An instrument table containing the equipment that nurses will need to have at their disposal, including gloves, local anesthesia, lubricant, biopsy fixative jars, forceps, and polypectomy snares. The table should also have dedicated spot lighting that is directly addressed on it.
- A trolley containing different caliber needles for EUS-guided fine-needle aspiration (19–25 gauge) and core needles and all the equipment necessary for specimen management (smears, biopsy fixative jars, alcohol, syringe with water and air). If the unit is equipped for interventional procedure, all the devices required should be available before the start of the procedure, closed to endoscopy room (cystotome, stents, guidewire, contrast medium).
- A trolley or distribution arm for anesthesia/emergency procedures, equipped and meeting agreed resuscitation standards as in standard or interventional endoscopic rooms.

1.7.3 Staffing

- Currently, two RNs are present during these procedures and are useful.

References

1. Byron Burlingame, MS, RN, CNOR. Operating room requirements for 2014 and beyond. www.fgiguidelines.org.
2. Calderwood AH, Chapman FJ, Cohen J, et al. Guidelines for safety in the gastrointestinal endoscopy unit. Gastrointest Endosc. 2014;79:363–72.
3. Blenkharn J. Sharps management and the disposal of clinical waste. Br J Nurs. 2009;18(860):862–4.
4. Decreto Legislativo 26 maggio 2000, n. 187 Attuazione della direttiva 97/43/EURATOM in materia di protezione sanitaria delle persone contro i pericoli delle radiazioni ionizzanti connesse ad esposizioni mediche. Modificato dall'art. 39, Legge 1 marzo 2002, n. 39.
5. Ordinanza concernente la radioprotezione relativa agli impianti a raggi X per uso medico (Ordinanza sui raggi X) 20 gennaio 1998 (Stato 14 aprile 1998).

6. Mulder CJJ, Jacobs MAJ, Leicester RJ, et al. Guidelines for designing a digestive disease endoscopy unit: report of the World Endoscopy Organization. Dig Endosc. 2013;25:365–75.
7. CEI 62-5, III edizione (UNI EN ISO 60601-1). Electromedical devices. Part 1: general rules for safety.
8. CEI 64-8, Sez.710 Section regulations for premises for medical use.
9. UNI EN ISO 11197 art.3.5 basic safety and essential requirements of power supply units for medical use.
10. European Council Directive 2007/47/CE on Medical Devices. https://eur-lex.europa.eu/LexUriServ/LexUriServ.do?uri=OJ:L:2007:247:0021:0055:en:PDF.

X-Rays in Endoscopy

2

Andrea Brameri

2.1 When Were X-Rays Discovered?

X-rays are a form of **electromagnetic radiation** characterized by a **wavelength** smaller than that of visible light. It is produced by making electrons collide with a metal target at high speed. The sudden deceleration of the free electrons excites the electrons of the metal which move into more energetic orbits and immediately jump back to their ground state or original orbit releasing X photons.

X-rays were accidentally discovered in 1895 by the German physicist **Wilhelm Conrad Röntgen** while doing his research on **cathode rays**: although the vacuum tube in which he produced the electric discharge was covered with heavy black paper, he noticed that a barium platinocyanide screen that happened to be lying nearby his tube was emitting a fluorescent glow at each discharge.

Röntgen concluded that the **fluorescence** was due to invisible radiation, even more penetrating than ultraviolet radiation, which he called an "X-ray" alluding to its unknown nature.

> The energy and ability of penetration of radiation are inversely proportional to the wavelength: so, X-rays characterized by longer wavelengths, i.e. closer to the ultraviolet band of the electromagnetic spectrum, are called "soft" as they are relatively little penetrating; those with a shorter wavelength and hence closer to or even overlapping the region of gamma rays are called "hard" as they are highly penetrating.

2.2 Benefits of X-Rays

X-rays are beneficial but also dangerous and a scientific explanation is given below.

The problem is that X-rays are a form of **ionizing radiation**.

When "normal" light, i.e. in the radiation spectrum visible to the human eye, hits an atom, it cannot change it in any significant way. But when X-rays hit an atom, they can knock some electrons out of their orbit and from an atom (which by its nature is neutral) an **ion**, that is, an electrically charged atom is created. The free electrons that were previously knocked out of their orbit then hit other atoms and create other ions.

The electric charge of an ion may lead to abnormal chemical reactions in living cells or break the DNA chain.

A cell with a damaged DNA filament may die or develop a mutation. If many body cells die, various types of diseases can develop. If the DNA of a cell is changed, it may become cancerous and hence proliferate autonomously. If the mutation occurs in a sperm cell or an egg cell, this may lead to congenital anomalies.

A. Brameri (✉)
Eurocolumbus Srl, Milan, Italy
e-mail: abrameri@eurocol.it

M. Mutignani et al. (eds.), *Endotherapy in Biliopancreatic Diseases: ERCP Meets EUS*,
https://doi.org/10.1007/978-3-030-42569-2_2

The major risk arising from ionizing radiation is repeated exposure over time: it is as if the radiation (normally identified with the word "dose") accumulated; therefore, the higher the dose and/or the longer the exposure time, the greater the risk, and it is therefore obvious that the subjects most at risk are healthcare operators.

The problems may involve:

- The eyes (in particular the cataract)
- The skin (e.g. skin tumours)
- Any other form of tumour correlated with exposure of the human body to ionizing radiation

2.3 Why X-Rays in Endoscopy?

During endoscopic procedures, the operator needs to understand where the guidewire or the catheter is positioned and what the right path to follow is.

Therefore, visually observing the catheter on the endoscope video and radiologically checking its position, the points of clinical interest can safely be reached.

2.4 Which Radiological Instruments Were Used in the Past?

At first, the endoscopist/gastroenterologist had to ask the radiologist (the only reference person and responsible for ionizing radiation in hospitals) if he or she could use a fluoroscopy instrument.

Generally, the radiologist made a room equipped with a "remote-controlled" fluoroscopy instrument available, which allowed continuously seeing the radiological images on a dedicated monitor.

Then, for the days when needing to work "with rays," the endoscopic trolley had to be transported from the gastroenterology department, often on the upper floors, to the radiology department, generally on the ground floor or in any case on a different floor from gastroenterology.

Clearly also the patient had to walk a similar path accompanied by the nurses, suffering all the discomforts along the way and tripling the time from a logistic point of view.

Doubtless, you could not work in peace in the radiology department as the radiology rooms were designed not to have a filtering area; the patients had to wait in the corridor in front of the radiology room, and also the medical staff had to pass through this corridor to enter the room. Moreover, the room was designed to do the most common abdominal examinations (e.g. enema and the stomach), and it was hence defined "dirty" and clearly not equipped like an operating theatre; it was not easy to sedate the patient—a routine procedure—and the endoscope could not be cleaned.

As you can see from the photo (Fig. 2.1), the equipment was very bulky and not suited to endoscopic needs as you could only work from one side of the table and, what's more, the aerial camera got in the way of the medical staff. In addition, the instrument was designed to make radiograms, and the scope was used only to "centre" the point of interest, and there was hence no need to obtain a quality "fluoroscopic" image, an unavoidable necessity in a gastroenterology operation.

2.5 Change

The first significant change in the way of working came about thanks to the ever greater importance this discipline assumed, and given the excellent results achieved, the number of operations increased exponentially. Endoscopists showed hospital administrations that it was no longer possible and logical—apart from being more costly—to transfer equipment and patients, and so they got the first C-arches that were interfaced with simple stretchers.

These C-arches were generally "second hand," often handed down from other depart-

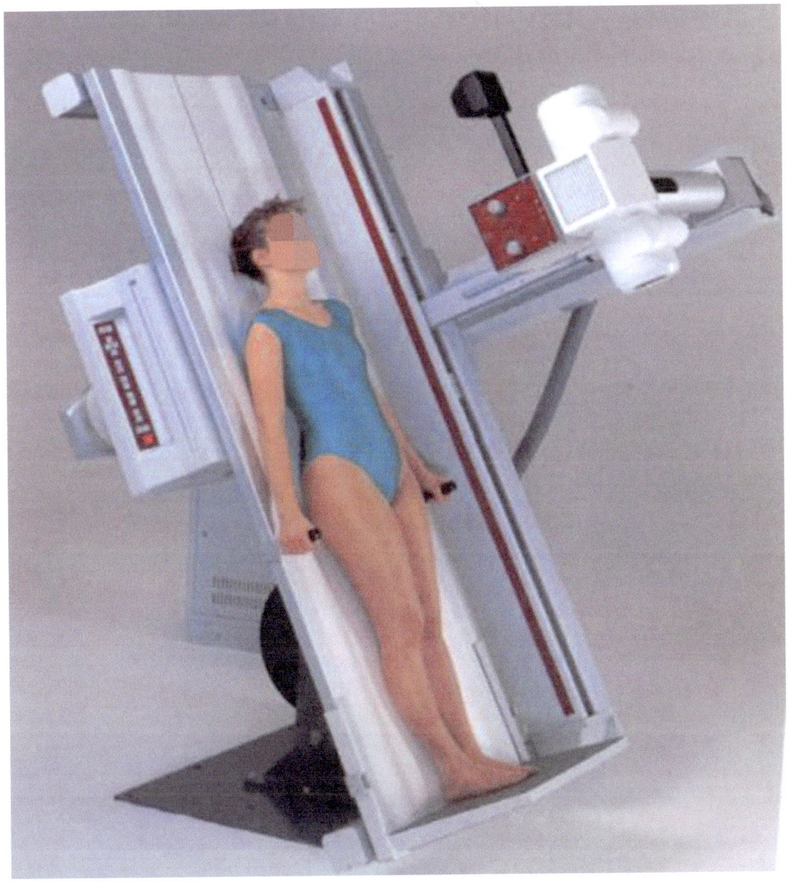

Fig. 2.1 One of the first available radiological equipment (not suitable for endoscopic procedure)

ments and equipped with a today outdated technology, i.e. with brightness intensifier and reduced field of vision (9″); little power, generally not more than 5 kW; and only just sufficient image quality.

The departments had to start getting to grips with the X-ray dose absorbed, the problem of obtaining a quality image also with large patients and the first problems of overheating of the radiological part.

Health physicists began checking the doses absorbed by the operators and carrying out quality controls on the instruments.

The epoch-making change however came when they started using stents, not only in the interventional and vascular cardiology field but also in endo/gastroenterology.

This led to the need to have dedicated equipped rooms and especially state-of-the-art instruments.

The new instruments must guarantee:

- An operating capacity equal to a mobile angiography system; it is hence essential that it be equipped with an active cooling system for the heat produced with control of the digital part of the instrument.
- Adequate power of at least 25 or 80 kW in order to be able to operate on any type of patient.
- When moving the arch, the possibility of not having to re-centre the point at which you were operating; this characteristic is called three-dimensional isocentric set-up.

- Motor-driven movement of the C-arch so that the technical operators do not enter the working field of the endoscopist: it is therefore preferable that the arch can be moved both by the instrument and through a remote console at the patient's bed.
- The safety of the patient through intelligent anticollision sensors that intervene before the obstacle is touched (Fig. 2.2).
- The best technology available on the market, namely, flat panel detector technology, i.e. with direct image formation no longer like on brightness intensifiers (BI-camera-cable-monitor) (drawings).
- The possibility of moving only the flat panel in order to move close to the patient or not; this is to be considered a preferential element (Fig. 2.3).
- Viewing the images on a large monitor, possibly hanging, 27″ with at least four million pixels or 31″ 4 K.
- The possibility of sending the radiological images to the endoscopic trolley monitor in order to have an immediate comparison with-

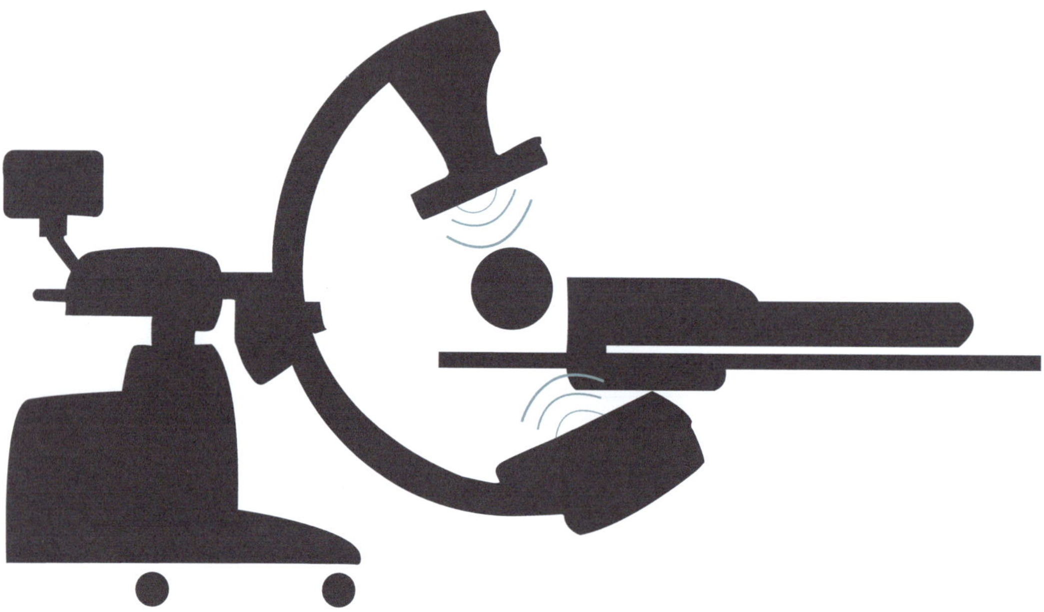

Fig. 2.2 Anticollision system avoids patient's injuries

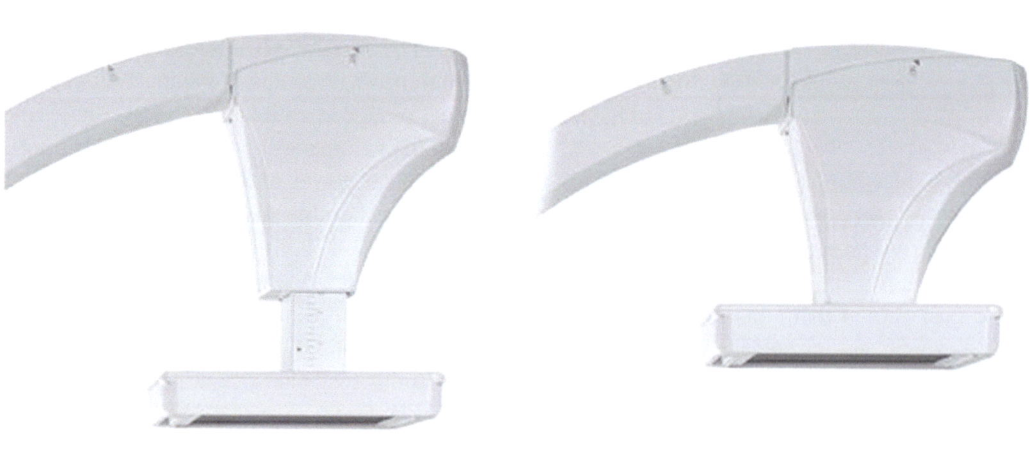

Fig. 2.3 Movable flat panel improves the capability of fluoroscopic view

out having to move the head and hence lose concentration on the point of interest.

- A real reduction in the X-ray dose through different X-ray filtration depending on the type of operation (insertion of motor filters on the collimator) (drawing) and new acquisition algorithms (acquisition in frequency) in real time; it is therefore advisable that the operating system be LINUX.
- The possibility of using FUSION software, i.e. the possibility of fusing images obtained through CAT with the images produced by the C-arch for greater certainty of the result to be achieved and reduction of the ionizing radiation emitted.

If endoscopy and gastroenterology departments could have these new technologies at their disposal, healthcare and the community would obtain major advantages as they would have equipment available that guarantees an operating ability and image quality comparable to angiographic or hemodynamic diagnostics with real dose reductions and reduced operating times.

3 Ultrasound Equipment

Anna Cominardi and Pietro Fusaroli

3.1 Fujifilm

Fujifilm's medical devices portfolio includes:

- **Sonart EUS**

  It allows the integration of ultrasonographic diagnosis and endoscopy systems. The SU-1 system (Fig. 3.1, Table 3.1) supports accurate diagnosis with a variety of imaging modes including:

  - *High-resolution B-mode*: SU-1 ultrasonic processor achieves high-precision ultrasonographic results and accurate evaluation of the affected area.
  - *Elastography.*
  - *Colour Doppler.*
  - *Contrast harmonic imaging (CHI):* images are created by extracting and emphasising higher harmonic signals generated by the injected contrast medium, assisting in the detection of tumours and abnormal growths.
  - *Tissue harmonic imaging (THI):* images are configured using high-harmonic components that are generated when ultrasound waves are transmitted through the body's tissue. It enables ultrasound image observation with reduced noise.

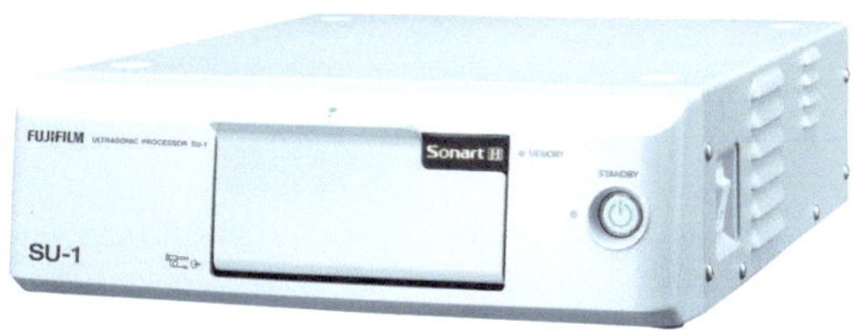

Fig. 3.1 Fujifilm endoscopic ultrasound processor

  - *Compound harmonic imaging (CH):* it visualises clear images in deep lying areas whilst maintaining high-resolution images in shallow lying areas to support accurate diagnoses.
  - *Sound speed correction:* images are recomposed using the estimated optimal sound speed inside the body.
  - **DICOM technology:** it achieves compatibility and improves workflow efficiency between imaging systems and other information systems.

In addition, echoendoscopes are provided with optical tools such as:

- **Super CCD technology**

  It provides brilliant images, which can facilitate procedures for detection and treatment of lesions.
- **HD technology**

  It offers detailed sharp pictures by using high-definition television (HDTV).

A. Cominardi · P. Fusaroli (✉)
University of Bologna, Bologna, Italy
e-mail: pietro.fusaroli@unibo.it

M. Mutignani et al. (eds.), *Endotherapy in Biliopancreatic Diseases: ERCP Meets EUS*,
https://doi.org/10.1007/978-3-030-42569-2_3

Table 3.1 Fujifilm endoscopic ultrasound processor specifications

Endoscopic ultrasonic processor SU-1 -H- SU-1 -S-		
Power supply	Power rating	AC 100–240 V
	Frequency rating	50 Hz/60 Hz
	Power consumption	2.0–1.2 A
Size	Dimensions	390 × 135 × 485 mm
	Weight	13 kg
Ultrasonography image display	Scanning method	Electronic scanning
	Probe types	Curved linear array/radial
	Scanning modes	B, M, CD, PD, PW, THI, CH
	Special modes[a]	Elastography/CHI
Received signal processing	Received gain correction	0–100, 2-step
	STC	6-step gain settings per depth
	Sound speed correction	Full screen ROI settings
	Dynamic range	40–100, 5-step
Display	PinP	Endoscopic/ultrasound imaging
	Observation screen	Hospital/date/time/patient
Applicable	Curved linear array	EG-580UT, EG-530UT2, EB-530US
	Radial	EG-580UR, EG-530UR2
Frequency		5 MHz, 7.5 MHz, 10 MHz, 12 MHz
Image input terminal	DVI image input terminal	1
Image output terminals	Video terminal	1
	S-video terminal	1
	RGB TV terminal	1
	DVI terminal (digital)	1
	DVI terminal (digital/analog)	1
	HD-SDI terminal	2
Sound output	RCA terminal	1
Control terminal	Remote terminal	2
	Remote terminal (input)	1
	RS-232C terminal	1
	Keyboard terminal	1
	Foot switch terminal	1
	Network terminal	1
Measurement function	Measurement items	Distance, perimeter, area, volume, flow speed
Storage	Data formats	JPEG, TIFF, DICOM, AVI
	Storage device	Internal/external memory (USB)
	Cine memory	Storage/playback
Accessories		Keyboard and foot switch

[a]CHI and elastography modes are available only in SU1-H-

– **Anti-blur function**

It automatically provides the clearest image by pressing the freeze button.

3.2 Olympus-Aloka

– **EU-ME2**

This ultrasound processor (Table 3.2) is compatible with a wide range of EUS scopes, including ultrasonic miniature probes. It offers:

- *Power flow*
- *Colour flow*
- *H-Flow*
- *PW Doppler*
- *Harmonic imaging* (tissue harmonic echo, contrast harmonic EUS)
- *Real-time elastography*

– **Aloka ProSound F75**

It is compatible with a wide range of EUS scopes and extracorporeal probes (Table 3.3).

Table 3.2 EU-ME2 specifications

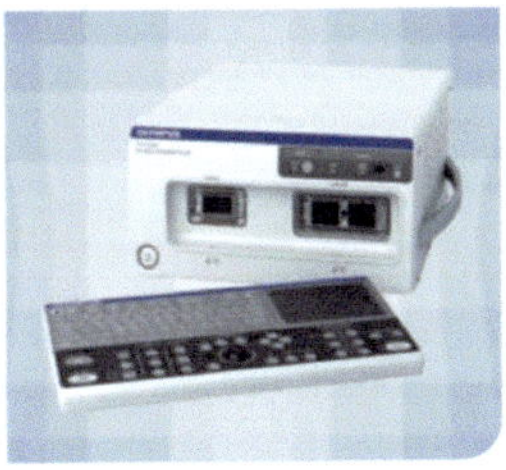

EU-ME2 PREMIER PLUS

Power supply	Voltage	100–240 V AC (for NTSC), 220–240 V AC (for PAL)	
	Voltage fluctuation	Within ±10%	
	Frequency		50/60 Hz
	Frequency fluctuation		Within ±1 Hz
	Consumption (electric power)		370 VA
Size	Dimensions	Main unit	371 (W) × 175 (H) × 480 (D) mm 445 (W) × 184 (H) × 495 (D) mm (max.)
		Keyboard	392 (W) × 39 (H) × 207 (D) mm
	Weight	Main unit	22.5 kg
		Keyboard	2.5 kg
Classification	Type of protection against electric shock	Class I	
	Degree of protection against electric shock of applied part	TYPE BF applied part Where no classification mark appears, the device is a TYPE BF applied part	
	Degree of protection against explosion	The ultrasound centre should be kept away from flammable gases	
TYPE BF applied part	This instrument can safely be applied to any part of the body except the heart		
EMC	This instrument complies with the standards listed as follows: IEC 60601-1-2: 2001, IEC 60601-2-37: 2007 CISPR 11 of emission: Group 1, Class B		
Ultrasound scanning format	Mechanical scanning, electronic scanning		
Mechanical scanning	Display mode	B-mode	
	Scanning	Radial scanning	
	Compatible equipment	Mechanical radial scanning ultrasound endoscope, miniature probe	
	Usable frequencies	C5, C7.5, C12, C20, 7.5, 12, 20 MHz	
	Display range	2, 3, 4, 6, 9, 12 cm	
	Image adjustment	Gain, contrast, STC, enhance	
	Display processing	Rotation	Rotatable (64 steps, clockwise/counterclockwise)
		Display area	Full circle, bottom sector, top sector, scroll
		Direction	Normal/inverse
	Cine memory	Maximum 160 frames, Cine review function	
	3D	3D display, MPR display	
	Measurement	Distance, area, circumstance	
Electronic scanning	Display mode	B-mode, FLOW mode, PW mode, THE mode, CH-EUS mode, elastography mode	
	Scanning	Radial scanning, curved linear array scanning	
	Compatible equipment	Electronic radial scanning ultrasound endoscope, Electronic curved linear array scanning ultrasound endoscope	
	Usable frequencies	5, 6, 7.5, 10, 12 MHz	
	Display range	2, 3, 4, 5, 6, 7, 8, 9, 12 cm	
	Image adjustment	Gain, contrast, STC, enhance, compound	
	Display processing	Display area	Radial: Full circle, bottom sector, top sector, scroll Curved linear array: convex
		Direction	Normal/inverse
		Display pattern	Single-screen/dual-screen
	Cine memory	Over 600 frames can be stored depending on the conditions Cine review function	
	Focus	Auto preset	Near/far
		Focus setting	Focus location adjustable, focus number adjustable
	FLOW mode	COLOR FLOW mode, POWER FLOW mode, H-FLOW mode	
	PW mode	B+PW, Color+PW, Power+PW, H-Flow+PW	
	Measurement	Distance, area, circumstance, PW measurement	
	THE (Tissue Harmonic Echo) mode *1, *2	THE-P, THE-R	
	CH-EUS mode *1, *2	Display pattern	CH-B, CH-Color
		Preset (CH agent type)	2 types, adjustable (middle or low)
		Frequency selection	2 types, adjustable (CH-R or CH-P)
		TIC analysis	Displays the change over time of the average brightness of each ROI
	ELST mode (elastography) *2	Pressurisation state guide	Strain graph, pressurisation bar
		Strain ratio	Displays the amounts of the strain and their ratio in two areas
Recording data	Data format	Still image	BMP, JPEG, 3DV
		Movie data *1, *2	AVI
Ancillary equipment	Keyboard		Keyboard with built-in trackball, LCD touch panel and LED backlit keys
	Recording device		Video printer (colour/monochrome), DVR
	Video system centre	Monitor display selection	Endoscopic/ultrasound image
		Picture-In-Picture	Displays the endoscopic image as PIP sub-display on the ultrasound image
		Patient data	Shares patient data with the video system centre

*1 Only available on EU-ME2 PREMIER/EU-ME2 PREMIER PLUS *2 Only available on EU-ME2 PREMIER PLUS

Table 3.3 Olympus endoscopic ultrasound processors

		Aloka ProSound F75	Aloka Alpha 7	EU ME2 series		
				EU-ME2 Premier Plus	EU-ME2 Premier	EU-ME2
Scanning mode	Mechanical radial scanning	–	–	✓		
	Electronic radial scanning	✓	✓	✓		
	Electronic convex scanning	✓	✓	✓		
Scope probe	Mechanical EUS	–	–	✓		
	Ultrasonic probe	–	–	✓		
	Electronic EUS	✓	✓	✓		
	Extracorporeal probe	✓	✓	–		
Function	B	✓	✓	✓		
	FLOW	✓	✓	✓		
	3D	–	–	✓		
	M	✓	✓	–		
	PW	✓	✓	✓		
	Tissue harmonic echo (THE)	✓	✓	✓		–
	Contrast harmonic echo (CHE)	✓	✓	✓		–
	Elastography	✓	–	✓		–
	Frequency	Electronic 5 MHz, 6 MHz, 7.5 MHz, 10 MHz, 12 MHz	Electronic 4 MHz, 5 MHz, 6.67 MHz, 8 MHz, 10 MHz, 13.3 MHz	Electronic 5 MHz, 6 MHz, 7.5 MHz, 10 MHz, 12 MHz Mechanical C5, C7.5, C12, C20 7.5 MHz, 12 MHz, 20 MHz, 30 MHz		
	Time intensity curve (TIC)	✓	✓	✓		–
Size probe	Processor	590(W) × 1000(D) × 1204–1675(H)	490(W) × 790(D) × 142–173(H)	371(W) × 480(D) × 175(H)		
	Keyboard	–	–	392(W) × 207(D) × 39(H)		
Weight	Processor	170 kg	108 kg	22.5 kg		
	Keyboard	–	–	2.5 kg		

However, it does not support ultrasonic miniature probes. It offers:

- *E-Flow*
- *Colour flow*
- *Power flow*
- *PW Doppler*
- *Harmonic imaging* (tissue harmonic echo, broadband harmonics, contrast echo, ExPHD)
- *Real-time elastography*

– **Aloka ProSound ALPHA7**

It is compatible with a wide range of EUS scopes and extracorporeal probes (Table 3.3). However, it does not support ultrasonic miniature probes. It offers:

- *Compound pulse wave generator:* it transmits preprogrammed waveforms to produce highly efficient, high-quality beams optimised for each mode of operation and transducer whilst also enabling highly sensitive transmission.
- *Full aperture apodisation:* it perfects the focus throughout the entire image.
- *Image optimiser:* automated adjustment of the image both in the B-mode and spectral Doppler.
- *DICOM compliant image capture.*
- *Broadband harmonics:* it allows the reduction of side lobes and multiple echoes offering significantly enhanced sensitivity and axial resolution for a new level of detail in the entire image.
- *Adaptive image processing (AIP):* it reduces speckle noise whilst maintaining the frame rate.
- *Directional eFLOW (D-eFLOW):* it allows enhanced spatial and time resolutions for greater detail of blood flow information, including directional flow.
- *3D automated volume measurement (AVM):* it calculates 3D volume
- *Advanced 3D/4D imaging functions:* such as multiplanar reconstruction (MPR), 3D automated volume measurement (AVM), multi-slice imaging (MSI) and Flow-3D.
- *Spatial compound imaging (SCI):* it enhances capability for depicting sidewall strictures and tubular cavities.

3.3 Pentax-Hitachi

Pentax echoendoscopes are compatible with a wide range of ultrasound processors (Fig. 3.2), including:

– **Noblus**

It allows:

- *HI-REZ:* it makes easier the study of tissue layers, it emphasised the margins of the

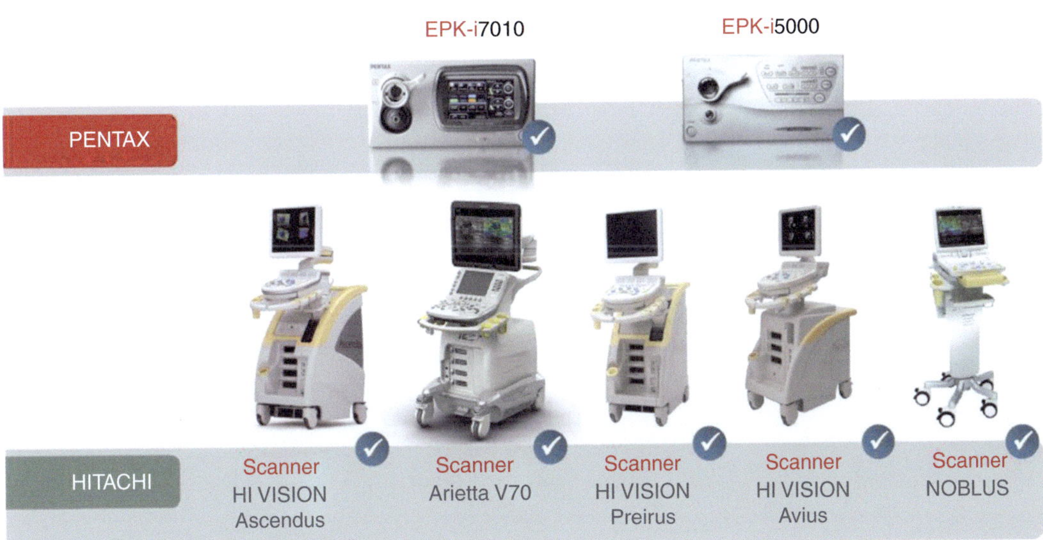

Fig. 3.2 Pentax-Hitachi ultrasound processors

organs (pancreatic and hepatic lobes) and allows high-quality visualisation of bioptic needle.
  - *HI-COM*: this technology overlaps images in real time allowing a reduction of noises and speckle artefacts.
  - *dTHI*: it allows to obtain higher space and contrast resolution images by the employment of depth ultrasound and resolution ultrasounds.
- **Avius HI VISION Series**
  - *HI Real-Time Elastography (RTE)*: it allows to differentiate malign and benign lesions providing strain graph display and strain histogram.
  - *Colour Doppler-CFM/colour flow imaging (CFI):* it measures flow velocity and direction, it helps to verify the presence of vessels during FNA/FNAB and it's a valid help in diagnosing malignancies.
  - *Fine flow-CFA:* it elaborates signal in order to visualise the smallest vessels.
  - *Contrast-enhanced ultrasonography-MDC dHCI Hitachi.*
  - *HI-REZ.*
  - *HI-COM.*
  - *dTHI.*
- **Arietta V70**
  - *Symphonic technology*
  - *CPWG:* connector's components are inside the transducer, reducing noises and creating high-resolution ultrasounds
  - *Multi-slice transductors:* it allows high-performance transduction of impulses with less energy dispersion, optimising images sensitivity and definition
  - *HI Real-Time Elastography (RTE)*
  - *Contrast-enhanced ultrasonography-MDC dHCI Hitachi*
  - *ITM:* it allows ongoing mapping of contrast flow
  - *HI-REZ*
  - *HI-COM*
  - *dTHI*

The ultrasound processors produced by the three main manufacturers that have been described so far are compatible with a variety of echoendoscopes (radial scanning, curved linear array and forward view). The main features of the echoendoscopes have been reported in Table 3.4.

Table 3.4 Comparison of the main features of echoendoscopes of Fujifilm, Olympus and Pentax

		Fujifilm		Olympus			Pentax		
		EG-580UR	EG-580UT	GF-UE160-AL5	GF-UCT180	TGF-UC180J	EG-3870UTK	EG-3270UK	EG-3670URK
Endoscopic functions	Viewing direction	0° (forward view)	40° (forward oblique)	100°/55° (forward/ oblique)	100°/55° (forward/oblique)	120°/0° (forward/ oblique)	120°/45° (forward/ oblique)	120°/50° (forward/ oblique)	130°/60° (forward/ oblique)
	Observation range	3–10 mm	3–100 mm	3–100 mm	3–100 mm	3–100 mm	5–100 mm	5–100 mm	4–100 mm
	Field of view	140°	140°	360°	180°	90°	120°	120°	140°
	Distal end diameter	11.4 mm	13.9 mm	11.8 mm	12.6 mm	12.6 mm	14.3 mm	12 mm	10.3 mm
	Flexible portion diameter	11.5 mm	12.4 mm	11.8 mm	12.6 mm	12.6 mm	12.8 mm	10.8 mm	13.4 mm
	Bending capability	Up 190°/down 90° Right 100°/left 100°	Up 150°/down 150° Right 120°/left 120°	Up 130°/down 90° Right 90°/left 90°	Up 130°/down 90° Right 90°/left 90°	Up 180°/down 90° Right 90°/left 90°	Up 130°/down 130° Right 120°/left 120°	Up 130°/down 130° Right 120°/left 120°	Up 130°/down 60°
	Working length	1250 mm	1250 mm	1250	1250	1245	1250 mm	1250 mm	1250 mm
	Overall length	1550 mm	1550 mm	1550 mm	1550 mm	1550 mm	1560 mm	1560 mm	1560 mm
	Working channel diameter	2.8 mm	3.8 mm	2.2 mm	3.7 mm	3.7 mm	3.8 mm	2.8 mm	2.4 mm
Ultrasonic functions	Scanning mode	Colour Doppler, power Doppler, pulse Doppler, B-mode, M-mode	Colour Doppler, power Doppler, pulse Doppler, B-mode, M-mode	Colour Doppler, power Doppler, tissue harmonic echo (THE), oblique view	Colour Doppler, power Doppler, contrast harmonic echo (CH-EUS)	Colour Doppler, power Doppler, real-time elastography, harmonic imaging	Colour Doppler, power Doppler, real-time elastography, harmonic imaging	Colour Doppler, power Doppler, real-time elastography, harmonic imaging	Colour Doppler, power Doppler, real-time elastography, harmonic imaging
	Scanning mode	Electronic radial scan	Electronic curved linear array scan	Electronic 360° radial array	Electronic curved linear array	Forward-viewing, electronic curved linear array	Electronic curved linear array	Electronic curved linear array	Electronic 360° radial array
	Scanning angle	360°	150°	360°	180°	180°	120°	120°	360°
	Frequency	5 MHz/7.5 MHz/ 10 MHz/12 MHz	5 MHz/7.5 MHz/ 10 MHz/12 MHz	5 MHz/6 MHz/ 7.5 MHz/10 MHz/ 12 MHz	5 MHz/6 MHz/ 7.5 MHz/10 MHz/ 12 MHz	5 MHz/6 MHz/ 7.5 MHz/10 MHz/ 12 MHz	5 MHz/10 MHz	5 MHz/10 MHz	5 MHz/10 MHz

Endoscopes

4

Arianna Massella and Paolo Bocus

4.1 Endoscopes

Since its introduction more than 40 years ago, endoscopic retrograde cholangiopancreatography (ERCP) has changed the treatment of biliopancreatic diseases. At the beginning, it was a diagnostic procedure, but over time due to the development of noninvasive imaging, it evolved to a therapeutic procedure. Such an evolution has required developments in technology and training to bring us to present ERCP.

Endoscopic ultrasound (EUS) was developed in the early 80s to overcome mainly difficulties by the radiological techniques of the time in visualizing the pancreas, located in retroperitoneal space and often covered by air. The first scope commercially available from 1986 was a fiber-optic radial device. In the early 1990s with the advent of the curved, linear-array echoendoscope began the era of interventional EUS (EUS-FNA). Over the years, many improvements have been achieved such as switchable frequencies, to allow more detailed visualization of GI wall layers and the conversion from a mechanical to a fully electronic instrument. This allowed to develop new functions such as Doppler, elastosonography, and the contrast enhanced echoendoscopy.

4.2 Duodenoscopes

The standard endoscope for ERCP is the side-viewing duodenoscope, equipped with a tip with four-way angulation capability, a side-positioned air/water nozzle, an instrument channel, and a forceps elevator adjacent to the instrument channel outlet that allows fine linear instrument position changes facilitating cannulation and placement of various devices.

Instrument channel diameter ranges from 2.2 to 5.5 mm. Duodenoscopes with 4.2 mm internal channel allowing to place biliary endoprostheses (10–11.5 Fr circumference) are the most used. Pediatric duodenoscopes with a 2.2 mm channel are available for examination in infants, while largest instrument channels (>5 mm) are found in so-called "mother/baby" scope system usedfor choledochoscopy and pancreatoscopy. However this system is difficult to manipulate and is now rarely used [1].

In certain situations where a traditional duodenoscope is not suitable (e.g., in patients with a Billroth II or a Roux-en-Y reconstruction), a forward-viewing endoscope may be tried instead [2]. Conventional endoscopes however provide a limited visualization of the ampullary region and are limited with respect to control of accessories during cannulation due to the absence of elevator.

A. Massella · P. Bocus (✉)
IRCCS "Sacro Cuore—Don Calabria",
Istituto di Ricovero e Cura a Carattere Scientifico, Ospedale Classificato e Presidio Ospedaliero Accreditato—Regione Veneto, Negrar di Valpolicella, Verona, Italy

M. Mutignani et al. (eds.), *Endotherapy in Biliopancreatic Diseases: ERCP Meets EUS*,
https://doi.org/10.1007/978-3-030-42569-2_4

In recent years, infections due to multidrug-resistant organisms (MDROs) have become a concern in health care, including in gastrointestinal endoscopy. Cases and serial outbreaks of MDROs infections associated with ERCP have been published from different countries from 2010 [3]. All the processes of cleaning, disinfection, and sterilization of duodenoscopes have been analyzed featuring different issues [4].

Major manufacturers developed tools to prevent infections such as detachable disposable distal cap. Post-procedure reprocessing is performed by detaching the disposable distal cap and cleaning and disinfecting the tip of the scope [5]. In addition, new adaptors that can be attached to the tip of the duodenoscope to inject a cleaning solution have been developed (Figs. 4.1, 4.2, and 4.3).

Four major manufacturers, Olympus (Olympus America, Center Valley, Pa), Pentax (Pentax of America, Montvale, NJ), Fujifilm endoscopy (Fujinon, Wayne, NJ), and Karl Storz Se & Co. (Tuttlingen, Germany—Fig. 4.4), produce duodenoscopes, and these are their major characteristics (Table 4.1).

4.3 Echoendoscopes

Endoscopic ultrasonography (EUS) combines endoscopy and intraluminal ultrasonography.

The new electronic instruments are connected with processors with considerable digital capabilities. Therefore, the technical peculiarities of the endoscopes of the same brand (i.e., NBI, FICE, Hi-scan) are contemporary available with the technical features of the most modern ultrasounds equipment (Doppler, power Doppler, color Doppler, tissue harmonic echo [THE], contrast harmonic EUS [CH-EUS], elastography, etc.).

The instruments for endoscopic ultrasound evaluation can be divided in:

- radial echoendoscopes for diagnostic purposes,
- linear echoendoscopes for diagnostic and interventional purposes.

Radial echoendoscopes consist of electronic radial-array transducers that orient the individual piezoelectric elements around the distal tip in a 360° radial array, producing an image in a plane perpendicular to the long axis of the echoendoscope that is very similar to the images provided by computed tomography. Radial-array echoendoscopes are used only for diagnostic EUS examinations because tissue sampling and therapeutic interventions are not possible due to the lack of visualization of needle or other devices track.

Linear echoendoscopes provide a plane of imaging parallel to the long axis of the scope with an image format that is similar to that obtained with transabdominal ultrasonography; only this type of probe allows real-time visualization of needles and other accessories introduced through the operative channel of the echoendoscope [6–8]. It allows to perform fine-needle aspiration or biopsy (FNA or FNAB), stent delivering, drainage, and locoregional treatments (i.e., celiac plexus block and neurolysis).

Three major manufacturers (Olympus, Pentax, Fujifilm) produce echoendoscopes. Their characteristics are summarized in the tables below (Figs. 4.5, 4.6, and 4.7, Tables 4.2 and 4.3).

4.4 EUS Processors

EUS processors consist of two parts: the first for the endoscopic view and the second one for the ultrasound view. These devices allow to capture, manipulate, and store EUS images. These platforms may be exclusively dedicated to EUS or may be compatible with transabdominal probes. Traditionally, a strict partnership has been created between the echoendoscope companies and well-known ultrasound processors manufacturers: Pentax radial and linear scopes are driven by a Hitachi platform, whereas Olympus echoendoscopes run from Aloka systems.

Table 4.1 Duodenoscopes

	Insertion tube outer diameter (mm)	Distal end outer diameter (mm)	Channel inner diameter	Working length (mm)	Field of view	Depth of field (mm)	Angulation range				Electronic capabilities	Single use distal tip	Remarks
							Up	Down	Right	Left			
Olympus TJF-Q180V	11.3	13.7	4.2	1240	100°/5° retro	5–60	120°	90°	110°	90°	NBI	No	V-System
Olympus TJF-Q190V	11.3	13.5	4.2	1240	100°/15° retro	5–60	120°	90°	110°	90°	NBI	Yes	OT, HFT, V-System
Fujinon ED-530XT	11.5	13.1	4.2	1250	100°/8° retro	4–60	130°	90°	110°	90°	FICE	No	
Fujinon ED-530XT8	11.5	13.1	4.2	1250	100°/8° retro	4–60	130°	90°	110°	90°	FICE	Yes	
Pentax ED34-i10T	11.6	13	4.2	1250	100°/10° retro	4–60	120°	90°	105°	90°	HISCAN	No	HD+, detachable cap, Pentax "CleanCap-system" (OE-A55)
Pentax ED34-i10T2	11.6	13.6	4.2	1250	100°/10° retro°	4–60	120°	90°	105°	90°	HISCAN	Yes	HD+, DEC, Disposable Elevator Cap (OE-A63)
Storz Silverscope	12.6	12.6	4.2	1260	140°	2–60	120°	90°	110°	90°	/	No	

OT One-Touch Connector, *FHT* High-Force Transmission, *HD+* High Definition New Chip, *DEC* Allows simplified reprocessing and increased cleaning capability, *Pentax "CleanCap-system"* Detachable distal end cap for a safe and quick mechanical cleaning of air and water channels

Table 4.2 Radial echoendoscopes

Radial	Insertion tube (mm)	Distal end (mm)	Working length (mm)	Channel inner diameter (mm)	Direction of viewing field	Ultrasound field of view	Depth of field	Frequency (MHz)	Doppler	CHE-EUS	Elastography	System compatibility
Olympus GF-UE160-AL5	11.8		1250	2.2	Forward oblique	360°	3–100	5/6/7.5/10/12	Yes	Yes	Yes	Hitachi-Aloka Olympus
Pentax EG-3670URK	12.1	10.3	1250	2.4	Forward	360°	4–100	5–10	Yes	Yes	Yes	Hitachi-Aloka
Fujinon EG-580UR	11.5	11.4	1250	2.8	Forward	360°	3–100	5/7.5/10/12	Yes	No	No	Fuji

Table 4.3 Linear echoendoscopes

Linear	Insertion tube (mm)	Distal end (mm)	Working length (mm)	Channel inner diameter (mm)	Direction of viewing field	Ultrasound field of view	Depth of field (mm)	Frequency (MHz)	Doppler	CHE-EUS	Elastography	System compatibility
Olympus GF-UCT180	12.6	14.6	1250	3.7	Forward oblique (55°)	180°	3–100	5/6/7.5/10/12	Yes	Yes	Yes	Hitachi-Aloka Olympus
Olympus TGF-UC180J	12.6	14.6	1245	3.7	Forward	90°	3–100	5/6/7.5/10/12	Yes	Yes	Yes	Hitachi-Aloka Olympus
Pentax EG-3270UK	10.8	12	1250	2.8	Forward oblique (50°)	180°	5–100	5–10	Yes	Yes	Yes	Hitachi-Aloka
Pentax EG-3870UTK	12.8	14.3	1250	3.8	Forward oblique (50°)	180°	5–100	5–10	Yes	Yes	Yes	Hitachi-Aloka
Fujinon EG-580UT	12.4	13.9	1250	3.8	Forward oblique (40°)	180°	3–100	5/7.5/10/12	Yes	No	No	Fuji

4.5 ERCP Instruments

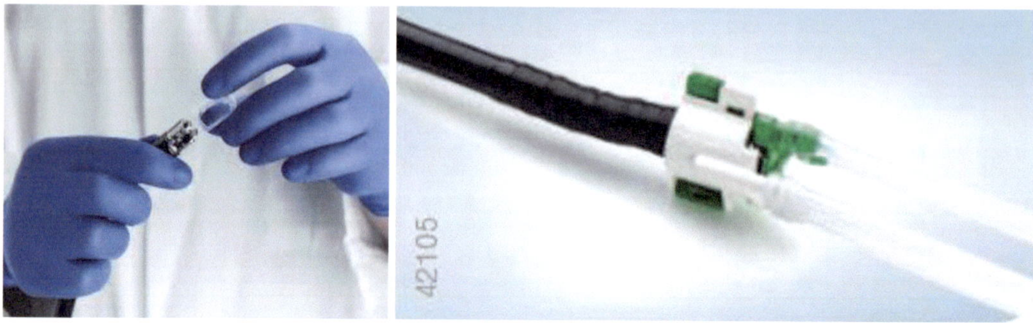

Fig. 4.1 Olympus TJF-Q190V. The single-use distal cover allows better access for reprocessing accessories during manual cleaning. The cover is transparent and is destroyed during removal, preventing unintended reuse. The new flushing adapter reduces the number of required flushing steps and ensures controlled distribution of detergent and disinfectant solution to the distal tip of the endoscope during manual reprocessing

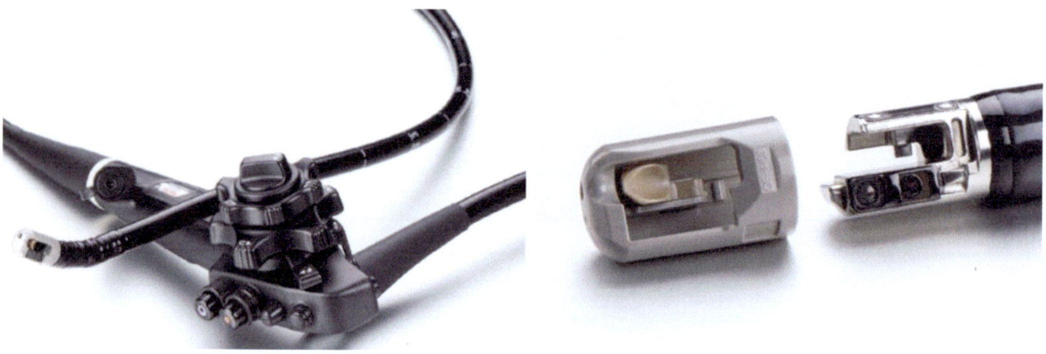

Fig. 4.2 Pentax ED34-i10T2. This video duodenoscope combines a sterile disposable elevator cap (DECTM) for single-patient use and simple disposal that advances cleaning capability of the duodenoscope. This is to help reduce risk of cross contamination

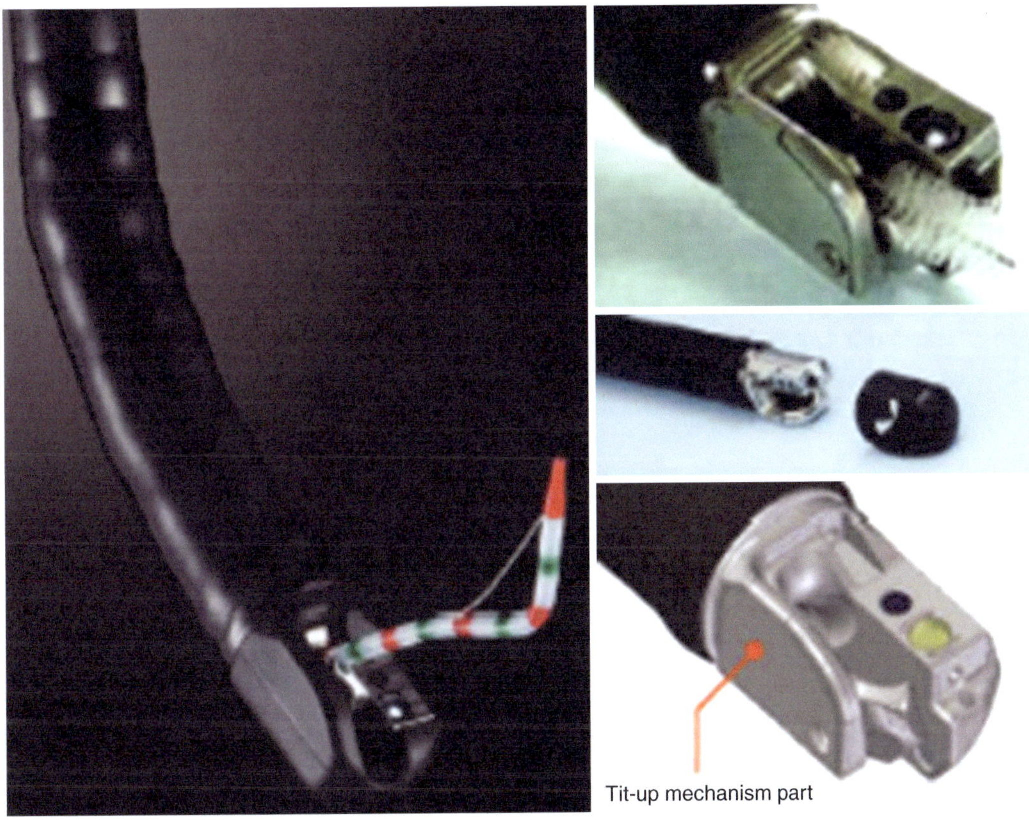

Fig. 4.3 Fujinon ED-530XT8. It is equipped with a disposable distal end cap that enables brushing of all channels and helps to improve the hygienic environment. A covered tilt-up mechanism of the forceps elevator maintains the elevator wire clean without any additional clearing procedure

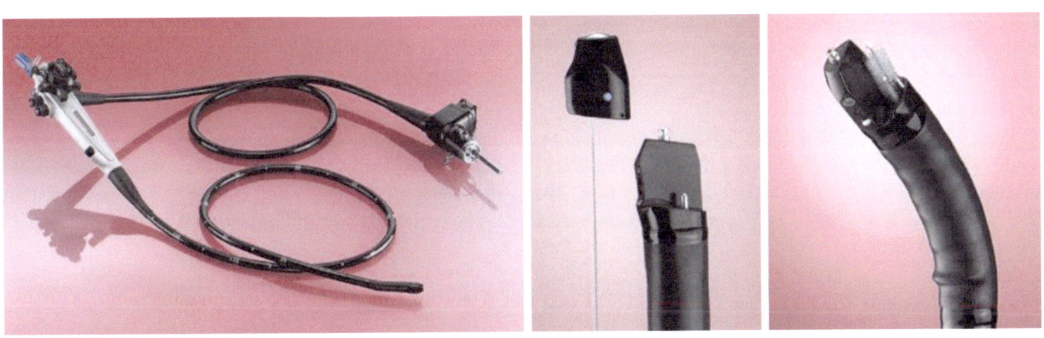

Fig. 4.4 Karl Storz 13885PKSK/NKSK duodenoscope. Removable and autoclavable Albarran module

4.6 EUS Instruments

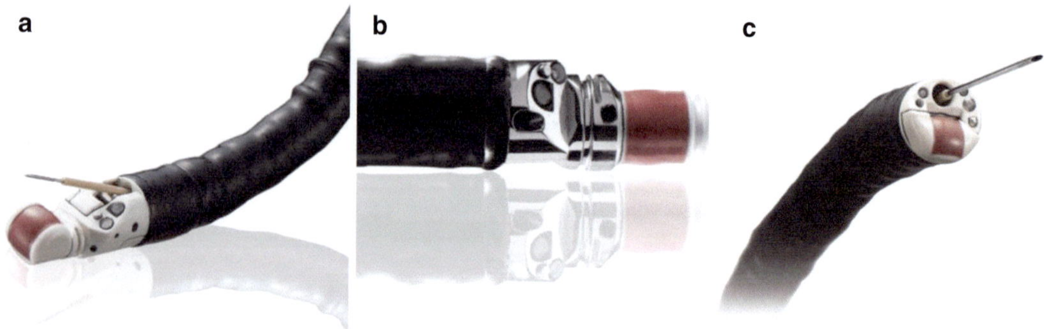

Fig. 4.5 The Olympus GF-UCT180 (**a**) delivers high-quality ultrasound images with greater B-mode imaging depth, offering safe control with a round transducer design and a short rigid distal end. Olympus GF-UE160-AL5 (**b**) radial ultrasound endoscope is a 360° radial-array scanning endoscope. Olympus TGF-UC180J (**c**) linear ultrasound endoscope. The forward-viewing ultrasound gastrovideoscope pioneers new opportunities in endoscopic ultrasound-guided treatment

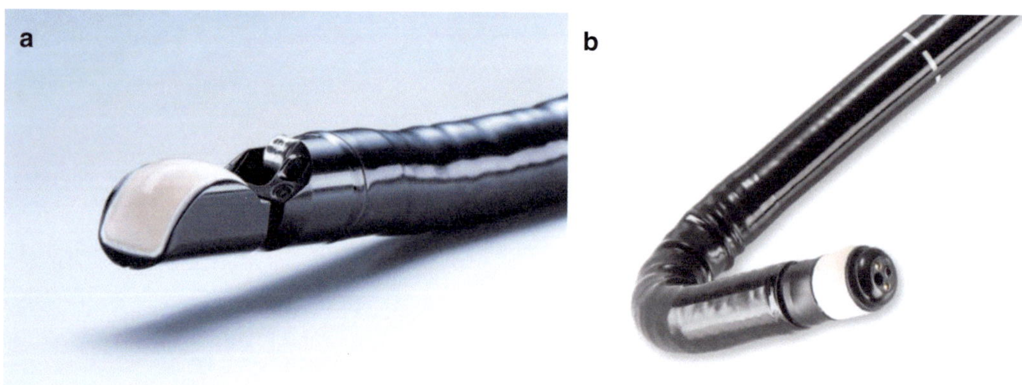

Fig. 4.6 Pentax EG-3870UTK (**a**) ultrasound video endoscope utilizes a curved, linear-array ultrasound transducer that provides a large 120° field of view. The EG-3670URK (**b**) features a 360°, electronic, radial-array ultrasound transducer, which generates high-resolution ultrasound images. Both are supported by various imaging modalities such as Hitachi Real-Time Tissue Elastography (HI-RTE) and Doppler function for a more accurate localization and targeting of lesions

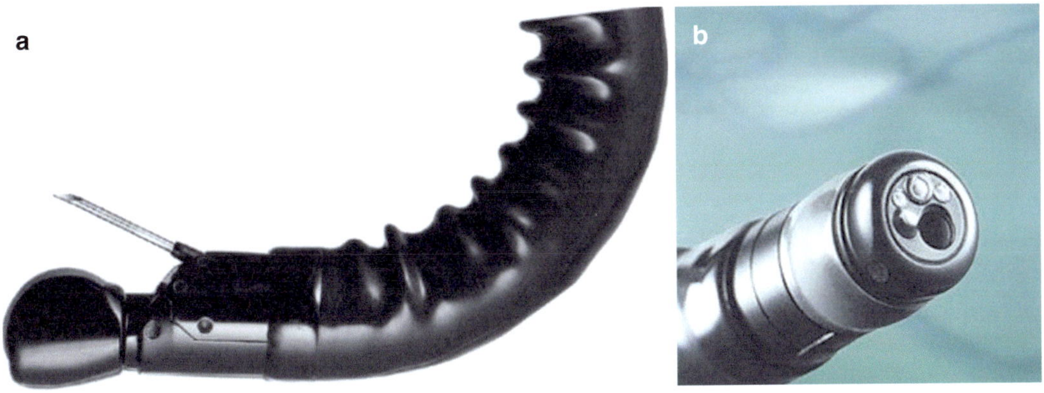

Fig. 4.7 Fujifilm EG-580UT (**a**) ultrasound endoscope with forceps elevator assist which enables convex scanning, developed for therapeutic interventions. With a working channel of 3.8 mm and equipped with an Albarran lever, it is the former scope, which also allows passage of therapeutic devices and needle position guide on the ultrasound image. Fujifilm EG-580 UR (**b**) with the thin outer diameter of 11.4 mm, the unique 190° bending, and the brilliant Super CCD image quality; the new EG-580UR allows to carry out endoscopic ultrasound examinations almost as simply as a traditional endoscopic examination. The 2.8 mm working channel enables a good suction ability and the use of a standard-size biopsy forceps. The electronic 360° radial scan ensures a reliable panoramic view

References

1. Baillie J, Byrne MF. ERCP preparation, positioning, and instrumentation. Tech Gastrointest Endosc. 2003;5(1):3–10.
2. Yao W, Huang Y, Chang H, et al. Endoscopic retrograde cholangiopancreatography using a dual-lumen endogastroscope for patients with Billroth II gastrectomy. Gastroenterol Res Pract. 2013;2013:146867.
3. Rauwers AW, Voor In 't Holt AF, Buijs JG, et al. High prevalence rate of digestive tract bacteria in duodenoscopes: a nationwide study. Gut. 2018;67:1637–45.
4. Beilenhoff U, Biering H, Blum R, et al. Prevention of multidrug-resistant infections from contaminated duodenoscopes: position Statement of the European Society of Gastrointestinal Endoscopy (ESGE) and European Society of Gastroenterology Nurses and Associates (ESGENA). Endoscopy. 2017;49:1098–106.
5. Humphries RM, McDonnell G. Superbugs on duodenoscopes: the challenge of cleaning and disinfection of reusable devices. J Clin Microbiol. 2015;53(10):3118–25.
6. Adler DG, Conway JD, Coff JM, et al. EUS accessories. Technology status evaluation report. Gastrointest Endosc. 2007;66:1076–81.
7. Ahmad N, Kochman ML. EUS instrumentation and accessories: a primer. Gastrointest Endosc. 2000;52:s2–5.
8. Murad FM, Komanduri S, Abu Dayyeh BK, et al. Echoendoscopes. Gastrointest Endosc. 2015;82(2):189–202.

5 ERCP Standard and Special Devices

Andrea Oliver Tal and Jörg G. Albert

Abbreviations

ERCP	Endoscopic retrograde cholangiopancreatography
MRCP	Magnetic resonance cholangiopancreatography
PDT	Photodynamic therapy
SEMS	Self-expanding metal stents

5.1 Introduction

The beginning of the endoscopic retrograde cholangiopancreatography (ERCP) era started in the 1970s when the first duodenoscopes were available and the cannulation of the bile duct system became feasible while sphincterotomy of the ampulla of Vater had been established [1]. ERCP has since become the gold standard for many therapeutic procedures of the biliopancreatic tract. Basic prerequisite was the development of a wide variety of cleverly designed auxiliary devices. Thereby, the complexity of ERCP and its instruments requested an ample investment in training and experience of the investigator [2]. During the last decades, a multitude of new techniques, devices and indications for ERCP have evolved, shifting the procedure from a diagnostic tool to a predominately therapeutic intervention that led ERCP to become the most common non-surgical treatment alternative for various biliopancreatic diseases [3]. In opposition, the quality of alternative radiological procedures for the imaging of the bile ducts, such as magnetic resonance cholangiopancreatography (MRCP) and endoscopic ultrasound, excelled and the need and justification for diagnostic ERCP has dramatically dwindled.

A. O. Tal (✉)
Gastroenterologie, Internistische Praxisgemeinschaft - IPG Hanau, Hanau, Germany

J. G. Albert
Hepatologie und Endokrinologie, Abteilung für Gastroenterologie, Robert-Bosch-Krankenhaus, Auerbachstraße, Stuttgart, Germany
e-mail: joerg.albert@rbk.de

5.2 Armamentarium for a Standard ERCP Procedure

A perfect ERCP may be performed with an optimum of technical equipment, high skill of the investigational team and all human resources available for pre-, intra- and post-procedural assistance of the team and patient. This chapter will immerse into the great multitude of standard and special instruments that are available for diagnostic and therapeutic ERCP.

M. Mutignani et al. (eds.), *Endotherapy in Biliopancreatic Diseases: ERCP Meets EUS*,
https://doi.org/10.1007/978-3-030-42569-2_5

5.2.1 Duodenoscopes

The duodenoscope is a side-viewing endoscope used to optimally visualize the papilla and to carry any device that is required for the purpose of the intervention. There are mostly so-called therapeutic duodenoscopes in use, with an outer diameter of about 12–14 mm and a working channel of 3.2–4.2 mm. Small duodenoscopes are mainly restricted for paediatric/neonatal applications. For the newborn (<1 year old), slim side-viewing endoscopes (7.5 mm outer diameter and 2 mm channel size, e.g. Olympus PJF-160 duodenoscope) are available. For children (>10–15 kg body weight), standard duodenoscopes with an outer diameter of 10 mm or more might be used.

The optical system of the endoscope is located on the side of the distal end, in contrast to the forward-viewing gastroscopes. Duodenoscopes contain a so-called Albarrán lever at the exit port of the working channel. This module is located parallel to the optics and helps to optimize the position of the devices that are passed through the working channel, and the angulation for cannulation and therapeutic interventions can be aligned precisely by moving this lever.

5.2.2 Cannulation Catheters

After positioning the duodenoscope in front of the papilla, cannulation catheters or sphincterotomes are used for intubation of the orifice. The majority of cannulation catheters are designed to gain access through the major papilla, although there are a few catheters that are specifically designed to facilitate minor papilla cannulation. These catheters have one or two lumens which offer the guidewire and/or contrast agent to reach the bile duct in order to succeed in biliary cannulation. Modified cannulas with three lumens for additional biopsy forceps are under evaluation [4]. A standard cannula is made from plastic material or Teflon and has a radiopaque tip with a diameter of 5 Fr (1.67 mm). A transparent material allows to visualize the guidewire in the endoscopic image. Many different models with different-shaped tips, lengths, diameters and materials may be purchased and can be useful under special circumstances (e.g. small bent tip for cannulation of the minor papilla).

5.2.3 Guidewires

Guidewires have become a cornerstone of ERCP as they are used for cannulation of the papilla and the biliary tree and for negotiating and traversing strictures [5, 6]. The guidewire-assisted cannulation of the papilla is actually proposed as first-line option by the European Society of Gastrointestinal Endoscopy [7]. Furthermore, guidewires are important when changing the instruments whilst uptaining the access to the occluded bile duct and can be used as a guardrail. The material composition of the respective guidewire grants a special property for attaining dedicated purposes. Monofilament guidewires are much more rigid than coiled wires as they are made of stainless steel. The structure of sheathed wires normally consists of a stiff inner radiopaque nitinol or stainless monofilament core that is covered by an outer polyurethane/PTFE/Teflon sheath. Coiled wires have a stiff core with an outer spiral coil. The guidewire's distal end is often coated with an hydrophilic material to facilitate the cannulation of the papilla [8]. The guidewires have coloured surfaces and radiopaque marks within the core, so that there are two possibilities of control: direct endoscopic or fluoroscopic visualization. The newest development over the last years was the establishment of the so-called short-wire systems [9]. The short wires propose handling and hygienic advantages. The design of these wires was driven by newly developed locking systems within the newest generations of duodenoscopes and by new designs of the catheters. Long guidewire systems (>400 cm) have to be handled by an additional assistant in most cases and may prolong exchange and investigation times. Handling of the long wire demands for an excellent communication between the investigator and the assistants. An unfortunate but typical undesirable effect of long wires might be that the team more frequently experiences dislocation of the guidewire, loss of access and that the guidewire might even touch the ground.

The short-guidewire systems have approximately twice the length of a duodenoscope and can be locked in their position, so that devices can be removed and replaced without displacement of the wire. Another benefit of the short-guidewire systems is the ability of an investigator-controlled guidewire cannulation. Other advantages might be shorter intervention time and less complications. Up to now, there is a variety of different long- and short-guidewire systems available with different materials, shapes, lengths and diameters. Even though there seem to be comparable rates of intra- and post-procedural complications, some models seem to increase the success rate of stricture cannulation while decreasing the procedure time (Table 5.1) [10].

In most instances, 0.025 or 0.032 in. guidewires are used, with 0.018 or 0.020 in. wires reserved for use in small catheters or minor papilla cannulation. Some 0.025 in. wires offer similar stability and flexibility to wires of bigger size and are therefore the standard size in many units. Further innovations could potentially lead to less ampullary trauma and post-ERCP pancreatic as well as to faster cannulation times.

5.2.4 Standard Sphincterotome, Pre-cut Sphincterotome and the Needle Knife

In comparison to a standard catheter, a sphincterotome has an electrosurgical cutting wire at the distal end of the catheter. For many therapeutic interventions, endoscopic sphincterotomy is required before starting the treatment. Thereby, after cannulating the papilla, the endoscopic sphincterotome is advanced into the bile duct orifice and the wire placed beside the biliary sphincter. For sphincteroplasty, i.e. large balloon dilation of the papilla, a balloon dilation is done after sphincterotomy. A numerous amount of different sphincterotomes with various characteristics are currently available (e.g. triple vs. dual lumen, different kinds of materials, angled vs. straight tip, short vs. long nose).

However, compared to the first sphincterotomes from 1974 [1], the fundamental principle has not changed: a sphincterotome is made of a monofil steel wire that is covered by a Teflon sheath. The wire runs outside this sheath for a few centimetres at the tip end of the sphincterotome and can indirectly be moved and tautened when in- or deflecting the tip end of the sphincterotome. Modern available sphincterotomes have more than one lumen for simultaneous use of guidewires and contrast agent.

When the cannulation of the papilla fails or is difficult, pre-cut sphincterotomes are sometimes used. With the pre-cut sphincterotome, the cutting wire directly ends at the front of the distal tip. In other instances, a needle knife is preferred [11, 12]. The needle knife has a retractable filament on its tip for electrosurgical cutting. The control handle of the catheter allows for projecting the metal filament out of the catheter, once the catheter is in position in the duodenal lumen. With the exposed needle in contact with

Table 5.1 Different kinds of short-wire systems

Characteristics	RX system	Fusion system	V-system
Type of endoscope	Standard	Standard	V-scope
Type of lock	External at the biopsy port	External at the biopsy port	Internal lock design
Type of device	Open channel tear-away	Close channel breakthrough	Close lumen device
Wire length (cm)	260	185	270
May be used with standard guidewires	Yes	Yes	Yes
0.025″/0.018″ wires can be used	No	Yes	Yes
Ability to flush wire channel	No	Yes	Yes
Intraductal exchange ability	No	Yes	No
Physician control of wire	Yes	Yes	Yes
Pushability of short-wire devices	++	+++	+++

the tissue, manual movement of the catheter and activation of the electrosurgical current permit cutting. The needle knife is recommended for use in expert hands only.

A detailed description of these techniques will be provided in Chaps. 16 and 17. A review of the literature including three meta-analyses seems to favour needle knife pre-cut as the preferred technique for difficult cannulations [7].

5.2.5 Balloon Catheters

Depending on the operator's preference, stone extraction balloon catheter or Dormia baskets are alternatives to remove bile duct stones [13]. However, balloon catheters can also be used to selectively contrast segmental bile ducts (occlusion cholangiography) with the contrast agent exiting above or below the balloon, depending on the device construction.

In contrast to stone extraction balloon catheters that are inflated with air, different types of balloon catheters are used for stricture dilatation or for the dilation of the papilla (sphincteroplasty). The latter techniques are based on hydrostatic pressure by injecting liquids (e.g. mixing sterile saline with contrast) with the help of a high-pressure inflation device. The balloon diameters typically range from 4 to 8 mm for stricture dilation in the biliary ducts and from 8 to 20 mm for sphincteroplasty. The diameters of the balloons always should respect the diameter of the normal adjacent bile duct to avoid a perforation.

Stone extraction balloon catheters are available with two and three lumens. One lumen is determined for taking the guide wire, one is for transporting the contrast agent to the orifice at the tip of the catheter and the third is for air insufflation of the balloon. Some experts prefer to use a balloon catheter for extraction of sludge, small, soft or fragmented concrements. The balloon-assisted stone extraction is recommended as the first-line treatment of stones given the ease of use, utility in occlusion cholangiography and the lack of risk of becoming entrapped in the duct [14].

5.2.6 Dormia Baskets

Stone extraction baskets (e.g. the Dormia basket) with mostly four or six wires come with a variety of wire configuration. They may be classified in cages for mechanical lithotripsy and cages for simple stone retrieval. Both are available from different suppliers, with different lengths, diameters, materials and specific characteristics (e.g. guidewire assisted or not). Most can be rotated to help to catch the stone. In guidewire-assisted stone retrieval, the guidewire can pass through either the basket's tip or an exit on the side of the catheter some centimetres below the basket. The former helps to cannulate the bile duct, whereas the latter is easing the catching of stones.

To successfully use a Dormia basket, the biliary orifice needs to be patent and large enough to allow for an exit of the stone. Otherwise, when the stone is too big for removal throughout the papilla's orifice, it can be disintegrated by mechanical lithotripsy. Thereby, the stone is caught by the dedicated lithotripsy basket. Subsequently, the stone can be fragmented by closing the basket with force that is applied through the outer metal coil of the catheter and the retraction of the basket's leading wire. By rotating a part of the handhold, the basket will be tightened step by step in direction of the coil until the stone bursts into smaller pieces which can then be retrieved (Chap. 41). Small and flexible baskets are available for the use in the pancreatic system.

5.2.7 Dilatation Catheters and Bougies

Dilatation catheters are mainly used in the presence of short (benign) bile duct stenosis. Biliary strictures in primary sclerosing cholangitis or anastomotic strictures of the bile duct after liver transplantation are typical examples. Furthermore, a balloon dilatation can be performed before stent insertion. Dilatation catheters can be precisely placed by using a guidewire and are expanded by using an integrated inflation device. Bougies are tapered stiff catheters that are advanced over a guidewire to dilate the stenosis. They are comparable to bougies that are used in the upper GI tract, but they are smaller, of course, and provide an outer diameter of 7, 8.5 and 10 French. They can be used for longer strictures in the distal common bile duct (CBD) or for strictures in an angulated bile duct segment.

5.2.8 Biopsy Forceps and Brush Cytology

When malignant strictures or biliary tumours are suspected, it is essential to obtain a specimen of adequate size with representative tissue. This is fundamental for the pathologist to establish the right diagnosis. Studies have demonstrated that potential malignancies can be misdiagnosed as false-negative caused by specimens containing insufficient cellularity [15]. The biopsy forceps and the brush are current standard for this purpose, but clinical results might be improved. They are easily used through the working channel under fluoroscopic guidance. Further methods and tools are under current investigation (e.g. molecular analysis of tissue, fluorescence in situ hybridization, confocal laser microscopy) and need to be evaluated within trials.

5.2.9 Lithotripsy

In case that mechanical lithotripsy techniques may not be used to fragment a stone, alternative options are available [16], such as electrohydraulic lithotripsy (EHL) and laser lithotripsy (ILL). Both demand for cholangioscopic visualization of the stone and close contact with the corresponding probe for successful fragmentation and subsequent duct clearance [17].

EHL probes can be applied through the working channel of cholangioscopes and positioned within contact or just before to the targeted stone. Through an electrohydraulic shock wave generator, shock waves of different frequency can be generated and applied [18]. Several laser lithotripsy variants have been developed over the last decades (neodymium-yttrium aluminium garnet, yttrium aluminium garnet, alexandrite and holmium-yttrium aluminium garnet). All of them need special laser systems to deliver laser therapy through specialized fibre probes. These can be applied and positioned concordant to EHL probes through the working channels of cholangioscopes by using guiding catheters. Under direct visualization and in contact with the targeted stone, laser therapy can then be applied until the stone bursts.

EHL and laser lithotripsy seem to be more effective than extracorporeal shock wave lithotripsy [19]. With these methods, bile duct clearance of biliary stones can be achieved in the vast majority of cases without great risks even in elderly patients [17, 20]. Cholangioscopy-guided laser lithotripsy increases the incidence of endoscopic clearance of large bile duct stones and decreases the need for surgery compared with conventional therapy alone [21].

5.2.10 Biliary Stenting

An adequate drainage of the biliopancreatic system is a fundamental requirement for living and the main goal of most ERCP interventions. For this purpose, the use of stents with different features has been established over the past decades. Initially the word stent was first used to describe a prosthesis that was used as spacer after root canal work by a dentist named Charles Stent in 1856 [22]. Today we use the word stent to describe implants inserted into a lumen or structure to maintain its patency or gain access. The use of stents has expanded to treat and palliate many conditions including malignant strictures, leaks, perforations, fistulas and bleedings. The main biliary stent categories can be divided into plastic stents and self-expanding metal stents (SEMS). A vast spectrum of different stent types is nowadays available ranging from several different materials, shapes, diameters and lengths to different flanges, stent tulips and coatings. Plastic stents and SEMS provide similar short-term results with respect to clinical success, morbidity, mortality and improvement in quality of life [23].

Plastic stents are cost-effective and easy to use and provide an effective drainage when used properly. It can be inserted in almost every part of the biliary tree via guidewire and released by so-called stent pusher catheters. Limitations are the necessity for stent exchange every 12 weeks as plastic stents tend to occlude due to their smaller inner diameter (5–10 Fr). Stents with similar features made of polyethylene and Teflon are available. In comparison, metal stents have larger diameters and therefore longer patency rates which could be demonstrated in several trials [24], but a superiority over a treatment with multiple plastic stents could not be seen throughout almost all indications [23].

In the beginning of the metal stent era, SEMS were mainly used for malignant strictures. Nowadays one can choose between uncovered and partially and fully covered removable biliary stents which led to an expansion of the indications. Metal stents are nowadays applied in a through-the-scope (TTS) technique. By using a special stent application catheter and a guidewire, the stent can be exactly placed under fluoroscopic control. Due to its radiopaque markings, the exact localization and its stepwise deployment can be seen while using the release mechanism respectively. Prospective trials show that successful treatment of benign strictures can be achieved by using SEMS with the same success rate compared to plastic stents but diminishing the number of interventions under certain circumstances [25]. For malignant strictures with a palliative condition, uncovered SEMS can be used, as a stent removal is not essential. Limitations for SEMS are intrahepatic strictures as well as hilar malignancies as a fully covered stent could lead to suspension of the gallbladder or biliary segments. Some studies show high migration rates resulting in no benefit over plastic stents.

To sum up, there are many different stent types. Recommendations of use are also available on the website of the endoscopic societies, e.g. the European Society of Gastrointestinal Endoscopy (www.ESGE.org) or the American Society for Gastrointestinal Endoscopy (www.asge.org).

5.2.11 Devices for ERCP in the Surgically Altered GI Tract

The success of ERCP in patients with surgically altered anatomy depends on multiple factors including the postoperative anatomy, expertise of the endoscopist and availability of specialized endoscopes and devices to perform endotherapy. In case of balloon-assisted enteroscopy plus ERCP, the working channel size and the length of the endoscope have to be respected in choosing the right instruments and for a successful intervention.

The Billroth II sphincterotome differs from the standard sphincterotome as the altered anatomy features an opposite position of the instrument in comparison to standard ERCP positioning. When ERCP is done in patients with a Roux-en-Y anastomosis (paediatric), colonoscopes or double balloon enteroscopes can be helpful [26], and the difference in working channel diameter and instrument length must be considered to choose the right device. In retrograde approach of the endoscope to the papilla, the papillotome will exit the endoscope with a position about 180° rotated. For this reason, the cutting wire of Billroth II sphincterotomes is located on the opposite side of the catheter's tip end. Three different types are available: Billroth II sphincterotome, Soehendra sphincterotome and the shark fin sphincterotome. Alternatively, a needle knife could be beneficial in Billroth II situations [27].

An exact description of altered techniques for sphincterotomy and therapeutic interventions will be given in Part VI of this book.

5.3 Special Devices for Therapeutic ERCP Interventions

5.3.1 Radiofrequency Ablation (RFA)

In 2009, the FDA approved an endoscopic RFA catheter for endoscopic treatment of palliative malignant biliary strictures [28]. The probe features two ring electrodes at the tip with a distance of 8 mm from each other and is designed to perform bipolar cautery in endoscopic surgical procedures. The catheter measures 8 French (2.6 mm) in diameter and 1.8 m in length and is positioned by guidewire under fluoroscopic guidance. The RFA catheter can be connected to a bipolar electrosurgical generator leading to a cylindrical necrosis around the ring electrodes. The extent of the necrotic area depends on the mode of the electrosurgical generator, power and duration of the application. Nevertheless, up to now, no randomized studies have been initiated to compare the corresponding standard of care for different malignant biliary strictures (e.g. stenting, chemotherapy, photodynamic therapy) with this treatment option. So it still remains unclear if RFA is an equal treatment option for palliative situations and should only be used within trials or individual situations as it bears potential risks [25].

5.3.2 Photodynamic Therapy (PDT)

PDT is an alternative palliative therapeutic option for the treatment of cholangiocarcinoma besides biliary stenting and chemotherapy [29, 30]. It is an expensive treatment that needs several compounds. Even though it is an easy to apply treatment, it can therefore only be recommended for the use in expert centres. PDT is a photochemotherapy in which a light-absorbing drug (photosensitizer) is injected and preferably taken up by tumour tissue. By emitting light to a targeted lesion, the photochemical process is initiated. Reactive oxygen variants lead to cell death and then trigger immune response eventually [31]. Photodynamic therapy is delivered through a fibre with a diffuser at its distal end. The diffuser can be inserted into a 10 Fr sheath of a plastic stent delivery system, for example, and placed at the level of the targeted lesion. Alternatively, some publications have been using cholangioscopy as a platform to administer PDT.

5.3.3 Cholangioscopy

Since the appearance of the first peroral cholangioscopy (POC) devices in 1976 [32], great technological progress has been made. Nowadays three main cholangioscopy techniques can be distinguished: a single-operator technique, a dual-operator “mother-baby” technique and a direct technique in which ultrathin gastroscopes are used to directly visualize the bile duct. All techniques have in common that they demand for continuous irrigation of the bile duct through an accessory channel to maintain good visualization during the examination.

The most used single-operator cholangioscope so far is named SpyGlass System (Boston Scientific). This system consists of a delivery catheter, a light source, a video monitor and an irrigation pump. The delivery catheter can be inserted through the working channel of therapeutic duodenoscopes and is positioned via guidewire assistance. The delivery catheter comprises four working channels: one for continuous irrigation, one for aspiration, one for the optical catheter and one for special biopsy forceps. The optical catheter has four-way tip manoeuvrability with a 30-degree view in each direction [33].

Direct “mother baby” cholangioscopes can be introduced through the working channel of therapeutic duodenoscopes into the bile duct under continuous fluid irrigation. Their limitation is their fragility and the need for two endoscopists. You can easily cause damages by tough movements with the Albarrán module.

The last technique to mention is the possibility of peroral cholangioscopy (POC) by the use of ultra-slim endoscopes [34]. These scopes are designed to directly enter the biliary system after a sphincterotomy or sphincteroplasty has been performed. However, these techniques struggle with the loss of stability due to loop formation in the stomach or the duodenum. Different anchoring techniques are on its way and seem to be promising (balloons, overtubes, e.g.).

This new era of direct mucosal visualization within the biliopancreatic system could potentially help to optimize the diagnosis of malignant lesions with new classification systems [35] and targeted biopsies [36]. Some investigators even describe new techniques as mucosal tumour excisions under direct visualization with cholangioscopy [37].

5.4 Conclusion

Endoscopic treatment of biliopancreatic disorders has been revolutionized since the first introduction about 50 years ago. The advance of techniques and devices has established ERCP as the main non-surgical therapeutic option. A vast number of different tools and instruments in indefinite variants help to manage treatment tasks. In fact, excellent devices are available from most established producers, and there might be no universal recommendation to choose one over the other product. For an expert in ERCP, it plays a key role to know the armamentarium by heart and to be familiar with alternative treatment options. Thereby, personal preferences of which catheter or guidewire would be optimal at what occasion are formed. Therefore, selection of devices is at the discretion of the investigator and depends on one's own experience in many situations. However, there are increasingly high-quality randomized trials available that help to choose the optimal approach and device for a treatment task. Gastroenterology societies' recommendations and endoscopic guidelines are available for many indications.

Key Points

- Ensure that all resources are ready for the planned therapeutic ERCP.
- Make sure that you and your team know the available ERCP armamentarium.
- Propose a plan for the use of every instrument and tool you want to use to your team before starting the procedure.
- Be familiar with the use of your instruments and tools before starting an ERCP.
- Think of all possible treatment options to reach your goal before starting the intervention.
- Know your own skill limitations and when to ask for help.
- Be prepared to manage complications as a team.

References

1. Classen M, Demling L. [Endoscopic sphincterotomy of the papilla of vater and extraction of stones from the choledochal duct (author's transl)]. Dtsch Med Wochenschr. 1974;99(11):496–7.
2. Keswani RN, et al. Association between endoscopist and center endoscopic retrograde cholangiopancreatography volume with procedure success and adverse outcomes: a systematic review and meta-analysis. Clin Gastroenterol Hepatol. 2017;15(12):1866–1875.e3.
3. Carr-Locke DL. Overview of the role of ERCP in the management of diseases of the biliary tract and the pancreas. Gastrointest Endosc. 2002;56(6 Suppl):S157–60.
4. Goetz M, Malek NP. Novel triple lumen catheter for ERCP tissue diagnosis. Endosc Int Open. 2018;6(8):E984–8.
5. Jacob L, Geenen JE. ERCP guide wires. Gastrointest Endosc. 1996;43(1):57–60.
6. Singhvi G, Dea SK. Guidewires in ERCP. Gastrointest Endosc. 2013;77(6):938–40.
7. Testoni PA, et al. Papillary cannulation and sphincterotomy techniques at ERCP: European Society of Gastrointestinal Endoscopy (ESGE) Clinical Guideline. Endoscopy. 2016;48(7):657–83.
8. Tse F, et al. Guide wire-assisted cannulation for the prevention of post-ERCP pancreatitis: a systematic review and meta-analysis. Endoscopy. 2013;45(8):605–18.
9. Reddy SC, Draganov PV. ERCP wire systems: the long and the short of it. World J Gastroenterol. 2009;15(1):55–60.
10. Albert JG, et al. A novel, stiff-shaft, flexible-tip guidewire for cannulation of biliary stricture during endoscopic retrograde cholangiopancreatography: a randomized trial. Endoscopy. 2014;46(10):857–61.
11. Kaffes AJ, et al. Early institution of pre-cutting for difficult biliary cannulation: a prospective study comparing conventional vs. a modified technique. Gastrointest Endosc. 2005;62(5):669–74.
12. Lim JU, et al. Early use of needle-knife fistulotomy is safe in situations where difficult biliary cannulation is expected. Dig Dis Sci. 2012;57(5):1384–90.
13. Ishiwatari H, et al. Balloon catheter versus basket catheter for endoscopic bile duct stone extraction: a multicenter randomized trial. Endoscopy. 2016;48(4):350–7.
14. Maple JT, et al. The role of endoscopy in the management of choledocholithiasis. Gastrointest Endosc. 2011;74(4):731–44.

15. Korc P, Sherman S. ERCP tissue sampling. Gastrointest Endosc. 2016;84(4):557–71.
16. Sauerbruch T, et al. Fragmentation of gallstones by extracorporeal shock waves. N Engl J Med. 1986;314(13):818–22.
17. Swahn F, et al. Ten years of Swedish experience with intraductal electrohydraulic lithotripsy and laser lithotripsy for the treatment of difficult bile duct stones: an effective and safe option for octogenarians. Surg Endosc. 2010;24(5):1011–6.
18. Kamiyama R, et al. Electrohydraulic lithotripsy for difficult bile duct stones under endoscopic retrograde cholangiopancreatography and peroral transluminal cholangioscopy guidance. Gut Liver. 2018;12(4):457–62.
19. Neuhaus H, et al. Randomized study of intracorporeal laser lithotripsy versus extracorporeal shock-wave lithotripsy for difficult bile duct stones. Gastrointest Endosc. 1998;47(5):327–34.
20. Finkelmeier F, et al. ERCP in elderly patients: increased risk of sedation adverse events but low frequency of post-ERCP pancreatitis. Gastrointest Endosc. 2015;82(6):1051–9.
21. Buxbaum J, et al. Randomized trial of cholangioscopy-guided laser lithotripsy versus conventional therapy for large bile duct stones (with videos). Gastrointest Endosc. 2018;87(4):1050–60.
22. Ring ME. How a dentist's name became a synonym for a life-saving device: the story of Dr. Charles Stent. J Hist Dent. 2001;49(2):77–80.
23. Dumonceau J-M, et al. Endoscopic biliary stenting: indications, choice of stents, and results: European Society of Gastrointestinal Endoscopy (ESGE) Clinical Guideline—updated October 2017. Endoscopy. 2018;50(9):910–30.
24. Blero D, Huberty V, Devière J. Novel biliary self-expanding metal stents: indications and applications. Expert Rev Gastroenterol Hepatol. 2015;9(3):359–67.
25. Tal AO, et al. Multiple plastic stents versus covered metal stent for treatment of anastomotic biliary strictures after liver transplantation: a prospective, randomized, multicenter trial. Gastrointest Endosc. 2017;86(6):1038–45.
26. Kim MH, et al. Endoscopic retrograde cholangiopancreatography and needle-knife sphincterotomy in patients with Billroth II gastrectomy: a comparative study of the forward-viewing endoscope and the side-viewing duodenoscope. Endoscopy. 1997;29(2):82–5.
27. Abdelhafez M, et al. Comparison of endoscopic sphincterotomy techniques after Billroth II gastrectomy using a novel mechanical simulator. Surg Endosc. 2017;31(12):5342–7.
28. Steel AW, et al. Endoscopically applied radiofrequency ablation appears to be safe in the treatment of malignant biliary obstruction. Gastrointest Endosc. 2011;73(1):149–53.
29. Kahaleh M, et al. Unresectable cholangiocarcinoma: comparison of survival in biliary stenting alone versus stenting with photodynamic therapy. Clin Gastroenterol Hepatol. 2008;6(3):290–7.
30. Ortner MA, et al. Photodynamic therapy of nonresectable cholangiocarcinoma. Gastroenterology. 1998;114(3):536–42.
31. Talreja JP, Kahaleh M. Photodynamic therapy for cholangiocarcinoma. Gut Liver. 2010;4(Suppl 1):S62–6.
32. Kawai K, et al. [A new endoscopic method: the peroral choledocho-pancreatoscopy (author's transl)]. Leber Magen Darm. 1976;6(2):121–4.
33. Kahaleh M, Xu M-M. Recent developments in choledochoscopy: technical and clinical advances. Clin Exp Gastroenterol. 2016;9:119–24.
34. Albert JG, et al. Peroral cholangioscopy for diagnosis and therapy of biliary tract disease using an ultra-slim gastroscope. Endoscopy. 2011;43(11):1004–9.
35. Robles-Medranda C, et al. Reliability and accuracy of a novel classification system using peroral cholangioscopy for the diagnosis of bile duct lesions. Endoscopy. 2018;50(11):1059–70.
36. Navaneethan U, et al. Single-operator cholangioscopy and targeted biopsies in the diagnosis of indeterminate biliary strictures: a systematic review. Gastrointest Endosc. 2015;82(4):608–614.e2.
37. Jung JH, Park SW, Shin E. Endoscopic mucosal resection for intra-ductal growing type intrahepatic cholangiocarcinoma under direct per-oral cholangioscopy. Dig Endosc. 2018;30(6):785–8.

EUS Standard Devices

6

Danilo Castellani, Ugo Germani, Gabrio Bassotti, and Raffaele Manta

6.1 EUS-FNA Devices

6.1.1 Overall Concepts

The introduction of EUS tissue acquisition 25 years ago was an important breakthrough in the endoscopic field, and the procedure has considerably evolved in the last decade. EUS-FNA is now considered as an integral part of the diagnostic and staging algorithm for the evaluation of benign and malignant diseases of both gastrointestinal tract and proximal organs, such as the lungs (Table 6.1).

In recent years, new fine-needle biopsy (FNB) has been developed to obtain samples with preserved tissue architecture suitable for histological evaluation. This FNB has either a special geometry of the cutting tip or a side slot in the distal portion of the needle. Conventional needles without these refinements are referred to as FNA needles [1] (Fig. 6.1).

All EUS-FNA needles have the same basic design and are for single use. They are composed of a hollow needle with a solid removable stylet, a semirigid protective sheath, and a handle with a port for stylet insertion or withdrawal and attachment of a vacuum syringe. The various commercially available FNA needles have different echogenicity under EUS guidance. The visibility of the needle tip is critical when performing FNA [2]. Needle tips are tailored for using different techniques, such as laser etching, mechanical dimpling, or sandblasting [3, 4]. A multicenter study evaluated and graded ten different EUS needles based on their echogenicity. A prototype needle with polymeric coating had significantly

Table 6.1 The potential uses for EUS-FNA

1. Pancreatic mass
2. Mediastinal lymph nodes (metastasis for esophageal and lung cancer)
3. Celiac lymph nodes in association with a known upper GI cancer or in a patient suspected of having lymphoma
4. Intra-abdominal lymph nodes in association with a known (or suspicion of) cancer
5. Perirectal lymph node/mass
6. Posterior mediastinal mass of unknown etiology
7. Intrapleural/intra-abdominal fluid
In addition to the lesions indicative for EUS-FNA mentioned above, the indications have been expanded to:
1. Peripancreatic mass
2. Submucosal masses
3. Small liver lesions
4. Left adrenal mass
5. Suspected recurrent cancers in and adjacent to surgical anastomosis

D. Castellani · U. Germani · R. Manta (✉)
Gastroenterology Unit, Perugia General Hospital, Perugia, Italy

G. Bassotti
Gastroenterology and Hepatology Section, Department of Medicine, University of Perugia Medical School, Perugia, Italy

M. Mutignani et al. (eds.), *Endotherapy in Biliopancreatic Diseases: ERCP Meets EUS*,
https://doi.org/10.1007/978-3-030-42569-2_6

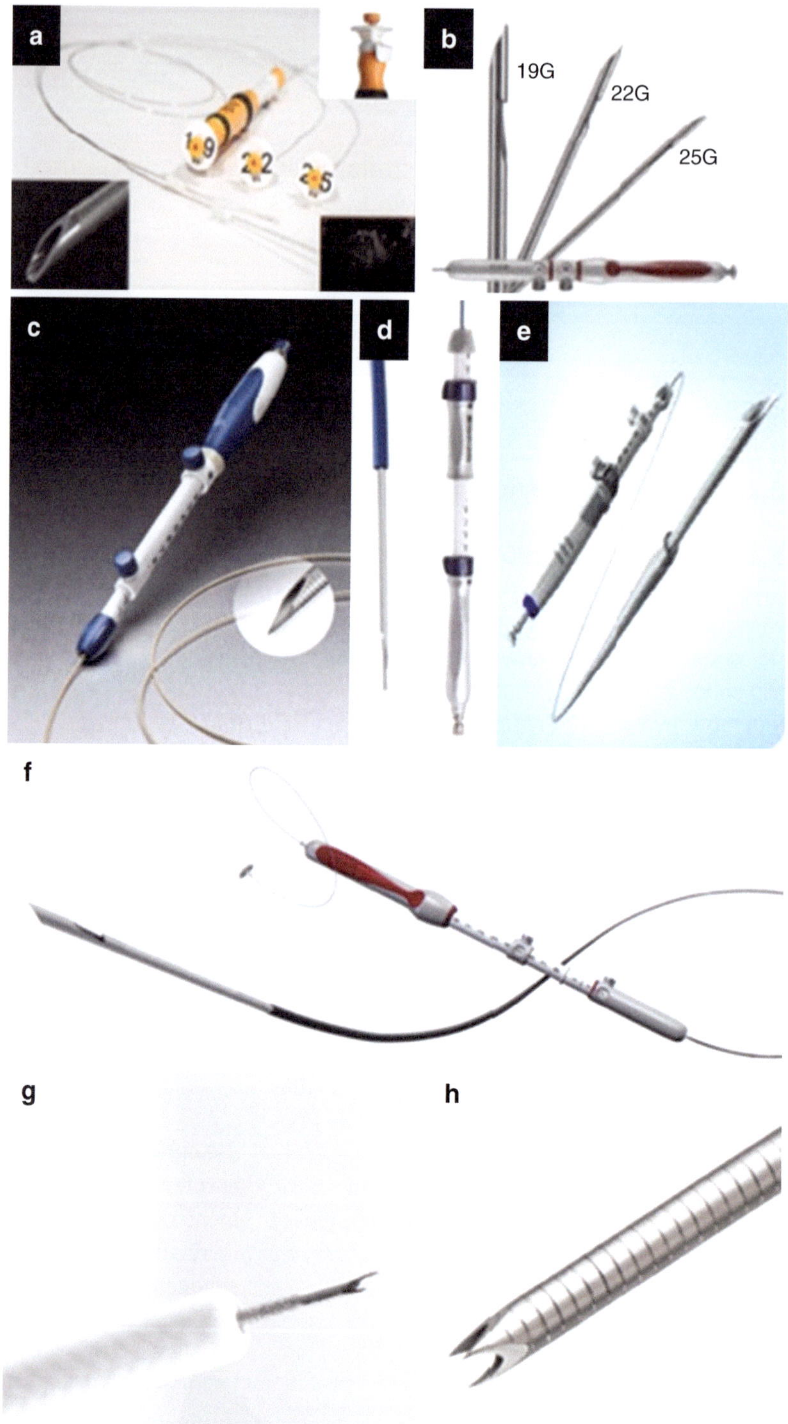

Fig. 6.1 FNA needles: (**a**) The BNX system with 19-gauge (G), 22-G, and 25-G needles (Medtronic). (**b**) The EchoTip ProCore needle (Cook Medical). (**c**) The nitinol-based Expect Flex 19-G fine aspiration needle (Boston Scientific). (**d**) ClearView FNA EUS Needles (ConMed). (**e**) The EZ Shot 3 Plus 19-G, 22-G, and 25-G (Olympus). FNB needles: (**f**) New 20-G EchoTip ProCore needle (Cook Medical). (**g**) BNX SharkCore (Medtronic) needle tip. (**h**) Acquire Endoscopic Ultrasound Fine Needle Biopsy Device (Boston Scientific)

higher overall ranking, indicating that this coating to the needle tip and shaft may enhance visualization [5].

The FNA needles are preloaded with a blunt stylet, which may protrude beyond the tip of the needle by 1–2 mm. Stylets enhance the rigidity of the needle during advancement through tissue to the target structure and protect the endoscope channel. Many manufacturers suggest withdrawing the stylet by a few millimeters before needle advancement to fully expose the sharp bevel at the needle tip. No data exist showing superiority of one stylet tip over another. In some devices, the stylet can be fixed in place within the needle by use of a Luer lock at the proximal end, whereas on other devices, the stylet is loosely held in place by a notched cap.

The device handle consists of several rigid plastic interlocking cylinders and is affixed to the echoendoscope by means of the Luer lock at the accessory channel port to enhance device stability during use. The handle assembly allows controlled and measured advancement of the needle from the protective sheath, the organ, or the structure of interest. Handles typically have markings at 1-cm intervals to monitor the depth of penetration of the needle, even though this distance can also be seen and measured endosonographically. Most needles can be advanced up to 9 cm. All devices come equipped with an adjustable "needle stopper" that limits advancement of the needle to a desired depth of insertion and prevents complete advancement during insertion and removal of the entire device into the echoendoscope as a safety precaution. The needle is advanced out of the sheath and into the target under direct ultrasound guidance. Once advanced into the target, the stylet is removed, and fluid, tissue, or both, can be aspirated, or therapeutic agents or contrast media are injected.

The EUS-FNA needles come with 10- or 20-cc syringes with locking mechanisms to hold the withdrawn plunger at different levels and maintain various amounts of suction. A stopcock attached to the tip of the syringe assists in creating and holding the vacuum. Once the needle tip is in the target lesion and the stylet is removed, the suction syringe is locked onto the needle handle, and the stopcock is opened for suction to be transmitted to the needle tip. When sampling of the target lesion is completed, suction is terminated by closing the stopcock or removing the suction syringe to avoid aspirating luminal contents as the needle is withdrawn from the target back into the needle sheath. When aspirating a cystic lesion, vacuum suction is used to aspirate fluid and to obtain cells from the cyst wall. Standard Luer lock syringes can also be used to manually create suction [6].

6.1.2 Types of Needles

Needles with a side hole at the tip have been developed as core biopsy needles, and numerous studies have investigated their efficacy. The EchoTip ProCore™ allowed diagnoses with fewer needle passes than conventional needles without side holes, but no significant difference in diagnostic adequacy and accuracy was reported [7, 8].

To date, four different needle sizes are available: 19-G (aspiration and core biopsy), 20-G (core biopsy), 22-G (standard size, aspiration, and core biopsy), and ultrathin 25-G needles. The most widely used needle for EUS-FNA is the 22-G needle [9], which is flexible and enables cytologic assessment without significant complications, although a 2% risk of acute pancreatitis was reported in a retrospective study [10]. For FNA of solid lesions, 25-G or 22-G needles are frequently used, while 22-G needles are usually used for cystic lesions [11]. Eight randomized clinical trials compared 22-G and 25-G needles in patients with solid masses and lymph nodes [12–15] or only with solid pancreatic masses [16–19]. One study showed a higher accuracy for the 25-G needle [13], whereas the others demonstrated no significant difference in diagnostic accuracy. Studies comparing FNA with 25-G and 22-G needles were also investigated in four meta-analyses [20–23] that provided conflicting results. The recent meta-analysis by Facciorusso et al. [20], comprising only randomized clinical trials, did not show significant differences between the needles in terms of sensitivity and specificity for pancreatic malignancy. On the other hand, Xu et al. [21] demonstrated higher sensitivity for 25-G needles with no significant difference in specificity for malignancy in patients with solid pancreatic masses.

The 19-G needles are more rigid, and consequently, transduodenal biopsies are more difficult [9]. These devices were developed to obtain larger amounts of material from the targeted lesions. However, compared to the 22-G needle, the 19-G needle has a higher rate of technical failure. One study showed that the 19-G needle had a higher diagnostic accuracy than the 22-G needle, but technical failures were not taken into consideration [24]. Twenty-five-G needles had the highest diagnostic accuracy for uncinate masses. In the case of pancreatic body and tail lesions, no significant difference between the three types of needle was found [25].

The use of nitinol for 19-G FNA needles has increased their flexibility. A multicenter study revealed no significant difference regarding diagnostic accuracy between the 22-G and the novel 19-G flexible needle made of nitinol, but histological core tissue was obtained in a larger number of patients by using the 19-G flexible needle [26]. Adequate samples in the case of liver biopsies were also obtained by the 19-G FNA [27–30]. Other studies have shown higher diagnostic yields with 19-G needles when performing subepithelial lesion (SEL) biopsies, which typically display lower diagnostic accuracy with 25-G and 22-G FNA needles [31].

EUS-guided tissue acquisition can be obtained by EUS-FNA or EUS-FNB. The needle-tip design is the distinguishing feature between FNA and FNB because the procedural techniques are comparable. Nevertheless, tissue histology has been proved to be important for the diagnosis of autoimmune pancreatitis [32], Hodgkin's lymphoma [31], and well-differentiated adenocarcinomas [33].

The initial commercially available EUS-FNB needle was the 19-G Tru-Cut. This needle had limited flexibility and consequently was replaced by the same manufacturer with the ProCore FNB needle, which is currently available in a range of sizes (19-G, 20-G, 22-G, 25-G). A multicenter randomized clinical trial showed that the ProCore 19-G needle was superior to the Tru-Cut needle, with a higher diagnostic accuracy (88% vs 62%; $P = 5.02$) [27]. A new variant of the ProCore needle (20-G) was introduced with a forward-facing direction of the side bevel. Two newly developed needles (SharkCore, Medtronic, Dublin, Ireland [34]; Acquire, Boston Scientific, Natick, MA, USA [35]) are designed with two or three opposing sharp points and a multifaceted bevel in the needle tip, aimed at capturing the core of tissue. According to the first results, the tissue acquisition was significantly higher than using standard aspiration needles, and diagnosis was possible with fewer needle passes [36, 37]. The same or a different needle of variable gauge can be reinserted through the delivery sheath to perform additional needle passes.

6.1.2.1 Access Needle

EUS-guided access to extraluminal structures, such as the bile duct, pancreatic duct, or pancreatic fluid collections, has been reported [38, 39]. A 19-G needle has been specifically designed for this particular application (EchoTip Ultra High Definition Ultrasound Access Needle, Cook Medical), which consists of a sharply beveled stylet used for puncture and then removed once access to the target has been obtained. After removal of the beveled stylet, the remaining needle tip is blunt, and this may prevent trauma and reduce the incidence of guidewire shearing. The needle diameter allows passage of a 0.035-inch guidewire.

6.1.2.2 Celiac Plexus Blockade and Neurolysis

Celiac plexus blockade (CPB) is performed to provide temporary pain relief, usually with injection of a local anesthetic agent combined with a steroid via an FNA needle. Celiac plexus neurolysis (CPN) involves the injection of a local anesthetic followed by injection of ethanol to permanently ablate nerve tissue [40]. Several reports have described the performance of these injections through available standard EUS-FNA needles [41–43]. A 20-G needle specifically designed for EUS-guided CPB and CPN (EchoTip Ultra Celiac Plexus Neurolysis Needle,

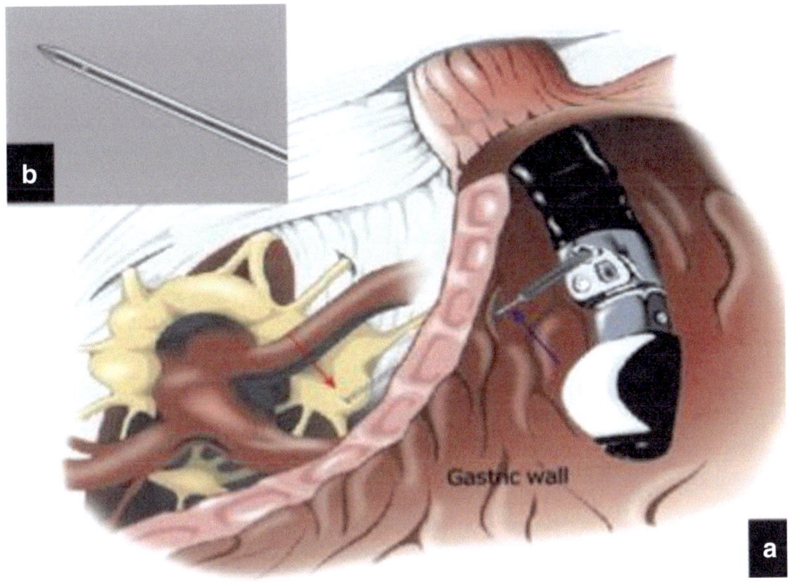

Fig. 6.2 (**a**) Endoscopic ultrasound-guided celiac plexus neurolysis. Red arrow: celiac ganglion; blue arrow: endoscopic ultrasound needle transfixing the gastric wall. (**b**) EchoTip Ultra Celiac Plexus Neurolysis Needle (Cook Medical). The needle has a sharp, conical tip with an array of side holes

Cook Medical) differs from other EUS needles by a solid, sharp, conical tip and an array of side holes for radial delivery of the desired agent into the region of the celiac plexus, the perineural space, or both (Fig. 6.2). However, studies comparing the efficacy of CPN using this device with standard EUS-FNA needles are lacking. Further improvements are expected in this field. For instance, intermediate-size needles (20-G or 21-G) might be more useful for combined cytol ogy and histology sampling or use of auxiliary devices inside the sheath of the 19-G needle. In the future, bulky scopes could be abandoned, and more flexible luminal robotic-driven devices can be used to access and puncture the targets.

6.1.3 EUS-FNA Technique

This technique involves the same preparation as for the other upper GI endoscopic examinations. Before EUS-FNA, it is recommended to check that the patient does not have any bleeding propensity or is receiving anticoagulant therapy. Sedation is required to avoid sudden movements, prevent injuries, and favor tolerability.

Lesions visualized with the scope withdrawn into a "straight or short use position" are more easily to be sampled. The best position is achieved when the path of the needle into the lesion does not require use of the elevator, although the latter is frequently employed to obtain the best needle direction. Once the lesion is visualized, the operator deflects the scope tip up against the lesion and aspirates air to minimize the distance between the lesion and the scope in order to perform more accurate EUS-FNA needle passage into the target lesion.

6.1.3.1 Application of Suction and Use of the Stylet

There is ample variation in clinical practice on the use of the stylet and application of suction. The capillary technique uses slow stylet withdrawal, while the needle is moving within the target lesion to generate a small amount of suction. Controversial diagnostic results for solid pancreatic masses have been reported with the use of suction, stylet withdrawal, and no suction. A trial comparing suction with no suction found higher diagnostic accuracy with suction (82.4% vs 72.1%; $p < 0.05$) [44]. Another trial found a higher sensitivity with the use of suction (0.86% vs 0.67%) [45]. In contrast, other studies reported increased sensitivity with slow stylet pull (capillary technique) with 25-G needles [46], and another showed no difference in outcomes between slow stylet pull and suction with 22-G needles [45, 46]. When performing lymph node aspiration, the addition of suction was found to increase the blood in the sample with no benefit in diagnostic yield [47].

Data of a systematic review evaluating the role of suction during EUS-FNA showed an advantage for its use in pancreatic masses, but not in lymph nodes [48]. The presence of the stylet within the needle at the time of the target puncture did not affect the adequacy of the samples or the diagnostic yield of malignancy [48]. In detail, two prospective randomized trials evaluating EUS-FNA of solid lesions reported no difference in bloodiness (25.1% vs 24.4% and 17% vs 14%) or in diagnostic yield of malignancy (40% vs 34.2% and 23% vs 28%), with and without a stylet, respectively [49, 50].

6.1.3.2 EUS-FNA/FNB Adverse Events

Overall, the rate of adverse events for EUS-FNA procedure is low [48]. Bleeding, bacteremia, and pancreatitis occur in less than 2% of all patients undergoing FNA [51, 52]. A systematic review assessing the morbidity and mortality associated with EUS-guided FNA demonstrated a 0.98% morbidity and 0.02% mortality rate [52].

Studies evaluating the safety of FNB devices have shown no significant difference in rates of adverse events as compared to FNA devices [53]. In a comparison of 22-G FNA and FNB devices used to sample solid pancreatic masses, the rate of adverse events was 1.7% and 5.2%, respectively [53].

6.1.4 Through-the-Needle Devices

Miniaturized devices such as a cytology brush, biopsy forceps, or confocal microscopy fiber-optic probes have been developed to be passed through 19-G EUS-FNA needles for evaluating both cystic and solid lesions [54, 55] (Fig. 6.3).

6.1.4.1 Cytology Brush

A cytology brush is available for dedicated use through echoendoscopes (EchoBrush, Cook Endoscopy) and comprises a disposable, modified EUS stylet with a 1 mm × 5 mm brush at its leading end that passes through the lumen of the Cook 19-G FNA needle. The device was used in several clinical studies to sample pancreatic cystic lesions [56–60]. In a study of 37 patients with pancreatic cysts at least 20 mm in maximal dimension, standard FNA using a 19-G FNA needle for aspiration of cyst contents was followed by EUS-guided brush cytology of the cyst interior using the EchoBrush [58]. The use of the cytology brush increased cytologic yield, with three (8%) cases of high-grade dysplasia identified only by brushing specimens. Another study compared the cytologic yield of the EchoBrush (47 patients) to EUS-FNA using a 22-G EUS-FNA needle (80 patients) in pancreatic cysts of varying size [57]. The use of the EchoBrush resulted in an adequate sample in 85.1% of cases compared with 66.3% for the EUS-FNA group.

6.1.4.2 Microforceps

Small biopsy forceps passed through 19-G needles have been developed for pathological diagnosis of pancreatic cystic lesions [61–63]. The use of mini-forceps through an FNA needle has been proven to be feasible and safe for pancreatic TA [64].

6.1.4.3 Needle-Based Confocal Laser Endomicroscopy Probe

Confocal laser endomicroscopy (CLE) is a novel endoscopic method that allows microscopy of the gastrointestinal mucosa during ongoing endoscopy, enabling real-time optical biopsy [65]. Technical advances allowed a confocal miniprobe to be passed through the biopsy channel of the endoscope [66].

Since probe-based confocal endomicroscopy has been miniaturized, needle-based confocal laser endomicroscopy (nCLE) has become available for clinical use. The nCLE miniprobe has 0.85-mm diameter and can be passed through a 19-G EUS-FNA needle [67]. Needle-based CLE was designed to allow in vivo histological images using fluorescent contrast. Therefore, nCLE could show which areas are most suspicious for malignancy and require biopsy [68]. EUS-guided nCLE seems to be a promising minimally invasive technique that might be used to improve the diagnostic accuracy of EUS-FNA. Optical needle biopsy could also be useful in reducing sampling

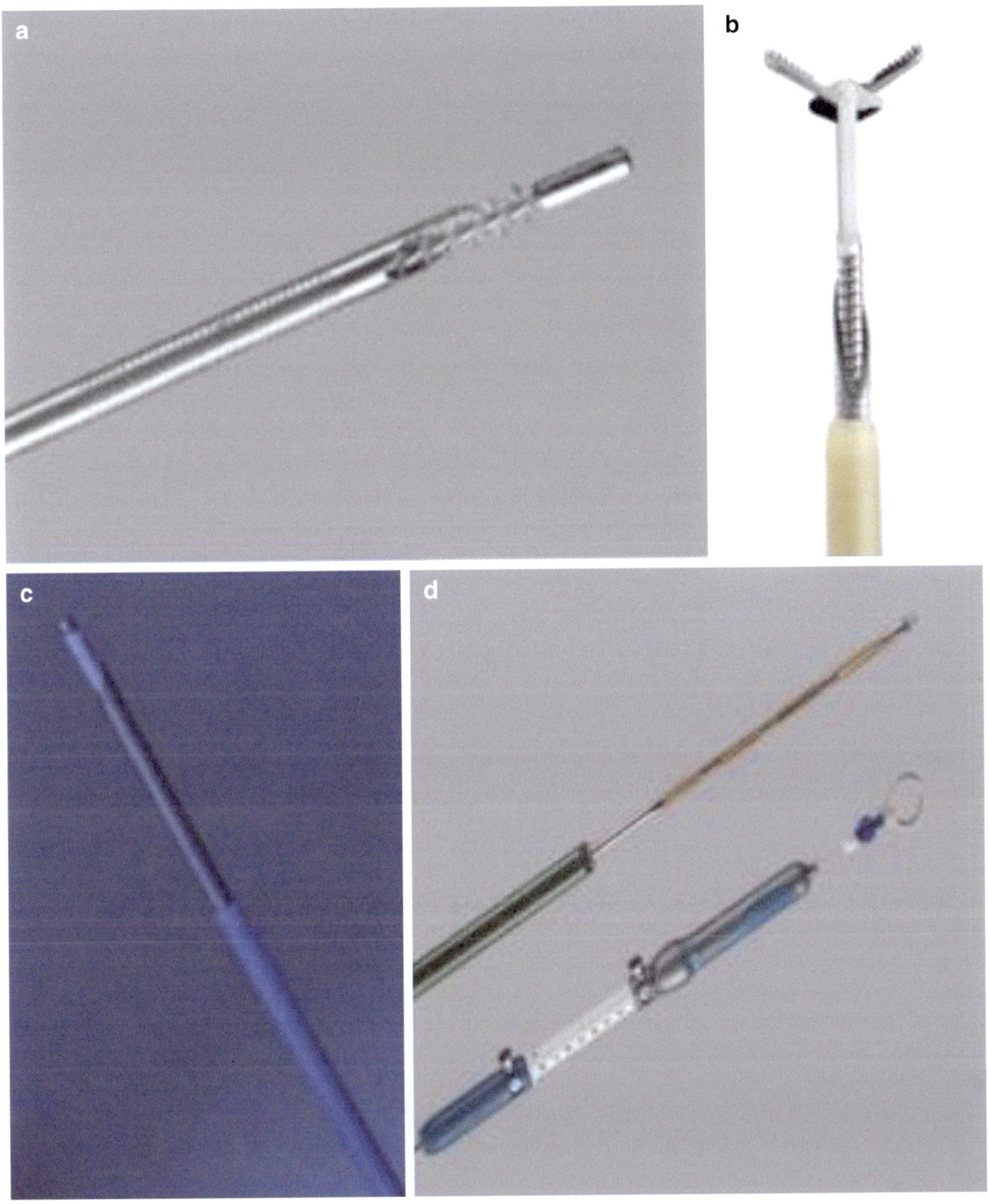

Fig. 6.3 Through-the-needle devices: (**a**) cytology brush (EchoBrush, Cook Endoscopy), (**b**) Moray microforceps (US Endoscopy), (**c**) AQ-Flex 19 (Mauna Kea Technologies) needle-based confocal laser endomicroscopy probe, (**d**) EchoTip fiducial needle (Cook Medical)

errors because it provides real-time microscopic details, especially in cystic masses.

The diagnosis of pancreatic cysts is sometimes difficult. Results of studies using nCLE have been very promising, and in the future, it may be used routinely for diagnosing pancreatic cysts as an adjunct to conventional EUS-FNA [69, 70]. Novel vascular patterns have been described, and a classification of nCLE patterns of pancreatic cystic lesions was reported, facilitating their diagnosis [71]. nCLE was found to be safe and feasible with high technical success [72]. However, these promising findings require validation in larger multicenter studies.

Feasibility and safety of nCLE for the assessment of solid pancreatic masses and lymph nodes were also assessed [73]. nCLE identified 77% of the cases in which malignancy was confirmed on histology. However, other studies are needed by using other contrast agents and targeted markers to improve diagnostic accuracy. Given the low negative predictive value of EUS-FNA, nCLE could help rule out malignancy after a previous inconclusive EUS-FNA [74]. The benefit of nCLE in the evaluation of solid pancreatic masses and lymph nodes is still unclear, and further studies are urged. This technique might also prove useful in the field of molecular imaging by allowing the in vivo visualization of pathophysiologic events in their natural environment [75–77].

Although it is unlikely that nCLE will replace EUS-FNA cytology for pancreatic masses and lymph nodes, it can be a complementary tool to FNA for diagnosis during EUS [78].

6.1.4.4 Fiducial Placement

EUS-guided fiducial placement is performed to assist image-guided radiation therapy (IGRT) [79]. The use of fiducial markers placed within pancreatic tumors resulted in less positional variation compared with the use of bony anatomy for IGRT [80]. At present, EUS-guided gold fiducial marker placement requires backloading of the fiducial into the tip of a 19-G or 22-G needle, followed by sealing of the needle tip with bone wax. This process is time-consuming and cumbersome and carries the risk of needle-tip injury. Dedicated EUS needles preloaded with fiducials have recently been developed. The EchoTip fiducial needle (Cook Medical) is a 22-G needle that is preloaded with four gold fiducials. In addition, Medtronic has developed 19-G and 22-G EUS fiducial needles that can be used with their BNX delivery system, with each needle containing two gold fiducials.

6.2 Interventional EUS

6.2.1 EUS-Guided Drainage of Intra-abdominal Fluid Collections

Historically, EUS-guided drainage of intra-abdominal fluid collections relied on the use of plastic and metal biliary stents designed for use with endoscopic retrograde cholangiopancreatography (ERCP). The AXIOS stent (Boston Scientific) is a lumen-apposing metal stent (LAMS) that is placed under EUS guidance [81]. This nitinol stent is fully covered, and it is available in diameters of 10 and 15 mm. The stent has two disk-shaped flanges, 10 mm apart each other, designed to achieve tissue apposition and decrease the risk of migration. The 10.8-Fr AXIOS stent delivery system has a hydrophilic coating and is advanced through the working channel of a therapeutic echoendoscope to the fluid collection over a previously placed guidewire after dilation of the transmural tract. Once into the fluid collection, the distal flange of the stent is deployed; the stent is then retracted so that the distal flange is pulled against the cyst wall. Therefore, the proximal flange is deployed within the lumen of the GI tract and the delivery system withdrawn. Tract dilation and use of a guidewire are not necessary with the AXIOS electrocautery enhanced system (Boston Scientific), which has a monopolar electrocautery element at the tip of the delivery system that can cut through the lumen wall (Fig. 6.4). The efficacy of the AXIOS stent has been evaluated in a multicenter study involving 33 patients with pancreatic fluid collections. Successful placement of the AXIOS stent was possible in 30 (91%) cases, with resolution of pancreatic fluid collections in 28 (84%) [82]. Stent migration was observed in a single patient. EUS-guided gallbladder drainage using the AXIOS stent has been reported in patients who were not fit for surgical approach [83–85]. In a multicenter, prospective trial on 30 patients, deployment of the stent into the gallbladder was successful in 90% of patients [85].

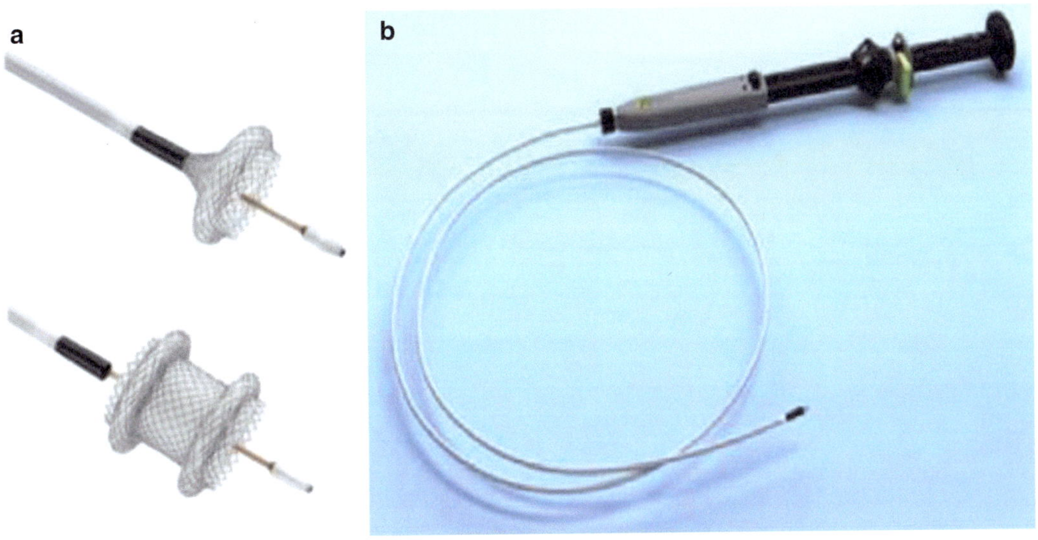

Fig. 6.4 The AXIOS stent (**a**) and Electrocautery Enhanced Delivery System (**b**) (Boston Scientific)

6.2.2 EUS-Guided Biliary Drainage

Endoscopic ultrasound-guided biliary drainage (EUS-BD) is being increasingly used as an alternative in patients with biliary obstruction who fail standard ERCP. There are two approaches for EUS-BD, one transgastric intrahepatic and the other transduodenal extrahepatic. Biliary drainage can be achieved by three different methods, transluminal biliary stenting, transpapillary rendezvous technique, and antegrade biliary stenting (Fig. 6.5). The choice of procedure depends on individual anatomy, underlying disease, and location of the biliary stricture. A recent meta-analysis showed cumulative technical success and adverse event rates of 90–94% and 16–23%, respectively. Development of new dedicated devices for EUS-BD would help refine the technical aspects and minimize the possibility of complications, making it a more promising procedure [86].

6.2.2.1 EUS-Guided Choledochoduodenostomy

EUS-guided choledochoduodenostomy (EUS-CDS), first described in 2001, consists of EUS transluminal stenting between the duodenal bulb (D1) and the extrahepatic bile duct [87].

Patients with distal bile duct obstruction and normal gastrointestinal anatomy may be candidates for this procedure. The extrahepatic bile duct is visualized through the D1 on EUS and usually punctured with a 19-G needle used for fine-needle aspiration (FNA). The tip is tapered to less than 3 Fr in diameter and is coaxial with a 0.025-inch guidewire. After puncturing the bile duct, the balloon catheter can be easily inserted without any dilation devices. A 4-mm balloon catheter is usually used to insert the stent device. During the procedure, the puncture angle must be adjusted so that the guidewire easily passes through toward the hilum. Bile is aspirated after puncture, and contrast medium is injected to obtain a cholangiogram. Thereafter, a guidewire is advanced into the bile duct and manipulated into the desired position. The fistulous tract is dilated using a bougie, balloon, or cautery dilator while maintaining the guidewire in place. A stent is then deployed through the dilated fistulous tract between the D1 and the extrahepatic bile duct.

In the majority of studies, a self-expandable metal stent has been used [39, 88–96]. A fully or partially covered tubular stent is often selected for EUS-CDS [97]. Metal stents longer than 4 cm have been used to prevent internal stent migration [98].

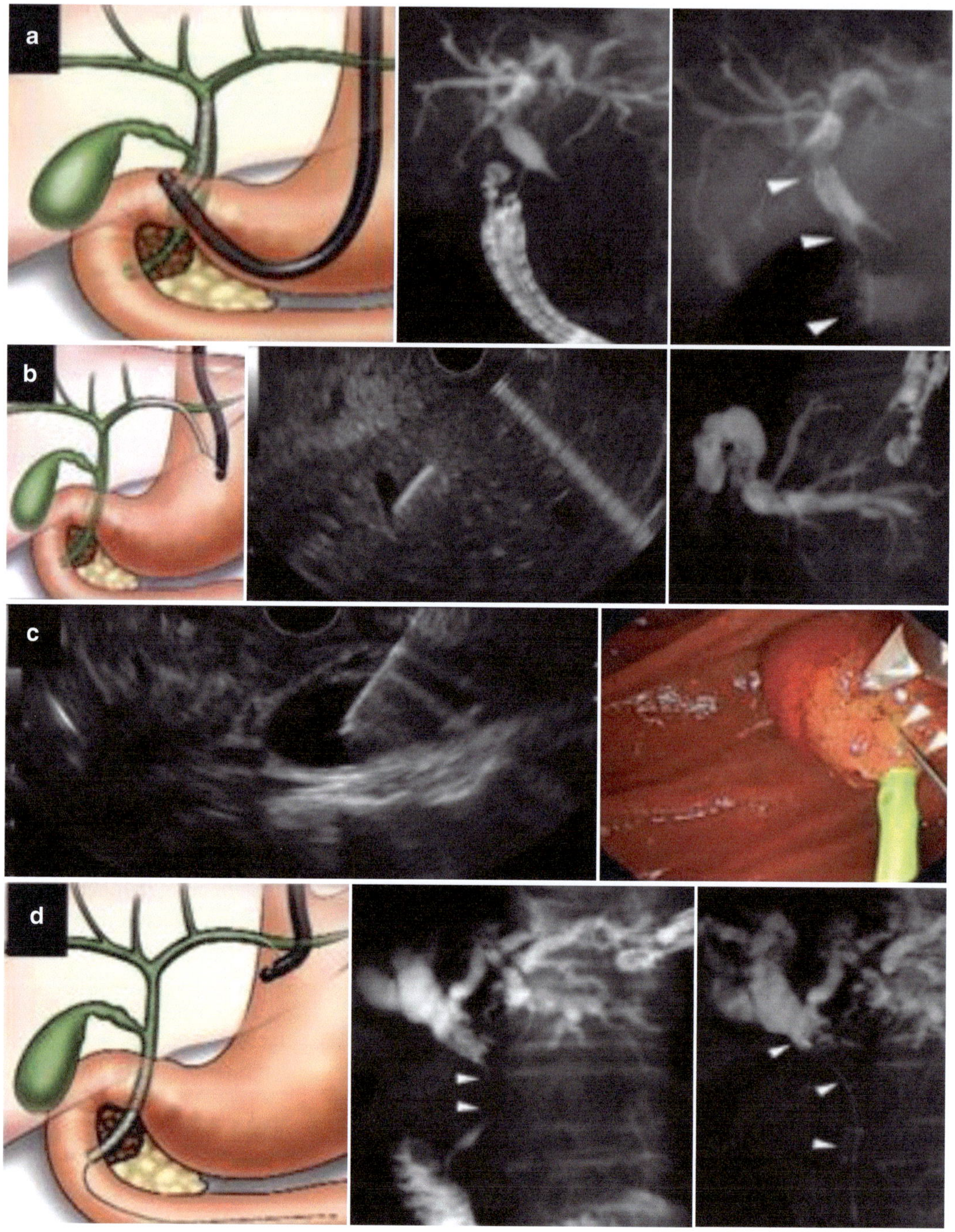

Fig. 6.5 EUS-guided biliary drainage: (**a**) Endoscopic ultrasound-guided choledochoduodenostomy (EUS-CDS), (**b**) endoscopic ultrasound-guided hepaticogastrostomy (EUS-HGS), (**c**) endoscopic ultrasound-guided rendezvous technique (EUS-RV), (**d**) endoscopic ultrasound-guided antegrade biliary stenting (EUS-ABS)

A recent study described the EUS-CDS procedure in 57 patients using a novel lumen-apposing metal stent (LAMS) [99]. The new LAMS achieved high technical and clinical success rates and other advantages, including avoidance of puncture and guidewire insertion, especially within the context of the Hot AXIOS system (XLumina Axios, Boston Scientific, Natick, MA, USA) [99].

6.2.2.2 EUS-Guided Hepaticogastrostomy

EUS-guided hepaticogastrostomy (EUS-HGS) is another transluminal stenting procedure, between the stomach and the left intrahepatic bile duct [100]. The presence of a dilated left intrahepatic bile duct is essential for this procedure, and it may have wider applications than the EUS-CDS procedure. For instance, while EUS-CDS is contraindicated in patients with surgically altered anatomy (e.g., Roux-en-Y or Whipple reconstruction) or duodenal obstruction as a result of tumor invasion, EUS-HGS can be carried out in these patients, as well as in those with distal bile duct obstruction. For hilar biliary obstruction, EUS-HGS is indicated as a rescue procedure in biliary reinterventions [101]. Massive ascites between the stomach and liver and unresectable gastric cancer are considered contraindications for EUS-HGS [102]. The left intrahepatic bile duct can be visualized through the gastric body. When a gastric body puncture is carried out, the intrahepatic bile duct of segment 3 (B3) is usually selected. The intrahepatic bile duct of segment 2 can be accessed through the esophagus, but such an approach may cause severe adverse events, such as mediastinitis or pneumomediastinum [102]. The angle of bile duct puncture is important for advancing the guidewire toward the hepatic hilum. Bile ducts that run from the upper left to the lower right on EUS images are considered the ideal puncture position. A bile duct diameter >5 mm and a 1–3-cm linear distance from the mural wall to the punctured bile duct wall on EUS may be suitable for successful EUS-HGS [103]. When sludge or debris in the bile duct makes difficult visualizing the B3, contrast-enhanced EUS may be useful [104]. As with EUS-CDS, a 0.025- or 0.035-inch guidewire is inserted through the 19-G FNA needle and manipulated to advance it toward the hepatic hilum. After the guidewire reaches the biliary system, the fistulous tract is dilated using a bougie, balloon, or cautery dilator, as described for EUS-CDS. Insertion of the stent device requires dilation of the bile duct and gastric wall. Then, a stent is deployed through the dilated fistulous tract between the gastric body and the B3. Fully covered or partially covered self-expandable metal stents were used in recent studies [102, 105].

Inward stent migration is a serious adverse event, especially soon after the procedure [106, 107]. A recent study reported that stent length ≥3 cm in the gastrointestinal lumen can prevent stent migration after deployment. Furthermore, a longer luminal length may be related to long-term stent patency. Therefore, metal stents longer than 10 cm may be suitable [105, 108]. A novel stent deployment maneuver has been reported to secure the deployed metal stent in a stable position and prevent stent migration [109]. Specifically, half of the metal stent was deployed within the bile duct under echoendoscopic and fluoroscopic guidance, and the remaining portion of the stent was deployed within the echoendoscope channel under fluoroscopic guidance. Subsequently, the echoendoscope was pulled out gently, and the stent was left in the HGS site [109].

6.2.2.3 EUS-Guided Rendezvous Technique

Firstly described in 2004 [110], in the EUS guided rendezvous technique (EUS-RV), the bile duct is accessed under EUS guidance with the creation of a temporary fistula, followed by guidewire advancement across the ampulla into the duodenum. Initially, conventional transpapillary biliary cannulation under guidance of the duodenoscope is attempted using the EUS-placed guidewire. EUS-RV is indicated in patients who failed ERCP but have endoscopic access to the ampulla or anastomosis site. Differently from the transluminal stenting, EUS-RV preserves the anatomical integrity of the biliary tree and avoids creation of a permanent fistula. Therefore, this procedure is particularly indicated for patients with resectable malignant biliary obstruction or benign biliary disorders (e.g., stone disease) [92]. The EUS-RV technique can be carried out by three different approaches: intrahepatic bile duct approach from the stomach, extrahepatic bile duct approach from the D1, and extrahepatic bile duct approach from the second portion of the duodenum (D2). The bile duct is accessed using a 19-G or 22-G FNA needle. After bile is aspirated, contrast is injected. Following cholangiography, a long guidewire is passed through the access needle into the bile duct and duodenum through the stricture and ampulla. Guidewire manipulation is the most challenging technical aspect of this procedure, and it is the key for success of EUS-RV [111, 112]. A hydrophilic guidewire was shown to be useful for passing the ampulla [113]. Recent studies showed that the extrahepatic bile duct approach from the D2 could improve the success rate of EUS-RV. However, this approach was not always feasible because of instability of the scope position [114, 115]. After the guidewire is manually manipulated to cross the ampulla and it is coiled within the duodenum, the needle and echoendoscope are withdrawn, leaving the guidewire in place. A duodenoscope is inserted alongside the guidewire, and the biliary tree is deeply cannulated with an ERCP catheter, using the EUS-placed guidewire to locate the biliary opening. Successful access to the bile duct allows completion of conventional ERCP in the usual procedure.

6.2.2.4 EUS-Guided Antegrade Biliary Stenting

EUS-guided antegrade biliary stenting (EUS-ABS) is a recently developed variation of EUS-BD described on 2008 [116]. A biliary stent is deployed in the intrahepatic bile duct accessed through the gastrointestinal lumen under EUS guidance. This technique is suitable in patients with an endoscopically inaccessible ampulla resulting from surgically altered anatomy or duodenal obstruction [117].

In EUS-ABS, the left intrahepatic bile duct is accessed from the gastric body or small intestine, with the creation of a temporary fistula between the gastrointestinal lumen and the intrahepatic bile duct. Similar to EUS-HGS, the left intrahepatic bile duct is punctured under EUS guidance, and a guidewire is inserted deeply into the biliary tree and is manipulated into the gastrointestinal lumen across the ampulla or anastomosis.

In EUS-ABS, a fistulous tract is temporarily created and unsealed after stent placement, with the minimal fistulous tract dilation reducing the risk of bile leakage. Recently developed, uncovered metal stents with a fine-gauge (5.7 or 6 Fr) stent delivery system can be deployed without fistulous tract dilation using a bougie or balloon dilator if an ERCP catheter can pass through the fistula [117–119]. The use of these stents in EUS-ABS may minimize bile leakage. A metal or plastic stent is inserted through the left intrahepatic bile duct into the malignant stricture site and deployed to cover the stricture in an anterograde manner. Metal stent deployment over the ampulla or anastomosis may reduce the risk of bile peritonitis by reducing the internal pressure of the biliary system [117]. The ideal location of the stent, whether covering or above the ampulla, is currently unclear.

6.2.2.5 EUS-BD Versus ERCP

EUS-BD is currently positioned as a rescue biliary drainage option after failed ERCP. One study at a tertiary care center found that EUS-BD was required in only three (0.6%) out of 524 patients with a native papilla undergoing therapeutic ERCP, concluding that EUS-BD should not replace ERCP [120]. A prospective study of 18 patients who underwent EUS-CDS as primary biliary intervention for malignant biliary obstruction after unsuccessful ERCP found that the technical and clinical success rates were 94% and 100%, respectively [121]. A retrospective cohort study comparing the clinical efficacy and safety of EUS-CDS and ERCP as first-line treatment for distal malignant biliary obstruction in 82 patients (26 EUS-CDS, 56 ERCP) found that mean procedure time was significantly shorter with EUS-CDS than with ERCP, although their clinical success and adverse event rates were similar [122]. Similar results were observed in another retrospective study [123]. It has been reported that the technical success and adverse event rates were similar when EUS-BD procedure was performed as first- or second-line approach [124]. The high rate of technical and clinical success of EUS-BD suggests that this method could represent a primary biliary drainage option in patients with ampulla covered by a duodenal stent or with surgically altered anatomy in the future. Nevertheless, standardization of the procedure and prospective comparative multicenter trials are still needed.

References

1. Polkowski M, Jenssen C, Kaye P, et al. Technical aspects of endoscopic ultrasound (EUS)-guided sampling in gastroenterology: European Society of Gastrointestinal Endoscopy (ESGE) Technical Guideline—March 2017. Endoscopy. 2017;49:989–1006.
2. Storm AC, Lee LS. Endoscopic ultrasound-guided techniques for diagnosing pancreatic mass lesions: can we do better? World J Gastroenterol. 2016;22:8658–69.
3. Culp WC, McCowan TC, Goertzen TC, et al. Relative ultrasonographic echogenicity of standard, dimpled, and polymeric-coated needles. J Vasc Interv Radiol. 2000;11:351–8.
4. Adler DG, Conway JD, Coffie JM, et al. EUS accessories. Gastrointest Endosc. 2007;66:1076–81.
5. Tang SJ, Vilmann AS, Saftoiu A, et al. EUS needle identification comparison and evaluation study (with videos). Gastrointest Endosc. 2016;84:424–3300.
6. ASGE Technology Committee, Hwang JH, et al. Devices for use with EUS. Video GIE. 2017;2(3):35–45.
7. Witt BL, Adler DG, Hilden K, et al. A comparative needle study: EUS FNA procedures using the HD ProCore™ and EchoTip® 22-gauge needle types. Diagn Cytopathol. 2013;41:1069–74.
8. Bang JY, Hawes R, Varadarajulu S. A meta-analysis comparing ProCore and standard fine-needle aspiration needles for endoscopic ultrasound-guided tissue acquisition. Endoscopy. 2016;48:339–49.
9. Vilmann P, Seicean A, Săftoiu A. Tips to overcome technical challenges in EUS-guided tissue acquisition. Gastrointest Endosc Clin N Am. 2014;24:109–24.
10. Yusuf TE, Ho S, Pavey DA, et al. Retrospective analysis of the utility of endoscopic ultrasound-guided fine-needle aspiration (EUS-FNA) in pancreatic masses, using a 22-gauge or 25-gauge needle system: a multicenter experience. Endoscopy. 2009;41:445–8.
11. Muniraj T, Aslanian HR. New developments in endoscopic ultrasound tissue acquisition. Gastrointest Endosc Clin N Am. 2017;27:585–99.
12. Gimeno-García AZ, Elwassief A, Paquin SC, et al. Endoscopic ultrasound-guided fine needle aspiration cytology and biopsy in the evaluation of lymphoma. Endosc Ultrasound. 2012;1:17–22.
13. Carrara S, Anderloni A, Jovani M, et al. A prospective randomized study comparing 25-G and 22-G needles of a new platform for endoscopic ultrasound-guided fine needle aspiration of solid masses. Dig Liver Dis. 2016;48:49–54.
14. Vilmann P, Săftoiu A, Hollerbach S, et al. Multicenter randomized controlled trial comparing the performance of 22 gauge versus 25 gauge EUS-FNA needles in solid masses. Scand J Gastroenterol. 2013;48:877–83.
15. Camellini L, Carlinfante G, Azzolini F, et al. A randomized clinical trial comparing 22G and 25G needles in endoscopic ultrasound-guided fine-needle aspiration of solid lesions. Endoscopy. 2011;43:709–15.
16. Lee JK, Lee KT, Choi ER, et al. A prospective, randomized trial comparing 25-gauge and 22-gauge needles for endoscopic ultrasound-guided fine needle aspiration of pancreatic masses. Scand J Gastroenterol. 2013;48:752–7.
17. Fabbri C, Polifemo AM, Luigiano C, et al. Endoscopic ultrasound-guided fine needle aspiration with 22- and 25-gauge needles in solid pancreatic masses: a prospective comparative study with randomisation of needle sequence. Dig Liver Dis. 2011;43:647–52.
18. Siddiqui UD, Rossi F, Rosenthal LS, et al. EUS-guided FNA of solid pancreatic masses: a prospective, randomized trial comparing 22-gauge and 25-gauge needles. Gastrointest Endosc. 2009;70:1093–7.
19. Lee JH, Stewart J, Ross WA, et al. Blinded prospective comparison of the performance of 22-gauge and 25-gauge needles in endoscopic ultrasound-guided fine needle aspiration of the pancreas and peri-pancreatic lesions. Dig Dis Sci. 2009;54:2274–81.
20. Facciorusso A, Stasi E, Di Maso M, et al. Endoscopic ultrasound-guided fine needle aspiration of pancreatic lesions with 22 versus 25 gauge needles: a meta-analysis. United European Gastroenterol J. 2017;5:846–53.
21. Xu MM, Jia HY, Yan LL, et al. Comparison of two different size needles in endoscopic ultrasound-guided fine-needle aspiration for diagnosing solid pancreatic lesions: a meta-analysis of prospective controlled trials. Medicine (Baltimore). 2017;96:e5802.
22. Madhoun MF, Wani SB, Rastogi A, et al. The diagnostic accuracy of 22-gauge and 25-gauge needles in endoscopic ultrasound-guided fine needle aspiration of solid pancreatic lesions: a meta-analysis. Endoscopy. 2013;45:86–92.
23. Affolter KE, Schmidt RL, Matynia AP, et al. Needle size has only a limited effect on outcomes in EUS-guided fine needle aspiration: a systematic review and meta-analysis. Dig Dis Sci. 2013;58:1026–34.
24. Song TJ, Kim JH, Lee SS, et al. The prospective randomized, controlled trial of endoscopic ultrasound-guided fine-needle aspiration using 22G and 19G

aspiration needles for solid pancreatic or peripancreatic masses. Am J Gastroenterol. 2010;105:1739–45.
25. Sakamoto H, Kitano M, Komaki T, et al. Prospective comparative study of the EUS guided 25-gauge FNA needle with the 19-gauge trucut needle and 22-gauge FNA needle in patients with solid pancreatic masses. J Gastroenterol Hepatol. 2009;24:384–90.
26. Varadarajulu S, Bang JY, Hebert-Magee S. Assessment of the technical performance of the flexible 19-gauge EUS-FNA needle. Gastrointest Endosc. 2012;76:336–43.
27. DeWitt J, Cho CM, Lin J, et al. Comparison of EUS-guided tissue acquisition using two different 19-gauge core biopsy needles: a multicenter, prospective, randomized, and blinded study. Endosc Int Open. 2015;3:E471–8.
28. Stavropoulos SN, Im GY, Jlayer Z, et al. High yield of same-session EUS-guided liver biopsy by 19-gauge FNA needle in patients undergoing EUS to exclude biliary obstruction. Gastrointest Endosc. 2012;75:310–8.
29. Diehl DL, Johal AS, Khara HS, et al. Endoscopic ultrasound-guided liver biopsy: a multicenter experience. Endosc Int Open. 2015;3:E210–5.
30. Pineda JJ, Diehl DL, Miao CL, et al. EUS-guided liver biopsy provides diagnostic samples comparable with those via the percutaneous or transjugular route. Gastrointest Endosc. 2016;83:360–5.
31. Kim GH, Cho YK, Kim EY, et al. Comparison of 22-gauge aspiration needle with 22-gauge biopsy needle in endoscopic ultrasonography-guided subepithelial tumor sampling. Scand J Gastroenterol. 2014;49:347–54.
32. Muniraj T, Sah RP, Chari ST. Autoimmune pancreatitis: an update. In: Pancreatitis: medical and surgical management. Chichester: Wiley; 2017. p. 152–60.
33. Karadsheh Z, Al-Haddad M. Endoscopic ultrasound guided fine needle tissue acquisition: where we stand in 2013? World J Gastroenterol. 2014;20:2176–85.
34. Adler DG, Witt B, Chadwick B, et al. Pathologic evaluation of a new endoscopic ultrasound needle designed to obtain core tissue samples: a pilot study. Endosc Ultrasound. 2016;5:178–83.
35. Bang JY, Hebert-Magee S, Hasan MK, et al. Endoscopic ultrasonography-guided biopsy using a Franseen needle design: initial assessment. Dig Endosc. 2017;29:338–46.
36. Kandel P, Tranesh G, Nassar A, et al. EUS-guided fine needle biopsy sampling using a novel fork-tip needle: a case-control study. Gastrointest Endosc. 2016;84:1034–9.
37. DiMaio CJ, Kolb JM, Benias PC, et al. Initial experience with a novel EUS-guided core biopsy needle (SharkCore): results of a large North American Multicenter Study. Endosc Int Open. 2016;4:E974–9.
38. Attam R, Arain M, Trikudanathan G, et al. EUS-guided pancreatic duct access and wire placement to facilitate dorsal duct cannulation after failed ERCP. Gastrointest Endosc. 2015;81:1260.
39. Khashab MA, Van der Merwe S, Kunda R, et al. Prospective international multicenter study on endoscopic ultrasound-guided biliary drainage for patients with malignant distal biliary obstruction after failed endoscopic retrograde cholangiopancreatography. Endosc Int Open. 2016;4:E487–96.
40. LeBlanc JK, Al-Haddad M, McHenry L, et al. A prospective, randomized study of EUS-guided celiac plexus neurolysis for pancreatic cancer: one injection or two? Gastrointest Endosc. 2011;74:1300–7.
41. Gress F, Schmitt C, Sherman S, et al. A prospective randomized comparison of endoscopic ultrasound- and computed tomography-guided celiac plexus block for managing chronic pancreatitis pain. Am J Gastroenterol. 1999;94:900–5.
42. Wiersema MJ, Wiersema LM. Endosonography-guided celiac plexus neurolysis. Gastrointest Endosc. 1996;44:656–62.
43. Kaufman M, Singh G, Das S, et al. Efficacy of endoscopic ultrasound-guided celiac plexus block and celiac plexus neurolysis for managing abdominal pain associated with chronic pancreatitis and pancreatic cancer. J Clin Gastroenterol. 2010;44:127–34.
44. Lee JK, Choi JH, Lee KH, et al. A prospective, comparative trial to optimize sampling techniques in EUS-guided FNA of solid pancreatic masses. Gastrointest Endosc. 2013;77:745–51.
45. Puri R, Vilmann P, Saftoiu A, et al. Randomized controlled trial of endoscopic ultrasound-guided fine-needle sampling with or without suction for better cytological diagnosis. Scand J Gastroenterol. 2009;44:499–504.
46. Nakai Y, Isayama H, Chang KJ, et al. Slow pull versus suction in endoscopic ultrasound-guided fine-needle aspiration of pancreatic solid masses. Dig Dis Sci. 2014;59:1578–85.
47. Wallace MB, Kennedy T, Durkalski V, et al. Randomized controlled trial of EUS-guided fine needle aspiration techniques for the detection of malignant lymphadenopathy. Gastrointest Endosc. 2001;54:441–7.
48. Wani S, Muthusamy VR, Komanduri S. EUS-guided tissue acquisition: an evidence-based approach (with videos). Gastrointest Endosc. 2014;80:939–59.e7.
49. Rastogi A, Wani S, Gupta N, et al. A prospective, single-blind, randomized, controlled trial of EUS-guided FNA with and without a stylet. Gastrointest Endosc. 2011;74:58–64.
50. Wani S, Gupta N, Gaddam S, et al. A comparative study of endoscopic ultrasound guided fine needle aspiration with and without a stylet. Dig Dis Sci. 2011;56:2409–14.
51. ASGE Standards of Practice Committee, Early DS, Acosta RD, Chandrasekhara V, et al. Adverse events associated with EUS and EUS with FNA. Gastrointest Endosc. 2013;77:839–43.
52. Wang KX, Ben QW, Jin ZD, et al. Assessment of morbidity and mortality associated with EUS-guided FNA: a systematic review. Gastrointest Endosc. 2011;73:283–90.

53. Lee YN, Moon JH, Kim HK, et al. Core biopsy needle versus standard aspiration needle for endoscopic ultrasound-guided sampling of solid pancreatic masses: a randomized parallel-group study. Endoscopy. 2014;46:1056–62.
54. Nakai Y, Iwashita T, Park DH, et al. Diagnosis of pancreatic cysts: EUS-guided, through-the-needle confocal laser-induced endomicroscopy and cystoscopy trial: DETECT study. Gastrointest Endosc. 2015;81:1204–14.
55. Stavropoulos SN, Abraham B, Friedel D, et al. Direct visualization of the wall of pancreatic cysts using the SPYGLASS optical probe: feasibility and preliminary results. Gastrointest Endosc. 2009;69:AB377.
56. Al-Haddad M, Raimondo M, Woodward T, et al. Safety and efficacy of cytology brushings versus standard FNA in evaluating cystic lesions of the pancreas: a pilot study. Gastrointest Endosc. 2007;65:894–8.
57. Lozano MD, Subtil JC, Miravalles TL, et al. EchoBrush may be superior to standard EUS-guided FNA in the evaluation of cystic lesions of the pancreas: preliminary experience. Cancer Cytopathol. 2011;119:209–14.
58. Al-Haddad M, Gill KR, Raimondo M, et al. Safety and efficacy of cytology brushings versus standard fine-needle aspiration in evaluating cystic pancreatic lesions: a controlled study. Endoscopy. 2010;42:127–32.
59. Bruno M, Bosco M, Carucci P, et al. Preliminary experience with a new cytology brush in EUS-guided FNA. Gastrointest Endosc. 2009;70:1220–4.
60. Thomas T, Bebb J, Mannath J, et al. EUS-guided pancreatic cyst brushing: a comparative study in a tertiary referral centre. JOP. 2010;11:163–9.
61. Samarasena JB, Nakai Y, Shinoura S, et al. EUS-guided, through-the-needle forceps biopsy: a novel tissue acquisition technique. Gastrointest Endosc. 2015;81:225–6.
62. Coman RM, Schlachterman A, Esnakula AK, et al. EUS-guided, through-the-needle forceps: clenching down the diagnosis. Gastrointest Endosc. 2016;84:372–3.
63. Shakhatreh MH, Naini SR, Brijbassie AA, et al. Use of a novel through-the-needle biopsy forceps in endoscopic ultrasound. Endosc Int Open. 2016;4:E439–42.
64. Nakai Y, Isayama H, Chang KJ, et al. A pilot study of EUS-guided through-the-needle forceps biopsy (with video). Gastrointest Endosc. 2016;84:158–62.
65. Kiesslich R, Burg J, Vieth M, et al. Confocal laser endoscopy for diagnosing intraepithelial neoplasias and colorectal cancer *in vivo*. Gastroenterology. 2004;127:706–13.
66. Kiesslich R, Neurath MF. Endomicroscopy is born—do we still need the pathologist? Gastrointest Endosc. 2007;66:150–3.
67. Bhutani MS, Koduru P, Joshi V, et al. EUS-guided needle-based confocal laser endomicroscopy: a novel technique with emerging applications. Gastroenterol Hepatol (N Y). 2015;11:235–40.
68. Deprez PH. Future directions in EUS-guided tissue acquisition. Gastrointest Endosc Clin N Am. 2014;24:143–9.
69. Napoléon B, Lemaistre AI, Pujol B, et al. A novel approach to the diagnosis of pancreatic serous cystadenoma: needle-based confocal laser endomicroscopy. Endoscopy. 2015;47:26–32.
70. Joshi V. NCLE (needle-based confocal laser endomicroscopy) in evaluation of indeterminate pancreatic cystic lesions: a single-center experience. Am J Gastroenterol. 2014;109(Suppl 2):S101–23.
71. Krishna SG, Brugge WR, Dewitt JM, et al. Needle-based confocal laser endomicroscopy for the diagnosis of pancreatic cystic lesions: an international external interobserver and intraobserver study (with videos). Gastrointest Endosc. 2017;86:644–5400.
72. Kadayifci A, Atar M, Basar O, et al. Needle-based confocal laser endomicroscopy for evaluation of cystic neoplasms of the pancreas. Dig Dis Sci. 2017;62:1346–53.
73. Karstensen JG, Cartana T, Klausen P, et al. Mo1430 pitfalls in the interpretation of pancreatic endoscopic ultrasound guided needle confocal LASER endomicroscopy. Gastrointest Endosc. 2014;79:AB433–4.
74. Giovannini M, Caillol F, Monges G, et al. Endoscopic ultrasound-guided needle-based confocal laser endomicroscopy in solid pancreatic masses. Endoscopy. 2016;48:892–8.
75. Nakai Y, Shinoura S, Ahluwalia A, et al. *In vivo* visualization of epidermal growth factor receptor and survivin expression in porcine pancreas using endoscopic ultrasound guided fine needle imaging with confocal laser-induced endomicroscopy. J Physiol Pharmacol. 2012;63:577–80.
76. Samarasena JB, Tarnawski AS, Shinoura S, et al. Mo1429 visualization of the gastric submucosal and myenteric neuronal network using endoscopic ultrasound (EUS) guided needle-based confocal LASER induced endomicroscopy and a novel EUS guided through-the-needle biopsy technique. Gastrointest Endosc. 2014;79:AB433.
77. Li H, Li Y, Cui L, et al. Monitoring pancreatic carcinogenesis by the molecular imaging of cathepsin E *in vivo* using confocal laser endomicroscopy. PLoS One. 2014;9:e106566.
78. Guo J, Bhutani MS, Giovannini M, et al. Can endoscopic ultrasound-guided needle-based confocal laser endomicroscopy replace fine-needle aspiration for pancreatic and mediastinal diseases? Endosc Ultrasound. 2017;6:376–81.
79. DiMaio CJ, Nagula S, Goodman KA, et al. EUS-guided fiducial placement for image-guided radiation therapy in GI malignancies by using a 22-gauge needle (with videos). Gastrointest Endosc. 2010;71:1204–10.
80. van der Horst A, Wognum S, Davila Fajardo R, et al. Interfractional position variation of pancreatic tumors quantified using intratumoral fiducial mark-

ers and daily cone beam computed tomography. Int J Radiat Oncol Biol Phys. 2013;87:202–8.

81. Binmoeller KF, Shah J. A novel lumen-apposing stent for transluminal drainage of nonadherent extraintestinal fluid collections. Endoscopy. 2011;43:337–42.
82. Shah RJ, Shah JN, Waxman I, et al. Safety and efficacy of endoscopic ultrasound-guided drainage of pancreatic fluid collections with lumen-apposing covered self-expanding metal stents. Clin Gastroenterol Hepatol. 2015;13:747–52.
83. Irani S, Baron TH, Grimm IS, et al. EUS-guided gallbladder drainage with a lumen-apposing metal stent (with video). Gastrointest Endosc. 2015;82:1110–5.
84. Teoh AY, Binmoeller KF, Lau JY. Single-step EUS-guided puncture and delivery of a lumen-apposing stent for gallbladder drainage using a novel cautery-tipped stent delivery system. Gastrointest Endosc. 2014;80:1171.
85. Walter D, Teoh AY, Itoi T, et al. EUS-guided gall bladder drainage with a lumen-apposing metal stent: a prospective long-term evaluation. Gut. 2016;65:6–8.
86. Minaga K, Kitano M. Recent advances in endoscopic ultrasound-guided biliary drainage. Dig Endosc. 2018;30(1):38–47.
87. Giovannini M, Moutardier V, Pesenti C, Bories E, Lelong B, Delpero JR. Endoscopic ultrasound-guided bilioduodenal anastomosis: a new technique for biliary drainage. Endoscopy. 2001;33:898–900.
88. Khan MA, Akbar A, Baron TH, et al. Endoscopic ultrasound-guided biliary drainage: a systematic review and meta-analysis. Dig Dis Sci. 2016;61:684–703.
89. Wang K, Zhu J, Xing L, Wang Y, Jin Z, Li Z. Assessment of efficacy and safety of EUS-guided biliary drainage: a systematic review. Gastrointest Endosc. 2016;83:1218–27.
90. Itoi T, Sofuni A, Itokawa F, et al. Endoscopic ultrasonography-guided biliary drainage. J Hepatobiliary Pancreat Sci. 2010;17:611–6.
91. Moole H, Bechtold ML, Forcione D, Puli SR. A meta-analysis and systematic review: success of endoscopic ultrasound guided biliary stenting in patients with inoperable malignant biliary strictures and a failed ERCP. Medicine. 2017;96:e5154.
92. Hara K, Yamao K, Mizuno N, et al. Endoscopic ultrasonography-guided biliary drainage: who, when, which, and how? World J Gastroenterol. 2016;22:1297–303.
93. Bruno MJ. Interventional endoscopic ultrasonography: where are we headed? Dig Endosc. 2017;29:503–11.
94. Iwashita T, Doi S, Yasuda I. Endoscopic ultrasound-guided biliary drainage: a review. Clin J Gastroenterol. 2014;7:94–102.
95. Chan SM, Teoh AY. Endoscopic ultrasound-guided biliary drainage: a review. Curr Treat Options Gastroenterol. 2015;13:171–84.
96. Ryozawa S, Fujita N, Irisawa A, Hirooka Y, Mine T. Current status of interventional endoscopic ultrasound. Dig Endosc. 2017;29:559–66.
97. Ogura T, Higuchi K. Technical tips of endoscopic ultrasound-guided choledochoduodenostomy. World J Gastroenterol. 2015;21:820–8.
98. Cho DH, Lee SS, Oh D, et al. Long-term outcomes of a newly developed hybrid metal stent for EUS-guided biliary drainage (with videos). Gastrointest Endosc. 2017;85:1067–75.
99. Kunda R, Pérez-Miranda M, Will U, et al. EUS-guided choledochoduodenostomy for malignant distal biliary obstruction using a lumen-apposing fully covered metal stent after failed ERCP. Surg Endosc. 2016;30:5002–8.
100. Burmester E, Niehaus J, Leineweber T, Huetteroth T. EUS-cholangio-drainage of the bile duct: report of 4 cases. Gastrointest Endosc. 2003;57:246–51.
101. Ogura T, Onda S, Takagi W, et al. Clinical utility of endoscopic ultrasound-guided biliary drainage as a rescue of re-intervention procedure for high-grade hilar stricture. J Gastroenterol Hepatol. 2017;32:163–8.
102. Ogura T, Higuchi K. Technical tips for endoscopic ultrasound-guided hepaticogastrostomy. World J Gastroenterol. 2016;22:3945–51.
103. Oh D, Park DH, Song TJ, et al. Optimal biliary access point and learning curve for endoscopic ultrasound-guided hepaticogastrostomy with transmural stenting. Ther Adv Gastroenterol. 2017;10:42–53.
104. Minaga K, Kitano M, Yoshikawa T, et al. Hepaticogastrostomy guided by real-time contrast-enhanced harmonic endoscopic ultrasonography: a novel technique. Endoscopy. 2016;48(Suppl 1):E228–9.
105. Nakai Y, Isayama H, Yamamoto N, et al. Safety and effectiveness of a long, partially covered metal stent for endoscopic ultrasound-guided hepaticogastrostomy in patients with malignant biliary obstruction. Endoscopy. 2016;48:1125–8.
106. Martins FP, Rossini LGB, Ferrari AP. Migration of a covered metallic stent following endoscopic ultrasound-guided hepaticogastrostomy. Endoscopy. 2010;42:E126–7.
107. Minaga K, Kitano M, Yamashita Y, Nakatani Y, Kudo M. Stent migration into the abdominal cavity after EUS-guided hepaticogastrostomy. Gastrointest Endosc. 2017;85:263–4.
108. Ogura T, Yamamoto K, Sano T, et al. Stent length is impact factor associated with stent patency in endoscopic ultrasound-guided hepaticogastrostomy. J Gastroenterol Hepatol. 2015;30:1748–52.
109. Paik WH, Park DH, Choi JH, et al. Simplified fistula dilation technique and modified stent deployment maneuver for EUS-guided hepaticogastrostomy. World J Gastroenterol. 2014;20:5051–9.
110. Mallery S, Matlock J, Freeman ML. EUS-guided rendezvous drainage of obstructed biliary and pan-

creatic ducts: report of 6 cases. Gastrointest Endosc. 2004;59:100–7.

111. Isayama H, Nakai Y, Kawakubo K, et al. The endoscopic ultrasonography-guided rendezvous technique for biliary cannulation: a technical review. J Hepatobiliary Pancreat Sci. 2013;20:413–20.
112. Kahaleh M, Hernandez AJ, Tokar J, Adams RB, Shami VM, Yeaton P. Interventional EUS-guided cholangiography: evaluation of a technique in evolution. Gastrointest Endosc. 2006;64:52–9.
113. Dhir V, Bhandari S, Bapat M, Maydeo A. Comparison of EUS-guided rendezvous and precut papillotomy techniques for biliary access (with videos). Gastrointest Endosc. 2012;75:354–9.
114. Iwashita T, Lee JG, Shinoura S, et al. Endoscopic ultrasound-guided rendezvous for biliary access after failed cannulation. Endoscopy. 2012;44:60–5.
115. Iwashita T, Yasuda I, Mukai T, et al. EUS-guided rendezvous for difficult biliary cannulation using a standardized algorithm: a multicenter prospective pilot study (with videos). Gastrointest Endosc. 2016;83:394–400.
116. Fujita N, Noda Y, Kobayashi G, et al. Temporary endosonography-guided biliary drainage for transgastrointestinal deployment of a self-expandable metallic stent. J Gastroenterol. 2008;43:637–40.
117. Iwashita T, Yasuda I, Mukai T, et al. Endoscopic ultrasound-guided antegrade biliary stenting for unresectable malignant biliary obstruction in patients with surgically altered anatomy: a single-center prospective pilot study. Dig Endosc. 2017;29:362–8.
118. Ogura T, Masuda D, Imoto A, et al. EUS-guided hepaticogastrostomy combined with fine-gauge antegrade stenting: a pilot study. Endoscopy. 2014;46:416–21.
119. Minaga K, Takenaka M, Miyata T, Ueda Y, Kitano M, Kudo M. Through-the-mesh technique after endoscopic ultrasonography-guided hepaticogastrostomy: a novel re-intervention method. Endoscopy. 2016;48:E369–70.
120. Holt BA, Hawes R, Hasan M, et al. Biliary drainage: role of EUS guidance. Gastrointest Endosc. 2016;83:160–5.
121. Hara K, Yamao K, Niwa Y, et al. Prospective clinical study of EUS-guided choledochoduodenostomy for malignant lower biliary tract obstruction. Am J Gastroenterol. 2011;106:1239–45.
122. Kawakubo K, Kawakami H, Kuwatani M, et al. Endoscopic ultrasound-guided choledochoduodenostomy vs. transpapillary stenting for distal biliary obstruction. Endoscopy. 2016;48:164–9.
123. Dhir V, Itoi T, Khashab MA, et al. Multicenter comparative evaluation of endoscopic placement of expandable metal stents for malignant distal common bile duct obstruction by ERCP or EUS-guided approach. Gastrointest Endosc. 2015;81:913–23.
124. Nakai Y, Isayama H, Yamamoto N, et al. Indications for endoscopic ultrasonography (EUS)-guided biliary intervention: does EUS always come after failed endoscopic retrograde cholangiopancreatography? Dig Endosc. 2017;29:218–25.

7 Deep Sedation and Anesthesia for Advanced Gastrointestinal Endoscopy: Challenging a Continuum

Aldo Cristalli and Andrea De Gasperi

7.1 Introduction

A consistent part of procedures requiring the presence of an anesthesiologist (more than 25% according to Goudra) [1] is now performed outside the operating room (OR) in Europe. A new acronym, NORA, *nonoperative room anesthesia*, has been proposed to describe a location often far from the main, traditional operating blocks (*remote environment anesthesia*) and usually within the gastroenterology or interventional radiology units [2–4]. The role of the anesthesiologist in the modern digestive endoscopy suite should be to match the often challenging requests of the advanced and complex interventional digestive endoscopic procedures with deeply sedated, prone-positioned, spontaneously breathing patients: this demanding task is usually performed in an unfamiliar *remote* location outside the "traditional" operative room (the endoscopic suite). This activity, which usually needs a quick turnover of often medically complicated, fragile, or elderly patients, has to be as safe as possible: the everyday expanding indications for the advanced complex endoscopic procedures (endoscopic retrograde cholangiopancreatography, ERCP, is an example) mandate a constant update of the anesthesiological periprocedural management, as recently addressed by a revised release of ASA guidelines for procedural anesthesia (2014) [3] and the very recent document dealing with moderate sedation [5]. Safety while offering to the patients sedation, comfort, and pain relief during complex endoscopic procedures is the first commitment of the anesthesiologist working in this setting. As recently stated by McAlevy and Levenick [6], sedation offered by anesthesiologists plays a crucial role in safety, efficiency, and patient satisfaction: with one estimated death per 200,000 to 300,000 anesthetics administered in this setting, the safety profile of deep sedation/general anesthesia is excellent; unfortunately, data dealing with the safety of anesthesiologist-administered sedation (specifically during ERCP) are scarce [7]. In this specific setting, deep sedation is frequently administered to patients in prone position without a secured airway: the most challenging "all-in-one" tasks to be matched by the anesthesiologist are to maintain a patent airway (using external manipulation), to check vital parameters (cardiovascular and respiratory variables and, if possible, information dealing with depth of anesthesia) [4–8], and to gain access to the airway in an emergency situation. This is why sedation and operative procedures are, in our opinion, to be managed by two different experts and trained professionals (the endoscopist and the anesthesiologist), each one involved and concentrated on his main task(s). Together with specifi-

A. Cristalli · A. De Gasperi (✉)
2° Servizio Anestesia e Rianimazione, ASST Grande Ospedale Metropolitano Niguarda, Milan, Italy
e-mail: andrea.degasperi@ospedaleniguarda.it

M. Mutignani et al. (eds.), *Endotherapy in Biliopancreatic Diseases: ERCP Meets EUS*,
https://doi.org/10.1007/978-3-030-42569-2_7

cally trained anesthesiologists, a well-designed and appropriately organized endoscopic suite layout should give a relevant contribution to a successful and safe procedure, comfortable for both the patient and the medical staff [8].

7.2 Sedation in Digestive Endoscopy: A Continuum from Deep Sedation to General Anesthesia

At the beginning of this activity, endoscopic procedures were considered minimally invasive and less risky than those scheduled in a conventional operating room. Requests for sedation were few, mainly for invasive diagnostics and/or for painful or lengthy procedures. In large part of the cases, light conscious sedation, usually managed by the proceduralist himself with the help of a trained nurse, was the rule. The ever-increasing complexity of the invasive procedures, where the diagnostic aspects are deeply entwined with therapeutic solutions, makes mandatory deep sedation or general anesthesia: boundaries between the two conditions are, as yet, far from being clear-cut [3, 5, 8, 9]. As stated by the many documents issued by the various scientific societies [3, 5, 8, 9], sedation is a continuum, from moderate to deep: while purposeful responses are present in "moderate" sedation, in "deep" sedation, response occurs (if it occurs!) only after painful or repeated stimulations, consciousness is drug-depressed, and ventilatory drive may be partially impaired: assistance (external airway manipulation) to maintain a patent airway is sometimes required, while cardiovascular function is usually stable. According to ASA definition [3, 5], also quoted by ASGO [8], general anesthesia is "a drug-induced loss of consciousness during which patients are not rousable, even by painful stimulation". The ability to independently maintain ventilatory function is often impaired. Assistance in maintaining a patent airway is sometimes needed, and positive pressure ventilation may be required because of depressed spontaneous ventilation or drug-induced depression of neuromuscular function. Cardiovascular function also may be impaired (Table 7.1 from ASA documents, reported also in ASGO guidelines) [3, 5, 8].

In the ESA document [9], to define sedation, a modified version of the five-level Ramsay scale level is proposed: level 5 is similar to, if not synonymous with, general anesthesia: *(1) level 1: fully awake, (2) level 2: drowsy, (3) level 3: apparently asleep but rousable by normal speech, (4) level 4: apparently asleep but responding to standardized physical stimuli (e.g., glabellar tap), and (5) level 5: asleep, but not responding to strong physical stimuli (comatose).* Level

Table 7.1 ASA definition of the continuum of depth of sedation (reproduced from ASA Continuum of Depth of Sedation: Definition of General Anesthesia and Levels of Sedation/Analgesia, with permission [3])

Continuum of Depth of Sedation: Definition of General Anesthesia and Levels of Sedation/Analgesia Committee of Origin: Quality Management and Departmental Administration (Approved by the ASA House of Delegates on October 13, 1999 and Last Amended on October 23, 2019)				
	Minimal sedation anxiolysis	*Moderate sedation/ analgesia ("conscious sedation")*	*Deep sedation/analgesia*	*General anesthesia*
Responsiveness	Normal response to verbal stimulation	Purposeful response to verbal or tactile stimulation	Purposeful response following repeated or painful stimulation	Unrousable even with painful stimulus
Airway	Unaffected	No intervention required	Intervention may be required	Intervention often required
Spontaneous ventilation	Unaffected	Adequate	May be inadequate	Frequently inadequate
Cardiovascular function	Unaffected	Usually maintained	Usually maintained	May be impaired

5 is the level required for ERCP. The ASA has defined four levels of sedation [3, 5], where level 4 corresponds to general anesthesia. In case of deeper levels of sedation (ASA levels 3 or 4, ESA 4 or 5), respiratory adverse events are possible and mandate prompt and appropriate management. As stated by the ESA 2018 document [9], management of transition from levels 3 to 4 may require specific knowledge and technical skills (advanced airway/cardiovascular resuscitation) that are in general only fully mastered by an anesthesiologist.

7.3 Location [10]

The number of NORAs has increased at a very rapid rate in the last few years and will undoubtedly increase even more in the next few years. The ever-expanding number of procedures anesthesiologists are asked to care for has to match the suite layout and the logistics (complex, sometimes bulky diagnostic technologies often deployed close to other diagnostic/therapeutic facilities peculiar for the endoscopic procedures) with complex patients, safety issues (including rescue maneuvers), and rapid turnover. Suites layout, equipment, monitoring systems, protocols, and staff should be finalized to maximize safety and working conditions while reducing risks.

In 2014, ASA guidelines specifically addressed how NORA locations are to be structured, organized, and equipped [3]: the document included standards to organize the anesthesia point outside the operating room (OR) to manage procedures requiring light sedation up to general anesthesia with tracheal intubation. The "OR safety standards" are to be "repositioned" and applied in the endoscopic suite. Aim of the document was to have in NORAs the same standards available in the traditional ORs, specifically addressing patient safety, monitoring, and equipment. Among the main requirements for NORA are:

1. Adherence to all applicable structural and safety codes.
2. Standards for anesthesia equipment, supplies, and patient monitoring as compared to the setting in the traditional operating rooms.
3. Room enough to accommodate the required anesthesia machines and facilities/supplies to allow a quick access to the patient and emergency/resuscitation equipment, including a defibrillator (if possible with external pacing wires) and difficult airway devices.
4. Wall oxygen (primary O_2 supply) and wall suction, both better in duplicate: mandatory by the nurse and the anesthesiologist to check both facilities (together with anesthesia machine and monitoring) before the start of the session.
5. Adequate illumination of the patient and of the vital signs monitor, without interfering with the endoscopist who must have a clear and complete vision on two monitor screens (X-ray and endoscopic images screens). The endoscopy screens should be positioned to have endoscopist's eye level three-quarters toward the top of the monitor screen. Monitors are usually placed at the opposite side of the patient, usually at a level above the head of the table, directly in front of the endoscopist.
6. An appropriate position of the anesthesia monitors is also relevant for the anesthesiologist's work, to ease the anesthesiologist's view of the monitor screen while working, particularly in case of airway manipulation (neck extension or jaw thrust in case of respiratory depression) during deep sedation and spontaneous ventilation with the patient in prone position (a usual setting during ERCP): the most ergonomic position should be, into our opinion, in front of the anesthesiologist.
7. Enough electric outlets/plugs to satisfy anesthesia machine, infusion pumps, vital signs monitors, and other supplies.
8. Isolated electric power or electric circuits with ground-fault electric interrupters (relevant in any wet location).
9. An appropriate postanesthesia care/recovery room: trained staff and basic monitoring equipment are mandatory to stabilize the patient after the procedure before a safe transfer to the ward.

An appropriate planning of the logistics and of the layout of an endoscopic suite is paramount [10]: room size and orientation, position of procedure table, position of the proceduralist and the anesthesiologist, and deployment of the endoscopic, radiologic, and anesthesia equipment should be planned and implemented according to the type of procedures and the possible rescue maneuvers the anesthesiologist might have to perform. Prone position is becoming a standard for ERCP, being mainly dictated by a more stable and ergonomic position for the endoscope and the endoscopist. However, the prone position could make the anesthesiologist less confident in airway management, particularly in case of acute respiratory depression. Many indications for ERCP are associated with a functional or mechanical gastric outlet obstruction, a condition able to increase the risk for periprocedural aspiration.

Aim of a "logic" endoscopy suite layout is to combine the maximum safety for the patient with an optimal ergonomic solution: a problematic access to the patient for the anesthesiologist (particularly to the patient's head in case of airway rescue maneuvers, included rapid shift from prone to supine position) should suggest to redesign the layout or might even change the usual anesthesia plan [10, 11] (Fig. 7.1).

7.4 The Anesthesia Staff

The average available locations are still far from being close to the ideal solution of the problem: even if the main goals of the anesthesiologist are patient safety and comfort, many other relevant issues are to be considered and implemented within the endoscopy suite, first of all the choice of adequately trained caregivers [12]. It has been documented that the number of adverse respiratory events—the most feared complication of a deep sedation or general anesthesia in nonintubated patients at remote locations—was doubled when compared to those recorded in operating rooms [11–13]. Metzner and Domino [11] warned about "oversedation and inadequate oxygenation/ventilation during monitored anesthesia care." The most recent good clinical practices documents and guidelines recommend the creation of a group of anesthesiologists expert and familiar with invasive endoscopic/radiologic procedures, the prone position, and the remote location. It has been demonstrated that anesthesiologists comfortable with this peculiar environment are more efficient than "occasional" practitioners [4, 14, 15] in terms of patient safety and work efficiency: this is mainly due to specific skills gained in (and for) this particular setting.

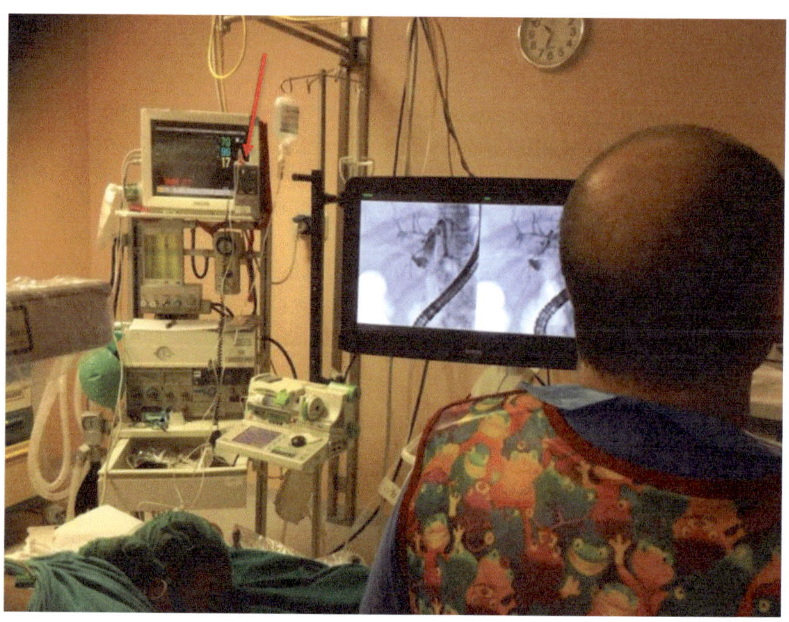

Fig. 7.1 Digestive endoscopy suite configuration at Niguarda Hospital. Note endoscopist position, patient position, cardiorespiratory monitoring, TIVA/TCI infusion pump, and anesthesia machine with emergency devices easily available. In this case, $ETCO_2$ monitoring is a stand-alone device (red arrow) (in other cases, $ETCO_2$ is integrated in the main monitor)

However, spread of competence, skills, and privileges for this activity has to be not only addressed but also developed and implemented in an anesthesia service, due to the non-infrequent urgent/emergent procedures for whom deep sedation might be requested at any time. Mean oxygen saturation (SaO_2) is higher when deep sedation or anesthesia is managed by a dedicated anesthesia pool or by anesthesiologists familiar with the endoscopic procedures: as already underlined, in modern anesthesia practice, diffusion of skills in this peculiar clinical setting is becoming crucial [14, 15]. With specific skills for NORA, anesthesiologists should be able to work more confidently in these "remote" but now frequently used locations with prone patients: procedures should be smoother, recovery time shorter, and safety higher, thus matching the quick turnover of patients, typical of the most demanding digestive endoscopic suites, with the mandatory safety requirements.

7.5 Drugs

The pharmacological armamentarium commonly used for deep sedation in digestive endoscopic setting includes benzodiazepines (BZD), opioids, propofol (PROP), and ketamine (KET). Dexmedetomidine (DEX) has recently been considered for sedation outside the ICU, and its use is now expanding in the USA and EU in NORAs: very recently, its use for sedations in NORAs has been approved also in Italy.

Benzodiazepines [16–19] (usually midazolam, less frequently diazepam) produce anxiolysis, sedation, and anterograde amnesia. BZD, devoided of analgetic properties, are frequently used in combination with opioids. Midazolam is now the most commonly drug used for conscious sedation and preanesthetic medication [5]. It has short onset of action (30–60 s), peak effect in 3–5 min, and duration of action up to 40 min. Site of metabolization is the liver; metabolites are active but quickly cleared, except in patients with end-stage liver disease, renal failure, and congestive heart failure. Diazepam has a longer duration of action and longer half-life (metabolites are active and slowly cleared by the liver). Half-life is prolonged in elderly patients, obese patients, and presence of hepatic dysfunction: delirium and agitation might be recorded in elderly patients [17, 18]. Both drugs have dose-dependent cardiorespiratory depressant properties, particularly in case of opioid co-administration. Side effects may be confusion or delirium, particularly in elderly patients. Flumazenil (FLU) is the specific benzodiazepines antagonist: repeated dose(s) after the initial dose (0.5 mg) might be needed in case of re-sedation, due to FLU half-life ranging from 40 to 100 min. Nausea, dizziness, and acute withdrawal symptoms may occur after FLU administration [5].

Opioids [16–19] (meperidine, remifentanil, fentanyl) are widely used for pain control, in addition to benzodiazepines or propofol. The most common choice in the gastroenterologic setting is *meperidine* (up to 0.5 kg mg/kg, single bolus), widely used by endoscopists together with benzodiazepines for light and moderate (conscious) sedation [14]. Its metabolite, normeperidine, is clinically active and has been reported to be associated with muscle twitching or, rarely, seizures. *Fentanyl* is considered safe according to its quick onset and rapid metabolism, and its use is now quite frequent. Respiratory depression is the most feared side effect: it is dose-dependent (>1.5 μg/kg) and can lead to apnea. Muscle rigidity (chest wall rigidity) and/or vocal cord closure might be associated with difficult mask ventilation. Nausea and vomiting are not infrequent. In spite of a very short recovery time, *remifentanil*, able to deepen sedation and to provide a good analgesia, has been associated with apnea requiring assisted ventilation (airway manipulation to keep patency sometimes may be not enough). Naloxone is the antagonist of choice (0.2–0.4 mg iv bolus) [5].

Propofol (PRO) [16–19] is a sedative-hypnotic drug used for induction and maintenance of deep sedation/general anesthesia, usually in combination with an opioid. Bolus induction of 1.5–2 mg/kg has a peak effect after 2 min, while the hypnotic action weans off after 2–8 min. Usually PRO is used as continuous infusion at 3–4.5 mg/kg/h (the average dosage used by the authors): bolus dose and maintenance infusion schedule are to be reduced in elderly patient. While the so-called "context-sensitive" half-life is close to 40 min, elimination half-life is 4–7 h. Recovery time at this dosage is usually in the range of 2–4 min. PRO has hepatic and extrahepatic (lung) metabolism, and inactive water-soluble metabolites are eliminated by the kidney. Following an induction dose, hypotension due to decreased systemic vascular resistances is the most common hemodynamic effect: heart rate usually does not change or is mildly reduced. Transient apnea (10 s) is frequently observed after the bolus dose of >1 mg/kg, together with relaxation of the upper pharyngeal muscles, reduced hypopharyngeal dimensions, and reduced laryngeal reflexes (then the use of neck extension or jaw thrust to counteract/prevent the hypoventilation: the endoscope in this setting might be considered a sort of supraglottic device).

Due to a reduced central respiratory drive, continuous infusion might reduce respiratory rate and tidal volume, resulting in reduced minute ventilation. In general, the favorable PK/PD profile, the short onset and recovery times, and the low rate of postprocedural nausea and vomiting make PRO the most (if not the only) drug used in various "sedation" settings, including complex digestive endoscopic procedures: to perform ERCP and its more complex variations, deep sedation (if not general anesthesia and endotracheal intubation, in selected cases) is increasingly required. In our opinion, the use of PRO should be reserved to anesthesiologists only, particularly in case of complex procedures (such as ERCP) and/or using the prone position. A wide body of literature however [9, 20–22] reports its safe use by non-anesthesiologists (non-anesthesiologist-administered propofol, NAAP). The unsatisfactory degree of sedation achieved with benzodiazepines and opioids combinations (usually midazolam and meperidine), together with the assumption that anesthesiologists represent an exaggerated economical burden, has pushed many gastroenterologists toward administration of sedatives and an anesthetic drug (the case for propofol) able to create conditions close to general anesthesia: this choice is in our opinion, and in spite of the favorable available literature, hazardous at best. A specific guideline was issued by ASA for the use of PRO by non-anesthesiologists [22]. PRO might have a narrow therapeutic index in not adequately trained professionals (particularly in case of airway rescue and severe hypoventilation), and its use together with other drugs such as benzodiazepines or opioids can induce too deep sedation, respiratory depression, hypoxia, and cardiovascular instability: all conditions which require breathing assistance (up to endotracheal intubation), since PRO has no antidote/antagonist. In the USA and several European Union countries, the use of PRO by non-anesthesiologists has been reported, although this practice still remains controversial at best (or sometimes banned). European guidelines on the non-anesthesiologists administration of propofol (NAAP) for endoscopy were published in December 2010 and later retracted: these guidelines have been rejected by many EU national societies of anesthesia (SIAARTI among them) [23, 24].

Ketamine [16–19] is a phencyclidine derivative: IV administration results in a rapid onset (peak effect of a bolus dose of 2 mg/kg is within 1 min) and short duration (10 min). The respiratory depression is minimal (even if a transient decrease in respiratory drive might occur); laryngeal reflexes are maintained as is CO_2 responsiveness: bronchial smooth muscle relaxation has been demonstrated. Heart rate, blood pressure, and systemic vascular resistances are usually increased due to a sympathetic nervous system stimulation. It produces dissociative anesthesia and may cause hallucinations when no benzodiazepines or other modulating drugs (trazodone is an example) are co-administered. It has good analgesic properties and has been utilized particularly for pediatric patients, due to the rapid onset of action. Unfortunately, it may be responsible for increased orotracheal secretions which may be controlled by an antisialogogue (atropine or glycopyrrolate).

Dexmedetomidine (DEX) [16–19] is an alpha2 centrally acting receptor agonist with sedative, anxiolytic, analgesic, and antisialogogue properties. It allows cooperation in spite of sedation. Bradycardia, hypotension, and reduced cardiac output might be present, particularly after the bolus dose. Minor modification in minute ventilation may be reported. Onset is slow (15 min); elimination half-life ranges from

2 to 3 h. Doses (both bolus and infusion maintenance) should be reduced in the elderly, in case of moderate-to-severe hepatic impairment, and in patients with reduced cardiac performance. For sedation in NORA, it could be used in association with propofol (to provide deeper sedation during endoscopic procedures), or with ketamine (reduced bradycardia and hypotension potentially associated with DEX, with a better modulation of secretion and reduced ketamine-related dissociation) [9] (Table 7.2).

Table 7.2 Drugs and average dosages used for sedation (from [17])

Drug	Sedative dose	Notes
Midazolam	1–2 mg IV, repeated PRN (0.025–0.1 mg/kg)	Frequently used in combination with fentanyl or for its amnestic properties when other agents are utilized as the primary sedative
Fentanyl	25–100 g IV, repeated PRN (0.25–1 g/kg)	Usually used in combination with other agents (e.g., midazolam, propofol)
Remifentanil	Bolus 0.5 g/kg IV followed by an infusion of 0.1 g/kg/min	Infusion can subsequently be titrated by 0.025 g/kg/min to 0.05 g/kg/min in 5 min intervals to achieve adequate sedation
Dexmedetomidine	Bolus 1 g/kg IV over 10 min, followed by an infusion of 0.2–0.7 g/kg/h	Reduce dose in the elderly and in patients with depressed cardiac function
Ketamine	0.2–0.8 mg/kg IV	Pretreat with antisialagogue Consider administration of midazolam to attenuate undesirable psychological effects
Diphenhydramine	12.5–50 mg IV	Useful as a substitute for midazolam in the elderly

7.6 Equipment

At least two reliable sources of oxygen (whenever possible, wall oxygen supplies) are mandatory: a secondary oxygen source for nasopharyngeal oxygenation via a dedicated cannula is more than advisable in case of desaturation while using the primary oxygenation source. Use of high-flow nasal devices (HFNO) [25] might be an updated and modern option, even if seldom, if ever, used at the moment in this setting (costs might become relevant). Adequate suction equipment (in duplicate), easily and quickly available for the anesthesiologist (separated from that used by the endoscopist); a portable breathing system with self-inflating balloon (AMBU); and a breathing system for rescue maneuvers compose the mandatory minimal safety set. A fully functional anesthesia machine should be available and properly checked before the start of every session, should a patient require endotracheal intubation and mechanical ventilation. Due to the systemic effect of the drugs used for deep sedation/general anesthesia (central depression), ability to rescue the patient from respiratory depression/cardiovascular impairment is mandatory. It is advisable to have an active gas scavenging system, in case of use of anesthetic vapors. If the location does not allow a safe use of anesthetic gases, intravenous administration of sedatives and anesthetic drugs (TIVA/TCI) is an appropriate choice [16]. NORA should have a proper illumination or adequate light sources [3]. Emergencies are possible in this setting, and rapid shift from prone to supine position of the patient is one of the most challenging and demanding maneuvers in case of severe desaturation and/or cardiovascular instability: rescue facilities are to be easily available and ready for the use [10]. Routine check before the start of the session is mandatory to avoid problematic situations in case of hyperacute critical conditions. A mobile anesthesia emergency cart with a defibrillator (external pacing would be advisable) together with standard devices for treating cardiac arrest and/or performing endotracheal intubation (difficult airway devices included) should be available.

7.7 Monitoring

Patient safety comes first and is the key word in this setting: considering the added risk of performing deep sedation/general anesthesia without an instrumented airway, monitoring must adhere to the full ASA/ESA standards [3, 5, 9], which include EKG, noninvasive (possibly automated) blood pressure measured at short intervals (every 5 min), pulse oximetry (possibly with an amplificated sound signal), and capnography (body temperature might be advisable, but not mandatory). Respiratory rate, derived from EKG or capnography, is advisable. Vital parameters are to be recorded in anesthesia charts at 5 min intervals. Impedance monitoring of respiratory rate requires adequate chest wall movements which can be reduced during deep sedation or in obese patients (Fig. 7.2).

Oxygen reserve index monitor is a new, noninvasive, promising function provided by the new generation of pulse oximeters. It gives an early warning in case of beginning hypoxia well before any changes in SpO_2 [26]. Capnography is now recommended as a standard monitor by ASA and ESA [3, 5, 9] for all patients undergoing deep sedation (and beyond). Although not always reliable in nonintubated patients mainly for technical (non-appropriate device) or "mechanical" reasons (dislodgement of the nasal device or too high oxygen flow, thus creating false-positive hypocapnia), capnography, when monitored with the appropriate device, is a reliable monitor of detecting depressed or depressing spontaneous respiratory activity, thus anticipating hypoxia, the major cause of increased morbidity and mortality in the endoscopic suites. As a matter of fact, even the most performing device to monitor peripheral oxygen saturation, pulse oximeter, has a significant delay in predicting respiratory arrest due to hypoxia. On the other hand, recovering from transient hypoxia to normal values after successful jaw thrust or left chin maneuvers (documented by deeper chest excursions and return of a normal capnogram curve) may require seconds to minutes. Interestingly enough, the majority of basic endoscopic procedures which last longer than 15–20 min and the totality of the advanced therapeutic procedures (ERCP, for instance) might shift from deep sedation to a depth equal to general anesthesia (see above). Depth of "sedation" has to be assessed continuously, together with vital parameters. Usually assessed in a subjective way, depth of sedation might in the very

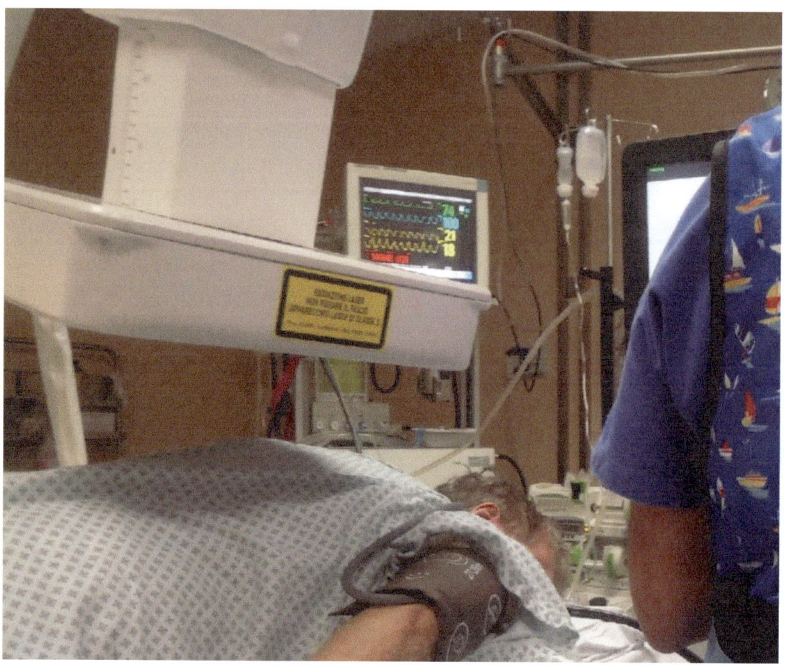

Fig. 7.2 Monitoring (heart rate, SaO_2, $ETCO_2$, respiratory rate, noninvasive blood pressure) during ERCP in prone position at Niguarda Hospital ($ETCO_2$ is integrated in the monitor)

near future rely upon dedicated devices (BIS®, ENTROPIA®, or SEDASYS® as examples) [9]. Even if not yet included among mandatory monitoring devices, depth of sedation monitors should be strongly considered to complete the safety monitoring standards: appropriate depth of sedation might help in optimizing sedative drugs administration, avoiding drug overuse, and futile, dangerous oversedation [9]. Then heart rate, noninvasive blood pressure, pulse oximetry (SaO_2), and $ETCO_2$ are the mandatory parameters to be monitored, starting before the procedure and checked with the patient awaken.

Basic monitoring (including EKG, SaO_2, NIBP) should be available in the postprocedural recovery room where the patient should be discharged from NORA: ad hoc trained and skilled nurses should be able to recognize (or better anticipate) complications and adverse events, possible in case of too deep postprocedural sedation. Among them are acute airway obstruction due to secretions and impaired cough reflex, respiratory depression with consequent hypoxia, and the risk of regurgitation and aspiration of gastric content. Mandatory for the nurse in charge is to provide first aid (safety position, oxygen delivery, jaw-thrust maneuver, suction of the secretions, mask ventilation) and to alert the anesthesiologist. A score for a safe discharge of the patients to the wards might be advisable (Aldrete score or White-Song score).

Pain should be appropriately controlled but always considered as an early warning: the endoscopists should be alerted, and in case of doubts, appropriate and immediate imaging is mandatory. The patient has to be discharged from the recovery room when conscious, verbally responsive, obeying orders, and with normal respiratory and circulatory patterns. Before the discharge and in case of doubts, the abdomen should be checked by the endoscopist for possible perforation.

7.8 Patient Assessment

Anesthesia for gastroenterologic procedures, as above alluded to, will increase in the next few years, becoming, from a sporadic activity, a relevant routine. In a busy digestive endoscopy service, due to the number of patients scheduled each day for endoscopic procedures (from 7 to 14 in authors' experience) and the different units the patients are sent from (surgical, medical, ICU, other institutions), the endoscopist has limited time to prepare an essential, focused medical history followed by a physical examination: unfortunately, the anesthesiologist faces the same problem. As very recently stated by many authors [6–9], a short but logical and possibly complete preprocedural assessment (challenging because pressed by the busy setting) is mandatory to reduce sedation adverse events [11, 13]. Respiratory problems associated with inadequate oxygenation and ventilation were the main cause of damaging events in US closed claims analysis and UK 4th National Audit Project during sedation outside the OR [13, 14]. Identification of the patients at risk is crucial for an adequate periprocedural management (including an appropriate planning and a specific monitoring). According to Tobin and Cotè [7], anesthesiologists should gather a short but relevant summary of the medical history, focusing mainly on fasting intervals, allergies, medications (in particular cardiovascular drugs, anticoagulants, and antiplatelet medications), significant organ dysfunctions (mainly the heart and lung but also central nervous system problems), and level of consciousness and/or its modifications. Relevant items to be addressed are history of snoring, obstructing sleep apnea syndrome (OSAS), COPD, asthma [7, 9], presence of arterial hypertension and treatment, chronic heart decompensation, angina, arrhythmias (in particular atrial fibrillation, AF), valvular disease (in particular aortic stenosis), cardiac interventions (in particular valve replacement or coronary arteries bypass surgery), coronary artery stents (aspirin has to be continued, unless a relevant risk of bleeding outweighs the risk of stent thrombosis), pacemakers (PM), or implantable cardioverter defibrillators (ICD) [27, 28]. Relevant is the definition of patient's efforts tolerance using the metabolic equivalents (METs, above or below 4, or the DASI,

Duke Activity Status Index) [27, 28]. Endocrine (diabetes and hypo- or hyperthyroidism), renal, and hepatic problems are to be known. Adverse events after general, locoregional anesthesia or deep sedation should be known. The physical examination should include lung auscultation, airway assessment (including teeth and dentures), problematic mouth opening (Mallampati classification), and history of radiation (marker of possible difficult laryngoscopy). According to ASA [5], routine blood tests may not be mandatory: it might be wise to have specific preprocedural tests in case of anemia (hemoglobin), diabetes (glycemia), renal failure (potassium), and liver failure (bilirubinemia). PT and aPTT could be relevant in case of anticoagulant medications. Even if no strict indication is available, it seems appropriate to have a recent ECG in patient over 60 years (50 YO in a very recent US paper) [7].

It is therefore mandatory to organize a timely access to the endoscopy service (same-day evaluation is unfortunately the rule but enough if wisely conducted) so that more problematic patients may undergo an anesthesiological-focused (even if short) assessment to plan the appropriate periprocedural pathway. In case of high-risk patients or in case of procedures which mandate ET and general anesthesia, assessment has to be done in advance, including the chance of an (rare but possible) admission in the ICU: preoperative risk stratification may add significant predictive value to the outcome of critical patients, even if the procedure is regarded as minimally invasive.

The ASA classification is reported by ESA 2018 preoperative evaluation guidelines [28] as a useful screening for limiting the administration of sedation for diagnostic procedures by endoscopists up to the ASA III patients. Obese patients might become a real problem during sedation. Noninvasive ventilation (NIV) is not always possible (dedicated masks are needed) and not safe enough. According to ASA [3, 5] and ESA [9], the following endoscopic procedures should be managed by anesthesiologists and in selected case considered for general anesthesia and endotracheal intubation:

1. Prolonged or therapeutic procedures requiring deep sedation
2. Anticipated intolerance to standard sedatives (benzodiazepines or narcotics)
3. Increased risk for adverse event because of severe comorbidity (ASA classes III and IV)
4. Increased risk for airway obstruction because of anatomic variant
5. Emergencies
6. Pediatric patients
7. (Morbid) Obese patients
8. Uncooperative or agitated patients
9. Refusal of acceptance of the procedure without anesthesia
10. Complex or long procedures (drainage of pseudopancreatic cysts with increased risk of aspiration, risk of bleeding, management of strictures, ERCP, endoscopic mucosal resection, endoscopic submucosal dissection): among these complex procedures are those sometimes requiring endotracheal intubation

Last but not least, an appropriate checklist before every procedure must include—apart from the noncompetent patient without the legal representative or in emergency—the informed consent, a keystone both for the endoscopist and for the anesthesiologist (in Italy, two separate informed consents are needed). Sedation might represent a major source of medicolegal claims [11, 13]. This is why the patient (and perhaps the relatives) should receive complete information about risk, benefit, and alternatives to the procedure, including the possibility to receive general anesthesia and ETI.

7.9 The Challenge

The increasing demand for deep sedation in patients candidates to advanced digestive endoscopy has induced relevant changes in the everyday work of a digestive endoscopic service. Complexities of the advanced endoscopic procedures are eased by an appropriately managed deep sedation performed by an anesthesiologist. This is why the involvement of anesthesia services in endoscopic activity has rapidly shifted from occasional assistances to scheduled daily services comparable to those available for the operating room: every effort should be done aiming at a safe and efficient working area. NORA is the organizational and logistical answer to an environment where standards of safety are to be redesigned according to specific needs: those of the endoscopist should match the anesthesia safety standards mandatory for any "operative/interventional environment" (in this case a procedural suite) to face possible cardiovascular and ventilatory emergencies. Monitoring standards should be the same available in the conventional ORs, while relevant efforts should aim at giving the personnel adequate training to prevent/reduce periprocedural adverse events. Nevertheless, these measures, while going toward an acceptable degree of procedural safety, still could miss the point. The main issue remains the difficult control of the airway [29–31]. As a matter of fact, all upper gastrointestinal procedures do not allow to "artificially" ventilate the patient until the endoscope is in place. Withdrawal of the endoscope could be possible, but sometimes not immediately, with potential life-threatening consequences. Routine endotracheal intubation provides optimal control of the airway but might be time-consuming and, according to a wide body of literature, not always mandatory: it should be reserved to extremely prolonged procedures; pediatric cases; critically ill individuals; morbidly obese patients; noncooperative, mentally disturbed subjects; or when the risk of aspiration is real [29]. Conditions at risk for aspiration and acute respiratory failure include delayed gastric emptying, gastric outlet obstruction, non-fasting state, drainage of large infected pancreatic pseudocysts, or acute upper gastrointestinal bleeding: the benefit in the latter situation remains, however, controversial [30]. To counterbalance the absence of secure airway, anesthesiologists have developed skills specific for deep sedation while keeping adequate spontaneous ventilation: in fact, hypoventilation and hypoxia are the most common complications potentially leading to cardiac arrest (in large part of the cases, when reported, secondary to profound hypoxemia) [30–32].

Virtually every gastrointestinal procedure is performed under the effect of sedative drugs. Large part of the diagnostic procedures requires mild intravenous sedation [5], usually under the direction of an endoscopist: among them are endoscopic ultrasound procedures (EUS, common even for outpatients with moderate sedation usually directed by the endoscopist), colonoscopies (CLS), and esophagogastroduodenoscopies (EGDS) with or without tissue biopsy; for advanced diagnostic or therapeutic procedures (ERCP or complex EUS are examples), deep sedation (or general anesthesia) is more appropriately managed by an anesthesiologist (in spite of part of markedly different opinions present in the literature) [32, 33]. Patients with proximal esophageal cancer and esophagotracheal fistula must be evaluated for possible endotracheal intubation.

Other endoscopic procedures usually performed with anesthesiological assistance are:

1. Percutaneous endoscopic gastrostomy (PEG), (usually performed in severely ill patients, may need deep sedation and analgesia).
2. Acute gastrointestinal bleeding is an emergency which requires anesthesiological skill, mainly in order to evaluate the patient who has often advanced liver disease with coagulopathy, low platelet count, and ascites. Risk of aspiration of blood is relevant, yet endotracheal intubation must be carefully evaluated according to the general status and possible outcome [30].
3. Resection of epithelial neoplasms (endoscopic mucosal resection, EMR) is a lengthy procedure requiring high precision and absence of movements: in most complex cases, general anesthesia with endotracheal intubation might be mandatory. The disease may be in proximity of the larynx. An advanced and longer form of EMR is endoscopic submucosal dissection (ESD), the en bloc resection of large lesion: general anesthesia is the rule.
4. ERCP is mainly a therapeutic procedure. It is a unique way to diagnose and treat disorders of the pancreas and biliary tract, ranging from choledocholithiasis to treatment of malignant

biliary obstruction. The endoscopist must reach the second portion of the duodenum to cannulate the ampulla of Vater, withdraw stones, and place stents within the biliary tract in case of benign or malignant strictures. In the early times, sedation was administered by endoscopists employing benzodiazepines and opiates: however, the length of the procedure, which may last more than 100 min; the need of immobility; and the pain caused by dilation of the biliary tract make the anesthesiological presence relevant (mandatory in our opinion). The procedure requires endoscopic as well as radiologic control, and the location must have appropriately located fluoroscopy equipment. This may leave little "operative" space for the anesthesiologist to guarantee adequate ventilation (see above). In addition, the room could be darkened to facilitate fluoroscopic imaging and its interpretation: should it be the case (less common nowadays), some form of illumination is among the safety standards for the anesthesiologist. The patient is usually in prone position, with the head turned toward the endoscopist: helpful for the endoscopist, this position may add some safety in case of aspiration in nonintubated patients but makes problematic any form of assisted ventilation (apart from airway manipulation as above described), not possible because of the presence of the endoscope. As already underlined, the main task of the anesthesiologist in this setting is to provide at the same time pain relief, comfort, and immobility of the patient (unconsciousness is the appropriate definition) while maintaining adequate oxygenation and ventilation. Considering that deep sedation is needed to perform an advanced procedure (as ERCP is), general anesthesia with spontaneous breathing is the right definition [29]: the level of sedation and not the sole presence of an artificial respiratory prosthesis makes the difference between sedation and general anesthesia, opening up to the need for depth of sedation monitoring in this setting to modulate drug-induced alteration of consciousness. As stated by Schumann [25] and already above underlined, "sedation is a continuum of altered consciousness, ranging from moderate to deep sedation and general anesthesia." As above alluded to, prone position might be a double-edged sword. As recently underlined [7], the prone position has not to be considered by default an independent predictor of sedation-related complications. In fact, it may confer more protection against aspiration, this position being in general at a lower risk if compared to the supine position: as an example, in prone position, airway obstruction occurs less frequently due to the tongue position, off the hard palate. When managed by an experienced anesthesiologist, and according to the literature, propofol deep sedation (quite often co-administered with opioid, in our experience almost always meperidine, 0.5 mg/kg, single bolus at the start of the procedure) and spontaneous ventilation have a favorable safety profile during ERCP and other advanced endoscopic procedures. According to Goudra and Singh [29], oxygen released by a nasal airway may become inadequate during deep sedation: the negative intraluminal pressure in the pharynx could be not counterbalanced by the tone of the upper airway musculature (the mechanism able to avoid in the awake patient the closure of the upper airway) (Fig. 7.3).

It has been demonstrated [29] that when the muscular valve called velopharyngeal mechanism collapses due to loss of muscular tone, a tight seal (created by soft palate and pharyngeal walls separating nasal and oral compartments) is anatomically formed, and no airflow from the nose becomes possible [Fig. 7.3 from Goudra and Singh (2017)] [29]. In addition, the obstruction of the oropharynx following retrolingual collapse blocks airflow from entering the larynx. This double block may be overcome by a nasopharyngeal device, for instance, a small silicone 18 or 20 F suction tube or a so-called nasal trumpet. This simple device, together with oxygen flow from the secondary oxygen source, if correctly positioned, allows a dramatic improvement of the

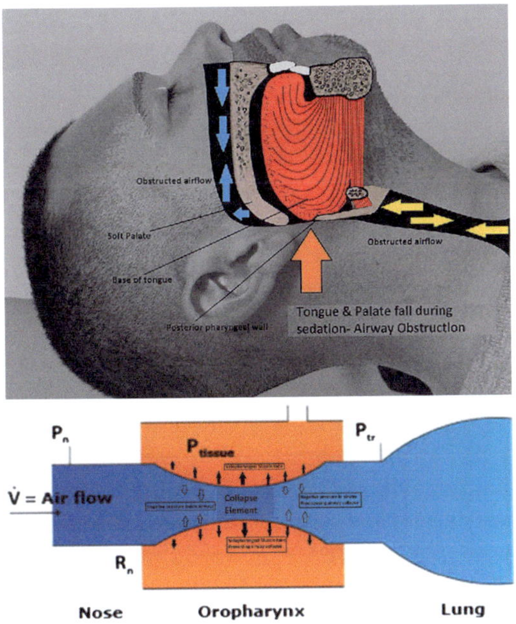

Fig. 7.3 The airways and the velopharyngeal mechanism during deep sedation (from [29])

hypoxemia: last but not least in this specific setting, the endoscope itself acts as a stent of the airway, preventing the collapse of the tissue at pharyngeal level [29].

Other simple tricks to be used in case of hypoxia are chin lift, jaw thrust, and neck extension: their efficacy can be limited by the prone position. These measures, alone or together, are usually successful together with O_2 administration (sometimes using the secondary source) in correcting dangerous hypoxia before asking the endoscopist to withdraw the endoscope and start with positive pressure ventilation or even the placement of an airway protection device such as laryngeal mask or endotracheal tube. It must be kept in mind that emergency endotracheal intubation in the peculiar setting of gastrointestinal endoscopic procedures, with the patient in the prone position, may be not easy at best: it might be wise, before starting with the procedure, to anticipate the way to turn the patients into the supine position in case of emergency.

In this setting, obese patients are worth for maximal alertness: orotracheal intubation has to be strongly considered above BMI > 30 kg/m^2. If the procedure is considered safe without intubation, it is advisable to keep the patients in supine or in semi-prone or lateral position (although many endoscopists might be uncomfortable with these positions), with extension of the atlanto-occipital joint, the well-known "sniffing the morning air." This is highly advisable in obese adults with obstructive sleep apnea syndrome (OSAS) [29]. A double oxygen source should be available; nasopharyngeal airway is recommended because displacement is less frequent. An additional risk of airway collapse in this setting is due to higher negative airway pressure and to increased amount of fat in the pharynx which diminishes the already narrow space between pharyngeal walls and reduces the stenting effect of the endoscope. Well before hypoxia might become threatening and positive pressure ventilation unavoidable, it is mandatory to ask the gastroenterologist to withdraw the endoscope and to proceed with ventilator assistance and/or tracheal intubation.

Research has developed different airway devices to provide additional oxygen supply: face mask, panoramic face mask, endoscopy mask, and dedicated endoscopic mask (Janus®). They represent the natural evolution of the face mask: all of them have a port for the endoscope; they fit the patient's face preventing leaks; some have a leak-proof cushioned seal along the facial contour to perform assisted/controlled positive pressure ventilation: an additional port for CO_2 monitoring may be available. The main limitation, common to all, is the inability to prevent airway obstruction or aspiration.

Other airway devices available are nasopharyngeal airway, gastrolaryngeal tube, and bite block. The nasopharyngeal airway [29] is a large nasopharyngeal tube (28F, 7 internal diameter) inserted through the nose. The concept is the same as for a smaller suction tube which goes beyond the velopharyngeal mechanism. The main differences are the size, which allows manual ventilation, and the correct timing for placement, since the patient should be sedated with suppression of the cough reflex. The gastrolaryngeal tube is recommended for complex procedures like ERCP and PEG. Its purpose is to secure the airway and prevent the regurgitation of gastric content. It increases the space for maneuvering the endoscope and allows positive pressure ventilation [29]. It should be utilized by experienced hands. The bite blocks are utilized by endoscopists in the oral cavity in order to avoid biting of the endoscope. Over the years, they have been modified in order to ease positive pressure ventilation and aspiration of oral secretions and prevent airway obstruction thanks to special devices like atraumatic airway flange or tongue depressor (Goudra's bite block, safety guard) [29]. With this kind of bite blockers, oxygen delivery and $EtCO_2$ monitoring are more reliable.

The variety of devices above discussed reflect the continuous research of optimal management of the airway and of the patient's and endoscopist's needs. Unfortunately, there is no ideal solution: the anesthesiologist may choose among different solutions with regard to the possible devices and strategies. As for the devices, all possible technical solutions are not always available for the caregiver, who has to find out the most suitable one for the specific setting/condition and the local availability. When doubts arise, it seems wise to ask an experienced colleague for help and/or advice. Four hands, two brains, and specific skills could be the best available solution: should help be unavailable, the best choice is to act according to one's capacity and experience.

7.10 Coming to a Conclusion: Sedation, the Proceduralist, and the Anesthesiologist

Many papers report of excellent results when intravenous sedation is administered by gastroenterologists [8, 32, 33]. There is wide-spread use of nurse-assisted (NAPS) or NAAP in many endoscopy suits in Europe. This is currently the case in all routine procedures performed for diagnostic purposes or of short duration. As already mentioned, most of the endoscopic procedures may require light sedation with midazolam and opioids and do not need the presence of an anesthesiologist. Even propofol sedation has been safely administered by endoscopists or qualified trained personnel [32, 33]. However, the European anesthesiology societies issued a consensus statement against the use of propofol by non-anesthesiologists [23, 24]. The current position of the BSG - for expample - is that NAAP services have been reported to be safe and effective, but the current UK position is that propofol administration should be the responsibility of a dedicated and appropriately trained anaesthetist [24]. Among the reasons that would propose NAAP is the minor expense for the hospital when sedation is administered by non-anesthesiologists [9]. Training curricula have been established by American and European societies. Trainees must be able to evaluate the patient, give adequate information, administer sedatives, monitor vital functions, ventilate the patient if necessary, and take care of him until the discharge. Unfortunately, there is paucity of training courses and still no validated methods to test competence. Moreover, we are convinced that deep sedation in the endoscopic setting is much better and more efficiently managed by an anesthesiologist. This might be, however, subject to local expertise of NAAP personel. Buxbaum [34], analyzing the different cost between anesthesiologist- and non-anesthesiologist-directed sedation, points out that the gastroenterologist-directed sedation (GDS) for ERCP has a major rate of failure due to excessive or insufficient sedative administration, and therefore, although anesthesiologist-directed sedation is more expensive, the additional cost is outweighed by the reduction of (expensive) alternative procedures (or redo) and shorter hospitalization. Buxbaum [34] stated that "routine use of anesthesia providers for routine endoscopies is not a cost." To increase safety while speeding up procedures, competent professionals able to solve specific problems are needed. If sedation is a continuum between light sedation and deep unconsciousness [3, 5, 8, 9] and if ERCP and similar complex procedures require a sedation level deep enough to equal the condition of general anesthesia while maintaining spontaneous breathing, a dedicated anesthesiologist is more than needed, allowing the endoscopists to concentrate on his demanding task without being "distracted" by problems (from ancillary to major adverse events) coming from the possible (adverse) effects of a (too) deep sedation.

Team working is better than "solo": team and not the "one man band" should become the standard.

References

1. Goudra BG, Alvarez A, Singh PM. Practical considerations in the development of a nonoperating room anesthesia practice. Curr Opin Anaesthesiol. 2016;29:526–30.
2. Cui W, Lee CZ. Chapter 38: Anesthesia for procedures in non-operating room locations. In: Miller anesthesia. Elsevier; 2016. p. 658–72.
3. ASA Statement on nonoperating room anesthetizing locations Committee of Origin: Standards and Practice Parameters (Approved by the ASA House of Delegates on October 19, 1994, and last amended on October 15, 2014).
4. Bhavani S. Non-operating room anesthesia in the endoscopy unit. Gastrointest Endosc Clin N Am. 2016;26:471–83.
5. Practice guidelines for moderate procedural sedation and analgesia 2018. A Report by the American Society of Anesthesiologists Task Force on Moderate Procedural Sedation and Analgesia, the American Association of Oral and Maxillofacial Surgeons, American College of Radiology, American Dental Association, American Society of Dentist Anesthesiologists, and Society of Interventional Radiology. Anesthesiology. 2018;128:437–79.
6. McAlevy ME, Levenick JM. Chapter 7: Anesthesia for upper GI endoscopy including advanced endoscopic procedures. In: Goudra BG, Singh PM, editors. Out of operating room anesthesia. A comprehensive review. Springer; 2017. p. 85–100.
7. Tobin CD, Cotè GA. Chapter 6: Sedation in ERCP. In: Baron T, Kozarek R, Carr-Locke D, editors. The ERCP book. 3rd ed. Elsevier; 2018. p. 49–53.
8. Early DS, Lightdale JR, Vargo JV, Acosta AR, Chandrasekhara V, Chathadi KV, et al. Guidelines for sedation and anesthesia in GI endoscopy. Gastrointest Endosc. 2018;87:327–37.
9. Hinkelbein J, Lamperti M, Akeson J, Santos J, Costa J, De Robertis E, et al. European Society of Anaesthesiology and European Board of Anaesthesiology guidelines for procedural sedation and analgesia in adults. Eur J Anaesthesiol. 2018;35:6–24.
10. Brauer BC, Edmundowicz SA. Chapter 2: The ERCP room. In: Baron T, Kozarek R, Carr-Locke D, editors. The ERCP book. 3rd ed. Elsevier; 2018.
11. Metzner J, Domino KB. Risks of anesthesia or sedation outside the operating room: the role of the anesthesia care provider. Curr Opin Anaesthesiol. 2010;23:523–31.
12. Goudra BG, Singh PM, Sinha AC. Anesthesia for ERCP: impact of anesthesiologist's experience on outcome and cost. Anesthesiol Res Pract. 2013;2013:570518.
13. Cotton P. Chapter 19: Medicolegal issues in ERCP. In: Baron T, Kozarek R, Carr-Locke D, editors. The ERCP book. 3rd ed. Elsevier; 2018. p. 99–108.
14. Han SJ, Lee TH, Park SH, Cho YS, Lee YN, Jung Y, Choi HJ, Chung IK, Cha SW, Moon JH, Cho YD, Kim SJ. Efficacy of midazolam- versus propofol-based sedations during therapeutic endoscopic retrograde cholangiopancreatography in patients aged over 80 years. Dig Endosc. 2017;29:369–76.
15. Da B, Buxbaum J. Training and competency in sedation practice in gastrointestinal endoscopy. Gastrointest Endosc Clin N Am. 2016;26:443–62.
16. Whitlock EL, Pardo MC. Chapter 14: Choice of anesthetic technique. In: Miller anesthesia. Elsevier; 2017. p. 213–9.
17. Artime CA. Chapter 1: Pharmacology of sedative drugs used in out of operating room anesthesia. In: Goudra BG, Singh PM, editors. Out of operating room anesthesia. A comprehensive review. Springer; 2017. p. 3–14.
18. Duggan EW, Schwock KL. Chapter 2: Pharmacology of anesthetic drugs used in out of operating room anesthesia. In: Goudra BG, Singh PM, editors. Out of operating room anesthesia. A comprehensive review. Springer; 2017. p. 15–36.
19. Charchaflieh JG, Ganatra M, Springer E. Chapter 3: Principles of delivery of sedatives and intravenous anesthetics in out of operating room anesthesia. In: Goudra BG, Singh PM, editors. Out of operating room anesthesia. A comprehensive review. Springer; 2017. p. 38–52.
20. Dumonceau JM, Riphaus A, Aparicio JR, Beilenhoff U, Knape JTA, Ortmann M, The NAAP Task Force Members. Non-anesthesiologist administration of propofol for gastrointestinal endoscopy: European Society of Gastrointestinal Endoscopy, European Society of Gastroenterology and Endoscopy Nurses and Associates Guideline—Updated June 2015. Endoscopy. 2015;47:1175–89.
21. Repici A, Pagano N, Hassan C, Carlino A, Rando G, Strangio G, et al. Balanced propofol sedation administered by nonanesthesiologists: the first Italian experience. World J Gastroenterol. 2011;17:3818–23.
22. Practice guidelines for sedation and analgesia by non-anesthesiologists—an updated report by the American Society of Anesthesiologists Task Force on Sedation and Analgesia by Non-Anesthesiologists. Anesthesiology. 2002;96:1004–17.

23. Perel A. Non-anesthesiologists should not be allowed to administer propofol for procedural sedation: a consensus statement of 21 European national societies of anesthesia. Eur J Anaesthesiol. 2011;28:580–4.
24. Sidhu R, Turnbull D, Newton M, et al. Deep sedation and anaesthesia in complex gastrointestinal endoscopy: a joint position statement endorsed by the British Society of Gastroenterology (BSG), Joint Advisory Group (JAG) and Royal College of Anaesthetists (RCoA). Frontline Gastroenterology 2019;10:141–47.
25. Schumann R, Natov NS, Rocuts-Martinez KA, Finkelman MA, Phan TV, Hegde SR, Knapp RM. High flow nasal oxygen availability for sedation decreases the use of general anesthesia during endoscopic retrograde cholangiopancreatography and endoscopic ultrasound. World J Gastroenterol. 2016;22(47):10398–405.
26. Scheeren TWL, Belda FJ, Perel A. The oxygen reserve index (ORI): a new tool to monitor oxygen therapy. J Clin Monit Comput. 2018;32:379–89.
27. Rossini R, Tarantini G, Musumeci G, Masiero G, Barbato E, Calabrò P, et al. A multidisciplinary approach on the perioperative antithrombotic management of patients with coronary stents undergoing surgery. Surgery after stenting 2. JACC Cardiovasc Interv. 2018;11:417–34.
28. De Hert S, Staender S, Fritsch G, Hinkelbein J, Afshari A, Bettelli G, Bock M, Chew MS, Coburn M, De Robertis E, Drinhaus H, Feldheiser A, Geldner G, Lahner D, Macas A, Neuhaus C, Rauch S, Santos-Ampuero MA, Solca M, Tanha N, Traskaite V, Wagner G, Wappler F. Pre-operative evaluation of adults undergoing elective noncardiac surgery: updated guideline from the European Society of Anaesthesiology. Eur J Anaesthesiol. 2018;35(6):407–65.
29. Goudra BG, Singh PM. Airway management during upper GI endoscopic procedures: state of the art review. Dig Dis Sci. 2017;62:45–53.
30. Koch DG, Arguelas MR, Fallon MB. Risk of aspiration pneumonia in suspected variceal hemorrhage: the value of prophylactic endotracheal intubation prior to endoscopy. Dig Dis Sci. 2007;52:2225–8.
31. Goudra BG, Nuzat A, Singh PM, Gouda GB, Carlin A, Manjunath AK. Cardiac arrest in patients undergoing gastrointestinal endoscopy: a retrospective analysis of 73029 procedures. Saudi J Gastroenterol. 2015;21:400–11.
32. Cheriyan DG, Byrne MF. Propofol use in endoscopic retrograde cholangiopancreatography and endoscopic ultrasound. World J Gastroenterol. 2014;20(18):5171–6.
33. Yang JF, Farooq P, Zwilling K, Patel D, Siddiqu AA. Effect and safety of propofol-mediated sedation for outpatient endoscopic retrograde cholangiopancreatography (ERCP). Dig Dis Sci. 2016;61:1686–91.
34. Buxbaum J, Roth N, Motamedi N, Lee T, Leonor P, Salem M, Gibbs D, Vargo J. Anesthetist-directed sedation favors success of advanced endoscopic procedures. Am J Gastroenterol. 2017;112:290–6.

Anatomy of the Biliary Tree

8

Giuseppe M. Ettorre and Roberto L. Meniconi

8.1 Overview

Hepatic (or bile) canaliculi are the smallest branches of the bile duct system in which the hepatocytes secrete the bile. They are formed by the lateral faces of the hepatocytes, draining the bile in a centripetal way into the hepatic ductules that are lined by epithelial cells. These ductules then join into larger ducts progressively forming lobular ductules; subsegmental and segmental ducts, which combine into sectorial ducts; and finally the left and right hepatic ducts (Fig. 8.1). According to the Couinaud model [1], the biliary system follows the same disposition of the portal system, being the bile ducts a part of the portal triad. The left and the right hepatic ducts join into the biliary confluence at the level of the hepatic hilum, and then the common hepatic duct joins the cystic duct to form the common bile duct which courses inferiorly and enters into the second portion of the duodenum either alone or after joining the pancreatic duct.

G. M. Ettorre (✉) · R. L. Meniconi
Division of General Surgery and Organ Transplantation, Azienda Ospedaliera San-Camillo Forlanini, Rome, Italy
e-mail: gmettorre@scamilloforlanini.rm.it

8.2 Intrahepatic Biliary Anatomy

According to the Brisbane 2000 terminology [2], the liver is divided into the right and left lobes by the Cantlie line. The right lobe is divided into anterior (segments 5 and 8) and posterior sectors (segments 6 and 7), whereas the left lobe is divided into medial (segment 4) and lateral (segments 2 and 3) sectors which are anatomically separated by the umbilical fissure. Similarly, segments 7 and 8 are also defined as superior segments, while segments 5 and 6 are inferior segments. The bile ducts draining each segment are considered third-order ducts. The sectoral bile ducts are second-order ducts with the main right and left hepatic ducts referred to as the first-order ducts [3]. Segment 1 is drained by several ducts joining both the right and left hepatic ducts close to the biliary confluence at the hilum.

8.2.1 Right Anterior Sectoral Ducts (Segments 5 and 8)

The right anterior sectoral duct is located intrahepatically and is formed by the joining of segments 5 and 8. It lies vertical, on the left of the anterior branch of the portal vein, and usually enters the right hepatic duct, along a longitudinal axis. In some cases, it receives bile ducts from segment 5 and the ventral part of segment 8, while the dorsal part of segment 8 is drained into

M. Mutignani et al. (eds.), *Endotherapy in Biliopancreatic Diseases: ERCP Meets EUS*,
https://doi.org/10.1007/978-3-030-42569-2_8

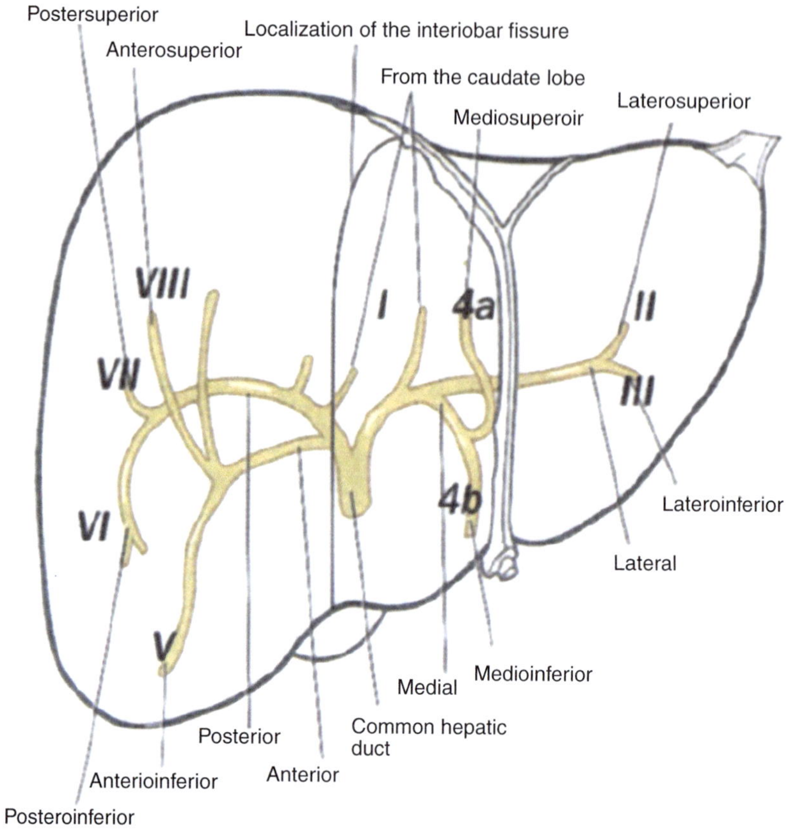

Fig. 8.1 Intrahepatic biliary anatomy according to the segmental Couinaud model of the liver. (From Karaliotas, Broelsch, Habib (eds.). Liver and biliary tract surgery. Embryological Anatomy to 3D-Imaging and Transplant Innovations. Springer: Vienna, 2007; with permission)

the right posterior sectoral duct. The right anterior sectoral duct may be absent: in these cases, bile ducts from segments 5 and 8 join separately the right hepatic duct. Rarely, the right anterior sectoral duct enters the left hepatic duct. A subvesical bile duct located in the gallbladder fossa may be present in up to one-third of cases and usually drains into the anterior sectoral duct or the right hepatic duct, without any communications with the gallbladder.

8.2.1.1 Segment 5

One or two ducts of segment 5 enter the right anterior sectoral duct. In some cases, bile ducts from segment 5 join directly the right hepatic duct, separately with bile ducts of segment 8, forming a right-sided confluence with the right posterior sectoral duct. When two or more bile ducts arising from segment 5 are present, one of them may enter the bile duct of the ventral part of segment 8.

8.2.1.2 Segment 8

Segment 8 is the most voluminous segment of the liver and is located in the upper part of the right liver, corresponding to the hepatic dome. It is divided in two parts, ventral and dorsal, each one drained by one or two bile ducts which course vertically. Normally, ventral and dorsal bile ducts of segment 8 join to form a common duct before entering the right anterior sectoral duct (Fig. 8.1). In the absence of the latter, this common duct from segment 8 enters directly the right hepatic duct, together with the bile duct of segment 5 and the right posterior sectoral duct (20% of cases). Sometimes, the ventral bile duct of segment 8 joins with the bile duct from segment 5 to form an incomplete right anterior sectoral duct, while the dorsal bile duct of segment 8 joins directly the right hepatic duct or the right posterior sectoral duct. Rarely, a bile duct from segment 9 (right paracaval region) joins the dorsal bile duct of segment 8.

8.2.2 Right Posterior Sectoral Ducts (Segments 6 and 7)

The right posterior sectoral duct drains bile from segments 6 and 7 and is generally oriented in a horizontal direction, passing superior to the anterior portal branch making a curve around it, known as the Hjortsjö crook [4], before joining the right anterior sectoral duct. However, the course of the right posterior duct is the most variable, as depicted in Fig. 8.2. In some cases, it joins a common duct formed by the union of the right anterior sectoral duct and the left hepatic duct, distally from the biliary confluence. Conversely, the right posterior sectoral duct may join the left hepatic duct into a common duct to form the biliary confluence with the right anterior sectoral duct. In rare cases, the right posterior sectoral duct may receive the cystic duct.

8.2.2.1 Segment 6

One or more bile ducts from segment 6 contribute to form the right posterior sectoral duct together with bile ducts of segment 7. Sometimes, the bile duct from segment 6 joins the right anterior sectoral duct. In other cases, it enters the common hepatic duct, distally: in such cases, the right hepatic duct is formed by the segmental duct of segment 7 and the right anterior sectoral duct. When two bile ducts of segment 6 are present, one can join the segmental duct of segment 7, while the other can join the right anterior sectoral duct.

8.2.2.2 Segment 7

Segment 7 is generally drained by one bile duct, which is formed by the union of smaller subsegmental ducts. It usually joins one or more segmental ducts from segment 6 to form the right posterior sectoral duct. Sometimes, the bile duct

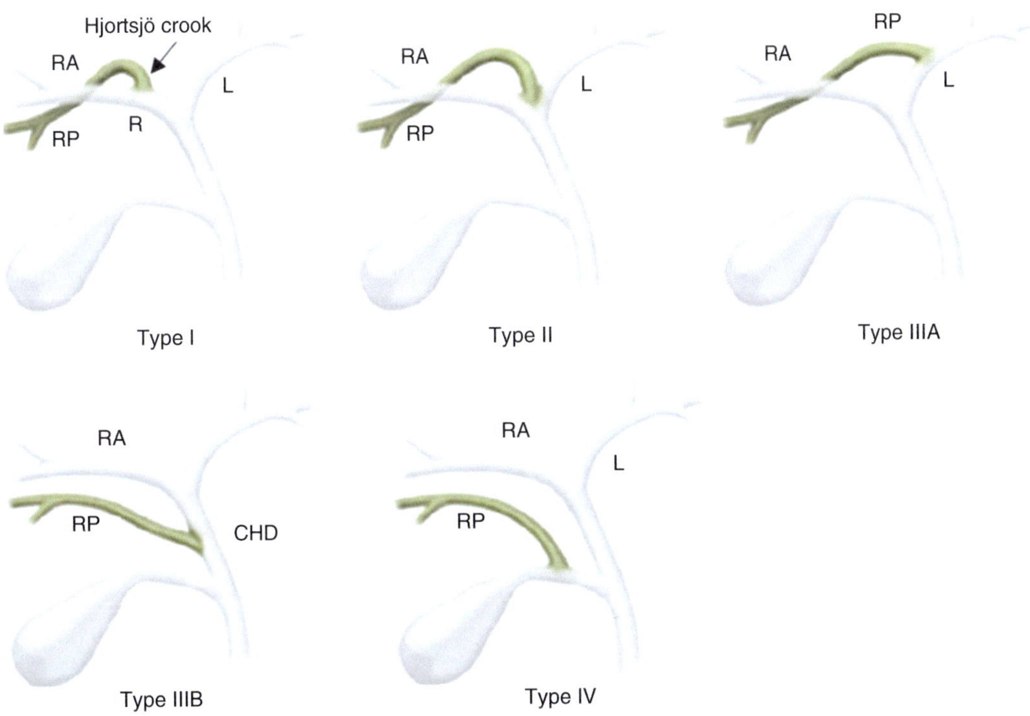

Fig. 8.2 Schematic representation of intrahepatic bile duct anatomy, focusing on the right posterior sectoral duct variations. Type I is conventional; type II is a trifurcation pattern with a common confluence of the right posterior and the right anterior sectoral ducts; type III is an abnormal right duct configuration including type IIIA in which the right posterior duct drains into the left hepatic duct and type IIIB in which the right posterior duct drains directly into the common hepatic duct; in type IV, the right posterior duct drains into the cystic duct. *RA* right anterior sectoral duct, *RP* right posterior sectoral duct, *R* right hepatic duct, *L* left hepatic duct, *CHD* common hepatic duct. (From Khaled M. Elsayes. Cross-sectional imaging of the abdomen and pelvis. Springer, 2015; with permission)

of segment 7 drains into the right anterior sector or enters the right hepatic duct.

8.2.3 Bile Ducts from Segments 2 and 3 (Left Lateral Sector)

Usually, bile ducts from the left lateral and medial sectors join each other within the umbilical fissure to form the left hepatic duct. The left lateral sector is generally drained by a biliary stem formed by bile ducts of segments 2 and 3 (Fig. 8.3). They follow generally the course of the portal branches. Usually, the segmental duct of segment 3 follows the left horn of the Rex recessus and joins the bile duct of segment 2 above its portal branch.

8.2.4 Bile Ducts from Segment 4 (Left Medial Sector)

The left medial sector is entirely represented by the segment 4 which is divided into two subsegments: superior (4a) and inferior (4b). Biliary drainage from segment 4 has a complex and variable pattern. In most cases, all ducts coming from segment 4 join to form a single duct of the left medial sector. As shown in Fig. 8.3, some variations can occur in bile duct anatomy of segment 4. In one-fourth of cases, two bile ducts drain separately the superior (4a) and inferior (4b) part of segment 4. Sometimes, the segmental bile duct of segment 4 can join a duct from segment 3. In rare occasions, bile duct from segment 4 drains separately into the common duct or very close to the biliary confluence. Finally, during its horizontal course at the base of segment 4, the left hepatic duct may receive small branches from segment 4b. This is the reason why the lowering of the hilar plate at this level should be done intraparenchimally in segment 4b, in order to avoid any injury to these small biliary branches.

8.2.5 Bile Ducts from Segments 1 and 9 (Right Paracaval Region)

Segment 1 represents the caudate lobe and is divided into a caudate lobe proper (between the

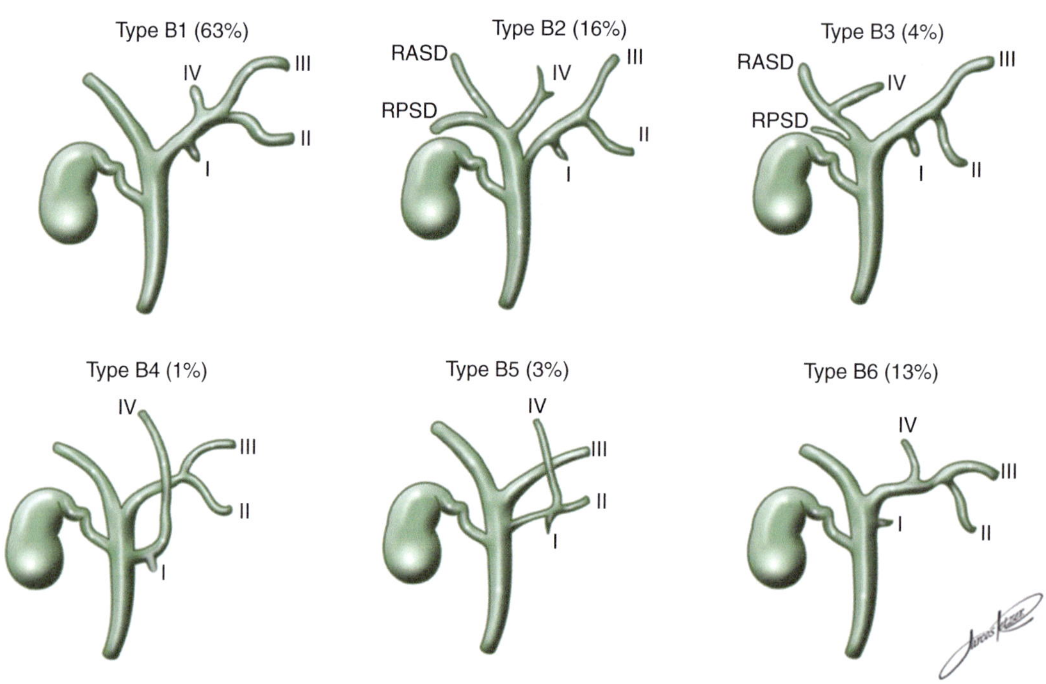

Fig. 8.3 Left hepatic duct anatomy and its main variations classified into six types based on biliary drainage of left-sided segments [6]. (From Chaib E, Kanas AF, Galvão FH, et al. Bile duct confluence: anatomic variations and its classification. Surg Radiol Anat. 2014 Mar;36(2):105–9; with permission)

inferior vena cava and the umbilical fissure) and the caudate process which connect the caudate lobe to the right hepatic lobe. This right paracaval region of the caudate lobe is also known as segment 9. Several bile ducts drain segment 1, from one to six branches, which enter both left and right hepatic ducts near to the biliary confluence. Sometimes, bile ducts from segments 1 drain only into the left hepatic duct (15% of cases) or the right hepatic duct (5% of cases). The bile ducts from segment 9 (two or three branches) generally join the right hepatic duct, the right posterior sectoral duct, or bile ducts from segments 6 or 7.

Bile ducts of segment 1 run generally posterior and above the portal branches, joining the bile duct on its posterior surface.

This anatomical pattern of the biliary drainage of segment 1 justifies the need to resect routinely the segment 1 and its biliary ducts in case of hilar biliary tumors.

8.3 Extrahepatic Biliary Anatomy

The extrahepatic biliary tree is formed by the left and right hepatic ducts, the biliary confluence (hilum region), the common hepatic duct, and the common bile duct. The gallbladder is considered as a part of the extrahepatic biliary system and is connected with the common hepatic duct by the cystic duct to form the common bile duct.

8.3.1 Right Hepatic Duct

The right hepatic duct drains all segments of the right lobe (5, 6, 7, and 8) and generally runs extrahepatically anterior to the right portal vein before joining the biliary confluence cephalad to the right portal vein. It is short (about 1 cm in length) and generally vertical, along the same axis of the common bile duct, and is formed by the confluence of the right anterior and posterior sectoral ducts. In some cases, it receives a duct from the segment 1.

The right hepatic duct can be absent in about 25% of cases, mostly when the anterior and posterior sectoral ducts enter the biliary confluence separately forming a triple confluence (see below) [5].

8.3.2 Left Hepatic Duct

The left hepatic duct drains bile from segments 2, 3, 4, and 1. It is longer than the right hepatic duct, with an average length of 2.5 cm, and runs horizontally in the hilum from left to right above the left portal vein, at the base of the quadrate lobe (segment 4), until joining the right hepatic duct to form the biliary confluence. The left hepatic duct is formed by the confluence of branches from segments 2, 3, and 4 within the umbilical fissure. The orientation of the left hepatic duct and the left portal vein is usually transversal at the hilum before entering the umbilical fissure where they course in a longitudinal fashion. This "normal" anatomy of the left hepatic duct is reported in 80% of cases, and its anatomical variations are less common than the right hepatic duct [5].

Sometimes, the left hepatic duct is absent, and bile from segments 2 and 3 is collected by a biliary stem which forms the biliary confluence with the right hepatic duct, while the bile duct from segment 4 joins the common bile duct separately. In 4% of patients, a right sectoral duct can join the left hepatic duct (3% posterior and 1% anterior). These main variations of left hepatic duct anatomy have been classified in six types by Huang et al. [6], as shown in Fig. 8.3.

The segment 1 usually drains into the left hepatic duct by one or more ducts, superior or inferior to the left portal vein.

8.3.3 Biliary Confluence

The biliary confluence is located extrahepatically and lies anterior to the origin of the right branch of the portal vein. It is covered by the hilar plate, a fibrotic sheath originating from Glisson's capsule, which continues with the hepatoduodenal ligament, and is usually formed by the confluence of the right and left hepatic ducts.

However, this classic junction is found only in 60% of cases, and the triple confluence is not

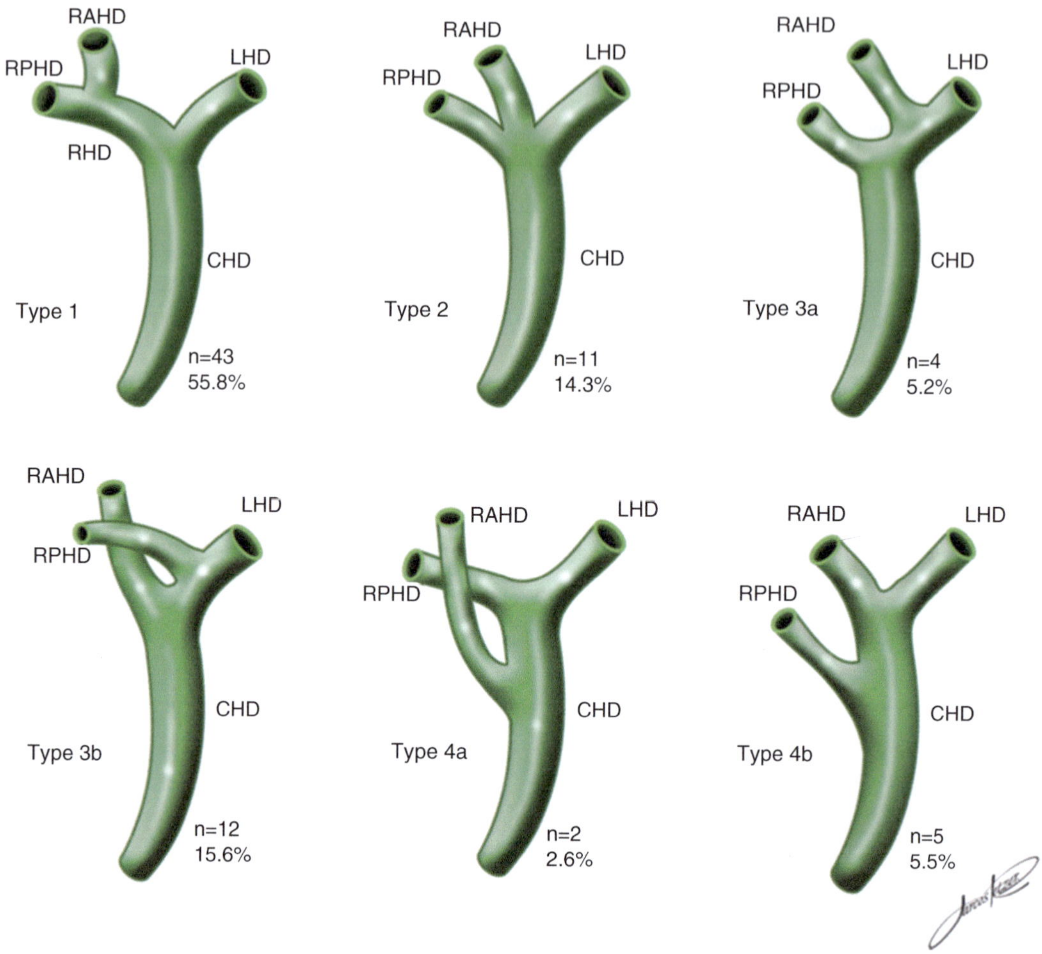

Fig. 8.4 Biliary confluence anatomy, classification, and frequency of its main variations (six types). *CHD* common hepatic duct, *LHD* left hepatic duct, *RAHD* right anterior hepatic duct, *RPHD* right posterior hepatic duct. (From Chaib E, Kanas AF, Galvão FH, et al. Bile duct confluence: anatomic variations and its classification. Surg Radiol Anat. 2014;36:105–9; with permission)

rare. This can be composed of the right anterior and posterior sectoral ducts, which join directly and separately to the confluence with the left hepatic duct to form the common hepatic duct (Fig. 8.4).

Other variations of the biliary confluence are shown in Fig. 8.4 and can be found as follows: the left hepatic duct can receive the right anterior or posterior (rare) sectoral ducts forming a common anonymous duct in which the other right sectoral duct enters distally at different distance from the confluence; in some cases, the right anterior or posterior sectoral duct joins distally the common hepatic duct below the normal confluence, forming an anatomical variation called "convergence étagée" by the French authors [7]; more rarely, the right posterior sectoral duct drains directly into the cystic duct, also known as "cystohepatic duct" (1–2% of cases) [8].

Very rarely, there are two right hepatic ducts and two left hepatic ducts forming a quadruple biliary confluence.

Such unusual variations of the biliary confluence are usually accompanied by portal and arterial variation in the *porta hepatis*.

Variations in confluence of the left and right hepatic ducts can also be found at different levels of the hepatic hilum or hepatoduodenal ligament:

the biliary confluence is generally extrahepatic, but an intrahepatic or a low biliary confluence may also be found.

Given the wide variability of the biliary confluence, the knowledge of these anatomical variations is extremely important for hepatobiliary surgeons, radiologists, and endoscopists, not only for diagnosis but also in the operative setting, from the simple cholecystectomy to the more complex cases of perihilar tumors.

8.3.4 Common Hepatic Duct and Common Bile Duct

Similar to the biliary confluence, the formation of the common hepatic duct can be variable. It generally drains all bile from the liver and is formed by the junction of the right and the left hepatic ducts at different levels, from the hilum to the low part of the hepatoduodenal ligament. As seen formerly, aberrant bile ducts from the right or left hemiliver can open directly into the common hepatic ducts: these anomalies are more frequent for the right-sided bile ducts (right posterior duct, aberrant duct from segment 6) than left-sided ducts (aberrant duct from segment 4). It is about 3 cm in length and merges with the cystic duct to form the common bile duct (or *ductus choledochus*).

The length of the common bile duct is variable (from 5 to 13 cm), depending on where the cystic duct joins the common hepatic duct. It lies anterior to the portal vein along the right free edge of the lesser omentum and descends behind the first portion of the duodenum and the posterior surface of the head of the pancreas in the pancreatic groove. At this level, the common bile duct is covered or embedded within the pancreatic tissue, before joining the main pancreatic duct to form the ampulla of Vater which enters the second portion of the duodenum on its posteromedial wall at the major papilla [9]. Rarely, other sites of major papilla location in the duodenum are between the second and third portion of the duodenum, or the third part of the duodenum (Fig. 8.5). Sometimes, the pancreatic and bile ducts enter the duodenum separately and share an opening at the duodenal papilla, the so-called double barrel.

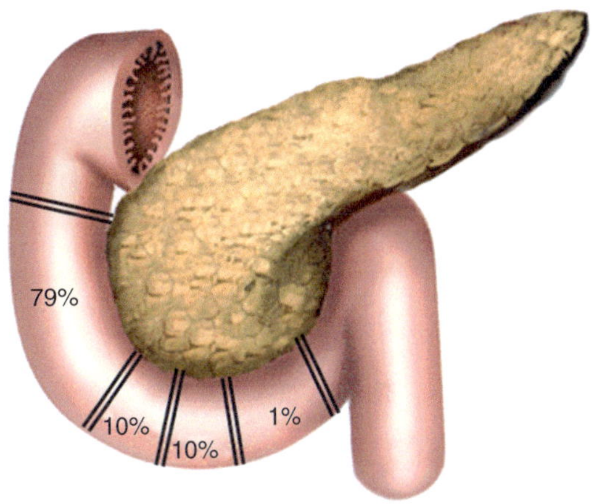

Fig. 8.5 Schematic representation and frequency of major papilla locations in the duodenum

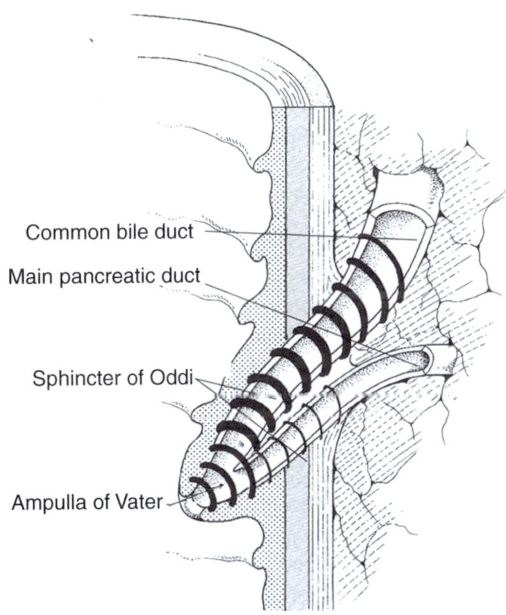

Fig. 8.6 Schematic view of the sphincter of Oddi

At the level of the ampulla of Vater, there is a neuromuscular structure named sphincter of Oddi which regulates the delivery of bile and pancreatic juice into the duodenum and prevents the reflux of duodenal contents into the biliary and pancreatic systems (Fig. 8.6). According to the Boyden classification [10], the sphincter of Oddi is divided in to three portions: (1) The *sphincter choledochus*, further divided into superior and inferior regions, represents the main part

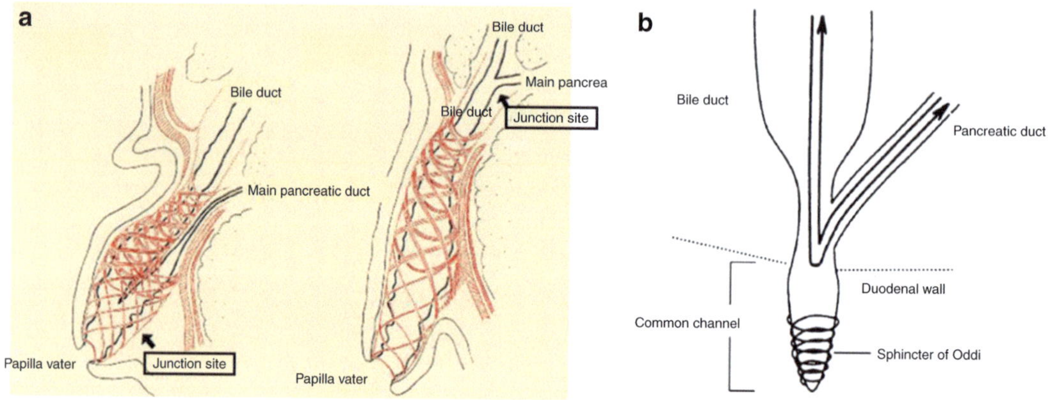

Fig. 8.7 Anatomical view of the sphincter of Oddi at the major papilla and the different locations of pancreatobiliary junction between healthy patients (within the duodenal wall) and patients with pancreatobiliary maljunction (outside the duodenal wall) (**a**). Pathophysiology of pancreatobiliary maljunction causing reflux of pancreatic juice into the common bile duct (**b**). (From Kamisawa T, Ando H, Suyama M, et al. Working Committee of Clinical Practice Guidelines for Pancreaticobiliary Maljunction; Japanese Study Group on Pancreaticobiliary Maljunction. Japanese clinical practice guidelines for pancreaticobiliary maljunction. J Gastroenterol. 2012;47:731–59; with permission)

of the sphincter complex and surrounds the terminus of the common bile duct in order to regulate the biliary flow while simultaneously preventing the reflux of pancreatic juices; (2) the *sphincter pancreaticus* is less important and is present in only one-third of individuals; and (3) the *sphincter ampullae* surrounds the ampulla of Vater or the terminus of the common bile duct when bile and pancreatic ducts do not join together into the ampulla.

In some cases, the common bile duct and the main pancreatic duct join outside the duodenal wall, usually forming a markedly long common channel: this congenital anomaly is defined as "pancreaticobiliary maljunction"; it is more frequent in Eastern countries and is associated with an increased incidence of biliary tract tumors or dilatations, as the action of sphincter of Oddi does not have a functional impact in this case, allowing pancreatic juice to reflux into the common bile duct (Fig. 8.7) [11].

8.3.5 Gallbladder and Cystic Duct

The gallbladder is a muscular piriform sac situated in the so-called cystic fossa, on the inferior aspect of the hepatic right lobe. Very rarely, the gallbladder is found on the left side of the liver or intrahepatically. In adults, it measures 7–10 cm in length and 4 cm in diameter and normally stores about 30 mL of bile, even it can hold up to 300 mL of fluid when distended. The gallbladder is divided in four parts: the fundus, body, infundibulum, and neck. The fundus is the blind-ending portion that appears to the inferior border of the liver at the level of the ninth costal cartilage. The body is the largest part of the gallbladder which runs on the left and continues in the infundibulum as it becomes the neck, making a curve on the right side of the main bile duct. On the right side of the neck, sometimes as a result of chronic dilatation, there may be a recess that projects toward the duodenum called the Hartmann pouch. The neck drains into the cystic duct which is 2–4 cm long and courses to the left of the neck joining the common hepatic duct to form the common bile duct at different levels of the hepatoduodenal ligament. As already described above, subvesical bile ducts (frequently termed incorrectly as "ducts of Luschka") may be present with a prevalence of 4% of cases, causing sometimes postcholecystectomy bile leak. Subvesical bile ducts consist in aberrant or

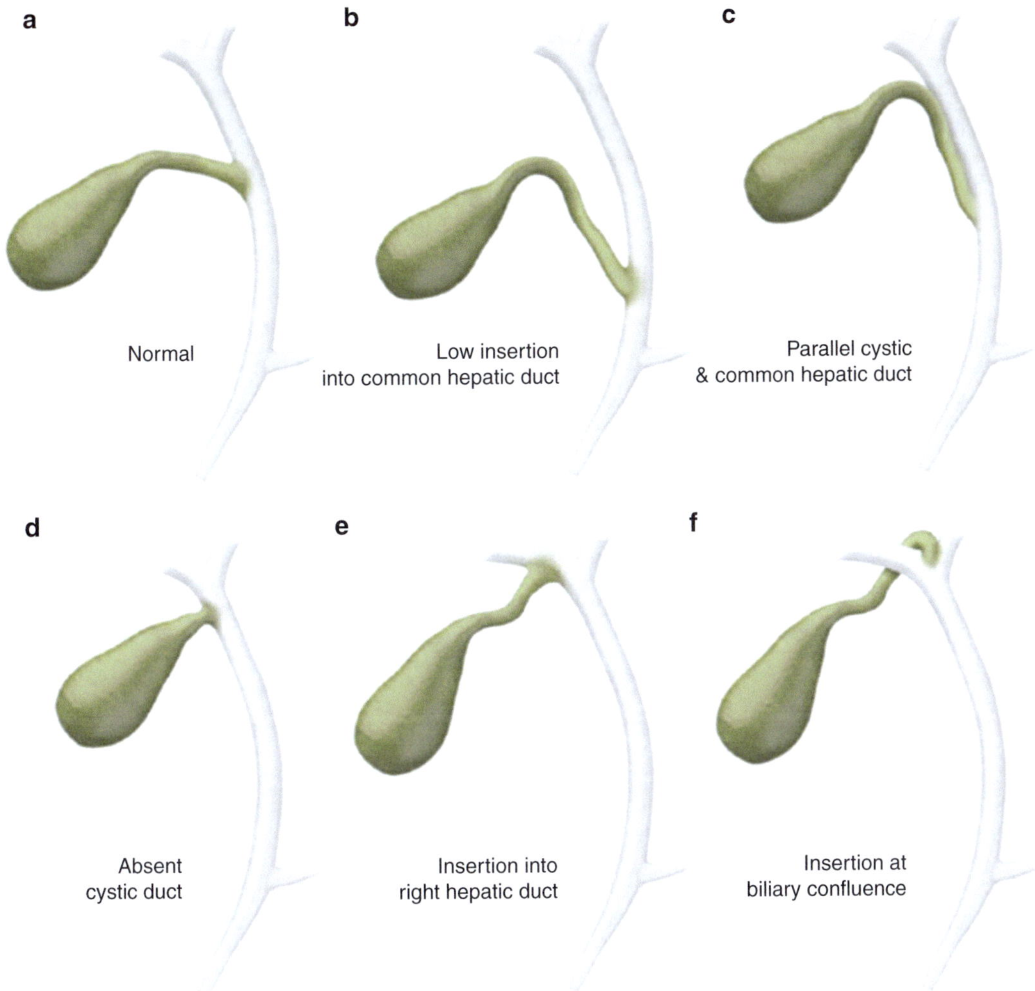

Fig. 8.8 Cystic duct variants (**a–f**). (From Khaled M. Elsayes. Cross-sectional imaging of the abdomen and pelvis. Springer, 2015; with permission)

accessory bile ducts located in the gallbladder fossa, generally without any communications with the gallbladder (with the exception of the so-called hepaticocholecystic duct which drains from the liver directly into the gallbladder) [12]. Rare variations of gallbladder anatomy include agenesis, multiple or bilobed gallbladders, and double cystic ducts. In some cases, the gallbladder is entirely covered by visceral peritoneum which forms a kind of "meso."

The cystic duct has some mucosal folds known as spiral valves of Heister. The insertion of the cystic duct into the common bile duct is variable and aberrant in up to 25% of cases (Fig. 8.8): in most cases, the cystic duct enters the middle one-third of the common bile duct, while a low or very low insertion is reported in about 10% of cases. Very rarely, the cystic duct is absent or inserts into the right or left hepatic ducts or at the biliary confluence. The typical course of the cystic duct is medial toward the right side of the common bile duct, but it can also run parallel to the common hepatic duct: in this case, there is an increased risk of biliary injury during cholecystectomy.

References

1. Couinaud C. Le foie. Etudes Anatomiques et chirurgicales. Edition Masson; 1957.
2. Belghiti J, Clavien PA, Gadzijev E. The Brisbane 2000 terminology of liver anatomy and resections. HPB. 2000;2:333–9.
3. Healey JE Jr, Schroy PC. Anatomy of the biliary ducts within the human liver; analysis of the prevailing pattern of branchings and the major variations of the biliary ducts. AMA Arch Surg. 1953;66:599–616.
4. Hjortsjö CH. The topography of the intrahepatic duct system. Acta Anat (Basel). 1951;11:599–615.
5. Hribernik M, Gadzijev EM, Mlakar B, Ravnik D. Variations of intrahepatic and proximal extrahepatic bile ducts. Hepatogastroenterology. 2003;50:342–8.
6. Huang TL, Cheng YF, Chen CL, et al. Variants of the bile ducts: clinical application in the potential donor of living-related hepatic transplantation. Transplant Proc. 1996;128:1669–70.
7. Hepp J, Pernod R, Hautefeuille P. Les lésions concernant la convergence radiculaire en chirurgie biliaire réparatrice. Ann Chir. 1966;20:382–411.
8. Chaib E, Kanas AF, Galvão FH, D'Albuquerque LA. Bile duct confluence: anatomic variations and its classification. Surg Radiol Anat. 2014;36(2):105–9.
9. Hollinshead WH. The lower part of the common bile duct: a review. Surg Clin North Am. 1957;37:939–52.
10. Boyden EA. The anatomy of the choledochoduodenal junction in man. Surg Gynecol Obstet. 1957;104:642–52.
11. Kamisawa T, Ando H, Suyama M, et al. Working Committee of Clinical Practice Guidelines for Pancreaticobiliary Maljunction; Japanese Study Group on Pancreaticobiliary Maljunction. Japanese clinical practice guidelines for pancreaticobiliary maljunction. J Gastroenterol. 2012;47:731–59.
12. Schnelldorfer T, Sarr MG, Adams DB. What is the duct of Luschka? A systematic review. J Gastrointest Surg. 2012;16:656–62.

Anatomy of the Pancreas

9

Marianna Arvanitakis

9.1 Introduction

Thorough knowledge of anatomy is a prerequisite for optimal management in therapeutic endoscopy. Nevertheless, 30 years ago, defining the anatomy of the pancreatic ducts was exclusively based on diagnostic endoscopic retrograde cholangiopancreatography (ERCP), or autopsy, making impossible to plan in advance any therapeutic decision. Magnetic resonance cholangiopancreatography (MRCP) has revolutionized the approach to biliary and pancreatic diseases by permitting precise and noninvasive imaging of the ducts, vessels, and their anatomic variants [1]. The knowledge of ductal anatomy before any therapeutic procedure allows the physician to plan the access and potential alternative routes to the ducts and to decrease the risk of complications. This chapter focuses on the structural anatomy of the pancreas and its ducts, including the most frequent anatomic variations.

M. Arvanitakis (✉)
Department of Gastroenterology, Erasme University Hospital, ULB, Brussels, Belgium
e-mail: marianna.arvanitaki@erasme.ulb.ac.be

9.2 Morphology of the Pancreas

The pancreas is a soft, lobular digestive gland, which is located in the retroperitoneum posterior to the stomach. It extends transversely from the duodenal curve to the hilum of the spleen and crosses the vertebral bodies at the level of L1–L3. It is approximately 15 cm in length and weighs 80 g.

The pancreas is divided into four parts (from right to left): the head with the uncinate process, a neck (or genu), a body, and a tail. The head is located in the loop of the duodenum, anterior to the inferior vena cava and the left renal vein. The common bile duct passes through the pancreatic head and then is directed posterior toward the liver. The uncinate process is a small portion of the inferior part of the head that is directed to the left and hooks around the superior mesenteric vessels. The neck links the head to the body of the pancreas and is located anterior to the portal vein and the superior mesenteric vessels. The close proximity of the neck of the pancreas to major blood vessels posteriorly limits the option for a wide surgical margin when pancreatectomy is done. The body lies parallel to the splenic artery, posterior to the distal portion of the stomach and anteriorly to the aorta, the left renal vein, and the left kidney. The tail lies between the layers of the splenorenal ligament within the splenic hilum [2–4] (Figs. 9.1 and 9.2).

M. Mutignani et al. (eds.), *Endotherapy in Biliopancreatic Diseases: ERCP Meets EUS*,
https://doi.org/10.1007/978-3-030-42569-2_9

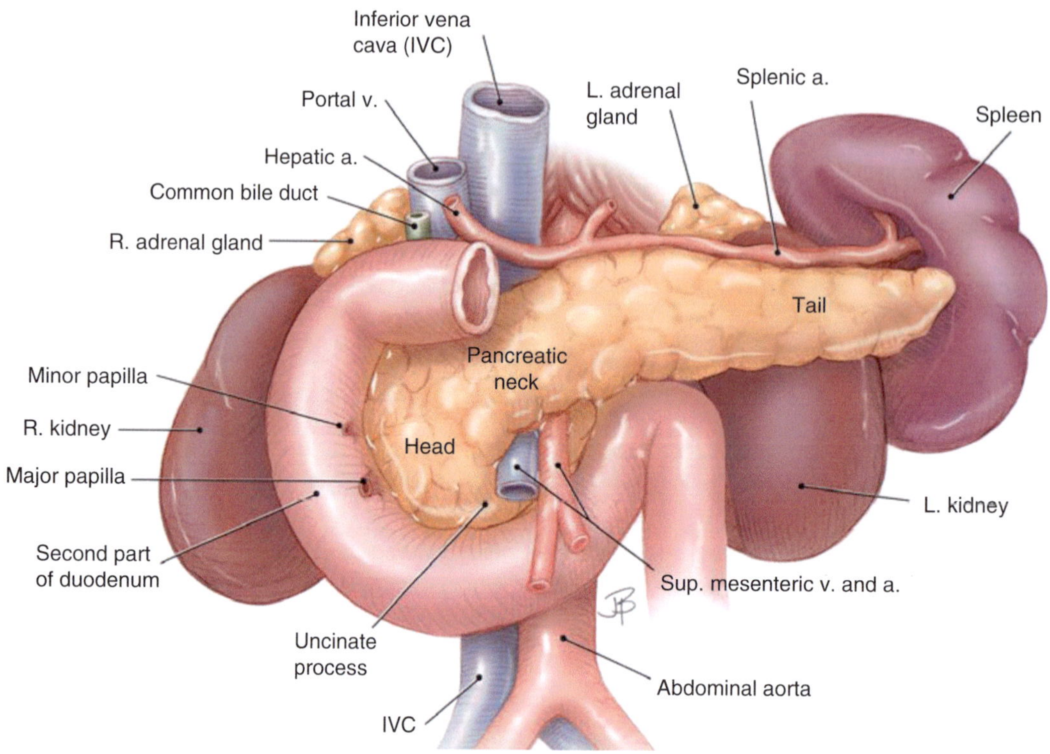

Fig. 9.1 Anatomic relationships of the pancreas with surrounding organs. (Image by Jennifer Parsons Brumbaugh; used with permission of the publisher) [3]

Fig. 9.2 CT scan of the upper abdomen at the level of the pancreas showing anatomic relationships

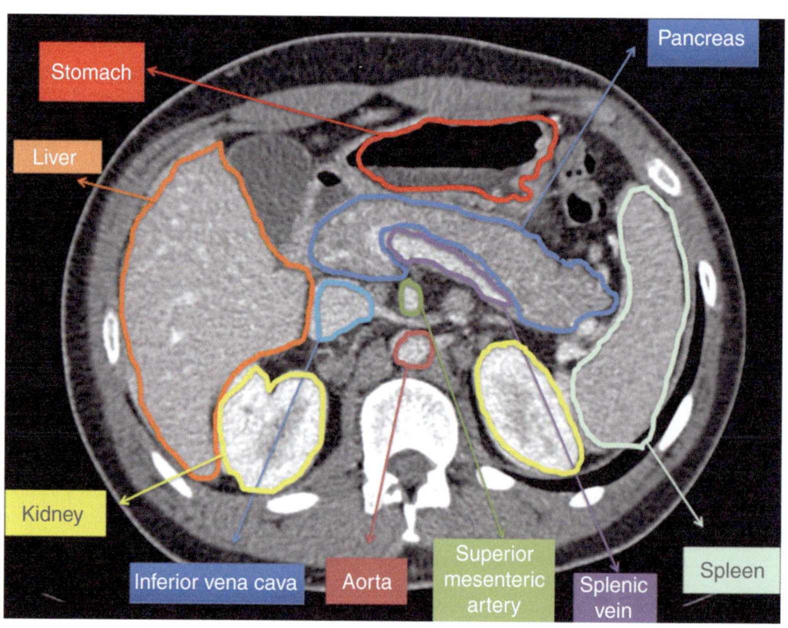

9.3 Blood Supply

The pancreas depends mainly on irrigation from the splenic artery for the body and tail and superior and inferior pancreaticoduodenal arteries for the head. The superior pancreaticoduodenal arteries, posterior and anterior, originate from the gastroduodenal artery. Similarly, the inferior pancreaticoduodenal arteries, posterior and anterior, originate from the superior mesenteric artery. All these branches communicate around the pancreas providing collateral circulation and a secure arterial supply. The splenic artery, a branch of the celiac trunk, provides the dorsal pancreatic artery, which irrigates the neck and posterior surface of the body, before it becomes the inferior pancreatic artery, which terminates at the tail of the pancreas. Several small arterial branches also originate from the splenic artery, along the superior length of the body and tail, while also giving rise to the multiple arcades of pancreatic arteries to supply the rest of the pancreas (Fig. 9.3a, b). The venous drainage follows a similar pattern as the corresponding arterial supply. The head of the pancreas is mainly drained by the four pancreaticoduodenal veins, whereas they enter into the

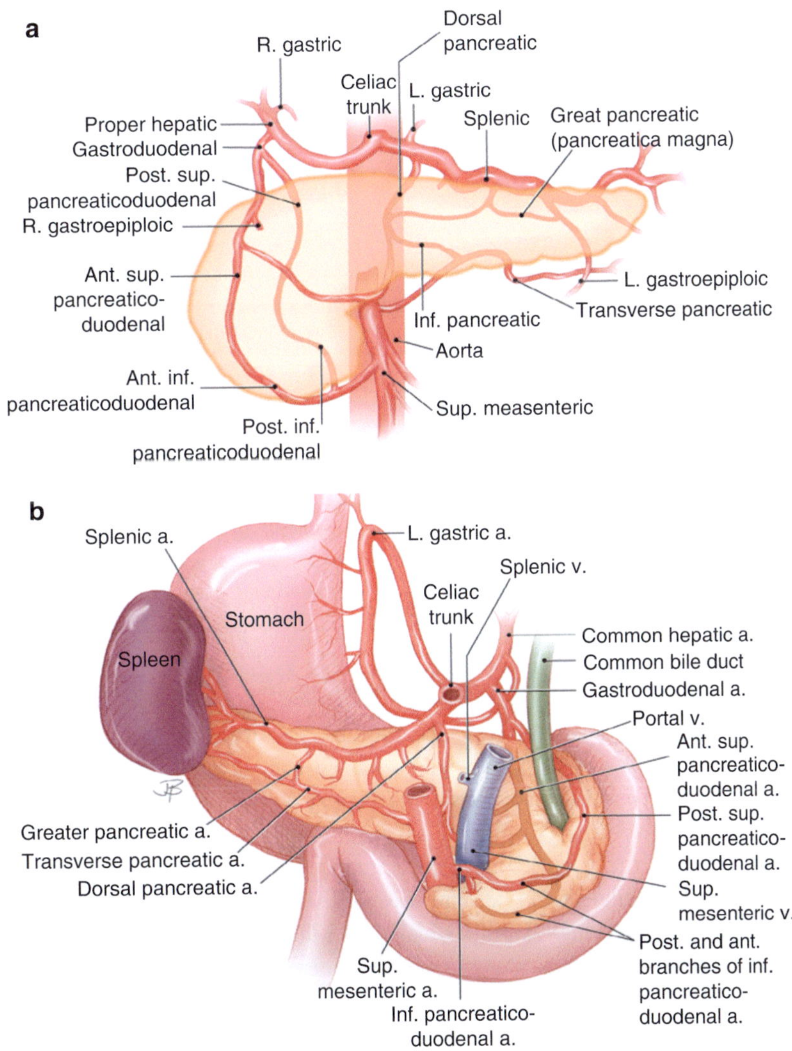

Fig. 9.3 The arterial blood supply to the pancreas. (**a**) Anterior view. (**b**) Posterior view. (Image by Jennifer Parsons Brumbaugh; used with permission of the publisher) [3]

superior mesenteric or the portal vein. The neck, body, and tail of the pancreas have venous drainage into the splenic vein [2–4].

9.4 Lymphatic Drainage and Innervation

Lymphatic drainage helps in collecting interstitial fluid containing pathogens, immune cells, cell products, and debris, which drain from vascular capillaries. Before being returned to the venous circulation, the fluid filters through a series of lymph nodes. In general, the lymphatic vessels follow the pancreatic blood vessels and are divided into the head/neck and the body/tail groups [5]. Lymph vessels from the body and tail of the pancreas mainly lead into the pancreaticosplenic nodes, although some may also lead directly to the preaortic lymph nodes. The neck and head regions of the pancreas have a more extensive drainage system, as lymph can travel through the nodes running alongside the pancreaticoduodenal, superior mesenteric, and hepatic arteries. Innervation depends mostly on the celiac and superior mesenteric artery plexus of the autonomous system located lateral to the aorta and the superior mesenteric artery [5].

9.5 Ductal Anatomy

9.5.1 Normal Ductal Anatomy

During embryological development, there is a clockwise rotation (posterior) of the duodenum and the stomach, leading to the formation of the pancreas by fusion of the ventral and dorsal parts draining in the duodenum through the major (ventral part) and minor papilla (dorsal part). This fusion leads to many variations in the connection. The caudal portion of the head of the pancreas (uncinate) and the major papilla, which drains the duct of Wirsung (or ventral pancreatic duct), are derived from the ventral part. The minor papilla that drains the duct of Santorini (or dorsal pancreatic duct) derives from the dorsal part [6].

The main pancreatic duct originates from the ventral pancreatic duct in the head and the dorsal pancreatic duct in the body and tail. The dorsal pancreatic duct joins the main pancreatic duct at a site 1–2 cm proximal to the ventral pancreatic duct. The main pancreatic duct traverses the gland from the tail to the head and, together with the bile duct, opens into the second part of the duodenum at the major duodenal papilla. The orifices of the main pancreatic duct and the common bile duct are usually located at the tip of the papilla. As the distal part of the biliary and pancreatic ducts approaches the duodenal wall, they become surrounded by smooth muscle fibers, which form the sphincter of Oddi, and extend to, respectively, the biliary and pancreatic sphincters. The word "ampulla" defines the dilated, jug-like appearance of the joining of the two ducts in the duodenal wall. Its length is variable, ranging from 1 to 12 mm, with an average length of 4.4 mm and a diameter varying from 1 to 4 mm (2.6 mm on average) [7]. In 60–80% of patients, the biliary and pancreatic ducts merge to form a common ampullary channel (2–15 mm, average 5 mm). Therefore, in a variable percentage of people, their opening at the major papilla can be separate, or a septum could be interposed between the two ducts [7]. The ampulla is found in the lower part of the head of the pancreas and protrudes for 5–10 mm in the medial aspect of the second part of the duodenum, forming the major papilla, which appears as an oval or hemispherical elevation. In some cases, it can be located in the genus inferior or even the third portion of the duodenum. The major papilla is covered by two triangular folds of duodenal mucosa: the hood, on the cranial side, and the frenulum, on the caudal side, which is not always clearly visible (Fig. 9.4a, b).

The dorsal duct drains the superior and anterior portion of the head, usually as a separate duct terminating at the minor papilla, which is located 10–15 mm above and to the right of the major papilla. In approximately 60–70% of the population, the dorsal and ventral ducts have fused, resulting in a communicating dual drainage of the main pancreatic duct, either with a patent or obliterated minor papilla (Fig. 9.5). Variations

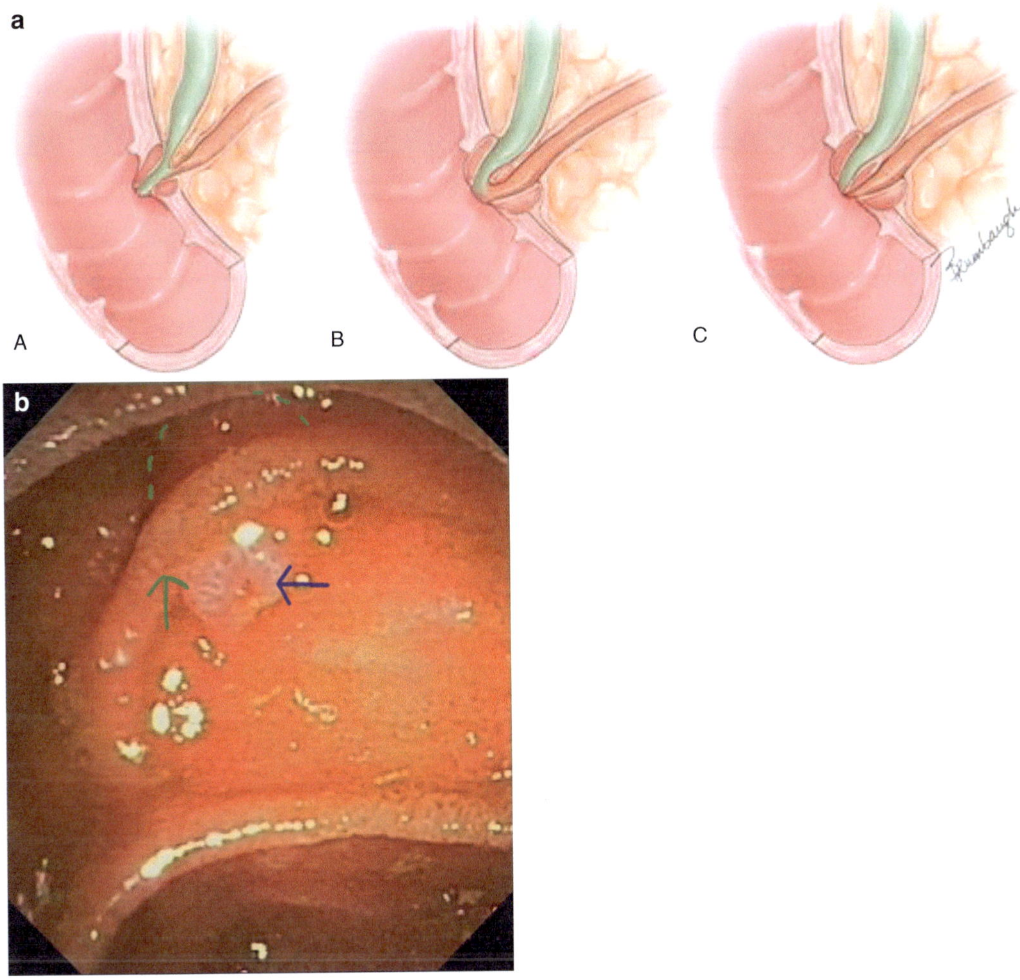

Fig. 9.4 (**a**) Anatomic variations in the union of the common bile duct and the main pancreatic duct at the major papilla (ampulla of Vater). The green duct represents the bile duct and the orange the main pancreatic duct (Image by Jennifer Parsons Brumbaugh; used with permission of the publisher) [3]. (**b**) Endoscopic image of the papilla (blue arrow, papillary orifice; green arrow, hood; dashed green line, delimitation of the ampulla)

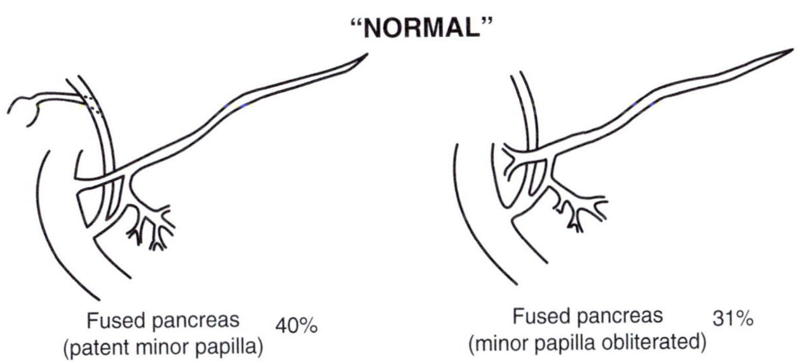

Fig. 9.5 Schematic illustration of normal pancreatic anatomy with fusion of ventral and dorsal duct [8]

during the embryological process regarding fusion of the dorsal and ventral pancreas can lead to various congenital variants of the pancreatic ducts [2].

9.5.2 Pancreas Divisum

Pancreas divisum is the most common congenital variation of the pancreas and results when the ventral and dorsal ducts fail to fuse together. This finding occurs with an incidence of 3–7% in patients who are undergoing ERCP and in approximately 9% of autopsy cases [8]. The body, tail, and part of the head of the pancreas (dorsal pancreas) drain through Santorini's duct (which becomes the main pancreatic duct) into the minor papilla, while another part of the head (ventral pancreas) drains through the short ventral duct into the major papilla. Most patients with pancreas divisum are asymptomatic, and pancreas divisum should not be considered a cause of acute or chronic pancreatitis, despite conclusions of previous publications, which were faltered by selection bias. On the other hand, patients with pancreas divisum can also present with chronic pancreatitis, eventually requiring endoscopic therapy [9] (Fig. 9.6a–c).

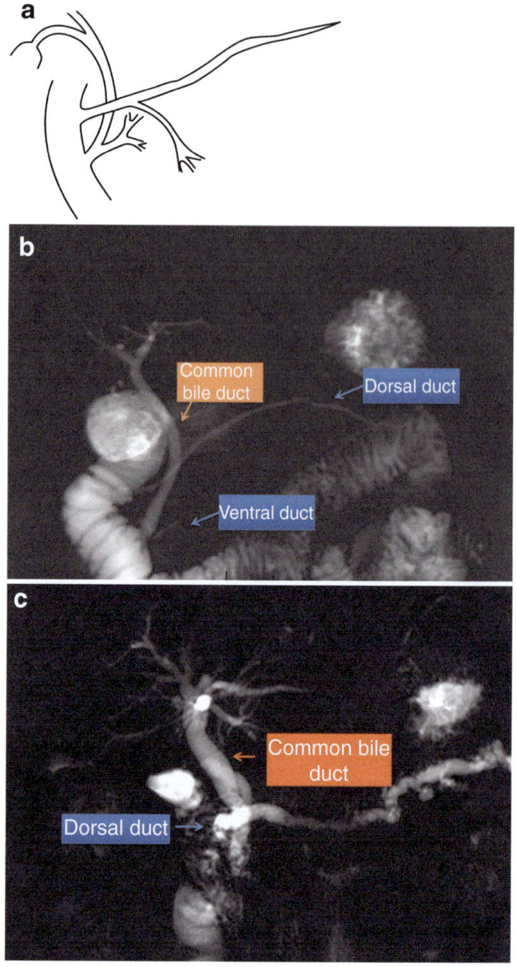

Fig. 9.6 (**a**) Schematic illustration of pancreas divisum [8]. (**b**) MRCP of a patient with anatomy of pancreas divisum; the crossing of the common bile duct from the dorsal duct is clearly visible. (**c**) MRCP of a patient with chronic pancreatitis, dilation of the dorsal pancreatic duct, and anatomy of pancreas divisum

9.5.3 Incomplete Pancreas Divisum

In incomplete pancreas divisum, a small branch of the ventral duct communicates with the dorsal duct. Approximately 15% of cases of pancreas divisum are of the incomplete type (Fig. 9.7).

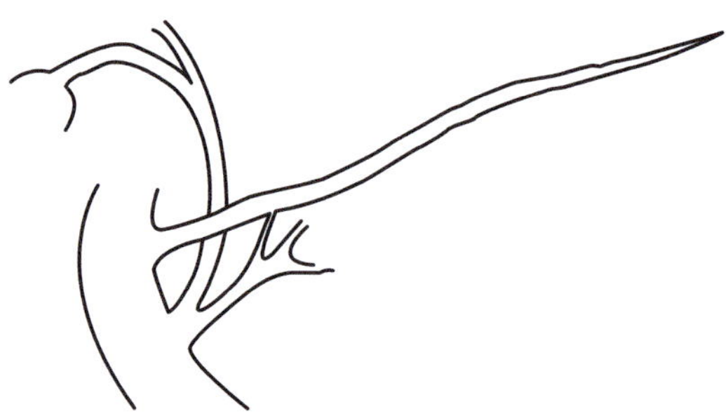

Fig. 9.7 Schematic illustration of incomplete pancreas divisum [8]

9.5.4 Abnormal Pancreatobiliary Junction

Abnormal pancreatobiliary junction (APBJ) is a rare congenital anomaly in which the pancreatic and biliary ducts join outside the duodenal wall, 15–20 mm proximal to the sphincter of Oddi, forming a long common channel [8]. The incidence of APBJ has been reported to be

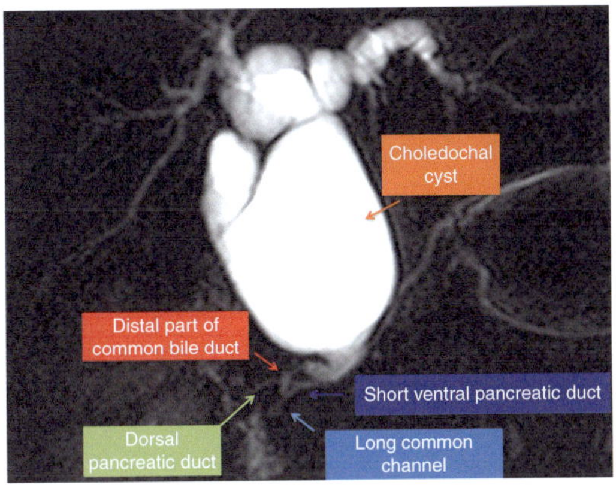

Fig. 9.8 MRCP of a patient with a type IV choledochal cyst, an abnormal pancreatobiliary junction with a long common channel, and a pancreas divisum anatomy

1.5–3.0% in patients who are undergoing endoscopic retrograde cholangiopancreatography (ERCP) [8]. APBJ is classified into two groups, with or without bile duct dilatation, and is seen in >90% of patients with type I and IV choledochal cysts [10] (Fig. 9.8). APBJ is commonly associated with carcinoma of the bile ducts and gallbladder. The reason for biliary carcinogenesis in such patients has been attributed to reflux and stasis of bile mixed with pancreatic juice in the biliary system.

9.5.5 Annular Pancreas

Annular pancreas is a rare congenital variation in which a ring of pancreatic tissue surrounds the duodenum. The annular pancreatic tissue forms a complete (25%) or partial (75%) ring around the descending duodenum (Fig. 9.9a, b). The incidence of annular pancreas has been reported to be 0.005–0.015% in autopsy cases in adults. The most widely accepted theory of etiopathogenesis is that the ventral bud is dividing early into two segments, one migrating posteriorly and the other anteriorly, thus encircling the duodenum. This anomaly can be discovered in asymptomatic patients. In other cases, annular pancreas is associated with duodenal stenosis, gastric outlet syndrome, postbulbar ulcerations, pancreatitis, or biliary obstruction [8].

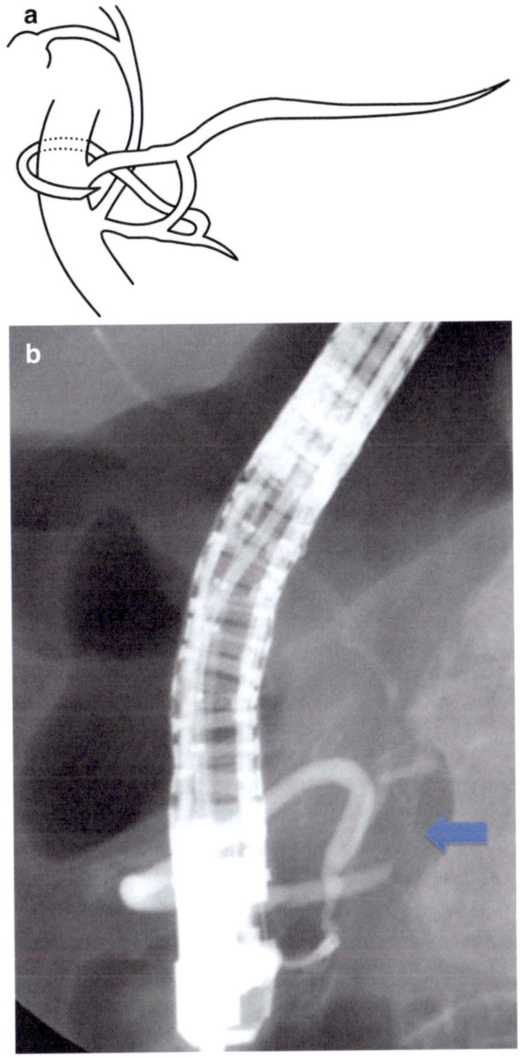

Fig. 9.9 (**a**) Schematic illustration of annular pancreas [8]. (**b**) ERCP of a patient with an anatomy of an annular pancreas and a stricture (arrow), which was confirmed to be due to pancreatic cancer

9.5.6 Ansa Pancreatica

Ansa pancreatica consists in a looping between the dorsal and ventral duct. It is characterized by the obliteration of the accessory duct at the proximal extremity, near its junction with the main pancreatic duct, and the replacement of this portion by an additional curved canal between the dorsal and the ventral ducts. Indeed, in the ansa pancreatica, the accessory duct arises from the main pancreatic duct and runs an arched course passing in front of the main duct, ending in the minor papilla [11] (Fig. 9.10a). A similar looping can be seen on the ventral pancreatic duct (Fig. 9.10b). Comparably to pancreas divisum, the association between ansa pancreatica and pancreatitis is speculative, but recognizing the anatomic variation is important for planning therapeutic ERCP in symptomatic patients [8].

9.5.7 Dominant Dorsal Duct

The term dominant dorsal duct includes all anatomic variations in which drainage of pancreatic juices is mainly provided by the dorsal duct through the minor papilla. In these cases, if endoscopic therapy is considered, the access should be done from the minor papilla. Therefore, pancreas divisum (complete or incomplete) and some forms of ansa pancreatica are considered as dominant dorsal ducts.

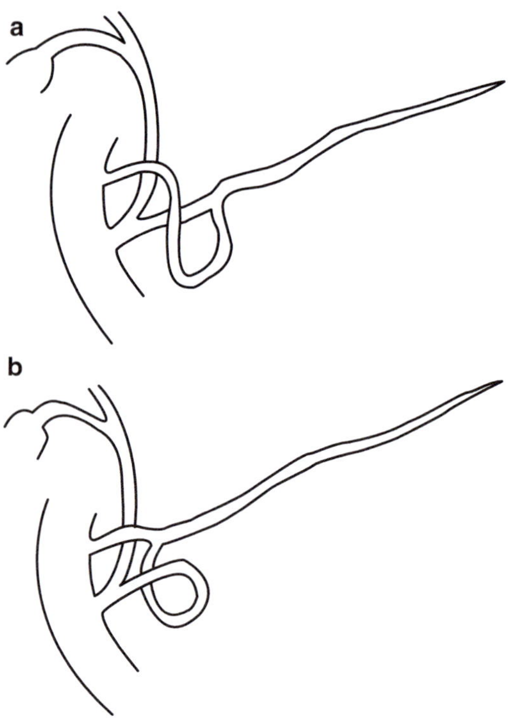

Fig. 9.10 Schematic illustration of ansa pancreatica anatomy of the dorsal duct (**a**) and the ventral duct (**b**) [8]

9.6 Conclusion

With the latest development in interventional endoscopy regarding pancreatic diseases, it is crucial to define a therapeutic plan before the procedure. With the development of MRCP, it has become possible to obtain a reliable cartography of the pancreatic ducts, as well as important features regarding the pancreatic disease (strictures, collections, leaks, etc.). Up to 20% of patients may have some common variant of ductal anatomy; therefore, pre-therapeutic planning is indispensable. In the case of pancreatic duct treatment, pre-procedural imaging allows the decision to access either the major papilla or the minor papilla (i.e., pancreas divisum, incomplete pancreas divisum, or ansa pancreatica) beforehand. This type of pre-procedural planning also highlights the message that in case of uncommon anatomy, the treatment should be done in centers able to provide all of the different techniques.

References

1. Manfredi R, Pozzi Mucelli R. Secretin-enhanced MR Imaging of the Pancreas. Radiology. 2016;279:29–43. https://doi.org/10.1148/radiol.2015140622.
2. Arvanitakis M, Deviere J, Cremer M, Le Moine O. Anatomy of the biliary and pancreatic ducts. In: Albert J, editor. Endoscopic retrograde cholangiopancretography (ERCP): current practice and future perspectives. Bremen: UNI-MED Verlag AG; 2015. p. 16–23.
3. Longecker D. Anatomy and histology of the pancreas. Pancreapedia: exocrine pancreas knowledge base. Version 1.0. March 21, 2014. https://doi.org/10.3998/panc.2014.3. https://www.pancreapedia.org/reviews/anatomy-and-histology-of-pancreas. Accessed 25 Sept 2018.
4. Hruban RH, Pitman MB, Klimstra DS. AFIP atlas of tumor pathology, Fourth Series. In: Fascicle tumors of the pancreas. American Registry of Pathology, Washington, DC in collaboration with the Armed Forces Institute of Pathology, Washington, DC; 2007.
5. Cesmebasi A, Malefant J, Patel SD, Du Plessis M, Renna S, Tubbs RS, Loukas M. The surgical anatomy of the lymphatic system of the pancreas. Clin Anat. 2015;28:527–37.
6. Yu J, Turner MA, Fulcher AS, Halvorsen RA. Congenital anomalies and normal variants of the pancreaticobiliary tract and the pancreas in adults:

part 2, pancreatic duct and pancreas. AJR Am J Roentgenol. 2006;187:1544–53.

7. Alessandrino F, Ivanovic AM, Yee EU, Radulovic D, Souza D, Mortele KJ. MDCT and MRI of the ampulla of Vater. Part I: technique optimization, normal anatomy, and epithelial neoplasms. Abdom Imaging. 2015;40:3274–91.
8. Delhaye M, Matos C, Deviere J. Acute relapsing pancreatitis. Congenital variants: diagnosis, treatment, outcome. JOP. 2001;2:373–81.
9. Delhaye M, Engelholm L, Cremer M. Pancreas divisum: congenital anatomic variant or anomaly? Contribution of endoscopic retrograde dorsal pancreatography. Gastroenterology. 1985;89:951–8.
10. Ten Hove A, de Meijer VE, Hulscher JBF, de Kleine RHJ. Meta analysis of risk of developing malignancy in congenital choledochal malformation. Br J Surg. 2018;105:482–90. https://doi.org/10.1002/bjs.10798.
11. Jarrar MS, Khenissi A, Ghrissi R, Hamila F, Letaief R. Ansa pancreatica: an anatomic variation and a rare cause of acute pancreatitis. Surg Radiol Anat. 2013;35:745–8.

CT: What We Need to Know to Start to Interpret Radiological Pictures

10

Marialavinia Catalano, Consolato Gullì, Alessandro Cina, Carmine Di Stasi, and Riccardo Manfredi

10.1 Computed Tomography Imaging Technique

CT examination is a diagnostic imaging modality in which X-rays pass through a thin axial section of the patient from various directions. At each point within the CT section, a mathematical image reconstruction calculates how much the beam is "attenuated" by the material it is passing through, resulting in the production of *attenuation coefficients* translated into "CT numbers" and finally converted into shades of grey displayed as a CT image [1]. Thereby, *Hounsfield units* (HU) are obtained from linear transformation of the measured attenuation coefficients in the form of simple numbers set on a scale (i.e. *Hounsfield scale*) which is based on the arbitrary definitions of air and water with the following values: (a) air as1000 HU and (b) water as 0 HU. Generally, most soft tissues occupy a narrow range in the scale presenting a value of about 50 HU [1]. In this regard, intravenous (IV) administration of iodinated contrast agents improves contrast resolution by allowing higher differentiation between tissues.

The introduction of multidetector computed tomography (MDCT) in late 1990s has improved volume coverage speed and spatial resolution, enabling more diagnostic information with less radiation in a shorter scanning time, contrast enhanced multiphasic imaging in a well-defined perfusion phase, three-dimensional reformatting due to isotropic voxels and better multiplanar reconstruction of biliary and pancreatic anatomy.

The timing of image acquisition is crucial in pancreatico-biliary imaging, and the choice of each imaging protocol usually corresponds to an appropriately designed clinical question. Generally, a baseline, unenhanced scan obtained from the hepatic dome may be useful to assess whether identifiable lesions are enhanced and to visualize hyperattenuating findings, such as hematomas, biliary stones or pancreatic calcifications that may be obscured once contrast material is injected.

At MDCT examination, pancreas-specific protocol is typically performed by using a thin-section (<1 mm), multiphase technique with images obtained in the early arterial phase, pancreatic phase and portal venous phase, with IV administration of iodinated contrast material injected at a rate of 3 mL/s.

Early arterial phase images (generally obtained with a delay of 20 s after the start of contrast material injection) assess good visualization of the aorta and peripancreatic arterial supply. *Pancreatic phase images* (40 s after the

M. Catalano · C. Gullì · A. Cina · C. Di Stasi
R. Manfredi (✉)
Department of Radiology, Università Cattolica del Sacro Cuore, Rome, Italy
e-mail: riccardo.manfredi@unicatt.it

M. Mutignani et al. (eds.), *Endotherapy in Biliopancreatic Diseases: ERCP Meets EUS*,
https://doi.org/10.1007/978-3-030-42569-2_10

start of contrast injection) show peak pancreatic parenchymal enhancement and thereby provide best tumour-to-parenchymal attenuation difference, since both hypo- and hypervascular pancreatic lesions may be well seen. *Portal venous phase images* (70 s after the start of contrast injection) assess optimal visualization of peripancreatic veins and may be useful to identify metastatic disease to the liver [2–4]. In addition, 10–20 min delayed images may be obtained when a cholangiocarcinoma (CC) is suspected [2], since such tumour commonly shows delayed enhancement due to contrast retention related to its fibrotic nature.

With regard to post-processing reformation methods, a variety of techniques have been described for pancreatic and biliary imaging [2, 4]. Thin-section imaging (<1 mm) allows higher-quality reformatted images obtained from isotropic source data. The most commonly used techniques are multiplanar reformations (MPR), curved multiplanar reformations (CMPR), maximum intensity projections (MIP) and minimum intensity projections (MinIP).

MPR is frequently used to generate orthogonal (coronal or sagittal) views. Coronal, oblique coronal and curved planar reformatted images enable the evaluation of the complex anatomy of the biliary tract. Oblique coronal reformations, sagittal MPR or CMPR along the main pancreatic duct (MPD) may demonstrate the relationship between tumour, MPD itself and adjacent structures [2, 4]. MIP consists of projecting the voxels with the highest attenuation value throughout the volume of interest onto a bidimensional image. This technique displays high-attenuation structures and, with regard to pancreatico-biliary imaging, is often used with positive CECT cholangiography or to evaluate the relationship between tumours and adjacent enhanced vascular structures [2, 4]. MinIP performs the opposite processing task and is a data reformation method which provides detection of low-density structures in a given volume, such as pancreatic and bile ducts, and is particularly useful on contrast enhanced images when the background parenchyma is bright [2].

In addition to standard CT examination, biliary imaging may be obtained with positive CECT cholangiography, which is performed by using positive contrast material introduced into the biliary tract through a percutaneous catheter or by ERCP or with IV administration of contrast agent which is excreted into the bile; the data are then reformatted to obtain MIP and volume rendering images [2]. The disadvantages of this technique may include the possibility of adverse reactions to biliary contrast media and poor biliary opacification due to liver dysfunction. Therefore, CECT cholangiography is currently less commonly performed than MR cholangiopancreatography (MRCP) and endoscopic retrograde cholangiopancreatography (ERCP) to provide precise depiction of the biliary system [2, 5, 6].

10.2 CT Imaging of the Biliary System

10.2.1 Choledocholithiasis

Choledocholithiasis (Fig. 10.1) refers to the presence of stones within the common bile duct (CBD). Although CT is not the preferred imaging modality for detection of choledocholithiasis, it is often requested in the emergency department for patients presenting nonspecific abdominal complaints [7]; however, its sensitivity may be limited due to stones which can be relatively isoattenuating to the surrounding bile.

Actually, when visible at CT, biliary stones may present heterogeneous appearance (e.g. showing calcified radiopaque components, cholesterol deposition which is slightly less radiopaque than bile, or presenting gas attenuation due to nitrogen locules). In addition, calculi often manifest angulated shapes and laminated appearance and may be bound anteriorly by a crescent-shaped collection of bile or gas; furthermore, they are commonly identified in the dependent portions of the biliary tract, on both CT and MR imaging [2]. In general, unenhanced CT scan helps identify calcified stones confirming their lack of contrast enhancement. Use of thin sections and coronal reconstructions can also improve detection. Moreover, after

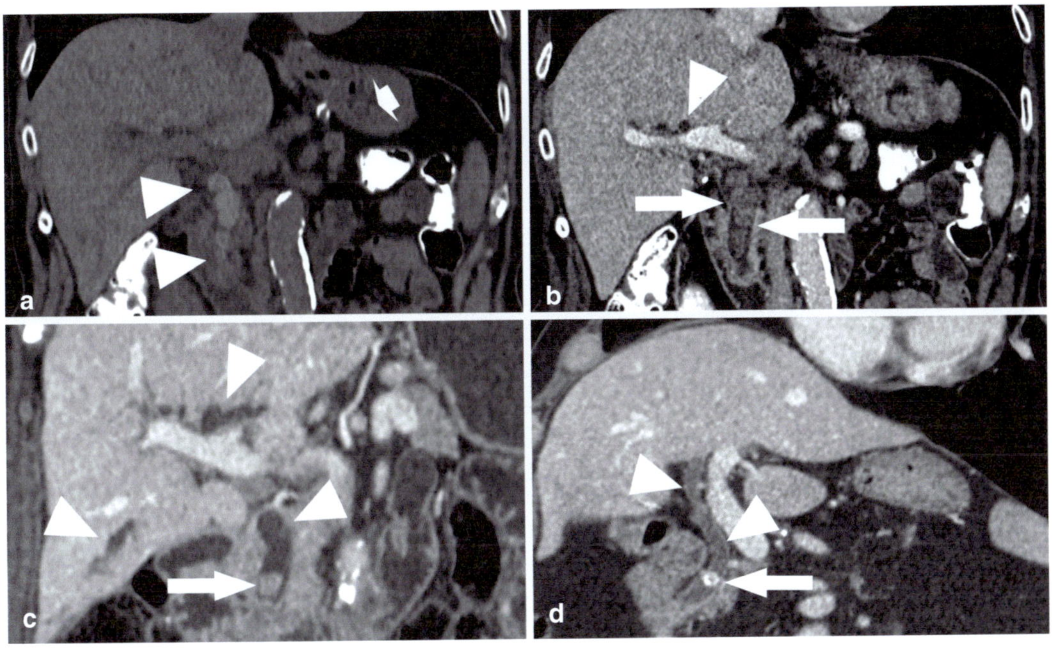

Fig. 10.1 Choledocholithiasis. (**a**, **b**) CBD stones in a 74-year-old woman. (**a**) Coronal nonenhanced CT image shows several hyperattenuating stones (arrowheads) within common hepatic duct and CBD which appears dilated. (**b**) Coronal contrast enhanced CT image shows upstream dilatation of the intrahepatic bile ducts (arrowhead) and mild mural enhancement of CBD (arrows), findings suggestive of cholangitis. (**c**) CBD stone in a 56-year-old man. Coronal contrast enhanced CT image shows a hyperattenuating stone (arrow) within the distal CBD associated with upstream dilatation of the intra- and extrahepatic biliary ducts (arrowheads) with imperceptible walls. (**d**) CBD stone in a 64-year-old woman. Coronal contrast enhanced CT image shows a hyperattenuating stone (arrow) within the CBD associated with dilated extrahepatic biliary ducts with the evidence of mural thickening and mild wall enhancement (arrowheads), findings that indicate cholangitis

IV administration of contrast agent, there may be coexisting findings of local inflammation, including periductal oedema, thickening of the biliary wall and mural enhancement, which should be carefully investigated to exclude the possibility of malignancy [2].

10.2.2 Mirizzi Syndrome

Mirizzi syndrome (Fig. 10.2) results from biliary obstruction caused by an impacted cystic duct stone leading to extrinsic compression of the common hepatic duct and subsequent obstructive jaundice. CT findings include an impacted gallstone in the gallbladder neck with upstream dilatation of the common hepatic duct and an abrupt change to normal calibre of the CBD distal to the gallstone [8].

10.2.3 Cholangitis: Biliary Tract Infection and Inflammation

10.2.3.1 Acute Cholangitis

Acute cholangitis is an acute biliary bacterial infection. The most common underlying aetiology is the obstruction of CBD by calculi. *Acute suppurative cholangitis* refers to the presence of pus in the biliary tree.

The most common CT finding of acute cholangitis is biliary obstruction, with dilatation of the CBD and segmental or diffuse ectasia of the intrahepatic biliary ducts. Both extra- and intrahepatic biliary ducts may show diffuse and concentric mural thickening (Fig. 10.1b, d), often associated with enhancement [7, 9]. Purulent bile may manifest increased attenuation [7]. At CECT, during the arterial phase, hepatic parenchymal enhancement may be inhomogeneous,

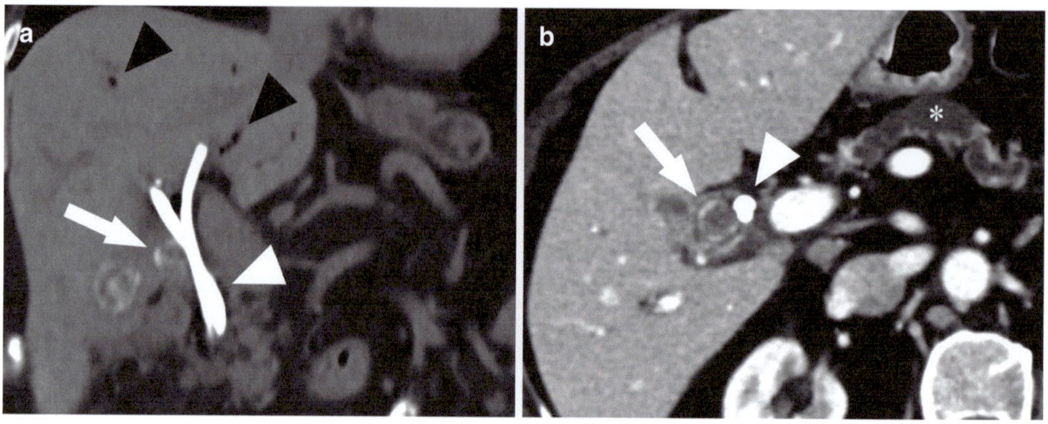

Fig. 10.2 Mirizzi syndrome in a 73-year-old man with dual biliary stent. (**a**) Coronal nonenhanced CT image shows several hyperattenuating gallstones and an impacted stone (arrow) in the gallbladder neck. Dual biliary stent (white arrowhead). Pneumobilia (black arrowheads) is seen in the intrahepatic biliary ducts due to the reflux of gas from duodenum related to the presence of the biliary stents. (**b**) Axial contrast enhanced CT image shows the impacted stone in the gallbladder neck (arrow) adjacent to the biliary stent (arrowhead). Pancreatic parenchymal atrophy with the evidence of marked dilatation of the MPD (∗) are also seen, findings suggestive of coexisting chronic pancreatitis

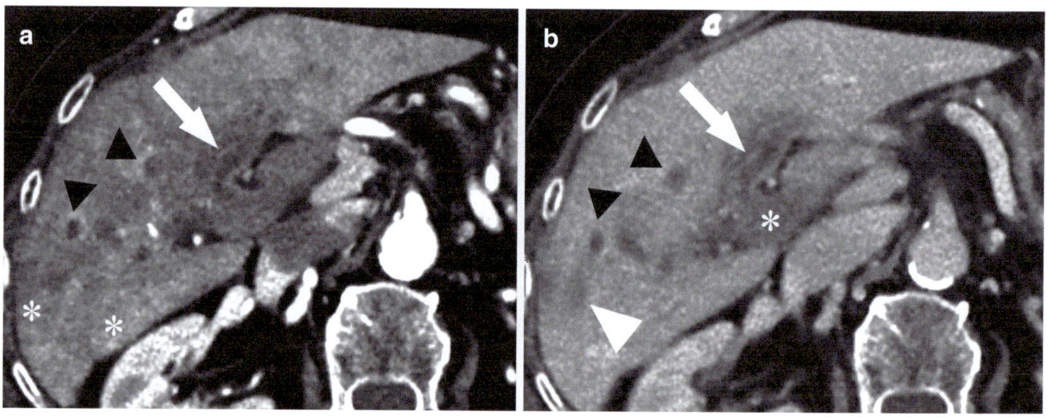

Fig. 10.3 Acute cholangitis. (**a**) Axial contrast enhanced arterial phase CT image shows inhomogeneous hepatic parenchymal enhancement (∗). (**b**) Axial contrast enhanced portal phase CT image shows portal vein thrombosis (∗) and an ill-defined hypoattenuating parenchymal collection, indicative of hepatic abscess (white arrowhead). (**a**, **b**) Intrahepatic biliary ductal dilatation (black arrowheads) and mural thickening with wall hyperenhancement of the dilated left biliary duct are also seen (white arrows)

patchy, nodular or wedge-shaped [10]. In addition to acute suppurative cholangitis, a number of life-threatening complications may result from acute cholangitis (Fig. 10.3), including pyogenic hepatic abscesses, portal vein thrombosis and biliary peritonitis [11]. A uni- or multiloculated hypoattenuating collection with peripheral rim enhancement is characteristic for abscess formation at CT.

10.2.3.2 Recurrent Pyogenic Cholangitis

Recurrent pyogenic cholangitis (RPC) is a progressive disease resulting from recurrent episodes of bacterial cholangitis. The aetiology is uncertain, although a possible role of chronic infestation with parasites such as *Clonorchis sinensis*, *Opisthorchis viverrini* or *Ascaris lumbricoides* has been postulated. Persistent inflammation results

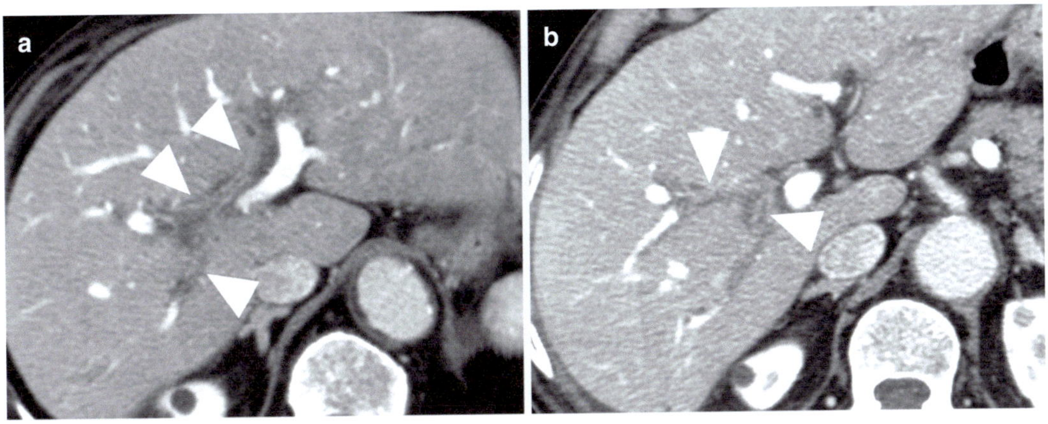

Fig. 10.4 Primary sclerosing cholangitis in a 51-year-old man. (**a**, **b**) Axial contrast enhanced portal phase CT images obtained at different levels show mild intrahepatic biliary ductal dilatation with the evidence of irregular beading, wall enhancement and periductal hypoattenuating oedema (arrowheads)

in intrahepatic bile ducts fibrosis, which leads to segmental strictures and dilatations with bile stasis, stones formation and subsequent recurrent infections [11]. Typical imaging findings of RPC include intra- and extrahepatic biliary ductal dilatation, with relative sparing of peripheral ducts. Intraductal stones occur in up to 80% of patients and usually appear hyperdense relative to the liver parenchyma. Pneumobilia can be commonly seen resulting from infection with gas-forming organisms or due to reflux of enteric gas from stones passage across the ampulla. Additionally, in acute exacerbations, biliary duct wall enhancement can be present, whereas liver parenchyma atrophy may occur in chronic stages [11, 12].

10.2.3.3 Primary Sclerosing Cholangitis

Primary sclerosing cholangitis (PSC) is a chronic cholestatic disease of unknown cause, characterized by inflammatory and obliterative fibrosis of the intra- and extrahepatic bile ducts. Wall thickening with bile ducts dilatation can be seen at CT (Fig. 10.4); however, only these findings are not sufficient for diagnosis of PSC [13]. Classical imaging features of PSC can be seen at MRCP/ERCP, including alternating multifocal strictures, mild segmental ectasia and irregular beading which typically involves both intra- and extrahepatic ducts, with peripheral pruning of the intrahepatic ducts. Additional imaging findings, on both CT and MR imaging, include hepatic perfusion abnormalities, marked enlargement of the caudate lobe and atrophy involving the lateral aspect of the left lobe [13, 14].

10.2.3.4 Autoimmune Pancreatitis-Related Cholangitis

Biliary involvement is frequently seen in patients with autoimmune pancreatitis with the distal CBD being most commonly affected (Fig. 10.5a, b), although both intra- and extrahepatic bile ducts may be involved, often presenting with multifocal strictures or mural thickening and enhancement. Thereby, the appearance may mimic primary sclerosing cholangitis. However, unlike PSC, biliary abnormalities associated with autoimmune pancreatitis usually resolve after corticosteroid therapy; thus, it is important to recognize them as they both demonstrate a favourable response to treatment [15].

10.2.4 Cholangiocarcinoma

Cholangiocarcinoma (CC) arises from the bile duct epithelium, and it is the most common malignancy of the biliary system.

Cholangiocarcinoma is classified by location as intrahepatic (ICC), perihilar (PCC, also known as Klatskin tumour) and distal (DCC). ICC arises distal to the second-order bile ducts [16]. PCC is

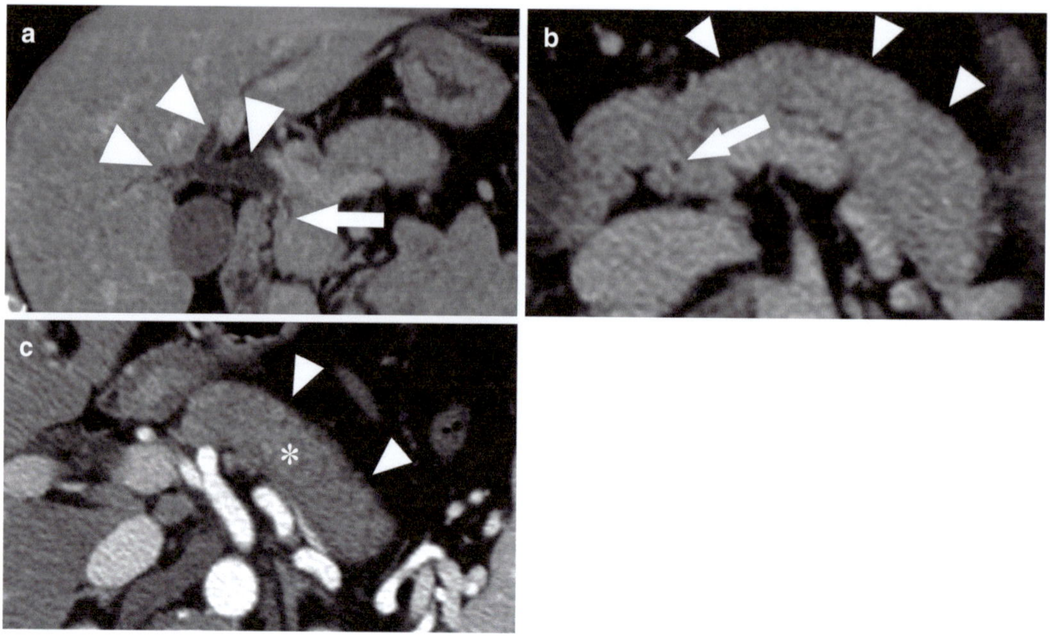

Fig. 10.5 Autoimmune pancreatitis and autoimmune pancreatitis-related cholangitis in a 39-year-old woman. (**a**) Coronal contrast enhanced portal phase CT image shows smooth and tapered narrowing of the intrapancreatic portion of the distal CBD (arrow) associated with upstream extra- and intrahepatic biliary ductal dilatation with evidence of mild wall enhancement (arrowheads). (**b**) Axial contrast enhanced portal phase CT image shows distal CBD with mild wall thickening and mural enhancement (arrow) and diffusely enlarged sausage-like pancreas (arrowheads). (**c**) Axial contrast enhanced pancreatic phase CT image at a more caudal level shows mildly heterogeneous pancreas (∗) with loss of normal pancreatic lobulation and a subtle low-attenuating peripancreatic halo (arrowheads)

proximal to the second biliary bifurcation, and DCC is distal to the cystic duct insertion [17]. The perihilar subtype accounts for 50–60% of all CC.

Morphologically, tumour growth can be described as (1) mass forming, (2) periductal infiltrating and (3) intraductal (least common, but with most favourable prognosis). CC of mixed mass-forming and periductal-infiltrating pattern is also frequently seen [18].

Intrahepatic cholangiocarcinoma is the second most common primary malignant hepatic tumour and is most often of the mass-forming type. At CT, mass-forming ICC usually appears with lobulated contours, irregular peripheral enhancement during arterial and portal venous phases (Fig. 10.6) and progressive central enhancement during delayed phase. Delayed enhancement is a characteristic finding of CC, consisting in contrast retention, and is directly proportional to the amount of interstitial space in the fibrous stroma, although, in presence of necrosis and mucin, it may be not seen. The sclerotic nature of the tumour can lead to capsular retraction; however, other hepatic malignancies such as metastasis, fibrolamellar hepatocellu-

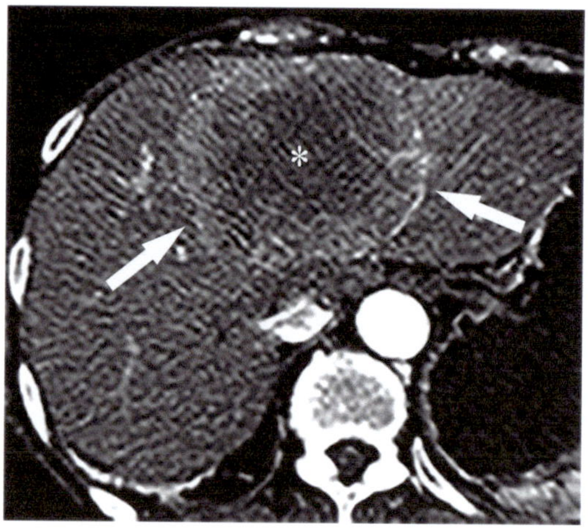

Fig. 10.6 Intrahepatic cholangiocarcinoma. Axial contrast enhanced arterial phase CT image shows a lobulated hypodense mass-forming intrahepatic cholangiocarcinoma (∗) with peripheral irregular enhancement (arrows)

lar carcinoma (HCC) and epithelioid hemangioendothelioma can also present this feature. Furthermore, peripheral satellite lesions are commonly seen [2, 19–22].

Vascular encasement is a common finding of CC, with segmental obstruction due to tumour infiltration and stenosis, rather than thrombosis, as seen with HCC. Other imaging findings include hepatic atrophy, which suggests vascular infiltration, and upstream bile duct dilatation [17]. The differential diagnoses to consider in all patients with underlying liver disease are sclerosing HCC and the rare combined HCC-cholangiocarcinoma.

Intraductal CC infrequently invades outside the duct and thus has a better prognosis, presenting as a papillary or polypoid mass [23], relatively hypoattenuating to hepatic parenchyma but with mild persistent enhancement, associated with typical upstream ductal dilatation (Fig. 10.7a, b).

Perihilar and *distal cholangiocarcinoma* commonly have a periductal-infiltrating morphology

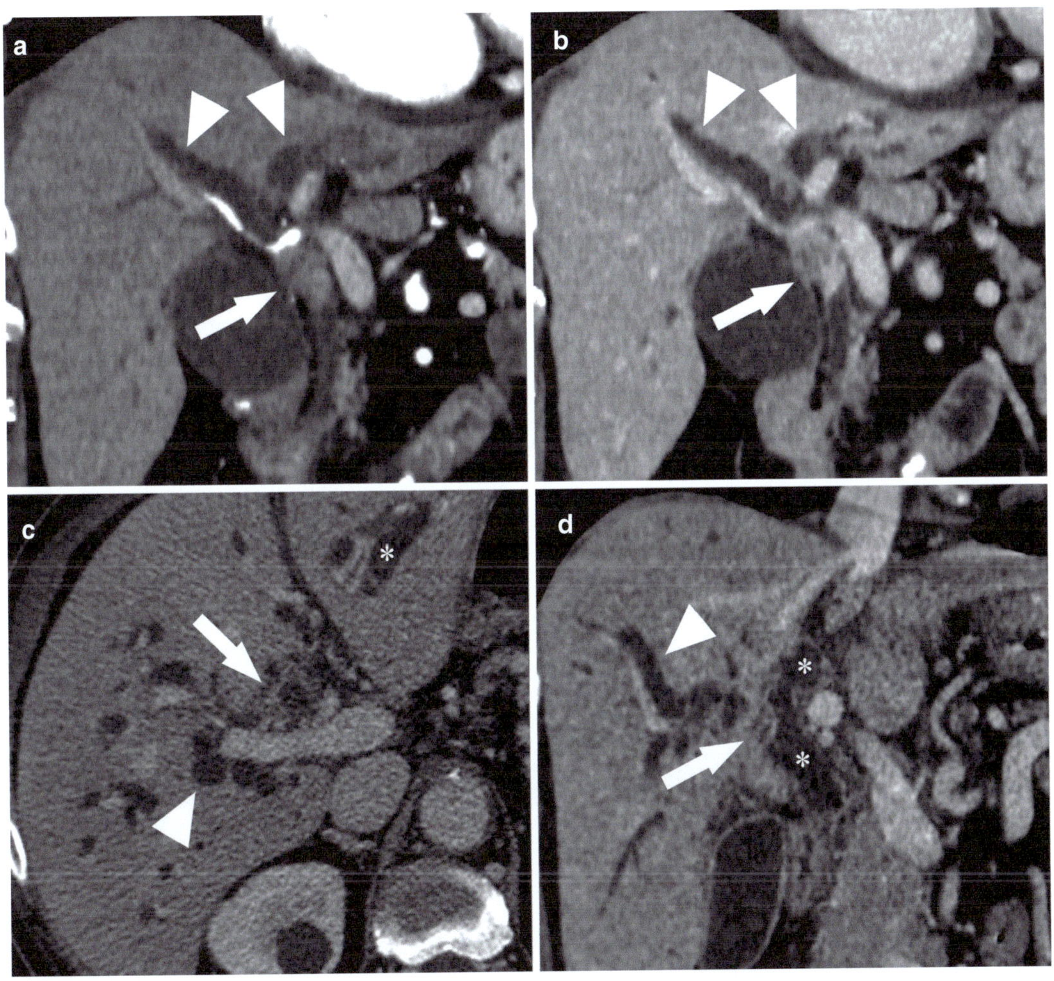

Fig. 10.7 Perihilar cholangiocarcinoma in two patients. (**a**, **b**) Coronal contrast enhanced CT images show intraductal cholangiocarcinoma (arrows), proximal to the primary biliary confluence and distal to the cystic duct, thereby perihilar in location, which appears hypoattenuating during the arterial phase (**a**) and manifests progressive increasing enhancement on the subsequent delayed phase (**b**); upstream intrahepatic biliary ductal dilatation is also seen (arrowheads). (**c**, **d**) Axial and coronal contrast enhanced CT images show periductal-infiltrating cholangiocarcinoma, perihilar in location, which appears as inhomogeneous ill-defined periductal tissue (arrows) with the evidence of irregular narrowing of the proximal right hepatic duct and disruption of the right secondary confluence, associated with upstream right intrahepatic biliary ductal dilatation (arrowheads). (**c**, **d**) Left intrahepatic biliary ductal dilatation and (**d**) extrahepatic ductal dilatation are also seen (∗)

(Fig. 10.7c, d), with bile duct wall thickening and arterial and delayed hyperenhancement, although mass-forming morphology may also occur in this location showing delayed enhancement [17, 22]. At CT, an abrupt change in calibre of the duct indicates the obstructing mass, which may or may not be seen, depending on tumour morphology [17]. Malignant biliary thickening is typically irregular, and upstream ductal ectasia usually presents a segmental, lobar or diffuse distribution, depending on the location of the obstruction. Note that lymphadenopathy in the porta hepatis may cause biliary dilatation at the confluence of the right and left intrahepatic ducts, mimicking a PCC; in this regard, CT examination can help locate the obstruction and determine the organ of origin of the malignant neoplasm.

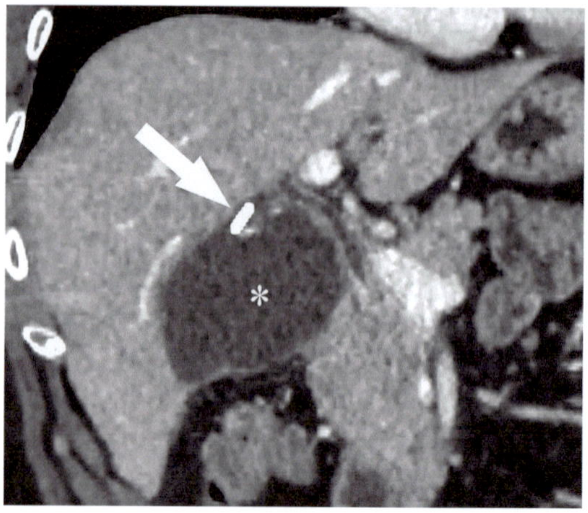

Fig. 10.8 Biloma post laparoscopic cholecystectomy in a 66-year-old man with right upper quadrant pain. Coronal contrast enhanced CT image shows a loculated well-defined extrahepatic fluid collection (*) adjacent to the clip of cholecystectomy (arrow); these findings are indicative of biloma

10.2.5 Biliary Injuries

10.2.5.1 Bile Leaks

Bile leaks are a rare complication of abdominal trauma being the gallbladder the most common location of biliary injury, followed by the extra- and intrahepatic bile ducts, respectively. Iatrogenic bile leaks may occur after open or laparoscopic cholecystectomy or after liver transplantation and pancreaticoduodenectomy, at sites of biliary anastomosis or biliary-enteric anastomosis. Additionally, bile leaks may occur after hepatic resection, liver biopsy and ablation of a liver lesion. Significant postoperative bile leaks have been reported more commonly with laparoscopic cholecystectomy than with open cholecystectomy (Fig. 10.8), resulting most frequently from slippage of the cystic duct ligature, from the gallbladder bed when the dissection plane is too deep and from incidental injury of accessory or anomalous bile ducts [24–27].

A *biloma*, or encapsulated extrabiliary bile collection, may result from biliary surgery, laparoscopic cholecystectomy, ERCP, radiofrequency ablation, percutaneous biliary drainage or transcatheter arterial chemoembolization [7].

At CT, free or loculated peri- or intrahepatic low-attenuation fluid collections seen after recent trauma or hepatobiliary surgery should raise suspicion for bile leak, although these nonspecific findings may be mistaken for more common posttraumatic and postoperative collections (e.g. seromas) [7, 28].

In addition to CT, hepatobiliary scintigraphy and MRCP with hepatobiliary contrast agents can help detect active or contained bile leaks. Thus, a multimodality imaging approach may be useful to determine the appropriate treatment [7, 28].

10.2.5.2 Biliary Necrosis

Biliary necrosis refers to destruction of the intrahepatic biliary duct epithelium usually caused by hepatic artery thrombosis which can be a serious complication of hepatic transplantation or may result from incidental artery ligation during cholecystectomy or from occlusion after transarterial chemoembolization. Additional causes of hepatic artery thrombosis can be atherosclerosis, embolic disease, hypercoagulable state, vasculitis and traumatic laceration [7]. CT findings of biliary necrosis include marked regional beaded intrahepatic biliary dilatation with low attenuation in the adjacent parallel liver parenchyma. Hypodense bile lakes or focal cavitations may be seen as a late sequela.

10.2.5.3 Hemobilia

Hemobilia refers to the presence of blood in the biliary tree. Possible causes include hepatic

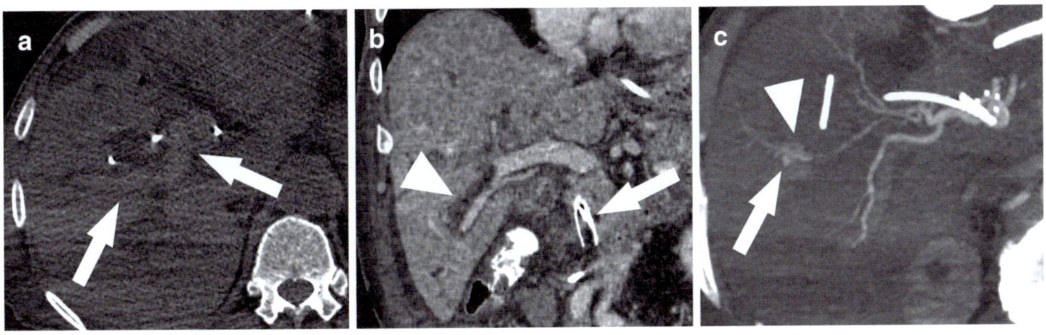

Fig. 10.9 Hemobilia in a 67-year-old man with gallbladder carcinoma infiltrating the extrahepatic biliary ducts and biliary stent, presenting with anaemia after percutaneous transhepatic biliary catheter placement. (**a**) Axial nonenhanced CT image shows hyperattenuating material in massively dilated intrahepatic biliary ducts (arrows) suggestive of acute haemorrhage. (**b**) Coronal contrast enhanced CT image shows marked intrahepatic biliary system dilatation (arrowhead); biliary stent is also seen (arrow). (**c**) Axial arterial phase maximum intensity projection CT image shows a well-defined millimetric focal outpouching (arrow), indicative of pseudoaneurysm, arising from a branch of the hepatic artery in the V hepatic segment, associated with IV contrast material leak (arrowhead). These findings are suggestive of pseudoaneurysm rupture with active arterial extravasation in the biliary tract

trauma, anticoagulation and hepatic artery aneurysm or pseudoaneurysm. Notably the incidence of hemobilia has increased, likely due to iatrogenic factors related to the increased number of diagnostic and therapeutic interventional hepatobiliary procedures being performed. At nonenhanced CT examination, high-attenuation layering material may be present in the gallbladder or biliary tree (Fig. 10.9). The differential diagnosis for high-attenuation bile includes biliary sludge, purulent bile, vicarious excretion of IV-iodinated contrast material, retained contrast agent from cholangiography and malignancy. In addition, arterial phase images may show active extravasation of blood into the biliary tract if the cause is an aneurysm or pseudoaneurysm [7].

10.3 CT Imaging of the Pancreas

10.3.1 Acute Pancreatitis

Acute pancreatitis is an acute inflammatory condition affecting the pancreas.

The Atlanta Classification [29] is the only widely accepted clinically based classification system used by clinicians and radiologists for the management of acute pancreatitis, which underwent revision in 2012 to incorporate the latest understanding of the disease [30].

At least two of the following three criteria are required for the diagnosis of acute pancreatitis: (a) abdominal pain suggestive of pancreatitis, (b) serum amylase or lipase level greater than three times the upper normal value, or (c) characteristic imaging findings [30].

Disease severity is stratified by organ failure, local and systemic complications. Local complications include a variety of pancreatic and peripancreatic collections. Additional local complications may include secondary infection of the collections or splenic and portal vein thrombosis, whereas systemic complications are an exacerbation of pre-existing co-morbid disease.

The disease course is divided into early and late phases. The *early phase* usually lasts up to 1 week. The *late phase* generally starts in the second week and occurs only in patients with moderately severe or severe pancreatitis [30].

Wide availability and excellent spatial resolution of CECT make it the most commonly used imaging tool for diagnosis, severity assessment and morphological classification of acute pancreatitis [31]; however, many patients meet the criteria for the diagnosis on the basis of symptoms and laboratory tests and may not require imaging initially. Additionally, the role of imaging is limited during the initial phase of disease, because early morphological changes may not correlate with clinical findings or may not help predict the subsequent clinical course [32]. Therefore, imaging may be performed early in the disease course when its causes are unclear or to evaluate suspected complications, whereas it is essential in the late phase for diagnosing and evaluating the evolution of necrotizing pancreatitis and its complications.

10.3.1.1 Interstitial Oedematous Pancreatitis Versus Necrotizing Pancreatitis

Two subcategories of acute pancreatitis are identified based on imaging findings: interstitial oedematous pancreatitis (IEP) and necrotizing pancreatitis.

IEP is more common and represents non-necrotizing inflammation of the pancreas. In IEP, the oedematous pancreas can appear enlarged and hypodense on unenhanced CT scan. Peripancreatic inflammation may manifest as an irregular pancreatic contour with peripancreatic fat stranding and a small amount of fluid in the anterior pararenal space. At CECT, parenchymal enhancement may be slightly heterogeneous or less avid due to interstitial oedema; however, there is no evidence of nonenhancing (i.e. necrotic) areas (Fig. 10.10a, b). In more severe IEP (Fig. 10.11a), surrounding nonnecrotic fluid collections may be seen [33, 34].

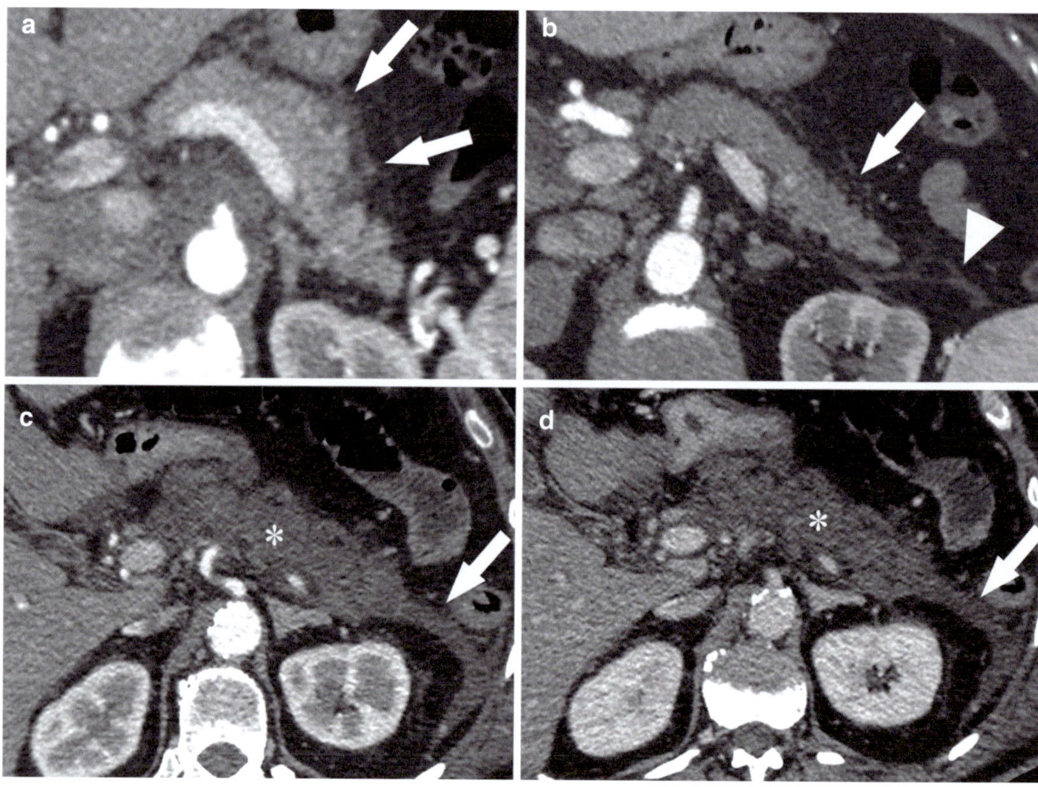

Fig. 10.10 Acute pancreatitis. (**a**) IEP in a 27-year-old woman. Axial contrast enhanced pancreatic phase CT image shows irregular pancreatic contours and peripancreatic inflammation (arrows) with normal pancreatic enhancement and no collections. (**b**) IEP in a 63-year-old man. Axial contrast enhanced pancreatic phase CT image shows normal pancreatic enhancement with mild peripancreatic fat stranding (arrow) and a small amount of fluid in the left anterior pararenal space (arrowhead). (**c**, **d**) Necrotizing pancreatitis in a 59-year-old man. Axial contrast enhanced CT images show a diffusely nonenhancing pancreas (*) during both pancreatic (**c**) and portal venous phase (**d**), findings indicative of necrosis. (**c**, **d**) A homogeneous fluid-attenuation collection is seen in the left anterior pararenal space (arrows), a finding that is consistent with ANC (due to the association with pancreatic parenchymal necrosis)

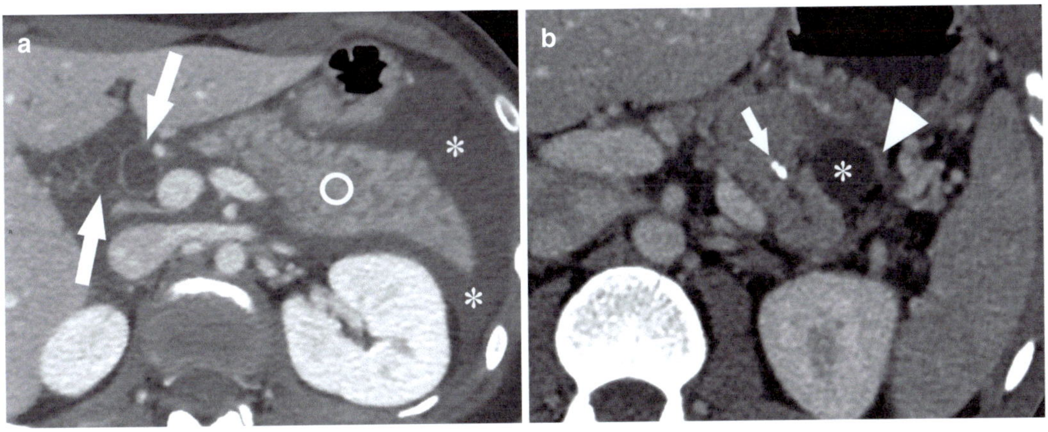

Fig. 10.11 APFC and pseudocyst. (**a**) IEP with APFC in a 33-year-old woman. Axial contrast enhanced CT image shows homogeneous nonencapsulated fluid collection in the peripancreatic and bilateral anterior pararenal spaces (*); these findings are consistent with APFC. Note diffusely enlarged pancreas with slightly inhomogeneous parenchymal enhancement but no evidence of necrotic areas (circle). Cystic ductal dilatation and CBD dilatation are also seen (arrows). (**b**) Pseudocyst in a 38-year-old man with alcohol-related pancreatitis. Axial contrast enhanced CT image shows a well-defined peripancreatic homogeneous low-attenuating collection (*) with a thin enhancing wall (arrowhead). A ductal calcification (arrow) can be also seen within the MPD, which appears slightly dilated

Necrotizing pancreatitis (Fig. 10.10c, d) accounts for 5–10% of cases of acute pancreatitis [30]. Three subtypes are described based on the area of necrotic involvement: (a) pancreatic, (b) peripancreatic and (c) combined (most common subtype).

At CT, pancreatic necrosis is suspected when any region of parenchyma displays an attenuation of less than 30 HU during the pancreatic parenchymal phase. In peripancreatic necrosis, the pancreas enhances normally, but the peripancreatic tissues show necrosis, with collections containing variable amounts of fluid and non-liquefied components. The combined subtype demonstrates necrotic pancreatic parenchyma, as well as heterogeneous peripancreatic collections [33, 35].

When imaging is performed within the first few days of disease onset, necrosis may be indistinguishable from IEP; in these cases, CECT performed 5–7 days later is more accurate for the diagnosis of necrotizing pancreatitis [30]. In addition to establishing the diagnosis, CT can be used to define the extent and severity of acute pancreatitis, with findings having been shown to correlate with the outcome [36, 37]. The modified CT severity index (MCTSI) includes extrapancreatic complications in the grading system and simplifies the evaluation of extent of parenchymal necrosis (Table 10.1) [37].

Table 10.1 Modified CT severity index [37]

Prognostic indicator	Points
Pancreatic inflammation	
– Normal pancreas	0
– Intrinsic pancreatic abnormalities with or without inflammatory changes in peripancreatic fat	2
– Pancreatic or peripancreatic fluid collection or peripancreatic fat necrosis	4
Pancreatic necrosis	
– None	0
– ≤30%	2
– >30%	4
Extrapancreatic complications (one or more of pleural effusion, ascites, vascular complications, parenchymal complications or gastrointestinal tract involvement)	2

The severity of pancreatitis is categorized as mild (0–2 points), moderate (4–6 points) or severe (8–10 points)

10.3.1.2 Pancreatic and Peripancreatic Collections

Four distinct collection subtypes are identified: *acute peripancreatic fluid collection* (APFC), *pancreatic pseudocyst*, *acute necrotic collection* (ANC) and *walled-off necrosis* (WON) (Table 10.2) [30, 33, 38]. The important distinctions for classifying collections are the time course (≤4 weeks or >4 weeks from pain onset) and the presence or absence of necrosis at imaging [30].

Table 10.2 Pancreatic and peripancreatic collections [30, 33, 38]

Collection	Time after pain onset (week)	Pancreatitis subtypes	Location	Imaging features
APFC	≤4	IEP	Extrapancreatic	Homogeneous, fluid attenuation, conforms to retroperitoneal structures, no wall
ANC	≤4	Necrotizing pancreatitis	Intra- and/or extrapancreatic	Inhomogeneous[a], non-liquefied components[b], no wall
Pseudocyst	>4	IEP	Extrapancreatic[c]	Homogeneous, fluid filled, circumscribed, encapsulated with wall
WON	>4	Necrotizing pancreatitis	Intra- and/or extrapancreatic	Inhomogeneous, non-liquefied components, encapsulated with wall

ANC acute necrotic collection, *APFC* Acute peripancreatic fluid collection, *IEP* interstitial oedematous pancreatitis, *WON* walled-off necrosis

[a]Early ANCs may be homogeneous; follow-up imaging performed in second week may help clarify status

[b]Includes solid-appearing components or fat globules within fluid

[c]Persistent pancreatic leak or disconnected duct may lead to intrapancreatic pseudocyst (uncommon)

APFCs occur during the first 4 weeks and are present only in patient with IEP. APFCs are peripancreatic in location, contain only fluid and are visualized at CT as homogeneous fluid-attenuation collections that lack a wall and tend to conform to the retroperitoneal spaces (Fig. 10.11a). If a similar-appearing collection is seen within the pancreatic parenchyma, it is by definition an ANC; thereby, the diagnosis is no longer IEP but necrotizing pancreatitis [30].

Pseudocysts lack an epithelial lining and thus are not true cysts. They typically evolve from acute peripancreatic fluid collections in the setting of IEP usually after 4 weeks, by developing a capsule. Pseudocysts appear as round-to-oval hypoattenuating collections with a well-defined enhancing wall at CECT and should contain only fluid with no non-liquefied components (Fig. 10.11b). If there is even a small area of fat or soft tissue attenuation in a fluid collection, the diagnosis is not pseudocyst but WON [30, 33]. In addition, pseudocysts may have a connection to the pancreatic ductal system, which is best seen at MRCP. A pseudocyst is typically peripancreatic in location, although it can rarely be intrapancreatic in cases of prior necrosectomy, resulting from pancreatic juice leakage from the disconnected pancreatic duct [30, 33].

ANCs arise within the first 4 weeks of necrotizing pancreatitis and are poorly organized nonencapsulated necrotic collections, often found in the lesser sac and pararenal spaces. They are often multiple, with a loculated appearance, and may extend into the pancreas within areas of parenchymal necrosis, or inferiorly as far as the pelvic sidewalls (Fig. 10.12a, b). ANCs show a variable amount of fluid and can be distinguished from APFCs by the presence of non-liquefied debris (i.e. solid-appearing hyperdense components or fat globules within the fluid). Any peripancreatic collection associated with pancreatic parenchymal necrosis should be termed an ANC, even if it is homogeneous and contains no non-liquefied debris [30, 33] (Fig. 10.10c, d). In the early phase of disease, the diagnosis of necrosis may be uncertain, and imaging performed in the second week is usually helpful for distinguishing an APFC from an ANC.

WON arises after 4 weeks in the setting of necrotizing pancreatitis, when ANCs mature by developing a thick wall (Fig. 10.12c, d). Like pseudocysts, WON contains fluid and shows thick enhancing walls. However, unlike pseudocysts, WON presents non-liquefied debris within the fluid such as necrotic fat and/or pancreatic tissue (Fig. 10.13). Generally, WON occurs in the peripancreatic space or can often manifest with a coalescent collection extending from the lesser sac to a portion of parenchyma [30].

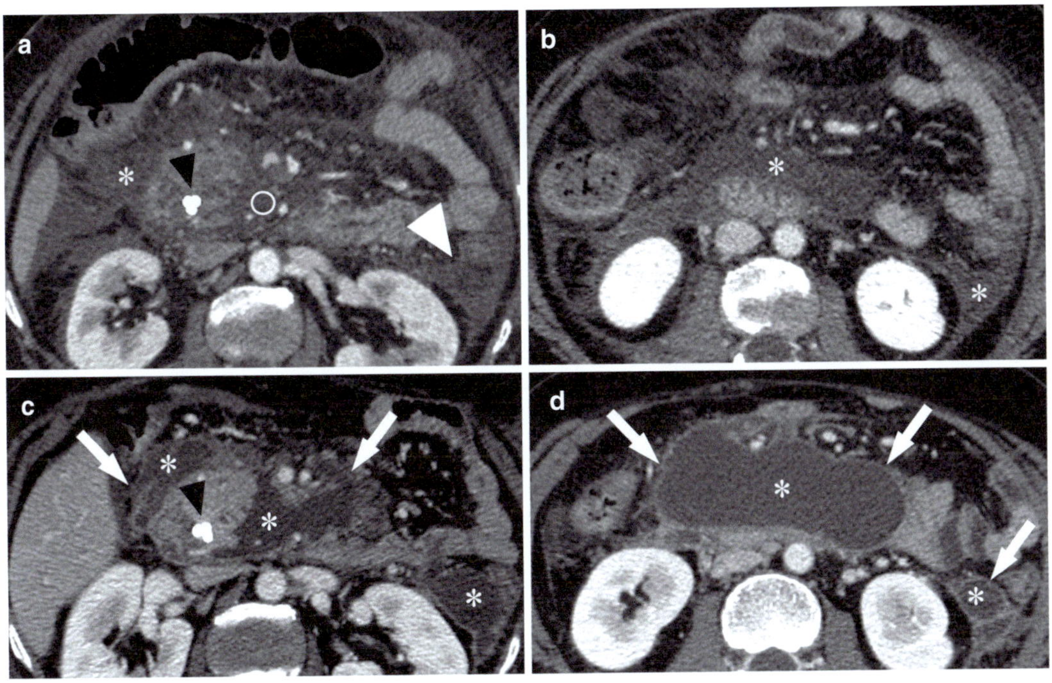

Fig. 10.12 ANC and WON. Evolution of necrotizing pancreatitis in a 44-year-old woman with biliary stent. (**a**) Axial contrast enhanced pancreatic phase CT image shows heterogeneous nonencapsulated fluid attenuating peripancreatic collection (∗) extending into the pancreas in an area of parenchymal necrosis (circle) and to the left anterior pararenal space (arrowhead). (**b**) Axial contrast enhanced portal venous phase CT image at a more caudal level shows the heterogeneous nonencapsulated fluid collection extending inferiorly in the anterior pararenal space (∗). These findings are consistent with ANC. (**c**, **d**) At follow-up imaging performed 1 month later, axial contrast enhanced portal venous phase CT images obtained at different levels show maturation of the collections (∗) by developing thick enhancing walls with irregular borders (arrows); these findings are suggestive of WON. (**a**, **c**) Biliary stent can also be seen (black arrowheads)

Additional imaging findings may include irregular borders and thick multiple septations. CECT may not readily distinguish solid from liquid content; for this purpose, MRI and transabdominal or endoscopic ultrasound (US) may be required for the distinction of WON from pseudocysts [30, 33, 34].

10.3.1.3 Infection and Other Local Complications

Any collection can be sterile or infected, although infection occurs more frequently in necrotic collections [30]. The only imaging finding of an infected collection is the presence of gas often appearing as multiple scattered small bubbles within the collection (Fig. 10.14a); wall enhancement is not a reliable indicator of infection, as it is invariably present in mature collections (i.e. pseudocysts and WON) [33, 35]. Infected collections may also manifest with gas bubbles due to a pancreatic-enteric fistula, which can result from necrotic collections erosion through the bowel wall. In addition, large abdominopelvic fluid collections may displace and compress adjacent organs (Fig. 10.13b).

Inflammatory reactions can lead to venous thrombosis, which is the most common vascular complication of pancreatitis, usually involving the splenic vein (Fig. 10.14b). Acute venous thrombo-

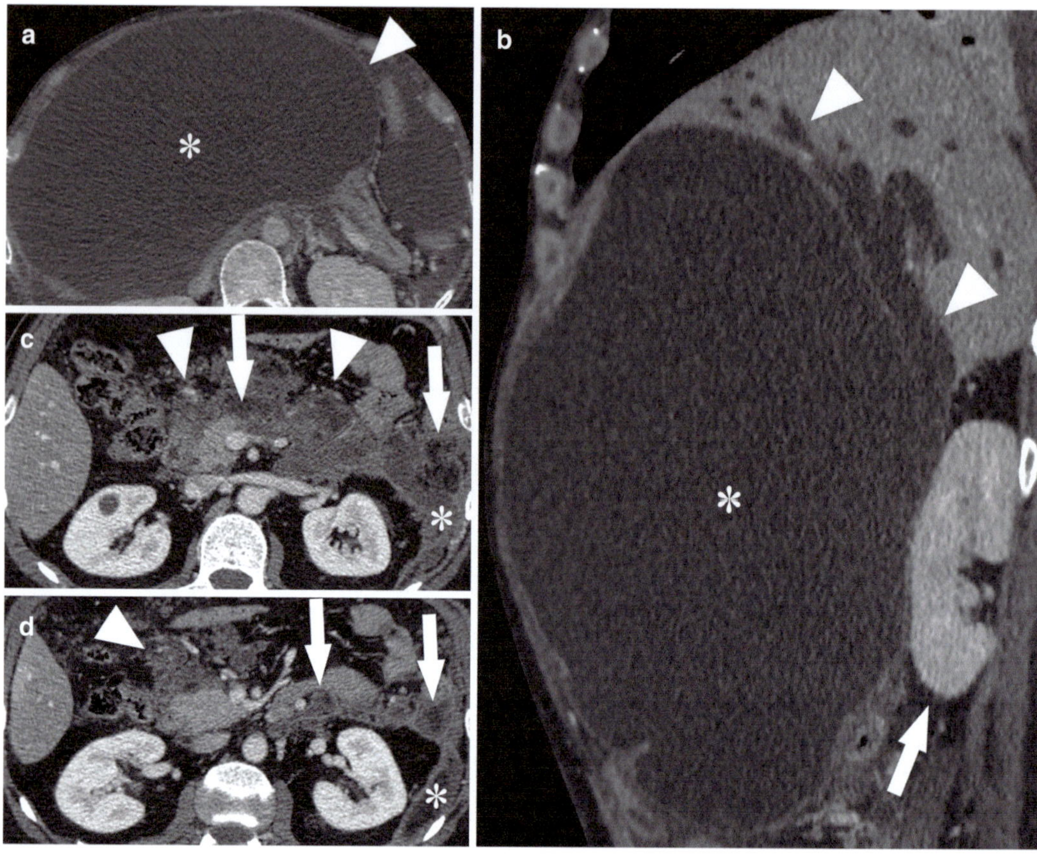

Fig. 10.13 Pseudocyst and WON. (**a**) Pseudocyst in a 42-year-old man. Axial contrast enhanced portal venous phase CT image shows a huge homogeneous peripancreatic fluid collection (∗) with no non-liquefied components and a thin enhancing wall (arrowhead). (**b**) Sagittal contrast enhanced portal venous phase CT image in the same patient shows the extent of the fluid collection (∗) which compresses the liver determining marked biliary ductal dilatation (arrowheads) and displaces posteriorly the adjacent right kidney (arrow). (**c**, **d**) WON in a 36-year-old man. Axial contrast enhanced CT image (**c**) and axial contrast enhanced CT image at a more caudal level (**d**) show organized inhomogeneous peripancreatic collection with enhancing walls (arrowheads) containing non-liquefied debris including fat tissue (arrows) and extending to the left anterior pararenal space (∗)

sis manifests with enlarged nonenhancing vessels at imaging, whereas chronic thrombosis presents with less well-visualized venous structures and multiple collateral vessels [35]. Pancreatic enzymes can also cause vessel erosion and lead to spontaneous arterial haemorrhage or pseudoaneurysm formation, with the splenic artery most frequently involved. At CT and MR imaging, a pseudoaneurysm appears as a focal outpouching of a vessel within the necrotic region (Fig. 10.14c, d). Spontaneous haemorrhage or resulting from pseudoaneurysms rupture usually manifests at CT as a region of high attenuation, typically in an area of necrosis.

A further complication of acute pancreatitis is the *disconnected pancreatic duct syndrome*, which results from necrosis of the central pancreas or from a therapeutic intervention that disrupts the MPD leading to a persistent leakage of pancreatic fluid. At CT or MR imaging, this condition is suggested by a large or growing collection around the pancreas, involving the neck or body of the gland and a viable upstream segment of the body or tail [34, 35].

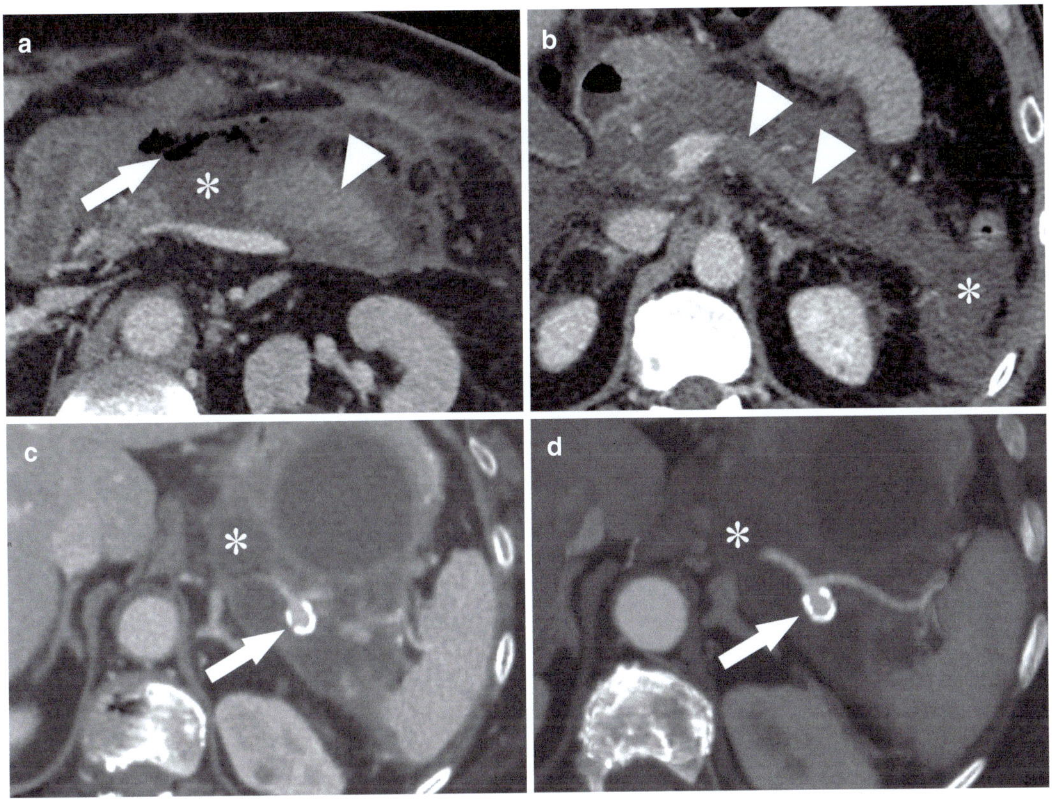

Fig. 10.14 Acute pancreatitis complications. (**a**) Seventy-two-year-old woman with acute pancreatitis. Axial contrast enhanced portal venous phase CT image shows pancreatic tail (arrowhead) and multiple gas foci (arrow) within a heterogeneous fluid attenuating peripancreatic collection (∗) with thick enhancing walls. These findings are suggestive of infected WON. (**b**) Sixty-four-year-old man with acute pancreatitis. Axial contrast enhanced portal venous phase CT image shows a hypoattenuating thrombus within the splenic vein (arrowheads). Heterogeneous peripancreatic non-organized fluid collection suggestive of ANC is also seen (∗). (**c**, **d**) Forty-one-year-old man with acute recurrent alcohol-related pancreatitis. (**c**) Axial contrast enhanced arterial phase CT image and (**d**) axial arterial phase maximum intensity projection CT image show a well-defined focal outpouching (arrows), indicative of pseudoaneurysm with calcified wall arising from the splenic artery within a heterogeneous peripancreatic thick-walled fluid collection consistent with WON (∗)

10.3.2 Chronic Pancreatitis

Chronic pancreatitis (CP) is defined by continuous or relapsing inflammation of the organ leading to irreversible morphological injury. Imaging plays a significant role in detecting parenchymal and ductal abnormalities in CP and helps in differentiating early from advanced phases of disease [39].

Unlike MR imaging, CT is unreliable in diagnosis of early CP, as it often shows no abnormalities [40]. However, CT examination is especially useful in detecting changes seen in advanced disease. Most common findings seen at CT in advanced CP include dilatation of MPD and its side branches; the ductal contour may be smooth or irregular. Additional findings include intraductal calcifications, seen in nearly half of the patients with CP, and parenchymal atrophy (Figs. 10.2b, 10.3, 10.4, 10.5, 10.6, 10.7, 10.8, 10.9, 10.10, 10.11, 10.12, 10.13, 10.14, and 10.15). However, parenchymal atrophy is a nonspecific feature as it can also be seen with normal aging [40].

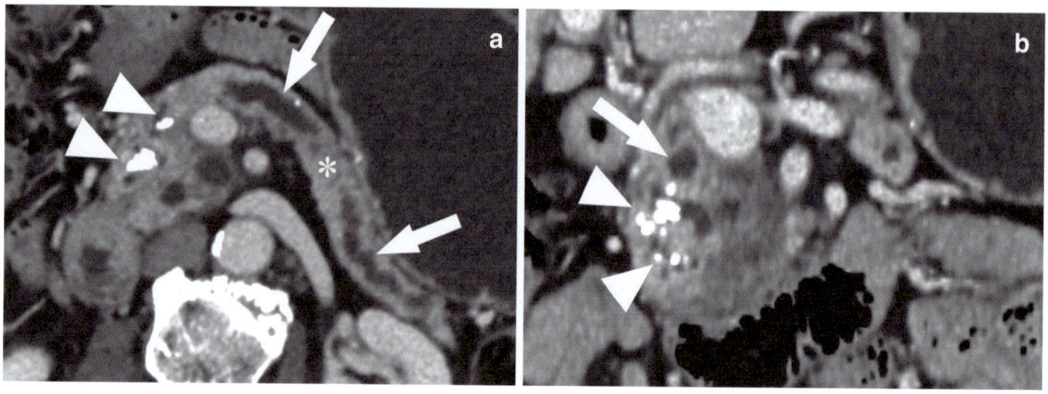

Fig. 10.15 Advanced-stage chronic pancreatitis. (**a**) Axial contrast enhanced portal venous phase CT image and (**b**) coronal contrast enhanced portal venous phase CT image show markedly dilated and tortuous MPD (arrows) with thick ductal calcifications involving the pancreatic head (arrowheads). (**a**) Parenchymal atrophy of the pancreatic body (i.e. reduction of the anteroposterior dimensions of the gland) is also seen (*)

10.3.2.1 Autoimmune Pancreatitis

Autoimmune pancreatitis is a distinct type of chronic pancreatitis characterized by periductal infiltration with IgG4-positive plasma cells, which leads to interlobular fibrosis and diffuse narrowing of the pancreatic duct.

Patients with autoimmune pancreatitis usually demonstrate a dramatic response to corticosteroid therapy; thus, it is important to recognize the disease and its imaging features [41].

Diffuse disease is the most common type, with a diffusely enlarged sausage-like pancreas and loss of its lobular contour (Fig. 10.5b, c). Focal disease is less common and manifests as a well-defined mass, often involving the pancreatic head and mimicking pancreatic adenocarcinoma, although, when present, upstream dilatation of the MPD is typically milder than in patients with pancreatic carcinoma [15, 40].

In patients with autoimmune pancreatitis, CECT often demonstrates decreased enhancement of the involved parenchyma on the pancreatic phase, while moderate enhancement is seen on the delayed phase, due to fibrosis. The presence of a hypoattenuating capsule-like rim or "halo" surrounding the affected areas is common and is believed to represent inflammatory cell infiltration (Fig. 10.5c). Diffuse or segmental narrowing of the MPD is typical and may be demonstrated at ERCP or MRCP. In addition, when the pancreatic head is involved, narrowing of the intrapancreatic portion of the CBD is typically seen (Fig. 10.5a, b) which may lead to upstream biliary dilatation and subsequent obstructive jaundice [15, 40].

10.3.2.2 Paraduodenal Pancreatitis

Paraduodenal pancreatitis (PDP) is a rare form of focal chronic pancreatitis involving the duodenal wall in the vicinity of the minor duodenal papilla, the adjacent pancreatic parenchyma and the pancreaticoduodenal "groove" [42], which is defined as a small potential space bordered by the pancreatic head, duodenum and CBD. The concept of PDP unifies several inflammatory entities with similar pathogenesis, anatomical location and clinical course including cystic dystrophy of the pancreas, paraduodenal wall cyst, groove pancreatitis, pancreatic duodenal hamartoma and myoadenomatosis [42, 43].

At imaging, PDP may present as a solid fibrotic mass (*solid variant*) around the minor papilla or as cystic changes within the thickened duodenal wall or the pancreaticoduodenal groove (*cystic variant*) [42, 44].

At CT examination, a hypoattenuating soft tissue may be seen in the groove, with increasing delayed enhancement due to fibrotic component (Fig. 10.16). The CBD can appear narrowed, although, in most cases, this narrowing is relatively smooth and tapered, with no evidence of irregularity or abrupt margins, as seen frequently in malignant strictures [42, 45].

Inflammatory changes involving the adjacent pancreatic parenchyma may result in a mass-like enlargement of the pancreatic head, making challenging the differentiation between PDP and pancreatic adenocarcinoma [45], particularly in cases of pancreatic carcinoma with fibrotic component, which presents delayed enhancement as seen with solid variant of PDP.

In recent years, MRI and MRCP have shown to contribute to the diagnosis of PDP [46, 47]; however, differentiating PDP from pancreatic head, ampullary or duodenal malignancy on the basis of imaging features is still difficult, and patients may frequently undergo fine needle aspiration biopsy, followed by pancreaticoduodenectomy because of the inability to completely exclude malignancy [45, 46].

10.3.3 Solid Pancreatic Lesions

10.3.3.1 Pancreatic Adenocarcinoma

Pancreatic adenocarcinoma is the most common malignant pancreatic tumour, affecting the head of the gland in 60–70% of cases and presenting a high mortality rate. CT is currently the established imaging technique for detecting and staging the tumour [48]; thus, all patients presenting suspicion of pancreatic cancer should undergo initial evaluation by CT, performed according to a dedicated pancreas-specific protocol [49]. MRI can be used as a problem-solving tool in equivocal CT cases, particularly when suspected tumours are not visible at CT, for characterization of CT-indeterminate liver lesions, or in cases of contrast allergy [50, 51].

At CT, arterial phase and pancreatic phase imaging allow optimal visualization of the peripancreatic arteries and the tumour, due to the highest difference in contrast enhancement between the parenchyma and the lesion

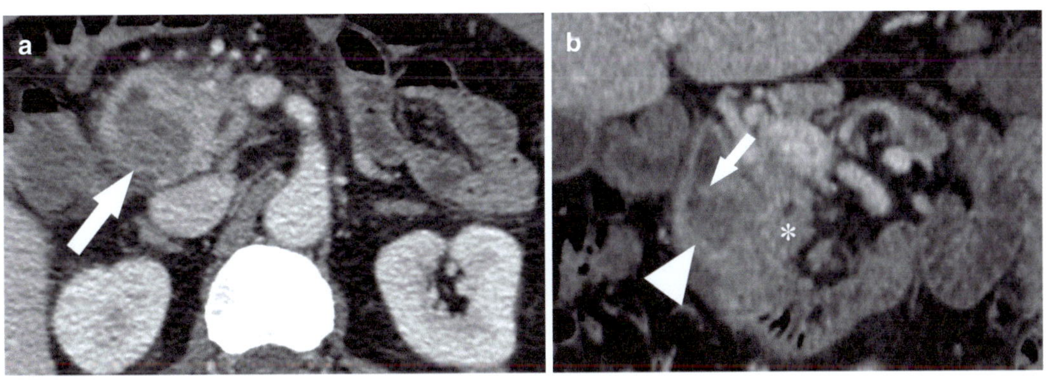

Fig. 10.16 Contrast enhanced CT images in a 45-year-old alcoholic man with vomiting and weight loss, depicting paraduodenal inflammatory changes. (**a**) Axial contrast enhanced portal venous phase CT image shows hypoenhancing soft tissue (arrow) within the medial wall of the descending duodenum, extending to the pancreaticoduodenal groove. (**b**) Coronal contrast enhanced portal venous phase CT image shows the soft tissue (arrowhead) determining submucosal duodenal contour bulge (arrow). Uncinate process (∗). There is no evidence of biliary duct or MPD dilatation. These findings are consistent with PDP (solid variant)

(Fig. 10.17a, b). Portal phase imaging is optimal for assessing the peripancreatic veins and detecting metastatic disease to the liver [4, 48, 52]. After IV contrast administration, most pancreatic adenocarcinomas are hypoattenuating; however, approximately 10% of these tumours may manifest isoattenuation relative to the background pancreatic parenchyma, especially in case of small lesions (2 cm or less). In these situations, secondary signs such as mass effect, contour abnormalities of the gland, abrupt ductal obstruction, distal parenchymal atrophy (Fig. 10.17c) and vascular invasion may be helpful for diagnosis [53, 54]. Dilatation of both CBD and MPD, known as the "double duct sign," may be seen in case of tumours occurring in the pancreatic head (Fig. 10.17d); whereas tumours in the pancreatic body may cause upstream MPD dilatation [55]. In addition, pancreatic adenocarcinomas may occasionally manifest cystic-necrotic degeneration [56]; the presence of calcifications is uncommon.

As the tumour grows, it typically infiltrates the peripancreatic structures and adjacent vasculature. Multiphase pancreatic protocol also allows the visualization of important arterial and venous structures, thereby providing an assessment of vascular invasion by the tumour [48].

The presence of a circumferential soft tissue cuff surrounding the peripancreatic vessels with loss of the perivascular fat plane suggests vascular invasion. The determination of the extent of vascular involvement is usually performed by identifying, with regard to the circular cross-section of a vessel, the degrees of circumferential contact (Figs. 10.17b and 10.18), with a sensitivity of 84% and a specificity of 98% for invasion if the tumour is contiguous with more than 50% of

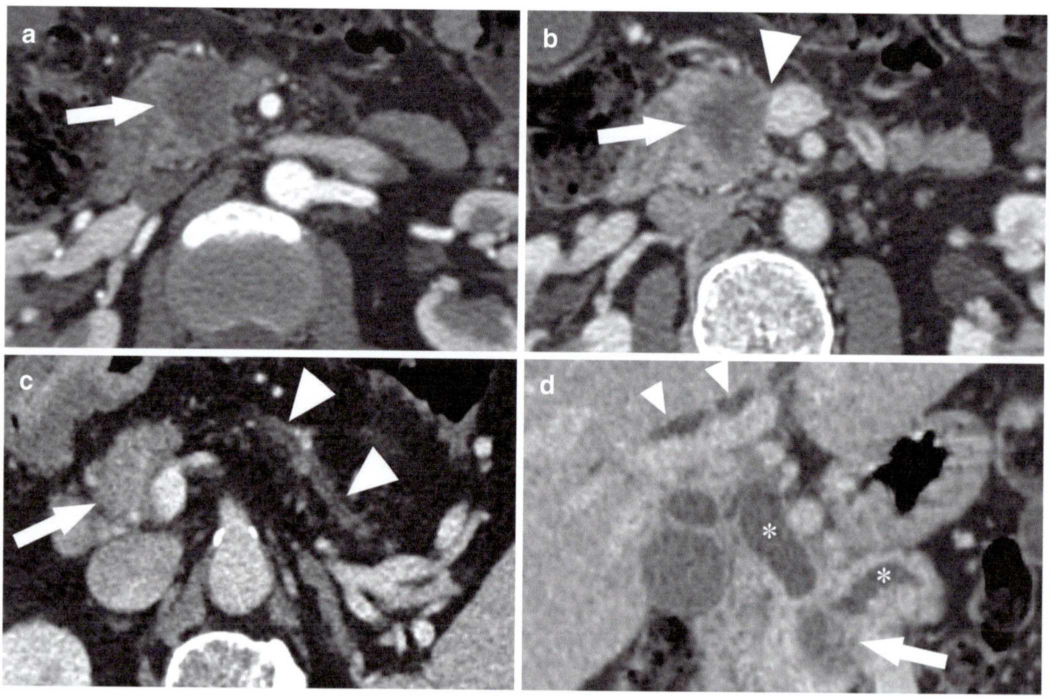

Fig. 10.17 Pancreatic head adenocarcinoma. (**a**, **b**) Pancreatic adenocarcinoma in a 53-year-old man. Axial contrast enhanced pancreatic phase CT image (**a**) and axial contrast enhanced portal venous phase CT image (**b**) show a hypoattenuating mass in the pancreatic head/uncinate process (arrows). (**b**) Solid tumour contact with the superior mesenteric vein <50% of the circumference of the vessel (arrowhead). (**c**) Pancreatic head adenocarcinoma in a 66-year-old woman. Axial contrast enhanced CT image shows pancreatic head mass (arrow) causing marked distal parenchymal atrophy (arrowheads). (**d**) Pancreatic adenocarcinoma in a 58-year-old man. Coronal contrast enhanced CT image shows hypoenhancing ill-defined mass (arrow) in the pancreatic head/uncinate process determining abrupt ductal obstruction with upstream dilatation of both CBD and MPD, known as "double duct sign" (∗). Intrahepatic biliary ductal dilatation is also seen (arrowheads)

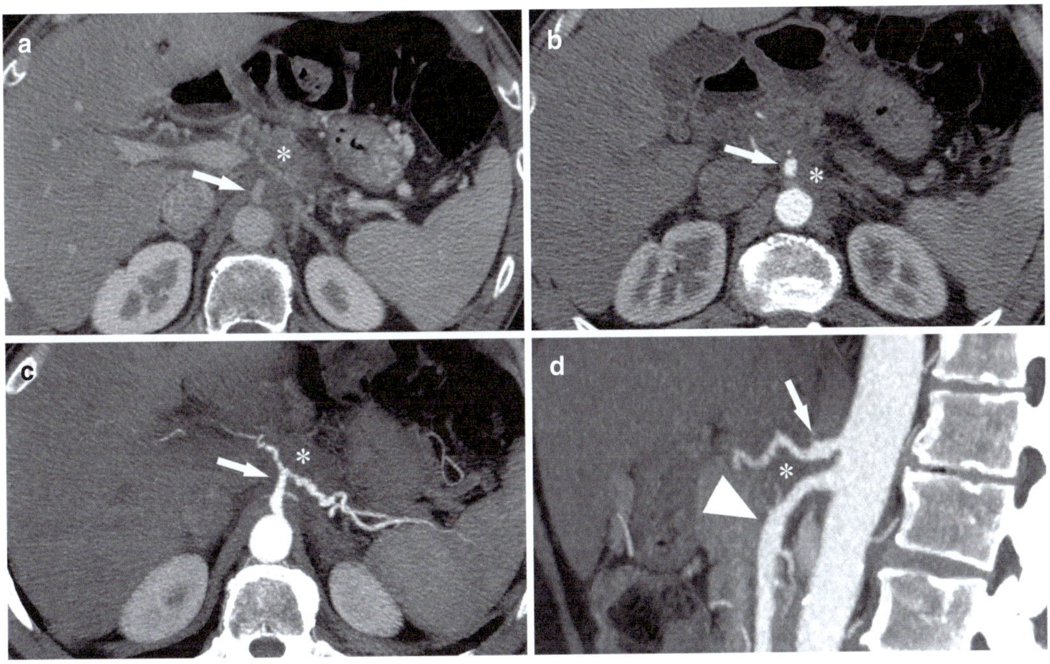

Fig. 10.18 Pancreatic adenocarcinoma in a 59-year-old woman. (**a**) Axial contrast enhanced CT image shows a hypoenhancing ill-defined pancreatic body cancer (∗), invading the celiac axis (arrow). (**b**) Axial contrast enhanced arterial phase image at a more caudal level shows the degree of tumour contact (∗) with the superior mesenteric artery (arrow), which is >50% of the circumference of the vessel. (**c**) Axial arterial phase maximum intensity projection CT image and (**d**) sagittal arterial phase maximum intensity projection CT image comprehensively assess the extent and the degree of major vascular involvement caused by the pancreatic cancer (∗). (**c, d**) Celiac axis (arrows). (**d**) Superior mesenteric artery (arrowhead)

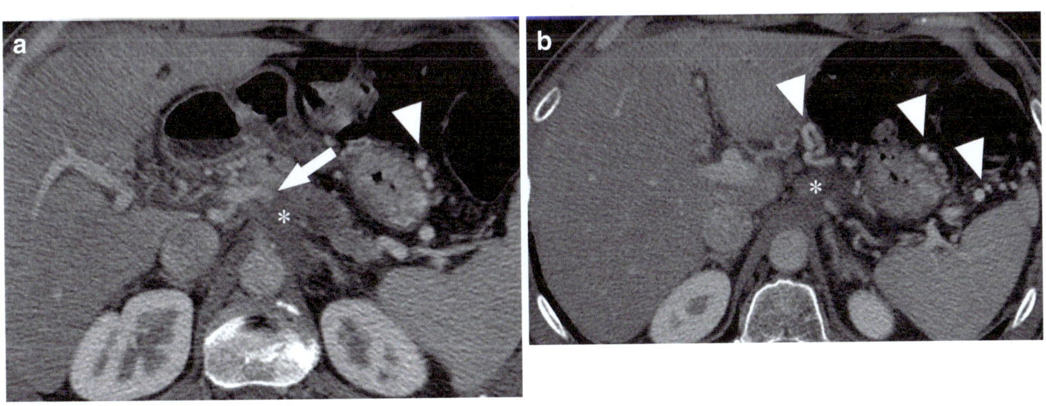

Fig. 10.19 Pancreatic adenocarcinoma in a 44-year-old man. (**a**) Axial contrast enhanced portal venous CT image and (**b**) axial contrast enhanced portal venous CT image at a more cranial level show hypoenhancing ill-defined pancreatic body cancer (∗). (**a**) Solid tumour contact with the superior mesenteric vein (arrow) with vessel contour irregularity. (**a, b**) Multiple collateral vessels are also seen (arrowheads). These findings suggest vascular invasion

the vessel circumference [57]. Vessel deformity, thrombosis and development of collateral vessels (Fig. 10.19) represent other features suggesting vascular invasion [58].

All of this information can improve the prediction of resectability; therefore, in addition to the detection of pancreatic adenocarcinoma, high-quality multiphase imaging can help distinguish between patients eligible for resection with curative intent and those with unresectable disease [48]. The current criteria for defining tumour resectability are shown in Table 10.3 [48, 49].

10.3.3.2 Pancreatic Neuroendocrine Tumours

Pancreatic neuroendocrine tumours (P-NETs) account for 1–5% of all pancreatic neoplasms and are classified into functioning and non-functioning tumours. In general, functioning tumours manifest early in the course of disease due to symptoms related to excessive hormone production, whereas non-functioning tumours usually tend to be large and malignant at the time of diagnosis [59, 60].

P-NETs present a rich vascular supply and, therefore, at CT, in the arterial phase, usually enhance more rapidly and intensely than the

Table 10.3 Criteria defining resectability status [48, 49]

Resectability status	Arterial	Venous
Resectable	No arterial tumour contact (celiac axis [CA], superior mesenteric artery [SMA] or common hepatic artery [CHA])	No tumour contact with the superior mesenteric vein (SMV) or portal vein (PV) or ≤180° contact without vein contour irregularity
Borderline resectable[a]	*Pancreatic head/uncinate process* • Solid tumour contact with CHA without extension to CA or hepatic artery bifurcation allowing for safe and complete resection and reconstruction • Solid tumour contact with the SMA of ≤180° • Solid tumour contact with variant arterial anatomy (e.g. accessory right hepatic artery, replaced right hepatic artery, replaced CHA and the origin of replaced or accessory artery) and the presence and degree of tumour contact should be noted if present as it may affect surgical planning *Pancreatic body/tail* • Solid tumour contact with the CA of ≤180° • Solid tumour contact with the CA of >180° without involvement of the aorta and with intact and uninvolved gastroduodenal artery, thereby permitting a modified Appleby procedure (some experts prefer these criteria to be in the unresectable category)	• Solid tumour contact with the SMV or PV of >180°, contact of ≤180° with contour irregularity of the vein or thrombosis of the vein but with suitable vessel proximal and distal to the site of involvement allowing for safe and complete resection and vein reconstruction • Solid tumour contact with the inferior vena cava (IVC)
Unresectable[a]	• Distant metastasis (including non-regional lymph node metastasis) *Head/uncinate process* • Solid tumour contact with SMA >180° • Solid tumour contact with the CA >180° • Solid tumour contact with the first jejunal SMA branch *Body and tail* • Solid tumour contact of >180° with the SMA or CA • Solid tumour contact with the CA and aortic involvement	*Head/uncinate process* • Unreconstructible SMV/PV due to tumour involvement or occlusion (can be due to tumour or bland thrombus) • Contact with most proximal draining jejunal branch into SMV *Body and tail* • Unreconstructible SMV/PV due to tumour involvement or occlusion (can be due to tumour or bland thrombus)

[a]Solid tumour contact may be replaced with increased hazy density/stranding of the fat surrounding the peripancreatic vessels (typically seen following neoadjuvant therapy); this finding should be reported on the staging and follow-up imaging. Decision on resectability status should be made in these patients, in consensus at multidisciplinary meetings/discussions [48]

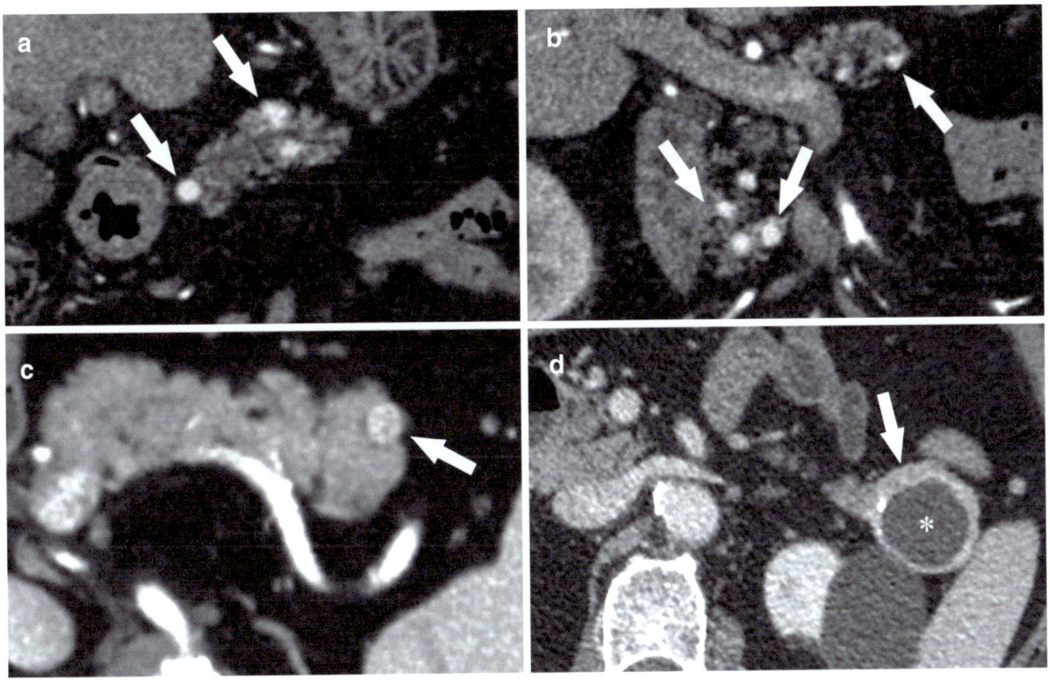

Fig. 10.20 Pancreatic neuroendocrine tumours. (**a**, **b**) Multiple P-NETs in an 83-year-old man. Coronal contrast enhanced arterial phase CT images show multiple hyperattenuating well-defined solid lesions (<1 cm in size) in the pancreatic body and pancreatic head/uncinate process (arrows). (**c**) Axial contrast enhanced pancreatic phase CT image in a 48-year-old woman shows a single well-defined hyperattenuating NET (arrow) localized in the pancreatic tail. (**d**) Axial contrast enhanced CT image in a 65-year-old woman shows a well-defined NET (4 cm in size) in the pancreatic tail, with central area of cystic degeneration (∗) and peripheral hyperattenuating solid tissue (arrow)

normal pancreas; this finding helps differentiate P-NETs from pancreatic adenocarcinomas, which commonly appear hypovascular. Homogeneous enhancement is typical for small tumours (less than 2 cm) which are often solid (Fig. 10.20a–c), whereas larger lesions tend to show heterogeneous enhancement, due to variable amounts of cystic-necrotic degeneration and calcification (Fig. 10.20d); in these cases, nonnecrotic or non-degenerated portions of the tumour may show avid enhancement [52, 55, 59].

References

1. Prokop M, Galanski M. Principles of CT, spiral CT, and multislice CT. In: Prokop M, Galanski M, editors. Spiral and multislice computed tomography of the body. New York: Thieme; 2011. p. 2–5.
2. Yeh BM, Liu PS, Soto JA, Corvera CA, Hussain HK. MR imaging and CT of the biliary tract. Radiographics. 2009;29:1669–88. https://doi.org/10.1148/rg.296095514.
3. Chaudhary V, Bano S. Imaging of the pancreas: recent advances. Indian J Endocrinol Metab. 2011;15:25. https://doi.org/10.4103/2230-8210.83060.
4. Lee ES. Imaging diagnosis of pancreatic cancer: a state-of-the-art review. World J Gastroenterol. 2014;20(24):7864. https://doi.org/10.3748/wjg.v20.i24.7864.
5. Hyodo T, Kumano S, Kushihata F, Okada M, Hirata M, Tsuda T, et al. CT and MR cholangiography: advantages and pitfalls in perioperative evaluation of biliary tree. Br J Radiol. 2012;85:887–96. https://doi.org/10.1259/bjr/21209407.
6. O'Connor OJ, O'Neill S, Maher MM. Imaging of biliary tract disease. AJR Am J Roentgenol. 2011;197:W551–8. https://doi.org/10.2214/AJR.10.4341.
7. Patel NB, Oto A, Thomas S. Multidetector CT of emergent biliary pathologic conditions. Radiographics. 2013;33:1867–88. https://doi.org/10.1148/rg.337125038.

8. Becker C, Hassler H, Terrier F. Preoperative diagnosis of the Mirizzi syndrome: limitations of sonography and computed tomography. AJR Am J Roentgenol. 1984;143:591–6. https://doi.org/10.2214/ajr.143.3.591.
9. Baron RL, Tublin ME, Peterson MS. Imaging the spectrum of biliary tract disease. Radiol. Clin. North Am. 2002;40:1325–54. https://doi.org/10.1016/s0033-8389(02)00045-3.
10. Arai K, Kawai K, Kohda W, Tatsu H, Matsui O, Nakahama T. Dynamic CT of acute cholangitis: early inhomogeneous enhancement of the liver. AJR Am J Roentgenol. 2003;181:115–8. https://doi.org/10.2214/ajr.181.1.1810115.
11. Catalano OA, Sahani DV, Forcione DG, Czermak B, Liu C-H, Soricelli A, et al. Biliary infections: spectrum of imaging findings and management. Radiographics. 2009;29:2059–80. https://doi.org/10.1148/rg.297095051.
12. Heffernan EJ, Geoghegan T, Munk PL, Ho SG, Harris AC. Recurrent pyogenic cholangitis: from imaging to intervention. AJR Am J Roentgenol. 2009;192:W28–35. https://doi.org/10.2214/ajr.08.1104.
13. Joshi A, Rajpal K, Kakadiya K, Bansal A. Role of CT and MRCP in evaluation of biliary tract obstruction. Curr Radiol Rep. 2014;2:72. https://doi.org/10.1007/s40134-014-0072-x.
14. Kawamoto S, Soyer PA, Fishman EK, Bluemke DA. Nonneoplastic liver disease: evaluation with CT and MR imaging. Radiographics. 1998;18:827–48. https://doi.org/10.1148/radiographics.18.4.9672968.
15. Vlachou PA, Khalili K, Jang H-J, Fischer S, Hirschfield GM, Kim TK. IgG4-related sclerosing disease: autoimmune pancreatitis and extrapancreatic manifestations. Radiographics. 2011;31:1379–402. https://doi.org/10.1148/rg.315105735.
16. Blechacz B, Komuta M, Roskams T, Gores GJ. Clinical diagnosis and staging of cholangiocarcinoma. Nat Rev Gastroenterol Hepatol. 2011;8:512–22. https://doi.org/10.1038/nrgastro.2011.131.
17. Mar WA, Shon AM, Lu Y, Yu JH, Berggruen SM, Guzman G, et al. Imaging spectrum of cholangiocarcinoma: role in diagnosis, staging, and posttreatment evaluation. Abdom Radiol. 2016;41:553–67. https://doi.org/10.1007/s00261-015-0583-9.
18. Yamasaki S. Intrahepatic cholangiocarcinoma: macroscopic type and stage classification. J Hepatobiliary Pancreat Surg. 2003;10:288–91. https://doi.org/10.1007/s00534-002-0732-8.
19. Valls C, Gumà A, Puig I, Sanchez A, Andía E, Serrano T, et al. Intrahepatic peripheral cholangiocarcinoma: CT evaluation. Abdom Imaging. 2000;25:490–6. https://doi.org/10.1007/s002610000079.
20. Ayuso J-R, Pagés M, Darnell A. Imaging bile duct tumors: staging. Abdom Imaging. 2013;38(5):1071–81. https://doi.org/10.1007/s00261-013-0021-9.
21. Kim TK, Choi BI, Han JK, Jang HJ, Cho SG, Han MC. Peripheral cholangiocarcinoma of the liver: two-phase spiral CT findings. Radiology. 1997;204:539–43. https://doi.org/10.1148/radiology.204.2.9240550.
22. Han JK, Choi BI, Kim AY, An SK, Lee JW, Kim TK, et al. Cholangiocarcinoma: pictorial essay of CT and cholangiographic findings. Radiographics. 2002;22:173–87. https://doi.org/10.1148/radiographics.22.1.g02ja15173.
23. Chung YE, Kim M-J, Park YN, Choi J-Y, Pyo JY, Kim YC, et al. Varying appearances of cholangiocarcinoma: radiologic-pathologic correlation. Radiographics. 2009;29:683–700. https://doi.org/10.1148/rg.293085729.
24. Albasini JLA, Aledo VS, Dexter SPL, Marton J, Martin IG, McMahon MJ. Bile leakage following laparoscopic cholecystectomy. Surg Endosc. 1995;9:1274–8. https://doi.org/10.1007/bf00190158.
25. Mungai F, Berti V, Colagrande S. Bile leak after elective laparoscopic cholecystectomy: role of MR imaging. J Radiol Case Rep. 2013;7:25–32. https://doi.org/10.3941/jrcr.v7i1.1261.
26. Hoeffel C, Azizi L, Lewin M, Laurent V, Aubé C, Arrivé L, et al. Normal and pathologic features of the postoperative biliary tract at 3D MR cholangiopancreatography and MR imaging. Radiographics. 2006;26:1603–20. https://doi.org/10.1148/rg.266055730.
27. Válek V, Kala Z, Kysela P. Biliary tree and cholecyst: post surgery imaging. Eur J Radiol. 2005;53:433–40. https://doi.org/10.1016/j.ejrad.2004.12.014.
28. Melamud K, LeBedis CA, Anderson SW, Soto JA. Biliary imaging: multimodality approach to imaging of biliary injuries and their complications. Radiographics. 2014;34:613–23. https://doi.org/10.1148/rg.343130011.
29. Bradley EL. A clinically based classification system for acute pancreatitis. Arch Surg. 1993;128:586. https://doi.org/10.1001/archsurg.1993.01420170122019.
30. Banks PA, Bollen TL, Dervenis C, Gooszen HG, Johnson CD, Sarr MG, et al. Classification of acute pancreatitis—2012: revision of the Atlanta classification and definitions by international consensus. Gut. 2012;62:102–11. https://doi.org/10.1136/gutjnl-2012-302779.
31. Manfredi R, Brizi MG, Canadè A, Vecchioli A, Marano P. Imaging of acute pancreatitis. Rays. 2001;26:135–42.
32. Spanier BWM, Nio Y, van der Hulst RWM, Tuynman HARE, Dijkgraaf MGW, Bruno MJ. Practice and yield of early CT scan in acute pancreatitis: a Dutch observational multicenter study. Pancreatology. 2010;10:222–8. https://doi.org/10.1159/000243731.
33. Foster BR, Jensen KK, Bakis G, Shaaban AM, Coakley FV. Revised Atlanta classification for acute pancreatitis: a pictorial essay. Radiographics. 2016;36:675–87. https://doi.org/10.1148/rg.2016150097.
34. Zhao K, Adam SZ, Keswani RN, Horowitz JM, Miller FH. Acute pancreatitis: revised Atlanta classification and the role of cross-sectional imaging. AJR

Am J Roentgenol. 2015;205:W32–41. https://doi.org/10.2214/ajr.14.14056.
35. Shyu JY, Sainani NI, Sahni VA, Chick JF, Chauhan NR, Conwell DL, et al. Necrotizing pancreatitis: diagnosis, imaging, and intervention. Radiographics. 2014;34:1218–39. https://doi.org/10.1148/rg.345130012.
36. Balthazar EJ, Robinson DL, Megibow AJ, Ranson JH. Acute pancreatitis: value of CT in establishing prognosis. Radiology. 1990;174:331–6. https://doi.org/10.1148/radiology.174.2.2296641.
37. Mortele KJ, Wiesner W, Intriere L, Shankar S, Zou KH, Kalantari BN, et al. A modified CT severity index for evaluating acute pancreatitis: improved correlation with patient outcome. AJR Am J Roentgenol. 2004;183:1261–5. https://doi.org/10.2214/ajr.183.5.1831261.
38. Thoeni RF. The revised Atlanta classification of acute pancreatitis: its importance for the radiologist and its effect on treatment. Radiology. 2012;262:751–64. https://doi.org/10.1148/radiol.11110947.
39. Manfredi R, Brizi MG, Masselli G, Gui B, Vecchioli A, Marano P. Imaging of chronic pancreatitis. Rays. 2001;26:143–9.
40. Busireddy KK, AlObaidy M, Ramalho M, Kalubowila J, Baodong L, Santagostino I, et al. Pancreatitis-imaging approach. World J Gastrointest Pathophysiol. 2014;5:252. https://doi.org/10.4291/wjgp.v5.i3.252.
41. Manfredi R, Graziani R, Cicero C, Frulloni L, Carbognin G, Mantovani W, et al. Autoimmune pancreatitis: CT patterns and their changes after steroid treatment. Radiology. 2008;247:435–43. https://doi.org/10.1148/radiol.2472070598.
42. Arora A, Dev A, Mukund A, Patidar Y, Bhatia V, Sarin SK. Paraduodenal pancreatitis. Clin Radiol. 2014;69:299–306. https://doi.org/10.1016/j.crad.2013.07.011.
43. Adsay NV, Zamboni G. Paraduodenal pancreatitis: a clinico-pathologically distinct entity unifying "cystic dystrophy of heterotopic pancreas," "para-duodenal wall cyst," and "groove pancreatitis". Semin Diagn Pathol. 2004;21:247–54. https://doi.org/10.1053/j.semdp.2005.07.005.
44. Itoh S, Yamakawa K, Shimamoto K, Endo T, Ishigaki T. CT findings in groove pancreatitis. J Comput Assist Tomogr. 1994;18:911–5. https://doi.org/10.1097/00004728-199411000-00011.
45. Raman SP, Salaria SN, Hruban RH, Fishman EK. Groove pancreatitis: spectrum of imaging findings and radiology-pathology correlation. AJR Am J Roentgenol. 2013;201:W29–39. https://doi.org/10.2214/ajr.12.9956.
46. Kalb B, Martin DR, Sarmiento JM, Erickson SH, Gober D, Tapper EB, et al. Paraduodenal pancreatitis: clinical performance of MR imaging in distinguishing from carcinoma. Radiology. 2013;269:475–81. https://doi.org/10.1148/radiol.13112056.
47. Boninsegna E, Manfredi R, Negrelli R, Avesani G, Mehrabi S, Pozzi Mucelli R. Pancreatic duct stenosis: differential diagnosis between malignant and benign conditions at secretin-enhanced MRCP. Clin Imaging. 2017;41:137–43. https://doi.org/10.1016/j.clinimag.2016.10.020.
48. Tempero MA, Malafa MP, Al-Hawary M, Asbun H, Bain A, Behrman SW, et al. Pancreatic adenocarcinoma, version 2.2017, NCCN clinical practice guidelines in oncology. J Natl Compr Cancer Netw. 2017;15:1028–61. https://doi.org/10.6004/jnccn.2017.0131.
49. Al-Hawary MM, Francis IR, Chari ST, Fishman EK, Hough DM, Lu DS, et al. Pancreatic ductal adenocarcinoma radiology reporting template: consensus statement of the Society of Abdominal Radiology and the American Pancreatic Association. Gastroenterology. 2014;146:291–304. https://doi.org/10.1053/j.gastro.2013.11.004.
50. Schima W, Ba-Ssalamah A, Goetzinger P, Scharitzer M, Koelblinger C. State-of-the-art magnetic resonance imaging of pancreatic cancer. Top Magn Reson Imaging. 2007;18:421–9. https://doi.org/10.1097/rmr.0b013e31816459e0.
51. Vachiranubhap B, Kim YH, Balci NC, Semelka RC. Magnetic resonance imaging of adenocarcinoma of the pancreas. Top Magn Reson Imaging. 2009;20:3–9. https://doi.org/10.1097/rmr.0b013e3181b48392.
52. Low G, Panu A, Millo N, Leen E. Multimodality imaging of neoplastic and nonneoplastic solid lesions of the pancreas. Radiographics. 2011;31:993–1015. https://doi.org/10.1148/rg.314105731.
53. Francis IR. Pancreatic adenocarcinoma: diagnosis and staging using multidetector-row computed tomography (MDCT) and magnetic resonance imaging (MRI). Cancer Imaging. 2007;7:S160–5. https://doi.org/10.1102/1470-7330.2007.9010.
54. Yoon SH, Lee JM, Cho JY, Lee KB, Kim JE, Moon SK, et al. Small (≤20 mm) pancreatic adenocarcinomas: analysis of enhancement patterns and secondary signs with multiphasic multidetector CT. Radiology. 2011;259:442–52. https://doi.org/10.1148/radiol.11101133.
55. de la Santa LG. Radiology of pancreatic neoplasms: an update. World J Gastrointest Oncol. 2014;6:330. https://doi.org/10.4251/wjgo.v6.i9.330.
56. Kosmahl M, Pauser U, Anlauf M, Klöppel G. Pancreatic ductal adenocarcinomas with cystic features: neither rare nor uniform. Mod Pathol. 2005;18:1157–64. https://doi.org/10.1038/modpathol.3800446.
57. Lu DS, Reber HA, Krasny RM, Kadell BM, Sayre J. Local staging of pancreatic cancer: criteria for unresectability of major vessels as revealed by pancreatic-phase, thin-section helical CT. Am J Roentgenol. 1997;168:1439–43. https://doi.org/10.2214/ajr.168.6.9168704.

58. Hough TJ, Raptopoulos V, Siewert B, Matthews JB. Teardrop superior mesenteric vein: CT sign for unresectable carcinoma of the pancreas. Am J Roentgenol. 1999;173:1509–12. https://doi.org/10.2214/ajr.173.6.10584793.
59. Noone TC, Hosey J, Firat Z, Semelka RC. Imaging and localization of islet-cell tumours of the pancreas on CT and MRI. Best Pract Res Clin Endocrinol Metab. 2005;19:195–211. https://doi.org/10.1016/j.beem.2004.11.01.
60. Graziani R, Brandalise A, Bellotti M, Manfredi R, Contro A, Falconi M, et al. Imaging of neuroendocrine gastroenteropancreatic tumours. Radiol Med. 2010;115:1047–64. https://doi.org/10.1007/s11547-010-0540-1.

MR: What We Need to Know to Start to Interpret Radiological Pictures

11

Martina Sbarra, Matteo Napoleone, Alessandro Cina, Carmine Di Stasi, Gennaro Restaino, and Riccardo Manfredi

11.1 Magnetic Resonance Cholangiopancreatography

Magnetic resonance (MR) with cholangiopancreatography imaging is a noninvasive technique that allows the simultaneous evaluation of the biliary and pancreatic duct systems and the pancreatic parenchyma. The main advantages of MR scans are the lack of ionizing radiation, the use of large field of view and the very high contrast resolution between different tissue types.

The combination of tissue-imaging sequences and MR cholangiopancreatography (MRCP) provides comprehensive information to evaluate the full range of biliary and pancreatic disorders.

11.1.1 Imaging Protocol

The standard MR protocol includes various sequences, such as T2- and T1-weigthed imaging with and without fat suppression technique, diffusion-weighted imaging (DWI) and dynamic contrast-enhanced imaging after intravenous injection of gadolinium chelates. The different tissue types are characterized by various signal intensity in each sequence. For example, the fluid-filled structures or cystic lesions generally appear very hyperintense (bright) on T2-weighted images, the biliary stones very hypointense (dark) in all sequences, and the solid lesions with high cellularity hyperintense on T2-weighted images and hypointense on T1-weighted images with variable enhancement after injection of contrast material (Fig. 11.1):

- *T2-weighted sequence* (single-shot fast spin echo, SSFSE) with longer echo times (≥60 ms) provides a sharp anatomic display of the common bile duct (CBD) and of the pancreatic duct on coronal plane and on axial plane images, respectively, and well depicts fluid-filled hyperintense lesions in or around pancreas [1] (Fig. 11.2a, b).
- *Balanced steady-state free procession (SSFP) sequence* with shorter echo and repetition times has a contrast T2-/T1-weighted. Unlike T2-weighted SSFSE sequence, it is not susceptible to flow-related artefacts that may mimic filling defects in the biliary tree. The easiest way to identify balanced SSFP sequence is to look for blood vessels and fluid-filled spaces that normally appear hyperintense (Fig. 11.2c).

Electronic Supplementary Material The online version of this chapter (https://doi.org/10.1007/978-3-030-42569-2_11) contains supplementary material, which is available to authorized users.

M. Sbarra · M. Napoleone · A. Cina · C. Di Stasi
G. Restaino · R. Manfredi (✉)
Department of Radiology, Università Cattolica del Sacro Cuore, Rome, Italy
e-mail: riccardo.manfredi@unicatt.it

M. Mutignani et al. (eds.), *Endotherapy in Biliopancreatic Diseases: ERCP Meets EUS*,
https://doi.org/10.1007/978-3-030-42569-2_11

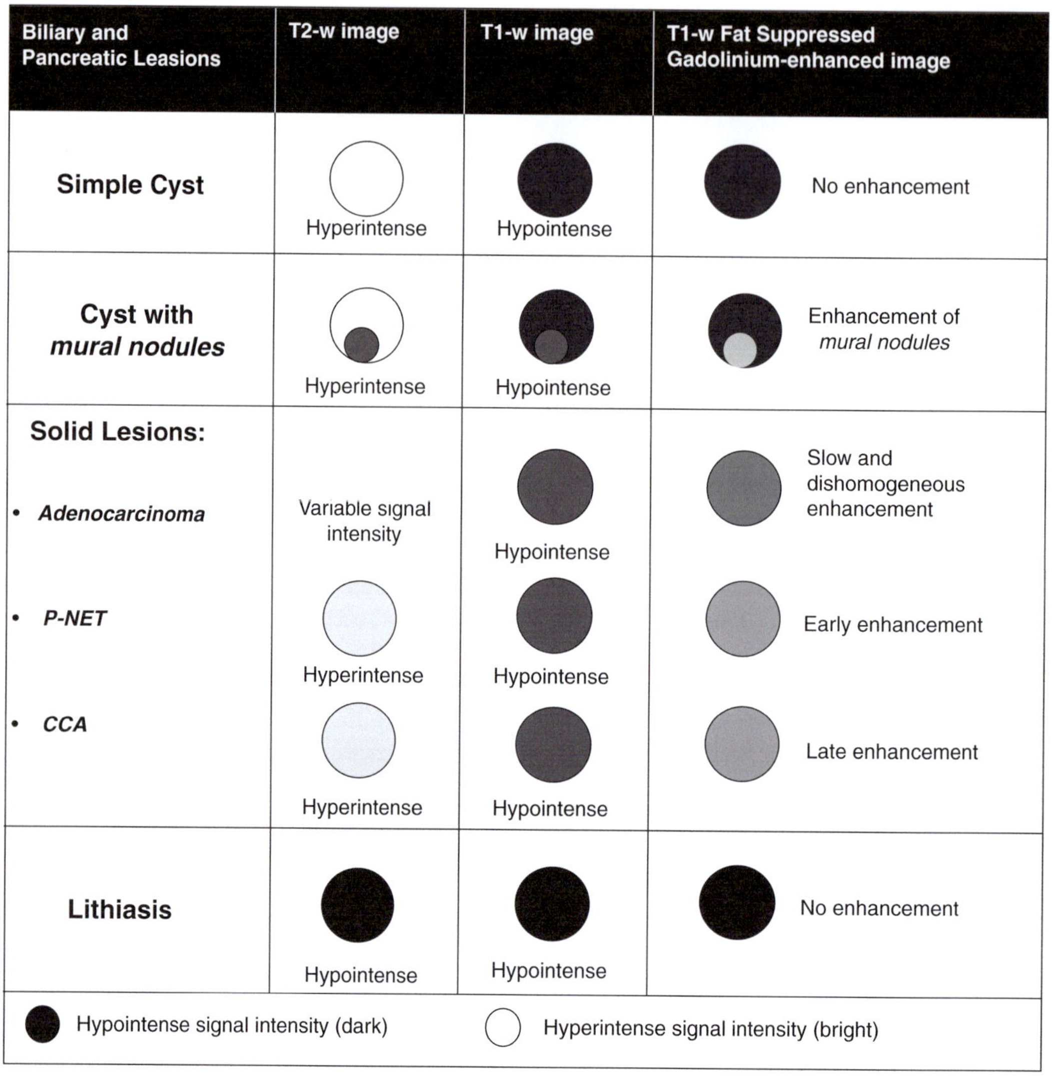

Fig. 11.1 MR signal intensity of the most common biliary and pancreatic lesions

- *T1-weighted sequence* (fast spoiled gradient echo, FSPGR) with shorter echo times (2.2 ms) is of paramount importance in the evaluation of the pancreatic parenchyma. The normal pancreas is a high signal structure compared to most pancreatic pathologies that are relatively hypointense [2]. Fat saturation is useful to improve the delineation of the pancreas that appears homogeneously brighter than the liver and the surrounding low-intensity fat [1] (Fig. 11.3a).
- *DWI* is typically performed by using a fat-suppressed T2-weighted sequence and exploits the random motion of water molecules in biologic tissues. The diffusion of water in tissues reflects at the same time a combination of tissue cellularity, tortuosity of extracellular spaces, integrity of cell membranes and viscosity of fluids [3]. Restricted diffusion structures result with high signal intensity (Fig. 11.2d).
- *T1-weighted sequence after gadolinium administration* (3D gradient echo sequences) is dynamically acquired with 40-s, 70-s and 180-s delay. Typically, the pancreas demonstrates a uniform enhancement in the capillary

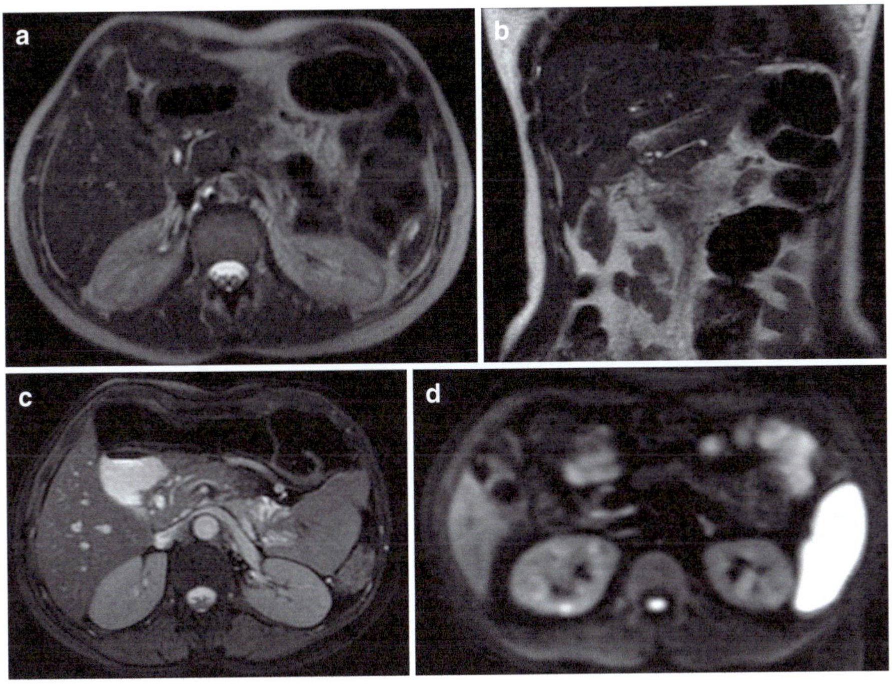

Fig. 11.2 Standard MR imaging protocol. (**a**) Axial T2-weighted sequence. (**b**) Coronal T2-weighted sequence. (**c**) Axial balanced SSFP sequence. (**d**) Axial DW image

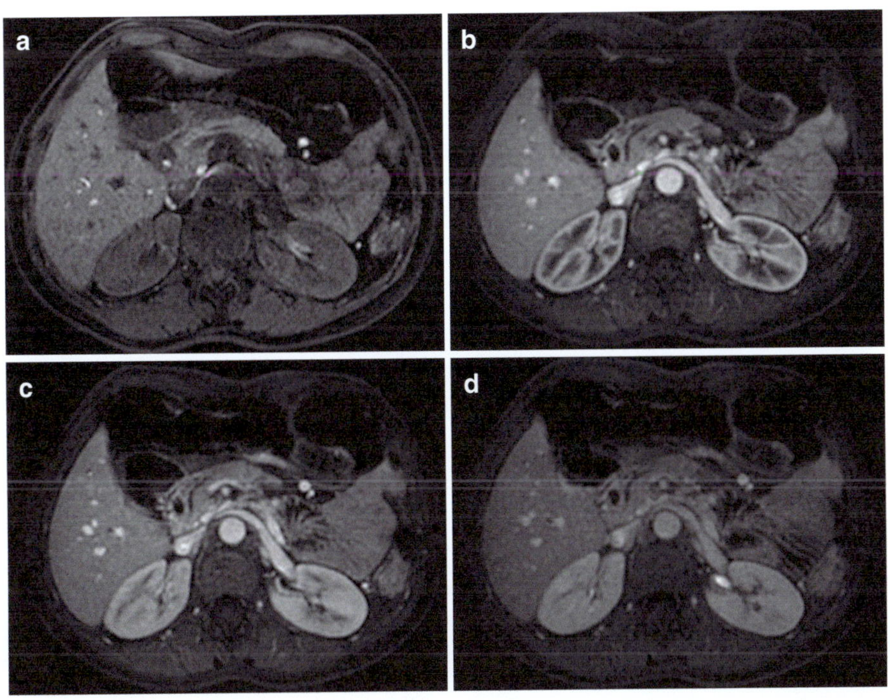

Fig. 11.3 Dynamic MR imaging during contrast agent administration. (**a**) Axial fat-suppressed T1-weighted sequence before gadolinium chelate administration and during (**b**) arterial (40-s delay), (**c**) nephrographic (70-s delay) and (**d**) pyelographic (180-s delay) phases

phase (40-s delay) [4]. The volumetric coverage and spatial and temporal resolution of fast gradient echo T1 sequences make possible the multiple post-processing reconstruction (Fig. 11.3b–d).

11.1.2 MRCP Technique

MR cholangiopancreatography (MRCP) is the imaging modality of choice to directly image the whole biliary and pancreatic duct systems without the need of contrast material agent administration.

This technique is based on heavily T2-weighted sequences with long echo times (>600 ms) that selectively displays static or slow-moving fluid-filled structures. Static and slow-moving fluids within biliary tree and pancreatic duct appear hyperintense, while surrounding tissue has lower signal intensity [5]. The result is an image that looks like those acquired by direct cholangiography in a totally noninvasive manner [6].

Two-dimensional (2D) or three-dimensional (3D) acquisitions may be performed to obtain MRCP images:

- *2D-MRCP* images are acquired on coronal oblique plane and can accurately demonstrate the whole extrahepatic biliary tract, the main pancreatic duct (MPD) and secondary ducts either in normal subjects or in dilated cases (Fig. 11.4). Since these sequences are virtually motion-independent, their quality is almost always diagnostic even in noncooperating patients. Because of the short acquisition time and there being no need for post-processing reconstruction, interpretation is immediately available. The main disadvantage is related to the two-dimensional nature, which may sometimes limit the visualization of thin ducts if they are projectively superimposed on other fluid structures. For this reason, improvements in MRCP technique can be made by using T2 shortening oral contrast agents (e.g. pineapple juice) that reduce signal from endoluminal gastric, duodenal or proximal jejunal fluid which may overlap and interfere with signal from the biliary system [6].
- *3D-MRCP* images are acquired on axial or coronal planes and provide a higher signal-to-noise ratio with the use of thinner contiguous slices (generally 4 mm thick) [1]. These thin

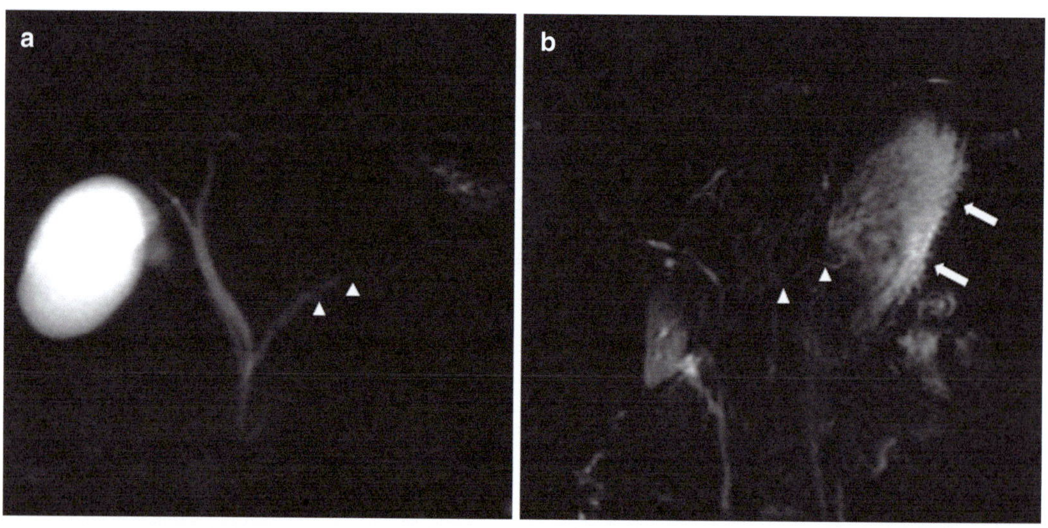

Fig. 11.4 2D-MRCP. (**a**) Coronal oblique image with the good visualization of the gallbladder, the whole extrahepatic biliary tract and the MPD (*arrowheads*). (**b**) Coronal oblique image with limited visualization of the MPD (*arrowheads*) due to endoluminal gastric fluid (*arrows*) projectively superimposed

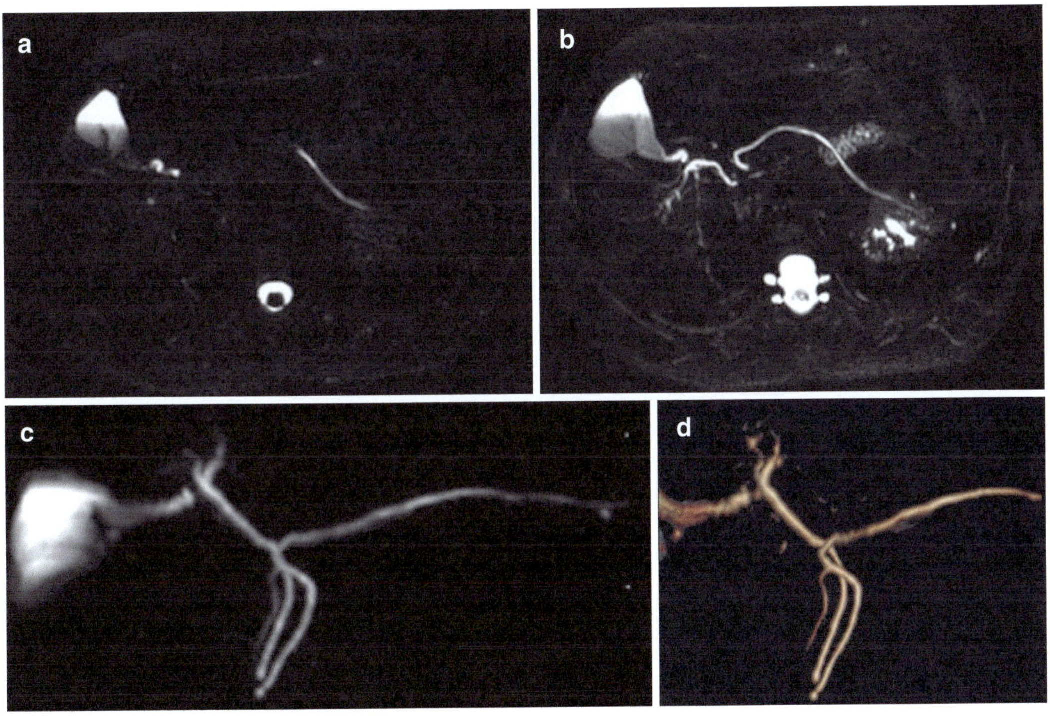

Fig. 11.5 3D-MRCP. (**a**) Axial 3D-MRCP image. (**b**) Axial multiplanar reconstruction image. (**c**) 3D-MIP (maximum intensity projection) image. (**d**) 3D-VR (volume rendering) image

slab sequences allow post-processing of the images for multiplanar reconstruction, maximum intensity projection and volume rendering [5] (Fig. 11.5). The 3D-MRCP should be performed for evaluating ductal-filling defects, visible as areas of decreased signal intensity, that may be missed with the 2D-MRCP thick-slab technique.

11.1.3 Secretin-Enhanced MRCP

Secretin-enhanced magnetic resonance cholangiopancreatography (S-MRCP), obtained after exogenous administration of secretin, has been suggested to improve sensitivity of MRCP in the visualization of pancreatic duct system [6].

Images are dynamically acquired in the coronal oblique plane with a temporal resolution of 30 s for 10 min. Secretin is responsible for both a physiological enlargement of the pancreatic duct system and an increase of the fluid content within the lumen of the pancreatic ducts. Its effect starts almost immediately after intravenous administration and peaks between 2 and 5 min. By 10 min, the calibre of the MPD should return to the baseline. Therefore, secretin-enhanced MRCP enables not only morphologic but also functional evaluation of the pancreas, providing information about the MPD flow dynamics and hydrodynamic changes [6, 7].

Moreover, this technique can indirectly assess the pancreatic exocrine reserve, evaluating the pancreatic output of juice through the duodenal papillae and duodenal filling [6–9]. According to the score described by Matos [8], the measurement of the duodenal filling may be performed in a semiquantitative manner: grade 0, no fluid signal in the duodenum; grade 1, fluid limited on duodenal bulb; grade 2, fluid filling up to the genu inferius; and grade 3 (normal), duodenal filling beyond the genu inferius (Video 11.1).

The main clinical indications for this imaging examination are recurrent acute pancreatitis, sphincter of Oddi dysfunction, anatomic variants, chronic pancreatitis and MPD stenosis [6].

11.2 MR Imaging of the Biliary System

11.2.1 Congenital Diseases of Biliary System

11.2.1.1 Choledochal Cysts

Choledochal cysts are rare congenital biliary tract anomalies characterized by cystic or fusiform dilations of part of the CBD and are often accompanied by intrahepatic bile duct dilation. Although they may be discovered at any age, 60% are diagnosed before the age of 10 years [10]. The aetiology is uncertain but is reported a close association with an anomalous pancreaticobiliary ductal union or dysfunction of the sphincter of Oddi.

According to Todani et al. [11, 12], the widely accepted classification system for choledochal cysts comprises five types: choledochal cyst (type I), diverticula originating from extrahepatic duct (type II), choledochocele (type III), multiple segmental cysts (type IV) and Caroli disease (type V) (Table 11.1).

Multiple imaging modalities can be used to diagnose choledochal cysts, including US, CT, MRCP, endoscopic retrograde cholangiopancreatography (ERCP) and percutaneous transhepatic cholangiography.

Table 11.1 Choledochal cysts according to Todani classification

Todani classification	
Classification	Characteristics
Type I, 77–87% (choledochal cyst)	(a) Diffuse dilatation of the entire common bile duct
	(b) Focal dilatation of the common bile duct
Type II, 3% (diverticulum)	Saccular outpouching arising from extrahepatic bile duct system
Type III, 5% (choledochocele)	Focal dilatation of the lower common bile duct that herniated into the lumen of the duodenum
Type IV 10% (multiple communicating intra- and extrahepatic cysts)	(a) Dilatation of the entire extrahepatic bile duct and the intrahepatic ducts
	(b) Dilatation involving only the extrahepatic bile duct
Type V (Caroli disease)	Dilatation of intrahepatic ducts with normal extrahepatic duct

The diagnosis of choledochal cyst is usually made with US, but information about the type of cyst, the length of the involved duct, the presence and location of protein plugs or calculi, the pancreaticobiliary junction and the length of the common channel is required, especially for preoperative planning. In the past few years, MRCP has increased its value as a less invasive option, demonstrating excellent overall detection rate for choledochal cysts. In addition, MRCP is helpful in detecting an abnormal pancreaticobiliary junction, which is seen in the majority of choledochal cysts [13].

These cysts appear as large fusiform or saccular masses, extrahepatic, intrahepatic or both, depending on the type of cyst, with a particularly strong signal on T2-weighted images (Fig. 11.6).

MRCP has replaced the more invasive techniques as the gold standard of diagnosis and should be safely used for diagnosis in both adult and paediatric patients. ERCP should be reserved in patients where therapeutic intervention is needed [14].

11.2.1.2 Anomalous Pancreaticobiliary Junction

Anomalous pancreaticobiliary junction is diagnosed when the union between the CBD and pancreatic duct is located far from the duodenum and the length of the common bile channel exceed 15 mm in adults and more than 5 mm in paediatric patients [5, 15]. This condition leads to a free reflux of bile within the lumen of Wirsung duct and pancreatic fluid within the lumen of the biliary tree [6]. This reflux is associated with high risk of pancreatitis and the development of biliary carcinoma [6]. On S-MRCP, the biliary reflux is well studied during dynamic acquisition as progressive CBD filling (Video 11.2).

11.2.2 Choledocholithiasis

The presence of a stone or stones within the CBD is known as choledocholithiasis.

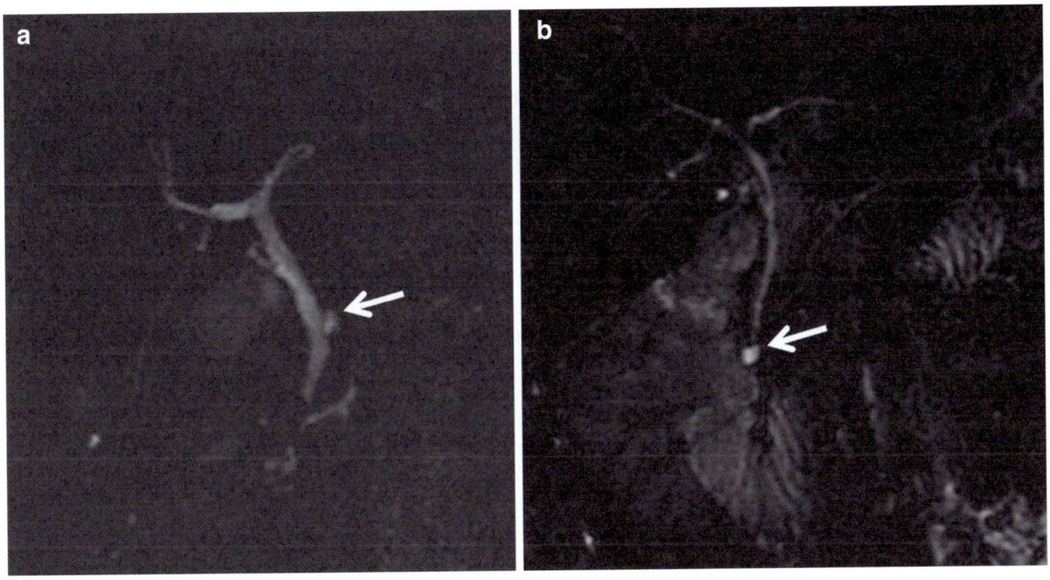

Fig. 11.6 Congenital choledochal cysts. (**a**) 2D-MRCP image shows a diverticulum (type II) that appears as a bright saccular outpouching (*arrow*) arising from sopra-duodenal extrahepatic bile duct. (**b**) S-MRCP image, 8 min delayed after administration of exogenous secretin, shows choledochocele (type III) that appears as a bright focal dilatation of the lower CBD (*arrow*) herniating into the lumen of the duodenum

US is usually the first investigation for biliary disease, but it has average sensitivity for the detection of biliary stones within the bile duct. Definitive diagnosis is made by advanced imaging, such as MR, particularly MRCP, ERCP and endoscopic ultrasound (EUS).

MRCP should be the method of choice for suspected cases of CBD stones, because it can show choledocholithiasis, in a totally noninvasive manner. MRCP has high diagnostic accuracy for the detection of choledocolithiasis, with high level of sensitivity (<90%) and specificity (>95%), as reported by Chen W. et al. [16].

Biliary stones are depicted as round or faceted filling defects within the biliary tree on thin cross-sectional T2-weighted imaging, surrounded by high-signal-intensity bile [17] (Figs. 11.7 and 11.8).

An impacted biliary stone will appear as a rounded filling defect with a crescent of bile. MRCP is also the preferred imaging modality for the assessment of intrahepatic stone burden.

Filling defects in the bile may arise, not only from bile duct calculi but also from the presence of gas, debris, haemorrhage and tumour. Aerobilia is seen as a nondependent filling defect on the axial images, while a signal void in the central part of the bile duct is due to flow phenomenon and may occur in dilated ducts and at the point of insertion of a large cystic duct [5].

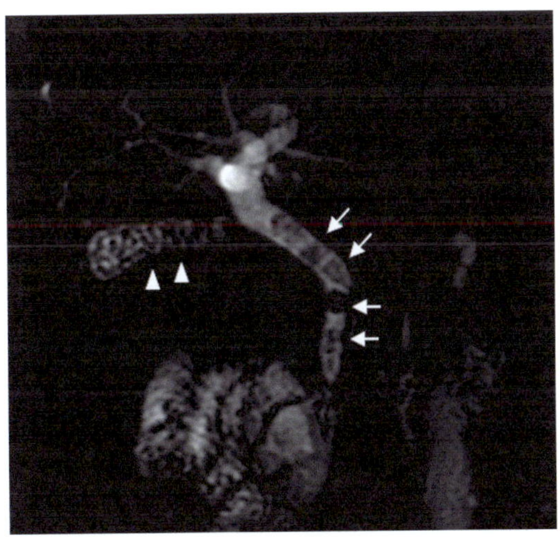

Fig. 11.7 Multiple biliary stones on 2D-MRCP image that appear as round hypointense (dark) filling defects localized within the CBD (*arrows*) and the gallbladder (*arrowheads*)

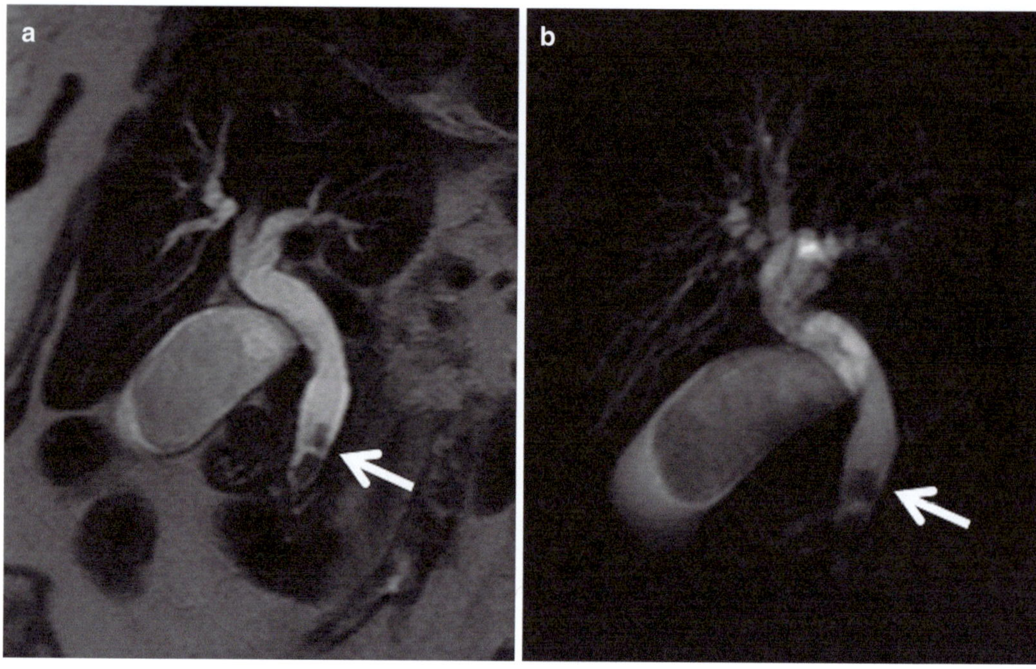

Fig. 11.8 Two hypointense biliary stones (*arrows*) in the distal part of the CBD on (**a**) coronal T2-weighted image and on (**b**) 2D-MRCP coronal oblique image

MRCP may allow for providing a higher spatial resolution than EUS, but is probably less sensitive than EUS for detecting CBD stones smaller than 6 mm [18].

11.2.3 Biliary Stricture

Biliary stricture is a fixed narrowing of a focal segment of the bile duct that results in proximal biliary dilatation. A wide spectrum of diseases, both benign and malignant, can result in the development of biliary strictures. It is important to differentiate malignant from benign strictures, since their treatment and prognosis vary.

US, CT and MR imaging play an important noninvasive role in the evaluation of suspected biliary stricture. MRCP is the best sequence for detecting strictures and may help to differentiate between benign and malignant causes.

Precontrast T1- and T2-weighted images are useful in the evaluation of the bile duct walls, peribiliary or periportal masses or collections and hepatic and pancreatic parenchymal diseases. Contrast-enhanced images aid in further characterization of the narrowed bile duct segment. Hepatocyte-specific MR contrast agents can be used and can help distinguish partial from complete biliary obstructions [19].

Unenhanced and contrast-enhanced MR imaging is extremely helpful in the evaluation of the narrowed bile duct segment and may suggest findings that are specific for a malignant cause. Kim et al. [20] show that a narrowed segment with the following MR imaging features is more likely to be malignant: hyperenhancement relative to the liver during the portal venous phase, length of over 12 mm, wall thickness greater than 3 mm, indistinct outer margin, luminal irregularity and asymmetry.

Biliary pseudostrictures on MRCP images may be present, and the most common causes of pseudostrictures include blooming artefact due to cholecystectomy clips and pulsation artefact from the hepatic artery (Fig. 11.9). In addition, MR imaging technique-related factors such as incomplete volume acquisition or incorrect reconstruction may also cause the appearance of a pseudostricture.

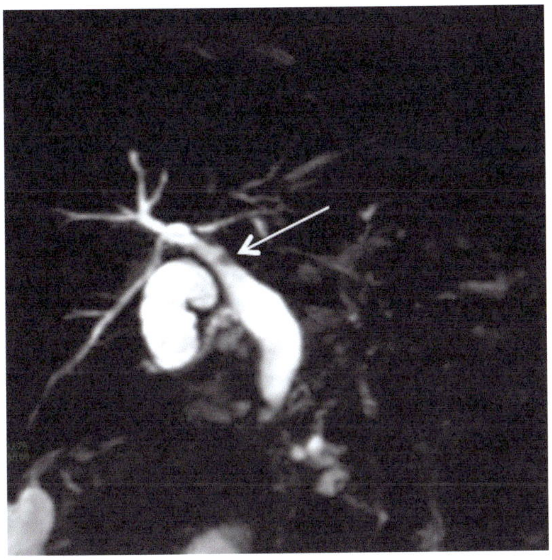

Fig. 11.9 Pseudostricture of the common hepatic duct, due to artefact from hepatic arterial pulsatile compression, that appears as an eccentric narrowing of the common hepatic duct (*arrow*) on MIP 3D-MRCP image

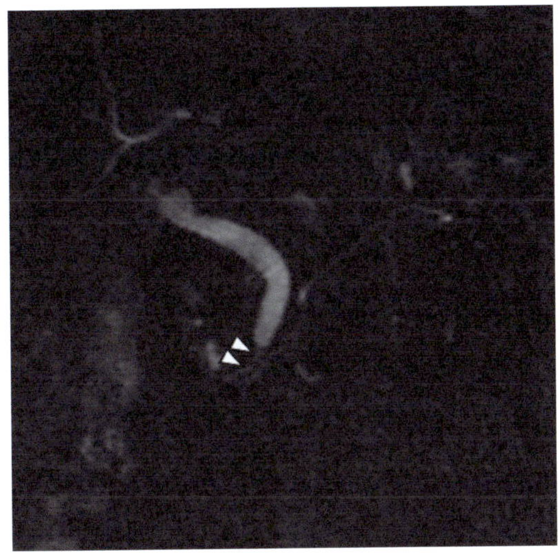

Fig. 11.10 Benign short-segment stricture (*arrowheads*) of the distal CBD with regular and smooth margins with moderate upstream dilation of the bile duct on 2D-MRCP image

11.2.3.1 Benign Biliary Stricture

Iatrogenic Causes

The most common benign biliary strictures are related to prior hepatobiliary surgery (up to 80–90% of cases), and cholecystectomy is the surgical technique that most commonly causes strictures of the extrahepatic bile ducts [19].

MRCP typically shows a short-segment smooth stricture of the common hepatic duct (CHD) or CBD with associated upstream biliary dilatation (Fig. 11.10).

However, MRCP may overestimate the length of the stricture, when the duct immediately distal to the stricture is not truly narrowed, but collapsed. After contrast material administration at MR imaging, the narrowed segment of the biliary duct commonly shows a thin and non-enhancing wall with smooth margins [19].

Primary Sclerosing Cholangitis

Primary sclerosing cholangitis (PSC) is an autoimmune chronic cholestatic disease, consisting of inflammatory and obliterative fibrosis of the intra- and extrahepatic bile ducts, that may progress to hepatic failure and cirrhosis.

MRCP is useful to evaluate the morphology of the bile ducts and to assess the parenchymal structure of the liver. At MRCP images, PSC typically has multifocal short-segment strictures of the intra- and extrahepatic ducts alternating with normal or mildly dilated ducts and peripheral pruning of the intrahepatic ducts. Hepatic parenchymal abnormalities are peripheral wedge-shaped or reticular T2-weighted bright lesions, hypertrophy of the caudate lobe and medial segment of the left lobe with atrophy of the lateral and posterior segments and large regenerating nodules. After contrast-enhanced administration, MR imaging may show enhancement of the thickened wall of the bile ducts, as well as multiple enhancing areas of fibrosis in the liver periphery [19].

11.2.3.2 Malignant Biliary Stricture

Cholangiocarcinoma

Cholangiocarcinoma (CCA) is the most common malignancy of the biliary system, and it is the second most common primary hepatic tumour after hepatocellular carcinoma [21]. It tends to have a poor prognosis and high morbidity. Several pathologic subtypes exist, but the most cholangiocarcinomas are adenocarcinoma subtype [22].

Classification is based on the anatomic location: perihilar (pCCA 60%, also known as

Klatskin tumour), extrahepatic (dCCA 20%) and intrahepatic (iCCA 20%) [23].

Intrahepatic cholangiocarcinoma is localized close to the second-degree bile ducts; perihilar cholangiocarcinoma is located to the area between the second-degree bile ducts and the insertion of the cystic duct into the CBD; distal cholangiocarcinoma is confined to the area between the origin of the cystic duct and ampulla of Vater [24].

The anatomic distribution of the tumour dictates the pattern of observed ductal distention and obstruction.

Imaging characteristics, behaviour and therapeutic strategies in CCA differ significantly, depending on the morphology and location of the tumour. There are three different growth patterns of CCA: (1) mass forming, (2) periductal infiltrating and (3) papillary or intraductal.

Diagnostic modalities used in the imaging of CCA include US, CT and MR with cholangiopancreatogaphy. According to current guidelines, MR is the modality of choice for the diagnosis and staging of CCA. A typical MR protocol for the assessment of CCA encompasses MRCP, conventional T1- and T2-weighted sequences as well as DWI and dynamic contrast-enhanced MR. Furthermore, MRI with hepatocyte-specific contrast agents is often performed for the assessment of CCA [25]:

- *MR Imaging of Mass-Forming Cholangiocarcinoma:* mass-forming CCA is often seen in iCCA, and it is a homogeneous mass with irregular but well-defined margin frequently associated with dilatation of the biliary trees in the tumour periphery [24]. It usually appears hyperintense on T2-weighted images and iso- or hypointense on T1-weighted images. Contrast enhancement of mass-forming iCCA is variable, and the most frequent pattern is peripheral enhancement on early images, which increases on late images. Both the peripheral and the centripetal enhancement may be more prominent at MR imaging than at CT. Contrast enhancement depends on the tumour size, structure and degree of central fibrosis; small tumours with less fibrotic tissue may show homogeneous enhancement, whereas large fibrotic tumours may only enhance in late images. The area of the tumour with early enhancement indicates active growth.
- *MR Imaging of Periductal Cholangiocarcinoma:* periductal growth is usually seen in pCCA and dCCA, and it is characterized by growth along a dilated or narrowed bile duct, without mass formation. The MR images, particularly the T2-weighted images, show diffuse periductal thickening and increased enhancement due to tumour infiltration, with an abnormally dilated or irregularly narrowed duct and peripheral ductal dilatation. Periductal CCA usually shows slow contrast enhancement, which is best seen in late contrast-enhanced images.
- *MRImagingofIntraductalCholangiocarcinoma:* intraductal cholangiocarcinoma has a variety of imaging features; the imaging patterns include diffuse and marked duct ectasia with a grossly visible papillary mass (similar to mass-forming CCA, intraductal CCA begins to enhance on early post-contrast images, with peak enhancement on late post-contrast images), diffuse and marked duct ectasia without a visible mass, localized ductal dilatation with an intraductal mass, intraductal soft-tissue material within a mildly dilated duct and focal stricture-like lesion with mild proximal ductal dilatation. MRCP is very suitable for the detection of intraductal CCA, with a higher diagnostic accuracy when compared to CT [25–27] (Fig. 11.11).

Ampullary Carcinoma

Ampullary carcinoma is a rare malignancy arising from the ampulla of Vater, and when suspicious malignant stricture of the distal CBD is detected, it should be taken into consideration. This tumour may appear at MR imaging as a small nodular mass, periductal thickening or bulging of duodenal papillae. The mass is isointense relative to the adjacent duodenal wall on T1-weighted images and shows variable signal intensity on T2-weighted images and delayed contrast enhancement [28]. MRCP may show marked abrupt dilatation of the distal CBD or the pancreatic duct without signs of pancreatitis or an obvious pancreatic mass or stones (Fig. 11.12).

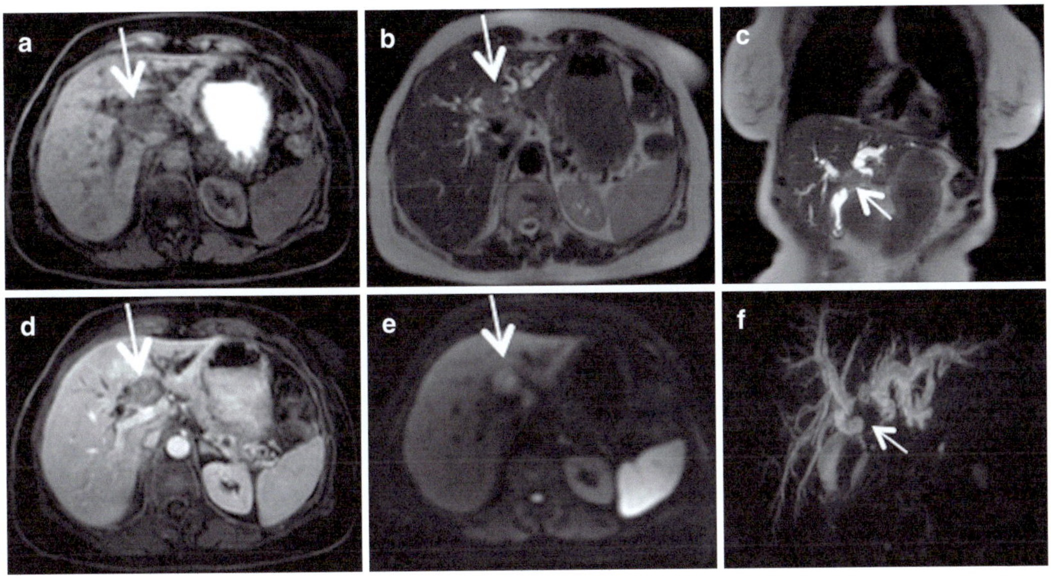

Fig. 11.11 Perihilar intraductal cholangiocarcinoma (Klatskin tumour, Bismuth type IIIB) that involves the confluence of the right and left hepatic ducts and extends to the bifurcation of the left hepatic duct. (**a**) Axial fat-suppressed T1-weighted image shows the biliary tumour (*arrow*) with hypointense signal intensity. (**b**, **c**) T2-weighted images on axial and coronal plane, respectively, show the hyperintense biliary tumour (*arrow*) with upstream dilation of the intrahepatic biliary ducts. (**d**) Fat-suppressed T1-weighted image after injection of paramagnetic contrast material (180-s delay) shows a delayed enhancement of the tumour (*arrow*), and (**e**) DWI a restricted diffusion of the lesion with bright signal intensity (*arrow*). (**f**) MIP 3D-MRCP shows the abrupt tapered end of the common hepatic duct at the stricture site (*arrow*) with associated marked upstream dilation of the intrahepatic right and left ducts

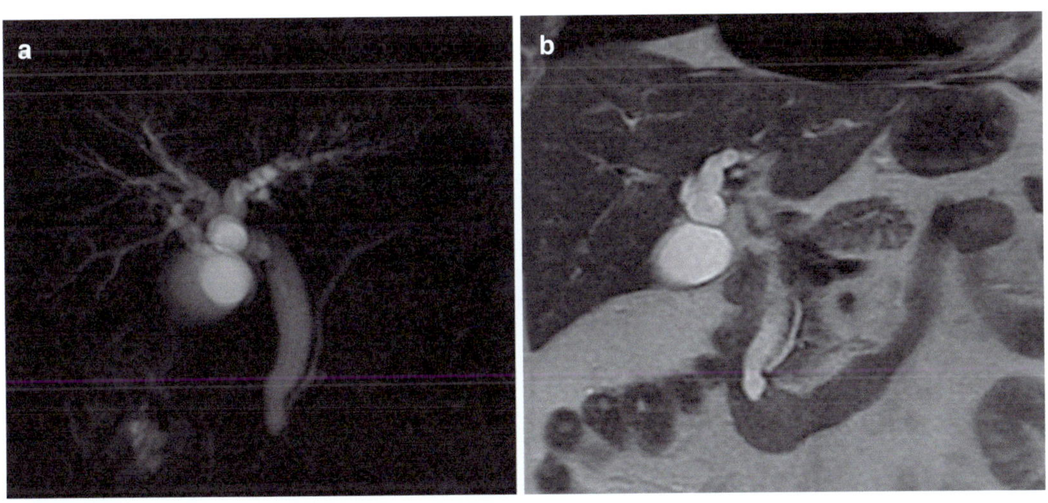

Fig. 11.12 Ampullary tumour with upstream abrupt dilation of the CBD on (**a**) 2D-MRCP image and on (**b**) coronal T2-weighted image

11.3 MR Imaging of the Pancreatic Ducts

11.3.1 Congenital Pancreatic Anomalies

11.3.1.1 Pancreas Divisum

Pancreas divisum is a congenital anomaly of the pancreas caused by lack of fusion between ventral and dorsal pancreatic ducts. At MRCP examination, the diagnosis of pancreas divisum can be suggested by the identification of two separate ducts entering the duodenum (Fig. 11.3). A coronal MRCP image can show (a) direct continuity of the dorsal pancreatic duct with the duct of Santorini which drains into the minor papilla and (b) a ventral duct that does not have connection with the dorsal duct, but joins with the distal bile duct entering the major papilla. Commonly, the ventral duct is short and very narrow, while the dorsal duct normally has a larger calibre [17]. S-MRCP improves the detection of pancreas divisum in 5–23% of patients, because it allows a more excellent assessment of the dorsal and ventral pancreatic duct and their relationship [6].

11.3.1.2 Santorinicele

Santorinicele is a cystic dilatation of distal dorsal duct just proximal to the minor papilla, due to obstruction and acquired or congenital weakness of the distal wall of the duct. When santorinicele occurs associated with pancreas divisum, it causes a relative stenosis of the minor papilla that may be clinically relevant, resulting in recurrent episode of acute pancreatitis (Fig. 11.3). S-MRCP allows a better evaluation of santorinicele [6, 29, 30] (Fig. 11.13).

11.3.1.3 Annular Pancreas

Annular pancreas is a rare anomaly, which occurs at a rate of 1 of every 2000 births. It is caused by a bifid ventral portion that encircles the duodenum and fuses with the dorsal pancreatic portion creating a ring around the duodenum [31]. On MR imaging, annular pancreas appears as high signal tissue on fat-suppressed T1-weighted sequences, completely or partially surrounding the second part of duodenum, with or without a small pancreatic duct (Fig. 11.14).

11.3.2 Pancreatitis

11.3.2.1 Acute Recurrent Pancreatitis

Acute recurrent pancreatitis (ARP) is diagnosed when patients have multiple episodes of acute pancreatitis [32].

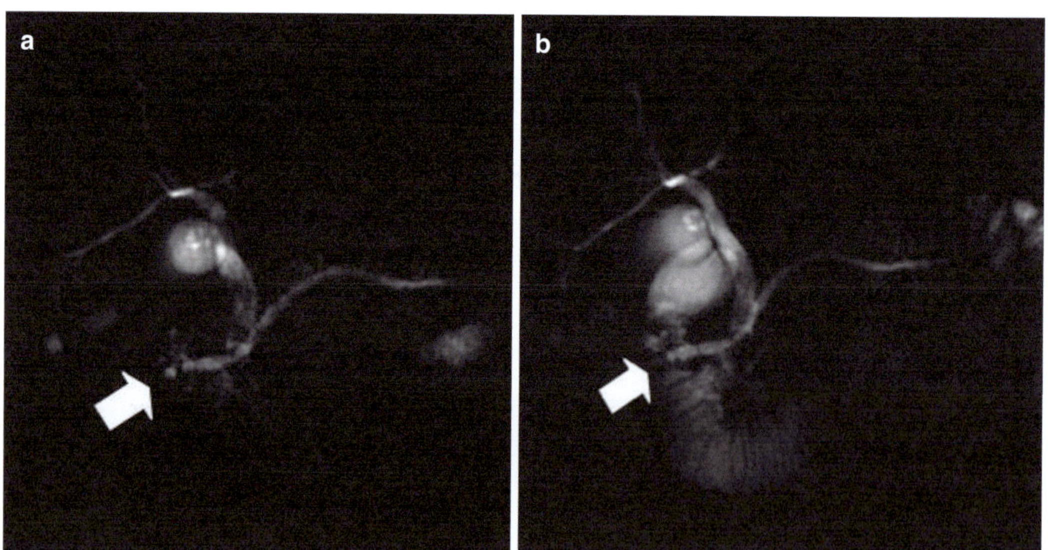

Fig. 11.13 Santorinicele (*arrow*) in pancreas divisum (**a**) before secretin administration and (**b**) after secretin administration, during S-MRCP examination

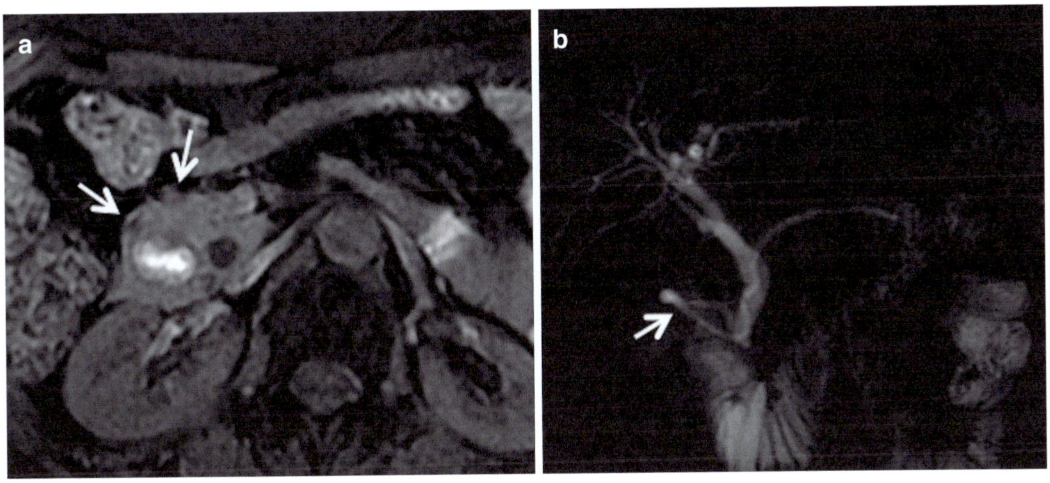

Fig. 11.14 Annular pancreas. (**a**) Fat-suppressed T1-weighted image shows the pancreatic parenchyma (*arrows*) completely encircling the second part of duodenum. (**b**) 2D-MRCP points out the pancreatic duct forming a ring around the duodenum (*arrow*)

In idiopathic ARP, when no cause is identified and the pancreatic duct is not dilated, S-MRCP is recommended as first-line imaging examination, in order to obtain better visualization of the pancreatic and biliary ducts.

More frequent causes of ARP are occulted microlithiasis, small lesions of the ampulla or pancreas, congenital anomalies of the pancreatic duct system (pancreas divisum, annular pancreas), biliary cystic diseases with anomalous pancreaticobiliary junction and sphincter of Oddi dysfunction [6, 33].

Table 11.2 Milwaukee classification of sphincter of Oddi dysfunction

Classification	Criteria
Type I	(a) Typical biliary pain (b) Elevated liver function test (×2 normal) on two or more occasions (c) Delayed drainage of contrast medium at ERCP (>45 min) (d) Dilated common bile duct diameter of >12 mm
Type II	(a) Typical biliary pain Plus one or more of B, C or D
Type III	(a) Typical biliary pain

Sphincter of Oddi Dysfunction

Sphincter of Oddi dysfunction (SOD) depends on abnormal contractility of the sphincter. Sphincter of Oddi manometry (SOM) is the goal standard to diagnose SOD and to select patients who benefits from endoscopic sphincterotomy [34].

According to Milwaukee classification, SOD has been classified in three categories, based on biliary pain, liver function tests, dilatation of MPD and delayed contrast medium at ERCP [6] (Table 11.2).

S-MRCP is a totally noninvasive diagnostic technique for investigating the sphincter of Oddi function. Therefore, ERCP and SOM are only needed in selected patients or difficult cases, for either therapeutic purposes or additional investigation, because they are both associated with high rate of post-procedure pancreatitis [33].

S-MRCP is an alternative approach to manometry in diagnosis SOD with a sensitivity of 37–57.1% and specificity of 85–100%, with better accuracy in type I–II sphincter of Oddi dysfunction in comparison with type III [34, 35]. The strength of S-MRCP is the lack of invasiveness. The difference between the basal and 10-min secretin-stimulated diameter of the MPD is evaluated as an indirect indicator of sphincter function. A persistent dilatation of the MPD, 10 min after administration of secretin, compared with baseline, is suspicious for sphincter of Oddi dysfunction (Video 11.3).

11.3.2.2 Chronic Pancreatitis

Chronic pancreatitis is a progressive fibrotic destruction of the glandular tissue as a result of different inflammatory processes. The diagnosis can be very challenging, and the real dilemma is to recognize and diagnose the disease in its early stage [33].

MR/MRCP is rapidly emerging as noninvasive important tool for the evaluation of pancreatic parenchymal and ductal abnormalities for the diagnosis, staging and evaluation of complications in chronic pancreatitis. In addition, the S-MRCP and DWI may be, respectively, possible to assess exocrine pancreatic function and to differentiate between focal chronic pancreatitis and cancer, all in noninvasive one session, with good sensitivity in early stage [36].

The staging of chronic pancreatitis is based on modified MRCP Cambridge Criteria [37] (Table 11.3).

MRI evaluates the parenchymal abnormalities, such as (a) reduction of the anteroposterior dimensions of the gland, (b) signal decrease on fat-suppressed T1-weighted images and (c) delayed perfusion of the glandular tissue [36].

MRCP also allows to detect the ductal abnormalities, such as (a) main pancreatic ductal dilatation associated with multiple stenosis and its loss of normal gentle taper and (b) dilated side branches, better seen after administration of secretin [36, 37] (Figs. 11.15 and 11.16). Calcified endoductal stones are difficult to diagnose at MR imaging. In fact, calcifications are better seen at non-enhanced CT examination (Fig. 11.16f).

Table 11.3 Modified MRCP Cambridge Criteria for chronic pancreatitis

Cambridge 1 (normal pancreas)	The side branches and main pancreatic ducts are normal
Cambridge 2 (equivocal findings)	Dilatation/obstruction of <3 side branches with a normal main pancreatic duct
Cambridge 3 (mild disease)	Dilatation/obstruction of ≥3 side branches with a normal main pancreatic duct
Cambridge 4 (moderate disease)	Include Cambridge 3 criteria plus stenosis and dilatation of the main pancreatic duct
Cambridge 5 (severe disease)	Include Cambridge 3 and 4 criteria plus additional obstructions, cysts, stenosis of the main pancreatic duct and calculi

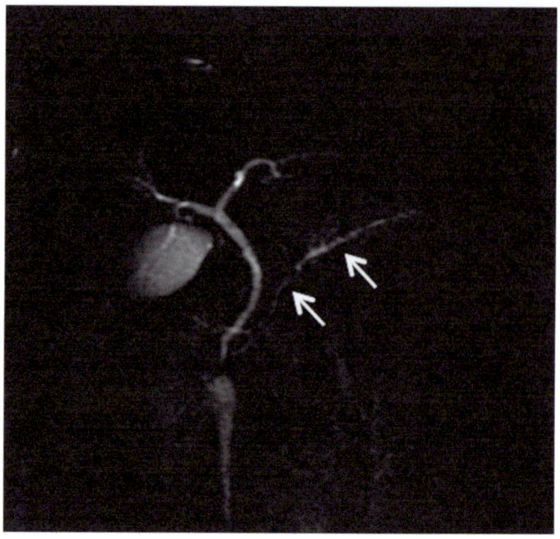

Fig. 11.15 Mild chronic pancreatitis (Cambridge 3) characterized by dilatation/obstruction of ≥3 side branches with a normal MPD (*arrows*) on 2D-MRCP image

S-MRCP may also be useful to assess hydrodynamically significant stenosis and pancreatic exocrine reserve by analysing the amount of pancreatic juice collected within the duodenal lumen [6, 38].

11.3.3 Solid Pancreatic Lesions

11.3.3.1 Pancreatic Adenocarcinoma

Adenocarcinoma is the most common malignant pancreatic tumour, affecting the head of the pancreas in 60–70% of cases. CT is the imaging technique of choice to detect and staging the tumour. MRI can be used as a problem-solving tool in equivocal CT cases: MRI may help rule out pitfalls such as inflammatory pseudotumour, focal lipomatosis, abscess or cystic tumours [39]. On imaging, pancreatic adenocarcinoma generally appears as hypovascular mass accompanied by secondary signs such as pancreatic duct cutoff, upstream ductal dilatation and parenchymal atrophy [40] (Fig. 11.17). An abrupt obstruction of the pancreatic duct in association with atrophy of the gland should

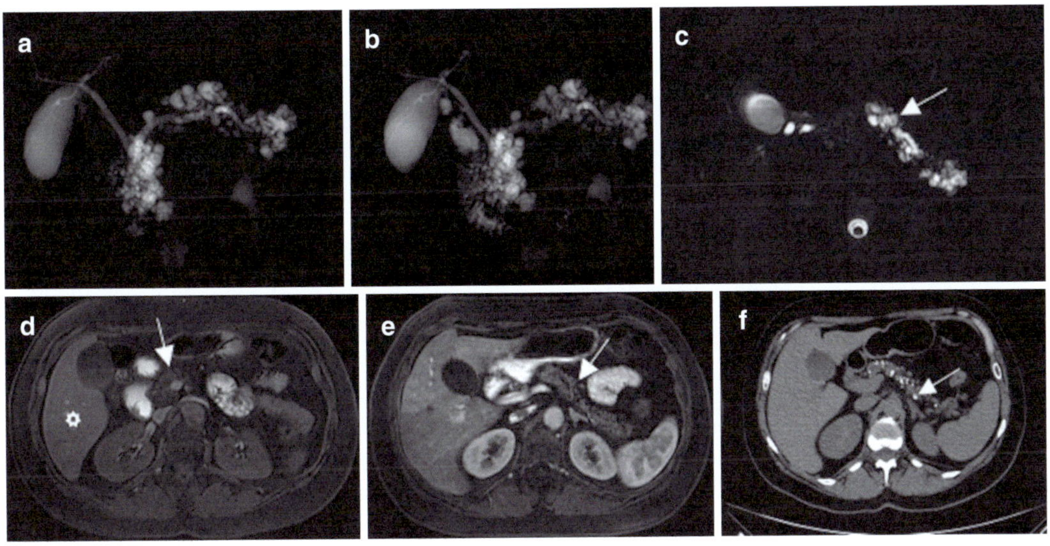

Fig. 11.16 Severe chronic pancreatitis (Cambridge 5), (**a**) S-MRCP before secretin administration with dilation/obstruction of >3 side branches and dilatation of MPD, (**b**) S-MRCP after secretin administration with reduced duodenal filling (grade 2) and reduced pancreatic duct compliance, (**c**) axial 3D-MRCP with evidence of small plugs (*arrow*) within dilated side branches, (**d**) axial fat-suppressed T1-weighted image with relative hypointensity of the pancreatic parenchyma (*arrow*) compared with the signal intensity of the liver (*asterisk*), (**e**) axial fat-suppressed T1-weighted image after gadolinium administration in arterial phase with reduced pancreatic enhancement and reduction of anteroposterior dimension of the gland, (**f**) axial non-enhanced CT image, with calcified endoductal stones

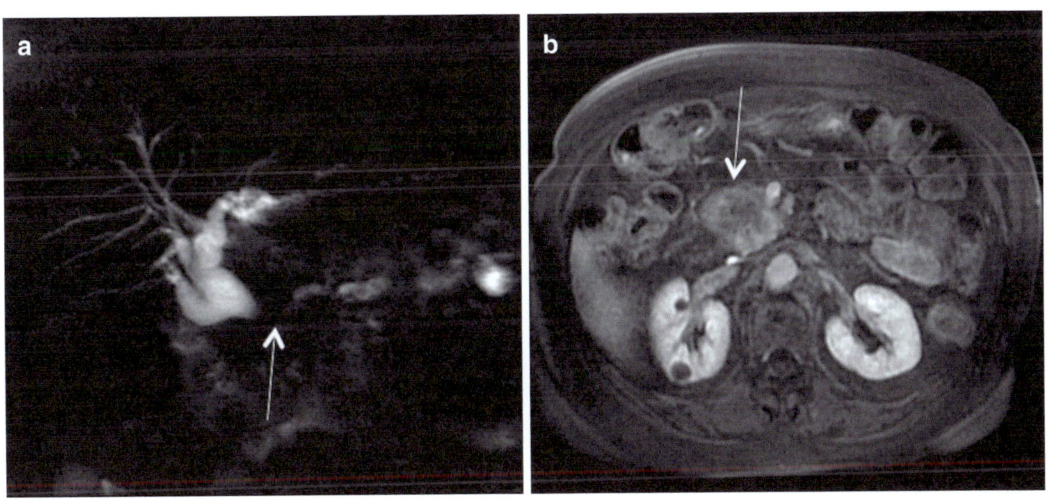

Fig. 11.17 Adenocarcinoma of the head of the pancreas that appears on (a) 2D-MRCP with the "double duct sign" (*arrow*) and in (**b**) fat-suppressed T1-weighted image as hypovascular mass (*arrow*) with inhomogeneous enhancement after paramagnetic contrast administration

arouse concern about the possible presence of pancreatic carcinoma [41]. If the lesion affects the head of the pancreas, on MRCP images the dilatation of pancreatic duct and/or CBD may be seen. Dilatation of both ducts is seen in approximately 75% of cases appearing as the "double duct sign" [5, 42]. If the double duct sign is present, the main differential diagnosis is between pancreatic adenocarcinoma and carcinoma of the ampulla of Vater.

MRI with the use of DWI may help in the identification of pancreatic lesions, even if small in size. On DWI images the lesion appears as hyperintense because of its restricted diffusion [43].

11.3.3.2 Pancreatic Neuroendocrine Tumours

Pancreatic neuroendocrine tumour (P-NET) is a rare pancreatic neoplasm with a better prognosis than adenocarcinoma. PNETs are unlikely to cause ampullary or ductal obstruction.

At MR imaging, they typically appear hypointense on fat-suppressed T1-weighted images and hyperintense on T2-weighted images. At contrast-enhanced MR imaging, PNETs are generally hypervascular relative to the normal pancreatic parenchyma [44, 45]. Only 24% of PNETs are hypovascular due to presence of stromal component. Others can appear as cystic lesions at imaging.

Multifocal lesions are typically associated with syndromic diseases (von Hippel-Lindau, VHL; multiple endocrine neoplasia, MEN).

11.3.4 Cystic Pancreatic Lesions

Cystic lesions of the pancreas have become a common incidental finding due to the expanding use of abdominal imaging. Despite significant developments in imaging technology MRCP and the advent of endoscopic ultrasound-guided fine needle aspiration (EUS-FNA), the detection and management of the pancreatic cystic lesions remains a significant clinical challenge [46]. The first diagnostic step is to differentiate between pancreatic pseudocyst and cystic neoplasm. If a pancreatic pseudocyst has been excluded, the second step is to determine the type and malignant potential of cystic neoplasm. Cystic pancreatic neoplasms represent approximately 10–15% of primary pancreatic cystic masses and are classified as intraductal papillary mucinous neoplasms, serous cystadenoma, mucinous cystic neoplasm and solid pseudopapillary tumour [46]. MR/MRCP is considered the noninvasive modality of choice for demonstrating the presence of cystic lesions and its morphologic features (uni- or multilocular), evaluating the location, size and number of lesions, establishing the presence of communication between the cystic lesion and the pancreatic duct and detecting any enhanced mural nodes or soft-tissue masses after administration of paramagnetic contrast material [47].

11.3.4.1 Pseudocyst

Pseudocyst is the most common pancreatic non-neoplastic cystic lesion associated with pancreatitis or trauma. It occurs in about 20–40% of patients with chronic pancreatitis and in 2–3% of those with acute pancreatitis [48]. Pseudocysts result from haemorrhagic fat necrosis and encapsulation of pancreatic secretions by granulation tissue. MR generally shows a unilocular cystic lesion, adjacent of any portion of the pancreas, that may contain a simple fluid content (hyperintense on T2-weighted images) or blood products and proteinaceous fluid (hyperintense on T1-weighted images) [49]. MRCP may demonstrate the communication of the pseudocyst with pancreatic ductal system. Over time pseudocyst become well circumscribed, with a thickened enhancing wall after administration of paramagnetic contrast material. The primary mimic of pseudocyst is MCN; in this cases serial follow-up imaging evaluation are helpful because pseudocyst reduces in size over time (Fig. 11.18).

11.3.4.2 Intraductal Papillary Mucinous Neoplasm

Intraductal papillary mucinous neoplasms (IPMNs) are mucinous cystic pancreatic neoplasms that originate from the mucinous epithelium of the pancreatic ductal system and are characterized by intraductal papillary growth and abundant mucin production, leading to ductal dilatation. IPMNs occur slightly more commonly in men, with a mean age of occurrence of 65 years [49].

IPMNs are classified into three types: main duct IPMN (MD-IPMN), branch duct IPMN (BD-IPMN) and mixed type:

- *MD-IPMN* appears at MRCP as a segmental or diffuse dilatation of the MPD of >5 mm with hyperintense T2 signal (Fig. 11.19). The mean frequency of invasive carcinoma and high-

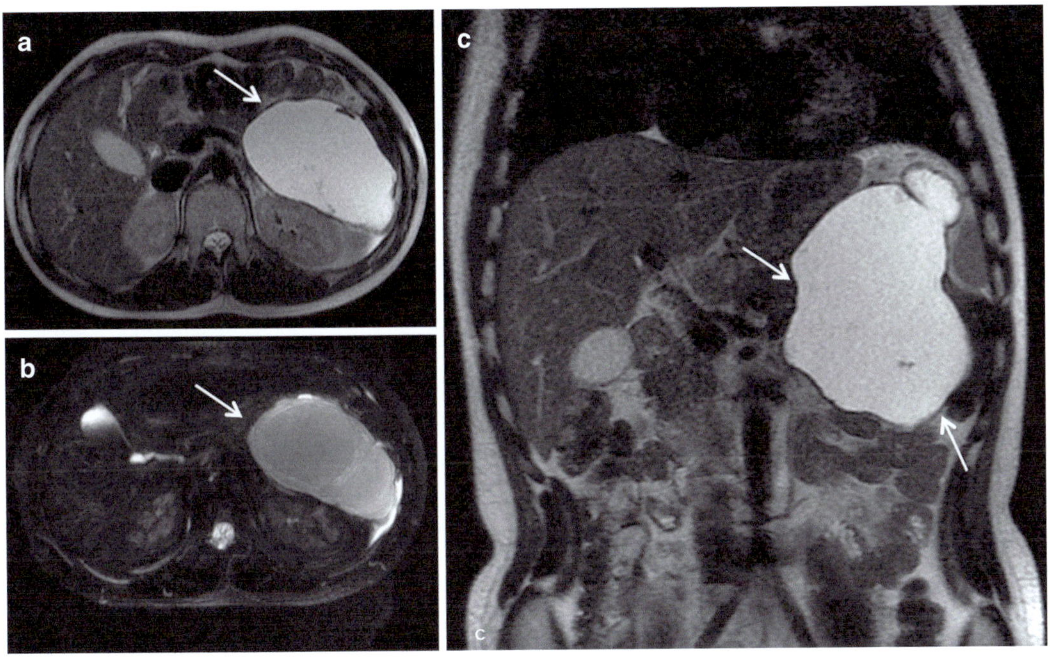

Fig. 11.18 Large pancreatic pseudocyst adjacent to the body/tail of the pancreas that appears as a unilocular bright fluid cystic lesion with mild thick wall (*arrows*) on (**a**) axial T2-weighted image, (**b**) axial 3D-MRCP and **c** coronal T2-weighted image

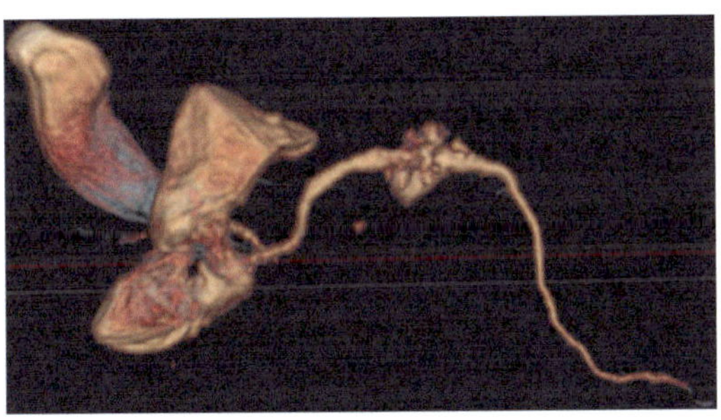

Fig. 11.19 MD-IPMN on VR 3D-MRCP image

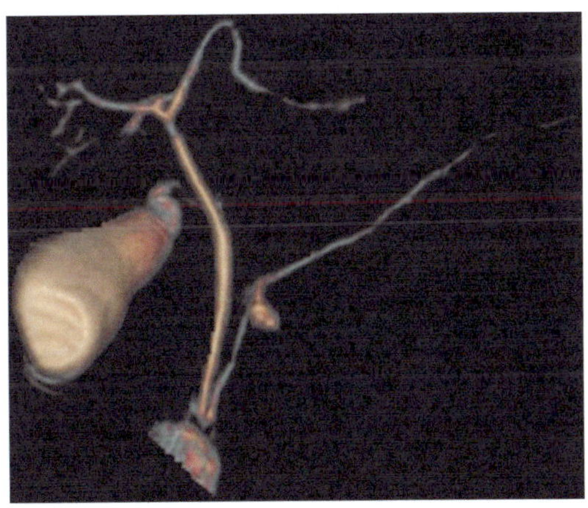

Fig. 11.20 Single BD-IPMN on VR 3D-MRCP image

grade dysplasia (HGD) is 61.6%, and the mean frequency of invasive IPMN is 41.3%. Surgical resection is strongly recommended for all patients with MPD >10 mm or with enhanced mural nodes [50]. MRCP is useful to exclude any other causes of MPD dilatation such as chronic pancreatitis or focal pancreatic lesion. In the diffuse dilatation type, without the presence of focal lesions, more careful evaluation is warranted, including ERCP. The endoscopic appearance of mucin extrusion from a widely patent papilla is diagnostic of IPMN.

– *BD-IPMN* appears at MRCP as small round or oval lobulated cystic lesion in communication with the MPD with a narrow neck at cyst-duct junction. They appear hyperintense on T2-weighted images and may have both a macrocystic and microcystic pattern with few or multiple septa inside (Fig. 11.20). BD-

IPMN are frequently multifocal and 5–10% involve the entire pancreas (Fig. 11.21). Because their malignant potential is relatively low (31.1% for invasive carcinoma and HGD; 18.5% for invasive cancer), conservative management with follow-up in patients who do not have worrisome features is recommended according to Tanaka et al. [50].

- The worrisome features [50] are cyst ≥3 cm, enhancing mural nodule <5 mm thickened enhanced cyst walls, MPD size 5–9 mm, elevated serum level of CA 19-9 and a rapid cyst growth >5 mm/2 years. If the lesions present any worrisome feature, EUS-FNA investigation should be done.

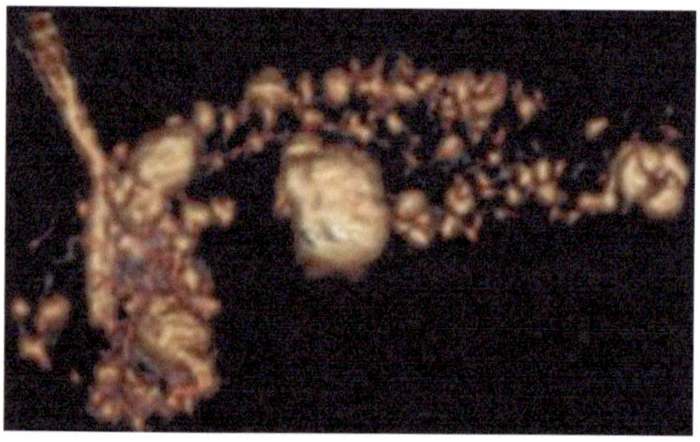

Fig. 11.21 Multifocal BD-IPMN on VR 3D-MRCP image

11.3.4.3 Serous Cystadenoma

Serous cystadenomas are benign in nearly all cases, indolent with slow growth and rarely symptomatic lesions [51]. They comprise approximately 20% of cystic lesions of the pancreas and more frequently occur in female between the sixth and seventh decades [48]. About 50% of these lesions are identified in the body and tail. The typical pattern is microcystic defined as multiple cysts measuring <2 cm separated by thin fibrous septa giving sometimes a honeycomb aspect. At MRI, microcystic serous cystadenoma appears as a cluster of tiny cyst with high T2 signal intensity, with intervening septa and a central stellate scar that may enhance on delayed contrast-enhanced MR images [49, 51, 52] (Fig. 11.22). MRCP shows no communication with pancreatic ductal system. In addition to the classic microcystic form, there are less common patterns: macro-/oligocystic, mixed and solid. In the oligocystic variant, the serous cysts are larger (≥2 cm), and the MR imaging appearance may mimic a mucinous cystadenoma. If there is no clear diagnosis after MRI, EUS should be performed. And if a doubt still remains, the association with FNA for cyst fluid analysis is necessary if technically feasible [49–51].

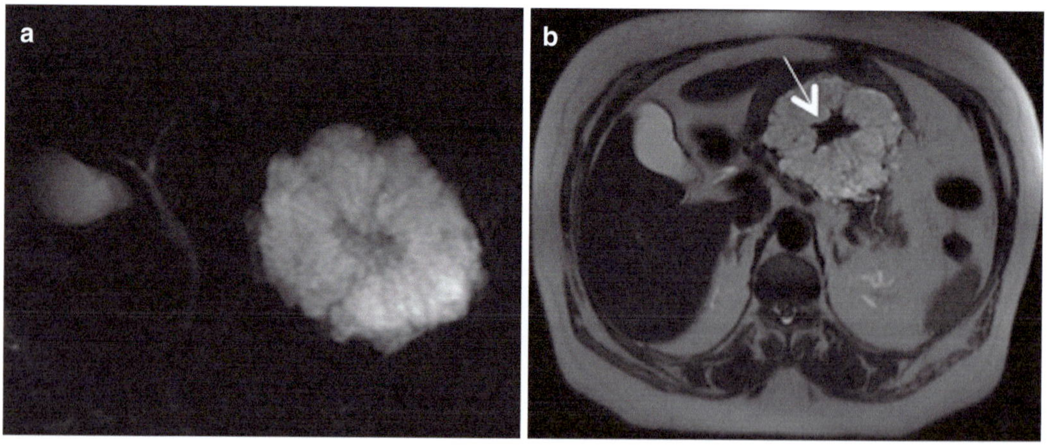

Fig. 11.22 Serous cystadenoma in the body/tail of the pancreas that on (**a**) 2D-MRCP image does not have communication with MPD and on (**b**) axial T2-weighted image appears as a hyperintense fluid lesion with microcystic pattern and a hypointense central stellate scar (*arrow*)

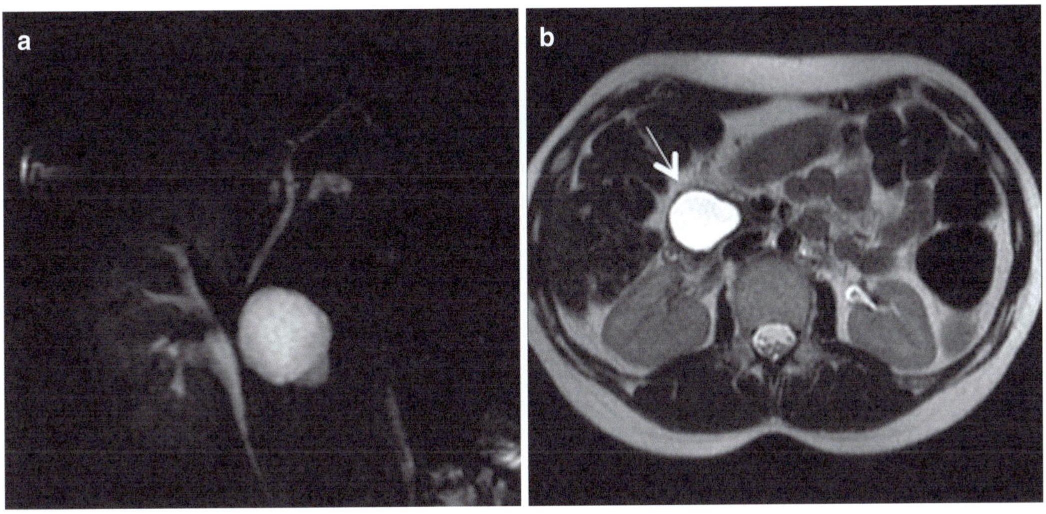

Fig. 11.23 Mucinous cystadenoma in the head of the pancreas that appears on (**a**) 2D-MRCP image and on (**b**) axial T2-weighted image as unilocular hyperintense fluid lesion (arrow) with no communication with the MPD

11.3.4.4 Mucinous Cystadenoma

Mucinous cystadenomas are benign pancreatic neoplasm, with a high-grade malignant potential. They comprise approximately 10% of cystic pancreatic lesion. The majority have been found in women with a mean age of 45 years, and they are generally located in the body and tail of the pancreas, without any communication with MPD [49–51].

At MR imaging mucinous cystadenoma appears as unilocular or mildly septate cystic lesion with thickened and delayed enhanced walls (Fig. 11.23). Despite of the mucinous fluid's content, they have homogenous low T1 signal and high T2 signal intensity. The presence of internal enhancing soft-tissue masses is indicative for adenocarcinoma. Generally, all of the lesions with an invasive carcinomas have a size of ≥4 cm and demonstrate soft-tissue nodularity [49, 52, 53].

11.3.4.5 Solid Pseudopapillary Tumour

Solid pseudopapillary tumour is an uncommon pancreatic neoplasm (5% of pancreatic cystic lesion) with low-grade malignant potential that occurs in young women (mean age, 28 years). The typical clinical presentation is abdominal pain with a palpable mass [48, 54]. Tumours may be solid or cystic with variable imaging characteristics. MRI generally shows a large (>6 cm), solitary and well-circumscribed lesion with no predilection of pancreatic localization. Areas of high T2 signal intensity correlate with cystic component, while areas of high T1 signal intensity are related to haemorrhagic degeneration. The haemorrhagic degeneration is one of the most specific MRI features of this lesion that may need a differential diagnosis with pseudocyst [54]. Enhancing soft-tissue components are uniformly present, allowing the differentiation from mucinous cystadenoma. Gradual accumulation of contrast material helps to differentiate solid pseudopapillary tumours from neuroendocrine tumours that have a typical arterial enhancement. Surgical resection is the treatment of choice.

References

1. Matos C, Cappeliez O, Winant C, Coppens E, Devière J, Metens T. MR imaging of the pancreas: a pictorial tour. Radiographics. 2002;22(1):e2.
2. Heyn C, Sue-Chue-Lam D, Jhaveri K, Haider MA. MRI of the pancreas: problem solving tool. J Magn Reson Imaging. 2012;36(5):1037–51.
3. Tang MY, Zhang XM, Chen TW, Huang XH. Various diffusion magnetic resonance imaging techniques for pancreatic cancer. World J Radiol. 2015;7(12):424–37.
4. Semelka RC, Kroeker MA, Shoenut JP, Kroeker R, Yaffe CS, Micflikier AB. Pancreatic disease: prospec-

tive comparison of CT, ERCP, and 1.5-T MR imaging with dynamic gadolinium enhancement and fat suppression. Radiology. 1991;181(3):785–91.

5. Griffin N, Charles-Edwards G, Grant LA. Magnetic resonance cholangiopancreatography: the ABC of MRCP. Insights Imaging. 2012;3(1):11–21.
6. Manfredi R, Pozzi Mucelli R. Secretin-enhanced MR imaging of the pancreas. Radiology. 2016;279(1):29–43.
7. Boninsegna E, Manfredi R, Negrelli R, Avesani G, Mehrabi S, Pozzi Mucelli R. Pancreatic duct stenosis: differential diagnosis between malignant and benign conditions at secretin-enhanced MRCP. Clin Imaging. 2017;41:137–43.
8. Matos C, Metens T, Devière J, Nicaise N, Braudé P, Van Yperen G, et al. Pancreatic duct: morphologic and functional evaluation with dynamic MR pancreatography after secretin stimulation. Radiology. 1997;203(2):435–41.
9. Cappeliez O, Delhaye M, Devière J, Le Moine O, Metens T, Nicaise N, et al. Chronic pancreatitis: evaluation of pancreatic exocrine function with MR pancreatography after secretin stimulation. Radiology. 2000;215(2):358–64.
10. Kim OH, Chung HJ, Choi BG. Imaging of the choledochal cyst. Radiographics. 1995;15(1):69–88.
11. Todani T, Watanabe Y, Narusue M, Tabuchi K, Okajima K. Congenital bile duct cysts: classification operative procedures, and review of thirty-seven cases including cancer arising from choledochal cyst. Am J Surg. 1977;134:263–9.
12. Kim MJ, Han SJ, Yoon CS, Kim JH, Oh JT, Chung KS, et al. Using MR cholangiopancreatography to reveal anomalous pancreaticobiliary ductal union in infants and children with choledochal cysts. Am J Roentgenol. 2002;179(1):209–14.
13. Lewis VA, Adam SZ, Nikolaidis P, Wood C, Wu JG, Yaghmai V, et al. Imaging of choledochal cysts. Abdom Imaging. 2015;40(6):1567–80.
14. Sacher VY, Davis JS, Sleeman D, Casillas J. Role of magnetic resonance cholangiopancreatography in diagnosing choledochal cysts: case series and review. World J Radiol. 2013;5(8):304–12.
15. Sugiyama M, Baba M, Atomi Y, Hanaoka H, Mizutani Y, Hachiya J. Diagnosis of anomalous pancreaticobiliary junction: value of magnetic resonance cholangiopancreatography. Surgery. 1998;123:391–7.
16. Chen W, Mo JJ, Lin L, Li CQ, Zhang JF. Diagnostic value of magnetic resonance cholangiopancreatography in choledocholithiasis. World J Gastroenterol. 2015;21:3351–60.
17. Patel HT, Shah AJ, Khandelwal SR, Patel HF, Patel MD. MR cholangiopancreatography at 3.0 T. Radiographics. 2009;29:1689–706.
18. Costi R, Gnocchi A, Di Mario F, Sarli L. Diagnosis and management of choledocholithiasis in the golden age of imaging, endoscopy and laparoscopy. World J Gastroenterol. 2014;20:13382–401.
19. Katabathina VS, Dasyam AK, Dasyam N, Hosseinzadeh K. Adult bile duct strictures: role of MR imaging and MR cholangiopancreatography in characterization. Radiographics. 2014;34:565–86.
20. Kim JY, Lee JM, Han JK, Kim SH, Lee JY, Choi JY, et al. Contrast-enhanced MRI combined with MR cholangiopancreatography for the evaluation of patients with biliary strictures: differentiation of malignant from benign bile duct strictures. J Magn Reson Imaging. 2007;26(2):304–12.
21. Blechacz B, Gores GJ. Cholangiocarcinoma: advances in pathogenesis, diagnosis, and treatment. Hepatology. 2008;48:308–21.
22. Bilgin M, Shaikh F, Semelka RC, Bilgin SS, Balci NC, Erdogan A. Magnetic resonance imaging of gallbladder and biliary system. Top Magn Reson Imaging. 2009;20(1):31–42.
23. Lowe RC. Epidemiology, pathogenesis and classification of cholangiocarcinoma. UpToDate 2019.
24. Razumilava N, Gores GJ. Classification, diagnosis, and management of cholangiocarcinoma. Clin Gastroenterol Hepatol. 2013;11:13–21.
25. Olthof SC, Othman A, Clasen S, Nikolaou K, Bongers M. Imaging of cholangiocarcinoma. Visc Med. 2016;32(6):402–10.
26. Chung YE, Kim MJ, Park YN, et al. Varying appearances of cholangiocarcinoma: radiologic-pathologic correlation. Radiographics. 2009;29(3):683–700.
27. Hossary SH, Zytoon AA, Eid M, Hamed A, Sharaan M, Ebrahim AA. MR cholangiopancreatography of the pancreas and biliary system: a review of the current applications. Curr Probl Diagn Radiol. 2014;43(1):1–13.
28. Kim JH, Kim MJ, Chung JJ, Lee WJ, Yoo HS, Lee JT. Differential diagnosis of periampullary carcinomas at MR imaging. Radiographics. 2002;22(6):1335–52.
29. Manfredi R, Costamagna G, Brizi MG, Spina S, Maresca G, Vecchioli A, et al. Pancreas divisum and "santorinicele": diagnosis with dynamic MR cholangiopancreatography with secretin stimulation. Radiology. 2000;217:403–8.
30. Boninsegna E, Manfredi R, Ventriglia A, Negrelli R, Pedrinolla B, Mehrabi S, et al. Santorinicele: secretin-enhanced magnetic resonance cholangiopancreatography findings before and after minor papilla sphincterotomy. Eur Radiol. 2015;25(8):2437–44.
31. Anupindi SA, Victoria T. Magnetic resonance cholangiopancreatography: techniques and applications. Magn Reson Imaging Clin N Am. 2008;16(3):453–66.
32. Levy MJ, Geenen JE. Idiopathic acute recurrent pancreatitis. Am J Gastroenterol. 2001;96(9):2540–55.
33. Larghi A, Petrone MC, Galasso D, Arcidiacono PG. Endoscopic ultrasound in the evaluation of pancreaticobiliary disorders. Dig Liver Dis. 2010;42:6–15.
34. Mariani A, Curioni S, Zanello A, Passaretti S, Masci E, Rossi M, et al. Secretin MRCP and endoscopic pancreatic manometry in the evaluation of sphincter of Oddi function: a comparative pilot study in patients with idiopathic recurrent pancreatitis. Gastrointest Endosc. 2003;58:847–52.
35. Pereira SP, Gillams A, Sgouros SN, Webster GJM, Hatfield ARW. Prospective comparison of secretin-

stimulated magnetic resonance cholangiopancreatography with manometry in the diagnosis of sphincter of Oddi dysfunction types II and III. Gut. 2007;56:809–13.
36. Choueiri NE, Balci NC, Alkaade S, Burton FR. Advanced imaging of chronic pancreatitis. Curr Gastroenterol Rep. 2010;12:114–20.
37. Balci NC, Bieneman BK, Bilgin M, Akduman IE, Fattahi R, Burton FR. Magnetic resonance imaging in pancreatitis. Top Magn Reson Imaging. 2009;20:25–30.
38. Manfredi R, Costamagna G, Brizi MG, Maresca G, Vecchioli A, Colagrande C, et al. Severe chronic pancreatitis versus suspected pancreatic disease: dynamic MR cholangiopancreatography after secretin stimulation. Radiology. 2000;214(3):849–55.
39. Schima W, Ba-Ssalamah A, Kölblinger C, Kulinna-Cosentini C, Puespoek A, Götzinger P. Pancreatic adenocarcinoma. Eur Radiol. 2007;17(3):638–49.
40. Yoon SH, Lee JM, Cho JY, Lee KB, Kim JE, Moon SK, et al. Small (≤ 20 mm) pancreatic adenocarcinomas: analysis of enhancement patterns and secondary signs with multiphasic multidetector CT. Radiology. 2011;259(2):442–52.
41. Leyendecker JR, Elsayes KM, Gratz BI, Brown JJ. MR cholangiopancreatography: spectrum of pancreatic duct abnormalities. AJR Am J Roentgenol. 2002;179(6):1465–71.
42. Ahualli J. The double duct sign. Radiology. 2007;244(1):314–5.
43. De Robertis R, Tinazzi Martini P, Demozzi E, Del Corso F, Bassi C, Perderzoli P, et al. Diffusion-weighted imaging of pancreatic cancer. World J Radiol. 2015;7(10):319–28.
44. Lewis RB, Lattin GE Jr, Paal E. Pancreatic endocrine tumors: radiologic-clinicopathologic correlation. Radiology. 2010;30(6):1445–64.
45. Graziani R, Brandalise A, Bellotti M, Manfredi R, Contro A, Falconi M, et al. Imaging of neuroendocrine gastroenteropancreatic tumours. Radiol Med. 2010;115(7):1047–64.
46. Draganov PV. Cystic neoplasm of the pancreas: a diagnostic challenge. World J Gastroenterol. 2009;15(1):48–54.
47. Manfredi R, Bonatti M, D'Onofrio M, Mehrabi S, Salvia R, Mantovani W, et al. Incidentally discovered benign pancreatic cystic neoplasms not communicating with the ductal system: MR/MRCP imaging appearance and evolution. Radiol Med. 2013;118(2):163–80.
48. Kucera JN, Kucera S, Perrin SD, Caracciolo JT, Schmulewitz N, Kedar RP. Cystic lesions of the pancreas: radiologic-endosonographic correlation. Radiographics. 2012;32(7):E283–301.
49. Kalb B, Sarmiento JM, Kooby DA, Adsay NV, Martin DR. MR imaging of cystic lesions of the pancreas. Radiographics. 2009;29(6):1749–65.
50. Tanaka M, Fernández-Del Castillo C, Kamisawa T, Jang JY, Levy P, Ohtsuka T, et al. Revisions of international consensus Fukuoka guidelines for the management of IPMN of the pancreas. Pancreatology. 2017;17(5):738–53.
51. Sahani VD, Kadavigere R, Saokar A, Fernandez-del Castillo C, Brugge WR, Hahn PF. Cystic pancreatic lesions: a simple imaging-based classification system for guiding management. Radiographics. 2005;25:1471–84.
52. Manfredi R, Ventriglia A, Mantovani W, Mehrabi S, Boninsegna E, Zamboni G, et al. Mucinous cystic neoplasms and serous cystadenomas arising in the body-tail of the pancreas: MR imaging characterization. Eur Radiol. 2015;25(4):940–9.
53. Di Paola V, Manfredi R, Mehrabi S, Cardobi N, Demozzi E, Belluardo S, et al. Pancreatic mucinous cystoadenomas and cystoadenocarcinomas: differential diagnosis by means of MRI. Br J Radiol. 2016;89(1057):20150536.
54. Ventriglia A, Manfredi R, Mehrabi S, Boninsegna E, Negrelli R, Pedrinolla B, et al. MRI features of solid pseudopapillary neoplasm of the pancreas. Abdom Radiol. 2014;39(6):1213–20.

12 Patient Management before and after EUS/ERCP

Katja S. Rothfuss and Jörg G. Albert

Careful analysis of the indication, patient condition and the planned proceeding of the endoscopy are mandatory for a successful procedure.

12.1 Pre-endoscopy Considerations

There are several considerations before starting the endoscopic procedure (Table 12.1). It is generally recommended to check the patient's past medical history including current medication, to do a complete physical examination and specific laboratory tests for preprocedure testing. If certain risk factors on the part of the patient are identified, further diagnostic examinations should be initiated, e.g. electrocardiogram (ECG), gastroscopy in patients with dysphagia or unclear anatomic conditions, further coagulation studies in case of suspected bleeding disorders, chest X-ray if decompensated heart failure is suspected, echocardiography if aortic stenosis is suspected and serum chemistry testing in patients with further comorbidities (endocrine, renal, hepatic, heart dysfunction). Risk factors are age dependent: critical incidents from sedation are more frequent in the elderly, but risk of post-ERCP pancreatitis is highest in younger patients and lower in elderly patients [1].

Table 12.1 Pre-endoscopy considerations

Patient selection	Indication	Is this procedure justified? What is the plan? Therapeutic vs. diagnostic procedure? Essential imaging results?
		Have alternative treatment options been considered?
	Comorbidities	Last meal of the patient?
		Intubation versus conscious sedation?
		Are there any spontaneous or iatrogenic coagulopathies present?
		Cardiopulmonary condition?
		Is the patient pregnant?
		In severe cholangitis emergency ERCP within 12 h
		Past medical history, past operations (biliodigestive anastomosis?)
Patient care	Prophylaxis of complications	Methods for pancreatitis prophylaxis (pancreatic duct stent, rectal indomethacin or diclofenac)?
		Prophylactic antibiotics indicated (e.g. PSC)?
	Radiation protection	Optimal positioning of the patient?
		Pelvic protection of the patient?
		Protection of the endoscopic team (e.g. eye protection, positioning of the team?)
		Low-dose imaging? Collimation?

K. S. Rothfuss (✉) · J. G. Albert
Department of Gastroenterology, Hepatology und Endocrinology, Robert-Bosch-Hospital, Stuttgart, Germany
e-mail: Katja.Rothfuss@rbk.de

M. Mutignani et al. (eds.), *Endotherapy in Biliopancreatic Diseases: ERCP Meets EUS*,
https://doi.org/10.1007/978-3-030-42569-2_12

For laboratory testing at least a complete blood count and coagulation studies (prothrombin time/ international normalized ratio (INR) and partial thromboplastin time (PTT)) are necessary, especially if interventions with high bleeding risk, e.g. ERCP with sphincterotomy, sphincterotomy + large balloon papillary dilatation, ampullectomy, EUS-guided fine needle aspiration biopsy of cysts and EUS-guided stent therapy, are intended. As sphincterotomy is declared a high-risk procedure, any anticoagulant therapy (except ASS) should be stopped well enough in advance. In case of an emergency ERCP (e.g. acute cholangitis) or in case of high thrombotic risk of the patient without the possibility to withdraw the dual antiplatelet therapy, small-calibre balloon sphincter dilatation or temporary biliary stent placement should be considered as an alternative to sphincterotomy.

In many patients anticoagulants and/or antiplatelet agents (APA) are needed to prevent or to treat cardiovascular disease. Weighing the risk of thrombosis in case of withdrawal of anticoagulants against the risk stratification of the endoscopic procedures should result in a well-balanced preprocedural decision. The assessment of the individual thrombotic risk of the patient, the haemorrhagic potential of the intervention and the urgency of the treatment have to be weighed against each other. Procedures with a low risk of bleeding (e.g. diagnostic ERCP and sole stent placement) don't require any APA or anticoagulation therapy adaptation. Oral anticoagulation therapy (warfarin) needs bridging with heparin only in high-risk cardiovascular conditions. High-risk vascular conditions (e.g. coronary artery stents) may require consultation of a cardiologist. For better evaluation and indication of the necessary ERCP, laboratory tests including bilirubin, alkaline phosphatase, G-GT, AST, ALT, lipase/ amylase and CrP are very helpful additionally to previously completed imaging results (ultrasound, CT or magnetic resonance cholangiopancreatography (MRCP)). ESGE recommends liver function tests and abdominal ultrasonography in suspected common bile duct stones and if ultrasound is insufficient complementary endoscopic ultrasonography (EUS) or MRCP [2].

12.2 Informed Consent

Informed written consent 24 h in advance is necessary not only on legal grounds but because ERCP carries an approximately 5% risk of major complications, including acute pancreatitis, post-sphincterotomy bleeding, sepsis and perforation. EUS-guided fine needle aspiration (EUS-FNA) of solid lesions carries only a **low bleeding risk** in contrast to EUS-guided therapy of cystic lesions or other kind of therapeutic procedures (e.g. EUS-guided biliary stenting) involving a **high-risk bleeding procedure** [3]. As part of the informed consent, the patient should be informed about risk factors, the fact that fluoroscopy might be needed, the specific benefits and possible alternatives of the endoscopic procedure. The patient should get to know the interventionalist befor the procedure, ideally some days before starting the intervention. If the procedure is not an emergency, the patient should be given 24 h time for consideration. Sedation is highly recommended during endoscopy also requiring informed consent with its benefits and adverse effects (allergic reaction, hypotension, hypoxemia despite careful monitoring and administration of oxygen, etc.). The informed consent process may vary from country to country just the same as the practice of sedation.

12.3 Conscious Sedation (see also Chap. 7)

The optimal sedation strategy should be preplanned before the endoscopic procedure and tailored to the patient based on specific risks, type and length of procedure. Meanwhile intravenous conscious propofol monotherapy has replaced "standard" combination sedation of short-acting benzodiazepines and opioids almost everywhere [4]. Propofol is more effective and safer in reaching and maintaining an adequate sedation level combined with a short recovery time. In Germany, most endoscopies are performed with moderate sedation and non-anesthesiologist-administered propofol (NAAP) services requiring a specialised nurse or doctor, having acquired adequate skills and knowledge through dedicated theoretical and practical training. The patient's American Society of Anesthesiologists (ASA) class, physical status, age, body mass index, Mallampati's classification and risk factors for obstructive sleep apnea (OSA) need to be assessed before each procedure. The ESGE recommends primary involvement of an anesthesiologist in patients of ASA class ≥3, with a Mallampati's class ≥3 or other conditions that put them at risk of airway obstruction [4]. At least one safe fixed venous line is required for i.v. sedation until full patient recovery.

12.4 Radiation Protection and Patient Position

Optimal positioning of the patient for ERCP is the **abdominal** or in other words **prone position** because of less radiation exposure during fluoroscopy and better recognition of (inadvertent) guidewire insertion of the pancreatic duct crossing the vertebral column apparent under fluoroscopy. EUS ideally is carried out in the **left lateral position** just the same as during gastroscopy. Both positions avoid aspiration of potential stomach contents and saliva. In intubated and mechanically ventilated patients the **supine position** is preferred due to facilitated airway access. Before starting ECRP it is particularly important to determine if the X-ray source is located below or above the patient. The patient's best position is as far as possible away from the X-ray tube and closest to the X-ray detector. Always administer the ALARA (As Low As Reasonable Achievable) principles by only using pulsed fluoroscopy with the lowest possible pulse rate, time-limited fluoroscopy, collimating X-rays to a small field of view, rather using "last image hold" function than doing radiographs and using magnification only if absolutely necessary. Certainly recording of overall fluoroscopy dose and fluoroscopy time is an essential part of every ERCP report.

Radiosensitive organs like the thyroid gland, breasts, gonads and eyes are kept out of the main X-ray beam whenever possible; this is particularly important in unfavourable oblique radiographic projections.

Pregnancy should also be excluded in women of childbearing age. In pregnant women and in children, there must be a very strong clinical indication only to perform EUS and/or ERCP with a therapeutic purpose by an experienced endoscopist. Whenever possible ERCP in pregnant women is probably best performed in the second trimester of pregnancy—if deferrable—with strictest recommendations to decrease radiation dose and adapted techniques like special cannulation techniques (guide wired without fluoroscopy, confirmation by bile aspiration, etc.). In pregnant women shielding the foetus by placing the radioprotective apron (RP shield) between the X-ray tube and the abdomen is recommended [5]. Because the prone position in advanced pregnancy is not possible, ERCP is done in left lateral position.

12.5 "Team-Time-Out"

The core endoscopy team should introduce themselves to the patient. Immediately before starting the procedure, a structured "team-time-out" (similar to the WHO surgical safety checklist) is required for an update of all endoscopic team members to check identification of the patient with its comorbidities, written consent form to the procedure and sedation, correct indication of the intended endoscopic procedure (including proper working equipment), the imminent tasks of every participant and the foreseeing of potential risks of the procedure. Is all necessary equipment present and ready to perform the planned EUS/ERCP?

12.6 Patient Management Before and During ERCP/EUS

Patients usually are kept fasting before the procedure; otherwise endoscopic view may be restricted and there is a high risk for aspiration of stomach contents. If there are food remains in the stomach despite fasting due to gastric emptying disorders, the procedure has to be cancelled, and the patient is kept fasting another day with additional prokinetic medication. In patients with suspected duodenal stenosis, the additional insertion of a nasogastric outlet tube at least 1 day before the procedure may be useful.

For some indications (primary sclerosing cholangitis (PSC), liver transplant patients) or procedures (incomplete biliary stenting, cholangioscopy, intraductal lithotripsy, pancreatic pseudocysts communicating with the main duct during ERCP, EUS-FNA of pancreatic cysts communicating with the main duct or located in the mediastinum, drainage of pancreatic pseudocysts), **antibiotic prophylaxis** prior to endoscopy is necessary.

For careful clinical **monitoring** commonly pulse oximetry, automated blood pressure measurement (at least every 3 min) and three-lead electrocardiogram monitoring is recommended. Routinely patients will receive oxygen per nasal oxygen tube (2 L) before, during and sometimes after sedation. Further equipment for airway management (a nasopharyngeal airway tube, the possibility of suction of secretion), resuscitation and endoscopy staff to be trained in advanced life support skills (e.g. tracheal intubation, defibrillation, etc.) is taken for granted.

In patients with automated implantable cardioverter-defibrillator, electromagnetic interference during electrocautery procedures (sphincterotomy) has to be taken into account. Tachyarrhythmia detection functions should be deactivated, or a magnet should be placed over the pulse generator; otherwise possibly defibrillation can be triggered. Consultation with a trained cardiology team should be carried out, and the device reprogrammed to its original state as soon as possible after the procedure.

The risk from **contrast agents**: An allergic reaction of the patient on contrast agents might be a risk factor. However, data are lacking on the extent of this complication and the value of medical prevention. No adverse events were observed in a series of patients undergoing ERCP (without any preprocedural prophylaxis) who had a prior history of reaction to contrast agent [6].

Avoiding post-**ERCP pancreatitis**, the rectal application of 100 mg diclofenac or 100 mg indomethacin is recommended before or immediately after ERCP in all patients without contraindications [7]. In high-risk patients, placement of a 5 Fr prophylactic pancreatic stent should be strongly considered.

12.7 Intra- and Postprocedural Considerations

Documentation of the procedure should be maintained throughout all phases of patient management in a monitoring protocol, including:

- Vital signs assessed at regular intervals (oxygen saturation, heart rate and blood pressure)
- Drugs (name, dosage), intravenous fluids (type, quantity) and oxygen (flow rate) administered
- Sedation-associated complications and their management

12.8 Monitoring After ERCP/EUS, Postprocedural Complications

Immediately after endoscopy patients should be continuously monitored in a post-anaesthesia care unit or in a monitoring unit observed by a qualified nurse until the patients are adequately awake and oriented again.

Following the procedure the patient is advised to continue to fast at least for a few hours if there is a **moderate to high risk for complications** such as pancreatitis or perforation.

Other complications include cardiopulmonary events, bleeding, drug reactions, cholangitis, cholecystitis and other miscellaneous adverse events (Table 12.2). See also Part IV (Chaps. 31, 32, 33, 34 and 35, complications) for an extensive discussion on complications following ERCP. Appropriate management requires recognition of an adverse event, its accurate definition and its prompt treatment.

Table 12.2 Risk factors of complication for ERCP based upon published data

Conditions/risk factors	Complications	Corrective measures
Related to the patient's condition and sedation		
Obesity Occlusion of intestinal tract Full stomach Pregnancy	Aspiration-pneumonia Difficult placement of the scope	Nasogastric tube Fasted for over 8 h Enteral feeding to be discontinued Prokinetic agents
Anticoagulation Antiplatelet agents Active coagulopathy	Bleeding (see Chap. 32)	Correction of INR (below 1.5) and platelet count (greater than 50/75,000 per mm^3)
Prosthetic cardiac valve History of previous endocarditis Cardiac transplant recipients with valvulopathy Congenital heart disease	Bacterial endocarditis	Antibiotic prophylaxis (based on amoxicillin)
Related to ERCP		
History of post-ERCP pancreatitis Female gender Absence of chronic pancreatitis Young age Sphincter Oddi dysfunction (SOD) Normal serum bilirubin Biliary balloon dilatation Moderate to difficult cannulation Pancreatic sphincterotomy *or* precut Repeated pancreatic opacification/acinarization Papillectomy	Pancreatitis (see Chap. 31)	Medical therapy (NSAIDs, etc.) Prophylactic pancreatic stent Meticulous endoscopic technique and use of the guidewire cannulation method Avoidance or report the procedure if nonessential/urgent
Precut sphincterotomy Difficult examination Altered anatomy (e.g. Billroth II) Ampullary stenosis (including SOD) Intramural injection	Perforation (see Chap. 33)	Reduce size of sphincterotomy Post-sphincterotomy cholangiogram (to control the absence of extravasation and late diagnosis) Meticulous progression through anastomosis and afferent limb Strict CO^2 insufflation
Suboptimal drainage (primary sclerosing cholangitis, hilar stricture) Jaundice and malignant stricture Stent placement	Infection/cholangitis	Antibioprophylaxis for transplant biliary stricture and patient with known or suspected biliary obstruction and incomplete drainage (cephalosporin)
Precut sphincterotomy Inexperienced endoscopist Cholangitis Bleeding during procedure Anticoagulation	Bleeding (see Chap. 32)	Use "endocut" mode/blended current for sphincterotomy [8] Endoscopic haemostatic therapy Protective stent placement
Children Pregnancy	Radiation	Avoid unnecessary magnification Pulsed and time-limited fluoroscopy Protect the radiosensitive organs and abdomen in pregnant women Experienced endoscopist

Typical risk factors for postprocedure complications (e.g., pancreatitis or bleeding) are difficulty in deep cannulation of the common bile duct, precut sphincterotomy, sphincter Oddi dysfunction (SOD), liver cirrhosis, periampullary diverticulum, pancreatic duct cannulation, ASA score > 3, BMI > 35 and intraprocedural sphincterotomy bleeding. In some studies, also younger age was an independent risk factor for complications [9, 10]. If no abdominal pain occurs after ERCP, patients are allowed to drink liquids and if well tolerated light food or normal diet the next day. Patients who are at **low risk of complications** (no sphincterotomy) usually start their normal diet 4–6 h after ERCP if no abdominal pain occurs. Observing the patient until the next day is justified in therapeutic interventions. The ESGE recommends testing of serum pancreatic enzymes 2–6 hours after ERCP in patients with post-procedural abdominal pain for early detection of post-ERCP pancreatitis and for further discharge management [7]. After difficult procedures optionally a blood count control for early detection of bleeding complication makes sense. Otherwise careful observation of stools is also recommended to exclude tarry stools indicating post-sphincterotomy bleeding. After sphincterotomy discontinuation of anticoagulation for another 5 days is recommended except with ASS. Mental deterioration or shivering can be early signs of sepsis or cholangitis, especially in elderly patients. Ideally the endoscopist achieves to do an afternoon ward round to visit his patients after the endoscopic procedure doing a clinical examination of the abdomen and checking the laboratory results.

12.9 Discharge

Minimum discharge criteria should be fulfilled before discharging a patient. The ESGE recommends that patients who have received combined sedation regimens, and all patients of ASA class >2, should upon discharge be accompanied by a responsible person and refrain for 24 h from driving, drinking alcohol, operating heavy machinery or engaging in legally binding decisions. Advice should be provided verbally and in written form to the patient and the accompanying person, including a 24-h contact phone number [4]. Certainly fulfilment of discharge criteria should be documented. Of course a detailed discussion of the results and medical advice with therapy recommendations should be offered to the patient.

12.10 Conclusion/Summary: Patient Management Before and After ERCP/EUS

- Informed consent 24 h before ERCP/EUS
- Laboratory tests before ERCP: blood count, INR, PTT, G-GT, AP, AST, ALT, lipase/amylase, CrP
- Imaging (ultrasound, EUS, CT, MRCP) available before ERCP? Do results justify ERCP?
- If necessary: gastroscopy before ERCP
- Antibiotics in cholangitis before ERCP
- Sedation with propofol under strict monitoring (pulse oximetry, blood pressure measurement and three-lead ECG), oxygen administration and monitoring protocol
- Post-ERCP pancreatitis prophylaxis with 100 mg indomethacin or diclofenac
- Postprocedural laboratory tests: blood count, lipase
- Follow-up and discharge

Key Points

- Always consider the legitimate indication for performing ERCP or interventional EUS, and ask yourself: "What if this patient has a serious complication, can I justify what I/we did?"
- Ensure that the therapeutic indication is the best of all alternatives.
- Be familiar with all general and specific risks of ERCP.
- Know your own skill limitations, when to ask for help and when to refer to a "high-volume centre".
- Be prepared to manage complications as a team.
- Document what you do (report must include fluoroscopy dose and time, monitoring protocol).
- Be aware that lawsuits mainly arise from situations where the indication was inappropriate or unclear, the consent was not informed and/or there was poor communication after the event.

References

1. Finkelmeier F, Tal A, Ajouaou M, Filmann N, Zeuzem S, Waidmann O, Albert JG. ERCP in old and very old patients—increased risk of sedation complications but low frequency of post-ERCP pancreatitis. Gastrointest Endosc. 2015. pii: S0016-5107(15)02392-5. https://doi.org/10.1016/j.gie.2015.04.032.
2. Manes G, et al. Endoscopic management of common bile duct stones: European Society of Gastrointestinal Endoscopy (ESGE) guideline. Endoscopy. 2019;51:472–91. https://doi.org/10.1055/a-0862-0346.
3. Denzer U, et al. S2k-Leitlinie Qualitätsanforderungen in der gastrointestinalen Endoskopie. Z Gastroenterol. 2015;53:1496–530. https://doi.org/10.1055/s-0041-109520.
4. Dumonceau JM, Riphaus A, Schreiber F, Vilmann P, Beilenhoff U, Aparicio JR, Vargo JJ, Manolaraki M, Wientjes C, Rácz I, Hassan C, Paspatis G. Non-anesthesiologist administration of propofol for gastrointestinal endoscopy: European Society of Gastrointestinal Endoscopy, European Society of Gastroenterology and Endoscopy Nurses and Associates Guideline—updated June 2015. Endoscopy. 2015;47(12):1175–89. https://doi.org/10.1055/s-0034-1393414. Epub 2015 Nov 12.
5. Dumonceau JM, Garcia-Fernandez FJ, Verdun FR, Carinou E, Donadille L, Damilakis J, Mouzas I, Paraskeva K, Ruiz-Lopez N, Struelens L, Tsapaki V, Vanhavere F, Valatas V, Sans-Merce M, European Society of Digestive Endoscopy. Radiation protection in digestive endoscopy: European Society of Digestive Endoscopy (ESGE) guideline. Endoscopy. 2012;44(4):408–21. https://doi.org/10.1055/s-0031-1291791. Epub 2012 Mar 21.
6. Draganov PV, Forsmark CE. Prospective evaluation of adverse reactions to iodine-containing contrast media after ERCP. Gastrointest Endosc. 2008;68(6):1098–101. https://doi.org/10.1016/j.gie.2008.07.031.
7. Dumonceau JM, et al. ERCP-related adverse events: European Society of Gastrointestinal Endoscopy (ESGE) Guideline. Endoscopy. 2020;52(2):127–49.
8. Rey JF, et al. European Society of Gastrointestinal Endoscopy (ESGE) guideline: the use of electrosurgical units. Endoscopy. 2010;42:764–71.
9. Coelho-Prabhu N, et al. Endoscopic retrograde cholangiopancreatography: utilisation and outcomes in a 10-year population-based cohort. BMJ Open. 2013;3:e002689.
10. Masci E, et al. Complications of diagnostic and therapeutic ERCP: a prospective multicenter study. Am J Gastroenterol. 2001;96:417.

Part II

ERCP: What and How

13 Cannulation Techniques

Lars Aabakken

Every ERCP procedure depends on the successful cannulation of the papilla. This, again, relies on the successful position of the duodenoscope in front of the papilla. These two components typically represent the initial challenges of anybody embarking on learning ERCP, despite the multitude of additional issues related to therapeutic and other measures involved.

13.1 Accessing the Papilla

Introduction of the side-viewing endoscopy is initially a confusing experience, partially because of the limited view, partially because of the unfamiliar effect of any navigational effort, given the background of forward-viewing instruments. However, with time the navigation becomes as automated as that of the colonoscope, so no reason to despair.

It is useful to remember the general moves of an upper endoscopy and mimic them throughout the insertion.

Start by passing the tongue, then ideally visualize the larynx that helps to stay in the midline, and know your level. Straighten the endoscope tip and slide through the sphincter; most of the time, it is smoother than a gastroscope despite the caliber, because the tip is partially rounded. If in trouble, try passing a catheter through the sphincter by visual control, and then follow that with the endoscope, elevator straight.

The esophagus is passed with straight tip, without much visual control. However, in some cases it may be relevant to check for varices, and that can easily be done if needed (to save a subsequent gastroscopy).

Once in the stomach, inflate a little air, suck out fluid content, and orient yourself. Usually you will rotate right, tip up, and slide along the greater curvature toward the pylorus. If you get lost, pull back to the cardia and retry. Approaching the pylorus, tip down to visualize it, and then back up again, aiming for the upper margin visually. Passing the pylorus is usually blind, but the mucosal appearance tells you it happened. Then orient yourself again, and navigate down the way you would with a gastroscope (tip up, right, rotate right, pull back). Fluoro control of this movement may be helpful in the beginning.

When you have straightened the endoscope, you usually end up at the lower end of D2. To visualize the papilla, pull back slowly with sideways movements (through rotation of the endoscope).

Usually the papilla is easily found (Fig. 13.1). Problems may arise with duodenal diverticula, with swollen duodenal folds due to acute pancreatitis, or malignant duodenal infiltration of the area. Look for the longitudinal fold below the

L. Aabakken (✉)
Department of Transplantation Medicine, Oslo University Hospital Rikshospitalet, Oslo, Norway
e-mail: larsaa@medisin.uio.no

M. Mutignani et al. (eds.), *Endotherapy in Biliopancreatic Diseases: ERCP Meets EUS*,
https://doi.org/10.1007/978-3-030-42569-2_13

papilla; it may be your guidance to hidden papillas, e.g., under a fold (Fig. 13.2). Fluoro-based position of the endoscope may guide in the hunt for the papilla in difficult cases.

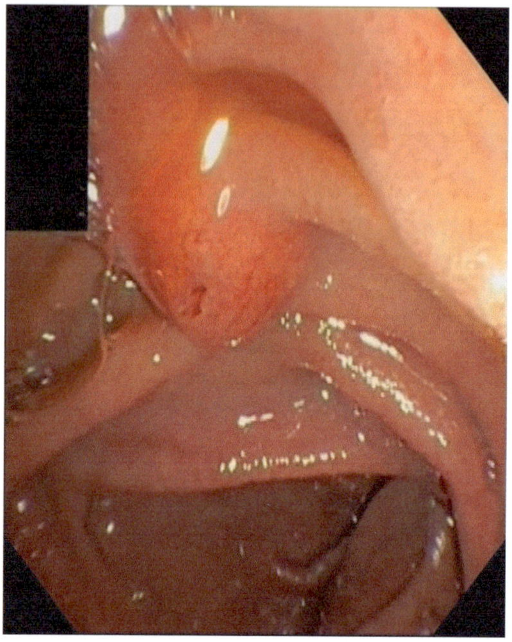

Fig. 13.1 Normal papilla

13.2 Pre-cannulation

A successful cannulation requires an optimal position of the endoscope tip. This involves the location, as well as the angulation of the access. Insert your catheter a little to understand where it will hit the papilla, and then readjust accordingly. Adjustments are done with both wheels, rotation of the endoscope, and push/pull on the endoscope. All movements should be minute and well controlled; coarse movements learned from luminal endoscopy will not work here.

Inspection of the papilla should also be performed prior to any cannulation attempt, to avoid traumatization that may complicate accurate cannula positioning. If needed, an obscuring fold can be lifted away with the catheter tip.

Usually the location of the orifice is in the center of the papillary bulge, and circular ridges can help locate it. Sometimes small mucosal prolapse may be present. If there is a "tip" of the bile duct protruding, this must be targeted and inverted by the catheter tip.

As for the direction of the cannulation, biliary access should be directed alongside the duodenal wall toward 11 o'clock, while pan-

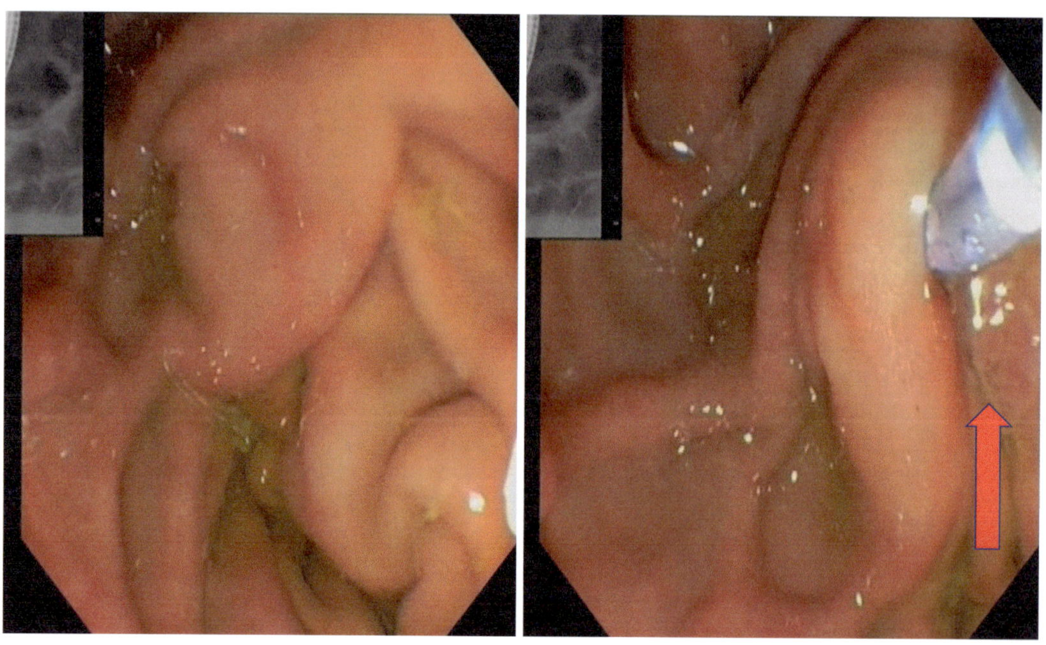

Fig. 13.2 Hidden papilla under a fold, exposed with the catheter tip (arrow)

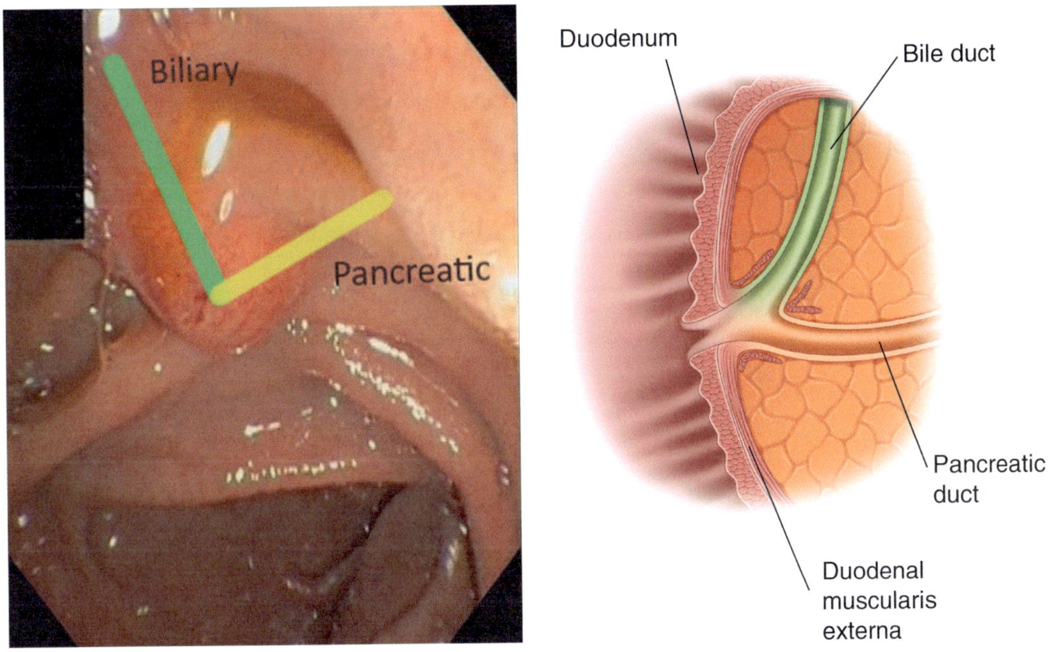

Fig. 13.3 Cannulation directions. Bile duct at 11, upward alongside the duodenal wall; the pancreas at 2–3 o'clock more perpendicular to the duodenal wall

creatic access is usually more perpendicular and toward 2–3 o'clock (Fig. 13.3).

13.3 Cannulation

For cannulation, a standard cannulation catheter or a wire sphincterotome may be used. The utility of using the (somewhat more expensive) sphincterotome is a possibility to introduce a graded bending of the catheter tip. This, in combination with rotation, adds to the directional flexibility during cannulation (Fig. 13.4). The majority of ERCPs also include a sphincterotomy, another reason to start with this accessory.

Introduce the catheter into the endoscope preloaded with a guidewire. To avoid blindly overinserting the catheter, close the elevator until the catheter hits it and stops, and then open to advance further. The standard cannulation starts with the insertion of the catheter tip gently into the orifice of the papilla. This is done with the catheter 10–15 mm out of the endoscope, then pushing it forward with tip up of the scope. Use the elevator to adjust as needed, but do not try cannulating by pushing the catheter. That is less controlled and with the elevator raised also entails a lot of friction.

With the tip inserted and in the right direction, gently advance the guidewire. This requires "fingerspitzgefühl" since any resistance should lead to retraction and another go. Micromovements of the catheter tip (in/out, angulation) may also be needed. Remember that inserting a bent sphincterotome too far inside will make you hit the roof of the bile duct and is counterproductive. Successful deep access of the targeted duct is ascertained by smooth movement of the guidewire and fluoro imaging verifying the correct direction. The duct of entry can usually be easily judged by the direction of the wire (Fig. 13.5).

When the wire is safely inside (10 cm or more), straighten the tip of the sphincterotome, and advance it over the wire into the duct before injecting contrast.

The distal part of the bile duct is not straight. Rather, it has a flat z-shape through the duodenal wall. That means that after the initial entry into the papilla upward toward 11, the direction should

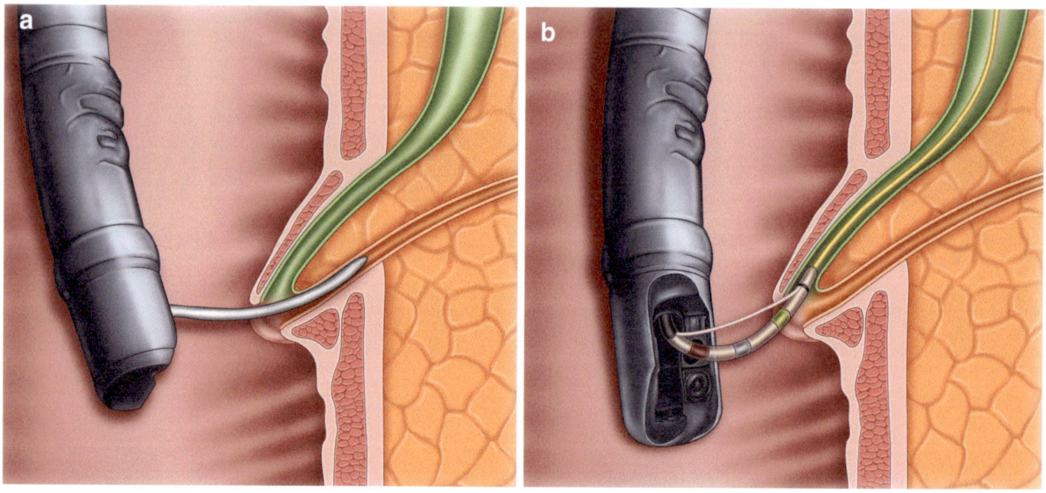

Fig. 13.4 Cannulating catheter versus sphincterotome angulation. The added angulation of the sphincterotome aids alignment with the bile duct. (**a**) cannulotome. (**b**) sphincterotome

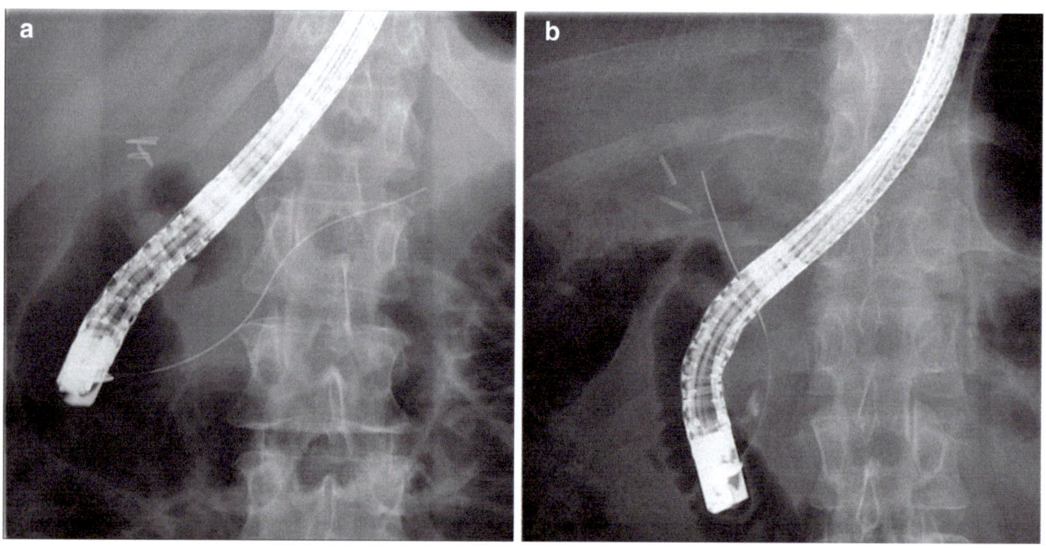

Fig. 13.5 (**a**) Pancreatic guidewire direction. (**b**) Biliary guidewire direction

be adjusted more perpendicular to the wall. Then, the direction of the duct again angles alongside the duodenum. This shape is accentuated if the papilla is hoisted upward by the sphincterotome; thus, this should be avoided.

Some prefer an angled-tip wire for cannulation, arguing that rotating the wire will facilitate access. This benefit has not been shown in comparative trials and comes down to personal preference.

Contrast injection at the level of the major papilla without deep access is usually avoided. However, in select cases a minimal injection can be useful to map the intramural passage of the ducts and help guidewire insertion. Filling of the pancreatic duct beyond the duodenal wall should be avoided.

13.3.1 Double-Wire Technique

Most ERCPs aim to access the bile duct. However, not infrequently your guidewire inadvertently end up in the pancreatic duct, as seen

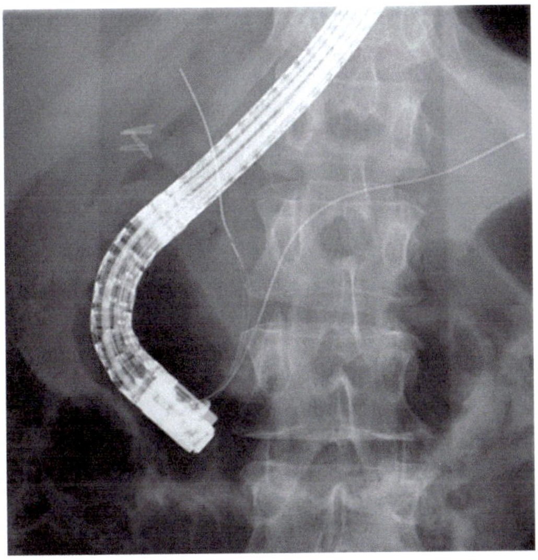

Fig. 13.6 Double-wire technique

on the fluoro image. If this happens repeatedly, one solution is to leave it there and resolve to the so-called double-wire technique (DWT).

With this technique, the pancreatic wire is left in place, and the catheter retracted and loaded with a second wire and then passed down again alongside the first wire. The pancreatic wire helps stabilize the papilla, straightens the transduodenal duct passage, and to some extent blocks the pancreatic access. Together, this often facilitates subsequent biliary access (Fig. 13.6). Aim to insert the catheter tip above the indwelling wire and point it up/left once inside. If this works, remove the pancreatic wire and continue working on the bile duct. If a lot of manipulation was done, consider placing a protective pancreatic stent before removing that wire.

13.3.2 When to Stop/Cut

Sometimes, cannulation is just difficult, for no apparent reason. At some point, it is necessary to stop, reassess the situation, and decide what to do differently. Take a few deep breaths, change whatever you are doing, or call a friend are all valid options. In a Scandinavian multicenter study, "difficult cannulation" was coined after 5 min, five attempts on the papilla, or two pancreatic guidewire passages. The risk of post-ERCP pancreatitis increased substantially in difficult cannulations.

Sometimes it is a valid option to stop and try another day (and/or with another endoscopist), particularly if there are special issues complicating the situation (luminal debris, uneasy patient, suboptimal accessories, etc.). If you decide to continue, either free hand precut or pancreatic sphincterotomy may be your next move. This is described elsewhere.

13.4 Special Situations

13.4.1 Previous Sphincterotomy

It is important to acknowledge previous ERCP procedures in a patient, to be prepared for specific issues (intubation, sedation, position, etc.) and also to know whether a previous sphincterotomy was done. Mostly this is readily appreciated endoscopically but not always. If the papilla is partially hidden under a fold, it may look native (Fig. 13.7), and the central orifice is the logical place to cannulate. This will, however, only lead to pancreatic access, while the wide open biliary orifice is separate and hidden.

13.4.2 Ampullary Tumor

Ampullary tumors, whether benign or malignant, distort the normal anatomy and may make cannulation challenging. Tumors often start bleeding on contact, so close scrutiny of the surface prior to probing with the catheter is key. If you are able to locate the ductal orifice, deep cannulation is often surprisingly easy. Conversely, some tumors are soft and/or necrotic, and you can enter the surface anywhere you want. In this situation, ERCP is likely to fail.

13.4.3 Impacted Stone

Small gallstones can get impacted at the level of the ampulla, with or without acute pancreatitis as

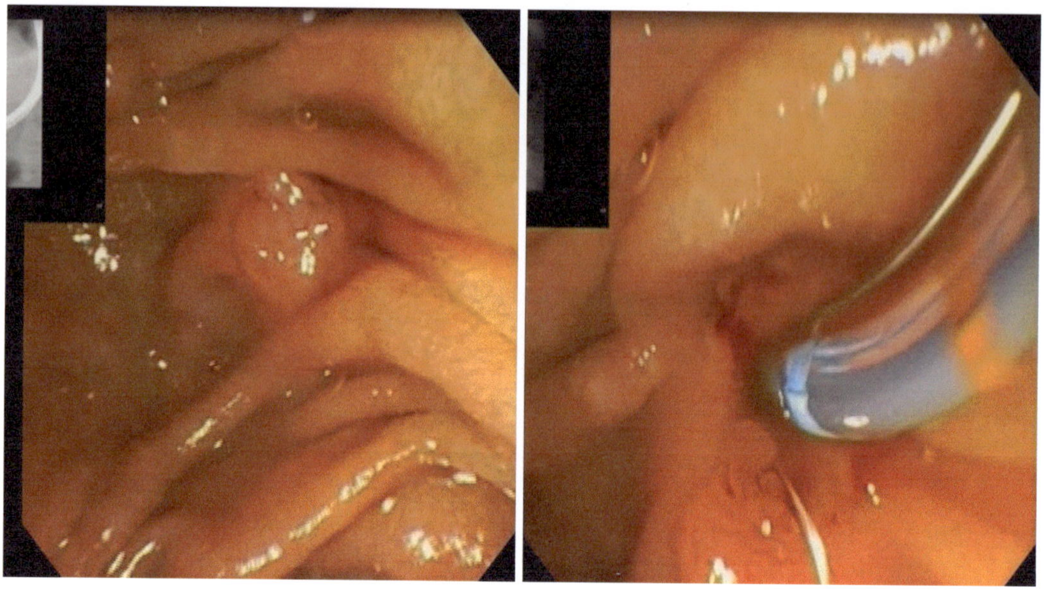

Fig. 13.7 Previous sphincterotomy. Cannulation on top of protruding papillary substance under fold

a consequence. Sometimes, you can view stone surface in the ostium; other times the shape, and the hardness on touch, gives the stone away. Try cannulation as normal, but if this fails, needle knife precut onto the stone is easy, safe, and effective. Just make sure there is actually a stone there (not just a bulging papilla)!

13.4.4 Diverticulum

Ampullary/periampullary diverticula may complicate ERCP. Diverticula may develop anywhere in the descending duodenum, so start looking elsewhere for the papilla. If it's nowhere to be found, look for a longitudinal fold entering a diverticulum from below. Typically the papilla will be at the 5 or 7 o'clock position, but sometimes it's found on a central ridge and occasionally somewhere else. Visualization and cannulation pose a challenge, but principles of above remain. Minute navigation, establish best angles, and probe carefully. A pancreatic wire should always be left in place to ease axis of cannulation. Sometimes, entering the diverticulum with the scope tip is the solution. Finally, clips, mini biopsy forceps, or fluid injection can sometimes flip a hidden papilla into the open.

13.4.5 Altered Anatomy

A number of GI surgical procedures change the access to the bile ducts if ERCP should be needed. Billroth II was for a long time the sole challenge, but recently, Whipple's procedures, Roux-en-Y hepaticojejunostomies, gastric resection, and bariatric gastric bypass all pose difficulties for the endoscopist. Details of these procedures span beyond the scope of this book, but with the advent of balloon enteroscopy, most anatomies are now accessible by the endoscopist. Moreover, percutaneous, EUS-guided, as well as surgical hybrid procedures may be the solution. Local expertise often mandates the procedure of choice.

Biliary Sphincterotomy and Precut

14

Vincenzo Cennamo, Marco Bassi, Stefano Landi, and Stefania Ghersi

14.1 Introduction

The role of the endoscopic retrograde cholangiopancreatography (ERCP) has changed over the years since this technological advance was introduced in the 1970s.

Thanks to the evolution of noninvasive diagnostic techniques such as computed tomography (CT), magnetic resonance cholangiopancreatography (MRCP), and endoscopic ultrasonography (EUS), indications for diagnostic ERCP should be reserved to selected cases like indeterminate biliary strictures for evaluation by tissue sample with or without cholangioscopic guidance.

Thus the ERCP has assumed an increasingly therapeutic role in biliopancreatic diseases, and endoscopic sphincterotomy (EST) of the biliary sphincter is needed for biliary interventions.

But the most important step in order to obtain a correct EST and a successful ERCP is to achieve a common bile duct cannulation, which remains a challenge even for the most experienced endoscopists.

Cannulation techniques have already been discussed in Chap. 13, but it is well known that, even in expert hands, failure to achieve deep biliary access occurs in 5–10% of cases [1].

V. Cennamo (✉) · M. Bassi · S. Landi · S. Ghersi
Unit of Gastroenterology and Operative Digestive Endoscopy, Maggiore-Bellaria Hospital, AUSL Bologna, Bologna, Italy
e-mail: vincenzo.cennamo@ausl.bologna.it

Failure to gain deep biliary access of a native papilla using standard techniques requires an alternative technique. In the 1980s, Singel was the first to introduce the technique of papillotomy precut using a needle-knife sphincterotome [2].

However, this technique still remains a challenge, even for the most experienced endoscopists, and it is important to understand the appropriate use and timing.

This chapter focuses on techniques, accessories, outcomes, and adverse events of biliary sphincterotomy and precut. We will also discuss the indications, contraindications, and evidence that support our recommendations.

14.2 Biliary Sphincterotomy

14.2.1 Technique and Devices

The approach to the papilla and different cannulation techniques are the same as for either diagnostic or therapeutic ERCP, which has already been discussed in Chap. 13.

Moreover, a therapeutic channel endoscope (4.2 mm diameter) has become standard in order to facilitate insertion of accessories and devices needed for operative interventions [3].

The use of the sphincterotome to reach the common bile duct is recommended for different reasons.

M. Mutignani et al. (eds.), *Endotherapy in Biliopancreatic Diseases: ERCP Meets EUS*,
https://doi.org/10.1007/978-3-030-42569-2_14

First of all, the sphincterotome, compared to standard catheters, offers the advantage of being more easily orientable. In addition, it avoids exchanges once the cannulation has been gained [3].

Studies showed significantly higher success rates for primary cannulation with sphincterotomes without significant differences in safety compared with standard catheters and also that guidewire-assisted cannulation increases the primary access rate and reduces the risk of post-ERCP pancreatitis (PEP) in comparison to the contrast-assisted cannulation approach [4–7].

There are several available types of sphincterotomes in terms of diameter and length of the tip, but also with different length and characteristics of the cutting wire. The choice of sphincterotome should be based on the individual anatomic situation as well as on the preferences of the endoscopist.

The more recent sphincterotomes are equipped with a lumen to insert a guidewire and an integrated hub for contrast injection; by this way it is possible to inject contrast without removing the guidewire so this can be helpful in cases of difficult cannulation [3] (Fig. 14.1).

Some sphincterotomes can also be preloaded with the guidewire; this makes it possible to perform the procedure more quickly and to use different types of guidewires with different lengths.

Indeed, short guidewire allows the endoscopist to reduce the length of over-the-wire exchange, to lock and to directly manipulate the wire.

The length of the cutting wire can also influence the success of the EST, for example, a short cutting wire (15–20 mm) can be precisely oriented, but it tends to be directed toward 2 o'clock, so the cut could be incorrect. On the other hand, a long cutting wire (30 mm) can lead to uncontrolled cutting ("zipper cut") and potentially increasing complications [3].

14.2.2 Procedure

Once the deep biliary cannulation has been achieved, confirmed by contrast injection, the guidewire should be led up to the proximal biliary system in order to make the subsequent maneuvers secure and stabilize the procedure.

It should be emphasized that a short and straight position of the duodenoscope facilitates the control of the device [8, 9].

Subsequently, bowing the tip of the sphincterotome facilitates its orientation toward 11 o'clock in the direction of the CBD. In this phase, it may be useful to straighten the tip and gently withdraw the endoscope so to overcome the distal part of CBD [3].

Moreover, the short wire systems allow us to fix the wire to the duodenoscope and improve stability.

When the sphincterotomy is performed, less than one-third (<5 mm) of cutting wire should be inserted into the papilla, so to cauterize only a

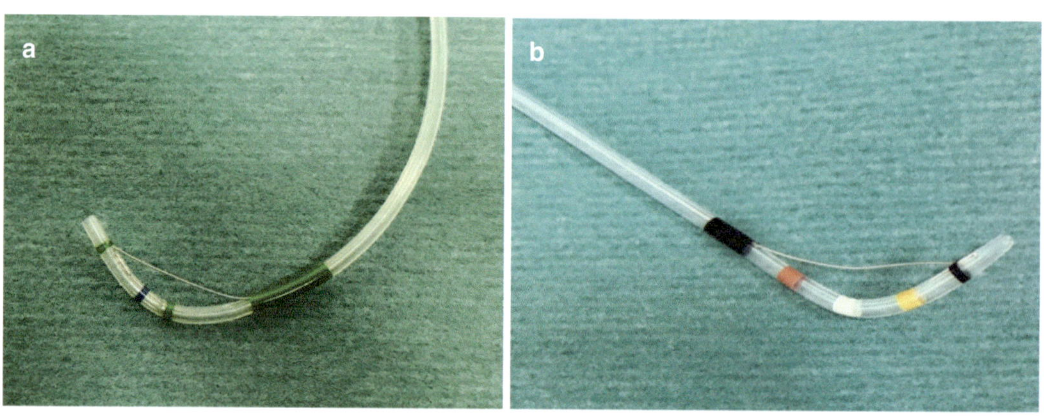

Fig. 14.1 Different types of sphincterotome. (**a**) A triple lumen sphincterotome with a cutting wire of 20 mm and a tip of 3 mm. (**b**) A triple lumen sphincterotome with a cutting wire of 25 mm

small part of tissue and prevent a quick and large incision ("zipper cut") [3].

The correct position of the sphincterotome can be identified by the presence of visible endoscopical markers on the distal part of the catheter.

The orientation of the cutting wire between the 11 and 1 o'clock reduces the possibility of complications such as perforation and bleeding, and, furthermore, it is appropriated to place the papilla on the left side, preferably along the 11 o'clock position, to make sure that the cut is correctly directed (Fig. 14.2).

This maneuver can be facilitated, in the most difficult cases, by rotating the right-left wheel to the left, while advancing the endoscope to the long position. Alternatively, the duodenoscope can be retracted during its rotation to the left with the movement of the wrist.

In patients with Billroth II anatomy (papilla is rotated 180° compared with native anatomy), it is recommended to use a rotatable push-type or sigmoid-shaped sphincterotome for EST, and the correct direction of the cutting wire in this situation is to 5 o'clock position [3].

Another discussed issue is the choice of electrosurgical current for EST [10–12].

The latest European guidelines recommend using mixed current for sphincterotomy rather than pure cutting alone because there is a decrease in the risk of slight bleeding. They also suggest using a current mode which provides an alternating phase of cutting and coagulation ("Endocut" ERBE, Tübingen, Germany, or "Pulsecut" Olympus, Tokyo, Giappone) instead of a mixed current conventional because it could be associated with minor episodes of uncontrolled cutting ("zipper cut") and a lower risk of bleeding at the time of sphincterotomy [10].

The use of this technology permits a stepwise cutting action that allows us a precise control of the direction and length of the incision, replacing the conventional mixed mode in which the current of cutting and coagulation are released together.

Endocut or Pulsecut can theoretically prevent the perforation of the upper part of the papilla, avoiding an uncontrolled cutting speed, thanks to their cutting automatic fractional. Therefore, the Endocut or Pulsecut modes have been associated with fewer "zipper cut" (uncontrolled cut) and bleeding at the time of sphincterotomy [13–17].

On the other hand, the pure cutting current has been associated with more episodes of bleeding [18], and, when it is used by less-experienced hands, there may be higher risks of bleeding and perforation, especially when a longer part of the cutting wire is inside the papilla.

The correct length of the EST may vary and depends on both the indication at the sphincterotomy and the diameter of the distal portion of the common bile duct.

Maintaining a slight pressure on the papillary roof is essential during cutting. This can be achieved by lifting the sphincterotome and arching it or by maneuvering the tip of the duodenoscope.

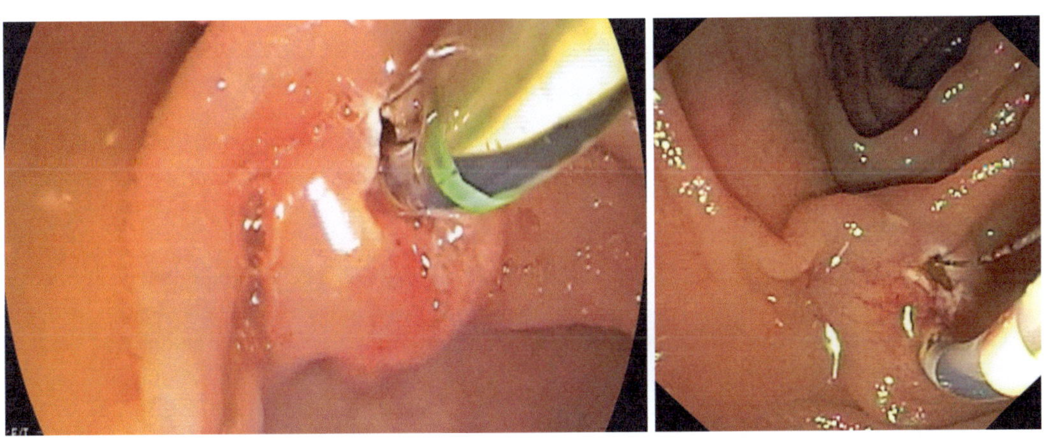

Fig. 14.2 During EST, the cut should be directed between 11 and 13 o'clock to minimize the risk of complications

As noted above, the cut should be continued only when the direction is between 11 and 1 o'clock. Furthermore, the correct movement of the device should be mainly controlled with the tip and the shaft of the endoscope.

The biliary sphincterotomy must be limited to junction point between the duodenal wall and the intraduodenal portion of the papilla of Vater although there are no clear endoscopic findings to identify this region [3].

However, even though there are no scientific data correlating the length of EST with the risk of complications, short EST can be used for stent placement in case of malignant biliary strictures, while more extensive EST with complete sphincter splitting should be used in case of sphincter of Oddi dysfunction (SOD) [3].

It should be emphasized that, if larger sphincterotomy is necessary, it is possible to dilate the orifice with a balloon catheter rather than extend it with a further cut [3].

The risk of adverse events is lower in patients with a dilated common bile duct and in the presence of ductal stones, especially when the papilla is large and protruding due to an impacted stone.

In special cases such as the treatment of recurrent bile duct stones or the reappearance of symptoms after SOD, it may be necessary an extension of a previous biliary sphincterotomy. In these situations, the technique does not differ from the one described above.

Large prospective studies have not correlated the extent of a previous EST with an increased risk of bleeding; however the risk of perforation or bleeding in these cases should be considered [19, 20].

14.2.3 Indications and Contraindications

The main indications and contraindications of biliary sphincterotomy are summarized in Table 14.1.

Consolidated indications for EST are the bile duct stones, acute cholangitis, severe biliary pancreatitis, facilitation of biliary stent placement, palliation of ampullary neoplasms, and treatment of SOD types I and II [3].

Table 14.1 Main indications and contraindications to biliary sphincterotomy

Indications	Contraindications
• Choledocholithiasis • Facilitation of biliary stent placement • Benign papillary stenosis or SOD (type I or II) • Malignant ampullary neoplasia in patients not suitable for surgery • Biliary leaks • Access for cannulation of the main pancreatic duct • Access for peroral choledochoscopy • Choledochocele, sump syndrome	• Uncooperative or unstable patient • Inability of the patient to provide informed consent • Uncorrected coagulopathy • A newly created gastrointestinal anastomosis

Choledocholithiasis remains today among the main indications for the execution of biliary sphincterotomy. This allows the endoscopic stones extraction by the use of basket or balloon catheters, with a success rate of not less than 90% [21, 22].

The success rate is increased by the use of additional techniques such as intracorporeal (intraductal) or extracorporeal lithotripsy [23].

To date, in order to remove biliary stones, biliary sphincterotomy can be considered safe, even in oldest old patients (>85 years of age) [24, 25].

Several studies have shown that in young patients EST can be performed safely before, during, or after laparoscopic cholecystectomy [19].

In this context, timing of EST should be coordinated between laparoscopic surgeons and endoscopists; often it depends on local expertise and access to the required interventions.

Biliary sphincterotomy is indicated in treatment of acute cholangitis due to choledocholithiasis or ductal stenosis with the possibility of removing ductal stones and placing biliary stents or drainage catheters.

An early EST (<72 h) should be performed in case of acute severe biliary pancreatitis, while it is mandatory performing an urgent EST (<24 h) in case of coexistence acute cholangitis regardless of pancreatitis severity [26, 27].

Another indication for biliary sphincterotomy is the initial treatment, before dilatation and/or stent placement, for biliary obstruction. Although sphincterotomy is not mandatory in these cases, it can facilitate stent placement, in particular for management of postoperative biliary strictures.

The role of EST in stent placement in case of malignant biliary obstruction is still unclear. Some studies have shown a lower risk of PEP onset, but an increased risk of post-ERCP bleeding in these patients [28].

A recent large randomized controlled trial showed no benefit of EST before implantation of self-expandable metal stents in patients with unresectable pancreatic cancer [29].

Biliary sphincterotomy has become the preferred treatment for patients with documented SOD (types I and II). In these patients, cannulation and EST may be more difficult because of the size of the papilla and a narrow orifice, so EST should be performed only by expert endoscopists to avoid excessive trauma of the papilla.

The increased risk of PEP can be significantly lowered by prophylactic placement of a 3-Fr or 5-Fr pancreatic stent [30, 31].

For other indications to EST present in Table 14.1, there is no strong evidence from the literature because data from randomized clinical trials are lacking.

Contraindications to ERCP and EST include an uncooperative or unstable patient, inability of the patient to provide informed consent, uncorrected coagulopathy, and passage of the endoscope through a newly created gastrointestinal anastomosis [3].

In case of contrast hypersensitivity, ERCP and EST could be performed, but prophylactic intravenous administration of corticosteroids may be considered [3].

Antiplatelet drugs such as clopidogrel and ticlopidine should be interrupted for at least 7 days before elective sphincterotomy; instead aspirin and other NSAIDs would not seem to be related to an increased risk of bleeding [3, 19].

Coagulopathy or bleeding disorders must be corrected before sphincterotomy. Child's A cirrhosis does not appear to be important predictor of bleeding [3, 19].

Finally, before executing an EST, it is very important to make sure to be in the correct position. Furthermore, to avoid to run into complications, the incision should be performed only if the cutting wire is correctly displayed and if the tip of the sphincterotome goes in the correct direction.

14.2.4 Adverse Events

In a large multicenter US study published by Freeman et al. [32], adverse event was reported in the 9.8% of the 2347 patients who underwent EST, and the acute pancreatitis was the most frequent major adverse event of EST (5.4% of all cases). Table 14.2 shows all the adverse events related to EST [19].

Definitive patient-related risk factors for PEP are suspected SOD, female gender, previous pancreatitis, difficulty cannulation, younger age, and repeated pancreatic injection, so these should be considered when patients are selected for EST.

The impact of prophylactic pancreatic stent placement on the prevention of PEP was recently reviewed. A meta-analysis of 1541 patients found that prophylactic pancreatic stent placement prevented PEP after ERCP compared with no pancreatic stent placement; similar findings

Table 14.2 Complications of endoscopic biliary sphincterotomy in 2347 patients from Freeman et al. [32]

Type of complication	Incidence (%)	Severe complication (%)	Fatal complication (%)
Pancreatitis	5.4	0.4	<0.1
Hemorrhage	2.0	0.5	0.1
Perforation	0.3	0.2	<0.1
Cholangitis	1.0	0.1	<0.1
Cholecystitis	0.5	0.1	<0.1
Miscellaneous	1.1	0.3	0.2
Total	9.8	1.6	0.4

were also noted from ten nonrandomized studies [33]. Therefore, pancreatic stent is strongly recommended in patients undergoing EST with risk factors for PEP.

Several prospective trials reported an incidence of EST-related bleeding, defined as the presence of melena, hematochezia, or hematemesis associated with a hemoglobin decrease of at least 2 g/dL or the need for blood transfusion, among 0.8–2% [19, 34–36]. Most bleedings appear within 24 h; however they can occur up to 1 week or more after the procedure. Risk factors for hemorrhage include coagulopathy before EST, therapeutic anticoagulation within 3 days after EST, cholangitis before EST, and bleeding during EST [19].

EST-related retroduodenal perforations are uncommon and mainly caused by "zipper cutting," which can be avoided by limited insertion of the cutting wire into the papilla and by the use of modern controlled-cut electrosurgical generators.

Studies reported a perforation rate related to EST of about 0.3% [19, 37]. Risk factors are SOD, a dilated common bile duct, and biliary stricture dilation [37].

Most cases are diagnosed during the procedure by observing the presence of free intra-abdominal air at radiological inspection or after the procedure by using the CT scan.

Presence of symptoms such as abdominal pain, signs of peritonitis, fever, or alteration of blood tests such as leukocytosis or increase in C-reactive protein should raise the suspicion of perforation.

Finally, EST-related colangitis is reported as a complication in about 1% of patients [19]. Nasobiliary catheters or endoprostheses should be placed when there is an incomplete bile duct clearance after EST, as well as antibiotic prophylaxis.

In conclusion, in particular in case of pancreatitis that is the most frequent adverse events in ERCP, it could be difficult to determine whether the complications are related to EST, bile duct cannulation, or additional therapeutic interventions in each patient, but it is important to know risk factors for individual complications and apply all possible preventive measures.

14.3 Precut

The term "precut" or "access papillotomy" generally refers to an incision of the papilla of Vater performed for the purpose of obtaining the deep cannulation of the bile duct. Since its introduction, which dates back to the 1980s [2], the technique has evolved a lot, and many variations and accessories have been introduced.

14.3.1 Devices

To perform a correct precut, it is essential to have adequate equipment. Usually, this type of procedure is performed using a needle-knife sphincterotome having a retractable electrosurgical wire, which can be maneuvered from the catheter handle, giving the possibility to lengthen or shorten it [38].

Needle-knife sphincterotomes are available in variable tip lengths (4–7 mm) and wire diameters and can be single, double, or triple lumen (Fig. 14.3) [38].

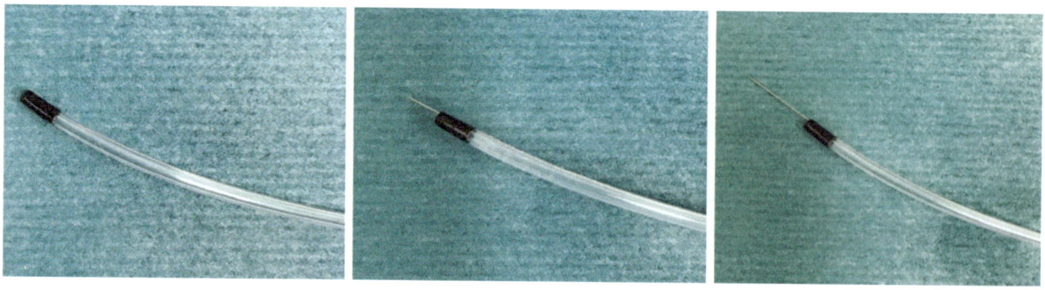

Fig. 14.3 A triple lumen needle-knife; the length of the cutting wire can be regulated according to different measures by the operator

Utilizing electrosurgical current, the wire is used to create an incision on the overlying mucosa through the movement of the elevator and/or the up-down wheel of endoscope.

The advantage of having a double or triple lumen is that of being able to preload the catheter with guidewires in order to inspect the incision area. During the precut, it is essential to use soft and hydrophilic guidewires; moreover, for this procedure it is recommended to use a current mode, which provides an alternating phase of cutting and coagulation. That allows stepwise cutting and precise control of the incision direction, depth, and length [38].

14.3.2 How and When

The fundamental principle of precut sphincterotomy (PS) is based on unroof the duodenal portion of the ampulla to expose the biliary orifice.

In order to deeply understand the different techniques of sphincterotomy precut, it is important to keep in mind the three-dimensionality of the ampullary region anatomy: (1) The terminal portion of both biliary and pancreatic ducts tapers before entering the medial wall of the duodenum. (2) The ampullary segment itself consists of the pancreatic, biliary, and ampullary sphincters that envelop the tapering biliary and pancreatic ducts in order to control the flow of their secretions. (3) The duodenal mucosa and submucosa overlay this ampullary segment [38].

Although there are several anatomical variants, often the ducts join to form a common channel of approximately 5 mm in length before entering the duodenum.

The pancreatic duct enters the ampulla in a straight fashion at the 1 o'clock position, while the biliary duct runs more superficially and parallel to the duodenal wall, where it enters the ampullae at the 11 to 12 o'clock position.

According to the classification proposed by the Mayo Clinic group [39], regardless of the instrumentation used, three different types of precut can be identified in relation to the starting point of the incision on the papilla (Table 14.3).

The most widely practiced precut method is the precut papillotomy (PP) (Fig. 14.4a). It is performed using needle-knife and making an incision upward from orifice to the roof of the papilla.

The endoscopist initiates the papillotomy by placing the needle-knife at upper portion of the papillary orifice, near the 12 o'clock position, and initiates the cut upward from the orifice or downward through the papillary sphincter. The incision is extended by cutting 1–2 mm increments with short pulses of cutting current (usually with a controlled generator) to de-roof the common biliary duct orifice [39].

The original description of the technique involved the use of an upward sweeping motion

Table 14.3 Type of precut techniques in accordance with Mayo Clinic precut sphincterotomy classification system [39]

Precut techniques
Precut papillotomy (PP)
Precut fistulotomy (PF)
Transpancreatic precut sphincterotomy (TPS)

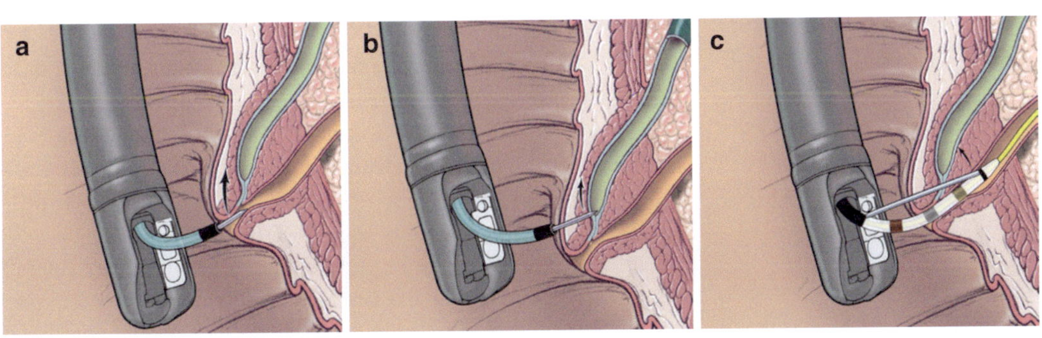

Fig. 14.4 Different precut techniques. (**a**) Precut papillotomy. (**b**) Precut fistulotomy. (**c**) Transpancreatic precut sphincterotomy. (Adapted from Da Vee T et al. [39])

with the elevator. However, improved control and safety can be achieved by loading the needle-knife by upward traction on the endoscope [40, 32].

Before proceeding with cutting, it is a good practice to try the movement few times with the needle retracted in order to be sure that position and movement are correct.

The direction of the cut is the most critical aspect of the procedure and determines its success or failure [41].

Once the cut is made, the biliary sphincter muscle is highlighted by separating the duodenal mucosa (it is identified by its whitish, onion-skin appearance). This maneuver can be facilitated by performing gentle aspirations (Fig. 14.5).

Eventually the precut area can be explored with a hydrophilic-tipped guidewire, which will subsequently serve to achieve the deep cannulation.

Once deep access has been achieved, the sphincterotomy can be completed by changing to a standard sphincterotome.

If cannulation cannot be performed and the patient is stable, the procedure can be repeated after 48–72 h in order to reduce edema and identify the biliary orifice more easily. So we suggest to postpone the procedure for 48–72 h in case of bleeding or excessive edema after precut. The success rate for repeat attempts ranges from 80% to 100% [42].

An alternative method to perform a precut is the precut fistulotomy (PF) (Fig. 14.4b). This technique should be preferred in case of large-stone impaction at the papillary orifice and in patients with a dilated intraduodenal segment of the bile duct [43].

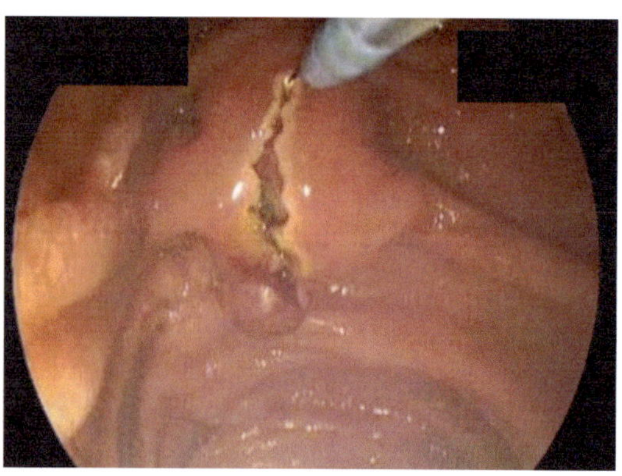

Fig. 14.5 Precut is a free-hand technique that requires a great skill by endoscopist

Moreover, it allows to avoid thermal damage on the pancreatic duct with theoretical reduction of pancreatitis risk [10].

This technique commonly employs a needle-knife to create an incision at the level of the intraduodenal segment of the CBD, which runs proximal to the major duodenal papilla.

The incision starts above the papillary orifice and is then extended upward in the cephalic direction or downward toward the papillary orifice. This approach leaves the papillary orifice intact, creates a fistulotomy for direct visualization of the CBD, and facilitates selective biliary cannulation (SBC) [39].

It is important to perform this maneuver by holding the direction between 11 and 12 o'clock to avoid complications such as retroperitoneal perforation.

The depth and direction of the incision are again achieved through the combined movement of the endoscope, large wheel, and elevator. The success rate of biliary cannulation using the PF technique is up to 98% [43].

In case of minimal bleeding during the precut procedure, it may be useful to irrigate the papillary area with epinephrine (1:20,000) to keep the field clean; on the contrary, it must be avoided a submucosal injection which could make CBD cannulation more complicated.

Another technique that is part of Mayo Clinic precut sphincterotomy classification system is the transpancreatic sphincterotomy (TPS) (Fig. 14.4c), this technique was reported for the first time by Goff in 1995, and it may be performed after attempts at SBC have led to guidewire passage into the PD [44–46].

The TPS technique uses a standard sphincterotome, which is oriented in the direction of the CBD at approximately the 11 o'clock position and is then inserted superficially into the PD. The incision is then made to expose the bile duct orifice or the bile duct itself. Once the pancreatic sphincter and major duodenal papilla are cut, biliary cannulation may be reattempted [39, 44, 47, 48].

Using this technique it is more easy to control the depth of incision with a theoretically lower of perforation, and it is not necessary to exchange the sphincterotome for a needle-knife device [49].

After a TPS it is useful to place a pancreatic stent to reduce risk of PEP [50].

As we have already pointed out several times, the biliary cannulation is one of the fundamental steps of ERCP.

Initial failure with standard technique can occur even in the most experienced hands, and, in these situations, alternative approaches are required.

Several studies suggest to move to an alternative technique after repeated failures to avoid traumatizing the papillary area with contrast injections and guidewire passages and increasing the risk of complication [19, 51–53].

An early PS has been proposed to reduce adverse events related to prolonged attempts at SBC. In a meta-analysis of 6 randomized controlled trials that included 966 ERCP patients published by our group [54], PS using various techniques were compared to persistent attempted cannulation using standard techniques. Overall biliary cannulation was similar at approximately 90%. A significantly lower PEP rate was seen in the early PS group, 2.5% vs. 5.3%, respectively.The overall adverse event rates, including bleeding, pancreatitis, cholangitis, and perforation, were not significantly different between the early PS group and the persistent attempt group (5.0% versus 6.3%, respectively). This suggests that, in experienced hands, persistent cannulation attempts and early implementation of PS have similar cannulation rates, but early PS reduces the incidence of PEP without adversely affecting the overall adverse event rate [39].

Current European guidelines suggest to take into consideration precut after the failure of at least five cannulation attempts or after at least 5 min [10].

However, precut techniques, in accordance with European guidelines, must be used only by endoscopists who achieve cannulation selective bile in more than 80% of cases with standard cannulation technique. The endoscopists who do not achieve this technical success should not perform the precut alone [10].

In conclusion, precut techniques should be used if the conventional cannulation technique fails, but always bearing in mind that they are not the only alternative techniques available because, for example, in case of repeated involuntary access to the pancreatic duct, the use of double-guidewire technique guide is recommended [10].

14.3.3 Adverse Events

Studies report a rate of complications of precuts between 2% and 34%, a rate that is generally higher than reported in patients undergoing standard sphincterotomy. A meta-analysis and a number of multivariate analyses have suggested that precutting is an independent risk factor for overall complications and particularly for PEP [19, 32, 51–53].

In 2003, Masci et al. published a meta-analysis of risk factors for PEP involving 7 studies and 7622 patients. From the meta-analysis emerged an incidence of PEP of 5.28% in patients undergoing a precut in comparison to 3.1% in other patients [53], but also that the repeated injections of the pancreatic duct are a risk factor for PEP.

Moreover, severe post-ERCP pancreatitis occurs disproportionately more often after precuts performed in the conventional way, without a pancreatic stent [19, 32, 51–53].

For this reason, if access to the pancreatic duct is easy to obtain, European guidelines suggest the placement of a pancreatic stent before the precut to prevent the risk of PEP and help the endoscopist in the procedure [10].

Focus on the risk of bleeding, studies report a rate of complication in patients who underwent precut between 1–2% and 48% if we consider the intra-procedural bleeding; however, these types of bleeding are often clinically insignificant [38].

A recent meta-analysis suggests that there is no significant difference in bleeding rates between early precut sphincterotomy (0–6.5%) and conventional techniques (0–5.9%) [55–57].

Most intra-procedural bleeding can be stopped by irrigation with solutions containing epinephrine (1:20,000), without resorting to aggressive hemostatic techniques that may obscure the anatomical landmarks and preclude successful cannulation after precut.

The risk of perforation after precut is between 0.1% and 0.8%, similar to standard sphincterotomy [57, 58].

Retroperitoneal perforation may occur if the precut is extended beyond the intramural portion of the bile duct, if the direction between 11 and 12 o'clock is not followed or the precut is too deep. The precut, being a free-hand technique, requires an excellent precision of the endoscopist to avoid complications. However, if a perforation is immediately recognized, it could be managed conservatively by biliary stent placement [38].

References

1. Sriram PV, Rao GV, Nageshwar Reddy D. The precut—when, where and how? A review. Endoscopy. 2003;35(8):S24–30.
2. Siegel JH. Precut papillotomy: a method to improve success of ERCP and papillotomy. Endoscopy. 1980;12:130–3.
3. Neuhaus H. Biliary sphincterotomy. In: Baron TH, Kozarek RA, Carr-Locke DL, editors. ERCP. 3rd ed. Philadelphia: Elsevier; 2019. p. 137–47.
4. Schwacha H, Allgaier HP, Deibert P, et al. A sphincterotome-based technique for selective transpapillary common bile duct cannulation. Gastrointest Endosc. 2000;52:387–91.
5. Cortas GA, Mehta SN, Abraham NS, et al. Selective cannulation of the common bile duct: a prospective randomized trial comparing standard catheters with sphincterotomes. Gastrointest Endosc. 1999;50:775–9.
6. Cheung J, Tsoi KK, Quan WL, et al. Guidewire versus conventional contrast cannulation of the common bile duct for the prevention of post-ERCP pancreatitis: a systematic review and meta-analysis. Gastrointest Endosc. 2009;70:1211–9.
7. Tse F, Yuan Y, Moayyedi P, et al. Guide wire-assisted cannulation for the prevention of post-ERCP pancreatitis: a systematic review and meta-analysis. Endoscopy. 2013;45:605–18.
8. Halttunen J, Kylänpää L. A prospective randomized study of thin versus regular-sized guide wire in wire-guided cannulation. Surg Endosc. 2013;27:1662–6.
9. Vihervaara H, Grönroos JM, Koivisto M, et al. Angled- or straight-tipped hydrophilic guidewire in biliary cannulation: a prospective, randomized, controlled trial. Surg Endosc. 2013;27:1281–6.
10. Testoni PA, Mariani A, Aabakken L, et al. Papillary cannulation and sphincterotomy techniques at ERCP: European Society of Gastrointestinal Endoscopy (ESGE) clinical guideline. Endoscopy. 2016;48:657–83.
11. Rey JF, Beilenhoff U, Neumann CS, et al. European Society of Gastrointestinal Endoscopy (ESGE) guideline: the use of electrosurgical units. Endoscopy. 2010;42:764–72.
12. Tokar JL, Barth BA, et al. Electrosurgical generators. Gastrointest Endosc. 2013;78:197–208.
13. Kohler A, Maier M, Benz C, et al. A new HF current generator with automatically controlled system (Endocut mode) for endoscopic sphincterotomy – preliminary experience. Endoscopy. 1998;30(4):351–5.
14. Akiho H, Sumida Y, Akahoshi K, et al. Safety advantage of endocut mode over endoscopic sphincterotomy for choledocholithiasis. World J Gastroenterol. 2006;12:2086–8.
15. Perini RF, Sadurski R, Cotton PB, et al. Post-sphincterotomy bleeding after the introduction of microprocessor controlled electrosurgery: does the new technology make the difference? Gastrointest Endosc. 2005;61:53–7.
16. Tanaka Y, Sato K, Tsuchida H, et al. A prospective randomized controlled study of endoscopic sphincterotomy with the endocut mode or conventional blended cut mode. J Clin Gastroenterol. 2015;49:127–31.
17. Parlak E, Koksal AS, Ozlas E, et al. Is there a safer electrosurgical current for endoscopic sphincterotomy in patients with liver cirrhosis? Wien Klin Wochenschr. 2016;128(15–16):573–8.
18. Verma D, Kapadia A, Adler DG. Pure versus mixed electrosurgical current for endoscopic biliary sphincterotomy: a meta-analysis of adverse outcomes. Gastrointest Endosc. 2007;66(2):283–90.
19. ERCP-related Adverse Events: European Society of Gastrointestinal Endoscopy (ESGE) Guideline. Endoscopy. 2020;52(2):127–149. PMID: 31863440 https://doi.org/10.1055/a-1075-4080.
20. Mavrogiannis C, Liatos C, Papanikolaou IS, et al. Safety of extension of a previous endoscopic sphincterotomy: a prospective study. Am J Gastroenterol. 2003;98(1):72–6.
21. Ogura T, Higuchi K. A review of treatment options for bile duct stones. Expert Rev Gastroenterol Hepatol. 2016;10:1271–8.
22. Easler JJ, Sherman S. Endoscopic retrograde cholangiopancreatography for the management of common bile duct stones and gallstone pancreatitis. Gastrointest Endosc Clin N Am. 2015;25:657–75.
23. Franzini TA, Moura RN, de Moura EG. Advances in therapeutic cholangioscopy. Gastroenterol Res Pract. 2016;2016:5249152.
24. Sugiyama M, Atomi Y. Endoscopic sphincterotomy for bile duct stones in patients 90 years of age and older. Gastrointest Endosc. 2000;52:187–91.
25. Sakai Y, Tsuyuguchi T, Hirata N. Can endoscopic sphincterotomy be performed safely in elderly

patients aged 80 years or older with pancreatic and biliary diseases? Hepato-Gastroenterology. 2013;60(126):1251–6.
26. Burstow MJ, Yunus RM, Hossain MB, et al. Meta-analysis of early endoscopic retrograde cholangiopancreatography (ERCP) ± endoscopic sphincterotomy (ES) versus conservative management for gallstone pancreatitis (GSP). Surg Laparosc Endosc Percutan Tech. 2015;25:185–203.
27. Da Costa DW, Schepers NJ, Römkens TE. Endoscopic sphincterotomy and cholecystectomy in acute biliary pancreatitis. Surgeon. 2016;14:99–108.
28. Cui PJ, Yao J, Zhao YJ, et al. Biliary stenting with or without sphincterotomy for malignant biliary obstruction: a meta-analysis. World J Gastroenterol. 2014;20:14033–9.
29. Hayashi T, Kawakami H, Osanai M, et al. No benefit of endoscopic sphincterotomy before biliary placement of self-expandable metal stents for unresectable pancreatic cancer. Clin Gastroenterol Hepatol. 2015;13:1151–8.
30. Choudhary A, Bechtold ML, Arif M, et al. Pancreatic stents for prophylaxis against post-ERCP pancreatitis: a meta-analysis and systematic review. Gastrointest Endosc. 2011;73:275–82.
31. Freeman ML. Preventing post-ERCP pancreatitis: update 2016. Curr Treat Options Gastroenterol. 2016;14:340–7.
32. Freeman ML, Guptta K, Howell DA, Robson KM. Precut (access) papillotmy—Uptodate. https://www.uptodate.com/contents/precut-access-papillotomy. Access 18 Dec 2018.
33. Mazaki T, Mado K, Masuda H, et al. Prophylactic pancreatic stent placement and post-ERCP pancreatitis: an updated meta-analysis. J Gastroenterol. 2014,49:343–55.
34. Ferreira LE, Baron TH. Post-sphincterotomy bleeding: who, what, when, and how. Am J Gastroenterol. 2007;102:2850–8.
35. Anderson MA, Fisher L, Jain R, et al. Complications of ERCP. Gastrointest Endosc. 2012;75: 467–73.
36. Parlak E, Dişibeyaz S, Köksal AŞ, et al. Factors affecting the success of endoscopic treatment of sphincterotomy bleeding. Clin Res Hepatol Gastroenterol. 2013;37:391–9.
37. Enns R, Eloubeidi MA, Mergener K, et al. ERCP-related perforations: risk factors and management. Endoscopy. 2002;34:293–8.
38. Sujievvan C, Gary M, Paul K. Access (precut) papillotomy. In: Baron TH, Kozarek RA, Carr-Locke DL, editors. ERCP. 3rd ed. Philadelphia: Elsevier; 2019. p. 123–31.
39. DaVee T, Garcia JA, Baron TH. Precut sphincterotomy for selective biliary duct cannulation during endoscopic retrograde cholangiopancreatography. Ann Gastroenterol. 2012;25(4):291–302.
40. Freeman ML. Precut (access) sphincterotomy. Tech Gastrointest Endosc. 1999;49(5):580–6.
41. Carr-Locke DL. Biliary access during endoscopic retrograde cholangiopancreatography. Can J Gastroenterol. 2004;18:251–4.
42. Mammen A, Haber G. Difficult biliary access: advanced cannulation and sphincterotomy technique. Gastrointest Endosc Clin N Am. 2015;25:619–30.
43. Freeman ML, Guda NM. ERCP cannulation: a review of reported techniques. Gastrointest Endosc. 2005;61:112–25.
44. Goff JS. Long-term experience with the transpancreatic sphincter pre-cut approach to biliary sphincterotomy. Gastrointest Endosc. 1999;50:642–5.
45. Goff JS. Common bile duct pre-cut sphincterotomy: transpancreatic sphincter approach. Gastrointest Endosc. 1995;41:502–5.
46. Akashi R, Kiyozumi T, Jinnouchi K, Yoshida M, Adachi Y, Sagara K. Pancreatic sphincter precutting to gain selective access to the common bile duct: a series of 172 patients. Endoscopy. 2004;36: 405–10.
47. Baron TH. Complications of endoscopic biliary sphincterotomy: the first cut is the deepest. Clin Gastroenterol Hepatol. 2004;2(11):968–70.
48. Weber A, Roesch T, Pointner S, et al. Transpancreatic precut sphincterotomy for cannulation of inaccessible common bile duct: a safe and successful technique. Pancreas. 2008;36:187–91.
49. Kapetanos D, Kokozidis G, Christodoulou D, et al. Case series of transpancreatic septotomy as precutting technique for difficult bile duct cannulation. Endoscopy. 2007;39:802–6.
50. Sakai Y, Tsuyuguchi T, Sugiyama H, et al. Transpancreatic precut papillotomy in patients with difficulty in selective biliary cannulation. Hepato-Gastroenterology. 2011;58:1853–8.
51. Loperfido S, Angelini G, Benedetti G, et al. Major early complications from diagnostic and therapeutic ERCP: a prospective multicenter study. Gastrointest Endosc. 1998;48:1–10.
52. Freeman ML, Guda NM. Prevention of post-ERCP pancreatitis: a comprehensive review. Gastrointest Endosc. 2004;59:845–64.
53. Masci E, Mariani A, Curioni S, Testoni PA. Risk factors for pancreatitis following endoscopic retrograde cholangiopancreatography: a meta-analysis. Endoscopy. 2003;35:830–4.
54. Cennamo V, Fuccio L, Zagari RM, et al. Can early precut implementation reduce endoscopic retrograde cholangiopancreatography-related complication risk? Meta-analysis of randomized controlled trials. Endoscopy. 2010;42:381–8.
55. Sundaralingam P, Masson P, Bourke MJ. Early precut sphincterotomy does not increase risk during endoscopic retrograde cholangiopancreatography in patients with difficult biliary access: a meta-analysis of randomized controlled trials. Clin Gastroenterol Hepatol. 2015;13:1722–9.
56. Navaneethan U, Konjeti R, Venkatesh PG, et al. Early precut sphincterotomy and the risk of endoscopic ret-

rograde cholangiopancreatography related complications: an updated meta-analysis. World J Gastrointest Endosc. 2014;6:200–8.
57. Choudhary A, Winn J, Siddique S, et al. Effect of precut sphincterotomy on post-endoscopic retrograde cholangiopancreatography pancreatitis: a systematic review and meta-analysis. World J Gastroenterol. 2014;20:4093–101.
58. Navaneethan U, Konjeti R, Lourdusamy V, et al. Precut sphincterotomy: efficacy for ductal access and the risk of adverse events. Gastrointest Endosc. 2015;81:924–31.

15 Pancreatic Sphincterotomy

Stefano Francesco Crinò, Laura Bernardoni, and Armando Gabbrielli

15.1 Introduction

Endoscopic sphincterotomy represents the first step of almost all endoscopic biliary and pancreatic procedures. It allows the widening of the papilla's orifice and sphincter providing the access to the biliary and pancreatic ducts. This procedure may itself represent a therapeutic maneuver (e.g., for the treatment of sphincter of Oddi dysfunctions) or be performed in concert with several other endoscopic procedures (stent placement, stone extraction, stenosis dilation, pancreatoscopy).

Historically, endoscopic sphincterotomy was firstly applied for the treatment of biliary disorders, and endoscopic management rapidly became the standard of care for these conditions. Differently, despite that the first case series of pancreatic sphincterotomy were reported in 1985, endoscopic therapy of pancreatic disorders spreads slower than biliary one. The less frequent pancreatic disorders to be treated, generally referred to as tertiary care centers, and the long-standing fear among endoscopists to induce pancreatitis while working and manipulating on the pancreatic side are probably the main reasons. Moreover, not so strong evidences as for biliary procedures support the indications for pancreatic sphincterotomy. Few studies and involving small number of patients have been published over the years, and indications as well as outcome or complications are not clearly outlined.

In this chapter we will focus on technical aspects of pancreatic sphincterotomy, both at the major and minor papilla, the latter in a dedicated section.

Electronic Supplementary Material The online version of this chapter (https://doi.org/10.1007/978-3-030-42569-2_15) contains supplementary material, which is available to authorized users.

S. F. Crinò · L. Bernardoni · A. Gabbrielli (✉)
Gastroenterology and Digestive Endoscopy Unit, The Pancreas Institute, G.B. Rossi University Hospital, Verona, Italy
e-mail: armando.gabbrielli@univr.it

15.2 Endoscopic Technique

15.2.1 Patient Preparation

As all endoscopic procedures, pancreatic sphincterotomy needs to be preceded by the acquisition of an informed consent with a clear explanation of potential risks and adverse events.

Preliminary laboratory tests should always include complete blood count and coagulation parameters. Administration of any anticoagulants must be discontinued for a sufficient time before the procedure and, if possible, for at least 3 days after [1]. The risk of bleeding associated with the

M. Mutignani et al. (eds.), *Endotherapy in Biliopancreatic Diseases: ERCP Meets EUS*,
https://doi.org/10.1007/978-3-030-42569-2_15

use of a thienopyridine (ticlopidine, clopidogrel, and prasugrel) has not been established. However, guidelines recommend these medications to be discontinued at least 5–7 days before endoscopic sphincterotomy [2]. Differently, use of aspirin or NSAIDs in the periprocedural period is safe and does not increase the risk of post-sphincterotomy bleeding.

Pancreatic sphincterotomy is considered to be a risk procedure for developing post-ERCP pancreatitis. Therefore, as recommended by the ASGE guidelines, rectal administration of NSAIDs (indomethacin or diclofenac) should be advocated before or immediately after the procedure [2]. For the same reason, despite a lower level of evidence, aggressive intravenous hydration with lactated Ringer's solution, when fluid overload risk is excluded, should be considered, especially in high-risk patients [3].

Data about the need of antibiotic prophylaxis prior to pancreatic sphincterotomy are scanty. Based on actual evidence, an antibiotic prophylaxis cannot be recommended as a routine practice.

Pancreatic sphincterotomy should be performed with the patient in prone or supine position to ensure a complete and comprehensive radiological view of the pancreatogram. If not contraindicated, intravenous administration of glucagon (0.5 mg) or hyoscine-butylbromide (40 mg) is suggested, as cannulation is often easier in an aperistaltic duodenum.

15.2.2 Pancreatic Duct Cannulation

Deep cannulation of the main pancreatic duct represents the first step to perform pancreatic sphincterotomy. Cannulation is generally attempted using a standard pull-type sphincterotome. The sphincterotome is essentially a catheter with an exposed cutting wire that can be pulled resulting in a bending of the tip. Several different sphincterotomes are commercially available. They differ from each other for the length of the cutting wire, the presence of additional lumens, and the length of the "nose" (e.g., the tip of the catheter beyond the cutting wire). Standard sphincterotomes can allow the passage of a 0.035-in. guidewire.

To achieve a selective pancreatic cannulation, it is crucial to understand the anatomy of the papilla of Vater. In a cross-section, the ampulla can be assimilated to a "doubled-eyed onion." The bile duct and the pancreatic duct run across the papilla in different directions. The bile duct courses from the papilla's orifice in an upward and leftward direction, with an acute angle in relation to the duodenal wall. Differently, the pancreatic duct runs more perpendicular to the duodenal wall and more to the right and downward. Sometimes, the biliary and pancreatic ducts merge in a common channel at the proximal portion of the ampulla. This channel has a length of 1–10 mm, and several folds of mucosa may hinder the advancement of the catheter. Cannulation therefore depends on finding the correct axis of the aimed duct. Due to the aforementioned anatomical principles, to obtain the axis of the main pancreatic duct with the tip of the sphincterotome is generally easier than the bile duct. Experts suggest to not bow the tip of the sphincterotome, to enter the catheter perpendicular to the duodenal wall. Then, the catheter should be advanced along the floor of the common channel by lowering the elevator of the duodenoscope. Lastly, to direct the tip of the sphincterotome toward the right, the small wheel of the duodenoscope should be gently turned left. After positioning the catheter tip in the presumed axis of the duct, there are two possibilities to ultimately assure a deep cannulation: (1) gently advance the guidewire into the duct while fluoroscopically following the path of the wire (that must go in a transverse direction toward the spine); (2) inject a little quantity of contrast to verify fluoroscopically the axis of the duct and its relation to the catheter tip. To limit the risk of pancreatitis, as little contrast as possible should be used. If a triple-lumen sphincterotome is employed, contrast injection and wire manipulation are simultaneously possible. Differently, with double-lumen sphincterotomes, contrast injection is possible only after guidewire removing.

In case of preferential access of the guidewire into the bile duct, it is possible to firstly perform standard biliary sphincterotomy. This will determine the exposition of the pancreatic orifice that can be subsequently easily identified and cannulated. The pancreatic orifice is generally observed at 5 o'clock position. In case of not immediate visualization, "wait and see" for few seconds may reveal transient opening of the orifice. This can be facilitated by gently transient aspiration of the duodenal air with the scope. In the early era of pancreatic sphincterotomy, prior biliary sphincterotomy was always advocated [4] (dual sphincterotomy) for the better exposure of pancreatic orifice and pancreatobiliary septum (resulting in easier pancreatic cannulation) and for the presumed lower risk of biliary complication (e.g., cholangitis secondary to biliary obstruction due to edema adjacent to the biliary orifice) [5]. However, there are poor and conflicting evidences about this topic [6, 7], and European Society of Gastrointestinal Endoscopy (ESGE) guidelines do not recommend routine biliary sphincterotomy for patients planned for pancreatic sphincterotomy and suggest to reserve dual sphincterotomy when coexisting bile duct obstruction or biliary sphincter of Oddi dysfunction (SOD) [8].

Deep cannulation of the main pancreatic duct should be always followed by contrast pancreatogram. Although accurate diagnostic imaging are generally available before ERCP (e.g., magnetic resonance pancreatogram) and indication for pancreatic intervention is already established, endoscopic pancreatogram confirms the correct position of the catheter inside the duct and provides important information about the ductal system morphology, necessary to direct subsequent choices (e.g., the length or caliber of the stent) (Fig. 15.1).

Once obtained a deep cannulation of the main pancreatic duct, two different techniques to perform pancreatic sphincterotomy are mainly used by expert endoscopists: the pull-type and the needle-knife sphincterotomy.

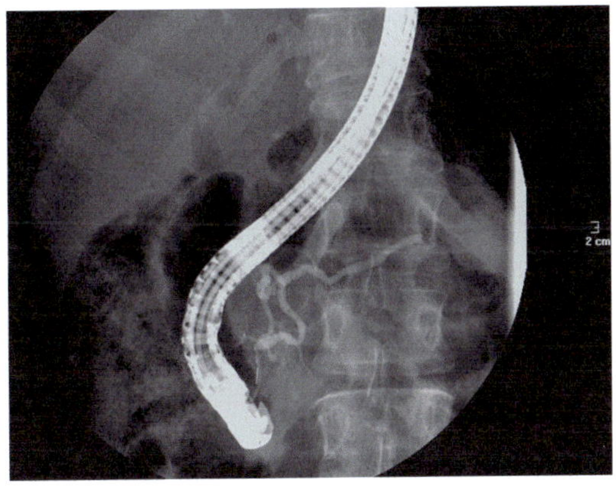

Fig. 15.1 Endoscopic pancreatography demonstrating an irregular course of the main pancreatic duct with "S" morphology

15.2.3 Pull-Type Sphincterotomy

Pull-type sphincterotomy represents the most popular technique. Principles involved are very much like those of biliary sphincterotomy. It is usually performed using the pull-type sphincterotome "over the wire." In other words, sphincterotomy is done while maintaining in place (deep in the pancreatic duct) the wire in order to ensure the cannulation during the procedure. For this technique, a hydrophilic-coated wire with soft and flexible tip should be preferred in order to prevent trauma to the main pancreatic duct or side branches. For the same reason, an angulated tip wire should be preferred. The wire-guided sphincterotomy is currently considered the standard of care for biliary and pancreatic sphincterotomy.

The cutting wire is gently pulled to ensure an adequate contact with the papilla's roof. Incision should be directed toward the 1 to 2 o'clock and performed with the distal part of the cutting wire (i.e., with most of the cutting wire outside the papilla's orifice). The procedure must be carried out in a stepwise fashion, gradually pulling and bowing the sphincterotome while proceeding with the incision. The length of incision generally ranges between 5 and 10 mm, depending on anatomic landmarks of the ampulla (i.e., the boundary between the papilla's infundibulum and the duodenal wall) and the diameter of the pancreatic duct. Completion of the incision can be verified by pulling through the incision a bended sphincterotome, determining the extroflexion of the remaining infundibulum and papillary roof (Video 15.1).

Sphincterotomy is performed by connecting the sphincterotome to an electrosurgical generator and delivering energy to the cutting wire. Most of the currently available electrosurgical unit offers pure cutting, pure coagulation, and mixed current. A mixed current can be delivered as blended (cutting and coagulating currents delivered together in one waveform) or alternated (cutting and coagulating currents are applied in turn in short bursts with an intermittent pause). In the latter (e.g., ENDO CUT by ERBE, Marietta Georgia, USA, or PulseCut by Olympus Europe, Hamburg, Germany), the cutting progression is fractionated in 1-mm segments signaled by an audible signal at the end of each segment. When compared with the conventional blended mode, the automatically fractionated cut reduce the risk of uncontrolled cutting and bleeding at the time of sphincterotomy [9] and could prevent perforation of the superior part of the papilla by avoiding an uncontrolled cutting speed. On the other hand, a pure cutting current induces less edema and is associated with lower rate of pancreatitis when compared with mixed current [10]. Moreover, pure cutting current is presumed to cause less fibrosis, diminishing the chance of developing future papillary stenosis. However, a meta-analysis confirmed that pure cutting current was associated with more episodes of mild bleeding, whether pancreatitis was similar with the two modes [11]. Nevertheless, the majority of evidences are about biliary sphincterotomy and no studies are available for pancreatic procedures. At our institution we routinely use an alternated mode (ENDO CUT), balancing the current discharge in favor of cutting.

15.2.4 Needle-Knife Sphincterotomy

For this technique, following pancreatic deep cannulation, a plastic stent is delivered over the wire. The stent is generally of small caliber (3 to 5 Fr) and serves as guide for the succeeding cut that is performed by using a needle-knife. The pancreatic sphincter is cut starting from the proximal portion of pancreatic sphincter "above" the stent, following its direction and proceeding for the maximum length in relation to anatomic landmarks. Some experts believe that prior biliary sphincterotomy is particularly helpful for needle-knife pancreatic sphincterotomy because of the exposure of the pancreatic orifice and the pancreatobiliary septum allows for easier pancreatic access and safer septotomy [4].

There are some limitations to this procedure. Precondition of this technique is the preliminary placement of pancreatic stent that may result in such a difficult procedure in the same situations, e.g., in the presence of chronic pancreatitis with intraductal calculi or when a tortuous or looping ductal conformation is observed. Moreover, despite that the plastic stent serves as a guide, the act of cutting is performed "hand-free." In theory this maneuver can be considered less safe and discomfortable for the endoscopist. However, a randomized trial comparing the pull-type and the needle-knife sphincterotomy was stopped early after an interim analysis showed that post-ERCP pancreatitis was significantly higher among patients undergoing sphincterotomy with a pull sphincterotome than a needle-knife [12]. The results of this study are in contrast with those previously reported [4, 13]. An explanation can be found in the high-risk population evaluated and in the previously performed sphincter of Oddi manometry, a procedure itself at risk of pancreatitis. Further prospective, specifically designed studies are needed to compare the outcomes of both techniques.

15.2.5 Precut Sphincterotomy

The precut technique refers to a maneuver to get the access to biliary or pancreatic duct when standard cannulation fails. However the need to resort to the precut for pancreatic access is lower than for biliary access, because standard cannulation of the pancreatic duct succeeds much more frequently. The technique is very similar to the biliary one and is generally reserved for those cases with impacted papillary stones blocking duct access. Once cannulation is achieved, pancreatic sphincterotomy is performed as aforementioned.

15.2.6 Post-sphincterotomy Plastic Stent Placement

Several randomized, controlled trials and meta-analyses have proven a significant reduction in incidence and severity of post-ERCP with prophylactic pancreatic duct stenting in high-risk patients [14]. Therefore, stent placement is recommended in patients who underwent pancreatic sphincterotomy. Once the sphincterotomy has been completed, a plastic stent is deployed and left in place usually for a short period of time (usually between 2–3 days and 2 weeks) in order to facilitate adequate drainage of the duct. The presence of the stent also prevents ductal obstruction related to the edema following sphincterotomy. Moreover, in case of post-sphincterotomy bleeding, the presence of the stent makes safer further hemostatic intervention (adrenaline injection or clip deploying). The choice of stent caliber should take into account the need of an adequate duct drainage and the probability of a spontaneous migration, thus obviating the need for a new endoscopic procedure to withdraw it. Thinner stents (3–4 Fr) are demonstrated to undergo spontaneous migration in about 90% [15, 16] and seem superior for post-ERCP prevention when compared with larger stents [17]. The length of the stent is usually chosen depending on duct morphology observed during the pancreatogram.

Some endoscopists postulated that leaving the stent in place for a longer time (more than 1 month) could prevent the onset of post-papillotomy stenosis by guaranteeing a complete healing of the sphincterotomy around the stent. On the other hand, a stent left in place for a longer time should determine ductal changes or get clogged with subsequent pancreatitis. This speculation, and any possible difference between different types of stent, can be answered only by future specifically designed randomized trials.

Table 15.1 Indications for pancreatic sphincterotomy as primary therapy or as precursor of further interventions

Primary therapy	Precursor of further interventions
Chronic pancreatitis with papillary stenosis	Chronic pancreatitis with ductal stricture or stone
Sphincter of Oddi dysfunction (type II or III)	Pancreatic duct insertion for drainage (e.g., pancreatic pseudocyst, pancreatic fistula)
Pancreatic fistula	Pancreatic duct insertion before surgery (i.e., pancreatic enucleation)
Intraductal papillary mucinous neoplasm (IPMN)-associated recurrent pancreatitis	Diagnostic or therapeutic pancreatoscopy

15.3 Indications for Pancreatic Sphincterotomy

Indications for pancreatic sphincterotomy can be classified according to the purpose of the procedure: pancreatic sphincterotomy as primary therapy and pancreatic sphincterotomy as precursor to other endotherapy (Table 15.1).

15.3.1 Pancreatic Sphincterotomy as Primary Therapy

The primary objective of pancreatic sphincterotomy is to eliminate the resistance to pancreatic juice outflow represented by the sphincter of Oddi, thus reducing intraductal pressure. In this setting, the following conditions can be identified: sphincter of Oddi dysfunction (SOD), chronic pancreatitis, intraductal papillary mucinous neoplasm (IPMN)-associated pancreatitis, and pancreatic fistula.

15.3.2 SOD

The term SOD refers to a transient functional obstruction of the biliary and/or pancreatic flow at the level of sphincter of Oddi, resulting in different grades of clinical manifestations. SOD has been classified according to the modified Milwaukee classification [18]. Firstly, SOD is differentiated between biliary-type and pancreatic-type and subsequently in three types according to the presence

Table 15.2 Contemporary (modified) Milwaukee classification criteria for biliary and pancreatic SOD

Presumptive SOD type	Definition
Biliary type I	Pain + abnormal hepatic enzymes + dilated CBD
Biliary type II	Pain + abnormal hepatic enzyme or dilated CBD
Biliary type III	Biliary-type pain alone
Pancreatic type I	Pain + abnormal pancreatic enzymes + dilated PD
Pancreatic type II	Pain + abnormal pancreatic enzyme or dilated PD
Pancreatic type III	Pancreatic-type pain alone

SOD sphincter of Oddi dysfunction, *CBD* common bile duct, *PD* pancreatic duct

of one, two, or three criteria (Table 15.2). Historically, the diagnosis of SOD was achieved by sphincter of Oddi manometry (SOM). To date SOM is not required for the diagnosis and management of patients with pancreatic SOD, thanks to the acquired knowledge from several clinical studies. Type I pancreatic SOD/idiopathic recurrent pancreatitis benefits from endoscopic sphincterotomy in the majority of cases [19, 20]. On the contrary, the EPISOD study definitely demonstrated that type III SOD does not benefit from endoscopic treatment [21]. Therefore, SOM could find a role only in patients with type II SOD. However, noninvasive diagnostic procedure can accurately predict a type II SOD. The study of Pereira et al. showed a 73% accuracy of secretin-enhanced MRCP [22] underlying a role in selecting patients who are most likely to benefit from sphincterotomy. Moreover, secretin stimulation to investigate idiopathic recurrent pancreatitis can be used also during endoscopic ultrasound (EUS) [23], revealing ductal or parenchymal abnormalities in about 80% of cases. Nevertheless, a recent survey demonstrated that the majority of endoscopist prefers to perform empiric sphincterotomy or endoscopic ultrasound-directed ERCP, for the belief that SOD II patients will ultimately undergo sphincterotomy [24]. Further studies are needed to investigate the role of minimally invasive diagnostic tools, such as secretin-enhanced magnetic resonance and endoscopic ultrasound.

When pancreatic sphincterotomy is performed for SOD treatment, dual sphincterotomy (biliary and pancreatic, in single or separated sessions) could be taken into account for the better clinical results reported [25]. For the same reason, pancreatic sphincterotomy may be indicated in those patients with biliary SOD (type I or II) not responding to biliary sphincterotomy alone.

15.3.3 Chronic Pancreatitis

In patients with symptomatic chronic pancreatitis, pancreatic sphincterotomy has been used as treatment with the purpose to reduce pancreatic ductal hypertension. Pancreatic sphincterotomy may be used alone or in concert with additional endotherapy according to the presence of ductal abnormalities distal to the papilla (ductal stenosis or presence of stones).

15.3.4 IPMN-Associated Recurrent Pancreatitis

IPMN may be associated with recurrent pancreatitis because of the obstruction of pancreatic duct by highly viscous mucus. A recent study reported the preliminary experience of pancreatic sphincterotomy in IPMN-associated recurrent pancreatitis in 16 patients [26]. This study has demonstrated that pancreatic sphincterotomy reduces the recurrence of pancreatitis episodes in about 80% of cases, both in main-duct and branches-duct IPMN. In this study, authors did not deliver a pancreatic stent after sphincterotomy because of the high risk of early obstruction by mucus. Post-ERCP pancreatitis was observed in one patient (6%). Currently, indication to pancreatic sphincterotomy for IPMN patients must be discussed in a multidisciplinary context and reserved for selected cases.

15.3.5 Post-distal Pancreatectomy Fistula

Pancreatic sphincterotomy has been proposed both as prevention and treatment of post-distal pancreatectomy fistula [27]. To date, we can assert that pancreatic sphincterotomy is not indicated as prevention procedure. Pancreatic fistula develops in about 20% of cases after distal pancreatectomy. Therefore about four out of five pancreatic sphincterotomy should be performed without reason.

Differently, pancreatic sphincterotomy with stent placement may be considered as treatment for those patients with post-distal pancreatectomy fistula not responding to conventional management [28]. Indeed, intraluminal pressure is lower than retroperitoneal one. Therefore, pancreatic sphincterotomy with stent placement can bring the flow of pancreatic juice back to the duodenum, leading the healing of the fistula. However, poor and sparse data are currently available, and further studies are needed to define its role in the management of this condition.

15.3.6 Pancreatic Sphincterotomy as Precursor of Other Endotherapy

Pancreatic sphincterotomy provides the gateway for any further pancreatic procedure. Therefore, it's indicated for chronic pancreatitis with ductal stenosis or stones, requiring stent placement, pneumatic dilation, or stone extraction, or for transpapillary drainage of fluid collection, and for pancreatic duct injury with bridge stent placement. Pancreatic stenting has been used as ductal shield before surgical enucleation of benign tumors (e.g., neuroendocrine neoplasms) [29]. However, available data are still scanty, and this procedure should be limited to controlled studies conducted at referral centers.

Despite that in these settings pancreatic sphincterotomy does not represent the primary therapy, it makes easier the manipulation of devices through the papilla and guarantees the ductal drainage at the end of endotherapy. Different chapters of this book are dedicated to these procedures.

15.4 Complications

Adverse events can be classified according to onset timing in early (within 72 h) and late (after 3 months). Post-ERCP pancreatitis is the most common complication of pancreatic sphincterotomy (7–15%) [4, 30]. The incidence of pancreatitis is strictly related to the indication of the procedure and the condition of the pancreas. In other words, when a healthy pancreas underwent sphincterotomy for recurrent pancreatitis or SOD, it is more likely it develops post-procedure pancreatitis because of the larger amount of normal parenchyma suitable for injury. Conversely, parenchymal hypotrophy, fibrosis, and scarring characterizing chronic pancreatitis offer the same protection against flogistic reaction. A recent large retrospective study showed 12.6% of post-ERCP pancreatitis of patient with SOD compared with 2.6% of patient with structural pathology [31].

Other adverse events are bleeding (about 1–2%), perforation (1%), and, rarely, cholangitis. Overall, adverse events rate range about 10–15%. However, when reading studies results should be considered that, in the majority of cases, pancreatic sphincterotomy is followed by several other interventions and is often difficult to understand which one is the responsible of pancreatitis onset.

The most common late adverse event is sphincterotomy stenosis. In the study of Kozarek et al., 56 patients underwent sphincterotomy, mainly for chronic pancreatitis [4]. Papillary stenosis occurred in 14% of cases. In patients with SOD, a higher rate of long-term endoscopic reintervention (about 40%) has been observed [31].

15.5 Minor Papilla Sphincterotomy

Minor papilla sphincterotomy is one of the most difficult procedures in pancreatobiliary endoscopy and requires a significant degree of technical expertise. In referral centers, deep cannulation is obtained in 86–93% of cases, independently to the used technique [32, 33]. Minor papilla sphincterotomy was demonstrated to be effective for the treatment of recurrent pancreatitis in patients with pancreas divisum [34, 35]. Moreover, a recent study showed a reduction of pancreatitis episodes after minor papilla sphincterotomy in patients with pancreas divisum and santorinicele (a cystic dilation of the distal portion of the dorsal duct) [36]. Furthermore, the minor papilla can be used as gateway when pancreatic therapy cannot be performed through the major papilla (e.g., in cases of ventral duct obstruction with dominant dorsal duct) [37].

Patient preparation tips and recommendations are the same as for the major papilla.

15.5.1 Minor Papilla Identification

The first challenge in minor papilla approach is its localization. Indeed, its size and position can be extremely variable, and a longitudinal fold (as generally observed in the major papilla) is absent. Usually, the size is about 5 mm and it is located 10–20 mm proximally and 5–10 mm anterior to the major papilla (Fig. 15.2). In other words, it should be searched in the above and right area than the major papilla. Generally, a long way position of the scope is preferable. This position can be achieved in two ways: by pushing the scope starting from the short way standard position or "in an antegrade way" by pushing the scope from the duodenal bulb to the second portion of the duodenum. In case of redundant folds, it should be necessary to lift the wall or displace the folds by using a sphincterotome or cannula, exploring all the surface of the region suspected to contain the accessory papilla.

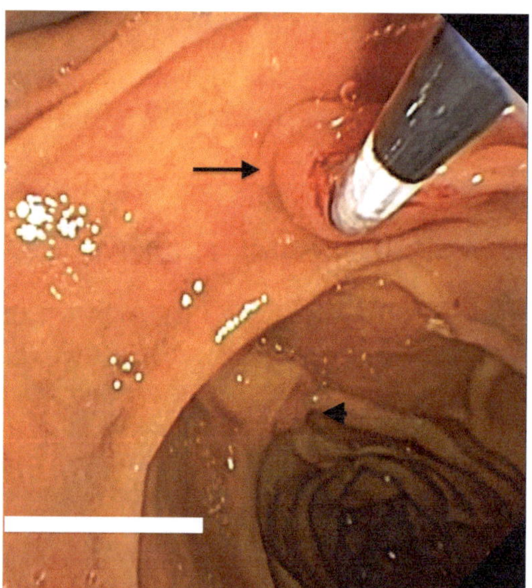

Fig. 15.2 The minor papilla (arrow) is generally located 1–2 cm proximally and 0.5–1 cm on the right to the major papilla (arrowhead)

To spray an amount of methylene blue on the duodenal mucosa may be useful to identify the papilla because it may highlight thin raised areas and frond-like mucosa [38].

Another technique to identify the minor papilla in difficult cases is the intravenous administration of secretin at a dose of 0.2 μg/kg (maximum of 16 μg). The stimulation of pancreatic secretion results in a dilation of the papilla's orifice with a visible flow of pancreatic juice into the duodenum (Video 15.2). It has been reported that secretin injection and the subsequent enlargement of the papilla's orifice can simplify cannulation as well [39].

As alternative to secretin that is expensive and not everywhere available, duodenal irrigation with acid solution (45 mL of 0.1 mol HCl) increased rate of dorsal duct cannulation in a small, randomized trial [40].

Finally, as rescue technique, an EUS-guided injection of contrast and methylene blue inside the pancreatic duct has been reported [41].

15.5.2 Dorsal Duct Cannulation

After identification of the minor papilla, a stable position of the scope must be obtained. The minor papilla is generally approached in a long way position in order to face the papilla and dorsal duct in a frontal axis (Fig. 15.3). This position helps to avoid wrong attempts of cannulation, which usually fail and induce papillary edema. Rarely, depending on the patient duodenum anatomy and papilla position, a very short position may be adequate.

A standard 0.035-in. guidewired or an ultratapered (4.4 Fr) 0.025-in. guidewired sphincterotome can be used. It must be kept in mind that first attempts of cannulation have the higher likelihood of success. Endoscopist must be very gentle while juxtaposing the sphincterotome to the papilla's orifice to prevent mucosal trauma and oozing.

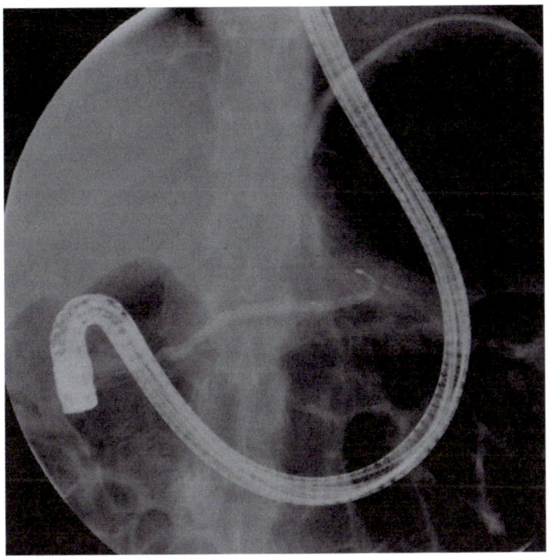

Fig. 15.3 The duodenoscope in long way position allows to face the minor papilla and the pancreatic dorsal duct with a straight axis

The minor papilla is very weak, and repeated cannulation attempts could alter its normal appearance and trigger sphincter's spasm, precluding the cannulation success. With this in mind, many expert endoscopists set the tip of the wire few millimeters outside of the sphincterotome trying to insert the tip of the wire into the papilla's orifice, without touching the papilla with the catheter. Then, while the endoscopist calibrates rotational movements of the duodenoscope axis or wheels, the wire is gently pushed to achieve deep cannulation (Video 15.2).

Differently, some other expert endoscopists prefer to inject a little quantity of contrast medium to define the anatomy and the axis of the Santorini duct prior to attempt deep cannulation with the guidewire, with the purpose to fluoroscopically direct the tip of the sphincterotome in the direction of the duct. From this point of view, we would underline the relevance of an accurate study of MRCP images by the endoscopist to check the pancreatic duct morphology.

In difficult cases, secretin administration can improve success rate as demonstrated in a randomized crossover trial [39]. In two large series, administration of secretin was utilized in 17–35% of cases [33, 42]. Moreover, a rendezvous procedure under EUS guidance has been proposed by inserting a guidewire into the pancreatic duct at the level of the pancreas body and pushes it through the minor papilla [43].

15.5.3 Pull-Type Sphincterotomy

Principles involved in sphincterotomy techniques are the same of those explained for the major papilla. When deep cannulation of the dorsal duct is achieved, a pull-type sphincterotome is inserted over the guidewire, and incision is performed in the 12 to 1 o'clock position. The length of the incision is generally about 5 mm but is strictly depending on patient anatomy. For the minor papilla, it is generally observed that the infundibulum became clearly visible only after deep cannulation, revealing the boundary for the sphincterotomy (Video 15.3).

15.5.4 Needle-Knife Sphincterotomy

As described for the major papilla, this technique is preceded by the insertion of a plastic stent. Then, incision is made with the knife over the stent.

15.5.5 Wire-Assisted Sphincterotomy

This technique is reserved for those cases where a deep cannulation is achieved with the guidewire, but the pull sphincterotome cannot be passed because of a stenotic orifice. Therefore, a knife is passed over or alongside the wire and the incision is made following the direction of the wire. After an initial cut with a needle-knife sphincterotome, the incision can be completed with a pull-type sphincterotome. Maple et al. [33] recently investigated this procedure in 32 patients. Authors found a higher percentage of post-ERCP pancreatitis when the wire-assisted sphincterotomy was performed compared with the pull-type (16% vs. 8%). Moreover, in our experience when a guidewire (even 0.021 in.) was deep inserted in the pancreatic duct, an ultra-tapered pull-type sphincterotomy was always possible to pass the papilla. In our opinion this procedure should be considered as a rescue technique for isolated cases.

15.5.6 Precut Sphincterotomy

It consists in a freehand needle-knife incision of the minor papilla to obtain succeeding cannulation. This procedure remains highly risky and must be performed only by expert endoscopist after a wise evaluation of the risk/benefit ratio.

15.5.7 Post-sphincterotomy Plastic Stent Placement

As well as for the major papilla, insertion of a plastic stent is always indicated after minor papilla sphincterotomy to reduce the risk of pancreatitis. With this purpose, the stent should be removed after few days to avoid stent-related ductal changes. The size (usually 5 or 7Fr) and the length of the stent depend on ductal caliber and morphology.

15.5.8 Complications

Post-ERCP pancreatitis is the most common adverse event following minor papilla sphincterotomy with a rate ranging from 8 to 12% [44, 45]. Bleeding is more frequently reported immediately after sphincterotomy whether clinically significant hemorrhage is rare (<2%). The incidence of perforation does not differ to the major papilla and is <1%. Overall adverse event rates were similar in those undergoing needle-knife and pull-type sphincterotome [45].

References

1. Freeman ML, Nelson DB, Sherman S, et al. Complications of endoscopic biliary sphincterotomy. N Engl J Med. 1996;335:909–18.
2. ASGE Standards of Practice Committee, Chandrasekhara V, Khashab MA, Muthusamy VR, et al. Adverse events associated with ERCP. Gastrointest Endosc. 2017;85(1):32–47.
3. Buxbaum J, Yan A, Yeh K, et al. Aggressive hydration with lactated Ringer's solution reduces pancreatitis after endoscopic retrograde cholangiopancreatography. Clin Gastroenterol Hepatol. 2014;12:303–307.e1.
4. Kozarek RA, Ball TJ, Patterson DJ, et al. Endoscopic pancreatic duct sphincterotomy: indications, technique, and analysis of results. Gastrointest Endosc. 1994;40:592–8.
5. Cremer M, Devière J, Delhaye M, et al. Stenting in severe chronic pancreatitis: results of medium-term follow-up in seventy-six patients. Endoscopy. 1991;23:171–6.
6. Kim MH, Myung SJ, Kim YS, et al. Routine biliary sphincterotomy may not be indispensable for endoscopic pancreatic sphincterotomy. Endoscopy. 1998;30:697–701.
7. Jakobs R, Reimann JF. Is there a need for dual sphincterotomy in patients with chronic pancreatitis? Endoscopy. 2003;35:250–1.
8. Testoni PA, Mariani A, Aabakken L, et al. Papillary cannulation and sphincterotomy techniques at ERCP: European Society of Gastrointestinal Endoscopy (ESGE) Clinical Guideline. Endoscopy. 2016;48(7):657–83.
9. Akiho H, Sumida Y, Akahoshi K, et al. Safety advantage of endocut mode over endoscopic sphincterotomy for choledocholithiasis. World J Gastroenterol. 2006;12:2086–8.
10. Elta GH, Barnett JL, Wille RT, et al. Pure cut electrocautery current for sphincterotomy causes less post-procedure pancreatitis than blended current. Gastrointest Endosc. 1998;47:149–53.
11. Verma D, Kapadia A, Adler DG. Pure versus mixed electrosurgical current for endoscopic biliary sphincterotomy: a meta-analysis of adverse outcomes. Gastrointest Endosc. 2007;66:283–90.
12. Varadarajulu S, Wilcox CM. Randomized trial comparing needle-knife and pull-sphincterotome techniques for pancreatic sphincterotomy in high-risk patients. Gastrointest Endosc. 2006;64(5):716–22.
13. Elton E, Howell DA, Parsons WG, et al. Endoscopic pancreatic sphincterotomy: indications, outcome, and a safe stentless technique. Gastrointest Endosc. 1998;47:240–9.
14. Mazaki T, Mado K, Masuda H, et al. Prophylactic pancreatic stent placement and post-ERCP pancreatitis: an updated meta-analysis. J Gastroenterol. 2014;49:343–55.
15. Pahk A, Rigaux J, Poreddy V, et al. Prophylactic pancreatic stents: does size matter? A comparison of 4-Fr and 5-Fr stents in reference to post-ERCP pancreatitis and migration rate. Dig Dis Sci. 2011;56(10):3058–64.
16. Lawrence C, Cotton PB, Romagnuolo J, et al. Small prophylactic pancreatic duct stents: an assessment of spontaneous passage and stent-induced ductal abnormalities. Endoscopy. 2007;39:1082–5.
17. Rashdan A, Fogel EL, McHenry L Jr, et al. Improved stent characteristics for prophylaxis of post-ERCP pancreatitis. Clin Gastroenterol Hepatol. 2004;2(4):322–9.
18. Seetharam P, Rodrigues G. Sphincter of Oddi and its dysfunction. Saudi J Gastroenterol. 2008;14(1):1–6.

19. Devereaux BM, Sherman S, Lehman GA. Sphincter of Oddi (pancreatic) hypertension and recurrent pancreatitis. Curr Gastroenterol Rep. 2002;4:153–9.
20. Thatcher BS, Sivak MV, Tedesco FJ, et al. Endoscopic sphincterotomy for suspected dysfunction of the sphincter of Oddi. Gastrointest Endosc. 1987;33:91–5.
21. Cotton PB, Durkalski V, Romagnuolo J, et al. Effect of endoscopic sphincterotomy for suspected sphincter of Oddi dysfunction on pain-related disability following cholecystectomy: the EPISOD randomized clinical trial. JAMA. 2014;311:2101–9.
22. Pereira SP, Gillams A, Sgouros SN, et al. Prospective comparison of secretin-stimulated magnetic resonance cholangiopancreatography with manometry in the diagnosis of sphincter of Oddi dysfunction types II and III. Gut. 2007;56(6):809–13.
23. Mariani A, Arcidiacono PG, Curioni S, et al. Diagnostic yield of ERCP and secretin-enhanced MRCP and EUS in patients with acute recurrent pancreatitis of unknown aetiology. Dig Liver Dis. 2009;41(10):753–8.
24. Watson RR, Klapman J, Komanduri S, et al. Wide disparities in attitudes and practices regarding Type II sphincter of Oddi dysfunction: a survey of expert U.S. endoscopists. Endosc Int Open. 2016;4(9):E941–6.
25. Park SH, Watkins JL, Fogel EL, et al. Long-term outcome of endoscopic dual pancreatobiliary sphincterotomy in patients with manometry-documented sphincter of Oddi dysfunction and normal pancreatogram. Gastrointest Endosc. 2003;57(4):483–91.
26. Bernardoni L, Crinò SF, De Conti G, et al. Preliminary experience with pancreatic sphincterotomy as treatment for intraductal papillary mucinous neoplasm-associated recurrent pancreatitis. Endosc Int Open. 2017;5(11):E1144–50.
27. Rieder B, Krampulz D, Adolf J, et al. Endoscopic pancreatic sphincterotomy and stenting for preoperative prophylaxis of pancreatic fistula after distal pancreatectomy. Gastrointest Endosc. 2010;72(3):536–42.
28. Goasguen N, Bourrier A, Ponsot P, et al. Endoscopic management of pancreatic fistula after distal pancreatectomy and enucleation. Am J Surg. 2009;197(6):715–20.
29. Shimura T, Suehiro T, Suzuki H, et al. Preoperative endoscopic pancreatic stenting for prophylaxis of pancreatic duct disruption during extirpation of a pancreatic head tumor. Am J Surg. 2007;194(4):553–5.
30. Esber E, Sherman S, Earle D, et al. Complications of major papilla pancreatic sphincterotomy: a review of 236 patients. Gastrointest Endosc. 1995;43:405A.
31. Dufault DL, Elmunzer BJ, Cotton PB, et al. Adverse events and reinterventions following pancreatic endoscopic sphincterotomy. Pancreas. 2018;47(7):880–3.
32. Lehman GA, Sherman S, Nisi R, et al. Pancreas divisum: results of minor papilla sphincterotomy. Gastrointest Endosc. 1993;39(1):1–8.
33. Maple JT, Keswani RN, Edmundowicz SA, et al. Wire-assisted access sphincterotomy of the minor papilla. Gastrointest Endosc. 2009;69(1):47–54.
34. Lans JI, Geenen JE, Johanson JF, et al. Endoscopic therapy in patients with pancreas divisum and acute pancreatitis: a prospective, randomized, controlled clinical trial. Gastrointest Endosc. 1992;38:430–4.
35. Mariani A, Di Leo M, Petrone MC, et al. Outcome of endotherapy for pancreas divisum in patients with acute recurrent pancreatitis. World J Gastroenterol. 2014;20(46):17468–75.
36. Crinò SF, Bernardoni L, Conti Bellocchi MC, et al. Efficacy of endoscopic minor papilla sphincterotomy for symptomatic santorinicele. Clin Gastroenterol Hepatol. 2017;15(2):303–6.
37. Brown NG, Howell DA, Brauer BC, et al. Minor papilla endotherapy in patients with ventral duct obstruction: identification and management. Gastrointest Endosc. 2017;85(2):365–70.
38. Park SH, de Bellis M, McHenry L, et al. Use of methylene blue to identify the minor papilla or its orifice in patients with pancreas divisum. Gastrointest Endosc. 2003;57:358–63.
39. Devereaux BM, Fein S, Purich E, et al. A new synthetic porcine secretin for facilitation of cannulation of the dorsal pancreatic duct at ERCP in patients with pancreas divisum: a multicenter, randomized, double-blind comparative study. Gastrointest Endosc. 2003;57:643–7.
40. Cai Q, Keilin S, Obideen K, et al. Intraduodenal hydrochloric acid infusion for facilitation of cannulation of the dorsal pancreatic duct at ERCP in patients with pancreas divisum: a preliminary study. Am J Gastroenterol. 2010;105:1450–1.
41. Dewitt J, McHenry L, Fogel E, et al. EUS-guided methylene blue pancreatography for minor papilla localization after unsuccessful ERCP. Gastrointest Endosc. 2004;59(1):133–6.
42. Benage D, McHenry R, Hawes RH, et al. Minor papilla cannulation and dorsal ductography in pancreas divisum. Gastrointest Endosc. 1990;36(6):553–7.
43. Bataille L, Deprez P. A new application for therapeutic EUS: main pancreatic duct drainage with a "pancreatic rendezvous technique". Gastrointest Endosc. 2002;55(6):740–3.
44. Gerke H, Byrne MF, Stiffler HL, et al. Outcome of endoscopic minor papillotomy in patients with symptomatic pancreas divisum. JOP. 2004;5:122–31.
45. Attwell A, Borak G, Hawes R, et al. Endoscopic pancreatic sphincterotomy for pancreas divisum by using a needle-knife or standard pull-type technique: safety and reintervention rates. Gastrointest Endosc. 2006;64:705–11.

16 Biliary Stones Extraction

Andrea Tringali

16.1 Introduction: "Difficult" Biliary Stones

The majority of common bile duct (CBD) stones can be considered "not difficult" since it can be removed with Fogarty balloon and/or Dormia basket following endoscopic sphincterotomy [1, 2]. When stone clearance of the biliary system is not possible with standard devices (balloon, basket), these stones are termed as "difficult," and further techniques are required (endoscopic papillary large balloon dilatation—EPLBD—mechanical lithotripsy, intraductal electrohydraulic/laser lithotripsy, or extracorporeal shock wave lithotripsy) [1].

"Difficult" biliary stones occur in 10–15% of the cases [3] and are usually large in diameter (>1.5 cm) and multiple (>5). Also stone shape (barrel-like), anatomical features of the bile ducts (strictures, narrowing, angulation), and location (cystic duct, intrahepatic) can make stones removal challenging. Altered anatomy increases ERCP difficulty but not the procedure of stones extraction itself.

Electronic Supplementary Material The online version of this chapter (https://doi.org/10.1007/978-3-030-42569-2_16) contains supplementary material, which is available to authorized users.

A. Tringali (✉)
Fondazione Policlinico Universitario A. Gemelli IRCCS. Digestive Endoscopy Unit, Rome, Italy

Centre for Endoscopic Research Therapeutics and Training (CERTT), Università Cattolica del Sacro Cuore, Rome, Italy
e-mail: andrea.tringali@unicatt.it

16.2 Bile Ducts Anatomy and Biliary Stones

Anatomical factors and stone location can affect the success in bile duct stones removal by ERCP.

16.2.1 Narrowing of the Distal Common Bile Duct

Extraction of CBD stones through the so-called "stemware-shaped" CBD [4] (Fig. 16.1a) requires mechanical lithotripsy (Fig. 16.1b) in 38% of the cases and conversion to a second-line procedure (PTC, temporary stenting, cholangioscopy, or surgery) in 58% of the cases, according to a retrospective series of 34 cases.

The absence of dilatation of the lower bile duct (DLBD) (diameter of the lower part of the extrahepatic bile duct <10 mm and its length > 10 mm, as measured by cholangiography) is another challenging anatomy when CBD stones extraction is attempted. EPLBD obtained stone clearance in all the 57 cases without DLBD included in a retrospective study [5]. When comparing EPLBD in

M. Mutignani et al. (eds.), *Endotherapy in Biliopancreatic Diseases: ERCP Meets EUS*,
https://doi.org/10.1007/978-3-030-42569-2_16

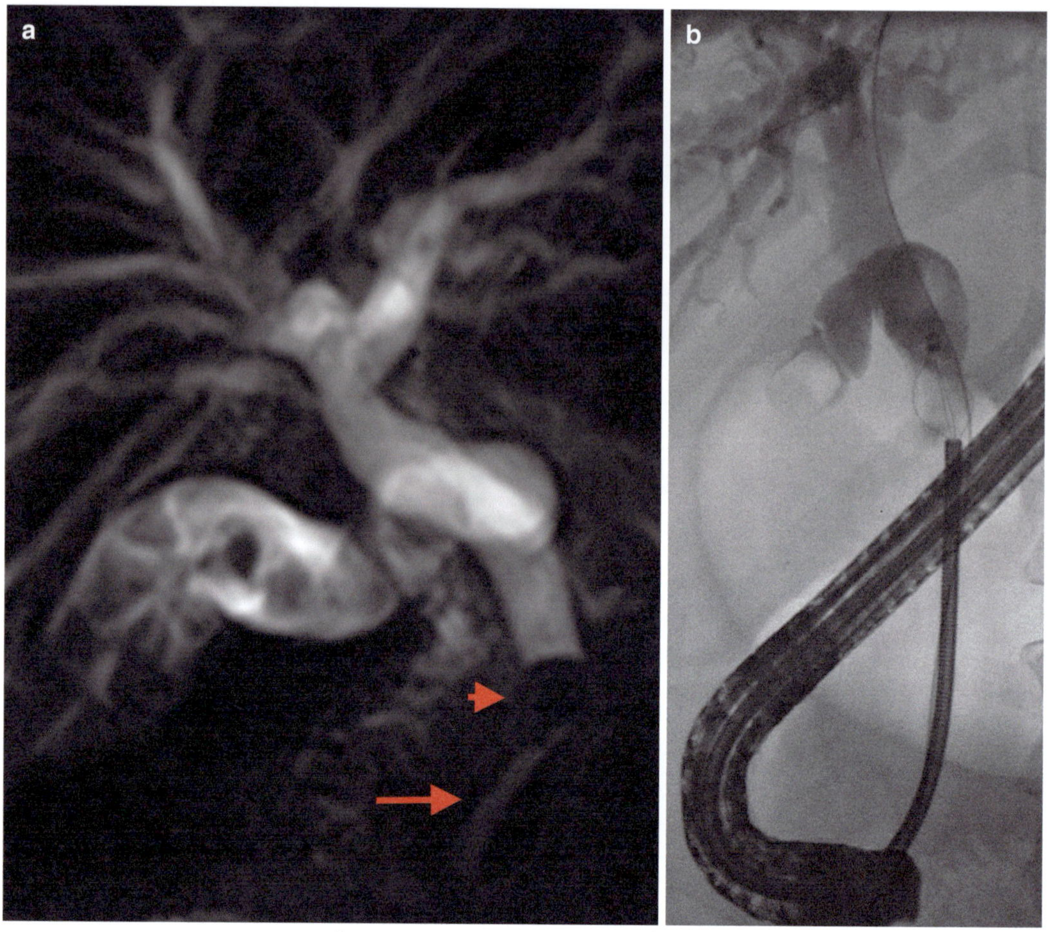

Fig. 16.1 A case of "stemware-shaped" bile duct diagnosed by magnetic resonance cholangiography; mismatch between distal bile duct (arrow) and stones diameter (arrowhead) is seen (**a**). Mechanical lithotripsy (**b**) is needed to fragment the stone

patients with and without DLBD, significant more time and more ERCP sessions were necessary to obtain stone clearance without DLBD, but the incidence of complications and the stone recurrence rate did not differ [5].

Discrepancy between stones diameter and the size of the distal common bile duct/sphincterotomy can be evaluated by the passage of an extraction balloon inflated at a fixed diameter.

16.2.2 Bile Duct Angulation

Kim et al. [6] prospectively evaluated risk factors for a difficult removal of CBD stones in 102 patients (46% with stones diameter ≥15 mm). Technical difficulty in CBD stones extraction were graded according to the number of attempts needed to completely clean the bile ducts by balloon or basket (easy, 1–2 attempts; moderately difficult, 3–8 attempts; difficult, > 8 attempts; failed, stones incompletely removed). A shorter length of the distal CBD arm (≤36 mm) and a more acute distal CBD angulation (≤135°) were found to be significant independent contributors to technical difficulty in the multivariate analysis. In such situations the sigmoid feature of the common bile duct makes handling of the devices challenging, and the possibility to pull the stone in the correct axis is limited.

16.2.3 Cystic Duct Stones

Cystic duct stones are usually impacted into the spiral valves of Heister; negotiating the cystic duct (usually not dilated) is challenging also by angled-tip, fully hydrophilic guidewires; grasping the stone, even if small, can be difficult due to the limited space.

16.2.4 Intrahepatic Stones

Stones located in the peripheral biliary ducts are difficult to remove especially if above a stricture or into an angled duct like the right posterior (segments VI–VII). Good-quality fluoroscopy is essential to negotiate intrahepatic ducts with an angled-tip fully hydrophilic guidewire which can be used to advance 5 French tapered devices (balloon or baskets over the wire).

16.3 Biliary Stones Extraction: Technical Points

16.3.1 The Sphincterotomy

A complete sphincterotomy (Video 16.1) is the first step to remove bile duct stones and to easily advance devices into the biliary ducts. The length of the sphincterotomy needs to be tailored according to the anatomy of the papillary infundibulum, which has different extension from papilla to papilla. For that reason the possibility to extract bile duct stones without prior fragmentation by lithotripsy needs to be evaluated according to the available extension of the sphincterotomy.

16.3.2 The Axis and the Traction

Endoscopic removal of bile duct stones needs a careful evaluation of the technique used to "pull" or "push" out the stones.

When *pulling* a balloon or a basket through the working channel the duodenoscope, the traction is not parallel to the axis of the bile duct, resulting in a breakdown strength through the angled part of the duodenoscope (Fig. 16.2).

Pushing out the stones can result in a more effective approach, especially to remove difficult bile duct stones. The endoscope is pushed and torqued clockwise (Video 16.2) providing the traction strength directly to the tip of the endoscope with an axis parallel to the bile duct (Fig. 16.3).

16.3.3 Fogarty Balloon or Dormia Basket?

Balloons and baskets resulted equally effective for stones ≤10 mm according to two randomized trials [7, 8].

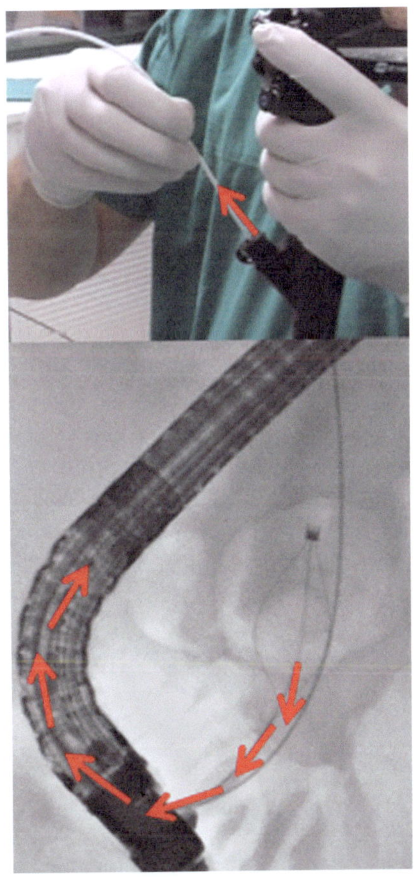

Fig. 16.2 Pulling a catheter through the working channel of the endoscope results in a breakdown strength through the angled part of the duodenoscope

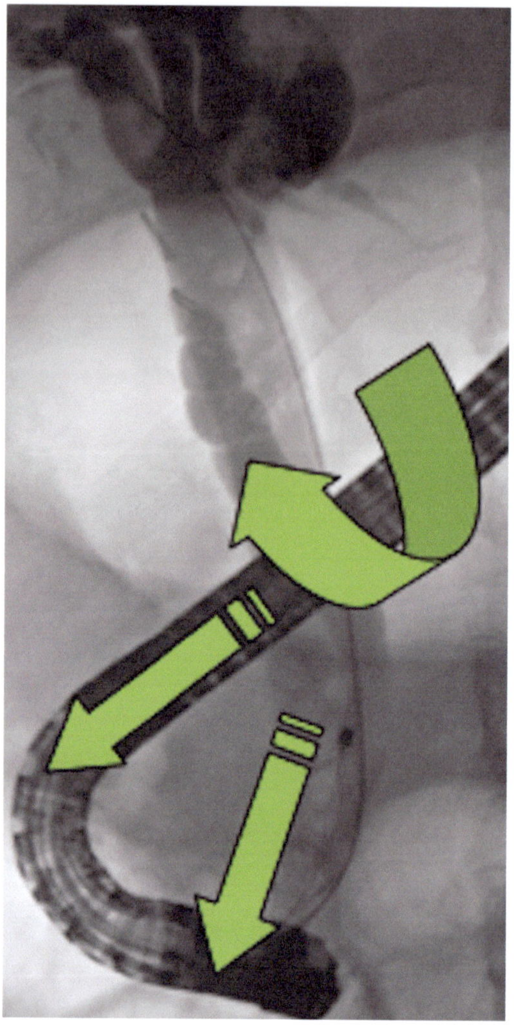

Fig. 16.3 Pushing and torquing clockwise the endoscope results in an effective transmission of the force to the tip of the endoscope

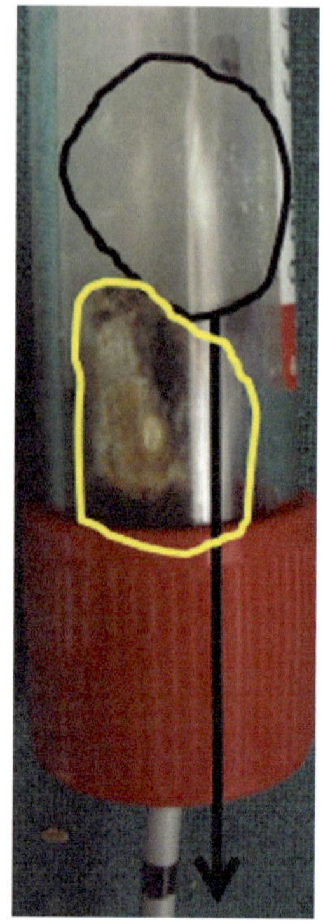

Fig. 16.4 The Fogarty balloon is compressed near the stone (yellow line) and the traction is applied on the side of the stone (arrow)

Fogarty balloons are inflated with air to avoid trauma to the bile ducts; air is compressed while the balloon is retracted over a stone and the resulting traction is eccentric (Fig. 16.4) and weak.

Dormia basket can grasp the stone, and the traction is transmitted in the middle of the stone (Fig. 16.5), making extraction very effective. Baskets are made of different materials (steel and nitinol). Nitinol has two main properties, memory shape (Fig. 16.6) and radial force (Fig. 16.7); these characteristics permit to firmly catch the stone. On the other hand, nitinol baskets are stiffer than others and some endoscopists consider them potentially traumatic. No studies compared different models of Dormia baskets.

The choice between balloon and baskets depends mainly from preference of the operator.

16.3.4 "Soft" and "Hard" Stones

Biliary stones have different consistency. Radiopaque stones are rare, but when encountered need to be considered extremely hard. In general bile duct stones migrated from the gallbladder are "hard," while recurrent bile duct stones are usually "soft." Dormia baskets of different size (Fig. 16.8) can be easily advanced over the wire to test stone consistency. To avoid entrapment of the basket over the stone, a small basket (i.e., 10 × 5 mm, 15 × 10 mm) can be used to scratch the stone and obtain a reduction in size before using a bigger basket to complete the extraction.

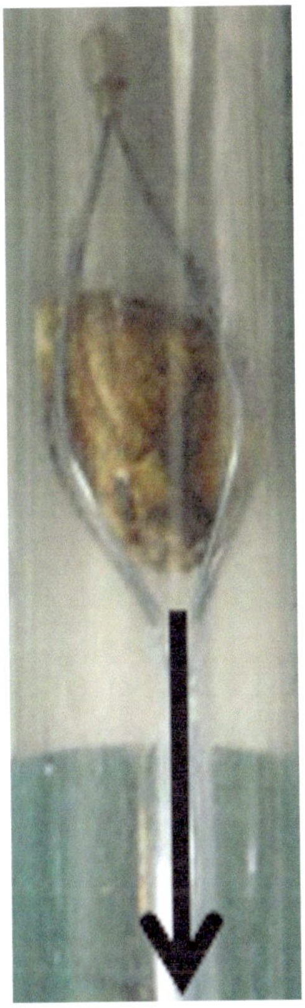

Fig. 16.5 The Dormia basket applies the traction in the middle of the stone (arrow)

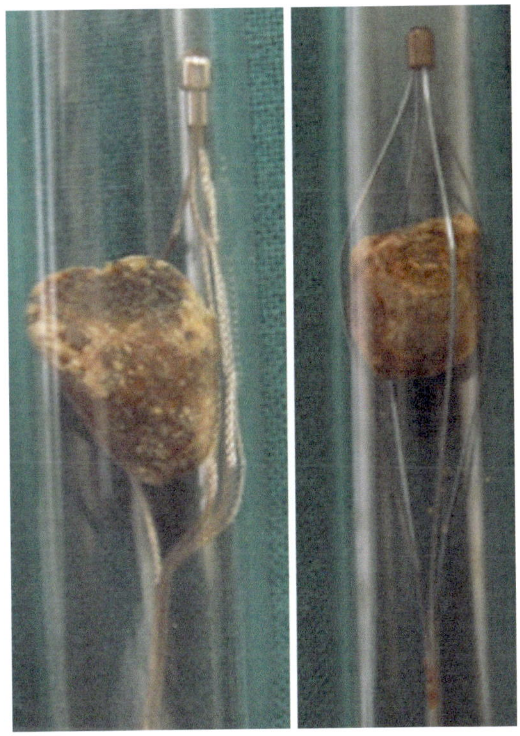

Fig. 16.7 Nitinol basket has radial force facilitating capture of the stone (right); stainless steel has a lower radial force (left)

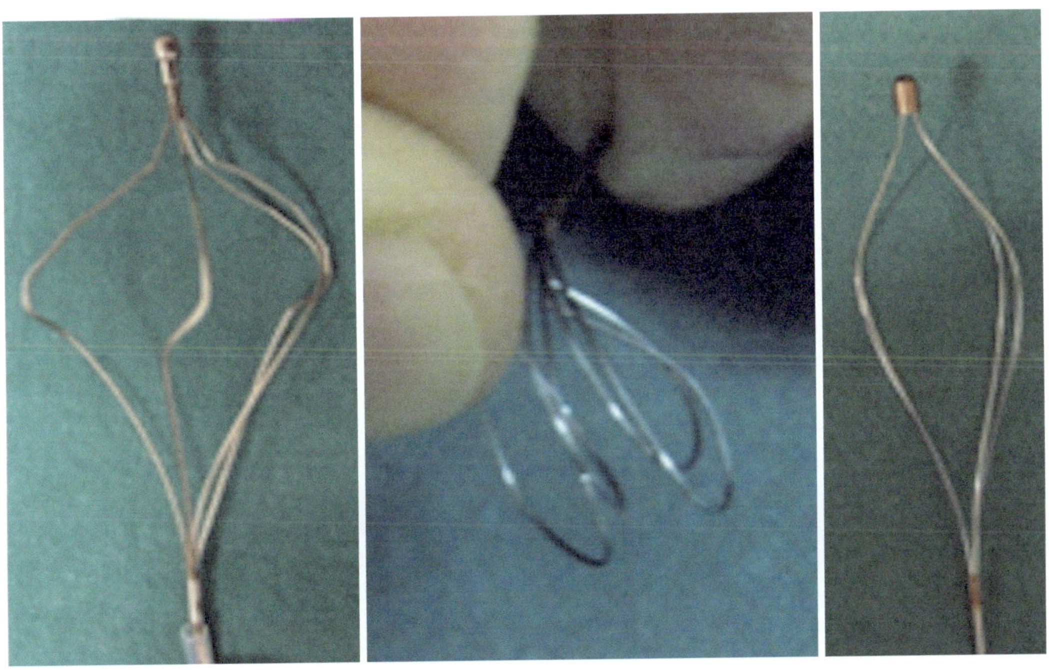

Fig. 16.6 Nitinol basket has memory shape (right), while stainless steel are easily deformed (left)

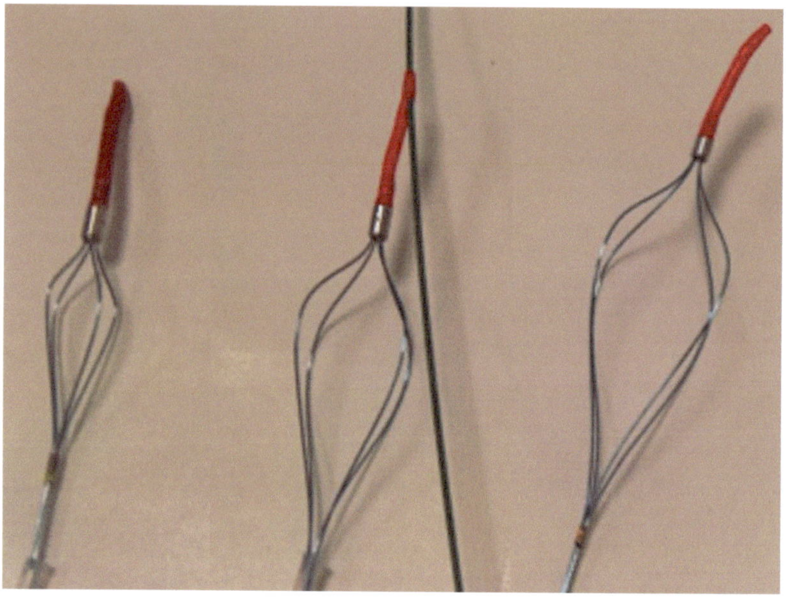

Fig. 16.8 Different sizes of nitinol Dormia baskets that can be advanced over the wire

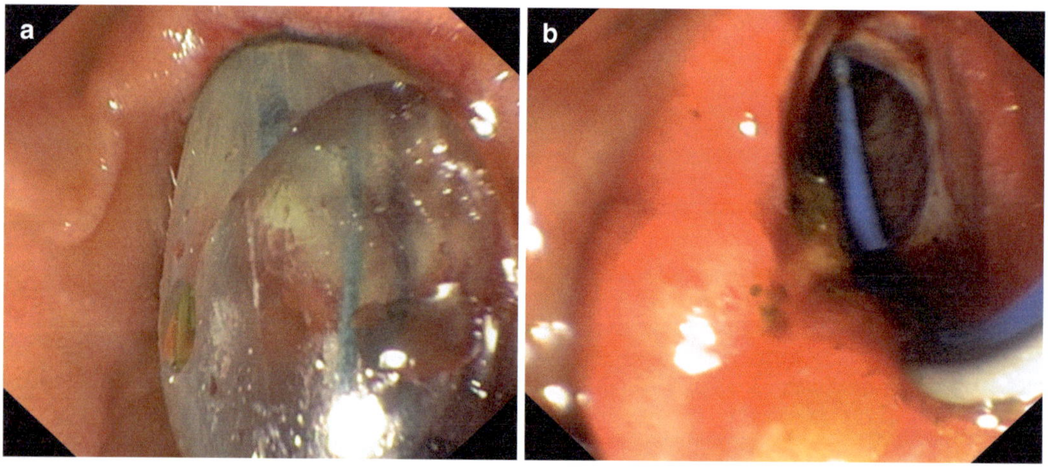

Fig. 16.9 Endoscopic papillary large balloon dilatation (**a**) results in a wide access to the bile duct (**b**)

16.3.5 Endoscopic Papillary Large Balloon Dilatation (EPLBD) and Mechanical Lithotripsy: When and How

EPLBD is a "large" (12–20 mm) dilatation of the ampulla (Fig. 16.9) after a complete or limited sphincterotomy. The technique was described in 2003 [9] and significantly reduced the need for the more complex mechanical lithotripsy [10, 11]. Balloon diameter is tailored according to bile duct diameter, and the balloon is slowly inflated until waist disappearance and is deflated 1 min later [10].

EPLBD is considered safe also in the presence of a periampullary diverticulum (Fig. 16.10) without increased complications [10].

Preferably EPLBD follows a limited sphincterotomy but can be performed also without sphincterotomy in patients with coagulopathy without increased risk of pancreatitis or bleeding [10].

The role of mechanical lithotripsy is today limited to the minority of stones that cannot be

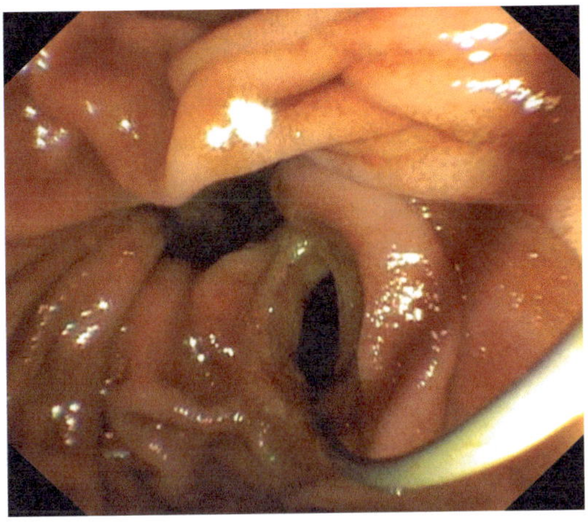

Fig. 16.10 Endoscopic papillary large balloon dilatation of a papilla on the rim of a duodenal diverticulum

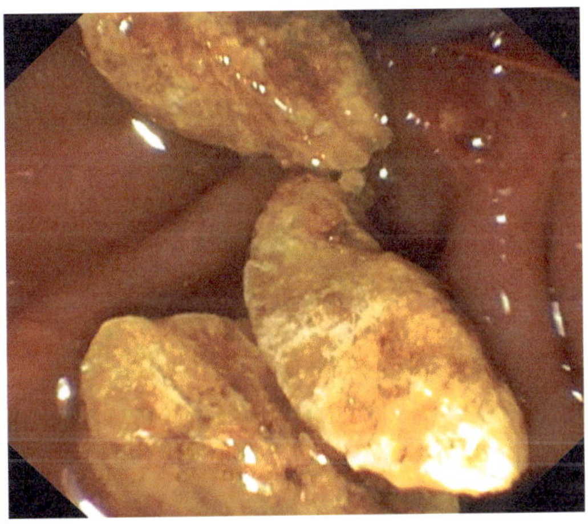

Fig. 16.11 Effective stone fragmentation after mechanical lithotripsy

extracted after EPLBD. Through the channel mechanical lithotripsy with dedicated Dormia baskets is effective (Figs. 16.1b and 16.11); handling of the stiff metal sheath and extraction of fragments are nevertheless facilitated by EPLBD. The main concern for mechanical lithotripsy are complications (trapped basket, traction wire fracture, duct perforation) which are rare [12], but difficult to manage.

In case of failed stones extraction after EPLBD, cholangioscopy-assisted lithotripsy is considered today a first-line choice with a low complications rate, despite the high costs.

Extracorporeal shock wave lithotripsy is less used today due to logistic problem (need for repeated ERCPs) and to the diffusion of cholangioscopy, which give the possibility to perform lithotripsy (laser/EHL) during the same ERCP procedure.

References

1. McHenry L, Lehman G. Difficult bile duct stones. Curr Treat Options Gastroenterol. 2006;9(2):123–32.
2. Trikudanathan G, Navaneethan U, Parsi MA. Endoscopic management of difficult common bile duct stones. World J Gastroenterol. 2013;19(2):165–73.
3. Strömberg C, Nilsson M. Nationwide study of the treatment of common bile duct stones in Sweden between 1965 and 2009. Br J Surg. 2011;98(12):1766–74.
4. Han JY, Lee DH, Jeong S, Choi HJ, Moon JH, Han JH, Kwon CI, Lee TH, Hyun JJ, Hwang JC, Koh DH. Clinical features and outcomes of endoscopic treatment for stones in stemware-shaped common bile ducts: a multicenter data analysis. Gut Liver. 2015;9(6):800–4.
5. Fujita Y, Iwasaki A, Sato T, Fujisawa T, Sekino Y, Hosono K, Matsuhashi N, Sakamaki K, Nakajima A, Kubota K. Feasibility of endoscopic papillary large balloon dilation in patients with difficult bile duct stones without dilatation of the lower part of the extrahepatic bile duct. Gut Liver. 2017;11(1):149–55.
6. Kim HJ, Choi HS, Park JH, Park DI, Cho YK, Sohn CI, Jeon WK, Kim BI, Choi SH. Factors influencing the technical difficulty of endoscopic clearance of bile duct stones. Gastrointest Endosc. 2007;66(6):1154–60.
7. Ishiwatari H, Kawakami H, Hisai H, Yane K, Onodera M, Eto K, Haba S, Okuda T, Ihara H, Kukitsu T, Matsumoto R, Kitaoka K, Sonoda T, Hayashi T. Balloon catheter versus basket catheter for endoscopic bile duct stone extraction: a multicenter randomized trial. Endoscopy. 2016;48(4):350–7.
8. Ozawa N, Yasuda I, Doi S, Iwashita T, Shimizu M, Mukai T, Nakashima M, Ban T, Kojima I, Matsuda K, Matsuda M, Ishida Y, Okabe Y, Ando N, Iwata K. Prospective randomized study of endoscopic biliary stone extraction using either a basket or a balloon catheter: the BasketBall study. J Gastroenterol. 2017;52(5):623–30.
9. Ersoz G, Tekesin O, Ozutemiz AO, Gunsar F. Biliary sphincterotomy plus dilation with a large balloon for bile duct stones that are difficult to extract. Gastrointest Endosc. 2003;57(2):156–9.
10. Kim TH, Kim JH, Seo DW, Lee DK, Reddy ND, Rerknimitr R, Ratanachu-Ek T, Khor CJ, Itoi T, Yasuda I, Isayama H, Lau JY, Wang HP, Chan HH, Hu B, Kozarek RA, Baron TH. International consensus

guidelines for endoscopic papillary large-balloon dilation. Gastrointest Endosc. 2016;83(1):37–47.
11. Williams E, Beckingham I, El Sayed G, Gurusamy K, Sturgess R, Webster G, Young T. Updated guideline on the management of common bile duct stones (CBDS). Gut. 2017;66(5):765–82.
12. Thomas M, Howell DA, Carr-Locke D, Mel Wilcox C, Chak A, Raijman I, Watkins JL, Schmalz MJ, Geenen JE, Catalano MF. Mechanical lithotripsy of pancreatic and biliary stones: complications and available treatment options collected from expert centers. Am J Gastroenterol. 2007;102(9):1896–902.

17 Intraductal Lithotripsy

Jörg G. Albert and Jan Peveling-Oberhag

17.1 Introduction

Intraductal lithotripsy is based on oral or percutaneous endoscopic access to the bile duct system. It is required in those cases in which the intraductal stone may not be removed by means of 'simple' ERCP. Laser lithotripsy (LL) and electrohydraulic lithotripsy (EHL) require cholangioscopy technique, as visualization of the stone is needed to guarantee effective destruction and to avoid damage to the bile duct wall. Stone destruction during ERCP can alternatively be achieved by mechanical lithotripsy using a metal basket which is consecutively closed to crush the stone.

Other alternatives, such as extracorporeal stone wave lithotripsy (ESWL), are less often used for destruction of incarcerated bile duct stones.

17.2 Mechanical Lithotripsy

Demling et al. introduced mechanical lithotripsy in 1982 using a basket, which is placed around the stone, and consecutively a metal sheath is advanced to forcefully close the basket and crush the stone [1]. Lithotripter baskets can be introduced into the bile duct with or without guide wire. The method is readily available as no cholangioscopy is required. However, in very hard stones, the basket wires may break or the wires may detach from the handle getting the basket stuck in the bile duct. In the latter case, emergency mechanical lithotripsy is required. Here, detached wires are connected to an emergency mechanical lithotripter to finally crush the stone. If this method fails, cholangioscopic methods as mentioned below or surgery is required to save the day. Impacted stones, stone diameter of >30 mm, and stone-to-bile duct diameter ratio >1 are associated with failure of mechanical lithotripsy [2]. Further features of "difficult biliary stones" besides stone size include altered patient anatomy, multiple stones, location in the intrahepatic or cystic duct, and barrel shape. Up to 10% of bile duct stones cannot be removed by standard techniques including mechanical lithotripsy [2, 3].

J. G. Albert (✉) · J. Peveling-Oberhag
Abteilung für Gastroenterologie, Hepatologie und Endokrinologie, Robert-Bosch-Krankenhaus, Stuttgart, Germany
e-mail: joerg.albert@rbk.de; Jan.peveling-oberhag@rbk.de

M. Mutignani et al. (eds.), *Endotherapy in Biliopancreatic Diseases: ERCP Meets EUS*,
https://doi.org/10.1007/978-3-030-42569-2_17

17.3 Cholangioscopy-Guided Lithotripsy

The primary advantage of cholangioscopy is the direct visualization of the biliary tree [4, 5]. It is mainly used to investigate indeterminate pancreaticobiliary strictures and manage difficult-to-treat stones (Figs. 17.1 and 17.2). The typical access for cholangioscopy is peroral but can also be transhepatic after a percutaneous transhepatic bile duct drainage has been established. Peroral access can be used either for retrograde or direct cholangioscopy. Generally, cholangioscopy has undergone a fast evolution in the last 10 years. Mother-baby scope systems requiring two separate operators have been taken over by single-operator cholangioscopy (SOC) systems. Especially the recent development of one-time-use catheter-based cholangioscopy with digital imaging (Spyglass Direct Visualization DS Boston Scientific) has made cholangioscopy available for a wide spectrum of users. The second access way is direct antegrade cholangioscopy with the use of an ultraslim endoscope. Retrograde SOC clearly has the advantage of improved user-friendliness as the technique largely resembles the typical procedure of instrument insertion during ERCP. However, direct cholangioscopy is able to use the existing endoscopy processor and the ultraslim endoscope can be hygienically reprocessed. Also, to date, optical resolution is superior, and a larger working channel allows for greater flexibility, has superior suction, and conserves introduced tools. A comparison of both techniques when used for stone extraction is listed in Table 17.1.

17.4 Cholangioscopy-Guided Laser Lithotripsy and Electrohydraulic Lithotripsy

17.4.1 Technical Background

EHL: Disintegration of calculi by a shock wave that results from an electric discharge. The probe is advanced to the stone through the working channel of an endoscope (CAVE: The EHL probe is very fragile and can be damaged by an acute angle of the cholangioscope). The position is monitored via direct endoscopic view and via X-ray. A controlled, very fast electric discharge centered at the tip of the EHL probe generates plasma sparks under water, which produce high-frequency hydraulic pressure waves. The hydraulic energy is absorbed by the bile duct stones and leads to their destruction. The effect is intensified under irrigation with electrolyte-containing fluids, such as normal saline instead of water.

LL: Disintegration of calculi by a shock wave that results from so-called nonlinear optical effects induced by laser light focused to a high power density (>100 billion W/cm^2). Pulsed dye lasers emit energy at a particular wavelength, which is delivered to the stone by optical fibers resulting in wave-mediated fragmentation. Different laser types are used such as pulsed solid-state lasers, e.g., yttrium aluminum garnet (Nd:YAG) or holmium:YAG, or pulsed dye lasers such as ash lamp-pulsed dye (coumarin), flash lamp-pulsed dye (rhodamine) with automatic stone recognition system, or frequency-doubled double-pulse Nd:YAG (FREDDY) system. More recently, holmium:YAG lasers have become the preferred option both in the United States and throughout Europe in the setting of cholangioscopic lithotripsy as they produce smaller stone fragments.

Stone removal using conventional methods, such as sphincterotomy and/or papillary balloon dilatation combined with a balloon retrieval catheter, basket catheter, or a mechanical lithotripter, are unsuccessful in 10–15% of cases [6, 7]. Part of the failure rate is due to the patient anatomy with difficult access to the papilla. The other part results from stone factors, such as large (>15 mm), multiple (>3), intrahepatic duct/cystic duct, barrel-shaped, or impacted stones.

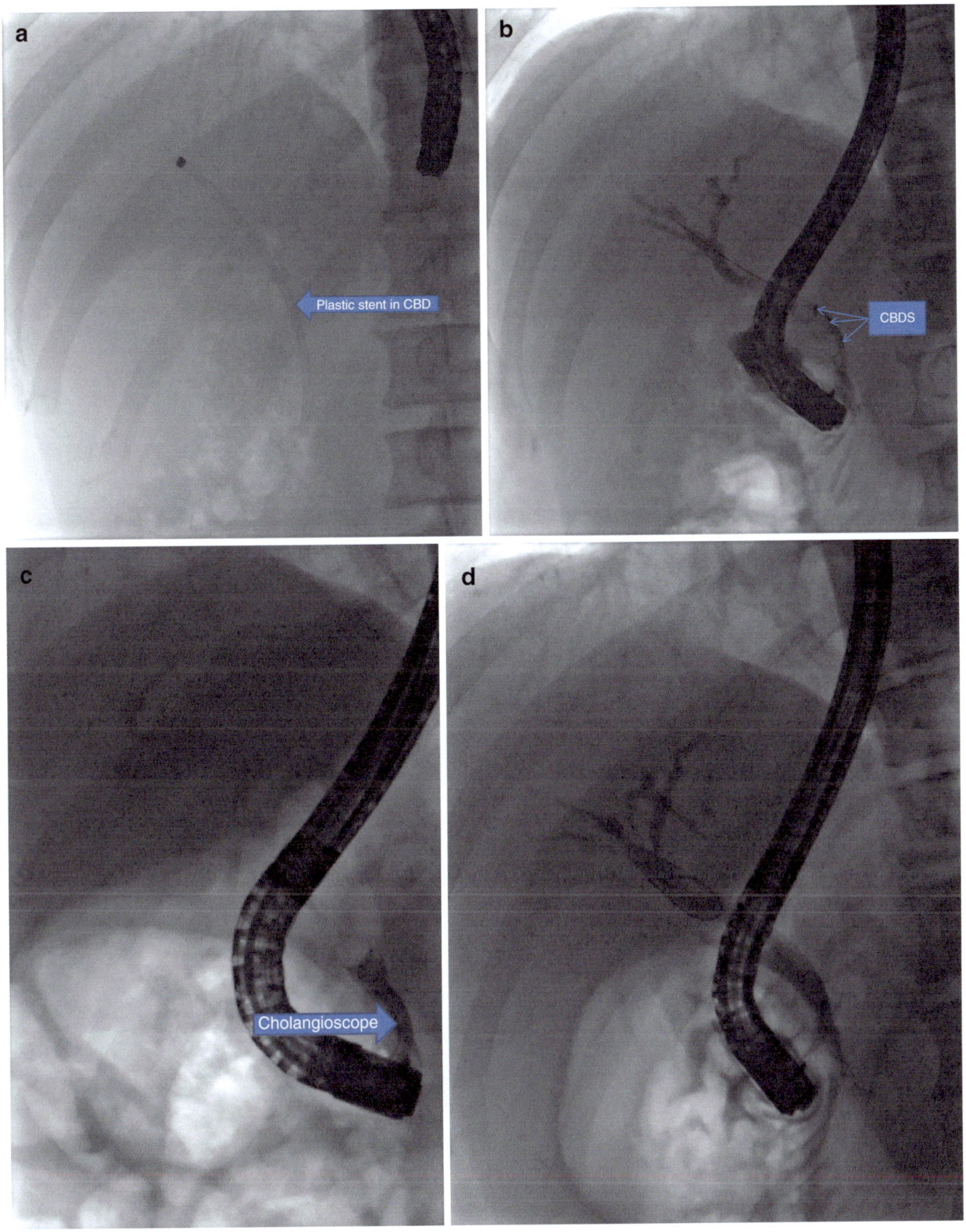

Fig. 17.1 Incarcerated stones of the distal common bile duct that could not be removed by conventional ERCP in a 49-year-old male patient. (**a**) Diverse attempts to remove the stone were not successful, and a plastic stent was placed to allow bile duct flow. (**b**) There were several stones incarcerated in the distal CBD. (**c**) With use of peroral retrograde cholangioscopy, intraductal EHL was performed …. (**d**) … and the stones were fragmented. (**e**) The EHL probe is placed on the stone. (**f**) … and the fragments after activating the EHL are visualized. (**g**) Finally, a fully covered metal stent (cSEMS) was placed for 6–8 weeks to allow for a completed healing of the inflamed CBD

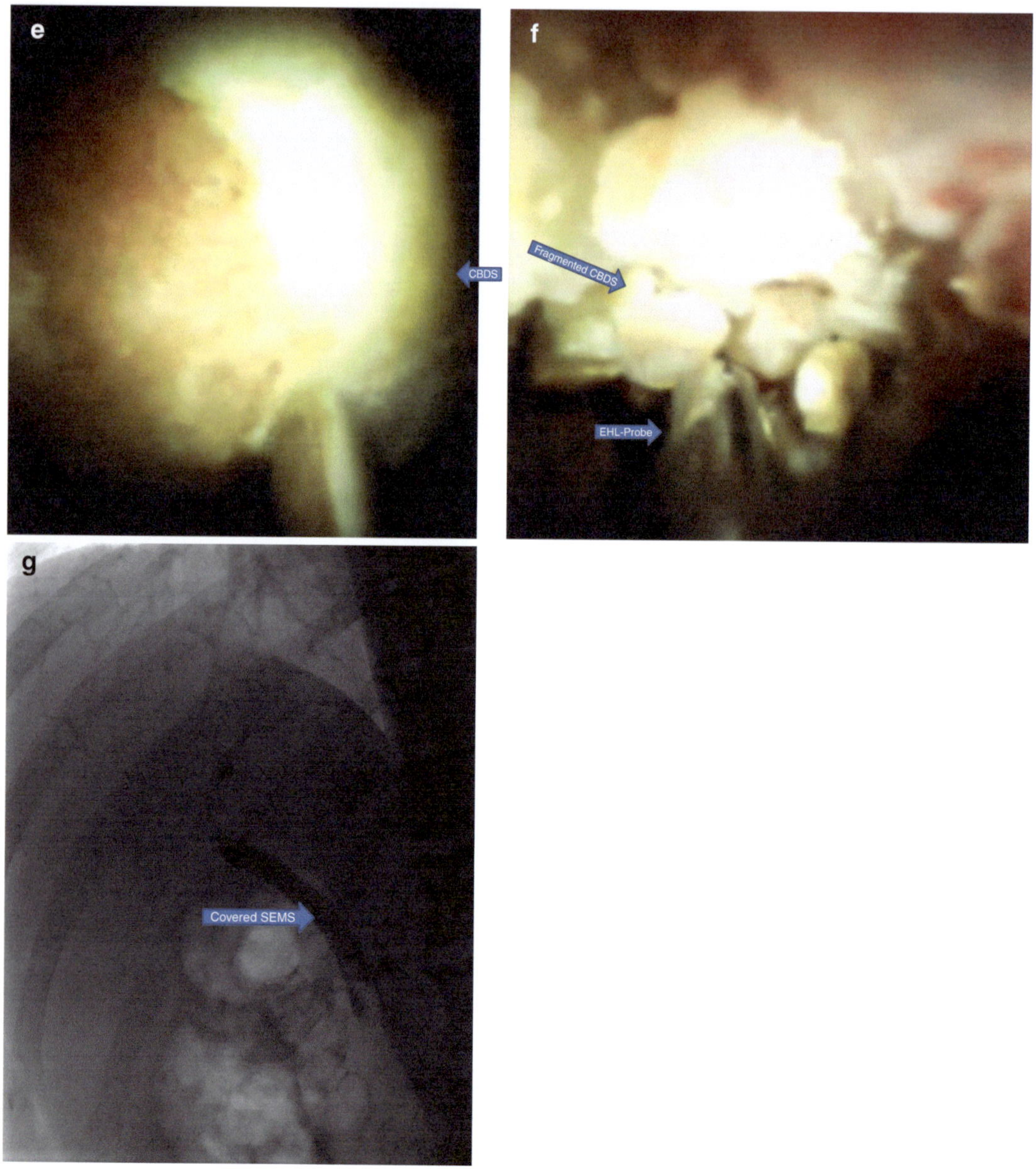

Fig. 17.1 (continued)

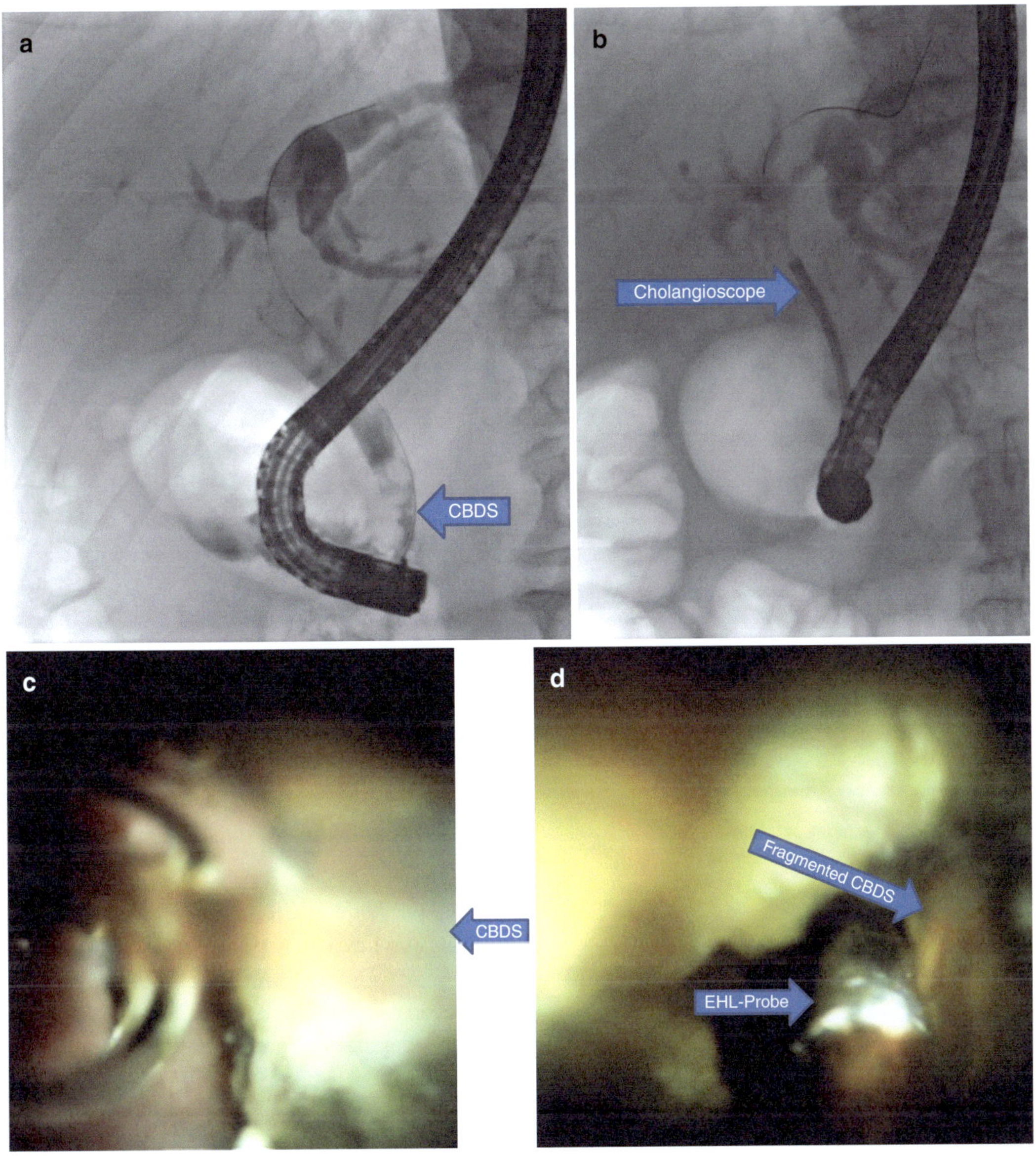

Fig. 17.2 Multiple stones of the distal common bile duct that could not be removed by mechanical lithotripsy in a 78-year-old male patient. (**a**) Several common bile duct stones up to 2 cm diameter. (**b**) Application of peroral retrograde cholangioscopy (Spyglass DS Boston Scientific). (**c**) Intraductal stones were visualized…. (**d**) … and the stones were fragmented using EHL. (**e**) The resulting multiple small stone fragments escape naturally through the papillotomy site

Cholangioscopic-guided lithotripsy is the method of choice to treat such "difficult stones."

Brewer Gutierrez et al. investigated the efficacy and safety of digital SOC with EHL and LL in an international, multicenter study of patients with difficult biliary stones [8]. The authors performed a retrospective analysis including 407 patients. Three hundred and six patients underwent EHL and 101 (24.8%) underwent LL. The mean procedure time was longer in the EHL group (73.9 min) than in the LL group (49.9 min; $P < 0.001$). The technical success rate was 97.3%. Adverse events occurred in 3.7% patients and the stone was incompletely removed from 6.6% of

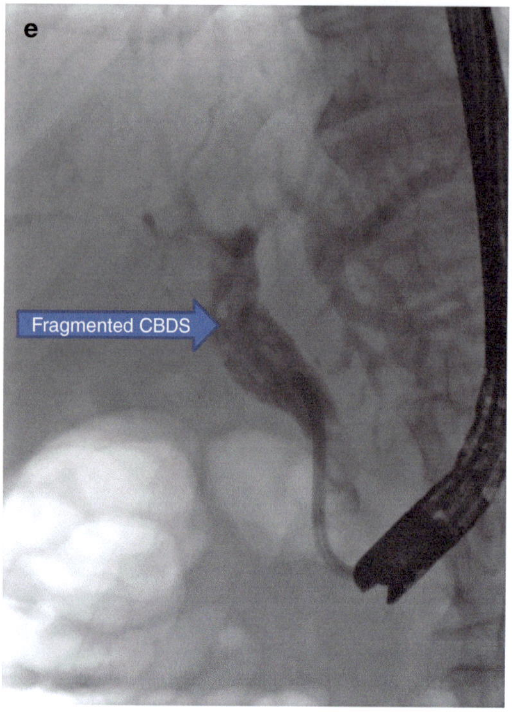

Fig. 17.2 (continued)

Table 17.1 Comparison of retrograde and antegrade access way for cholangioscopic lithotripsy

	Retrograde cholangioscopy	Direct cholangioscopy
User-friendliness/ easy insertion	++	–
Optical resolution	–	+
Diameter of working channel	–	+
Costs of probe/ endoscope	–	–
Costing of generator	–	n/a

patients. Adverse events consisted of mainly cholangitis and abdominal pain and one patient with bile duct perforation. Five percent of patients require additional treatment with surgery and/or extracorporeal shock wave lithotripsy to clear the duct.

Buxbaum et al. performed a randomized trial comparing cholangioscopy-guided LL using a holmium laser system with conventional therapy of large bile duct stones [9]. Patients with bile duct stones >1 cm in diameter were randomized in a 2:1 ratio to cholangioscopy-guided LL versus conventional therapy only. The primary endpoint was endoscopic clearance of the stones. Endoscopic clearance was achieved in 93% treated with LL and 67% treated with conventional therapy only ($P = 0.009$). Mean procedure time was longer in the LL group (120.7 vs. 81.2 min, $P = 0.0008$). Adverse events were similar in the two treatment groups (OR, 0.8; 95% CI, 0.1–5.0). EHL and LL are compared in Table 17.2.

Table 17.2 Comparison of EHL and LL for cholangioscopic lithotripsy

	EHL	LL
Environment	Fluid submersion	
Technical background	High-energy shock wave	Laser light
Diameter of probe	0.66–1.1 mm	0.5–1.0 mm
Costs of probe	(+)	(+)
Costs of generator	+	+++

17.5 General Tips and Tricks for Successful Lithotripsy

Antibiotic prophylaxis is recommended for all endoscopic lithotripsy procedures to avoid cholangitis as well as pulmonary infections through silent aspiration as procedure times are long and a deep level of sedation is usually needed.

Endoscopic papillary large balloon dilatation generally improves conventional biliary stone clearance [10, 11]. Also for cholangioscopy the accessibility of the bile duct for the cholangioscope is markedly improved. Therefore, endoscopic papillary large balloon dilatation can be recommended for lithotripsy.

When aiming to capture the stone for basket mechanical lithotripsy, it is advisable to open the basket below the stone. The success rate to catch the stone is decreased by 33% when the basket is opened above the target [12].

For mechanical lithotripsy it is very important to avoid sharp angles between the endoscope and the bile duct before advancing the metal sheath of the lithotripter, as strong forces apply and bile duct as well as the duodenal wall can be damaged.

EHL and LL probes are very thin and rather fragile. It is important to relax the duodenoscopic angle and the Albarrán lever when advancing the probe into the bile duct.

17.6 Conclusion

The majority of bile duct stones can be destructed and removed using conventional ERCP techniques. Mechanical lithotripsy is easy to use and readily available but may fail with impacted stones, stone diameter of >30 mm, and stone-to-bile duct diameter ratio >1. Cholangioscopic-guided EHL or LL can be used for such "difficult stones." EHL and LL are usually not available in small endoscopic centers. It is therefore recommended to refer patients with the abovementioned criteria to high-volume endoscopic centers after biliary stenting.

References

1. Riemann JF, Seuberth K, Demling L. Clinical application of a new mechanical lithotripter for smashing common bile duct stones. Endoscopy. 1982;14(6):226–30. Epub 1982/11/01.
2. Lee SH, Park JK, Yoon WJ, Lee JK, Ryu JK, Kim YT, et al. How to predict the outcome of endoscopic mechanical lithotripsy in patients with difficult bile duct stones? Scand J Gastroenterol. 2007;42(8):1006–10. Epub 2007/07/07.
3. Schneider MU, Matek W, Bauer R, Domschke W. Mechanical lithotripsy of bile duct stones in 209 patients—effect of technical advances. Endoscopy. 1988;20(5):248–53. Epub 1988/09/01.
4. Farnik H, Weigt J, Malfertheiner P, Grutzmann A, Gossner L, Friedrich-Rust M, et al. A multicenter study on the role of direct retrograde cholangioscopy in patients with inconclusive endoscopic retrograde cholangiography. Endoscopy. 2014;46(1):16–21. Epub 2013/12/20.
5. Korrapati P, Ciolino J, Wani S, Shah J, Watson R, Muthusamy VR, et al. The efficacy of peroral cholangioscopy for difficult bile duct stones and indeterminate strictures: a systematic review and meta-analysis. Endosc Int Open. 2016;4(3):E263–75. Epub 2016/03/24.
6. Stefanidis G, Christodoulou C, Manolakopoulos S, Chuttani R. Endoscopic extraction of large common bile duct stones: a review article. World J Gastrointest Endosc. 2012;4(5):167–79. Epub 2012/05/25.
7. Trikudanathan G, Arain MA, Attam R, Freeman ML. Advances in the endoscopic management of common bile duct stones. Nat Rev Gastroenterol Hepatol. 2014;11(9):535–44. Epub 2014/05/28.
8. Brewer Gutierrez OI, Bekkali NLH, Raijman I, Sturgess R, Sejpal DV, Aridi HD, et al. Efficacy and safety of digital single-operator cholangioscopy for difficult biliary stones. Clin Gastroenterol Hepatol. 2018;16(6):918–26.e1. Epub 2017/10/28.
9. Buxbaum J, Sahakian A, Ko C, Jayaram P, Lane C, Yu CY, et al. Randomized trial of cholangioscopy-guided laser lithotripsy versus conventional therapy for large bile duct stones (with videos). Gastrointest Endosc. 2018;87(4):1050–60. Epub 2017/09/04.
10. Karsenti D, Coron E, Vanbiervliet G, Privat J, Kull E, Bichard P, et al. Complete endoscopic sphincterotomy with vs. without large-balloon dilation for the removal of large bile duct stones: randomized multicenter study. Endoscopy. 2017;49(10):968–76. Epub 2017/07/29.
11. Yang XM, Hu B. Endoscopic sphincterotomy plus large-balloon dilation vs endoscopic sphincterotomy for choledocholithiasis: a meta-analysis. World J Gastroenterol. 2013;19(48):9453–60. Epub 2014/01/11.
12. Shi D, Yu CG. Comparison of two capture methods for endoscopic removal of large common bile duct stones. J Laparoendosc Adv Surg Tech A. 2014;24(7):457–61. Epub 2014/07/06.

18 Biliary and Pancreatic ESWL

Lorenzo Dioscoridi, Francesco Pugliese, Edoardo Forti, Alberto Tringali, Marcello Cintolo, Giulia Bonato, and Massimiliano Mutignani

18.1 General Principles About ESWL

ESWL is based on the principle of shock wave energy [1]. Whenever energy is abruptly released in an enclosed space, shock waves are generated. The passage of these shock waves through substances of different acoustic impedance generates compressive stress on the boundary surface. This stress eventually overcomes the tensile strength of the object (in the present case, biliary and pancreatic calculi), and the anterior surface of the calculi crumbles as a result. The shock waves cross to the posterior surface of the calculi and some of them are reflected back and cause further fragmentation. Modern lithotripsy machines consist of the following basic components:

1. *Shock wave generator*

   The first-generation lithotripters utilized electrohydraulic energy or piezoelectric crystals for shock wave generation. The newer third-generation lithotripter utilizes the principle of electromagnetic shock wave generation from an electromagnetic coil. These shock waves are focused on a target (calculi) using an acoustic lens or cylindrical reflector.
2. *Focusing system*

   Shock waves are focused to the focal point or target in the body. This focal path is conical in shape and all the waves are concentrated at the apex of the cone, which is called the focal point. During ESWL, the focal point targets the calculi. Targeted focusing reduces collateral tissue damage and minimizes the complications.
3. *Localization*

   Localization of the calculi is basically done by fluoroscopy or ultrasound. All the newer lithotripters are equipped with both these facilities.
4. *Coupling device*

   The generated shock waves are transmitted through a coupling device to the skin surface and then through the body tissue to the calculi. The first lithotripters used a "water bath" for this purpose. The newer machines use a small water-filled cushion covered with a silicone membrane to transmit the shock waves to the patient's skin.

When shock waves traverse the stone, cavitation occurs at the surface, and the changes in acoustic impedance release compressive and tensile forces, resulting in fragmentation.

L. Dioscoridi (✉) · F. Pugliese · A. Tringali
M. Cintolo · E. Forti · G. Bonato · M. Mutignani
Digestive and Interventional Endoscopy Unit, ASST Grande Ospedale Metropolitano Niguarda, Niguarda-Ca' Granda Hospital, Milan, Italy
e-mail: lorenzo.dioscoridi@ospedaleniguarda.it

M. Mutignani et al. (eds.), *Endotherapy in Biliopancreatic Diseases: ERCP Meets EUS*,
https://doi.org/10.1007/978-3-030-42569-2_18

In our experience, we use a third-generation lithotripter (Siemens) equipped with electromagnetic coil, a cylindrical reflector, both fluoroscopy and ultrasound, and a water-filled cushion as coupling device.

18.2 Technical Principles of ESWL

Here, we describe the main steps to basically perform pancreatic and biliary ESWL:

1. The patient must remain fasten from 6 h before the procedure. He lies down in supine or prone position with complete monitoring of vital parameters (minimal required are oxygen saturation and cardiac frequency). ECG monitoring does not interfere with the procedure (check the electrodes' position before the beginning). O_2 therapy and correct placement of eventual nose-biliary/pancreatic drains must be checked before starting the procedure. A urinary cathetering is not mandatory. A peripheral venous access must be in site before the beginning of the procedure.
2. A baseline X-ray is always performed to check if the stones are radiologically visible, to localize them, and to check the position of eventual nose-biliary/pancreatic drains. If they are not visible, firstly the XR projection has to be varied (sometimes they can be on the same plane of the vertebral column); secondly iodine contrast medium could be injected through the nose-biliary/pancreatic drain to indirectly localize the stones (*minus* findings). Ultrasound localization can be alternatively used. The patient's position must be modified according to the best view of the calculi (sustaining devices can be placed to fix the patient's position). From now on, patient's position must not be modified and the patient must remain firm with regular breathing.
3. The stones are punctated to obtain the limited field of ESWL action. The more in the center of the field they are, the more effective the ESWL will be. Punctature is better performed in two projections (frontal and lateral) to maximize the ESWL action. Ultrasound punctuation can also be used: it let to obtain a more precise and direct ESWL action than XR punctuation.
4. The therapeutic position is reached at this point: the coupling device descends automatically to the patient anterior abdominal wall. It is important to put water gel on the cushion to improve the signal power. A last fluoroscopic check can be done before starting the procedure. From now on, only the area of shock wave action can be studied.
5. We begin the procedure starting with a low energy (0.1 J) that automatically increases till 1 J in a period of 250 shock waves. We start conscient sedation at this time (the first steps are not painful at all) using intravenous midazolam and meperidine. We adjust the sedation according to the grade of discomfort of the patient. A referral image from point 2 could help to adjust the therapeutical position at the beginning and during the procedure.
6. During ESWL, the results of our action can be checked by fluoroscopy or ultrasounds. In our experience, this check is performed every 1000 W. We gradually increase the energy of ESWL trying to reach the maximum potence (around 4.5 J) in the first 1000 W according to the stones' dimension and the patient's discomfort. Moreover, if a nose-biliary/pancreatic drain is present, sterile saline solution injection during all the session would improve the shock wave action. Consider that saline solution injection usually worsens the patient's discomfort.
7. At the end of the procedure, the machine is put in the rest position. A post-procedural XR or ultrasound is always performed. Sometimes a small skin excoriation is visible.
8. The patient generally returns to the ward and starts a light diet 3–4 h after the procedure.

In our experience (around 30 patients per year), we performed from one to three sessions of ESWL, on consecutive days or at a medium interval of 1 week depending on the symptoms presented by the patient. We suggest to concentrate on a single stone for each session. In our center, ERCP is generally performed before ESWL to perform sphincterotomy and/or position a nose-pancreatic/biliary drain (Figs. 18.1, 18.2, 18.3, and 18.4).

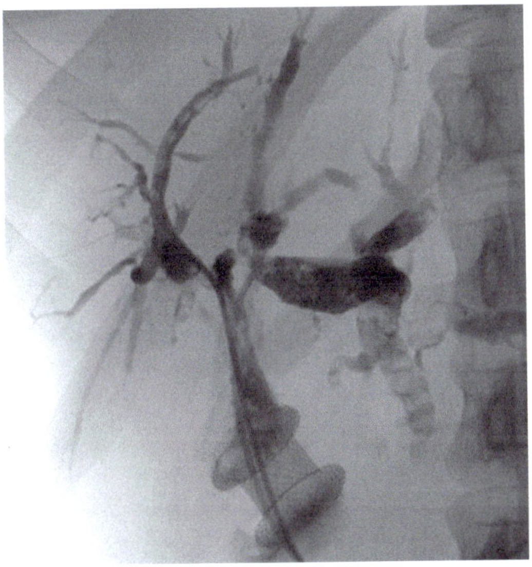

Fig. 18.1 Multiple intrahepatic biliary stones after hepaticojejunostomy. The patient underwent three consecutive ESWL sessions (5000 W, 4 J, 90 W for each session) and a subsequent ERC to remove all the fragmented stones

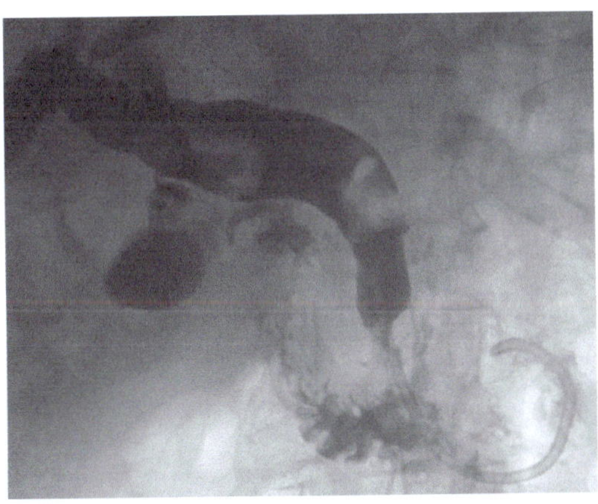

Fig. 18.2 Huge stones of the common bile duct after total gastrectomy. The patient underwent three consecutive sessions of ESWL (5000 W, 4,5 J, 90 W for each session), and the fragmented stones were pushed out using the percutaneous access

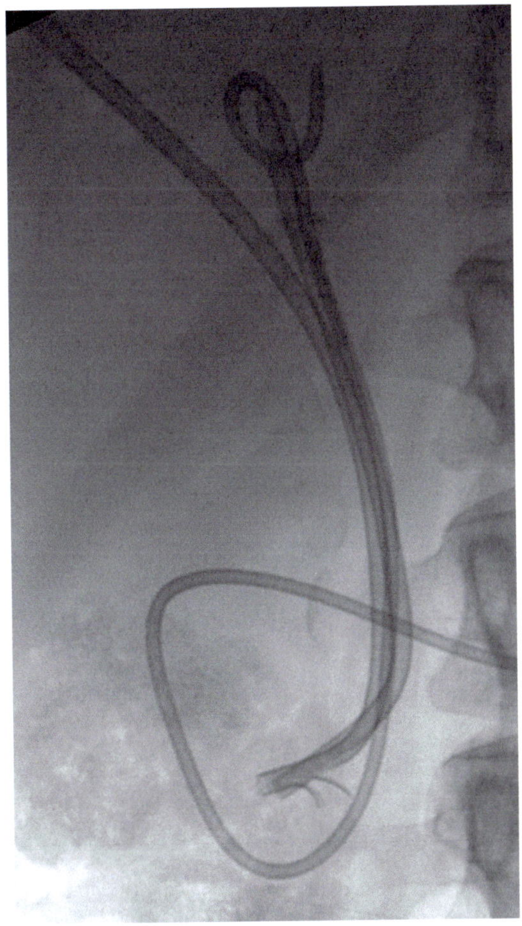

Fig. 18.3 An example of biliary stones directly visible at fluoroscopy. The patient underwent three consecutive sessions of ESWL (5000 W, 4,5 J, 90 W for each session). However, the fragmentation was minimal and the multiple attempts of ERCP failed. The patient was sent to surgery

18.3 Specific Issues on Pancreatic ESWL

It is mainly used in case of chronic calcified pancreatitis (CCP).

CCP is a disease of varied etiology that is associated with the development of pancreatic ductal calculi, which result in upstream hypertension, increased parenchymal pressure, and ischemia [2]. Pain is the dominant feature of both alcoholic and nonalcoholic CCP [3]. Decompression of the duct by clearing the stones leads to relief of pain in many patients. Small pancreatic duct

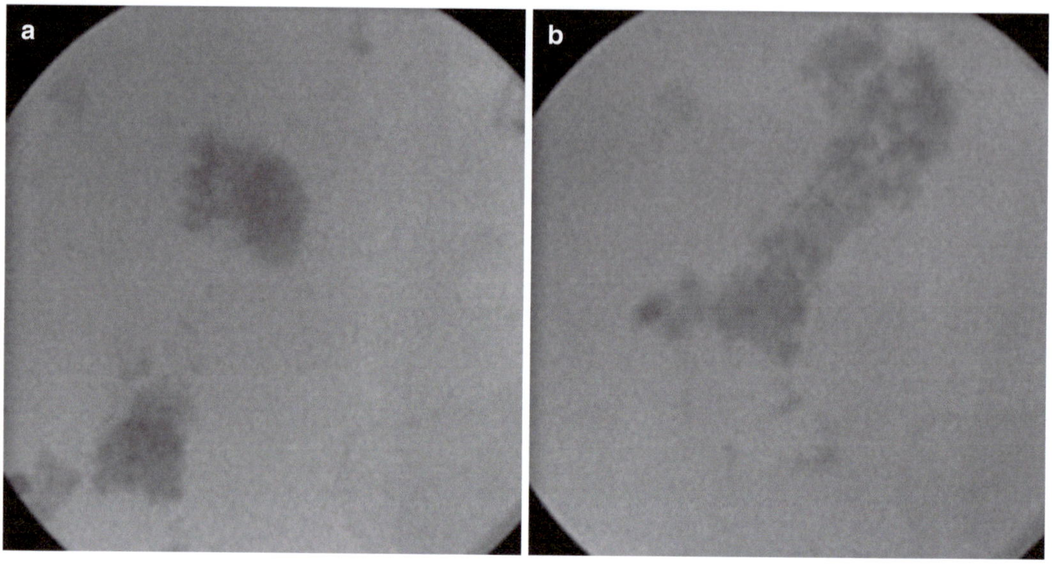

Fig. 18.4 Pancreatic stones obstructing the main pancreatic duct in chronic pancreatitis. This obstruction caused upper abdominal pain (badly controlled by maximal antalgic therapy) and onset of steatorrhea. The patient underwent one session of ESWL (5000 W, 4,5 J, 90 W) and subsequent ERCP. (**a**) Before ESWL; (**b**) after ESWL. At the subsequent ERCP, the fragmented stones appeared to be expelled (**a** previous ERCP, almost 2 years before, was performed with pancreatic sphincterotomy)

(PD) stones can be extracted by the routine technique of endoscopic pancreatic sphincterotomy and basketing [3]. Stones >5 mm in diameter are often impacted in the main pancreatic duct and require fragmentation to facilitate their expulsion [4]. ESWL has been successfully used at many centers for fragmentation of large PD calculi followed by spontaneous or endoscopic clearance with resultant relief in pain [2–5].

ESWL is indicated in all patients of CCP with large PD calculi (>5 mm) that are not amenable to routine endotherapy—where pain is the predominant symptom [4–7]. The aim is to break the calculi to fragments of ≤3 mm, so that they can be removed by subsequent endoscopic retrograde cholangiopancreatography (ERCP) [2–7]. Calculi in the head and body are targeted during ESWL. The procedure is safe and effective also in pediatric patients [3].

ESWL is not indicated in patients with extensive calculi in the head, body, and tail of the pancreas or in patients with isolated calculi in the tail area because increased chance of collateral damage to the spleen is high [4]. Patients with multiple stricture, head mass, pancreatic ascites, or pseudocysts are not treated by ESWL [6, 7]. Cholangitis or coagulopathy due to biliary stricture is treated before subjecting the patient to ESWL [2, 3].

Fragmentation of PD calculi using ESWL allows for natural passage of calculi and facilitates in endoscopic removal of stones [8]. Few studies suggest to use intravenous secretin administration during ESWL to improve the subsequent endoscopic clearance [7, 8]. Furthermore, reduction of pain and improvement of exocrine and endocrine function have been observed after the use of ESWL [6–8]. Effect of ESWL on quality of life improvement was assessed in recent studies [4–8]. All these studies showed an improved quality of life (defined as subjective appreciation of feeling better per patient) with the use of ESWL [4–8]. Improved endocrine function with the use of ESWL in CCP has been assessed by the amount of antidiabetic medications used or by comparing the number of patients with diabetes before and after the ESWL management [6–8]. Improvement of exocrine function has been assessed by monitoring the weight of the patient or steatorrhea before and after ESWL [7–9].

A mean of three sessions is indicated for pancreatic ESWL [9, 10]. ERCP is not always associated [6–11]. On one side, it can be performed before ESWL to do pancreatic sphincterotomy or to positionate a pancreatic plastic stent/nose-pancreatic stent with the distal edge ahead of the stone. On the other side, it can be performed after ESWL to clear completely the duct and/or to insert a plastic/metallic stent in case of associated stricture or ESWL insuccess.

There is ambiguity regarding the use of ESWL alone versus ESWL combined with endoscopic procedures to manage the patients with CCP. There was only one randomized controlled trial performed by Dumonceau et al. [11] comparing the percentage of patients with pain relapse in both the groups. It concluded that combining ESWL with systematic endoscopy added to the cost of patient care without improving the pancreatic pain outcome.

Pancreatic ESWL has been relatively a safe procedure. Although it had no contribution to mortality, it was associated with post-ESWL pancreatitis in 4.2% [12–15]. The mostly described one is pancreatitis of different grades [15]. Some studies recommend the use of intrarectal indomethacin suppository before ESWL to reduce this risk. Other described complications are hepatic hematoma [12], splenic rupture [13], and abscess [14].

The number of patients requiring surgery for CCP has reduced as a result of ESWL therapy [8, 10, 16–18]. Based on the aforementioned results and prior studies, ESWL is a safe and effective way of managing CCP. It should specifically be indicated when the PD calculi size is greater than 5 mm, in the presence of PD strictures, impacted PD calculi, and failure of endoscopic methods of PD stone extraction.

Pancreatic ESWL was performed also to assist the removal of pancreatic calcified entrapped stents [9].

Many controlled studies confirm the good results of pancreatic ESWL in CCP for stone clearance, main pancreatic duct drainage, and pain relief especially in patients in whom stones were removed completely at initial therapy [2–12, 16–21] (Figs. 18.5, 18.6, 18.7, 18.8, and 18.9).

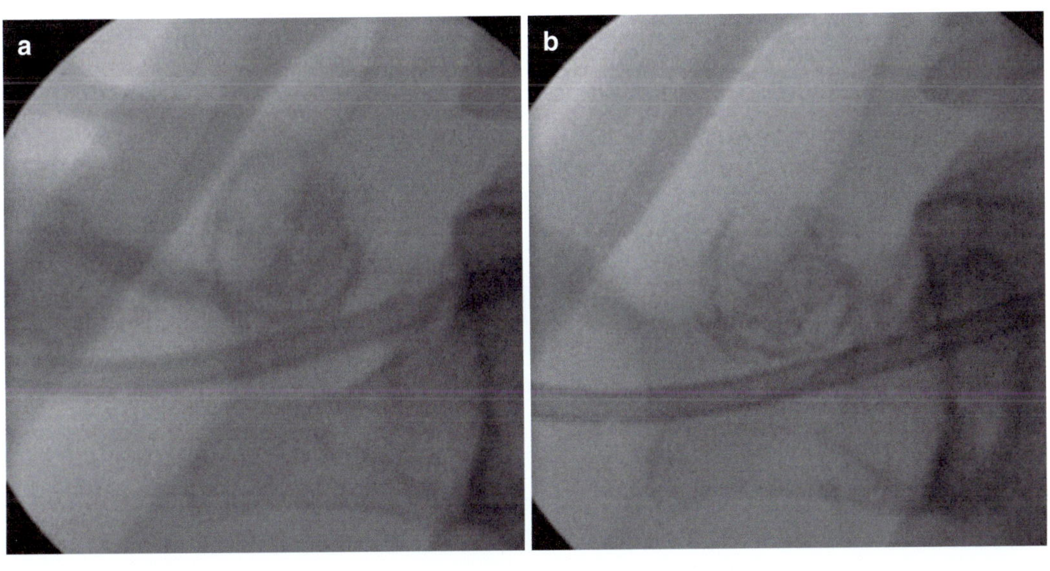

Fig. 18.5 A 10 mm pancreatic stone in chronic pancreatitis. At a first ERCP, pancreatic sphincterotomy and plastic pancreatic stenting were performed. One session of ESWL (5000 W, 4,5 J, 90 W) was subsequently performed. (**a**) The stone before ESWL showed integrated circumferential calcification; (**b**) after ESWL, the circumferential calcification was broken. At the second ERCP, the stone was easily fragmented due to a reduction of consistency

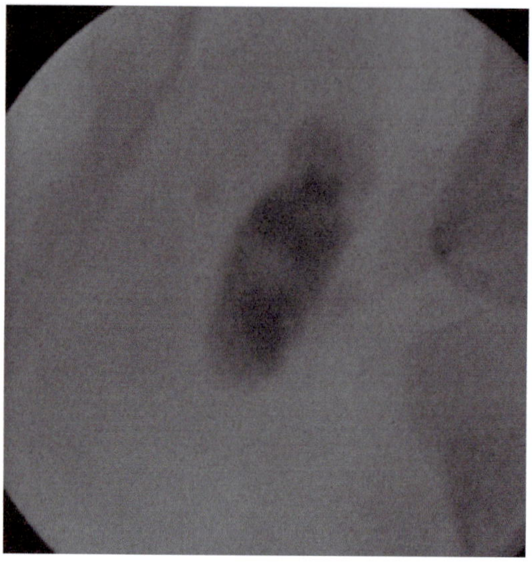

Fig. 18.6 An example of fluoroscopic view of pancreatic stone during ESWL. We recommend to perform XR check at certain interval during the session

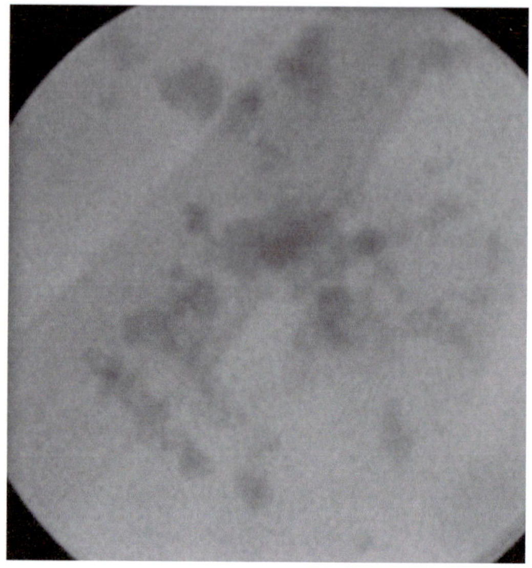

Fig. 18.7 Multiple pancreatic stones in chronic pancreatitis. Only the ones along the main pancreatic duct must be targeted by ESWL. The peripheral ones are not responsible for symptoms

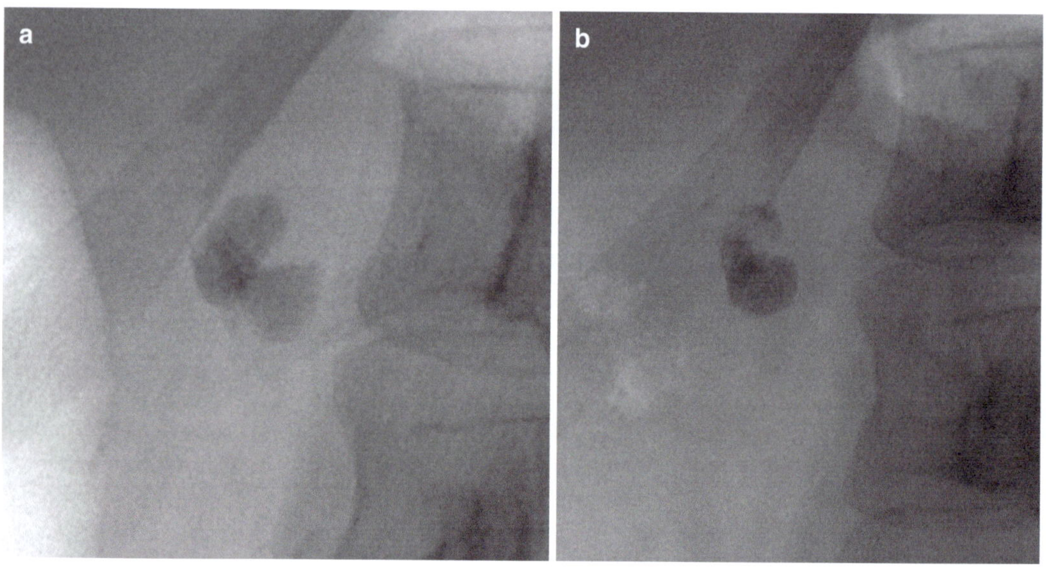

Fig. 18.8 Two pancreatic stones obstructing the main pancreatic duct in chronic pancreatitis. The first session of ESWL was focused on one of them (5000 W, 4,5 J, 90 W). This guaranteed the fragmentation of this one. (**a**) Before ESWL; (**b**) after ESWL. The patient underwent a second ESWL session and a subsequent ERCP with a complete clearance of the main pancreatic duct

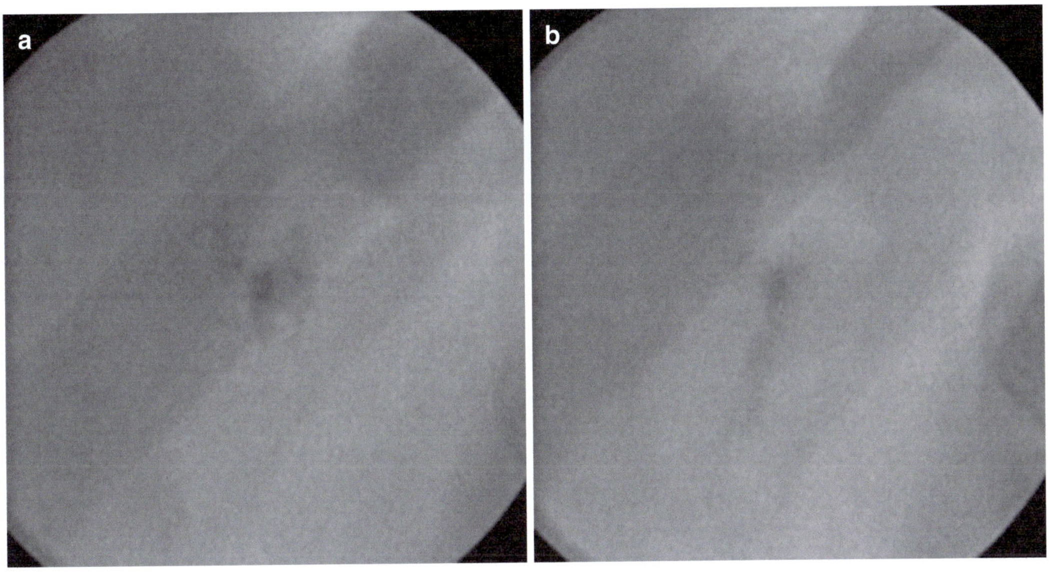

Fig. 18.9 A 6 mm pancreatic stone incuneated in the Santorini duct of a pancreas divisum. (**a**) the stone at the beginning of the ESWL session (3500 W, 3,5 J, 90 W); (**b**) at the end of the ESWL, the stone appeared to be completely destroyed

18.4 Specific Tools on Biliary ESWL

It is generally indicated for difficult CBD stones and includes large stones (>15 mm diameter) and impacted stones in patients with narrow distal CBD and/or difficult anatomy [22–25].

Large stones can either be fragmented or the CBD passage dilated to facilitate extraction. Fragmentation of large CBD stones can be carried out.

ESWL is indicated in all patients with large CBD calculi that are not extractable by routine techniques of sphincterotomy followed by basket or balloon trawl [22, 23]. It is especially useful for patients with post-cholecystectomy retained stones, isolated or primary CBD stones, and in those who refuse or are unfit for surgery [24]. Acute cholangitis and coagulopathy are relative contraindications and ESWL can be performed once these conditions are treated. Biliary ESWL was proposed also for gallbladder stones and compared with laparoscopic cholecystectomy: however, the risks of the procedure are not justified by the high risk of recurrence if the gallbladder was not surgically asported [25].

Biliary ESWL is generally less diffuse than pancreatic one. It was first used to treat bile duct stones in 1985, after its success and safety in treating renal calculi had been well established. Sauerbruch et al. [22] demonstrated the efficacy of ESWL in achieving common bile duct stone disintegration in more than 90% of patients with minimal side effects. Tandan et al. [23] reported excellent results using this method for intrahepatic bile duct stone after choledochal cyst resection; this was the first report showing the effectiveness of ESWL on biliary stones after choledochal cyst surgery. Intrahepatic bile ducts were filled with debris in that case, because of the occlusion of the biliodigestive anastomosis by impacted stones. In another report, Binmoeller et al. [24] were not successful in using ESWL because they were unable to maintain focus on the intrahepatic duct stones, as the shock waves caused them to move. They concluded that this approach is useful only in special cases, e.g., cases of impacted intrahepatic bile duct stones or immobile stones, such as ureteral calculi. Tandan et al. [23] recommended at least five sessions for the complete clearance of bile ducts.

When stones are located in the bile duct, a nasobiliary catheter is usually needed for contrast administration [22–28]. The major drawback of ESWL is the time-consuming process which requires one or more sessions of treatment, the insertion of a nasobiliary catheter in the interval and repeated endoscopic retrograde cholangiography (ERC) for fragment extraction. Complete clearance rate of common duct stones following ESWL ranges between 83% and 93% [28–31]. The majority of patients will require endoscopic extraction of the bile duct stone fragments following ESWL, although approximately 6–10% of stones may subsequently pass spontaneously following treatment [28–30]. Following ESWL, patients subsequently undergo ERC in which residual stone fragments are extracted using baskets. ESWL was effective in the clearance of stones in 80–90% in the available series [22–31]. Complications are observed in 30–40% of patients. Biliary colic is the most common complication; biliary obstruction or pancreatitis is developed in about 5% of patients. Moreover, ESWL for choledocholithiasis is associated with short-term morbidity in about 14% of patients, including pain, hemobilia, cholangitis, sepsis, hematomas, pancreatitis, hematuria, and paralytic ileus.

A high success rate, negligible complications, and noninvasive nature of the procedure make ESWL a useful tool for removing large CBD stones.

18.5 Conclusions

In summary, ESWL is a safe and efficacious treatment modality in managing CCP patients with MPD stones >5 mm who did not get adequate pain relief with conservative management. It demonstrates significant pain relief, improved quality of life, and pancreatic ductal clearance. It can be used alone or in addition to endoscopic therapies to improve the drainage from PD. It has a relatively safe side effect profile. The ESWL might improve exocrine function of the pancreas manifested by either constant or increased body weight in majority of the patients. Endocrine function is not significantly different before and after the ESWL management in patients with CCP.

A high success rate with low complication rate makes ESWL a useful tool also for removing large and/or difficult CBD stones (>15 mm) in specific cases.

References

1. Chaussy C, Schmiedt E, Jocham D, Brendel W, Forssmann B, Walther V. First clinical experience with extracorporeally induced destruction of kidney stones by shock waves. J Urol. 1982;127:417–20.
2. Tandan M, Reddy DN, Santosh D, Vinod K, Ramchandani M, Rajesh G, Rama K, Lakhtakia S, Banerjee R, Pratap N, Venkat Rao G. Extracorporeal shock wave lithotripsy and endotherapy for pancreatic calculi-a large single center experience. Indian J Gastroenterol. 2010;29:143–8.
3. Ong WC, Tandan M, Reddy V, Rao GV, Reddy N. Multiple main pancreatic duct stones in tropical pancreatitis: safe clearance with extracorporeal shockwave lithotripsy. J Gastroenterol Hepatol. 2006;21:1514–8.
4. Guda NM, Partington S, Freeman ML. Extracorporeal shock wave lithotripsy in the management of chronic calcific pancreatitis: a meta-analysis. JOP. 2005;6:6–12.
5. Delhaye M, Vandermeeren A, Baize M, Cremer M. Extracorporeal shock-wave lithotripsy of pancreatic calculi. Gastroenterology. 1992;102:610–20.
6. Costamagna G, Gabbrielli A, Mutignani M, Perri V, Pandolfi M, Boscaini M, Crucitti F. Extracorporeal shock wave lithotripsy of pancreatic stones in chronic pancreatitis: immediate and medium-term results. Gastrointest Endosc. 1997;46:231–6.
7. Neuhaus H. Fragmentation of pancreatic stones by extracorporeal shock wave lithotripsy. Endoscopy. 1991;23:161–5.
8. Kozarek RA, Brandabur JJ, Ball TJ, Gluck M, Patterson DJ, Attia F, France R, Traverso LW, Koslowski P, Gibbons RP. Clinical outcomes in patients who undergo extracorporeal shock wave lithotripsy for chronic calcific pancreatitis. Gastrointest Endosc. 2002;56:496–500.

9. Lehman GA. Role of ERCP and other endoscopic modalities in chronic pancreatitis. Gastrointest Endosc. 2002;56:S237–40.
10. Adamek HE, Jakobs R, Buttmann A, Adamek MU, Schneider AR, Riemann JF. Long term follow up of patients with chronic pancreatitis and pancreatic stones treated with extracorporeal shock wave lithotripsy. Gut. 1999;45:402–5.
11. Dumonceau JM, Costamagna G, Tringali A, Vahedi K, Delhaye M, Hittelet A, Spera G, Giostra E, Mutignani M, De Maertelaer V, Devière J. Treatment for painful calcified chronic pancreatitis: extracorporeal shock wave lithotripsy versus endoscopic treatment: a randomised controlled trial. Gut. 2007;56:545–52.
12. Hirata N, Kushida Y, Ohguri T, Wakasugi S, Kojima T, Fujita R. Hepatic subcapsular hematoma after extracorporeal shock wave lithotripsy (ESWL) for pancreatic stones. J Gastroenterol. 1999;34:713–6.
13. Leifsson BG, Borgström A, Ahlgren G. Splenic rupture following ESWL for a pancreatic duct calculus. Dig Surg. 2001;18:229–30.
14. Plaisier PW, den Hoed PT. Splenic abscess after lithotripsy of pancreatic duct stones. Dig Surg. 2001;18:231–2.
15. Karakayali F, Sevmiş S, Ayvaz I, Tekin I, Boyvat F, Moray G. Acute necrotizing pancreatitis as a rare complication of extracorporeal shock wave lithotripsy. Int J Urol. 2006;13:613–5.
16. Farnbacher MJ, Schoen C, Rabenstein T, Benninger J, Hahn EG, Schneider HT. Pancreatic duct stones in chronic pancreatitis: criteria for treatment intensity and success. Gastrointest Endosc. 2002;56:501–6.
17. Delhaye M, Arvanitakis M, Bali M, Matos C, Devière J. Endoscopic therapy for chronic pancreatitis. Scand J Surg. 2005;94:143–53.
18. Inui K, Tazuma S, Yamaguchi T, Ohara H, Tsuji T, Miyagawa H, Igarashi Y, Nakamura Y, Atomi Y. Treatment of pancreatic stones with extracorporeal shock wave lithotripsy: results of a multicenter survey. Pancreas. 2005;30:26–30.
19. Ohara H, Hoshino M, Hayakawa T, Kamiya Y, Miyaji M, Takeuchi T, Okayama Y, Gotoh K. Single application extracorporeal shock wave lithotripsy is the first choice for patients with pancreatic duct stones. Am J Gastroenterol. 1996;91:1388–94.
20. Darisetty S, Tandan M, Reddy DN, Kotla R, Gupta R, Ramchandani M, Lakhtakia S, Rao GV, Banerjee R. Epidural anesthesia is effective for extracorporeal shock wave lithotripsy of pancreatic and biliary calculi. World J Gastrointest Surg. 2010;2:165–8.
21. Schneider HT, May A, Benninger J, Rabenstein T, Hahn EG, Katalinic A, Ell C. Piezoelectric shock wave lithotripsy of pancreatic duct stones. Am J Gastroenterol. 1994;89:2042–8.
22. Sauerbruch T, Stern M. Fragmentation of bile duct stones by extracorporeal shock waves. A new approach to biliary calculi after failure of routine endoscopic measures. Gastroenterology. 1989;96:146–52.
23. Tandan M, Reddy DN, Santosh D, Reddy V, Koppuju V, Lakhtakia S, Gupta R, Ramchandani M, Rao GV. Extracorporeal shock wave lithotripsy of large difficult common bile duct stones: efficacy and analysis of factors that favor stone fragmentation. J Gastroenterol Hepatol. 2009;24:1370–4.
24. Binmoeller KF, Schafer TW. Endoscopic management of bile duct stones. J Clin Gastroenterol. 2001;32:106–18.
25. Ellis RD, Jenkins AP, Thompson RP, Ede RJ. Clearance of refractory bile duct stones with extracorporeal shockwave lithotripsy. Gut. 2000;47:728–31.
26. Hochberger J, Tex S, Maiss J, Hahn EG. Management of difficult common bile duct stones. Gastrointest Endosc Clin N Am. 2003;13:623–34.
27. Adamek HE, Maier M, Jakobs R, Wessbecher FR, Neuhauser T, Riemann JF. Management of retained bile duct stones: a prospective open trial comparing extracorporeal and intracorporeal lithotripsy. Gastrointest Endosc. 1996;44:40–7.
28. Binmoeller KF, Brückner M, Thonke F, Soehendra N. Treatment of difficult bile duct stones using mechanical, electrohydraulic and extracorporeal shock wave lithotripsy. Endoscopy. 1993;25:201–6.
29. Neuhaus H, Zillinger C, Born P, Ott R, Allescher H, Rösch T, Classen M. Randomized study of intracorporeal laser lithotripsy versus extracorporeal shock-wave lithotripsy for difficult bile duct stones. Gastrointest Endosc. 1998;47:327–34.
30. Kocdor MA, Bora S, Terzi C, Ozman I, Tankut E. Extracorporeal shock wave lithotripsy for retained common bile duct stones. Minim Invasive Ther Allied Technol. 2000;9:371–4.
31. Kratzer W, Mason RA, Grammer S, Preclik G, Beckh K, Adler G. Difficult bile duct stone recurrence after endoscopy and extracorporeal shockwave lithotripsy. Hepato-Gastroenterology. 1998;45:910–6.

19 Biliary Stenting

Edoardo Forti, Giulia Bonato, and Massimiliano Mutignani

19.1 Introduction

Biliary stenting is one of the most valuable and versatile tools for managing pancreato-biliary disorders. Plastic endoprosthesis has been firstly described in 1979 for palliative treatment of obstructive jaundice [1]. Since then, technological advancement led to the development of various types of biliary stents, with higher performance, and their use in clinical practice has been progressively increasing.

Main indications for biliary stenting include malignant and benign biliary obstruction and postsurgical biliary leaks; in selected cases, stent insertion can be effective in bleeding control of hemobilia from iatrogenic trauma, portal hypertensive biliopathy, and post-ERCP perforations, and it can have an ancillary role in difficult common bile duct stone management [2].

19.2 Plastic Stents

Plastic stents (PS) are widely used in cases of biliary obstruction of either malignant or benign etiology, due to their availability, ease to use, and low cost. Unfortunately, these devices show much lower patency times as compared with self-expandable metal stents, due to the smaller inner diameter which facilitates the formation of biliary sludge and bacterial biofilm.

Plastic stents are usually made of polyethylene or polytetrafluoroethylene (PTFE or Teflon). Although pilot studies on in vitro models suggested a superiority of Teflon over polyethylene, multiple RCT did not find significant differences among PTFE and polyethylene in terms of stent patency [3, 4] and ease of implantation [5]. Plastic stents must be radiopaque: it allows to correctly place the PS under fluoroscopy and check the presence and location of the stent during the follow-up. Many lengths, caliber, and shapes are currently available: size can vary between 3 Fr and 11.5 Fr in caliber (being the 3Fr and the 5Fr mostly used for the pancreatic duct) and from 5 to 15 cm in length. Stents can be straight, softly curved, or with single/double pigtail configuration. Every feature has been developed with a specific purpose: for example, in cases of tight strictures, a gently curved design and a tapered tip potentially facilitate stent insertion. Pigtails and flaps are systems created in order to minimize the risk of migration, but, to date, there are no evidences supporting differences in migration rate among different shapes or stent designs [6]. The only factor significantly associated with longer patency times seems to be a wider diameter (i.e., 10Fr). In our experience,

E. Forti · G. Bonato · M. Mutignani (✉)
Digestive and Interventional Endoscopy Unit, ASST Grande Ospedale Metropolitano Niguarda, Niguarda-Ca' Granda Hospital, Milan, Italy
e-mail: edoardo.forti@ospedaleniguarda.it; giulia.bonato@unimi.it; Massimiliano.mutignani@ospedaleniguarda.it

M. Mutignani et al. (eds.), *Endotherapy in Biliopancreatic Diseases: ERCP Meets EUS*, https://doi.org/10.1007/978-3-030-42569-2_19

however, pigtail design shows shorter patency time and should be reserved for fluid collection and intrahepatic biliary stone treatment.

19.3 Self-Expandable Metal Stents

Self-expandable metal stents have been developed in the late 1980s [7, 8]. At first their use was described for palliation of malignant strictures, but now they find indication in a variety of benign conditions as well. SEMSs are made of a metal wire shaped into a cylindrical mesh, and this design is responsible for the main property of those devices: self-expansion after deployment. This feature allows much higher diameters as compared with plastic stents, thus enhancing consistently patency rates and times. Two mechanical properties are crucial in determining the stent's behavior in the bile duct, namely, radial force and axial force [9]. Radial force is the expansive force opposed to the stricture compression; a high radial force improves patency and guarantees a better adherence to the duct wall, thus reducing the risk of migration. Axial force is responsible for the attitude of restraightening of a SEMS when it is bent; this physical property needs to be as low as possible since it is inversely related to flexibility. If too strong, axial force could lead to excessive compression to adjacent structures such as the main pancreatic duct, thus increasing the risk of pancreatitis [9].

Many shapes and sizes are available: diameter can vary from 6 to 10 mm and length from 40 to 120 mm; in exceptional cases, stents 20 mm in diameter can be used off-label. In terms of wire-weaving methods for SEMS, the wire is braided as a wire crossover structure or is cut by laser (also known as lasercut stents), the latter resulting in more difficulties during removal, if the SEMS is uncovered. Currently, SEMSs are usually made of nitinol or Platinol, the former being a combination of nickel plus titanium while the latter a combination of platinum and titanium; stainless steel has almost been abandoned for its lower elasticity, higher occlusion rate, and shorter time to occlusion [10, 11]. SEMS can be covered with polyurethane or silicone; this feature has been developed in order to reduce the risk of stent occlusion. Indeed, in the last two decades, many studies revealed a high need of re-intervention with uncovered stents, mainly for stent occlusion due to the inward growth of tumor or tissue hyperplasia through the mesh. Membrane cover has been proven to reduce the burden of such complication [12]; in addition, it allows stent removal. On the other hand, stent migration is much more frequent for covered SEMS, as shown by a wide body of evidence. In order to minimize the risk of migration, partially covered metal stents with both extremities uncovered as anti-migration systems have been developed, although data on their outcomes in comparison with fully covered metal stents are sparse. Uncovered SEMS still finds indication in palliative treatment of malignant biliary obstruction, especially in case of long intrahepatic strictures, when risk of occluding secondary bile ducts is high.

Technique:

- *Preliminary stricture assessment*: preliminary evaluation with second-level imaging of the biliary tree (i.e., MRI or CT scan) can be useful in order to establish length and width of the stricture, as well as the number and type of the involved ducts. This step is necessary to choose the appropriate strategy, to employ stents as short as possible, thus reducing bile stasis and avoiding premature stent occlusion (Fig. 19.1); moreover, in intrahepatic stenting, excessive length of the prosthesis could result in the occlusion of side branches (Figs. 19.2 and 19.3). In some cases of malignant hilar obstruction with severe stricture of one or more hepatic ducts, it may be wiser to avoid injection of contrast medium into the intrahepatic biliary tree in order to avert secondary cholangitis. In such cases one can inject contrast medium only in the distal portion of the main biliary duct.
- *Guidewire insertion*: deep cannulation of the biliary duct with a wire is necessary to guide the delivery system in place. There are several different guidewires available for this purpose. Wires can be straight-tipped or angle-tipped.

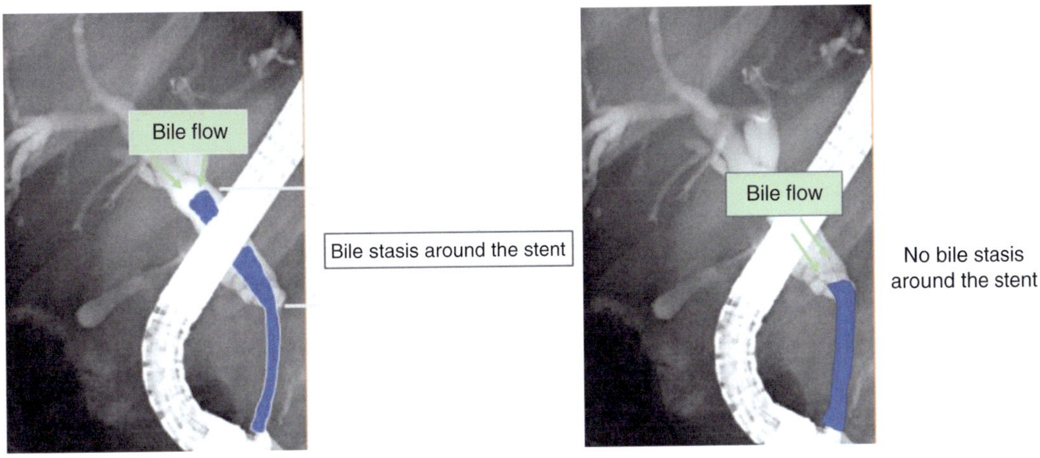

Fig. 19.1 Stents should be as short as possible, in order to reduce bile stasis and avoid premature stent occlusion

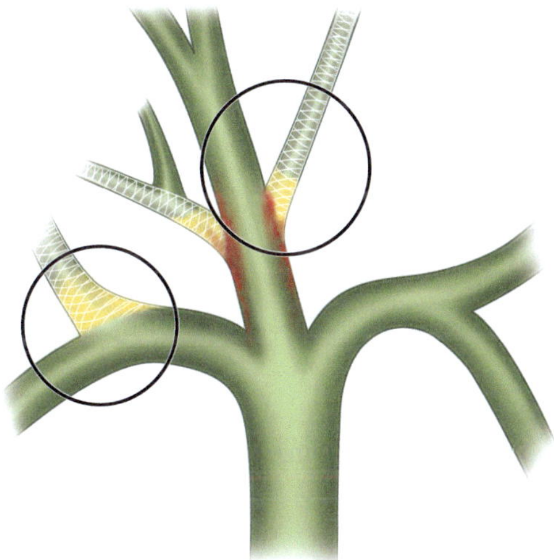

Fig. 19.2 Uncovered SEMS length is also crucial in intrahepatic stenting; excessive length of the stent could cause occlusion of side branches of the biliary tree by both hyperplastic tissue (in red) and biliary sludge/stones (in yellow)

Partially and fully hydrophilic wires are both widely used, and the choice between the two depends on the endoscopist's preference. In our experience fully hydrophilic wires, although much more difficult to handle, increase significantly successful cannulation in challenging cases; angled-tip wires can be crucial when selective cannulation of intrahepatic ducts is needed. Stiff wires should usually be preferred because too "floppy" wires often turn out to be unable to overpass the stricture or, alternatively, they do not confer enough axial force (strength) to the delivery system during the stent insertion phase. On the other hand, floppy wires can be useful to cannulate angled strictures or intrahepatic ducts. Thus, endoscopists can take advantage of multiple wires during a single procedure, for example, starting with a straight, stiff wire while cannulating the papilla; then switching to a more flexible, angled wire for complex or kinked strictures; and then switching back to a more stable wire once the stent needs to be inserted.

With regard to wire diameter, 0.035 in. is usually the optimal diameter in biliary stenting. Nevertheless, in very selected cases of tight strictures, thinner wires such as 0.025 in. or even 0.018 in. can be considered.

- *Endoscopic sphincterotomy*: the role of endoscopic biliary sphincterotomy (ES) prior to biliary stent's placement is still debated. This procedure is routinely performed by most endoscopists since it is thought to facilitate deployment of biliary stent and, potentially, lower the risk of post-endoscopic retrograde cholangiopancreatography pancreatitis (PEP). On the other hand, sphincterotomy increases procedure duration and implies some well-known risks such as bleeding and perforation. Many studies aimed to assess this issue, with heterogeneous results [13–15]. A meta-analysis by Cui on biliary

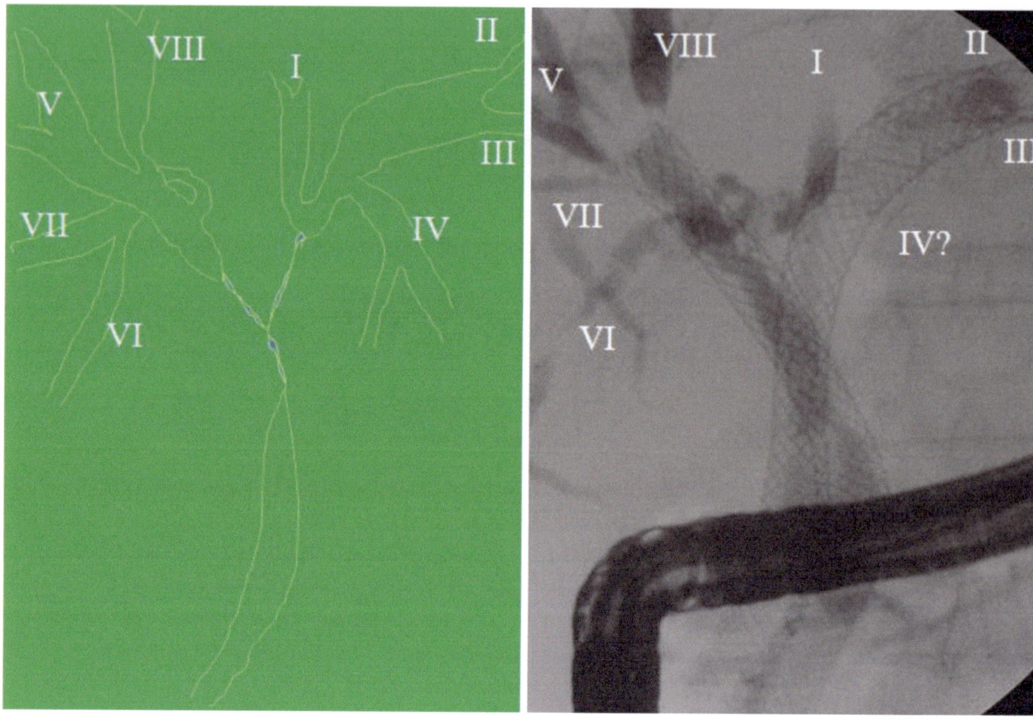

Fig. 19.3 Worsening effect on a hilar neoplastic stricture due to too long uncovered SEMS, 3 months after insertion. On the left side, draw to simplify the anatomy of the biliary tree

stenting for malignant obstruction reported a significantly lower incidence of PEP but higher incidence of post-procedural bleeding if sphincterotomy was performed, while technical success in stent insertion was not influenced by sphincterotomy [13]. However, the two main factors affecting risk of pancreatitis following biliary stenting seem to be the clinical scenario (pancreatic cancer vs. other indications) and the type of stent used (plastic versus SEMS). ES brings actual benefits in cases of biliary obstruction, both benign and malignant, if the main pancreatic duct is not involved; indeed, ES decreases the risk of PEP by reducing tension at the pancreatic duct orifice [14, 15]. In our view, when a SEMS is placed trans-papillary, sometimes ES can be insufficient to prevent compression on the main pancreatic duct which can be responsible for delayed abdominal pain (usually 12–24 h after ERCP or when restarting feeding); such event can be effectively treated by inserting a plastic stent in the main pancreatic duct.

In contrast, no differences were noticed in biliary obstruction from pancreatic cancer when the main pancreatic duct is invaded by the tumor; in such an event, there is little risk of pancreatitis, and ES can be avoided.

- *Stent insertion*: plastic stents are loaded on a guide catheter, over the guidewire, and then pushed with the pusher catheter. Guide catheter size depends on stent's diameter: usually, 8.5Fr stents are loaded over 5Fr catheter, 10 or 11.5 Fr over 6Fr catheter. This is particularly useful for tight strictures as the guide catheter facilitates stent introduction through the stenosis by reducing the gap between stricture's and stent's diameter. Self-expandable metal stent is mounted on an inner catheter and constrained by an outer catheter. This delivery system is

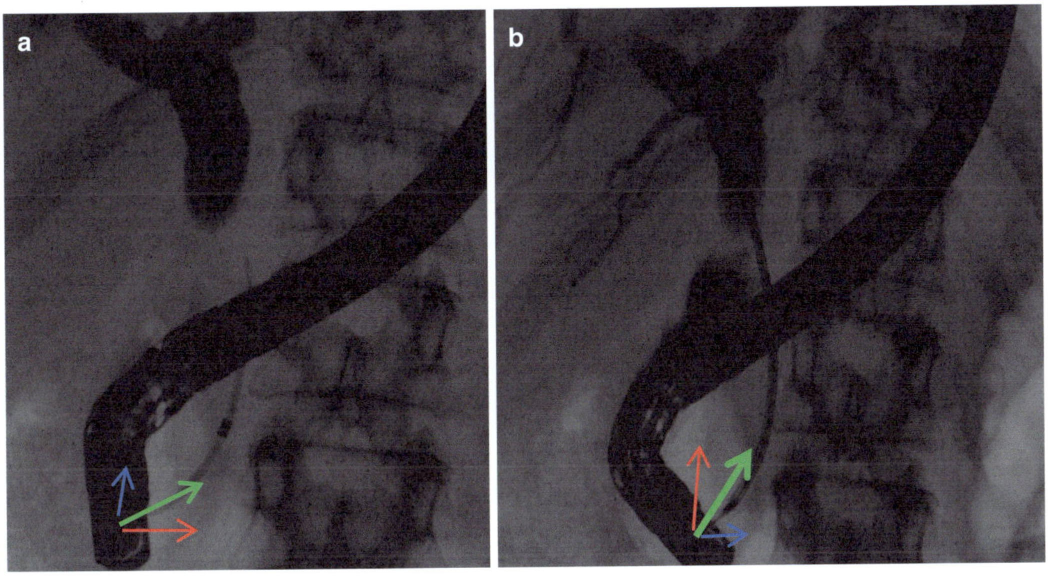

Fig. 19.4 (**a**) During stent insertion, endoscope's tip must be oriented perpendicularly to the common biliary duct (**b**) in order to increase the force to pushing up the stent

loaded over the guidewire and pushed up into the bile duct.

In this phase, the endoscope's tip must be oriented perpendicularly to the main biliary duct in order to increase the force to pushing up the stent (Fig. 19.4). Then, the operator will push the prosthesis across the stricture and will release it with its middle part across the stric ture in order to guarantee a good balance between the forces that push it upward and the forces that push it downward, thus minimizing the risk of displacement. Two techniques can be useful to effectively push the stent:

- Standard technique: pushing directly the catheter with the right hand.
- Arising the elevator in order to firmly fix the catheter and then applying pressure on the duodenoscope by pulling it in the backward and rightward direction. This variant confers more strength and can be employed when the standard technique fails, for example, in cases of severe strictures of the main bile duct.

In cases of unsuccessful attempt to overpass the stricture with the delivery set or the stent itself, it may be necessary to dilate the stricture in order to permit stent's insertion. Dilation modalities include mechanical dilation (e.g., using a dilation catheter) and pneumatic dilation (e.g., using balloon dilation catheter); such techniques are similarly effective, although the latter brings a higher risk of tissue trauma and injury. For further details on this topic, see chapter on *stricture dilation*. In very exceptional cases, such as extremely hard strictures, some off-label techniques have been successfully performed by our team, such as dilation using the Soehendra mechanical lithotriptor (® Cook Medical) or the electrocautery of the stricture's tissue using a Cystotome (® Cook medical). However, data about safety and efficacy of such methods are still lacking.

- *Stent releasing*: this step is slightly different for plastic stent and metal stent.
  - For plastic stent the releasing phase consists of two distinct steps: first, withdraw the guide catheter while holding the push-

ing catheter in order to keep the stent in place; then, withdraw the pushing catheter (if the two catheters were removed simultaneously, stent may be accidentally displaced).

- Release of self-expandable metal stents is done as follows: open partially the delivery set in order to release the proximal edge of the SEMS. Slightly retrieve the delivery set under fluoroscopy till the stricture has been engaged. When the stent is warped by the stricture with the proximal portion very adjacent to the stricture, the releasing process can be completed.

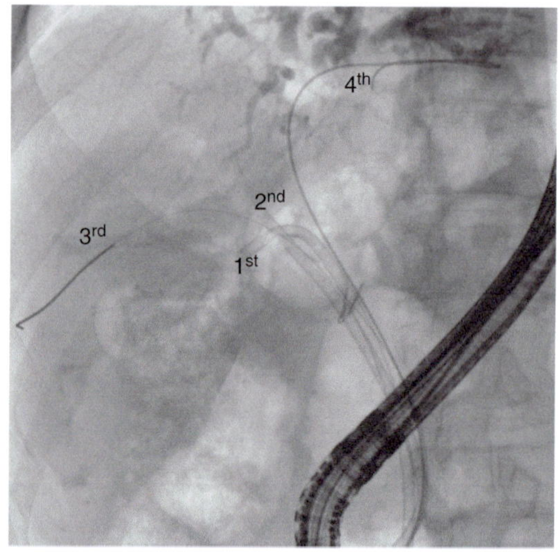

Fig. 19.5 First, position all the guidewires into the ducts that need to be stented, and, after that, start stent insertion from the most tight stricture or the most angled duct, which could result unapproachable later as indicated by the numbers in the image

19.4 Multiple Biliary Stenting

Special considerations are required for multiple biliary stenting with either self-expandable metal stents or plastic stents.

Multiple SEMS insertion: this technique may be required in cases of benign or malignant strictures with intrahepatic or hilar involvement. In such situations, a careful preemptive evaluation is crucial to decide which ducts need to be stented. The most important trick to facilitate deployment of subsequent SEMSs is to firstly position all the guidewires into the ducts that need to be stented and, after that, start stent insertion from the most tight stricture or the most angled duct, which could result unapproachable later (Fig. 19.5). While inserting the first stent, the operator must maintain the other guidewires in the correct position by holding them. After deploying the first SEMS, all the subsequent steps need to be carried out quickly because the progressive dilation of the stent may obstruct the insertion of the subsequent ones (Fig. 19.6).

Multiple plastic stenting (MPS): endoscopic placement of multiple plastic stents has become a widely accepted procedure for treating postoperative biliary strictures and benign pancreatic strictures [16]. This procedure involves four steps: (1) evaluate stricture's caliber by mechanical dilation; (2) insert a 5Fr or 6Fr guide catheter over a wire; (3) stent and deploy plastic stent; (4) repeat step 2 and 3 inserting as many stents as possible according to the tightness of the stricture. When multiple plastic stents need to be inserted side by side, endoscopists should keep in mind that some stents show tendency to crush when the second stent is inserted, mainly because of excessive friction between the two devices. This event can only be prevented by choosing, in this setting, stents with low frictional force.

Subsequent ERCP and placement of an increasing number of stents will be scheduled, usually every 3 months. Placement of new stents can be achieved in two ways: the firstly described technique involves removal of all the stents and placement of a greater number of new stents. The latter, proposed in order to decrease costs and procedural time, has been called the "dirty" technique, and it consists in inserting new stents leaving the former in place: even if the older ones may be predictably occluded, the new ones should compensate for them and allow a normal bile flow.

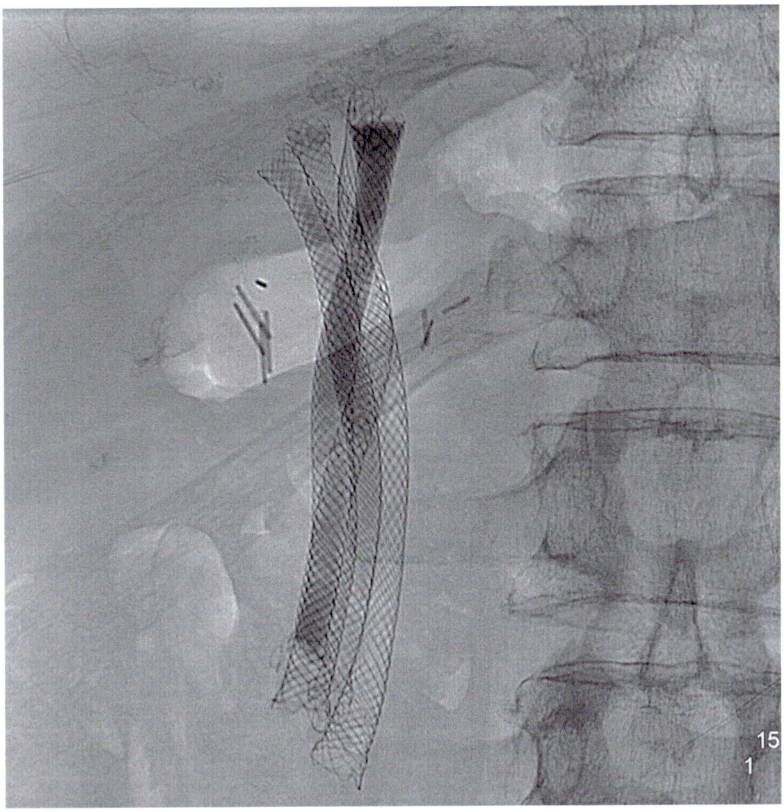

Fig. 19.6 Use of multiple self-expandable metal stents for palliative management of a malignant hilar stricture

Usually this approach requires multiple sessions to reach an adequate number of stents, but it has a major benefit allowing a gradual dilation of the stricture, thus leading to excellent long-term efficacy and lower recurrence rates (Fig. 19.7).

At the time of stents' removal, PS can be pulled out all together using a polypectomy snare. For this maneuver we suggest to pull tight the polypectomy catheter in order to bend the proximal end of the stent, thus decreasing the risk of injury during the retrieval through the pylorus.

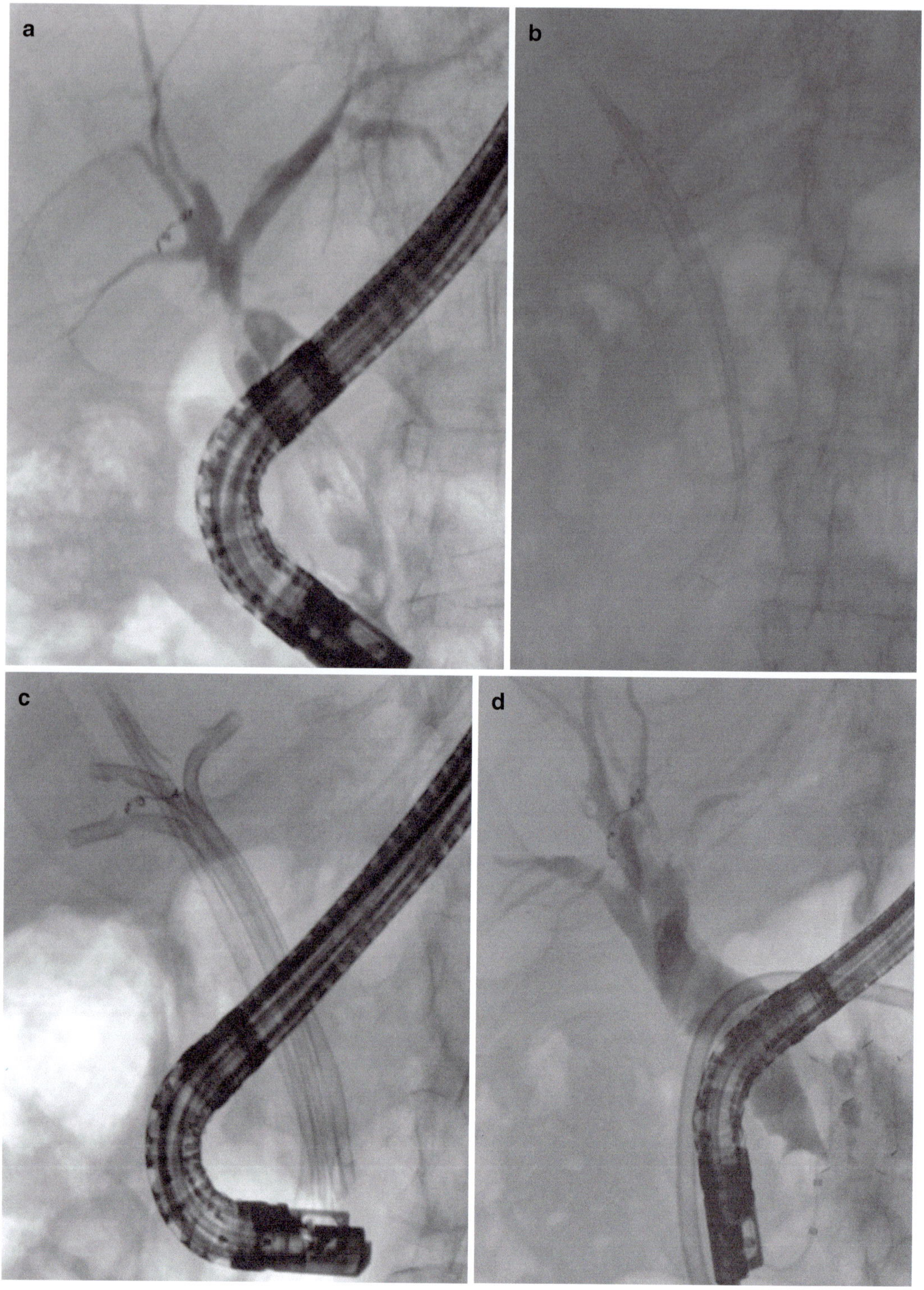

Fig. 19.7 Postoperative biliary stricture (**a**) treated with multiple sessions of multiple plastic stent insertion (**b**, **c**) led to complete resolution of the stricture (**d**)

References

1. Soehendra N, Reynders-Frederix V. [Palliative biliary duct drainage. A new method for endoscopic introduction of a new drain]. Dtsch Med Wochenschr. 1979;104(6):206–7.
2. Yang J, Peng JY, Chen W. Endoscopic biliary stenting for irretrievable common bile duct stones: indications, advantages, disadvantages, and follow-up results. Surgeon. 2012;10(4):211–7. https://doi.org/10.1016/j.surge.2012.04.003.
3. England RE, Martin DF, Morris J, et al. A prospective randomized multicenter trial comparing 10 Fr Teflon Tannenbaum stents with 10 Fr polyethylene Cotton-Leung stents in patients with malignant common duct strictures. Gut. 2000;46(3):395–400.
4. Catalano MF, Geenen JE, Lehman GA, et al. "Tannenbaum" Teflon stents versus traditional polyethilene stents for treatment of malignant biliary stricture. Gastrointest Endosc. 2002;55(3):354–8.
5. Van Berkel AM, Boland C, Redekop WK, et al. A prospective randomized trial of Teflon versus polyethylene stents for distal malignant biliary obstruction. Endoscopy. 1998;30(8):681–6.
6. Kwon CI, Kim G, Jeong S, et al. The stent patency and migration rate of different shaped plastic stents in bile flow phantom model and in vivo animal bile duct dilation model. Dig Dis Sci. 2017;62:1246–55. https://doi.org/10.1007/s10620-017-4514-1.
7. Neuhaus H, Hagenmuller F, Classen M. Self-expanding biliary stents: preliminary clinical experience. Endoscopy. 1989;21:225–8.
8. Huibregtse K, Cheng J, Coene PP, Fockens P, Tytgat GN. Endoscopic placement of expandable metal stents for biliary strictures—a preliminary report on experience with 33 patients. Endoscopy. 1989;21:280–2.
9. Isayama H, Nakai Y, Hamada T, et al. Understanding the mechanical forces of self-expandable metal stents in the biliary ducts. Curr Gastroenterol Rep. 2016;18:64.
10. Luigiano C, Ferrara F, Cennamo V, et al. A comparison of uncovered metal stents for the palliation of patients with malignant biliary obstruction: nitinol vs stainless steel. Dig Liv Dis. 2012;44(2):128–33.
11. Isayama H, Mukai T, Itoi T, et al. Comparison of partially covered nitinol stents with partially covered stainless stents as a historical control in a multicenter study of distal malignant biliary obstruction: the WATCH study. Gastrointest Endosc. 2012;76(1):84–92.
12. Tringali A, Hassan C, Rota M, et al. Covered vs uncovered self-expandable metal stents for malignant distal biliary strictures: a systematic review and meta-analysis. Endoscopy. 2018;50(6):631–41.
13. Cui PJ, Yao J, Zhao YJ, et al. Biliary stenting with or without sphincterotomy for malignant biliary obstruction: a meta-analysis. World J Gastroenterol. 2014;20(38):14033–9. https://doi.org/10.3748/wjg.v20.i38.14033.
14. Okano N, Igarashi Y, Kishimoto Y, et al. Necessity for endoscopic sphincterotomy for biliary stenting in cases of malignant biliary obstruction. Dig Endosc. 2013;25(Suppl 2):122–5.
15. Sofi AA, Nawras A, Alaradi OH, et al. Does endoscopic sphincterotomy reduce the risk of post-ERCP pancreatitis after biliary stenting? A systematic review and meta-analysis. Dig Endosc. 2016;28:394–404.
16. Costamagna G, Bulajic M, Tringali A, et al. Multiple stenting of refractory pancreatic duct strictures in severe chronic pancreatitis: long-term results. Endoscopy. 2006;38(3):254–9.

Endoscopic Papillectomy

20

Laura Bernardoni, Stefano Francesco Crinò, and Armando Gabbrielli

Neoplasms of the ampulla of Vater account for only 0.5% of all gastrointestinal malignancies. Although ampullary carcinomas are rare neoplasms, they occur more frequently in the ampullary region than elsewhere in the small intestine. The cancer of the ampulla is a rare disease with an incidence of less than 1 per 100,000; in autopsy series, ampullary neoplasms are seen in 0.06–0.21% of the general population [1]. Ampullary adenoma is an uncommon pathology in general population, most frequent in the setting of familial adenomatous polyposis (FAP).

FAP syndrome is a high penetrance autosomal dominant disease defined by numerous adenomatous polyps of the gastrointestinal mucosa, with an incidence of approximately 1 in 7000 to 1 in 30,000 births, characterized by mutation of APC gene. The duodenum is the second most common site for the adenomatous polyps of FAP to arise, and it occurs in 30–70% of patients with FAP. Duodenal/periampullary carcinoma is the second leading cause of death in patients with FAP, after colorectal cancer, with the lifetime risk of development of duodenal malignancy similar to that of colorectal carcinoma at approximately 100%. Duodenal adenomas of FAP most commonly arise in the second and third (vertical and horizontal) parts of the duodenum [2].

Ampullary adenoma follows adenoma-to-carcinoma sequence, similar to colorectal cancer, so early diagnosis and endoscopic therapy are mandatory in premalignant staging. In FAP patients the adenoma-to-carcinoma sequence is slower, so endoscopic or surgical removal is unnecessary for the adenoma, and in asymptomatic FAP patients with a small lesion, surveillance of the ampulloma with biopsies is reasonable [3, 4].

20.1 Clinical Features

Ampullary lesions can be symptomatic or asymptomatic, found incidentally during upper endoscopy or an imaging test.

Obstructive jaundice is the most common presenting symptom of ampullary cancer (85%), caused by compression of the distal bile duct by the tumor. In benign neoplasms jaundice is intermittent. Gallstones are present in one-third of patients, which may lead to misdiagnosis. Presence of jaundice is associated with advanced stage of disease and increased risk of tumor recurrence after resection [5]. Other common

Electronic Supplementary Material The online version of this chapter (https://doi.org/10.1007/978-3-030-42569-2_20) contains supplementary material, which is available to authorized users.

L. Bernardoni (✉) · S. F. Crinò · A. Gabbrielli
Gastroenterology and Digestive Endoscopy Unit, The Pancreas Institute, G.B. Rossi University Hospital, Verona, Italy
e-mail: laura.bernardoni@aovr.veneto.it

M. Mutignani et al. (eds.), *Endotherapy in Biliopancreatic Diseases: ERCP Meets EUS*,
https://doi.org/10.1007/978-3-030-42569-2_20

symptoms include weight loss, fatigue, and abdominal pain which are present in more than half of patients. Acute pancreatitis is less frequent, but ampullary cancer should be ruled out in this case. Up to one-third of patients have chronic, frequently occult, gastrointestinal blood loss, but occasionally frank bleeding may occur. Rarely, large lesions may produce gastric outlet obstruction [1].

20.2 Classification and Staging

The ampulla of Vater represents the common junction of the distal common bile duct and the main pancreatic duct of Wirsung as it enters into the second portion of the duodenum. It is surrounded by smooth muscle fibers known as the sphincter of Oddi. The smooth muscle fibers are interspersed with glandular tissue which secretes directly into the ampulla [6]. Cancers can arise from anywhere along the ampulla of Vater and are therefore at risk for direct extension into the sphincter of Oddi, duodenum, and/or pancreas. The variable 3D pattern of spread and nonuniform histopathologic grossing practices make the proper staging of ampullary carcinoma, especially with regard to the T category of the tumor, node, and metastasis (TNM) system, particularly challenging [7] (Table 20.1).

Three distinct categories of carcinomas are recognized, after the correlation of gross and microscopic features:

1. Intra-ampullary neoplasms, characterized by a prominent intraluminal growth of the preinvasive neoplasms, which frequently protrude into the duodenal lumen from a patulous orifice of the papilla of Vater.
2. Periampullary, with prominent exophytic, ulcerous-vegetating components on the duodenal surface of the ampulla. The ulcerating part frequently corresponds to the invasive component, whereas the vegetating part represents the preinvasive component.
3. Mixed exophytic and mixed ulcerated lesions [1].

Table 20.1 Comparison of the seventh and eighth editions of the AJCC/UICC classification and staging systems for ampullary carcinoma

Seventh edition		Eighth edition	
T			
T1	Limited to ampulla or sphincter of Oddi	T1a	Limited to sphincter of Oddi
		T1b	Invasion into the duodenal submucosa
T2	Invasion into the duodenal wall	T2	Invasion into the duodenal muscularis propria
T3	Invasion into the pancreas	T3a	Invasion into the pancreas ≤ 0.5 cm
		T3b	Invasion into the pancreas > 0.5 cm or duodenal subserosa
T4	Invasion into peripancreatic soft tissue or other adjacent organs	T4	Involvement of celiac or superior mesenteric artery
N			
N0	No lymph node involvement	N0	No lymph node involvement
N1	Lymph node involvement	N1	Metastasis in 1–3 lymph nodes
		N2	Metastasis in ≥ 4 lymph nodes
AJCC stage			
IA	T1, N0, M0	IA	T1a, N0, M0
IB	T2, N0, M0	IB	T1b–2, N0, M0
IIA	T3, N0, M0	IIA	T3a, N0, M0
IIB	T1–3, N1, M0	IIB	T3b, N0, M0
III	T4, any N, M0	IIIA	T1a–T3, N1, M0
		IIIB	Any T, N2, M0 T4, any N, M0
IV	Any T, any N, M1	IV	Any T, any N, M1

20.3 Indication of Endoscopic Papillectomy

The indications for endoscopic papillectomy (EP) are based on features that can predict a complete tumor removal, while minimizing complications related to the procedure. Currently the indications are not fully established and are far from a consensus.

The main criteria for EP include the lesion size (up to 5 cm) and no evidence of intraductal tumor growth or malignancy in endoscopic findings, such as ulceration, spontaneous bleeding, and friability [8]. However, the indications for EP are expanding. For example, the endoscopic piecemeal resection technique is used to remove tumors that can't be removed "en bloc" and provided increasing resections, when properly performed. The ductal invasion extending less than 1 cm does not seem to be an absolute contraindication for endoscopic papillectomy, because the tumor can be exposed by endoscopic maneuvers, such as the use of an extractor balloon into the lumen, and thus it can be completely resected with a polypectomy snare [9]. The cancer arising within an adenoma without invasion of the duodenal muscularis propria and pancreas, or common bile duct and main pancreatic duct, is liable to resection by endoscopic papillectomy. However, in some situations, endoscopic papillectomy can be used as a macrobiopsy procedure for a simple local tumoral staging, if the resection margins are compromised [10].

In patients with ampullary adenoma (T1-N0-M0 for TNM classification), EP can be a therapeutic option in appropriately selected patients.

In patients affected by ampullary adenocarcinoma must be considered surgical resection or only palliative therapy must be considered in joundice patients affected by ampullary adenocarcinoma.

20.4 Staging

Papillectomy represented the resection of adenoma of the papilla, limited to the mucosa and submucosa of the duodenal wall, tissue around the bile duct, and the pancreatic duct orifices.

Papillectomy cannot remove tissue inside common bile duct or pancreatic duct for a long stretch, so staging of adenoma before papillectomy is very important. Abdominal MRI, EUS, or intraductal US (IDUS) can be useful for demonstrate invasion of common bile duct and pancreatic duct, to exclude pancreatic abnormalities (such as pancreas divisum) or metastatic lymph node [11]. Ductal dilation is significant predictor of malignancy in ampullary adenoma [12].

EUS has been shown to be superior to CT, magnetic resonance imaging, or transabdominal US for tumor staging. Magnetic resonance imaging has been found to be superior to EUS for nodal staging for these patients.

It is uncertain whether all patients with ampullary adenomas should undergo EUS before therapy. Some experts propose that lesions <1 cm in diameter or those that do not have obvious signs of malignancy (ulceration, induration, bleeding) do not require US evaluation before endoscopic removal. If available, EUS examination should be considered for larger lesions or those with features concerning for malignancy before endoscopic or surgical resection is performed [13]. IDUS (intraductal ultrasound) is superior to EUS for tumor visualization, but for intricate use and increased risk, clinical utility is unclear. IDUS may be better than EUS for detailed imaging of the anatomy of the ampulla of Vater because it has a higher ultrasound frequency and obtains images in a perpendicular direction to the duct. In a recently published study of 48 patients with ampullary tumors, EUS and IDUS showed the same (85%) overall diagnostic accuracy. The diagnosis of foci of adenocarcinoma or focal invasion of the duodenal wall layer presented difficulties with both modalities. If the clinical suspect for invasive cancer is low (asymptomatic patient without biliary and pancreatic duct dilation at MRI and endoscopic benign appearance), EUS don't impact the endoscopic papillectomy [14].

Endoscopic inspection with a side-viewing endoscope is essential to distinguish different causes of prominent ampulla. Endoscopic features of noncancerous lesions include regular margins, absence of ulceration, spontaneous bleeding, and soft consistency (Fig. 20.1).

Histopathologic diagnosis of benign adenoma by endoscopic biopsy is recommended before papillectomy to confirm the diagnosis of adenoma; forceps biopsies have high sensitivity (>90%) to confirm the presence of adenoma but a lower sensitivity and accuracy for grade of dysplasia/adenocarcinoma [15]. During biopsy it is safer to avoid pancreatic or bile duct orifice to reduce the possibility of acute pancreatitis or cholangitis.

Diagnostic (adenoma and carcinoma diagnosis) rates for ampullary biopsies of 45–80% have

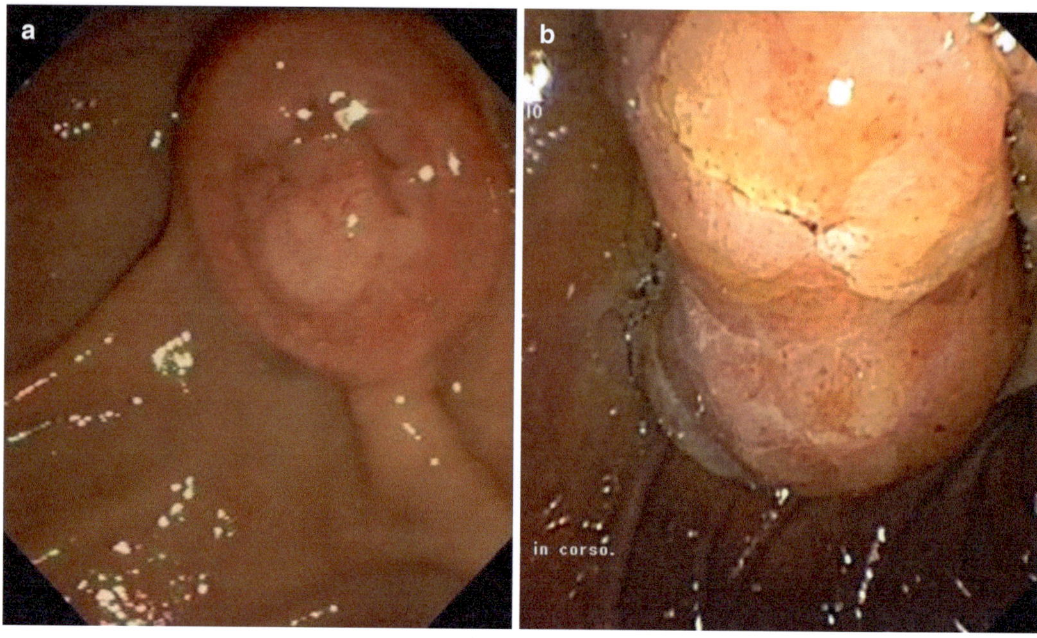

Fig. 20.1 Neoplasia of the papilla. (**a**) A little ampulloma inside the papilla. (**b**) A big ampulloma that involves major papilla

been reported, with false-negative results in 16–60% of patients with carcinoma. The rate of false-negative biopsies may be minimized by sampling within 10 days after sphincterotomy or obtaining at least 6 biopsy specimens. Biopsy of flat lesions that involve more than onefold can result in submucosal fibrosis, potentially impeding subsequent endoscopic resection. Orienting the forceps parallel to the folds while taking the tissue gently from between the folds may decrease the risk of subsequent fibrosis [13].

Evaluation of the papilla with new techniques such as NBI is still not standardized, but NBI can be usefull for enhancement of tumor margin of the duodenal papilla [16].

20.5 Techniques

Binmoeller et al. [17] in 1993 was the first to report endoscopic resection with curative intent. The principal concerns to date regarding endoscopic ampullectomy are the difficulty of resecting a lesion in the proximal duodenum at the junction of the biliary and pancreatic duct orifices compared with a simple polypectomy, incomplete removal of the lesion, post-procedure complications, and insufficient treatment of tumors with undetected malignant foci or intraductal invasion.

Techniques of endoscopic removal of ampullary adenomas remain not standardized because of the small number of formal investigations of this practice (Table 20.2). The term ampullectomy refers to removal of the entire ampulla of Vater and is a surgical term for procedures that require surgical reimplantation of the distal common bile duct and pancreatic duct within the duodenal wall. Technically, when endoscopic resection of lesions at the major papilla are performed, only tissue from the papilla can be removed endoscopically, and thus the term papillectomy is more appropriate than the term ampullectomy, although the two often are used interchangeably in the literature.

Complete en bloc excision of the entire neoplasm should be the goal with conventional papillary adenomas. To this end complete papillectomy to the plane of the duodenal wall should always be considered to minimize recur-

Table 20.2 Steps of endoscopic papillectomy

Inspection	Inspect the ampulla for firmness, ulceration, induration, and friability
Cannulation of pancreatic and biliary ducts	Use sphincterotome and hydrophilic guide wire to • Assess for intraductal invasion or stricturing • Injection with epinephrine/saline solution reserved for flat periampullary lesions
Resection	• Grasp adenomatous tissue at the base with polypectomy snare • Apply 45–60 W blended electrosurgical current (ERBE setting) • Perform piecemeal resection for lesions unamenable to en bloc resection (often >2 cm) (another point) Mind that the sample can progress and be lost distally
Ablation	Adjunctive therapy for residual tumor with APC (setting of 45–60 J)
Stenting	Place 5–7 Fr stent into the pancreatic duct • Place a biliary stent in poorly draining ducts despite sphincterotomy
Sphincterotomy	• Pancreatic sphincterotomy is not mandatory • Biliary sphincterotomy performed either routinely or in the absence of free bile flow
Final observation	Observe the site for evidence of bleeding. If present, inject 1:10,000 epinephrine or use clip if you see bleeding vessel

rence. For lesions with extrapapillary extension, the goal should be to remove the lesion in as few pieces as safely possible, and again the papilla itself should be excised as one. En bloc resection has many advantages including more accurate histological assessment and negligible recurrence. It should be remembered that endoscopic ampullectomy is an advanced therapeutic intervention and that the endoscopist must have sufficient training and expertise to undertake the procedure. Repeat intervention for partially resected lesions is often difficult with an increased risk due to submucosal fibrosis and disruption of the underlying anatomy [18].

Endoscopic papillectomy should be performed in the X-ray room with patient in prone position and with anesthesiologist assistance for deep sedation; before start of procedure, intravenous antiperistaltic agent is used to reduce the possibility of distal migration of resected adenoma. Carbon dioxide insufflation can be an advantage in the event of duodenal perforation [19].

Whether or not submucosal injection should be used to lift ampullary tumors during endoscopic snare papillectomy is still unclear.

Fluids injected into the submucosa have included saline solution, epinephrine, and viscous materials such as hydroxypropyl methylcellulose. Volumes of injected fluid are not standardized and vary widely among published studies. It is important to note that ampullary lesions are tethered down by the biliary and pancreatic ducts and may not lift with submucosal injection. In addition, the surrounding normal mucosa that does lift may form a sort of "mushroom" around the ampullary adenoma. This "mushroom" may partially depress the central aspect of the tumor, which may preclude adequate snare placement and complete excision. Some authors have not used submucosal injection, and currently there are insufficient data to conclude that this is a mandatory step in the procedure [13].

A prospective multicenter study concluded that although the recurrence rate was similar between the simple snare papillectomy group and submucosal injection papillectomy group, submucosal injection papillectomy group showed no advantage over simple snare papillectomy group in terms of achieving complete resection or decreasing the frequency of post-papillectomy adverse events, such as bleeding [20].

Another group indicated that submucosal injection before endoscopic papillectomy of ampullary tumor was related to more frequent residual tumor and shorter recurrence-free survival and did not reduce post-procedural adverse events [21].

Preresection sphincterotomy is not indicated because it adds a supplemental risk of bleeding or perforation, can modify anatomy of the adenoma and duodenal wall, and makes histopathological evaluation difficult. In case of jaundice, we suggest that the patient should be treated directly by a papillectomy or insertion of biliary stent, to reduce the risk of fibrosis of biliary sphincterotomy.

Conventional snares ranging from 10 to 27 mm of diameter are usually used. The adenoma together with the papilla is grasped and excised snaring the tumor from the cephalic to the caudal side: the snare apex is placed at the superior margin of the ampulloma and slowly opens, while the snare goes out to the endoscope. For this reason oval and soft snare has a better conformation to perform papillectomy. Spiral snares can firmly grasp flat lesion compared with the single-wire snare. A gentle movement of the snare with the elevator can assess the mobility of tumor and the absence of deep invasion of the duodenal wall.

After a satisfactory catching of adenoma with snare, electrosurgical current is used to cut the papilla. There is no established consensus regarding power and the mode of electrosurgical current used for papillectomy [22]. Pure cutting current can avoid edema caused by coagulation reducing the incidence of post-procedure pancreatitis (Video 20.1).

En bloc resection is fundamental for treatment of tumor and correct staging, to establish the presence of neoplastic cells in lateral or deep margin of resection. If the size of the lesion could not allow en bloc resection, we prefer to start the resection from the papilla and then remove the remaining adenoma with piecemeal technique such as a duodenal polyp during the same session.

If a small remnant lesion is suspected, we can remove it with small snare, biopsy forceps, or adjunct thermal ablation with APC because it does not cause a deep damage to the duodenal wall. APC ablation can control immediate bleeding, prevent post-procedural bleeding, or ablate suspected microscopic remnant tumor [23].

The ductal invasion less than 1 cm is not an absolute contraindication for papillectomy because the tumor can be exposed by endoscopic maneuvers such as the use of extractor balloon and it can be completely resected with snare.

To recover surgical specimen, we can use the snare or the suction trap.

Surgical specimen of the papilla should be sent for histological examination in *fresco*; in piecemeal resection other pieces could be sent in formalin.

After resection, detection of pancreatic orifice is mandatory because placement of pancreatic stent can reduce the risk of acute pancreatitis after papillectomy (do not forget that the pancreas is completely normal and very reactive), allow to perform local hemostatic therapy for post-procedural bleeding, and reduce the fibrotic stenosis of the duct. Pancreatic stent of different diameters or length is used according to the duct morphology (5, 7, or 10 F, length 5 cm). In patients with pancreas divisum, pancreatic stenting is not indicated (Fig. 20.2).

A recent meta-analysis showed that prophylactic pancreatic stenting after pancreatic sphincterotomy decreased the odds of post-procedure pancreatitis (OR, 0.71; 95% CI, 0.36–1.40; $p = 0.325$) as well as late papillary stenosis (OR, 0.35; 95% CI, 0.07–1.75; $p = 0.200$; I 2 = 0%) and increased the odds of bleeding (OR, 1.32; 95% CI, 0.50–3.46; $p = 0.572$; I 2 = 0%) and perforation (OR, 2.25; 95% CI, 0.33–15.50; $p = 0.412$; I 2 = 0%) but not significantly [24]. Chang et al. investigated the efficacy of prophylactic pancreatic stent placement for preventing post-procedure pancreatitis in patients undergoing endoscopic papillectomy; there was no difference in the development of post-procedure pancreatitis between the stent group and the no stent group (6/54, 10.5% and 2/28, 7.14%, respectively; $p = 1.00$). These data suggest that routine prophylactic pancreatic duct stent placement in all patients undergoing endoscopic papillectomy may not be necessary and large-scale prospective studies are required to identify the subgroup of patients who would benefit [25].

A hydrophilic guide wire should be used gently to obtain deep cannulation of the pancreatic duct. The pancreatic orifice should be searched at 5 o'clock.

Pancreatic duct identification after resection may be facilitated by injecting methylene blue into the pancreatic duct before resection, and this

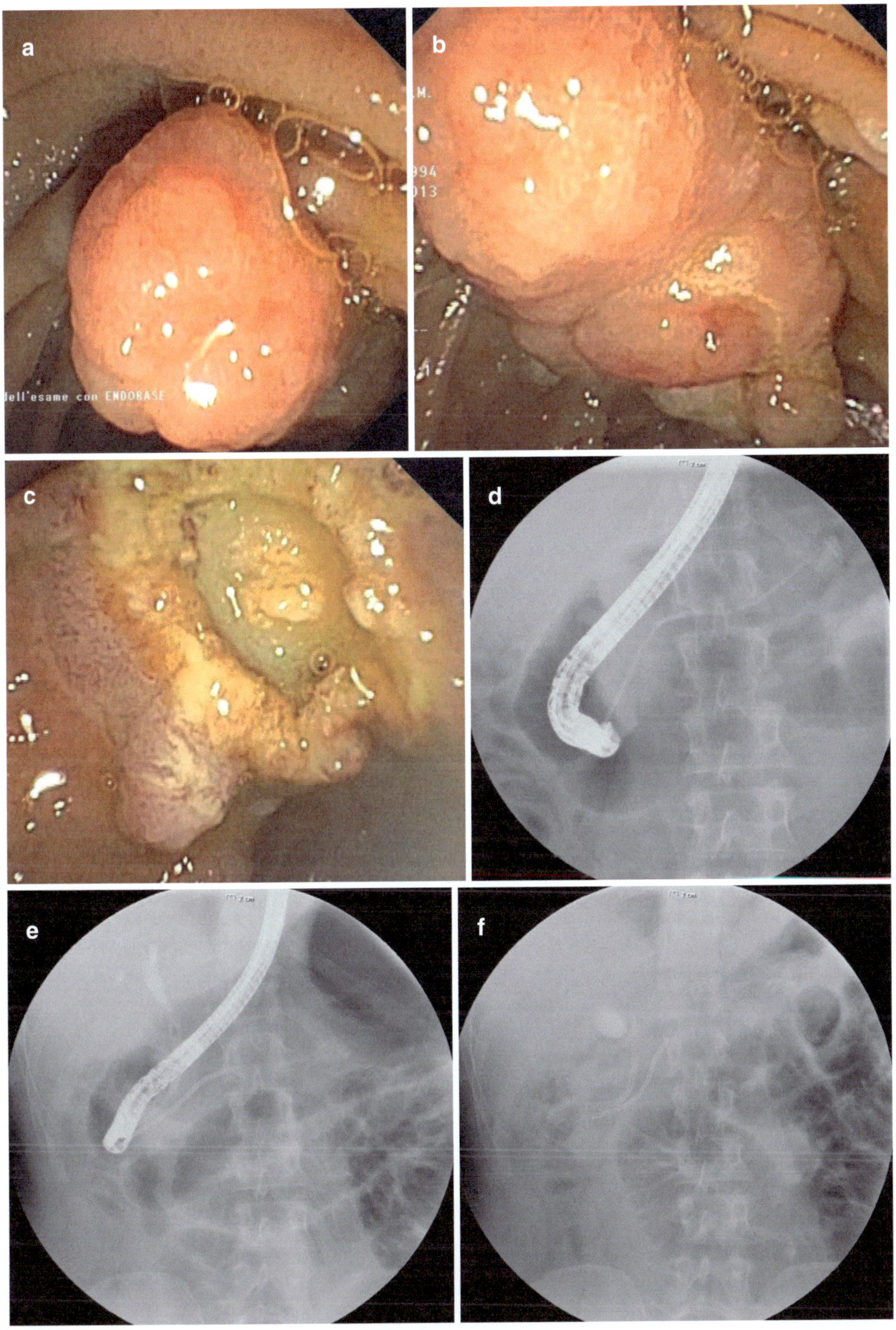

Fig. 20.2 Endoscopic papillectomy steps. (**a**, **b**) Ampullary neoplasm view with duodenoscope of the proximal part and of entire ampullary neoplasm. (**c**) Base of resection after cutting neoplasm with main pancreatic duct orifice in the center. (**d–g**) Biliary and pancreatic stent insertion after resection. (**h**, **i**) Specimen of ampulla after resection with evidence of main pancreatic duct. (**j**, **k**) Specimen after coloring with ink to evaluate deep margin and orientation of specimen

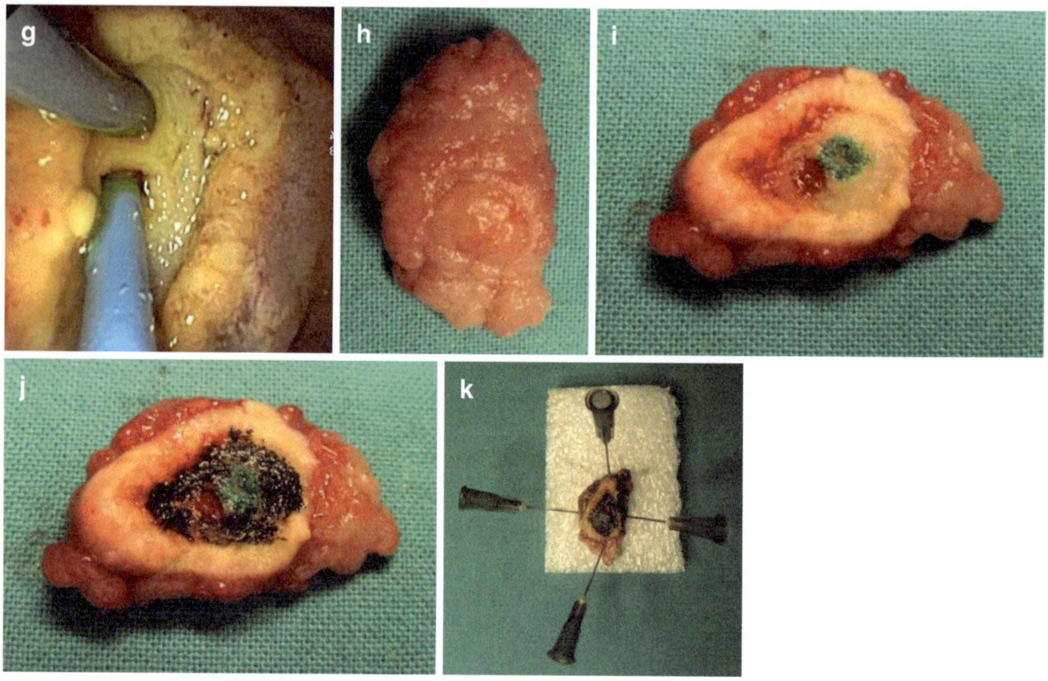

Fig. 20.2 (continued)

could decrease the risk for post-procedure pancreatitis [26].

Pancreatic sphincterotomy could be performed alone or associated with pancreatic stent insertion [27].

Cannulation of common bile duct after papillectomy is not a debate because cholangitis is a rare complication of papillectomy. Bile orifice should be searched at 11 o'clock, near the apex of papillectomy. If bile duct clearance of contrast medium is slow, biliary sphincterotomy and/or biliary stent insertion (10 Fr, 5–7 cm) is indicated.

After resection patient keeps fasting for 24 h, so new therapeutic endoscopy is possible in case of early complications (Video 20.2).

20.6 Complications

In published series the most common complications after endoscopic papillectomy are bleeding (0–25%) and pancreatitis (0–25%). Less commonly reported complications include perforation, cholangitis, and stenosis of the pancreatic or biliary orifice. Procedure-related mortality after papillectomy has been reported but is rare, occurring in 2 of 706 reported cases (0.3%) [28] (Table 20.3).

Table 20.3 Complication of papillectomy

Complications	Reported rate (%)	Measure to reduce risk
Acute pancreatitis	4–20	Pancreatic stenting Rectal indomethacin
Bleeding	2–30	Submucosal epinephrine injection
Perforation	0–4	Assess mobility
Cholangitis	1–2	Biliary stent
Papillary stenosis	1–2	Post-resection biliary and/or pancreatic sphincterotomy Biliary and pancreatic stent

Acute bleeding can usually be managed by typical endoscopic hemostatic techniques. If bleeding after papillectomy is suspected, duodenoscope is mandatory for therapeutic endoscopy. If bleeding occurs, the presence of pancreatic and biliary stent makes the therapeutic endoscopy safer for potential damage of hemostatic accessories like clip, coagulation forceps, APC, and Hemospray on the ducts (Video 20.3). In the absence of stent after papillectomy, ERCP in the X-ray room is indicated to stop bleeding and guarantee the patency of pancreatic and bile duct. Clots often cause cholangitis, so cholangiogram and clot removal from common bile duct with Fogarty balloon are mandatory; in these cases biliary plastic stent insertion is indicated.

Whenever possible, placement of a prophylactic pancreatic duct stent is recommended to reduce the incidence and severity of post-papillectomy pancreatitis.

A careful inspection of the resection defect must always be undertaken to assess for areas of deep resection. Endoscopic features are less reliable at determining deep resection than in other sites, and so a high clinical index of suspicion must be maintained during post-procedural clinical assessment. The absence of free intraperitoneal or subdiaphragmatic air on plain X-rays at the end of the procedure does not exclude perforation which is usually retroperitoneal. Ongoing pain should prompt radiological assessment and, if required, surgical review. Computed tomography (preferably with oral contrast) is more sensitive and is required if symptoms continue. Multidisciplinary management between medical and surgical teams is necessary to achieve the best possible clinical outcome. Not all cases of perforation require surgical intervention, and select cases may be managed with gut rest and intravenous antibiotics [29].

After receiving the final report on histological findings of the resected tumor, the need for further treatment can be determinate.

A high-grade dysplasia or carcinoma in situ recommended additional surgery. However close follow-up with periodic endoscopy with biopsies may be sufficient in cases of focal high-grade dysplasia or carcinoma in situ which was removed completely when the patient was unfit for surgery or refuses surgery. In patients with positive resection margin related to low-grade dysplasia, further endoscopic resection or adjunct thermal ablation can be applied. APC, a no-contact thermal ablation mode, is safer for the treatment of residual adenoma.

In case of persistent intraductal growth (Fig. 20.3), biliary or pancreatic duct, intraductal radiofrequency ablation (RFA) can be used for treatment and eradication of dysplasia. In these circumstances a biliary fully covered metal stent insertion is indicated after the treatment (Fig. 20.4).

Treatment success was achieved in 92% if RFA is associated to other procedures; the rate of neoplasia eradication after one single RFA session was obtained in 70% of patients.

A short duration of the RFA application (30 s) and a limitation in the power used (10 W) should be selected as the settings of choice because the treatment is delivered over the ampullary orifice, thus making the risk of pancreatitis very high. Because of these considerations, both diclofenac

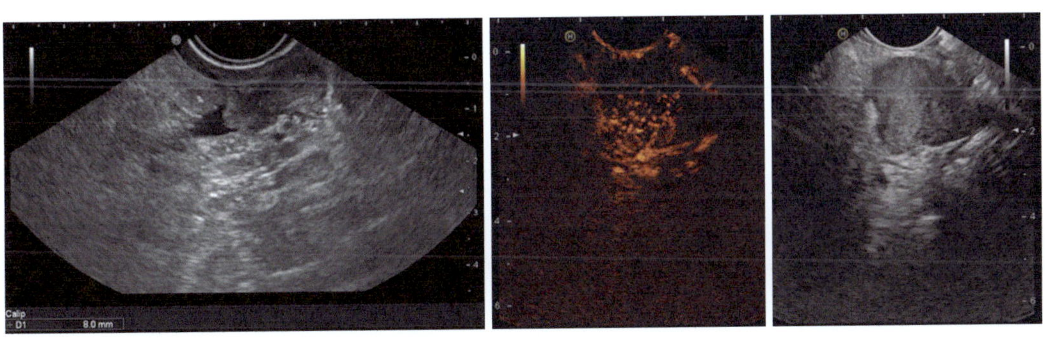

Fig. 20.3 Common bile duct invasion at EUS. (**a**) Ampullary neoplasm grows inside common bile duct for 8 mm. (**b**–**c**) Echogenic material inside biliary tract takes contrast rapresenting ampulloma endoductal ingrowth

100 mg suppository and pancreatic stent placement should be recommended in these patients. Adverse events of RFA range from 40 to 43% (ductal strictures are more frequent complications; retroduodenal abscess, mild pancreatitis, and self-limited bleeding are signaled in literature). Endoscopic follow up is mandatory every 3 months in the first year to confirm complete ablation or to identify disease recurrence [30, 31].

20.7 Surveillance

Recurrence rates reported in literature after papillectomy ranged from 2 to 33% [32].

Risk factors for recurrence include FAP and lesions with high-grade dysplasia; size has not been definitively linked to increased likelihood of recurrence [33]. Technical factors also are likely important including incomplete excision and lack

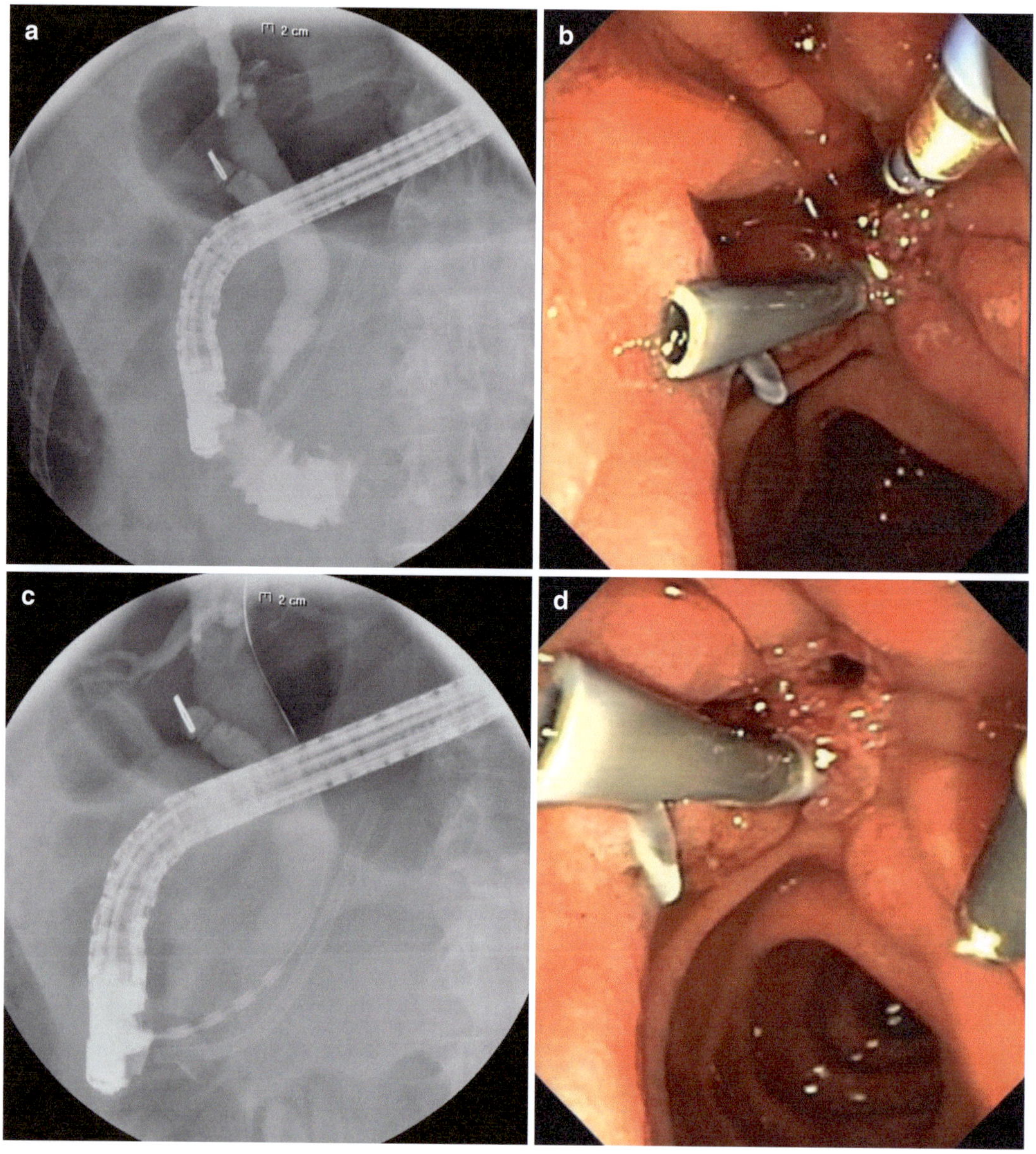

Fig. 20.4 (**a**) Radiological view of ampulloma in-growth inside distal part of common bile duct. (**b–d**) Introduction of radiofrequency catheter in common bile duct. (**e**) Fully covered metal stent insertion in common bile duct

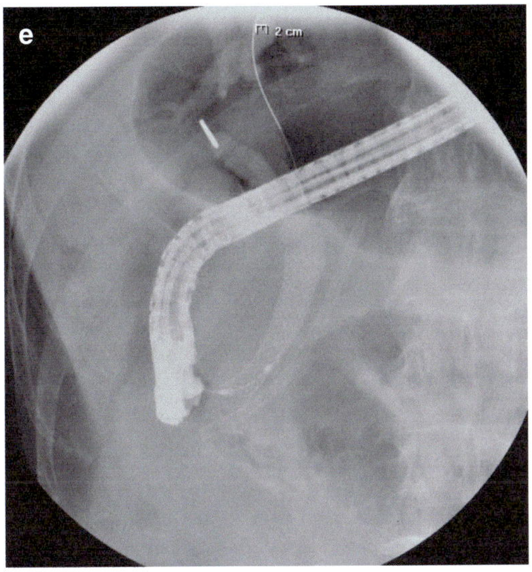

Fig. 20.4 (continued)

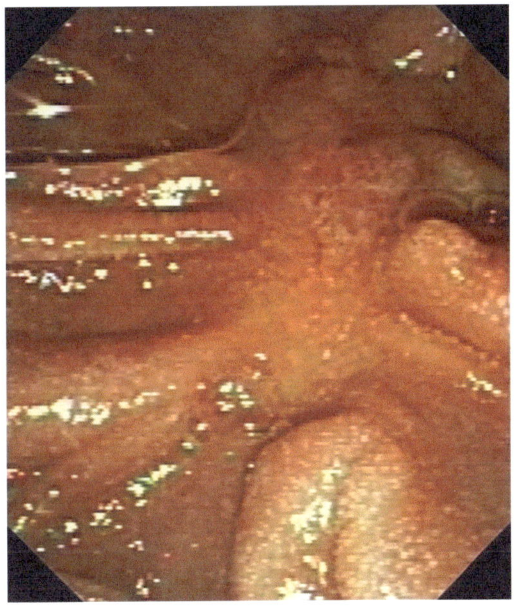

Fig. 20.5 A 6-month follow-up after endoscopic papillectomy without adenoma residual

of use of thermal ablation for any residual tissue, although there are no standardized guidelines for post-papillectomy surveillance [34]. A complete endoscopic resection is defined as the absence of endoscopically visible and histologically proven residual adenoma.

After papillectomy, first scheduled follow-up endoscopy is at 3 months to remove pancreatic and/or biliary stent and to check for any adenoma residuals. If there is a residual, this is generally diminutive and easily excised (or ablated if excision is not possible) (Fig. 20.5).

In cases with complete resection of ampullary adenoma, follow-up endoscopy with ERCP and multiple biopsies is recommended at 3, 6, and 12 months after resection and then at yearly intervals for 5 years on obtaining a negative biopsy [35]. In cases of incomplete excision, or those in which thermal ablation is performed, endoscopic examination should be performed every 1–3 months until complete resection is proven. Cases in which resection shows that patients have focal cancer in the main adenoma or carcinoma in situ can be followed with cautious routine endoscopic surveillance [36]. However, cases with incomplete resection of cancer should be considered for radical surgery because of the risk of lymph node metastasis.

References

1. Panzeri F, Crippa S, Castelli P, et al. Management of ampullary neoplasms: a tailored approach between endoscopy and surgery. World J Gastroenterol. 2015;21(26):7970–87.
2. Dinarvand P, Davaro EP, Doan JV, et al. Familial adenomatous polyposis syndrome: an update and review of extraintestinal manifestations. Arch Pathol Lab Med. 2019;143(11):1382–98.
3. Moozar KL, Madlensky L, Berk T, et al. Slow progression of periampullary neoplasia in familial adenomatous polyposis. J Gastroint Surg. 2002;6:831–7.
4. Matsumoto T, et al. Natural history of ampullary adenoma in familial adenomatous polyposis: reconfirmation of benign nature during extended surveillance. Am J Gastroenterol. 2000;95(6):1557–62.
5. Kamisawa T, Tu Y, Egawa N, et al. Clinicopathologic features of ampullary carcinoma without jaundice. J Clin Gastroenterol. 2006;40:162–6.
6. Avisse C, Flament JB, Delattre JF. Ampulla of vater. Anatomic, embryologic, and surgical aspects. Surg Clin N Am. 2000;80:201–12.
7. Adsay NV, Bagci P, Tajiri T, et al. Pathologic staging of pancreatic, ampullary, biliary, and gallbladder cancers: pitfalls and practical limitations of the current AJCC/UICC TNM staging system and opportunities for improvement. Semin Diagn Pathol. 2012;29:127–41.
8. Ardengh JC, Kemp R, Lima-Filho ÉR, et al. Endoscopic papillectomy: the limits of the indication,

technique and results. World J Gastrointest Endosc. 2015;7(10):987–94.

9. Kim JH, Kim JH, Han JH, et al. Is endoscopic papillectomy safe for ampullary adenomas with high-grade dysplasia? Ann Surg Oncol. 2009;16:2547–54.
10. Yoon LY, Moon JH, Choi HJ, et al. Wire-guided endoscopic snare retrieval of proximally migrated pancreatic stents after endoscopic papillectomy for ampullary adenoma. Gut Liver. 2011;5:532–5.
11. Hirooka Y. EUS/IDUS and endoscopic papillectomy. Dig Endosc. 2004;16(Suppl):S176–7.
12. Kim HN, Kim KM, Shin JU. Prediction of carcinoma after resection in subjects with ampullary adenomas on endoscopic biopsy. J Clin Gastroenterol. 2013;47(4):346–51.
13. Chathadi KV, Khashab MA. The role of endoscopy in ampullary and duodenal adenomas. Gastrointest Endosc. 2015;82:773–81.
14. Han J, Lee DW, Kim HG. Recent advances in endoscopic papillectomy for ampulla of Vater tumors: endoscopic ultrasonography, intraductal ultrasonography, and pancreatic stent placement. Clin Endosc. 2015;48:24–30.
15. Yamamoto K. Discrepancy between the preprocedure biopsy and final diagnosis in endoscopic papillectomy of ampullary tumors. J Gastroenterol Hepatol. 2015;237.
16. Itoi T, Tsuji S, Sofuni A, Itokawa F. A novel approach emphasizing preoperative margin enhancement of tumor of the major duodenal papilla with narrow-band imaging in comparison to indigo carmine chromoendoscopy (with videos). Gastrointest Endosc. 2009;69(1):136–41.
17. Binmoeller KF, Boaventura S, Ramsperger K, et al. Endoscopic snare excision of benign adenomas of the papilla of Vater. Gastrointest Endosc. 1993;39:127–31.
18. Klein A, Tutticci N, Bourke MJ. Endoscopic resection of advanced and laterally spreading duodenal papillary tumors. Dig Endosc. 2016;28(2):121–30.
19. Chathadi KV, Khashab MA, Acosta RD. The role of endoscopy in ampullary and duodenal adenomas. Gastrointest Endosc. 2015;82(5):773–8.
20. Hyun JJ, Lee TH, Park JS, et al. A prospective multicenter study of submucosal injection to improve endoscopic snare papillectomy for ampullary adenoma. Gastrointest Endosc. 2017;85(4):746–55.
21. Chung KH, Lee SH, Choi JH, et al. Effect of submucosal injection in endoscopic papillectomy of ampullary tumor: propensity-score matching analysis. United European Gastroenterol J. 2018;6(4):576–85.
22. Van Gossum A, Cozzoli A, Adler M, et al. Colonoscopic snare polypectomy: analysis of 1485 resections comparing two types of current. Gastrointest Endosc. 1992;38:472–5.
23. Nam K, Song TJ, Kim RE, et al. Usefulness of argon plasma coagulation ablation subsequent to endoscopic snare papillectomy for ampullary adenoma. Dig Endosc. 2018;30(4):485–92.
24. Wang Y, Qi M, Hao Y, Hong J. The efficacy of prophylactic pancreatic stents against complications of post-endoscopic papillectomy or endoscopic ampullectomy: a systematic review and meta-analysis. Ther Adv Gastroenterol. 2019;26:12.
25. Chang WI, Min YW, Yun HS, et al. Prophylactic pancreatic stent placement for endoscopic duodenal ampullectomy: a single-center retrospective study. Gut Liver. 2014;8(3):306–12.
26. Poinclouxa L, Scanzia J, Gouttea M, et al. Pancreatic intubation facilitated by methylene blue injection decreases the risk for postpapillectomy acute pancreatitis. Eur J Gastroenterol Hepatol. 2014;26(9):990–5.
27. Lee TY, Cheon YK, Shim CS, et al. Endoscopic wire-guided papillectomy vs. conventional papillectomy for ampullary tumors: a prospective comparative pilot study. J Gastroenterol Hepatol. 2016;31(4):897–902.
28. El Hajj II, Coté GA. Endoscopic diagnosis and management of ampullary lesions. Gastrointest Endosc Clin N Am. 2013;23:95–109.
29. Bassan M, Bourke M. Endoscopic ampullectomy: a practical guide. J Interv Gastroenterol. 2012;2(1):23–30.
30. Larghi A, Rimbaş M, Tringali A, et al. Endoscopic radiofrequency biliary ablation treatment: a comprehensive review. Dig Endosc. 2019;31:245–55.
31. Rustagi T, Irani S, Reddy N, et al. Radiofrequency ablation for intraductal extension of ampullary neoplasm. Gastrointest Endosc. 2017;86(1):170–6.
32. Albores-Saavedra J, Schwartz AM, Batich K, et al. Cancers of the ampulla of Vater: demographics, morphology, and survival based on 5,625 cases from the SEER program. J Surg Oncol. 2009;100:598–605.
33. Meneghetti AT, Safadi B, Stewart L, et al. Local resection of ampullary tumors. J Gastrointest Surg. 2005;9:1300–6.
34. Patel R, Varadarajulu S, Mel Wilcox C. Endoscopic ampullectomy. Techniques and outcomes. J Clin Gastroenterol. 2012;46(1):8–15.
35. Catalano FS, Linder JD, Chak A, et al. Endoscopic management of adenoma of the major duodenal papilla. Gastrointest Endosc. 2004;59:225–32.
36. Yoom YS, Kim MH, Kim NJ, et al. Focal early stage cancer in ampullary adenoma: surgery or endoscopic papillectomy? Gastrointest Endosc. 2007;66:701–7.

Ductoscopy

21

Manuel Pagitz and Jörg G. Albert

With the introduction of high-resolution endoscopy, the previous standard, i.e. radiography, took the back seat in diagnosing gastrointestinal disease, and gastroscopy replaced gastrography, while small bowel enterography was progressively substituted by small bowel endoscopy techniques. However, ductography is still the mainstay of visualizing endoscopic interventions in biliopancreatic disease, and ductoscopy is used as an auxiliary technique in indeterminate findings. However, it might be possible that ductography is replaced by ductoscopy of the biliopancreatic system at some point of time in the near future.

The advantage of cholangioscopy lies within the possibilities to take biopsies under direct endoscopic vision, to perform intraductal treatment, e.g. laser lithotripsy, electro-hydraulic lithotripsy (EHL), laser tumour ablation and argon plasma coagulation (APC), and to apply cholangioscopy-guided virtual histology. With improved technology and better safety profiles, indications for performing biliopancreatic ductoscopy are widened.

M. Pagitz (✉) · J. G. Albert
Abteilung für Gastroenterologie, Hepatologie und Endokrinologie, Robert-Bosch-Krankenhaus, Stuttgart, Germany
e-mail: Manuel.Pagitz@rbk.de; joerg.albert@rbk.de

21.1 History and Technical Background

Anterograde ductoscopy requires establishing a percutaneous channel that enables the endoscope to pass. First attempts of anterograde (percutaneous) cholangioscopy were made in the 1970s using fibrescopes that had been designed for bronchoscopy or urological examinations.

Retrograde ductoscopy has either been realized by using miniature endoscopes that are advanced over the working channel of a conventional duodenoscope ("mother/baby" cholangioscopy) or by directly approaching and intubating the papilla with an ultra-slim endoscope. Peroral (or retrograde) cholangioscopy (POC) was introduced into clinical practice in 1976, with using a mother/baby approach. A year later, the first cholangioscopy using a routine forward-viewing endoscope was reported. Yet a broader implementation into the clinical routine was limited by technical issues as well as a high demand of time and skill of the endoscopist. These limitations have gradually been overcome since. Poor image quality of fibre endoscopes significantly improved after introduction of video endoscopes and digital techniques. Image enhancement techniques such as narrowband imaging were implemented into video cholangioscopes. Miniaturization of the optics and light channel left space over for air and water irrigation channels as well as instrumentation channels for

M. Mutignani et al. (eds.), *Endotherapy in Biliopancreatic Diseases: ERCP Meets EUS*,
https://doi.org/10.1007/978-3-030-42569-2_21

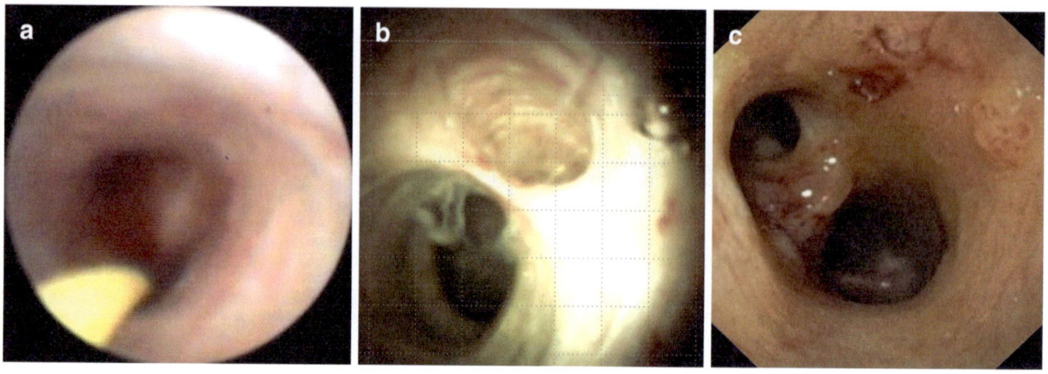

Fig. 21.1 (**a**) Fibre-optic imaging of the common bile duct. (**b**) Digitally enhanced imaging. (**c**) Video endoscope

interventional use. The number of investigators in mother/baby techniques was optimized by introducing single-operator mother/baby scopes, like, e.g. the SpyGlass® system introduced in 2005 [1], Fig. 21.1.

21.1.1 Technical Details

Modern endoscopes for ductoscopy come from a broad range of manufacturers who offer different solutions with varying technical details. In summary, the most important technical aspects to consider are:

- Direct retrograde cholangioscopy vs. mother/baby system
- Outer diameter and working channel diameter
- One or two investigators required
- Imaging quality: fibre optic, digitally enhanced, video endoscopy
- Irrigation capability vs. gas insufflation

Endoscopes for direct retrograde access are handicapped by the anatomical conditions: the endoscope might recoil within the stomach, and passing the small calibre endoscope through the pylorus might be difficult [2, 3]. More challenging still might be to overcome the angulation in the duodenum, thereby turning the endoscope to a cranial direction for the advancement into the biliary orifice. Using conventional ultra-slim gastroscopes for this purpose requires appropriate anatomic conditions as well as a versed investigator and often auxiliary tools (i.e. anchoring balloon) to assist in intubating the Vaterian papilla. Furthermore, manoeuvring in the duct is more difficult due to reduced stiffness and insufficient shoring in the duodenum (and can require the use of a balloon too). Ultra-slim gastroscopes are not dedicated for cholangioscopy, and they are experimentally used for this purpose. New inventions like the prototype CHF-Y0010 (Olympus Tokio, Japan) try to reduce these shortcomings with a more stiff construction of the body of the endoscope, an ultrashort tip of the endoscope and a dual deflection ability of the tip within one plane for better duodenal shoring [4].

Biliary access is alleviated with a mother/baby system: the angulation in the duodenum and the twisting of the endoscope in the stomach are corrected by the position of the mother endoscope. However, the outer diameter is important, and the "baby" has to fit into the "mother's" working channel. A current example of a reusable cholangioscope for mother-baby application is the CHF B 290 (Olympus Tokio, Japan).

Working channel diameter is crucial when interventions are required. Special miniaturized equipment is necessary for some systems with small working channels (like EHL probes, etc.). For biopsy forceps smaller working channels can correlate with smaller biopsy samples.

In clinical routine the necessity of a second versed investigator is a relevant time and cost issue. The mother/baby systems usually require two investigators. An example for a modification removing the need of a second investigator is the SpyGlass® system where the "baby" scope is secured at the "mother" scope so that an experienced investigator can use one hand to hold the "mother" and the other hand to handle the "baby" or vice versa.

Varying optical methods deliver varying imaging qualities. Fibre-optic scopes are quite fragile and offer very limited imaging qualities. Electronic scopes enhance and modify optic information and can therefore greatly increase imaging quality depending on various factors like positioning of the video chip, software specifications, image processor and quality of the necessary separate light source.

Another technical issue in direct regard to miniaturization is the irrigation capacity. Most fibre- or electronic scopes lack a separate irrigation system resulting in decreased clarity. Systems like SpyGlass® or SAMBA as well as conventional ultra-slim gastroscopes offer dedicated irrigation and aspiration channels. The prototype CHF-Y0010, for example, allows irrigation of saline or CO_2.

Other technical aspects like field of view, imaging enhancements (e.g. narrowband imaging) or length play a secondary role. Table 21.1 delineates currently available cholangioscopes and their specifications.

21.2 Current Indications for Biliary Ductoscopy

- To clarify aetiology of indeterminate biliary stricture or lesion
- To treat large bile duct stones or to exclude residual stones in large diameter CBD
- To facilitate the access of excluded/obstructed bile duct segments
- To remove foreign body from the CBD like recovering dislocated biliary stents ("rescue" indication) Fig. 21.2.

21.2.1 Indeterminate Biliary Strictures

If preliminary diagnostics (CT, E/MRCP, laboratory tests, etc.) do not resolve the aetiology of biliary stricture, the character of the obstruction ("indeterminate biliary stricture") might be clarified by cholangioscopy. Visual criteria to differentiate between malignant and benign lesions are not yet standardized. However, in line with experience of other endoscopic diagnostics (not only in the intestine but including bronchoscopy and urological endoscopy), some criteria are highly suggestive for malignancy. This can include aberrant tumour vessels, production of mucus or suspect papillary or nodular structures. Image enhancement techniques can be used (like chromocholangioscopy or with some endoscopes light-enhancing imaging, such as narrowband imaging) but have as of now quite limited experience and are also not standardized yet.

Therefore histological procession is necessary for a definite diagnosis. While standard ERCP can produce histologic results (using cytology brushings or fluoroscopically guided forceps biopsy), cholangioscopy enables visually controlled tissue sampling (in addition to the visual clinical impression of the lesion). Keep in mind that smaller forceps produce smaller samples which can lead to false-negative results.

Furthermore, cholangioscopy can help to differentiate between different aetiologies of post-transplant strictures in liver-transplant patients. Especially using image enhancement strategies, differentiation between ischemic lesions, ulcers and scar tissue is improved [5].

21.2.2 Bile Duct Stones

In diagnosis of biliary stones, sonography is our leading method of diagnostic. Yet external sonography is often impaired due to meteorism or other conditions decreasing image quality. In distal biliary duct stones, endosonography can provide the diagnosis, but still small stones can elude the diagnostics. For intervention an ERCP is usually performed. Large stones can elude fluoroscopic detection when totally obstructing a duct near a furcation and therefore blocking the contrast agent without a clue of an interruption of the duct. In patients suffering of primary sclerosing

Table 21.1 Examples of available cholangioscopes

	SpyGlass® system	CHF-Y0010	The short-access mother/baby (SAMBA) cholangioscopy system	Polyscope	Conventional ultra-slim gastroscope
Manufacturer	Boston Scientific	Olympus, Tokyo	Karl Storz, Tuttlingen, Germany	PolyDiagnost, Germany	Diverse
Cholangioscopy technique	"Mother/baby"—Standard duodenoscope	Direct retrograde cholangioscopy	"Mother/baby"—Dedicated duodenoscope	"Mother/baby"—Standard duodenoscope	Direct retrograde cholangioscopy
Assist	Duodenoscope	Balloon assisted (20–30%)	Duodenoscope	Duodenoscope	Balloon assisted (80–90%)
Outer diameter (mm)	3.33	5.2	3.4	2.7	5–7 mm
Working channel (mm)	1.2	2.2 and 0.8	1.5	1.2	Often 2.0–2.2
Investigators	One or two investigators	One investigator	Two investigators	Two investigators	One investigator
Imaging	Digitally enhanced visualization	Video endoscopy	Fibre optic	Fibre optic	Video endoscopy
Irrigation/ insufflation	Sterile saline irrigation	Sterile saline irrigation CO_2 insufflation option	Sterile saline irrigation	Sterile saline irrigation	Sterile saline irrigation CO_2 insufflation
Tip deflection	Up/down Left/right	Tip: Up/down Second up/down	Up/down	Down	Up/down Left/right
Cost/availability	Single use	Prototype cholangioscope	Special duodenoscope needed	Single use	Common

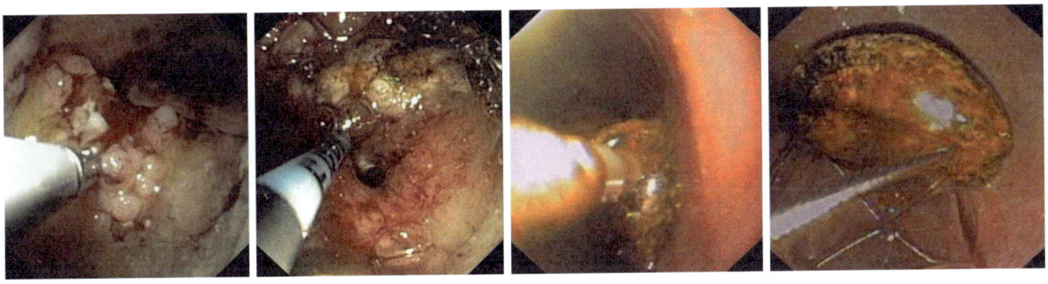

Fig. 21.2 Interventions at direct retrograde cholangioscopy: Taking biopsies with a conventional biopsy forceps, argon plasma coagulation of a mucin-producing tumour of the intrahepatic bile ducts, electro-hydraulic lithotripsy, stone extraction with a stone removal basket (from left to right)

cholangitis, for example, the co-morbid strictures can lead to a significant under-detection of biliary stones.

Cholangioscopy is able to reveal missed stones, and in special situations where clinical aspects suggest a stone disease but other diagnostics fail to reveal them, cholangioscopy should be performed according to risk-benefit evaluation.

The more common use of cholangioscopy in biliary stones, however, is the fragmentation of large or incarcerated duct stones especially after conventional approaches failed. Two methods are available: electro-hydraulic lithotripsy (EHL) or laser lithotripsy. EHL requires irrigation of water (sterile saline); the laser probe is usually thinner and easier to use in intrahepatic stones. Performed by an experienced investigator, success rates are high even in a single session; severe adverse events are rare.

21.2.3 Other Indications for Cholangioscopy

There are a lot of further situation where cholangioscopy can improve treatment, yet these settings are less common than the above-mentioned. They include evaluation of the distal bile duct in neoplasms of the papilla, evaluation of cystic biliary lesions, ablative therapies for intraductal neoplasms (argon plasma coagulation, brachytherapy, Nd:YAG laser ablation, etc.), evaluation of haemobilia and "rescue" therapies, e.g. for proximally dislocated stents, adverse events after transarterial chemoembolization.

21.3 Indications for Pancreatoscopy

- To disintegrate symptomatic pancreatic stones
- To evaluate the extent and localization of IPMN prior to surgery
- To clarify aetiology of indeterminate pancreatic stricture

Methods and specifications in pancreatoscopy are the same as in cholangioscopy. Yet years of experience with ERCP showed the potential severe adverse events when manipulating near the pancreas. Pancreatitis is not an uncommon adverse event, and severe necrotic pancreatitis is associated with relevant morbidity and mortality. Therefore indication for pancreatoscopy is more restrictive than for cholangioscopy. The ductus wirsungianus has to be dilated for a secure pancreatoscopy (Fig. 21.3).

21.4 Retrograde Cholangioscopy

21.4.1 Sphincter Management

In most cases sphincterotomy is needed prior to ductoscopy as most scopes are too large to pass the sphincter of Oddi. Ultra-slim fibrescopes can sometimes be inserted (usually wire-guided) without sphincterotomy, but with good non-invasive diagnostics available purely diagnostic cholangioscopy without interventional intention (including aiming for a biopsy) is not often intended. Most commonly during a preliminary

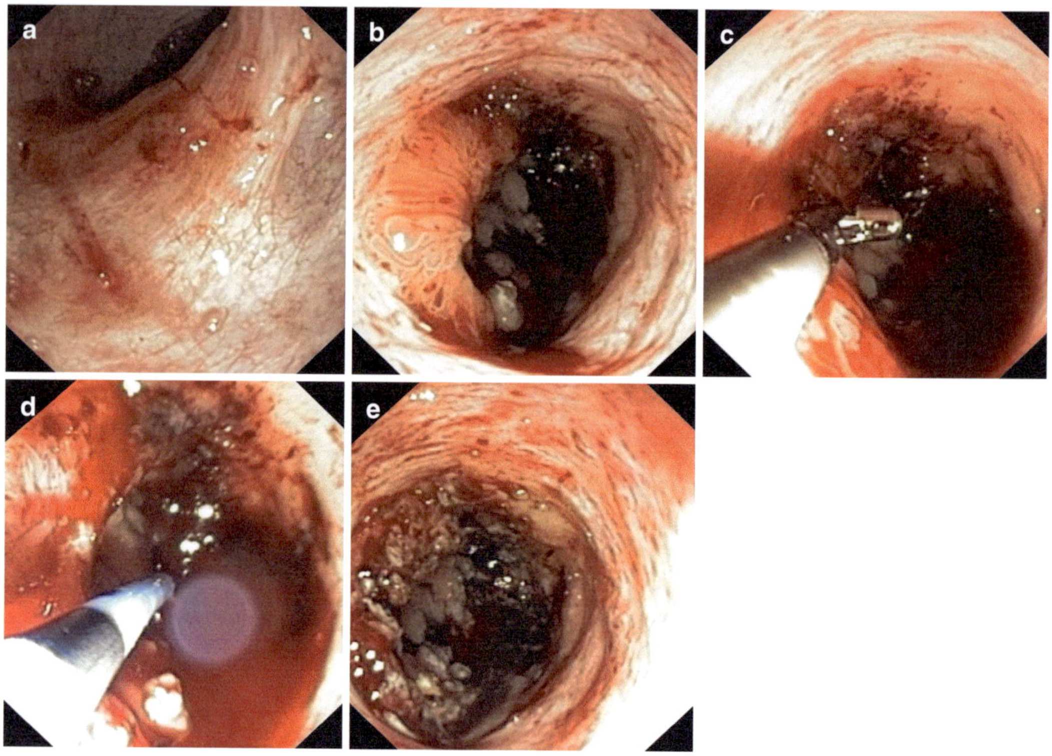

Fig. 21.3 Pancreatoscopy. (**a**) Hemosuccus pancreaticus in a 89-year-old female patient. Retrograde pancreatoscopy reveals normal pancreatic duct at the level of the pancreatic head. (**b**) Villous tissue proliferation with some bleeding from a central vessel is visualized. (**c**) A biopsy forceps is used to obtain histopathological analysis of the tissue. (**d**) Argon plasma coagulation of the bleeding site with successful termination of the bleeding from the pancreatic duct. (**e**) The bleeding was stopped and did not return with a follow-up of almost 2 years after the event

ERCP, a wide sphincterotomy is provided. Sometimes sphincteroplasty using papillary balloon dilatation is used exclusively or in addition to sphincterotomy. In some cases it can be helpful to place a stiff guidewire far into the biliary system during ERCP.

21.4.2 Cannulation and Manoeuvrability

Using mother/baby systems, cannulation is a standard procedure while performing ERCP. Using direct scopes can lead to challenges in papillary cannulation and impaired feed inside the ducts. One issue is the correct placement of antegrade optics regarding the papilla of Vater. Insufficient stiffness and looping of the endoscope in the stomach or duodenum can sometimes cause the attempted ductoscopy to technically fail. Using overtubes or balloons can reduce looping and increase rates of cannulation (compared to free cannulation technique) and effectiveness of intraductal manoeuvrability.

Using an anchor balloon, over the preliminary applied guidewire, the balloon catheter is inserted into an intrahepatic duct (or near a stricture) and inflated acting as an anchor, so that the cholangioscope can be more easily inserted. Drawback of the anchor balloon is the necessity to remove it through the working channel if an intervention is to be performed, therefore risking dislocation of the endoscope.

Using a balloon-assisted overtube—as in regular single- or double-balloon enteroscopy—prevents the formation of loops and can sometimes lead to a better positioning in front of the papilla.

21.4.3 Safety

Ductoscopy with diagnostic and therapeutic intention is generally safe. Risk of cholangitis is increased. Some severe adverse events happen during the preliminary ERCP where complications such as bleeding or perforation can occur. The required and usually larger sphincterotomy aggravates this risk. Bleeding and perforation due to ductoscopy itself are uncommon. Interventions like EHL can increase the risk.

As mentioned before, each ERCP has a risk of causing pancreatitis. A larger cholangioscope and a smaller sphincterotomy can increase risk for acute pancreatitis.

Risk rate of infection, especially cholangitis after cholangioscopy, differs greatly between the authors but is reported as up to 14%. Especially, patients with PSC are at an increased risk for acute or chronic infection due to the larger sphincterotomy. A peri-interventional antibiotic therapy is recommended.

As with other upper endoscopic investigations, there is a theoretical risk of aspiration pneumonia, especially when larger amounts of saline irrigation are used.

Air embolisms as a fatal complication have been reported for various endoscopic procedures (esophagogastroduodenoscopy, colonoscopy, ERCP, EUS, etc.) as well as in cholangioscopy. It was assumed that using CO_2 insufflation eliminates the risk of air embolisms [6]. CO_2 is significantly better soluble in blood than nitrogen and thereby better tolerated, yet clinically serious embolic outcomes have been described using CO_2 during direct peroral cholangioscopy [7]. One aspect seems to be the fact that especially some gastroscopes have a continuous baseline CO_2 insufflation that leads to higher applied volumes of gas. Some authors recommend using only saline solution at a possible cost of image quality.

21.4.4 Limitations

Retrograde cholangioscopy is subject to a few limitations, especially anatomic circumstances whether inherent (e.g. pancreas divisum, intramural diverticula, etc.) or acquired (post-surgery situs, juxtapapillary diverticula, etc.) hindering cannulation of the papilla.

Furthermore a minimal diameter of the bile ducts is required in order to manoeuvre the cholangioscope. High-grade stenosis can hinder passage to proximal regions.

Even more than in ERCP, at least one experienced investigator is needed (two in case of two-operator systems); therefore issues of time and cost limit the use of retrograde cholangioscopy further. Newer technologies however decrease that limitation a bit especially regarding optimization of single-operator systems.

21.5 Anterograde (Percutaneous) Cholangioscopy

Whenever retrograde access is hampered but cholangioscopy indicated, the percutaneous access route may be the optimal alternative. Using continuous cross-sectional imaging (e.g. ultrasound or CT), the intrahepatic bile ducts are located and punctured with a tiny hollow needle (Fig. 21.4). Contrast agent is injected as soon as a safe intraductal access is accomplished and cholangiography realized. For cholangioscopy, several sessions of PTC (percutaneous transhepatic cholangiography) are required to stepwise increase the diameter of the access. Conventional Seldinger technique is used to dilate the access tract and to insert the appropriate catheter. With accomplishing an outer diameter of about 16 or 18 Fr, a 5 mm endoscope can fit through the channel. Therefore, a sheath introducer with an adequate inner diameter of at least 5 mm is introduced into the hepatic parenchyma over the wire and the cholangioscope advanced through the sheath after removing the wire.

Anterograde cholangioscopy usually shows—due to the short route and direct access of the CBD—good manoeuvrability and feed. However, the inversion of the endoscope for arriving at bile ducts of other segments may be cumbersome or impossible. Combining

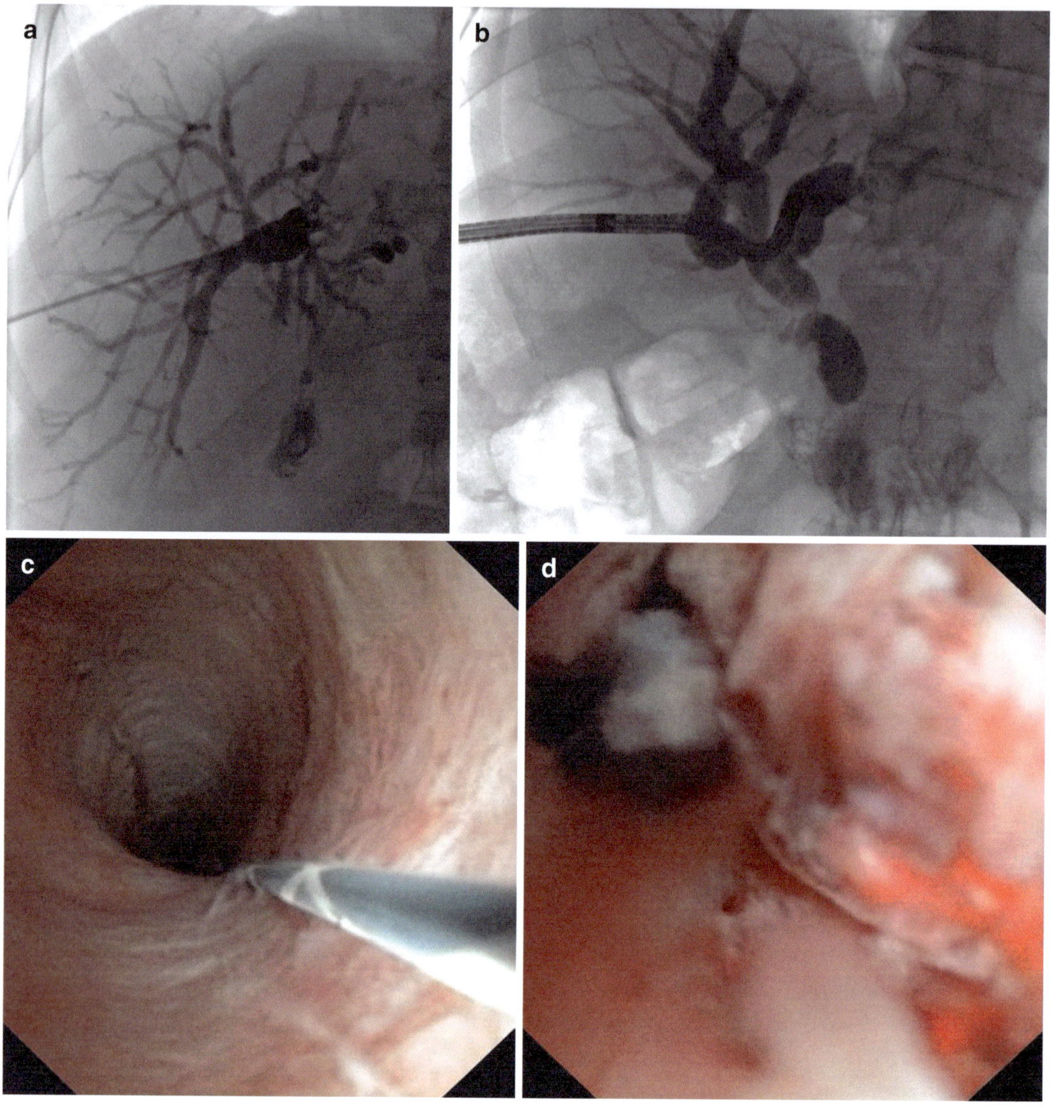

Fig. 21.4 (**a**) Percutaneous transhepatic cholangiography in a patient with a hilar tumour obstruction of the intrahepatic bile ducts. (**b**) Anterograde percutaneous cholangioscopy coming from the right liver. (**c**) Endoscopic image from a video cholangioscope for anterograde percutaneous cholangioscopy. Water submersion technique. (**d**) Tumour obstruction of the proximal CBD in the same patient

anterograde cholangioscopy with conventional peroral endoscopy can lead to rendezvous techniques to overcome difficult anatomic structures (e.g. positioning a guidewire anterograde through the papilla and internalizing a drainage).

Anterograde cholangioscopy can be performed without much discomfort. Local anaesthesia is sufficient; usually no systemic sedation is needed. Therefore very old, frail or moribund patients may benefit from a primary anterograde access rather than undergoing peroral endoscopy.

21.5.1 Limitations

Anterograde approaches are also limited: intrahepatic ducts have to be large enough for the scope to fit, ascites leads to high-risk puncture, and multifocal stenoses can prevent further advancement.

21.5.2 Safety of Anterograde Cholangioscopy

Due to route of access, possible risks of anterograde and retrograde cholangioscopy differ in regard to transhepatic puncture versus peroral endoscopy and sphincterotomy. Percutaneous transhepatic cholangiography itself is a low-risk procedure but with higher complication rates than conventional ERCP (possibly selection bias occurs). Possible risks of PTC include acute bleeding (haemobilia, possibly life -threatening in arteriobiliary fistulas, hemoperitoneum, hematoma), infections (abscess, peritonitis, cholangitis, sepsis), intestinal perforation or pneumothorax.

References

1. Rösch W, Koch H, Demling L. Peroral cholangioscopy. Endoscopy. 1976;8:172–5.
2. Farnik H, Weigt J, Malfertheiner P, Grützmann A, Gossner L, Friedrich-Rust M, Zeuzem S, Sarrazin C, Albert JG. A multicenter study on the role of direct retrograde cholangioscopy in patients with inconclusive endoscopic retrograde cholangiography. Endoscopy. 2014;46(1):16–21. https://doi.org/10.1055/s-0033-1359043.
3. Albert JG, Friedrich-Rust M, Elhendawy M, Trojan J, Zeuzem S, Sarrazin C. Peroral cholangioscopy for diagnosis and therapy of biliary tract disease using an ultra-slim gastroscope. Endoscopy. 2011;43:1004–9.
4. Beyna T, Farnik H, Sarrazin C, Gerges C, Neuhaus H, Albert JG. Direct retrograde cholangioscopy with a new prototype double-bending cholangioscope. Endoscopy. 2016;48(10):929–33. https://doi.org/10.1055/s-0042-110,395. Epub 2016 Jul 19.
5. Sethi A, Tyberg A, Slivka A, Adler DG, Desai AP, Sejpal DV, Pleskow DK, Bertani H, Gan S-I, Shah R, Arnelo U, Tarnasky PR, Banerjee S, Itoi T, Moon JH, Kim DC, Gaidhane M, Raijman I, Peterson BT, Gress FG, Kahaleh M. Digital single-operator cholangioscopy (DSOC) improves interobserver agreement (IOA) and accuracy for evaluation of indeterminate biliary strictures. J Clin. Gastroenterol. 1.
6. Lo SK, Fujii-Lau LL, Enestvedt BK, Hwang JH, Konda V, Manfredi MA, Maple JT, Murad FM, Pannala R, Woods KL, Banerjee S. The use of carbon dioxide in gastrointestinal endoscopy. Gastrointest Endosc. 2016;83(5):857–65.
7. Donepudi S, Chavalitdhamrong D, Pu L, Draganov PV. Air embolism complicating gastrointestinal endoscopy: a systematic review. World J Gastrointest Endosc. 2013;5(8):359–65.

Intraductal Ablation Techniques

22

Brian C. Brauer

22.1 Introduction

Biliary and pancreatic malignancies often present with biliary obstruction. While surgical resection affords the only opportunity for cure, a majority presents with advanced unresectable disease [1, 2]. Chemotherapy and/or chemoradiation has been the mainstay of therapy for most of these tumors. In recent years, intraductal ablation techniques have been introduced. These techniques provide adjunctive therapy to standard of care, may have a role in select patients who are not surgically resectable, and may provide some benefit in select patients. Radiofrequency ablation (RFA), photodynamic therapy (PDT), and argon plasma coagulation (APC) will be described in more detail in this chapter.

Electronic Supplementary Material The online version of this chapter (https://doi.org/10.1007/978-3-030-42569-2_22) contains supplementary material, which is available to authorized users.

B. C. Brauer (✉)
Division of Gastroenterology and Hepatology, University of Colorado Anschutz Medical Campus, Aurora, CO, USA
e-mail: Brian.brauer@ucdenver.edu

22.2 Radiofrequency Ablation

While radiofrequency ablation sounds like a highly technical term, it is actually used daily in the endoscopy practice. Standard electrosurgery generators used in the endoscopy practice and in surgery are considered radiofrequency ablation, which refers to the use of alternating current at high frequencies, usually greater than 100 kHz. The application of radiofrequency ablation for malignant tumors has been used for over 20 years via the surgical and percutaneous routes, primarily for liver malignancies. Heat generated by the high frequency of alternating current results in coagulative necrosis of tissue around the probe [3].

In recent years, a RFA probe has been developed for over-the-wire intraductal ablation during ERCP (Habib™ EndoHPB, EMcision/Boston Scientific, Marlborough, MA). The catheter is an 8 Fr catheter 180 cm long with two electrodes at the tip measuring 8 mm each in length and will accommodate a guidewire up to 0.035″ in diameter (Fig. 22.1a, b). The catheter requires a proprietary cable to connect to an electrosurgical unit but utilizes existing electrosurgical units. Recommended settings are a bipolar power of 7–10 W for a maximum duration of 90 s. Many electrosurgical generators can be programmed to automatically deliver 7–10 W for the duration of 90 s (Fig. 22.2). The manufacturer should be contacted for program

M. Mutignani et al. (eds.), *Endotherapy in Biliopancreatic Diseases: ERCP Meets EUS*,
https://doi.org/10.1007/978-3-030-42569-2_22

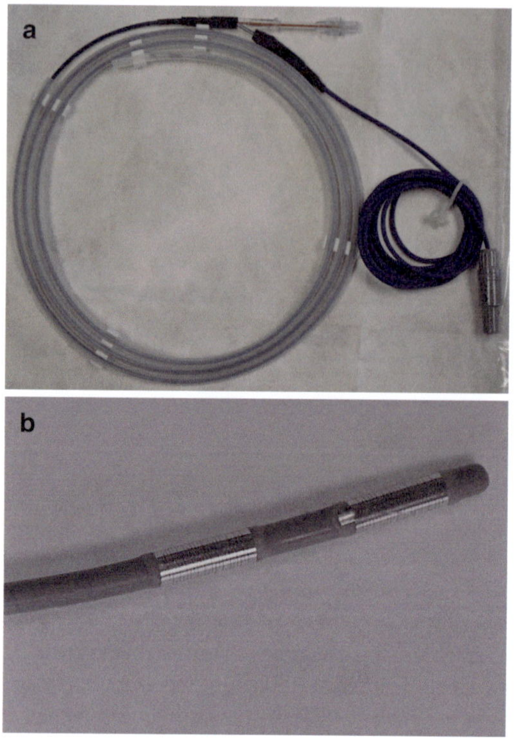

Fig. 22.1 (**a**) Habib biliary catheter as supplied in dispensing coil. (**b**) Close-up of tip showing two radiopaque bands

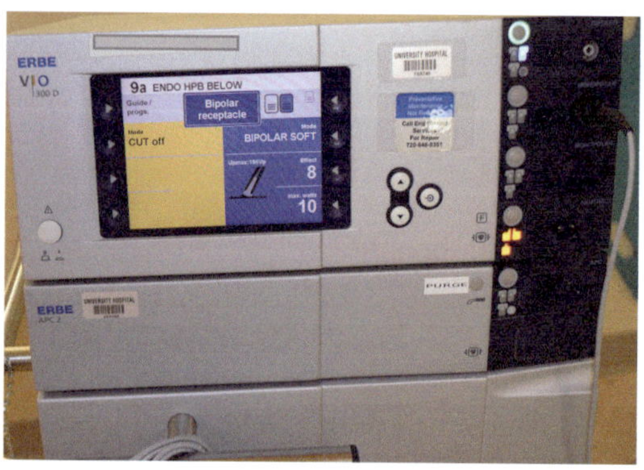

Fig. 22.2 Preprogrammed settings on an Erbe VIO 300D electrosurgical generator (Erbe USA, Marietta, GA, USA)

settings for specific electrosurgical units and to ensure the correct adapter cable is utilized. A power setting of 7–8 W is recommended for intrahepatic strictures upstream of the bifurcation, while a power of 10 W is recommended for strictures within the extrahepatic duct downstream of the bifurcation. Technique varies among experts, and many treat all areas at 10 W. RFA is indicated for treatment of biliary and pancreatic tumors prior to stent insertion and to clear occluded metal stents.

A second manufacturer, STARmed, Gyeonggi-do, South Korea, has the ELRA™ probe available in Europe and Asia, with anticipated availability in the USA soon. It is a 7 Fr by 175 cm long catheter, with available electrode exposure lengths of 11, 18, 22, and 33 mm. Unlike the Habib, it requires the use of a proprietary generator.

The technique for RFA use is quite straightforward. The technique described applies to the Habib catheter as it is the only catheter available in the USA at the time of submission. Standard ERCP biliary access is obtained and a 0.035″ guidewire is advanced across the stricture. A working channel at least 3.2 mm in diameter is required for passage of the catheter. A nonconductive hydrophilic tip wire is recommended. Smaller diameter wires may be used, but a 0.035″ wire is optimal given the stiffness of the catheter. Dilation is not recommended, but small diameter dilation can be performed if the stricture is too tight to allow easy catheter passage. A good test is passage of an extraction balloon catheter: if the extraction balloon passes easily, then passage of the 8 Fr RFA catheter should be successful. A biliary sphincterotomy is not absolutely required but will ease passage of the 8 Fr catheter across the papilla and minimize trauma to the pancreatic orifice.

The generator should be prepared and an appropriate adaptor cable should be connected. The RFA catheter is then removed from the package and the dispensing coil is removed. The catheter is then passed over the guidewire and placed fluoroscopically into proper position. If treating more than one area, the upstream portion is treated first, proceeding sequentially along the length of the stricture . The catheter is placed with the target area to be treated between the two electrodes (Fig. 22.3, Video 22.1). The catheter is then connected to the adapter cable, and bipolar current is applied at a maximum of 10 W for a

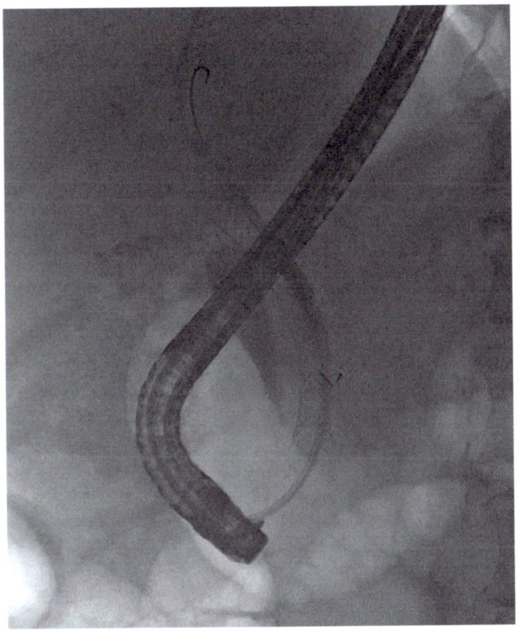

Fig. 22.3 RFA catheter within occluded stent

maximum duration of 90 s for extrahepatic strictures and 7–8 W for intrahepatic strictures. The catheter should remain in this location for 1 min after treatment to allow cooling and can then be withdrawn. If more than one area is to be treated, the catheter is withdrawn by 2 cm along the length of the stricture, and subsequent treatments are applied in the exact same manner.

Following treatment, the duct should be swept with a balloon catheter to remove any debris. Stenting should be performed if a stent is not already in place. For strictures within a metallic stent, placement of additional stent(s) is performed at the discretion of the endoscopist; one author suggests placement of a stent within the metallic stent if less than 80% of tumor burden is eradicated [4–6] based on cholangiography following ablation and balloon sweep.

RFA is well tolerated overall. Common side effects include abdominal pain, mild bleeding, and pancreatitis [4, 5]. Improved stent patency has been shown in some studies, and one small study showed improved survival in pancreatic cancer patients [7]. Therapy may be repeated, especially for clearing occluded metal stents. No specific guidelines or recommendations exist.

22.3 Photodynamic Therapy

Photodynamic therapy is a more technically and logistically complex procedure involving intravenous injection of a photosensitizer followed by endoscopic laser application. The photosensitizer is retained by malignant cells. Laser activation results in release of toxic oxygen radicals which result in apoptosis and tumor necrosis. The only FDA-approved photosensitizer is porfimer sodium (Photofrin®, Pinnacle Biologics, Bannockburn IL). In Europe, temoporfin or *meta*-tetrahydroxyphenylchlorin (Foscan®) is the primary photosensitizer. Porfimer sodium is not FDA approved for the use in cholangiocarcinoma or other pancreaticobiliary malignancies, so PDT of the bile duct is an off-label use. The photosensitizer is injected 48 h prior to laser therapy.

The target lesion is treated with red laser light that is then delivered at 630 nm with a dose of 180–200 J/cm^2, fluence of 0.250 W/cm^2 for 450–750 s [8]. The most commonly used laser in the USA is the Diomed diode laser (Diomed, Andover, MA) paired with a 3.0-m-length fiber with a 2.5 cm diffuser (Pioneer Optics, Windsor Locks, CT) which also has fluoroscopically visible marker. Other lengths of catheters are also available and vary depending on location and manufacturer. PDT is usually delivered via cholangioscopy but may be delivered through catheter without the use of cholangioscopy.

Porfimer sodium is administered 2 mg/kg IV 48 h prior to planned PDT. To perform PDT, the affected segments are accessed via ERCP and dilated adequately to traverse with a 10 Fr cholangioscope. The target lesion is then accessed with a cholangioscope or fluoroscopically (Fig. 22.4a). The guidewire is exchanged for the cholangioscope, and the margins of the tumor are documented. If more than one diffuser length is available, the size that most closely corresponds with the length of the lesion should be chosen. Once the target area to be treated is determined, the guidewire is withdrawn and the diffuser fiber placed through the cholangioscope channel and positioned within the target lesion. Laser energy is then applied at 180–200 J/cm^2 at a fluence of

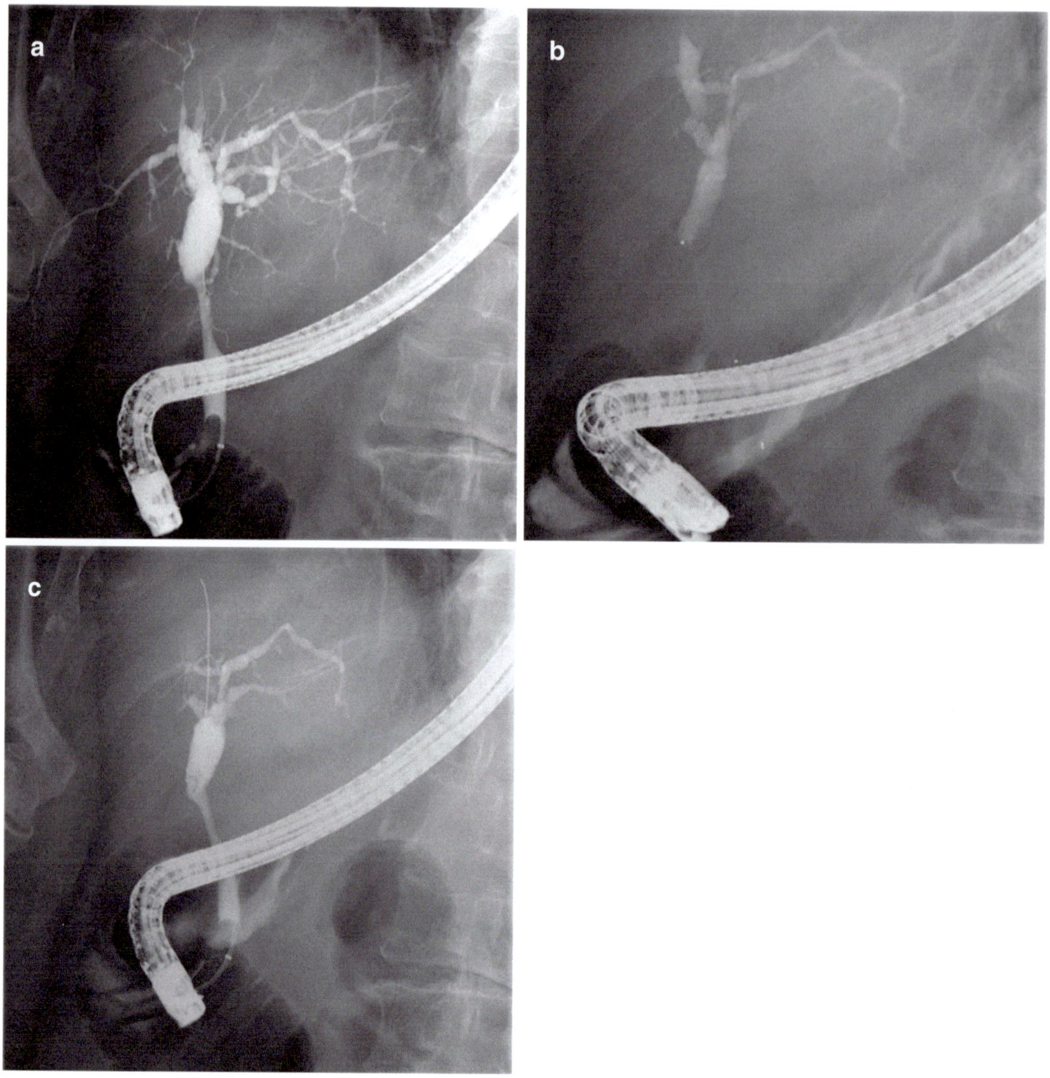

Fig. 22.4 (**a**) Malignant-appearing stricture of common bile duct. (**b**) Radiopaque markers of PDT diffuser fiber at the level of the stricture using fluoroscopic guidance. (**c**) Cholangiogram posttreatment

0.025 W/cm^2 for 450–750 s. It is recommended that no more than three segments be treated in one session [5]. Stenting is required following PDT as there is a high risk of cholangitis due to edema created by the therapy. Prophylactic antibiotics should be administered for 5–7 days following treatment of hilar strictures.

Application of PDT can also be performed without the use of cholangioscopy. Its application requires defining the target lesion with fluoroscopy. An ERCP cannula is then used to deliver the diffuser fiber. Multiple catheters can be used, but steerable tip cannulas work well to direct the fiber into the target lesion. Fluoroscopic markers allow for placement of the diffuser within the target lesion (Fig. 22.4b, c).

The main side effect of PDT is phototoxicity. Strict avoidance of sun exposure is required for 4–6 weeks following PDT. Photosensitive reactions can occur in noncompliant patients. Although a detailed review of outcomes of ablative therapies is beyond the scope of this chapter, studies have demonstrated an increase in median survival and quality of life [5].

22.4 Argon Plasma Coagulation (APC)

Argon plasma coagulation (APC) involves the passage of high-frequency alternating current through an argon gas medium. While argon is usually inert, at higher energies, the gas will ionize and conduct electricity. The ionized argon creates a plasma which can transit current without direct contact to the tissue. APC is not FDA approved for the use in the bile duct. Its use therefore is off-label.

Several electrosurgical unit manufacturers make APC systems. The settings vary between manufacturers, and as APC is not approved in the bile duct, no standardized settings exist. APC should be reserved for inoperable biliary tumors with poor alternatives to APC available.

We reported the use of APC in a refractory intraductal papillary biliary neoplasm, in which the patient kept having bouts of cholangitis due to intense mucin production. Even with stents in place, the stents would occlude and result in cholangitis. It was decided to perform APC to curb the recurrent bouts of cholangitis. Using a standard diagnostic gastroscope, the markedly dilated bile duct was directly intubated. Irrigation with 1% *N*-acetylcysteine was performed. Argon plasma coagulation was then performed at 15–25 W. The patient underwent two ablation sessions which was well tolerated but expired from complications of underlying cirrhosis 1 month later [9]. Other reports of APC using an ultraslim gastroscope for ablation of biliary tumors have been reported [10].

Most APC catheters are on the order of 7 Fr in diameter, and therefore require a 2.8 mm working channel. A standard diagnostic gastroscope or larger is required to accommodate the catheter. A small diameter probe is available measuring 4.5 Fr that can be accommodated in a pediatric diameter endoscope with a working channel of 2.2 mm (APC™ probe, OD 1.5 mm, Erbe USA, Marietta, GA). APC cannot be performed through mother-daughter cholangioscopy systems or catheter-based systems due to the small working channel of 1.0–1.2 mm. Any configuration catheter can be used, but a circumferential fire probe works well in this setting as it will transmit current to the area closest to the probe, obviating the need for precise catheter orientation (Fig. 22.5).

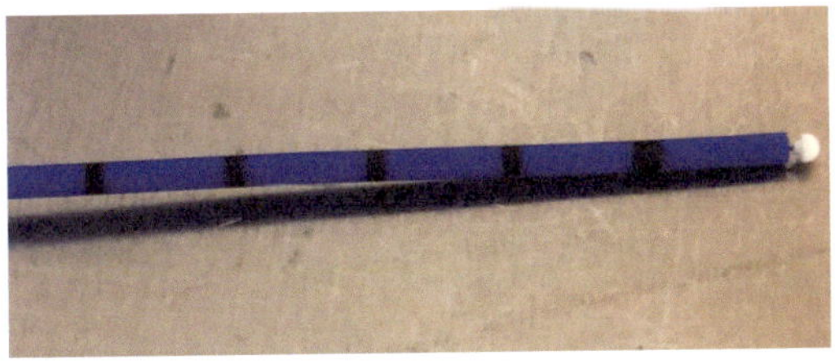

Fig. 22.5 Circumferential fire APC catheter

When performing direct cholangioscopy with a gastroscope, it is imperative to use saline or carbon dioxide insufflation, as reports of air embolism have been reported during ERCP [11]. Insufflation directly within the duct increases the chance of translocation of air into the vascular bed. A biliary sphincterotomy is required for passage of these larger diameter scopes, unless the papilla is patulous such as in the setting of intraductal papillary mucinous neoplasm.

Prophylactic antibiotics should be administered prior to direct cholangioscopy, and we recommend oral antibiotics for 5–7 days post-procedure.

22.5 Summary

Intraductal ablation technologies offer a palliative alternative or adjunct therapy in patients with unresectable biliary neoplasms and malignant biliary strictures. RFA is FDA approved; PDT and APC are not FDA approved. PDT, despite not being FDA approved, has data to support its endoscopic use dating back to the early 2000s. APC has much more limited data and should be reserved for select cases where RFA or PDT are not available or contraindicated. When using any technology off-label, it is important to disclose to the patient that it is an off-label use and to thoroughly discuss risks, benefits, and alternatives.

All ablative technologies are considered adjunct therapies to standard of care and are not a substitute for conventional therapies such as surgical resection, chemotherapy, and radiation therapy. A careful discussion with other providers and a multidisciplinary approach are key to providing the best care for the patient and allowing the best outcomes with ablative technologies. Oncology clinical trials have very strict inclusion and exclusion criteria, and ensuring adjunctive therapies do not interfere with other treatment plans is vital. Likewise, it is important to have the support of surgeons in borderline resectable patients who may become surgical candidates after appropriate response to therapy.

Although intraductal ablation options are limited at this time, it is likely that improved technologies will be available in the future.

References

1. Vincent A, Herman J, Schulick R, Hruban RH, Groggoins M. Pancreatic cancer. Lancet. 2011;378:607–20.
2. Ramirez-Merino N, Aix SO, Cortez-Funes H. Chemotherapy for cholangiocarcinoma: an update. World J Gastrointest Oncol. 2013;5:171–6.
3. Khan AS, Fowler CJ, Chapman WC. Current surgical treatment strategies for hepatocellular carcinoma in North America. World J Gastroenterol. 2014;20:15007–17.
4. Kadayifci A, Atar M, Forcione DG, et al. Radiofrequency ablation for the management of occluded biliary metal stents. Endoscopy. 2016;48:1096–101.
5. Patel J, Rizk N, Kahaleh M. Role of photodynamic therapy and intraductal radiofrequency ablation in cholangiocarcinoma. Best Pract Res Clin Gastroenterol. 2015;29:309–18.
6. Lais H, Sengoz C, Gonenc M. Endobiliary radiofrequency ablation for malignant biliary obstruction. Hepatobiliary Pancreat Dis Int. 2013;12:423–7.
7. Kallis Y, Phillips N, Steel A, et al. Analysis of endoscopic radiofrequency ablation of biliary malignant strictures in pancreatic cancer suggests potential survival benefit. Dig Dis Sci. 2015;60:3449–55.
8. Talreja JP, DeGaetani M, Ellen K, et al. Photodynamic therapy in unresectable cholangiocarcinoma: not for the uncommitted. Clin Endosc. 2013;46:390–4.
9. Brauer BC, Fukami N, Chen YK. Direct cholangioscopy with narrow-band imaging, chromoendoscopy, and argon-plasma coagulation of intraductal papillary mucinous neoplasm of the bile duct. Gastrointest Endosc. 2008;67:574–6.
10. Larghi A, Waxman I. Endoscopic direct cholangioscopy by using an ultra-slim upper endoscope: a feasibility study. Gastrointest Endosc. 2006;63:853–7.
11. Finsterer J, Stöllberger C, Bastovansky A. Cardiac and cerebral air embolism from endoscopic retrograde cholangio-pancreatography. Eur J Gastroenterol Hepatol. 2010;22:1157–62.

Stent Removal (Plastic and Metal) 23

Feng Li, Prabhleen Chahal,
and Manuel Perez-Miranda

23.1 Indications for Removal

Removal of biliary stents becomes necessary with resolution of benign disease or stent malfunction. Benign indications such as choledocholithiasis or bile leaks may require stent placement, but stents should be removed at the end of therapy or resolution of disease. Conditions leading to stent malfunction can include intimal hyperplasia, stenosis of proximal portion, tumor ingrowth, sludge, migration, and malposition. Malfunction of biliary stents leads to complications such as recurrent obstruction, cholangitis requiring removal, or replacement for decompression of the bile duct.

In a prospective study of plastic biliary stents (PBS) in distal biliary malignant obstruction, PBS patency averaged 68 days (range 32–175 days) [1]. Another study comparing patency rates of two types of PBS in malignant obstruction demonstrated a median patency of 133 (95% CI 92, 174) to 181 (95% CI 59, 303) days [2]. On average 70% of PBS will be occluded by 6 months [1, 2].

A large meta-analysis of patients with malignant biliary obstruction demonstrated that compared to PBS, self-expandable metal stents (SEMS) had lower occlusion rate, less therapeutic failure, less need for reintervention, and lower cholangitis incidence [3]. A systematic review article evaluating stent placement for benign extrahepatic biliary strictures demonstrated mean patency duration of covered SEMS ranging from 20 to 35 months (range 7–57 months) [4].

In general, uncovered SEMS should only be placed in patients with malignancy where retrieval is not anticipated given the difficulty in removal.

F. Li · P. Chahal
Cleveland Clinic, Ohio State University,
Columbus, OH, USA

M. Perez-Miranda (✉)
Hospital Universitario Rio Hortega, Valladolid, Spain

23.2 Removal Techniques of Biliary Stents

Removal of PBS and covered SEMS is usually uncomplicated. Rates of successful removal of PBS and covered SEMS range from 95 to 100% [5, 6]. On the other hand, uncovered SEMS are much more difficult to remove compared to covered SEMS.

Certain factors can make removal of stents more difficult. Proximal migration of a PBS can make stent retrieval more challenging. For example, migration upstream above a stenosis, migration into a deep biliary branch, and impaction of the stent into the bile duct wall may complicate removal. Despite these challenges, success rates of endoscopic removal of proximally migrated PBS still exceed 70% [6].

M. Mutignani et al. (eds.), *Endotherapy in Biliopancreatic Diseases: ERCP Meets EUS*,
https://doi.org/10.1007/978-3-030-42569-2_23

Factors contributing to difficult removal of SEMS include:

- Stent type: Uncovered SEMS are much more difficult to remove compared to covered SEMS and in certain cases may be unable to be removed endoscopically. Surgical removal may be necessary in these cases to avoid further complications such as bowel/ductal perforation or enteric fistulas [7].
- Duration of placement: In a case series of 19 patients undergoing SEMS removal, a longer duration of stent placement was associated with failure of stent removal [5].
- Tissue ingrowth: Tumors or tissue may grow into the lumen of uncovered stents, leading to obstruction of the stent but also leading to the stent becoming embedded. This is typically seen in uncovered SEMS and not covered SEMS, although in partially covered SEMS, tissue ingrowth may also be seen in the uncovered portions. Tissue ingrowth embeds the stent and this may preclude removal of the stent.

Standard method for stent removal: The standard method of removal of PBS and covered SEMS involves advancing a side-viewing duodenoscope to the second portion of the duodenum. The distal end of the stent is grasped with a polypectomy snare or foreign body forceps (such as a raptor grasper or rat-tooth forceps). After the stent is grasped, it can be removed by pulling through the working channel of the duodenoscope, or the duodenoscope itself can be pulled out of the patient to remove the stent.

23.3 Removal of Proximally Migrated Stents

In the event of proximal migration, removal of biliary stents can be more complicated, requiring other techniques:

- The indirect grasping technique has been described for removal of proximally migrated stents. A grasping device, such as a forceps, is advanced through the papilla into the bile duct and is used to grasp the distal end of the stent (typically under fluoroscopic guidance), allowing the stent to be pulled distally into the duodenum.
- The lasso technique involves cannulation of the bile duct with a wire either within the stent lumen [8] or alongside the stent [9]. A polypectomy snare is then advanced over the wire into the duct to grasp the stent, which is then pulled out over the wire. This advantage of this technique is that it preserves access to the bile duct after removal of the stent although care should be taken to maintain wire access to the duct when the stent is being pulled.
- The Soehendra stent retriever is a metal wire-guided spiral device. It is advanced over the wire and screwed into the distal end of the biliary stent. Once attached to the stent, it can be pulled out over the wire [10]. Various sizes of retrieval devices are used for stents ranging in size from 5 Fr, 7 Fr, 8.5 Fr, 10 Fr, to 11.5 Fr [11].
- Fogarty balloons or dilation balloons have been used for extraction of both PBS and covered SEMS. For removal of PBS 10 Fr or higher in diameter, a 4 mm dilating balloon can be inserted into the stent over the guidewire, inflated, and then pulled out of the duct with the stent, leaving the wire in place [12]. The balloon may also be advanced over a wire that is alongside the PBS and a similar technique used to drag the stent out. For removal of covered SEMS, a similar technique can be applied.
- Stent in stent technique: Tumor ingrowth can preclude removal of an uncovered metal stent. Adapting a technique for removal of embedded esophageal stents [13], a covered metal biliary stent can be placed within an uncovered metal biliary stent that needs to be removed. The covered metal stent induces pressure necrosis of the ingrown tissue, allowing both stents to be removed. In prior case reports, the covered stent was left in place for 2–4 weeks prior to attempting removal of both stents [14, 15].

Distal migration of a SEMS can lead to impaction on the contralateral duodenal wall. This can cause complications including stent obstruction (leading to jaundice and cholangitis), bleeding, or even duodenal perforation. APC may be used to cut the stent, allowing the remaining portion to be more easily removed from the bile duct. Ideal settings for APC for this indication are not standardized but a voltage of 60–80 W and flow of 1.5 L/min has been reported in the literature [5]. In a case series of eight patients undergoing stent trimming by APC, all were successful, and no complications other than one case of self-limited bleeding requiring transfusion was reported [5].

Endoscopic removal of uncovered SEMS is challenging. Standard methods, such as with a snare or rat-tooth forceps, may be unsuccessful [16]. Techniques to remove uncovered SEMS have been described in case reports. In some cases, uncovered SEMS were removed piecemeal using a hot biopsy forceps [16] or an endoscopic suture cutting device [17] to break apart individual wires of the stent which are then able to be removed piecemeal. In cases where the uncovered stent had migrated distally and impacted on the duodenal wall, APC was used to cut stent shorter, and a snare was able to be used to extract the remaining portion of the stent [16].

23.4 Complications from Stent Removal

Complications from stent removal are rare but can include bleeding [16], pancreatitis [18], and abdominal pain [19].

23.5 Indications for Removal of Pancreatic Stents

Pancreatic stents are typically placed in the management of benign diseases such as strictures or stones in the setting of chronic pancreatitis and therefore need to be removed following completion of therapy. Because pancreatic stents are smaller in caliber compared to biliary stents, they should be removed or replaced sooner. Indications for removal include stent occlusion or migration.

Almost all pancreatic stents placed for chronic pancreatitis will be occluded by 3 months [20]. Stent migration may also occur, both proximally and distally, necessitating removal if proximally migrated. Stents placed for prophylaxis of post-ERCP pancreatitis only have a single external flange and are designed to migrate out of the pancreatic duct spontaneously, which occurs in approximately 88% of patients by 30 days [21]. It is recommended to check an abdominal X-ray to confirm migration out of the pancreatic duct 7–10 days after placement and endoscopic removal if still not migrated by 14 days [21].

Covered SEMS may also be placed into the pancreatic duct and are recommended to be replaced at 2–3 month intervals. A prospective study evaluating fully covered SEMS for chronic pancreatitis-associated pancreatic duct strictures in 32 patients demonstrated no stent-induced pancreatitis or migration, and follow-up ERCP at 3 months demonstrated resolution of stricture on pancreatogram [22].

23.6 Removal Techniques of Pancreatic Stents

The standard removal techniques with snare or foreign body forceps that are used for removal of biliary stents can also be applied to removal of pancreatic stents.

23.7 Removal of Migrated Pancreatic Stents

Proximal migration of a stent into the pancreatic duct can be very challenging to manage, sometimes requiring surgery for removal. Successful endoscopic removal of proximally migrated pancreatic stents is approximately 78% in case series [23]. In the majority of reports, stent removal was successful with either a basket to capture the stent or a balloon inflated proximally and dragging the stent outward. The lasso technique (described above), in which a snare is advanced up a wire that is placed through or alongside the stent, may also be adapted to this situation. While these techniques are similar to those used in the removal of biliary stents, more care needs to be taken with removal of pancreatic stents due to the smaller caliber of the pancreatic duct.

With newly mother-daughter scope systems such as the SpyGlass system (Boston Scientific), direct visualization of the bile duct or pancreatic can be achieved. Once the stent is visualized, a SpyForceps (Boston Scientific) can be used to grasp the stent and remove it [24]. Alternatively, the SpyGlass can be used to allow for wire cannulation of the migrated stent and then this can allow for removal of the stent using other tools such as the Soehendra stent retriever [25]. Once wire access is achieved, other techniques such as the lasso technique described above may also be used.

23.8 Complications of Pancreatic Stent Removal

Complications from endoscopic removal of pancreatic duct stents are rare including pancreatic duct disruption, stent fragmentation, and pancreatitis [23]. These may occur in up to 4% of patients in a case series of 33 patients. Another series describing removal of retained pancreatic duct stents showed a post-ERCP pancreatitis rate of approximately 3% [26].

23.9 Conclusion

While removal of biliary and pancreatic duct stents is typically uncomplicated, certain situations (such as proximal migration) may necessitate nonstandard techniques for success. It is important for the endoscopist to be familiar with the indications, techniques, and risks of stent removal.

References

1. Costamagna G, Mutignani M, Rotondano G, Cipolletta L, Ghezzo L, Foco A, et al. Hydrophilic hydromer-coated polyurethane stents versus uncoated stents in malignant biliary obstruction: a randomized trial. Gastrointest Endosc. 2000;51(1):8–11.
2. England RE, Martin DF, Morris J, Sheridan MB, Frost R, Freeman A, et al. A prospective randomised multicentre trial comparing 10 Fr Teflon Tannenbaum stents with 10 Fr polyethylene Cotton-Leung stents in patients with malignant common duct strictures. Gut. 2000;46(3):395–400.
3. Sawas T, Al Halabi S, Parsi MA, Vargo JJ. Self-expandable metal stents versus plastic stents for malignant biliary obstruction: a meta-analysis. Gastrointest Endosc. 2015;82(2):256–67.e7.
4. van Boeckel PG, Vleggaar FP, Siersema PD. Plastic or metal stents for benign extrahepatic biliary strictures: a systematic review. BMC Gastroenterol. 2009;9:96.
5. Ishii K, Itoi T, Sofuni A, Itokawa F, Tsuchiya T, Kurihara T, et al. Endoscopic removal and trimming of distal self-expandable metallic biliary stents. World J Gastroenterol. 2011;17(21):2652–7.
6. Katsinelos P, Kountouras J, Paroutoglou G, Chatzimavroudis G, Paikos D, Zavos C, et al. Migration of plastic biliary stents and endoscopic retrieval: an experience of three referral centers. Surg Laparosc Endosc Percutan Tech. 2009;19(3):217–21.
7. Diller R, Senninger N, Kautz G, Tubergen D. Stent migration necessitating surgical intervention. Surg Endosc. 2003;17(11):1803–7.
8. Sherman S, Hawes RH, Uzer MF, Smith MT, Lehman GA. Endoscopic stent exchange using a guide wire and mini-snare. Gastrointest Endosc. 1993;39(6): 794–9.
9. Vila JJ, Marcos K, Manuel PM. Retrieval of proximally migrated pancreatic stents. Video J Encycl GI Endosc. 2013;1(2):584–7.
10. Soehendra N, Maydeo A, Eckmann B, Brückner M, Ch Nam V, Grimm H. A new technique for replacing an obstructed biliary endoprosthesis. Endoscopy. 1990;22(06):271–2.
11. Soehendra Stent Retriever Cook Medical; 2019. https://www.cookmedical.com/products/esc_ssr_webds/.
12. Martin DF. Wire guided balloon assisted endoscopic biliary stent exchange. Gut. 1991;32(12):1562.
13. Hirdes MMC, Siersema PD, Houben MHMG, Weusten BLAM, Vleggaar FP. Stent-in-stent technique for removal of embedded esophageal self-expanding metal stents. Am J Gastroenterol. 2010;106:286.
14. Arias Dachary FJ, Chioccioli C, Deprez PH. Application of the "covered-stent-in-uncovered-stent" technique for easy and safe removal of embedded biliary uncovered SEMS with tissue ingrowth. Endoscopy. 2010;42(S 02):E304–E5.
15. Tan DM, Lillemoe KD, Fogel EL. A new technique for endoscopic removal of uncovered biliary self-expandable metal stents: stent-in-stent technique with a fully covered biliary stent. Gastrointest Endosc. 2012;75(4):923–5.
16. Kahaleh M, Tokar J, Le T, Yeaton P. Removal of self-expandable metallic wall stents. Gastrointest Endosc. 2004;60(4):640–4.
17. Levy MJ, Wiersema MJ. Endoscopic removal of a biliary wallstent with a suture-cutting device in a patient

with primary pancreatic lymphoma. Endoscopy. 2002;34(10):835–7.

18. Sakai Y, Tsuyuguchi T, Ishihara T, Sugiyama H, Eto R, Fujimoto T, et al. Cholangiopancreatography troubleshooting: the usefulness of endoscopic retrieval of migrated biliary and pancreatic stents. Hepatobiliary Pancreat Dis Int. 2009;8(6):632–7.
19. Mahajan A, Ho H, Sauer B, Phillips MS, Shami VM, Ellen K, et al. Temporary placement of fully covered self-expandable metal stents in benign biliary strictures: midterm evaluation (with video). Gastrointest Endosc. 2009;70(2):303–9.
20. Buscaglia JM, DiMaio CJ, Pollack MJ, Shin EJ, Harris MD, Richards R, et al. Are large side holes associated with reduced rates of pancreatic stent occlusion? Results of a prospective study. JOP. 2009;10:496–500.
21. Lawrence C, Cotton PB, Romagnuolo J, Payne KM, Rawls E, Hawes RH. Small prophylactic pancreatic duct stents: an assessment of spontaneous passage and stent-induced ductal abnormalities. Endoscopy. 2007;39(12):1082–5.
22. Moon S-H, Kim M-H, Park DH, Song TJ, Eum J, Lee SS, et al. Modified fully covered self-expandable metal stents with antimigration features for benign pancreatic-duct strictures in advanced chronic pancreatitis, with a focus on the safety profile and reducing migration. Gastrointest Endosc. 2010;72(1):86–91.
23. Price LH, Brandabur JJ, Kozarek RA, Gluck M, Traverso WL, Irani S. Good stents gone bad: endoscopic treatment of proximally migrated pancreatic duct stents. Gastrointest Endosc. 2009;70(1):174–9.
24. Rahimi A, Ejtehadi F. SpyGlass pancreatoscopy and successful retrieval of a proximally migrated pancreatic stent; unusual case and technical tips. Middle East J Dig Dis. 2016;8(3):232–4.
25. Maydeo A, Bhandari S, Bapat M, Mathew P, Kwek A. Sp848 Spyglass pancreatoscopy-guided cannulation and retrieval of a deeply migrated pancreatic duct stent. Gastrointest Endosc. 2011;73(4):AB107.
26. Moffatt DC, Cote GA, Fogel EL, Watkins JL, McHenry L, Lehman GA, et al. Acute pancreatitis after removal of retained prophylactic pancreatic stents. Gastrointest Endosc. 2011;73(5):980–6.

24 ERCP in Altered Anatomy

Stefanos M. Dokas

24.1 Surgical Reconstruction

Postoperative anatomy, in biliopancreatic access terms, can be divided in to three major groups. The first group comprises postoperative anatomy featuring an intact papilla for both biliary and pancreatic orifices (Table 24.1), the second group involves postoperative reconstructions with biliojejunal and pancreaticojejunal anastomoses and includes all forms of pancreatoduodenectomy (Table 24.2), and the third group is a mixed group where an intact, native papilla for pancreatic access coexists with biliojejunal anastomosis (Table 24.3).

Table 24.1 Postoperative reconstruction with native papilla for both ducts

Esophagectomy with gastric pull-up
Sleeve gastrectomy
Billroth I and Billroth II reconstruction
Roux-en-Y gastrojejunostomy and esophagojejunostomy
Roux-en-Y gastric bypass (RYGB) for obesity
Biliopancreatic diversion

S. M. Dokas (✉)
Endoscopy Department, St. Luke's Private Hospital, Thessaloniki, Greece
e-mail: altair@med.auth.gr

Table 24.2 Postoperative reconstruction with biliojejunal/pancreaticojejunal anastomosis

Pancreaticoduodenectomy (Whipple's procedure), both classic and pylorus preserving
Choledochoduodenostomy

Table 24.3 Biliojejunal anastomosis with native papilla for pancreatic access

Roux-en-Y hepaticojejunostomy
Roux-en-Y liver transplantation

24.2 Increased Incidence of Biliopancreatic Disease Requiring ERCP

Roux-en-Y anastomosis is probably the main surgical reconstruction used to connect the biliopancreatic system to the intestine, with an afferent jejunal limb. The afferent limb may be short (~50 cm) or long (>100 cm), and the papilla may or may not be preserved. This kind of reconstruction gives rise to a wide variety of postoperative anatomy of the biliary and the pancreatic ducts.

The short limb Roux reconstruction is usually employed during partial or total gastrectomy and preserves the papilla. After pancreaticoduodenectomy, the papilla is not preserved, and two separate anastomoses (biliary and pancreatic) are created. After liver transplantation the papilla is preserved only for the pancreatic orifice, and a biliojejunal anastomosis is created. Long limb

M. Mutignani et al. (eds.), *Endotherapy in Biliopancreatic Diseases: ERCP Meets EUS*,
https://doi.org/10.1007/978-3-030-42569-2_24

Roux anastomosis is used to induce malabsorption when performed in the context of bariatric operations and features an intact papilla.

Stricture of the postoperative biliary or pancreatic anastomosis is a common long-term complication requiring intervention [1]. Rapid weight loss after bariatric surgery, on the other hand, predisposes to gallstone formation, and intervention is required to treat common bile duct stones [2]. Moreover, RYGB may create a predisposition for primary common bile duct formation as noted in one study [3]. Indeed, the need for biliopancreatic interventions in post-gastrectomy patients is relatively high. Although percutaneous or surgical methods can be employed to treat such conditions, the endoscopic approach is less invasive and more appealing.

24.3 Preparation for ERCP

Prior to ERCP certain essential prerequisites should be addressed. ERCP in altered anatomy is technically demanding [4] and carries significantly more risks compared to ERCP in native anatomy. In particular, the risk of small bowel perforation is higher, while all other potential post-ERCP complications remain unchanged. At the same time, the need for endoscopic re-intervention in altered anatomy should be set at a minimum. Therefore, referring candidates for ERCP at high-volume centers is probably the best thing to do if local experience in advanced ERCP is limited.

A thorough review of each patient history is crucial. Indication for ERCP should be absolute and interventions best avoided in obscure/gray zone cases. Patients and family should also be aware of possible risks, and a signed informed consent form is a sine qua non, as in every ERCP.

A review of the surgical reconstruction in each patient is mandatory. If the surgical report is at hand, it will certainly assist in understanding and recognizing anatomical landmarks during the procedure. Discussion with the surgeon who operated the patient or other surgical colleagues may help if there are still unclear issues.

Scope selection is of pivotal role, as wrong endoscope choice leads to time waste and adds frustration to the endoscopist and the team. A scout endoscopy with a standard diagnostic gastroscope before ERCP may help identify postoperative anatomy and should be performed whenever the surgical report is missing. An assessment of the length and mobility of the intestine is performed at the same time; this may critically influence the selection of the scope. A rough guide to endoscope selection for commonly encountered postoperative rearrangements is found in Table 24.4.

ERCP under general anesthesia should be preferred over conscious sedation to achieve the best

Table 24.4 Endoscope selection according to postoperative anatomy (DAE - device assisted enteroscopy)

Postoperative anatomy	Recommended Endoscope
Billroth I, sleeve gastrectomy, esophagectomy with gastric pull-up, Choledochoduodenostomy	Duodenoscope
Billroth II	Duodenoscope Forward-viewing scope (gastro–/colonoscope) with transparent cap DAE
Whipple's procedure	Forward-viewing scope (gastro–/colonoscope) with transparent cap Duodenoscope (in short limb rearrangement) DAE
Roux-en-Y gastrectomy/RYGB	DAE Colonoscope EUS guided, direct or indirect methods Via gastrostomy methods Laparoscopy-assisted ERCP w. duodenoscope
Biliopancreatic diversion	Laparoscopy-assisted ERCP w. duodenoscope

operative conditions and accommodate prolonged procedure time which is expected in these cases. CO_2 insufflation should be the rule, as in every ERCP. Finally, specific endoscopes, specialized catheters, and equipment required for the scheduled intervention should be readily available in the ERCP suite.

24.4 Reaching the Papilla and/or Ductal Anastomosis

ERCP after Billroth I reconstruction, choledochoduodenostomy, sleeve gastrectomy, or esophagectomy with gastric pull-up is performed with the standard duodenoscope. Especially for Billroth I, but also for esophagectomy, the duodenoscope may not be as stable as in normal anatomy; nevertheless, the intervention is usually carried out with similar success rate. A semi-long or long position of the duodenoscope may provide extra stability when needed [5].

In Billroth II anatomy, the procedure should be performed with a duodenoscope as a first choice instrument. The usually short afferent limb and the elevator are the main reasons for this. The elevator helps with cannulation and all subsequent interventions (Fig. 24.1). Yet this comes at a price, as the risk of perforation is significantly elevated when compared with forward-viewing endoscopes such as gastroscopes or pediatric colonoscopes. A careful assessment of published studies, though, reveals a declining trend regarding perforations over the years, reaching less than 2% in recent studies. This may reflect higher skill acquisition and/or increased familiarity with the procedure [6–9].

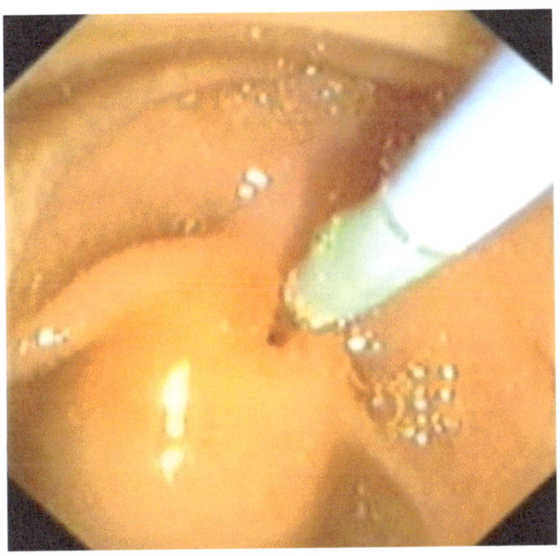

Fig. 24.1 Native papilla in Billroth II anatomy. Straight (diagnostic) catheter exiting duodenoscope

The afferent loop may be at the lesser (antiperistaltic) or the greater curvature (isoperistaltic) of the stomach, and there is no sure way of predicting the correct limb. The anastomosis is a preferred site of perforation, and the afferent loop may be hard to intubate, especially if it is stitched on top of the gastric suture as a protective measure, thus creating a very acute and fixed angle. Peristalsis of the afferent loop moves toward the lens, and bilious fluid is present when biliary obstruction is absent. When the afferent loop is intubated, the scope crosses the spine soon after exiting the stomach under fluoroscopy. Conversely, if the scope is seen heading toward the left lower quadrant, the efferent loop is intubated. Sometimes, an extra anastomosis is encountered. The Braun anastomosis is a side to side jejunojejunal anastomosis fairly close to the stomach. The rationale behind it is to decrease the bile reflux in the stomach and prevent alkaline gastritis. The presence of this anastomosis sometimes disorients the endoscopist. The correct limb is the one with abundant bile and peristalsis moving toward the lens, while fluoroscopically a course toward the right upper quadrant is followed. Air in a blind stump at the right hypochondrium during fluoroscopy is another sign of the correct direction. Contrast injection through a catheter may also help identify the duodenal stump. The distance from the stomach to the papilla is shorter in the retrocolic and longer in the antecolic rearrangement. Successful papilla identification in Billroth II anatomy with a duodenoscope is reported in a range from 62.5% [10] to 100% [11]. In real life, the truth lies in between [9, 12].

Straight-viewing endoscopes equipped with transparent cap provide better viewing when negotiating acute bends and stability in front of the papilla. Moreover, manipulation of the papilla with the cap during cannulation improves position and increases cannulation rates [10, 13, 14]. In any case, manual compression of the abdomen whenever there is sharp angulation or loop formation may assist in scope advancement. Scouting the anatomy with a gastroscope prior to using a duodenoscope is another alternative. Upon reaching the papilla, a guidewire is left in place, and the duodenoscope is inserted alongside or over the wire. This helps identifying the afferent loop and monitoring progress fluoroscopically [15].

In a recent systematic review, the success rates of afferent loop intubation and selective cannulation rate for each type of endoscope were duodenoscope 98.2% and 95.3%, forward-viewing endoscopes 97.4% and 95.2%, and balloon-assisted enteroscopes 95.4% and 97.5%, respectively. The rate of bowel perforation was slightly higher in side-viewing endoscopy (3.6%) and balloon-assisted enteroscopy (4.1%) compared with forward-viewing endoscopy (1.7%) [16]. If the papilla cannot be reached with the duodenoscope, the gastroscope, or the pediatric colonoscope, enteroscopy techniques is the next logical step.

In Whipple's procedure, the second portion of the duodenum including the head of the pancreas is removed, so there is no papilla. In the classic Whipple, there is an end to side gastrojejunostomy (similar to Billroth II), whereas in the pylorus-preserving variation, the jejunostomy is performed right after the pylorus. Both biliary and pancreatic ducts are anastomosed to the jejunum rendering cannulation much easier. Since there is no particular need for the elevator, it seems wiser to start with a straight-viewing scope such a pediatric/adult colonoscope or even a gastroscope. A transparent cap helps in navigating through the intestine. Pneumobilia, in a patent hepaticojejunostomy, is also a valuable guide during scope insertion. Alternatively, the biliary anastomosis may be reached with the therapeutic duodenoscope as well as with deep enteroscopy techniques.

The pancreatic anastomosis is usually at the very end of the blind stump, whereas the biliary anastomosis is located a few centimeters proximally. Variations may exist as sometimes the pancreatic anastomosis is done in an end to side manner and is located before the blind stump but always after the biliary anastomosis. Rarely, the two anastomoses are performed on separate Roux limbs. When the two hepatic ducts are separately anastomosed, one encounters two biliary openings.

The size of the anastomosis in relation to the size of the bile duct determines the degree of fibrosis and the need for dilation, especially if there are stones present. The pancreatic anastomosis is quite difficult to locate and cannulate [17]. Flat tissue around it is a clue of vicinity. Secretin injection along with methylene blue spraying for identification may be used as done for the minor papilla. All cannulations are performed with straight catheters.

The Roux rearrangement (Fig. 24.2), be it after gastrectomy or RYGB, is the most difficult to tackle. This is due to the long distance to traverse before reaching the papilla. Given the fact that distance from mouth to stomach is around 40 cm, the distance of the Roux limb is at least 50–70 cm and many times longer, and finally the length of the biliopancreatic limb is another 50 cm or more, one understands that reaching the papilla requires at least 150 cm of shaft without looping. With the duodenoscope it is almost impossible to accomplish the task. The only exception is after total gastrectomy where distances are shortened, and often a duodenoscope can traverse the distance. ERCP can be performed

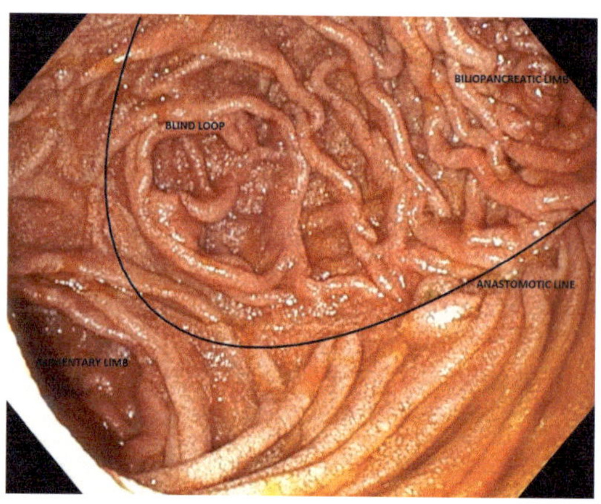

Fig. 24.2 Endoscopic view of a side to side Roux anastomosis. Anastomosis line, alimentary, Roux, and blind limb marked on image. The blind loop is absent in end to side reconstruction

with the help of various long forward-viewing endoscopes or more complex procedures either transluminally or transmurally depending on the postoperative anatomy.

The pediatric colonoscope is usually the first choice although success in reaching the papilla is low. If available, the best option is to use enteroscopy techniques. All deep enteroscopy techniques are referred to under the general term device-assisted enteroscopy (DAE) and, in the case of ERCP, device-assisted ERCP (DAERCP) and will be addressed to subsequently. Cannulation and interventions are performed as in Billroth II anatomy.

Should intraluminal efforts prove fruitless, transmural interventions may be employed, usually, but not restricted to Roux-en-Y gastric bypass. These approaches are either EUS guided or surgically assisted. EUS-guided techniques may be applied directly, to decompress the desired duct with EUS-guided transmural stents, or indirectly to allow access to the papilla after creating an anastomosis usually between the remnant and the excluded stomach after RYGB. Laparoscopy-assisted options apply here as well.

ERCP after biliopancreatic diversion is possible only with laparoscopy-assisted techniques.

24.5 Device-Assisted ERCP, DAERCP

Especially for Roux-en-Y gastrectomy, but also in post-Billroth II or post-Whipple's, whenever duodenoscopes and traditional front-viewing endoscopes fail to reach the papilla, mostly due to distance issues, DAE has provided endoscopists with a valuable and safe alternative. Latest advances in enteroscopy include wireless small bowel capsule endoscopy (SBCE) which is a strictly diagnostic procedure and double-balloon (DBE), single-balloon (SBE), and spiral enteroscopy (SPE) which all offer the possibility to perform various interventions.

Mainly DBE (Fujinon) and SBE (Olympus) but also SPE have been used to traverse the small bowel with intent to perform ERCP. Properties and capabilities of each system are reviewed elsewhere [18, 19]. Both SBE and DBE are highly effective methods in reaching the papilla in surgically altered anatomy. Many studies have shown this. Standard, long enteroscopes used for balloon-assisted small bowel endoscopy require customized, long catheters and wires for endotherapy, and the market availability for these catheters is low. Shorter (~150 cm) enteroscopes that can accommodate standard ERCP catheters are commercially available from both manufacturers. These models are equipped with a 3.2 mm working channel through which most endotherapy is possible with standard length catheters. Long enteroscopes are superior to short enteroscopes in reaching the papilla in case of Roux reconstruction without gastrectomy or in peritoneal dissemination [20]. Successfully reaching the papilla with DBE is reported ranging from 75 to 97.1% in Roux-en-Y gastrectomy series [21–24]. The success in reaching the papilla in Billroth II or post-Whipple's anatomy is even higher [25]. Conversely, in long Roux rearrangement (RYGB), the success in reaching the papilla is significantly lower, at the range of 71%, as shown from a large multicentric study including all forms of DAE specifically in RYGB [23].

Single-balloon enteroscopy has similar effectiveness in reaching the papilla. Local availability and expertise are the main determinants in scope choice [23, 25–27].

Spiral endoscopy with the Spirus overtube is no longer commercially available. The Olympus Corporation after acquiring the Spirus overtube has developed its own dedicated system with a built-in motorized system called PowerSpiral. This system is commercially available since early 2019 and studies are underway. ERCP in surgically altered anatomy with the Spirus overtube has been attempted with success, but a limited number of studies have been published [28, 29].

24.6 EUS-Guided Methods

As mentioned earlier, EUS-guided techniques may be applied directly to relieve ductal obstruction or indirectly to facilitate scope passage to the duodenum.

EUS-guided hepaticoentero-/gastrostomy is equally successful, in terms of biliary drainage, compared with percutaneous transhepatic drainage, but superior in terms of post-procedural pain and need for re-interventions [30]. The method has application both in malignant and benign obstruction not only to achieve decompression but also to provide definitive therapy in benign disease [31] although further studies are necessary. EUS-guided therapy may be performed transgastrically, directly at the pancreatic duct to treat stenosis of the pancreaticojejunostomy with good success rate and accepted complications [32, 33].

Specifically in RYGB, EUS-guided gastrogastrostomy is a valuable adjunct in performing ERCP. The technique consists of several steps with intent to create a gastrogastrostomy between the small gastric pouch and the excluded stomach. Through the gastrogastrostomy, a duodenoscope is passed and a standard ERCP is performed. Initially, the excluded stomach is identified with a linear echoendoscope and punctured with a 19-gauge EUS needle. Contrast injection confirms the intragastric position of the needle. Afterward more water with contrast and CO_2 are injected to distend the gastric cavity, and a long guidewire is coiled inside the excluded stomach. The tract is then dilated with a 6 mm balloon. Finally, a short lumen-apposing metal stent (LAMS) is inserted to secure the connection. The stent is dilated to 18 mm to permit the passage of a duodenoscope to perform ERCP as in native anatomy [34]. The stent may be retrieved several weeks later, and the fistula can be sutured with endoscopic suturing. This last step may pose difficulties as the working space inside the small gastric pouch is very confined. More studies are needed before adopting this technique.

24.7 Alternatives in RYGB/ ERCP via Gastrostomy

The creation of a Russell-type gastrostomy by EUS guidance [35, 36] or after reaching the excluded stomach with enteroscopy techniques [37], and subsequent exchange for an esophageal stent, allows the performance of standard ERCP with a duodenoscope through the stent, after balloon dilation. All the above steps are performed in the same session. At the end, the stent is again exchanged for a gastrostomy tube. Similarly, a surgical gastrostomy may be dilated after maturation to allow the insertion of a conventional duodenoscope, although this procedure is time-consuming and not suited for interventions in a timely manner [38].

24.8 Laparoscopy-Assisted ERCP

Laparoscopy-assisted ERCP may be attempted in all long limb Roux reconstructions, when less invasive methods to reach the papilla have failed. Furthermore, it is the only way of performing ERCP after biliopancreatic diversion [39, 40]. It may be the best choice whenever there is an indication for concomitant cholecystectomy [3]. In RYGB, the excluded stomach is punctured and a 15 mm trocar is inserted and secured. Through the trocar, a standard therapeutic duodenoscope is passed and ERCP may be carried out as in native anatomy. In non-bariatric Roux reconstructions, including biliopancreatic diversion, laparoscopy-assisted ERCP may be performed with a duodenoscope through a trocar inserted in a jejunal loop close to the papilla. ERCP is performed in an inverted fashion, as in all caudally approached papillae.

24.9 Cannulation, Sphincterotomy, and Other Interventions

Whenever the papilla is approached orally (Billroth I, sleeve gastrectomy, transgastric ERCP in RYGB), cannulation and sphincterotomy are performed the same way as in native anatomy. Whenever the papilla is approached caudally, as in all other surgical rearrangements described above, all anatomic formations are seen from the opposite position. This means that the bile duct is at the 5–6 o'clock direction and the pancreatic duct toward the 7 o'clock position. The presence of the elevator on the duodenoscope, in every case, facilitates cannulation and further interventions.

Cannulation of the desired duct is best achieved with a straight (diagnostic) catheter pointing at the direction of the duct (Fig. 24.3a). The exit point of the working channel varies in the front-viewing scopes used for papillary access in altered anatomy. Rotation of the shaft of the endoscope helps adjusting for better alignment toward the desired duct. One can use the wire-guided cannulation method which has been shown to reduce the incidence of post-ERCP pancreatitis, at least in native anatomy, or instead try with the classic injection first method in order to understand the anatomy and advance the catheter accordingly so as to achieve deep cannulation. The selected catheter may be manually reshaped to point to a more favorable direction. In the absence of papilla, the ductal anastomosis is cannulated with a diagnostic catheter.

Rotatable catheters or sphincterotomes may prove very helpful in cannulation. The advantage of a rotatable sphincterotome is obviously that a single instrument is used both for cannulation and sphincterotomy. The pancreatic guidewire technique can also be applied if the pancreatic duct is repeatedly entered. Finally, needle knife pre-cutting (in skilled hands) when all other techniques fail and/or percutaneous transhepatic rendezvous are other options for cannulating the bile duct.

Sphincterotomy is done in the direction of the duct. Several methods have been described in the literature. Besides the rotatable sphincterotome, a variety of modified sphincterotomes (S-shaped, shark fin, sigmoid type) have been used, and many are commercially available (Fig. 24.3b). Needle knife sphincterotomy over a plastic biliary stent is another popular and safe way of per-

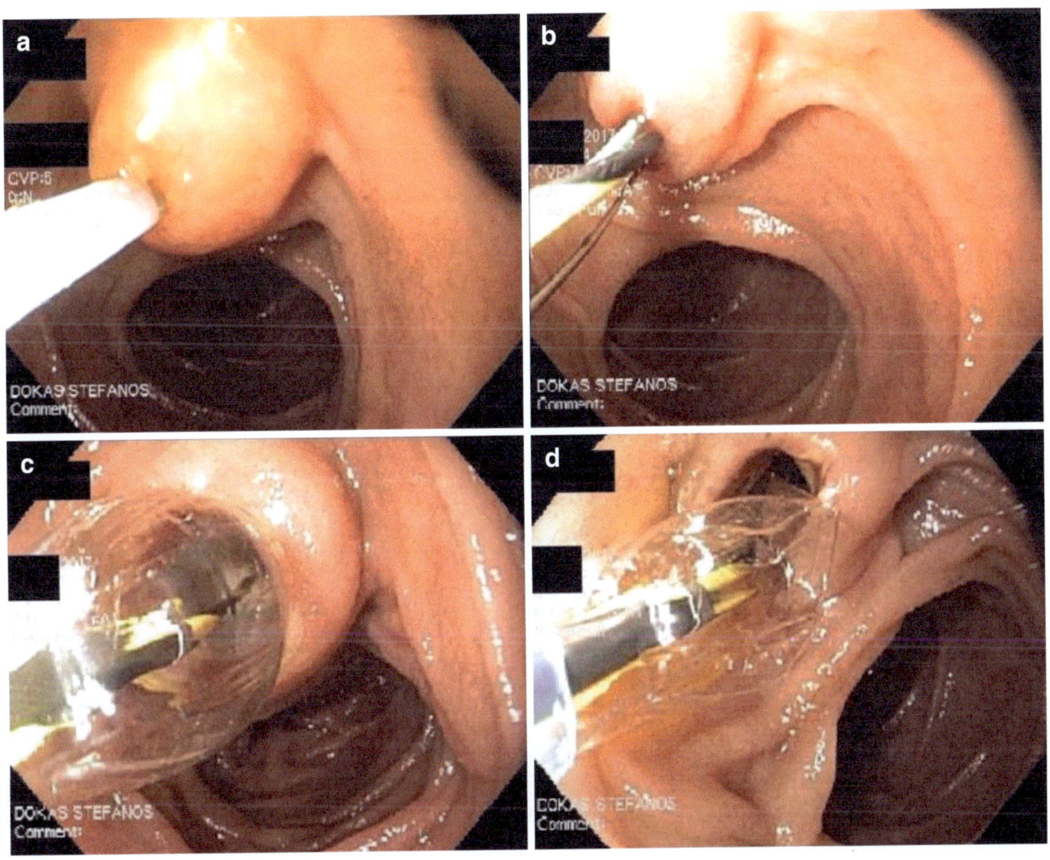

Fig. 24.3 Billroth II ERCP with a diagnostic gastroscope. (**a**) Cannulation with a straight catheter. (**b**) Endoscopic sphincterotomy with a Billroth II sphincterotome over the wire. (**c**) Large balloon papillary dilation after a small sphincterotomy. (**d**) Opening of the papilla after the dilation, dark stone visible inside the duct

forming sphincterotomy, always cutting above the stent without deeper injury. Finally, a small sphincterotomy followed by large balloon dilation of the papilla is probably the safest approach especially when dealing with large biliary stones (Figs. 24.3c, d and 24.4).

Specialized, longer cannulas and sphincterotomes are necessary if DAERCP with long shaft enteroscope is to be performed. The usual wires are not long enough for wire exchange, so dedicated 600-cm-long wires should be available for wire exchange. If not available, water-assisted wire exchange of a 450-cm-long, fully hydrophilic, wire may be attempted. Metal stent insertion is impossible through the working channel of long shaft enteroscope. Stent insertion, over a stiff wire, through the overtube, after scope withdrawal may be an alternative in this situation. Monitoring is solely radiological of course. Stone extraction is done the same way as in standard

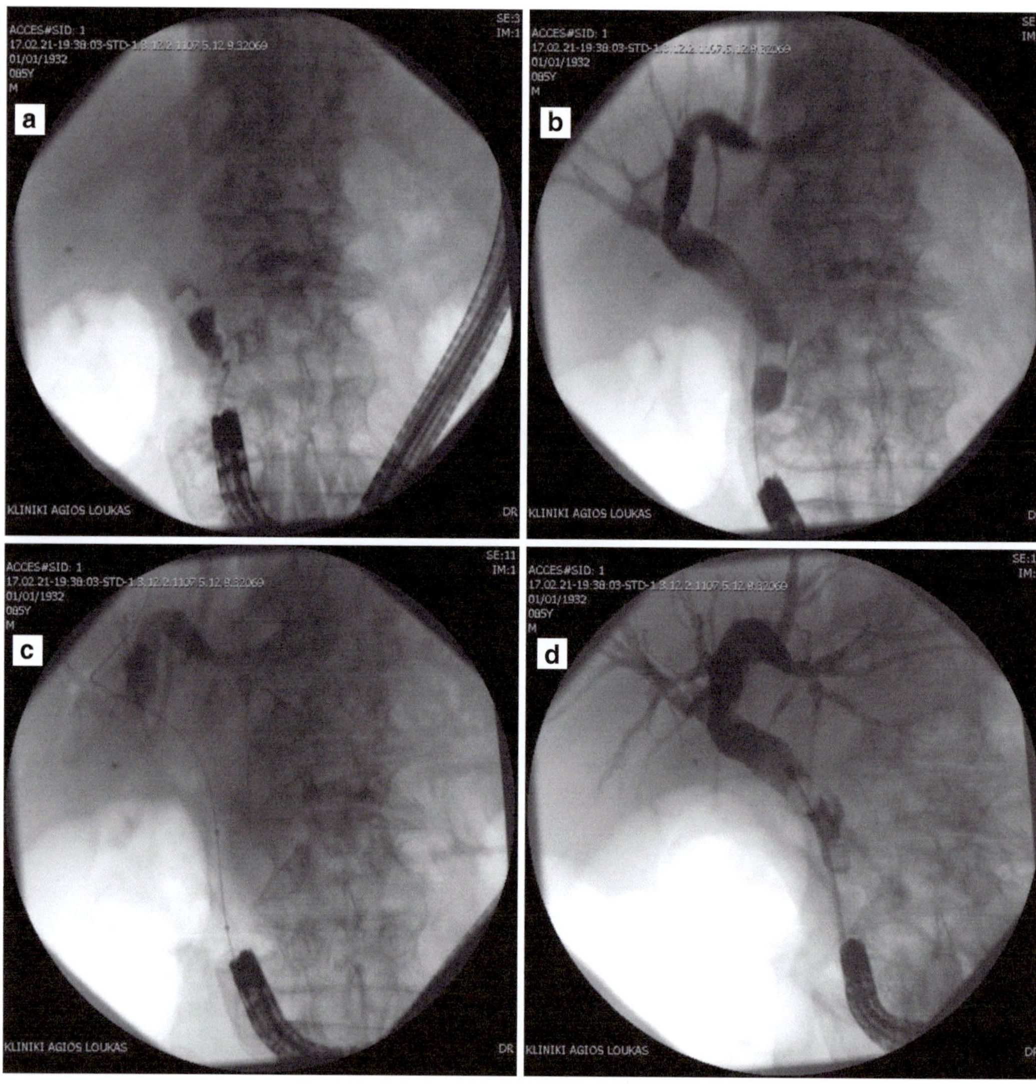

Fig. 24.4 ERCP with a diagnostic gastroscope – fluoroscopy from Fig. 24.3. (**a**) Initial injection inside the common bile duct. Cuboid stone close to the papilla and classic Billroth II position of the scope. (**b**) Cholangiogram—wire inside the bile duct. (**c**) Large balloon papillary dilation (plain water, no contrast). (**d**) Inflated balloon above the stone prior to extraction

ERCP. Longer stone extraction balloons and dormia baskets are necessary for long shaft enteroscopes.

24.10 Adverse Events

ERCP is the endoscopic intervention associated with the highest risk for complications. The usual complications include post-ERCP acute pancreatitis, hemorrhage, cholangitis, and perforation. In the surgically altered anatomy realm, perforations are the most frequently encountered complications. Perforations usually occur at the anastomoses or in any other site as a result of excess force applied at any fixed, angulated loop. Forward-viewing instruments are safer to navigate with when compared with duodenoscopes, resulting in fewer perforations. Care should be taken not to induce barotrauma when using balloon-assisted enteroscopy. The isolated loop between the duodenal stump and the inflated balloon should not be overinflated even with CO_2 insufflation [41].

24.11 Conclusion

ERCP in surgically altered anatomy is a challenging procedure. Clear understanding of the postoperative anatomy, careful planning of the intervention in terms of scope and accessory selection, and thinking ahead of possible hurdles are essential for a successful outcome. Skilled, high-volume endoscopists are best suited for these cases. Experience and familiarity with deep enteroscopy techniques and EUS are essential in order to achieve the highest success rates. Surgical assistance may be needed in certain cases to complete the planned treatment.

References

1. House MG, Cameron JL, Schulick RD, Campbell KA, Sauter PK, Coleman J, et al. Incidence and outcome of biliary strictures after pancreaticoduodenectomy. Ann Surg. 2006;243(5):571–6; discussion 6–8. https://doi.org/10.1097/01.sla.0000216285.07069.fc. 00000658-200605000-00001 [pii].
2. Hamdan K, Somers S, Chand M. Management of late postoperative complications of bariatric surgery. Br J Surg. 2011;98(10):1345–55. https://doi.org/10.1002/bjs.7568.
3. Habenicht Yancey K, McCormack LK, McNatt SS, Powell MS, Fernandez AZ, Westcott CJ. Laparoscopic-assisted transgastric ERCP: a single-institution experience. J Obes. 2018;2018:8275965. https://doi.org/10.1155/2018/8275965.
4. Schutz SM. Grading the degree of difficulty of ERCP procedures. Gastroenterol Hepatol (N Y). 2011;7(10):674–6.
5. Lichtenstein DR. Post-surgical anatomy and ERCP. Tech Gastrointest Endosc. 2007;9(2):114–24. https://doi.org/10.1016/j.tgie.2007.03.001.
6. Park TY, Kang JS, Song TJ, Lee SS, Lee H, Choi JS, et al. Outcomes of ERCP in Billroth II gastrectomy patients. Gastrointest Endosc. 2016;83(6):1193–201. https://doi.org/10.1016/j.gie.2015.10.036. S0016-5107(15)03052-7 [pii].
7. Faylona JM, Qadir A, Chan AC, Lau JY, Chung SC. Small-bowel perforations related to endoscopic retrograde cholangiopancreatography (ERCP) in patients with Billroth II gastrectomy. Endoscopy. 1999;31(7):546–9. https://doi.org/10.1055/s-1999-61.
8. Cicek B, Parlak E, Disibeyaz S, Koksal AS, Sahin B. Endoscopic retrograde cholangiopancreatography in patients with Billroth II gastroenterostomy. J Gastroenterol Hepatol. 2007;22(8):1210–3. https://doi.org/10.1111/j.1440-1746.2006.04765.x. JGH4765 [pii].
9. Bove V, Tringali A, Familiari P, Gigante G, Boskoski I, Perri V, et al. ERCP in patients with prior Billroth II gastrectomy: report of 30 years' experience. Endoscopy. 2015;47(7):611–6. https://doi.org/10.1055/s-0034-1391567.
10. Wang F, Xu B, Li Q, Zhang X, Jiang G, Ge X, et al. Endoscopic retrograde cholangiopancreatography in patients with surgically altered anatomy: one single center's experience. Medicine (Baltimore). 2016;95(52):e5743. https://doi.org/10.1097/MD.0000000000005743. 00005792-201612300-00042 [pii].
11. Kim KH, Kim TN. Endoscopic papillary large balloon dilation for the retrieval of bile duct stones after prior Billroth II gastrectomy. Saudi J Gastroenterol. 2014;20(2):128–33. https://doi.org/10.4103/1319-3767.129478. SaudiJGastroenterol_2014_20_2_128_129478 [pii].
12. Wu WG, Mei JW, Zhao MN, Zhang WJ, Gu J, Tao YJ, et al. Use of the conventional side-viewing duodenoscope for successful endoscopic retrograde cholangiopancreatography in postgastrectomy patients. J Clin Gastroenterol. 2016;50(3):244–51. https://doi.org/10.1097/MCG.0000000000000442.
13. Park CH, Lee WS, Joo YE, Kim HS, Choi SK, Rew JS. Cap-assisted ERCP in patients with a Billroth II gastrectomy. Gastrointest Endosc. 2007;66(3):612–5. https://doi.org/10.1016/j.gie.2007.04.024. S0016-5107(07)01897-4 [pii].

14. Testoni PA, Mariani A, Aabakken L, Arvanitakis M, Bories E, Costamagna G, et al. Papillary cannulation and sphincterotomy techniques at ERCP: European Society of Gastrointestinal Endoscopy (ESGE) Clinical Guideline. Endoscopy. 2016;48(7):657–83. https://doi.org/10.1055/s-0042-108641.
15. Garcia-Cano J. A simple technique to aid intubation of the duodenoscope in the afferent limb of Billroth II gastrectomies for endoscopic retrograde cholangiopancreatography. Endoscopy. 2008;40(Suppl 2):E21–2. https://doi.org/10.1055/s-2007-966950.
16. Park TY, Song TJ. Recent advances in endoscopic retrograde cholangiopancreatography in Billroth II gastrectomy patients: a systematic review. World J Gastroenterol. 2019;25(24):3091–107. https://doi.org/10.3748/wjg.v25.i24.3091.
17. Chahal P, Baron TH, Topazian MD, Petersen BT, Levy MJ, Gostout CJ. Endoscopic retrograde cholangiopancreatography in post-Whipple patients. Endoscopy. 2006;38(12):1241–5. https://doi.org/10.1055/s-2006-945003.
18. Rondonotti E, Spada C, Adler S, May A, Despott EJ, Koulaouzidis A, et al. Small-bowel capsule endoscopy and device-assisted enteroscopy for diagnosis and treatment of small-bowel disorders: European Society of Gastrointestinal Endoscopy (ESGE) Technical Review. Endoscopy. 2018;50(4):423–46. https://doi.org/10.1055/a-0576-0566.
19. Chauhan SS, Manfredi MA, Abu Dayyeh BK, Enestvedt BK, Fujii-Lau LL, Komanduri S, et al. Enteroscopy. Gastrointest Endosc. 2015;82(6):975–90. https://doi.org/10.1016/j.gie.2015.06.012. S0016-5107(15)02539-0 [pii].
20. Kawaguchi Y, Yamauchi H, Kida M, Okuwaki K, Iwai T, Uehara K, et al. Failure factors to reach the blind end using a short-type single-balloon enteroscope for ERCP with Roux-en-Y reconstruction: a multicenter retrospective study. Gastroenterol Res Pract. 2019:3536487. https://doi.org/10.1155/2019/3536487.
21. Katanuma A, Isayama H. Current status of endoscopic retrograde cholangiopancreatography in patients with surgically altered anatomy in Japan: questionnaire survey and important discussion points at Endoscopic Forum Japan 2013. Dig Endosc. 2014;26(Suppl 2):109–15. https://doi.org/10.1111/den.12247.
22. Osoegawa T, Motomura Y, Akahoshi K, Higuchi N, Tanaka Y, Hisano T, et al. Improved techniques for double-balloon-enteroscopy-assisted endoscopic retrograde cholangiopancreatography. World J Gastroenterol. 2012;18(46):6843–9. https://doi.org/10.3748/wjg.v18.i46.6843.
23. Shah RJ, Smolkin M, Yen R, Ross A, Kozarek RA, Howell DA, et al. A multicenter, U.S. experience of single-balloon, double-balloon, and rotational overtube-assisted enteroscopy ERCP in patients with surgically altered pancreaticobiliary anatomy (with video). Gastrointest Endosc. 2013;77(4):593–600. https://doi.org/10.1016/j.gie.2012.10.015. S0016-5107(12)02851-9 [pii].
24. Shimatani M, Hatanaka H, Kogure H, Tsutsumi K, Kawashima H, Hanada K, et al. Diagnostic and therapeutic endoscopic retrograde cholangiography using a short-type double-balloon endoscope in patients with altered gastrointestinal anatomy: a multicenter prospective study in Japan. Am J Gastroenterol. 2016;111(12):1750–8. https://doi.org/10.1038/ajg.2016.420. ajg2016420 [pii].
25. Yane K, Katanuma A, Maguchi H, Takahashi K, Kin T, Ikarashi S, et al. Short-type single-balloon enteroscope-assisted ERCP in postsurgical altered anatomy: potential factors affecting procedural failure. Endoscopy. 2017;49(1):69–74. https://doi.org/10.1055/s-0042-118301.
26. Obana T, Fujita N, Ito K, Noda Y, Kobayashi G, Horaguchi J, et al. Therapeutic endoscopic retrograde cholangiography using a single-balloon enteroscope in patients with Roux-en-Y anastomosis. Dig Endosc. 2013;25(6):601–7. https://doi.org/10.1111/den.12039.
27. Kawamura T, Mandai K, Uno K, Yasuda K. Does single-balloon enteroscopy contribute to successful endoscopic retrograde cholangiopancreatography in patients with surgically altered gastrointestinal anatomy? ISRN Gastroenterol. 2013;2013:214958. https://doi.org/10.1155/2013/214958.
28. Ali MF, Modayil R, Gurram KC, Brathwaite CEM, Friedel D, Stavropoulos SN. Spiral enteroscopy-assisted ERCP in bariatric-length Roux-en-Y anatomy: a large single-center series and review of the literature (with video). Gastrointest Endosc. 2018;87(5):1241–7. https://doi.org/10.1016/j.gie.2017.12.024. S0016-5107(18)30010-5 [pii].
29. Lennon AM, Kapoor S, Khashab M, Corless E, Amateau S, Dunbar K, et al. Spiral assisted ERCP is equivalent to single balloon assisted ERCP in patients with Roux-en-Y anatomy. Dig Dis Sci. 2012;57(5):1391–8. https://doi.org/10.1007/s10620-011-2000-8.
30. Sharaiha RZ, Kumta NA, Desai AP, DeFilippis EM, Gabr M, Sarkisian AM, et al. Endoscopic ultrasound-guided biliary drainage versus percutaneous transhepatic biliary drainage: predictors of successful outcome in patients who fail endoscopic retrograde cholangiopancreatography. Surg Endosc. 2016;30(12):5500–5. https://doi.org/10.1007/s00464-016-4913-y. 10.1007/s00464-016-4913-y [pii].
31. James TW, Fan YC, Baron TH. EUS-guided hepaticoenterostomy as a portal to allow definitive antegrade treatment of benign biliary diseases in patients with surgically altered anatomy. Gastrointest Endosc. 2018;88(3):547–54. https://doi.org/10.1016/j.gie.2018.04.2353. S0016-5107(18)32664-6 [pii].
32. Francois E, Kahaleh M, Giovannini M, Matos C, Deviere J. EUS-guided pancreaticogastrostomy. Gastrointest Endosc. 2002;56(1):128–33. https://doi.org/10.1067/mge.2002.125547. S0016-5107(02)00024-X [pii].
33. Chen YI, Levy MJ, Moreels TG, Hajijeva G, Will U, Artifon EL, et al. An international multicenter

study comparing EUS-guided pancreatic duct drainage with enteroscopy-assisted endoscopic retrograde pancreatography after Whipple surgery. Gastrointest Endosc. 2017;85(1):170–7. https://doi.org/10.1016/j.gie.2016.07.031. S0016-5107(16)30382-0 [pii].
34. Kedia P, Sharaiha RZ, Kumta NA, Kahaleh M. Internal EUS-directed transgastric ERCP (EDGE): game over. Gastroenterology. 2014;147(3):566–8. https://doi.org/10.1053/j.gastro.2014.05.045. S0016-5085(14)00849-X [pii].
35. Kedia P, Kumta NA, Widmer J, Sundararajan S, Cerefice M, Gaidhane M, et al. Endoscopic ultrasound-directed transgastric ERCP (EDGE) for Roux-en-Y anatomy: a novel technique. Endoscopy. 2015;47(2):159–63. https://doi.org/10.1055/s-0034-1390771.
36. Thompson CC, Ryou MK, Kumar N, Slattery J, Aihara H, Ryan MB. Single-session EUS-guided transgastric ERCP in the gastric bypass patient. Gastrointest Endosc. 2014;80(3):517. https://doi.org/10.1016/j.gie.2014.06.011. S0016-5107(14)01844-6 [pii].
37. Law R, Wong Kee Song LM, Petersen BT, Baron TH. Single-session ERCP in patients with previous Roux-en-Y gastric bypass using percutaneous-assisted transprosthetic endoscopic therapy: a case series. Endoscopy. 2013;45(8):671–5. https://doi.org/10.1055/s-0033-1344029.
38. Baron TH, Vickers SM. Surgical gastrostomy placement as access for diagnostic and therapeutic ERCP. Gastrointest Endosc. 1998;48(6):640–1. https://doi.org/10.1016/s0016-5107(98)70052-5. S0016-5107(98)70052-5 [pii].
39. Mutignani M, Marchese M, Tringali A, Tacchino RM, Matera D, Foco M, et al. Laparoscopy-assisted ERCP after biliopancreatic diversion. Obes Surg. 2007;17(2):251–4. https://doi.org/10.1007/s11695-007-9026-1.
40. Marchesini JCD, Noda RW, Haida VM, Medeiros R, Sadowski S, Galvao Neto M, et al. Transenteric ERCP for treatment of choledocholithiasis after duodenal switch. Surg Laparosc Endosc Percutan Tech. 2017;27(3):e28–30. https://doi.org/10.1097/SLE.0000000000000397.
41. Azeem N, Tabibian JH, Baron TH, Orhurhu V, Rosen CB, Petersen BT, et al. Use of a single-balloon enteroscope compared with variable-stiffness colonoscopes for endoscopic retrograde cholangiography in liver transplant patients with Roux-en-Y biliary anastomosis. Gastrointest Endosc. 2013;77(4):568–77. https://doi.org/10.1016/j.gie.2012.11.031. S0016-5107(12)02981-1 [pii].

25 PTC and PTC-ERCP Rendezvous Procedures

Jörg G. Albert

Abbreviations

CT	Computed tomography
ERC	Endoscopic retrograde cholangiography
ERCP	Endoscopic retrograde cholangiopancreatography
ESGE	European Society of Gastrointestinal Endoscopy
EUS-CD	Endoscopic ultrasound cholangiodrainage
MRCP	Magnetic resonance cholangiopancreatography
MRI	Magnetic resonance imaging
PTCD	Percutaneous transhepatic cholangiodrainage
US	Percutaneous ultrasound

25.1 Introduction

Percutaneous transhepatic cholangiography and cholangiodrainage (PTCD) offers an alternative access route to the bile duct system to endoscopic retrograde cholangiography (ERC) by creating a percutaneous bile fistula. In comparison to endoscopic retrograde cholangiography (ERC), PTCD is an antegrade drainage method that follows the bile flow direction, establishing a non-anatomical entry to the bile duct system. Historically, PTC was initiated in the 1960s and predates introduction of ERC in the mid-1970s. Worldwide, PTC is applied at variable frequency; some interventionalists prefer it over ERC, e.g. in some parts of Asia; however most often PTCD is regarded as a second-line alternative to ERC in many situations. Indications for PTC include impossibility of an endoscopic intervention in obstructive bile duct disease, e.g. in bowel obstruction, or previously failed endoscopic intervention.

Rendezvous techniques are used as a salvage technique after failed ERC or anticipating a complex intervention that might not be resolved by sole ERC. The reason for PTC-endoscopic rendezvous might be limited accessibility of the bile duct system by ERC, i.e. failed bile duct cannulation or failing to traverse a bile duct stricture, or difficulty to approach the biliary orifice in postoperative altered anatomy. A main advantage of PTC over ERCP is the opportunity to drain obstructed bile duct segments externally, even if the obstructing stricture is not passed by the draining catheter, as PTC uses a percutaneous antegrade access route, Table 25.1.

There are some basic differences in comparing PTCD vs. ERC (Table 25.2).

J. G. Albert (✉)
Hepatologie und Endokrinologie, Abteilung für Gastroenterologie, Robert-Bosch-Krankenhaus, Auerbachstraße, Stuttgart, Germany
e-mail: joerg.albert@rbk.de

M. Mutignani et al. (eds.), *Endotherapy in Biliopancreatic Diseases: ERCP Meets EUS*,
https://doi.org/10.1007/978-3-030-42569-2_25

Table 25.1 Comparison of biliary access techniques

	ERC	PTC	EUS-CD
Access route	Anatomic	Non-anatomic	Non-anatomic
Access distance	Long (>1 m)	Short (<1 m)	Long (>1 m)
Complexity	High	Intermediate	High
Complication rate	<10%	Ca. 10%	>10%
External drainage possible	No	Yes	No
Success rate	90–95%	95% (often after failed ERC)	70–80%

ERCP endoscopic retrograde cholangiography, *PTC* percutaneous transhepatic cholangiography, *EUS-CD* endoscopic ultrasound cholangiodrainage

25.2 Technique of PTCD

Percutaneous transhepatic biliary drainage can be differentiated as an external drainage, external/internal drainage or internal drainage, depending on the outcome of the procedure, the type of catheter and its position within the biliary tree (Fig. 25.1). In case that the catheter may not pass the obstruction site, it is placed with the tip in an intrahepatic or an extrahepatic bile duct above the site of obstruction (Fig. 25.1a). External drainage may offer advantages over internal drainage, since the pressure gradient for drainage from the intrahepatic ducts to an external system may be greater

Table 25.2 Differences of PTCD vs. ERCP in therapy of bile duct obstruction

	PTCD	ERC
Access route	Limited selection of access route ('from branch to trunk')	Selection of bile duct branch potentially feasible ('from trunk to branches')
Repeating interventions	Easy to repeat interventions as soon as biliary access is established by percutaneous interventions	Repeated interventions are easy to perform as long as endoscopic approach to the biliary orifice is easy and bile duct access/papillotomy is done
	Risk of establishing biliary access is higher than sequential interventions, and abandoning the external-internal catheter for internal drainage signifies de novo risk profile in case of necessity of recurrent bile duct access	
Surgically altered anatomy	No limitation	Access complicated
Complication rate	Morbidity (major complications) ca. 5% Mortality ca. 2%	Morbidity (minor + major complications) <10% Mortality <1%

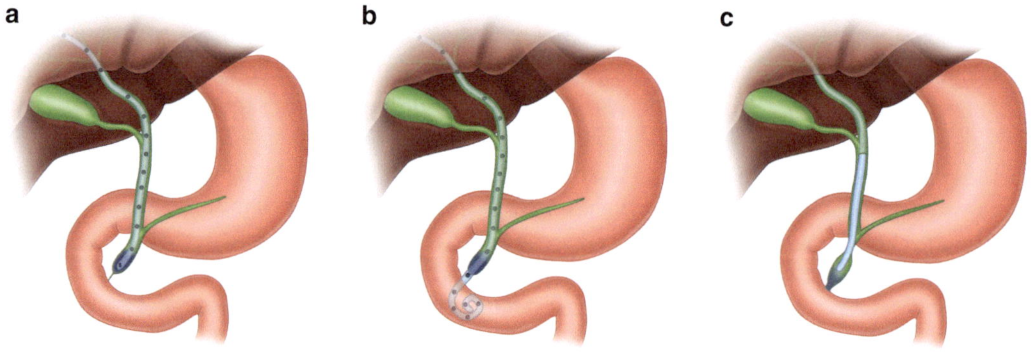

Fig. 25.1 External drainage (**a**), external-internal drainage (**b**) and internal drainage (**c**) by PTCD. (Adapted from: Percutaneous transhepatic biliary drainage in the management of biliary obstruction. Author links open overlay panel Philip J. Weyman M. D., Ronald G. Evens M.D. Current Problems in Diagnostic Radiology. Volume 11, Issue 3, May–June 1982, Pages 4-55. https://doi.org/10.1016/0363-0188(82)90018-4)

than the gradient for drainage into the intestine, and external drainage volumes can also be monitored easily. Sometimes decompression by external drainage may result in an improved outcome of difficult to navigate bile duct strictures in a second attempt. Its main disadvantage is the risk of dislodgement and the loss of nutrients: hyponatremia and dehydration can occur in patients with inadequate oral or intravenous replacement, and the loss of bile salts may result in malabsorption and wasting in the long term.

In most instances, external drainage is regarded a temporarily solution, and following decompression of the intrahepatic bile duct system, internalization of the catheter might be achieved in a second interventional session.

If an external-internal drainage situation is achieved (Fig. 25.1b), the catheter is placed into the intestine percutaneously, with the catheter side holes located above and below the obstruction site. While maintaining access to the biliary tree, the outflow of bile in to the intestines is re-established. Risk of dislodgement of the catheter is minimized as the catheter is sufficiently long to sustain a stable position.

An internal stent may be placed via the PTCD to bridge the obstructing lesion with removing the percutaneous catheter immediately after releasing the perfectly placed stent, thereby abandoning the external access (Fig. 25.1c). Internal drainage is attractive because all external catheters are removed and has cosmetic and psychological advantages for the patient. However, as soon as stents are occluded, additional interventions are required. Removal of all externally placed devices is possible in case that a free bile flow into the intestines has been established. Otherwise a biliary fistula with bile leakage into the peritoneal space can occur.

25.3 Patient Preparation

Attention to any pre-interventional diagnostic test available increases the probability of a successful intervention, and the therapeutic planning is based on a thorough visualization of the bile duct system by imaging. The clotting time should be sufficient, i.e. the platelet count should be greater than 75 × 10^9/L and the INR below 1.8. Cholangitis needs immediate antibiotic treatment, and in patients without previous evidence of cholangitis, we routinely use a broad-spectrum antibiotic such as ampicillin or ceftriaxone as a prophylactic treatment. A pre-procedure visit at the patient's bedside to discuss the risks and benefits of PTBD is an integral part of patient preparation.

25.4 Procedure of PTCD

Before starting the procedure, the therapeutic aim is planned based on cross-sectional imaging findings, i.e. percutaneous ultrasound (US) and/or CT/MRI and, ideally, MRCP. We prefer sonographically guided PTCD, with a continuous free-hand sonography guidance until puncturing a peripheric bile duct is attained. Any PTC procedure is performed under sterile conditions. The standard position is the midaxillary line approach for PTC; alternative puncture routes are chosen according to the anatomical situation and the location of the obstructing lesion or any treatment envisaged. Prior to PTC, the right lateral costophrenic angle should be localized in deep inspiration and the skin marked at this point to avoid transpleural fistulae. When PTCD is well planned, injection of contrast may be minimized, and a small amount of contrast medium is sufficient to opacify the intrahepatic ducts, without performing a complete diagnostic examination. This is particularly important in patients with pre-existing cholangitis or sepsis, as overdistention of the ducts can aggravate sepsis.

25.5 PTCD-ERCP Rendezvous

Non-surgical treatment of biliary obstruction was formerly a domain of percutaneous drainage [1, 2]. Only later, after replacing most indications for biliary drainage by endoscopic technique, it was identified to assist endoscopic access in impeded transpapillary intubation [3]. Naturally, PTCD-ERC rendezvous procedures require to master both endoscopic and percutaneous techniques. A firm grasp of the anatomy and pathology of the biliary tract, the necessary background of the interventional procedures and materials used and the willingness to function as part of a therapeutic team are mandatory for a successful intervention. Before any intervention, a diagnostic non-invasive clarification of the nature and the anatomic level of the bile duct obstruction are executed, e.g. MRCP, percutaneous ultrasonography and/or cross-sectional imaging.

Endoscopic rendezvous includes all procedures with antegrade introduction of a guidewire that might be caught by advancing it transpapillary to the duodenum. A combination of PTC and endoscopy, EUS-CD and intraoperative cholangiography plus endoscopic rendezvous have been reported [4, 5].

For PTCD-ERCP rendezvous, after puncturing a peripheric intrahepatic bile duct, a (hydrophilic) guidewire is advanced to the duodenum through a guiding catheter. The guidewire should feature a length of at least 100 cm. Hereupon, ERCP is performed. The guidewire, visualized in the duodenum, is grasped with a polypectomy snare and pulled retrograde through the accessory channel of the duodenoscope. A double lumen papillotome is then advanced over the guidewire, positioned at the papilla, and the sphincterotomy may be completed or any stent advanced transpapillary through the endoscope. The procedure is considered successful if biliary tract obstruction was completely resolved.

25.6 Indication for PTCD-ERCP Rendezvous

In case that sole endoscopic intervention failed or it might be foreseen that single-stage intervention might not be feasible, percutaneous access offers an alternative to enable repeated interventions and to combine percutaneous and endoscopic treatment modalities.

Rendezvous procedures might improve success rates of biliary drainage in unsuccessful ERCP (Fig. 25.2). In patients with superinfected bilioma in combination with distal bile duct obstruction, a combined draining of bile and bilioma by establishing a PTCD through the bilioma is most helpful and may also bridge and dilate the stricture site. Therefore, PTCD-ERC rendezvous within the bilioma is a valuable option: the percu-

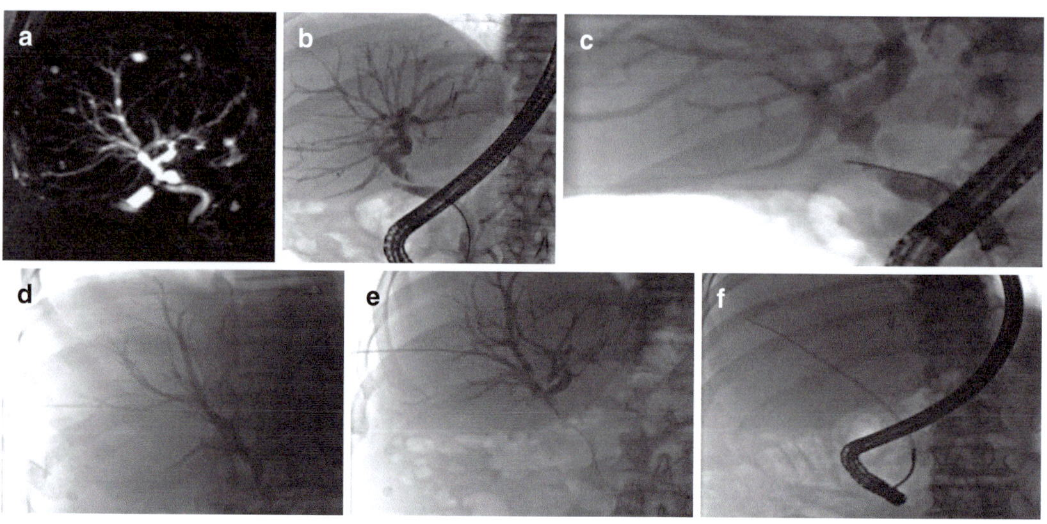

Fig. 25.2 (**a**, **b**, **c**) Anastomotic stricture in a patient with end-to-side choledocho-choledochal anastomosis after liver transplantation and with small biliary septic liver abscesses. (**a**) MRCP with delineation of the stricture. ERCP failed in repeated interventions (**b**, **c**) for eccentric anastomotic stricture. (**d**, **e**, **f**) After percutaneous access of the biliary tract, the guidewire was easily advanced into the duodenum and grabbed by the endoscope that had been placed at the duodenum, and a stent was advanced transpapillary across the stricture by way of endoscopy. The percutaneously placed catheter and guidewire were removed within the same session

taneously introduced guidewire may be caught by a snare or basket that has been transpapillary advanced into the bilioma through the duodenoscope. Thereby, a percutaneous, transhepatic, trans-bilioma biliary drainage could be established (Fig. 25.3) [4].

In patients with difficult to treat malignant or benign disease, PTCD might offer safe biliary drainage between repeating interventions. Combination of endoscopic and percutaneous interventions might help to achieve successful treatment (Fig. 25.4). In a large series, among a total of 812 patients, rendezvous was performed in 47 (6%), 31 (66%) of whom were diagnosed with complete transection of the bile duct (Amsterdam type D/Strasberg type E injury). The primary success rate of rendezvous was 94% [6]. In multisegmental obstruction in extensive hilar cholangiocarcinoma, complete drainage of the biliary tree is often not possible or practical. In these cases the configuration of the obstruction may guide the drainage plan, i.e. imaging such as MRCP should be performed before ERCP.

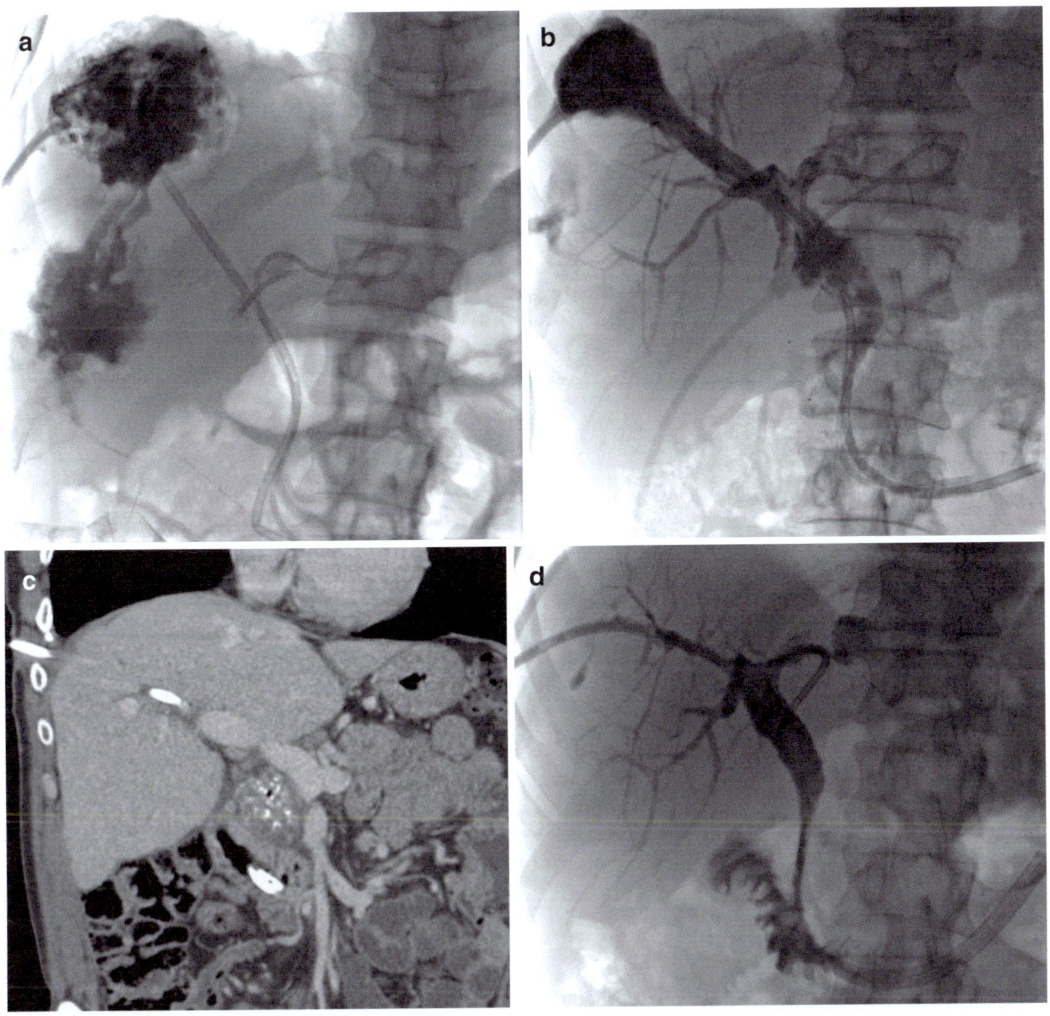

Fig. 25.3 (**a**) Infected bilioma in a patient with ischemic-type bile duct strictures. By percutaneous endoscopic rendezvous within the bilioma/abscess, a percutaneous transhepatic trans-bilioma biliary drainage could be established. (**b**) Over the course of several months, the bilioma was shrinking. (**c**) Finally, the bilioma was completely restored. (**d**) The PTCD could finally be removed after the bile duct stricture has resolved

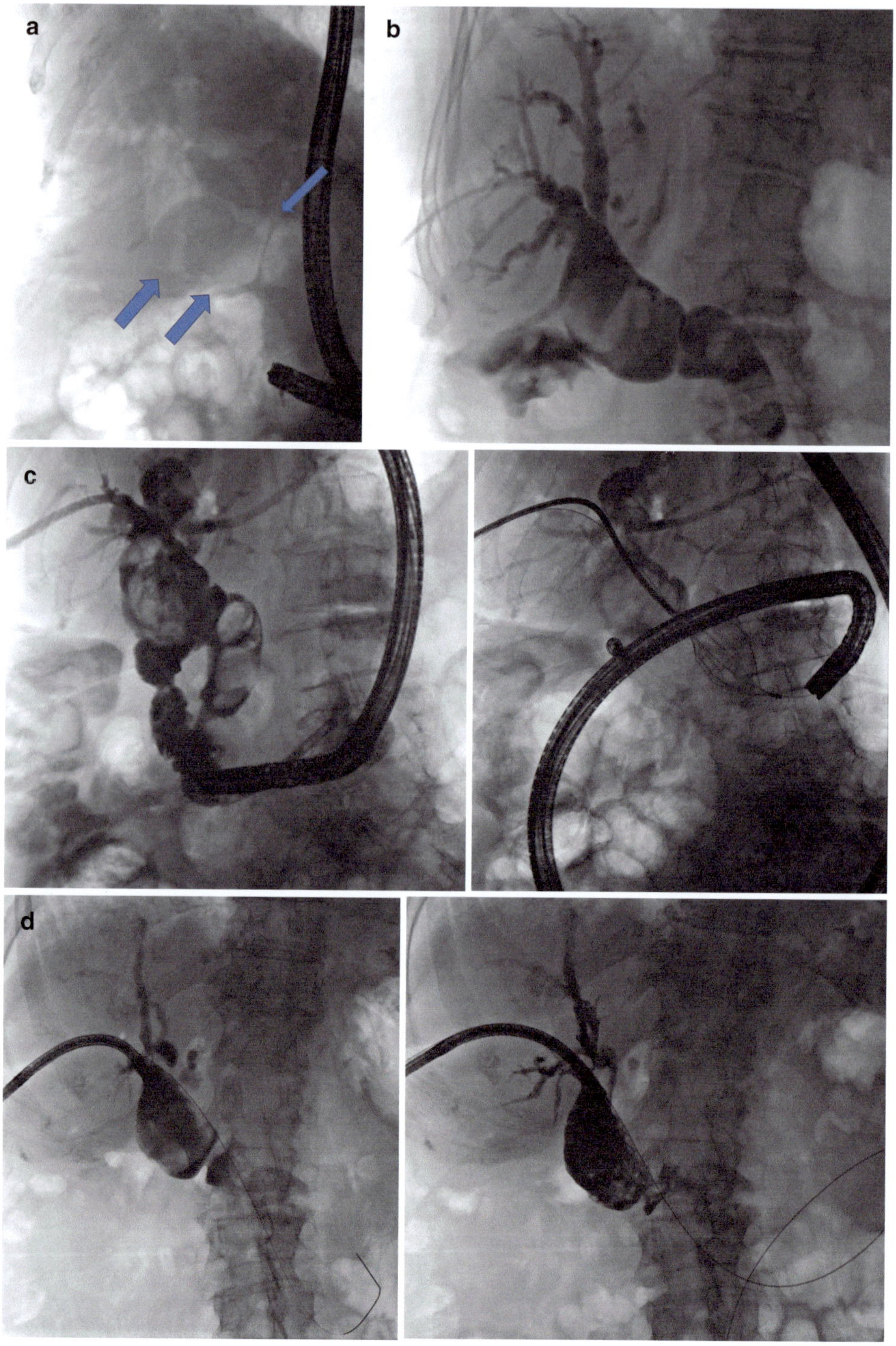

Fig. 25.4 (**a**) Grossly enlarged common bile duct at fluoroscopy (large arrows) before accessing the bile duct system in an 85-year-old patient with two episodes of biliary pancreatitis. Comorbidities included Billroth II surgery and choledochotomy with a stricture of the CBD (small arrow), obesity and lung fibrosis with long-term oxygen supply. (**b**) First, percutaneous biliary access was established to prevent any further pancreatitis and to maintain bile drainage in subsequent interventions. (**c**) (i and ii) Stone removal was achieved by a combined percutaneous and transpapillary approach within a rendezvous procedure. (**d**) (i and ii) The large proximally located CBD stones were fragmented with electro-hydraulic lithotripsy under cholangioscopic surveillance. (**e**) Finally, all stones and stone fragments were cleared and the percutaneous drainage catheter could be abandoned

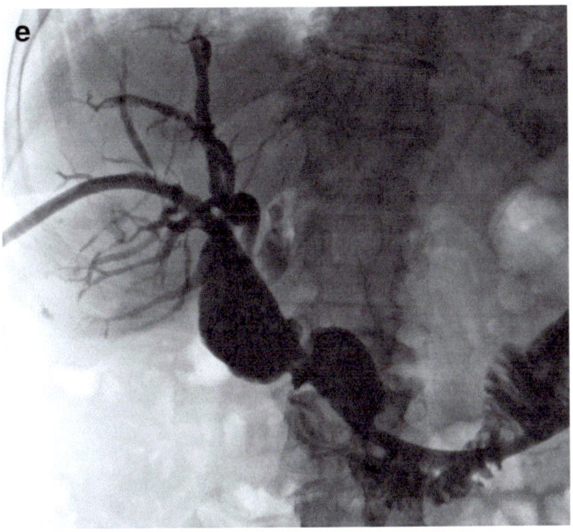

Fig. 25.4 (continued)

In sum, ERC-PTC rendezvous is a complex procedure to resolve difficult to treat bile duct obstruction and/or infection [7]. With a tailored approach, the interventionalists are able to drain externally or internally and may excellently treat infected bilioma with downstream bile duct obstruction. A dedicated team is required therefore.

References

1. Dooley JS, Dick R, Olney J, Sherlock S. Nonsurgical treatment of biliary obstruction. Lancet. 1979;2(8151):1040–4.
2. Cameron JL, Gayler BW, Zuidema GD. The use of silastic transhepatic stents in benign and malignant biliary strictures. Ann Surg. 1978;188(4):552–61.
3. Shorvon PJ, Cotton PB, Mason RR, Siegel JH, Hatfield ARW. Percutaneous transhepatic assistance for duodenoscopic sphincterotomy. Gut. 1985;26:1373–6.
4. Albert JG, Finkelmeier F, Friedrich-Rust M, Kronenberger B, Trojan J, Zeuzem S, Sarrazin C. Identifying indications for percutaneous (PTC) vs. endoscopic ultrasound (EUS)—guided "rendezvous" procedure in biliary obstruction and incomplete endoscopic retrograde cholangiography (ERC). Z Gastroenterol. 2014;52(10):1157–63.
5. Swahn F, Regnér S, Enochsson L, Lundell L, Permert J, Nilsson M, Thorlacius H, Arnelo U. Endoscopic retrograde cholangiopancreatography with rendezvous cannulation reduces pancreatic injury. World J Gastroenterol. 2013;19(36):6026–34. https://doi.org/10.3748/wjg.v19.i36.6026.
6. Schreuder AM, Booij KAC, de Reuver PR, van Delden OM, van Lienden KP, Besselink MG, Busch OR, Gouma DJ, Rauws EAJ, van Gulik TM. Percutaneous-endoscopic rendezvous procedure for the management of bile duct injuries after cholecystectomy: short- and long-term outcomes. Endoscopy. 2018;50(6):577–87. https://doi.org/10.1055/s-0043-123935.
7. Speer AG, Cotton PB, Russell RC, Mason RR, Hatfield AR, Leung JW, MacRae KD, Houghton J, Lennon CA. Randomised trial of endoscopic versus percutaneous stent insertion in malignant obstructive jaundice. Lancet. 1987;2(8550):57–62.

Part III

EUS: What and How

26 EUS Diagnostic Puncture

Paolo Giorgio Arcidiacono and Livia Archibugi

EUS diagnostic puncture or EUS-guided tissue acquisition (EUS-TA) has been performed for the first time in the early 1990s, by Prof. Peter Vilmann [1] being the pioneer on this technique, and has greatly evolved throughout these past years, with the development of new techniques and devices. This helped raise the sensitivity and specificity of this procedure, being nowadays 85–89% and 96–99%, respectively, for pancreatic lesions [2–4]. It is currently performed as a routine procedure for outpatients and is being increasingly used as it is able to give an accurate diagnosis with a very low risk of side effects.

EUS-TA is performed with linear scopes, as radial ones, depending on the device, either do not have a working channel or the different orientation of the probe in regard to working channel hampers the safe visualization of the tract needle during the biopsy.

Electronic Supplementary Material The online version of this chapter (https://doi.org/10.1007/978-3-030-42569-2_26) contains supplementary material, which is available to authorized users.

P. G. Arcidiacono (✉) · L. Archibugi
Pancreato-Biliary Endoscopy and Endosonography Division, Pancreas Translational and Clinical Research Center, San Raffaele Scientific Institute IRCCS, Vita-Salute San Raffaele University, Milan, Italy
e-mail: arcidiacono.paologiorgio@hsr.it

26.1 Indications

In order to correctly and safely perform the procedure, the first thing to think of is the indication. Although risk of complications for EUS diagnostic puncture is relatively low (about 0.2–2%) [5], we are performing an invasive procedure, and the benefit we'll get from the EUS diagnostic puncture has to outreach the risk of complications.

Main indications to perform an EUS diagnostic puncture are either to confirm a suspected neoplasia and determine its nature (e.g., puncturing a pancreatic cyst) or its staging (e.g., puncturing a suspected node), or for a differential diagnosis between a benign and a malignant neoplasia, or to assess the presence of an infection (e.g., in a walled-off pancreatic necrosis).

26.1.1 What Can I Puncture?

Ideally, anything inside the gastrointestinal wall or bronchial wall or close enough to it that is reachable with a needle passing through the scope for example, mediastinal masses or pulmonary lesions; abdominal organs like the pancreas, the liver, the bile duct, and the gallbladder; less frequently, left adrenal gland lesions or splenic lesions or suspected peritoneal carcinomatosis; other lesions through the rectal wall; or even ascites in case of small volumes not easily reached percutaneously.

M. Mutignani et al. (eds.), *Endotherapy in Biliopancreatic Diseases: ERCP Meets EUS*,
https://doi.org/10.1007/978-3-030-42569-2_26

EUS-TA is considered better than transabdominal US-guided or CT-guided biopsies as there is less tissue to go through and therefore a lower risk of complications and seeding [6].

Based on ESGE guidelines from 2017 [6] on EUS sampling, in case of:

- **Pancreatic solid lesions**, we should perform EUS-TA as first-line procedure when a pathological diagnosis is required. In case of metastatic disease, a percutaneous approach on the metastasis is recommended.
- High suspicion of **malignant disease** with a first negative or inconclusive result, we should either re-evaluate the slides or repeat EUS-TA or go to surgery.
- **Pancreatic cystic lesions** ≤10 mm, we do not require EUS-TA, unless high-risk stigmata are present.
- **Pancreatic cystic lesions** ≥10 mm, we should perform EUS-FNA to perform biochemical analyses of the fluid with dosage of amylase and carcinoembryonic antigen (CEA) and cytopathological examination in case the diagnosis will change the management of the patient. In these cases, in the occurrence of a small volume of the cyst, the priority goes to the dosage of intracystic CEA. In cases of very low amount of liquid, it is suggested to puncture the wall and perform an analysis for KRAS mutation.
- **Indeterminate biliary strictures**, we can perform EUS-FNA as an alternative or in combination with ERCP sampling. It is nevertheless still debated whether, in case of unresectable biliary malignancy amenable of liver transplantation, this can be considered a safe technique. In fact, in case of liver transplantation, the immunosuppressive therapy could lead to a high risk of spread of an eventual seeding [7].
- **Esophageal cancer**, we should perform FNA for the evaluation of regional lymph nodes in T1/T2 adenocarcinoma and distant nodes suspected for metastasis or left liver lesions or peritoneal carcinomatosis.
- **Lymphadenopathy of unknown origin**, we should perform FNA in case no superficial lymphadenopathy is revealed and easily accessible and in case sampling will affect the patient management.
- **Solid liver masses** that are suspected for being **metastasis**, we should perform FNA if this will change patient's management only if the lesion is not or poorly percutaneously accessible or if it has already been sampled percutaneously with inconclusive results or in case of lesions not previously visualized during cross-sectional imaging.
- **Ampullary lesions**, we can consider performing EUS sampling.
- **Subepithelial lesions**, we can perform EUS sampling in case a bite-on-bite biopsy has not retrieved a diagnosis only, in case of asymptomatic hypoechoic lesions ≥2 cm in the stomach if surveillance is considered, or when we are considering targeted therapy for a suspected GIST, when we suspect a carcinoma, neuroendocrine tumor, lymphoma, or intramural metastasis. There is no indication to perform EUS sampling in case of necessary surgery for symptomatic lesions, <2 cm lesions of the stomach or esophagus, pathognomonic EUS appearance of duplication cyst or lipoma, patient not candidate for a treatment, or esophageal subepithelial cysts.
- **Diffuse esophageal/gastric/rectal wall thickening**, after standard biopsies have failed to retrieve a diagnosis, we should perform EUS sampling aiming at a core biopsy, with flow cytometry performed in case of suspected GI lymphoma.

26.2 Contraindications

In terms of safety, strictly depending also on the experience of the operator and balancing the risks and benefits of the procedure, EUS-TA is usually contraindicated in case of:

- Coagulopathy with INR >1.5 or platelet count <50,000/mmc, although no reliable data on the topic exist, these are reasonable rules used in common clinical practice for invasive techniques at higher risk of bleeding.

- Antithrombotic therapy as referred by the British Society of Gastroenterology and ESGE guidelines [8], with anticoagulants and P2Y12 receptor antagonists, which should be stopped with adequate advance. Acetylsalicylic acid (ASS) does not need to be discontinued.
- For lesions of the adrenal gland, a pheochromocytoma needs to be excluded before performing EUS-TA. In fact, in case of a pheochromocytoma, with performing a puncture there is a high risk of abrupt release of catecholamine that can put the patient in serious danger.
- Pancreatic lesion (especially cystic lesions) situated >10 mm from the transducer [9], although this is strictly dependent on the operator's experience.

Again, contraindications are not absolute and strictly depend on the need of the diagnosis and the experience of the operator and have to be clearly discussed with the patients.

26.3 Starting the Exam

In general, it is advisable to first perform a complete evaluation of all the explorable abdominal and/or thoracic organs, evaluate the lesion closely and from different positions, and leave the puncture as the final part of the exam. This is mostly for two reasons:

1. You might decide that the puncture is not necessary anymore (e.g., when the diagnosis is clear enough just by looking at the lesion or when something else arises from the evaluation of abdominal organs).
2. When you puncture a lesion, you might:
   - Alter the ability of evaluating that lesion (e.g., if you aspirate the fluid from a cyst you will alter its dimension and might alter the echogenicity of the lesion, e.g., causing a bleeding into the cyst lumen or the formation of a hematoma in the gastrointestinal wall)
   - Cause a complication that will require an abrupt interruption of the exam and therefore prevent you from completing the examination.

26.4 Scope Positioning to Perform Puncture

The right position of the scope is crucial in order to perform a proper puncture. Once identified the lesion we intend to puncture, we need to study the best position to puncture it. The aim has to be:

- Puncture it from the closest position (the less tissue to go through, the less probable a complication will happen)—so, e.g., a pancreatic lesion of the head might be punctured from the duodenal bulb or the second portion of the duodenum.
- Find the most stable position: remember that you are exploring a body with a tube inserted in a hollow organ and that the human body is made mostly of soft tissue not perfectly stable; if you push against a wall with a needle, either your needle goes through the wall or your scope will be pushed away from the wall and you might not reach the lesion. If you have to puncture a pancreatic mass, remember that the stomach has a big lumen, a thicker wall to be penetrated, and wall layers able to slide one onto each other; also the stomach wall is more mobile compared to the duodenum. Therefore, from the stomach, the puncture might be less easily performed, while the second portion of the duodenum, with its thinner walls and more fixed position, can offer a preferable access to the lesion. On the other hand, the second portion of the duodenum, especially during the retraction of the scope and if no balloon or rigid scope is used, might be a less stable position.
- Avoid vessels as much as possible: this will reduce the risk of bleeding and the risk of having a bloody sampling.
- Avoid, if possible, pancreatic and bile ducts: this will reduce the risk of post-procedural pancreatitis and cholangitis.

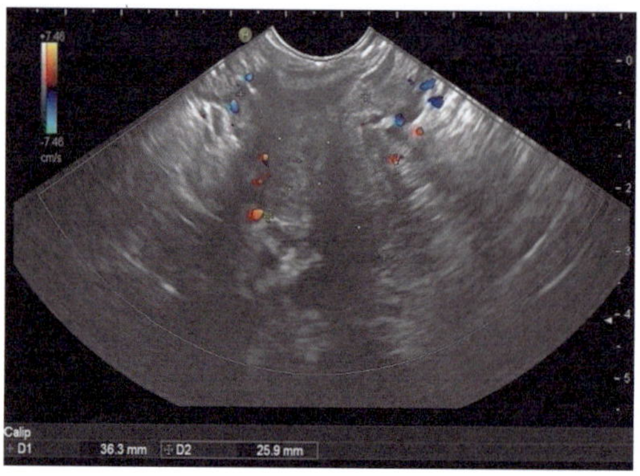

Fig. 26.1 Vessels around a lesion. Color Doppler identifies vessels near the target lesion, especially those in the tract of the needle toward the target lesion. A pulsative Doppler helps differentiating an artery (high speed, pulsative/spiky flow) from a vein (low speed, Doppler with waves, no spikes)

Passing the needle through the operating channel, you have to keep in mind that the torsion of the scope might limit the passage of the needle; this could be more frequent in case of small working channel instruments or with big size needs that are more rigid and therefore could block in the distal part of the working channel. Therefore, it is sometimes better to maintain the proper position of the scope with the handles blocked only after the passage of the needle sheath inside the operating channel and the anchorage of the needle handle onto the scope. On the other hand, this should be balanced with the fact that in particularly difficult positions, it is better to pass the needle with the handles blocked in order to maintain the position (Fig. 26.1).

26.5 Puncturing: How to Perform It Step-by-Step

1. Remember to explore everything before performing the EUS-TA; don't go straight to the lesion to puncture it.
2. Identify the target lesion and move the endoscope until the lesion is in the center of the image.
3. Antibiotic prophylaxis: if you are going to sample a cystic lesion → fluoroquinolones or beta-lactam; if you are going to sample a solid mass or a lymph node, no antibiotic is needed [5].
4. Find the best position (see tips mentioned previously in the *Scope Positioning to Perform Puncture* paragraph).
5. Use the color Doppler to check for vessels.
6. Remove the valve at the entrance of the scope working channel.
7. Have somebody pass you the needle (make sure the needle is in position 0 in order to avoid having the needle tip uncovered, which might damage the working channel of the scope).
8. Pass the needle sheath inside the working channel of the scope, and, once it is all in, tighten the needle handle onto the entrance of the scope working channel (another important issue is to lock the protection catheter at 0 position in order to have the possibility to easy lock the needle to the luer lock of the working channel).
9. Check again the scope position, and identify again the target lesion: focusing on the needle might have moved the scope and have you lost the proper position.
10. Once the position is found, block the up-down/left-right handles on the scope.
11. Release half-way the elevator.
12. Untighten the sheath handle, and advance it until you see it against the GI wall in the ultrasonographic view.
13. Move the elevator and the scope so that the elevator is in the most closed way possible but still centering the lesion. Why so? The more closed the elevator, the wider the angle between the scope and the needle and, therefore, the more stable the puncture will be.
14. *Based on the type of needle you are using you might need to* retract the stylet for a few mm (in case you are using the stylet) to uncover the sharp part of the needle.
15. Untighten the needle blockage handle, and slowly advance the needle making sure it's under ultrasonographic view. If not, gently turn the scope on both sides until you clearly see the needle. You must always keep the needle under sonographic view for the whole EUS-TA in order to evaluate how deep you are going and that you are clearly centering the lesion.

16. Where to aim? For cystic lesions aim at the center; for solid lesions you can either aim at the center or, as some might suggest, aim at some more peripheral part of the lesion where there is less chance to encounter necrosis.
17. Advance the needle until you reach what you were aiming: since you have to go through a gastrointestinal wall made of many different layers comprehending also a muscular layer, this passage might need some fast, firm, and determined stroke to take advantage of the sharp part of the needle.
18. Advance the stylet inside the needle so that the tissue of the gastrointestinal wall that has been cut and got inside the needle is actually pushed outside the needle (in case you are using the stylet): in this way you'll allow more "space" for the tissue of the lesion you are aiming at.
19. At this point:
    - In case of use of syringe negative pressure: ask your assistant to completely remove the stylet, and apply the syringe (once the vacuum inside of it it's been created).
    - In case of use of "slow-pull technique": ask your assistant, while you advance and retract the needle, to slowly retract the stylet until this is almost all out of the needle (see later for which one to use).
20. When puncturing a solid lesion, movement of the needle inside and outside the lesion has to be fast and firm when getting in, slow when getting out.
21. How many times you have to move the needle in and out inside the lesion depends on the operator experience (usually 15–20).
22. Once done with the movement of the first passage, firmly retract the needle to the "0" position, and tighten up the handle to block it.
23. Untighten the needle handle from the scope working channel and have your assistant remove the needle from the scope.
24. To express the sampling from the needle, either flush with air or saline or reinsert the stylet inside the needle.

26.6 Choosing the Needle

Compared to just a few years ago, nowadays many types of needles are quickly becoming available. They differ in:

- Size (19, 20, 22, or 25 gauge).
- Shape of the tip → this is what changes between an FNA and FNB needle. FNB needles have a special cutting tip or side slot made to cut the tissue and preserve the architecture of the lesion. The ability of evaluating the architecture is, in fact, what distinguishes a cytological examination from a histological examination. All other needles with no special tip are considered FNA needles.
- Visibility in ultrasound: some needles are designed with dimples or other features on the distal part to increase echogenicity.
- Flexibility: new needles in nitinol are less stiff and give the possibility to use 19G needles more easily.

Is there one recommended needle? The answer is not really; it really depends on your experience and the availability of a high-quality cytopathology department at your center. Yet, guidelines [5] give us some suggestions based on what we are going to puncture:

- **Pancreatic or other solid masses and lymph nodes** → 22G or 25G, either FNA or FNB.
- **Core tissue specimen** → 19G FNA or FNB needles or 22G FNB.
- **Pancreatic cystic lesions (with no solid component)** → 19G or 22G, empty the cyst with a single pass.
- **Pancreatic cystic lesions (with solid component)** → sample the solid component just like other solid lesions.
- **Suspected autoimmune pancreatitis** → 19G FNB.

Although a large-caliber needle might be more attractive as it provides a specimen with a more conserved architecture and therefore suitable for histological examination and the first thought is "large-caliber needle = bigger specimen = better diagnosis," we need to keep in mind two things:

- Large-caliber needles are more stiff. When the scope is in the duodenum, the passage of a large-caliber needle through the working channel can be difficult and can damage the scope.
- FNB is more useful for gastrointestinal subepithelial lesions, while is not necessary for other solid lesions.
- An FNB needle can provide material with a preserved architecture, but if our aim is to have more cells because we aim at a DNA evaluation (see paragraph *Future Perspectives in EUS Diagnostic Punctures*), FNA needles seem to retrieve a larger amount of DNA compared to histological slides (Figs. 26.2, 26.3, and 26.4).

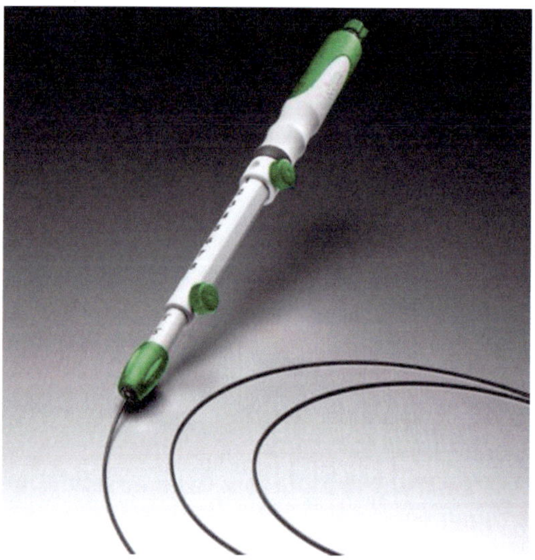

Fig. 26.2 Example of FNB needle. (Copyright of Boston Scientific)

26.7 Additional Tips and Tricks to Get More and Higher-Quality Material

- For solid masses and LNs, current guidelines suggest the use suction with a 10 mL syringe, although new studies are showing the benefits of using a slow-pull technique [10].
- Neutralize residual negative pressure before withdrawing the needle from the lesion closing the stopcock of the syringe and removing the syringe from the needle handle.
- The use of the stylet is suggested or even mandatory (depending on the type of needle) when performing FNB, while for FNA there is no clear indication whether to keep the stylet in or not, but it depends on the operator's preference.
- "Wet suction": pre-flushing the needle with saline in order to replace the air inside with a liquid that is less compressible and therefore more able to transmit the negative pressure from one side of the needle (syringe or stylet) to the tip. This seems to improve sample adequacy.
- "Stylet slow-pull": consists in the slow removal of the stylet (speed of removal not standardized) which creates a minimal negative pressure inside the needle. It's estimated that this creates a 5% of the force generated with the syringe. It is still debatable whether this technique is better compared to the standard technique with the syringe.
- Whether to leave the stylet in while performing the sampling depends on the endosonographer's preference; in fact, the potential advantages are to prevent clogs or contamination with GI cells or easier and controlled expressing from the needle, but potential disadvantages are the risk to damage the needle

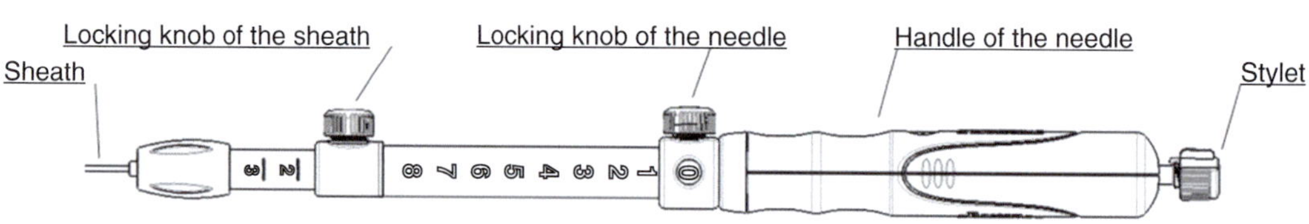

Fig. 26.3 Parts of the needle. (Copyright of Boston Scientific)

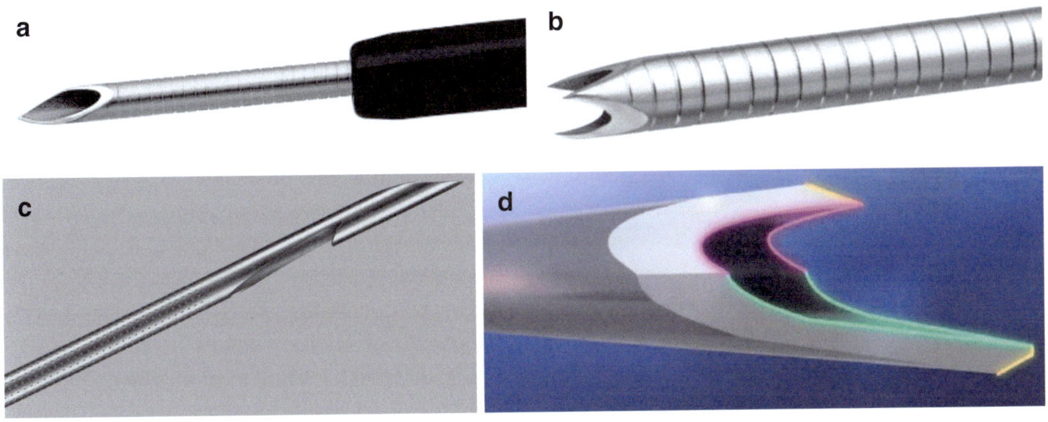

Fig. 26.4 Types of needle varying based on the "tip": (**a**) Chiba (e.g., Boston Scientific SlimLine). (**b**) Franseen (e.g., Boston Scientific Aquire). (**c**) Westcott (e.g., Cook Medical ProCore). (**d**) ForkTip (e.g., Medtronic SharkCore). (Copyright of Boston Scientific, Cook Medical and Medtronic)

during stylet manipulation, to increase needle stiffness, and to increase procedure time.

- "Fanning" the needle throughout the lesion for solid lesions and LNs: this means to change the direction of the back-and-forth movement during the same pass, progressively closing or opening the elevator (Fig. 26.3). This allows, for each pass, to target multiple areas within the same lesion.
- "ROSE": rapid on-site cytological evaluation consists in a rapid evaluation of the adequacy of tissue sample by a technician or a cytopathologist, with a first diagnostic orientation of the acquired tissue rapidly evaluated at the microscope. From a recent survey, this is available only in about half of European centers as it is more expensive and it is not clear yet whether this increases diagnostic accuracy or not. From guidelines it is generally suggested that if:
  - ROSE is available → stop when the cytopathologist/technique is satisfied.
  - ROSE is unavailable → 3–4 passes with FNA needle or 2–3 with FNB.
- Have a good communication with the cytopathology department in order to share useful information about your diagnostic hypothesis. This will help the pathologists to be guided in some direction or another and perform a more accurate diagnosis.
- For cystic lesions, if you are an experienced endosonographer and already in the past the cytological evaluation was poor, one additional tip could be to try to "scratch" the opposite wall with the needle while performing EUS-TA or try to perform a biopsy of the cystic wall with FNB needles; be aware that this technique might increase the risk of bleeding (Fig. 26.5).

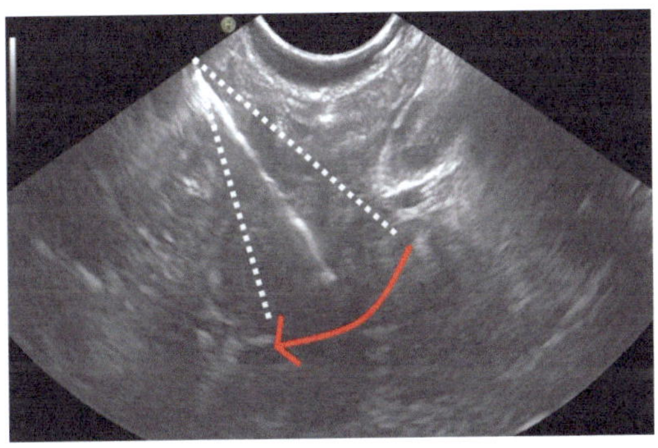

Fig. 26.5 Fanning technique

26.8 Cytopathology

26.8.1 Cytology or Histology?

This depends on the suspected diagnosis (pancreatic adenocarcinoma vs neuroendocrine tumor; GIST, etc.) and on the availability of ROSE or expert pathologist at your center.

This topic is extensively discussed in Part VII.

26.9 Markers in Pancreatic Cystic Fluid

The main purpose of cyst fluid evaluation is the differential diagnosis between pancreatic cystic lesions.

As reported before, in a cyst fluid, main analyses to be performed are amylase, CEA, and cytological evaluation.

Amylase level can exclude pancreatic pseudocysts (amylase <250 U/L) with a sensitivity of 0.44 and a specificity of 0.98, but cannot differentiate between other non-mucinous and mucinous cysts [9].

CEA level of ≥192 ng/ml can distinguish mucinous from non-mucinous cysts with a sensitivity of 52–78% and a specificity of 63–91% [9].

Currently, although used in some trials, there is no sufficient evidence to support the use of other tumoral markers such as Ca 19.9, Ca 125, Ca 72.4, Ca 15.3, or others [9]. An interesting and inexpensive marker to distinguish mucinous vs non-mucinous cysts seems to be the dosage of glucose in the cyst fluid, as lower levels of glucose are associated to mucinous cysts [11].

DNA markers such as mutation in GNAS and KRAS evaluated with next-generation sequencing (NGS) seem promising in identifying mucinous cysts [12]. Other interesting diagnostic molecular markers seem to be TP53, SMAD4, and CDKN2 [13].

Compared to what was thought in the past, differential diagnosis between mucinous cystic neoplasms (MCN) and IPMN based on CEA, amylase levels, and/or cytopathology is not possible.

Differential diagnosis between the cystic lesions of the pancreas has to be established combining cyst morphology, cystic fluid markers, and cytology.

26.10 Complications

Complications are explained in detail in Part IV.

26.11 What to Remember After the Puncture

- Observe the patients: performing an EUS diagnostic puncture means the patient underwent an invasive procedure with risk of complications which occur mostly in the first hours after the procedure; currently there is no standard post-procedural management of the patient undergoing EUS-TA, and this strictly depends on local protocols.
- If you punctured a cyst and aspirated the whole fluid emptying the cyst, don't be surprised if the cyst is smaller at next follow-up exam.

26.12 Future Perspectives in EUS Diagnostic Punctures

EUS is becoming a leading technique in the evaluation and tissue acquisition of many different organs for its ability to reach sites that were not thought to be easily reached unless with invasive techniques at high risk of complications. Great interest is now given to the discovery of new devices to increase EUS-TA diagnostic yield, and in the upcoming future, new techniques will be included in the routine practice. So let's see what the future holds for us.

26.12.1 Confocal Laser Endomicroscopy (CLE)

It is a technique developed in the early 2000, based on tissue illumination with a low-power laser with subsequent detection of the fluorescence of light reflected from the tissue through a pinhole. It was firstly adopted for the evaluation of gastrointestinal mucosa and later, with the development of new devices, also for biliary and pancreatic tissue. It is now mostly adopted for the evaluation of pancreatic cystic neoplasms, where a through-the-needle probe is passed through a 19G needle inside a cystic lesion, in order to evaluate the wall of the cyst.

This gives high-resolution images with great magnification that are almost comparable to an in vivo microscopy analysis of the cyst and helps differentiate the nature of the cyst. Although it has been adopted for many years now, data on this technique are still lacking, mostly for its high cost.

26.12.2 Microbiopsy Forceps

Moray micro forceps (US Endoscopy, Mentor, Ohio, USA) can be passed through a 19G working channel and allow, with a jaw opening width of 4.3 mm, to perform a biopsy of the cyst wall with a subsequent histological evaluation. It is also being tested in solid pancreatic lesions with success, but the experience on both cystic and solid lesion is still scarce, but new interesting studies on the topic are on the way.

26.12.3 Cytology Brush

This device is a brush designed to go through a 19G EUS needle, introduced in the market only few years ago. The EchoBrush (ECHO-19-CB; Cook Medical, Bloomington, Ind) allowed direct sampling of cystic pancreatic epithelium under EUS guidance and could therefore increase diagnostic accuracy in the differential diagnosis of pancreatic cystic neoplasms. The rate of complications due to the use of this device was although high, and, therefore, its utility has not been investigated further more (Fig. 26.6).

26.12.4 Fine Needle Vein Puncture

This technique allows to evaluate circulating tumor cells (CTCs) and free-circulating tumor DNA/RNA in the bloodstream (portal vein) in order to perform a "liquid biopsy." CTCs and tumor DNA/RNA enter the bloodstream early during the course of the disease and this technique can help with an early detection and monitoring of cancer therapy, also aiding in an early identification of mutations that confer resistance to therapy. It is carried out with a 19G needle reaching the portal vein transhepatically, where you can find higher levels of pancreatic adenocarcinoma cells compared to peripheral blood samples.

In general, for cancer therapy, there is high expectation on tumor genotyping and molecular profiling in order to plan a "personalized medicine." One example for pancreatic cancer is the evaluation of somatic BRCA mutations which seem to identify a group of patients who responds, as for patients carrying a germline BRCA mutation, better to platinum-based chemotherapy.

In conclusion, EUS diagnostic puncture is nowadays a routine technique that retrieves crucial information for patient's management.

In order to perform it properly, there are many steps that need to be followed and that we hope to have exhaustively explained in the chapter.

The field is in constant expansion, but there is still a lot to do: we still need to know which technique or needle is the best to obtain an accurate diagnosis; we need to understand if and how the

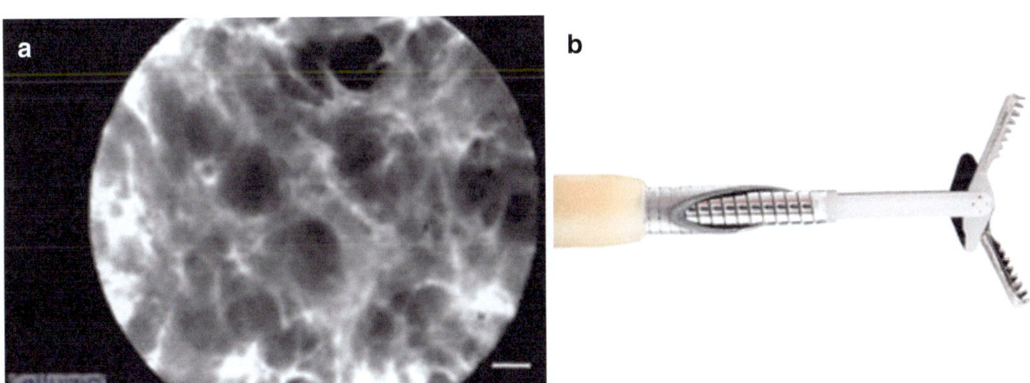

Fig. 26.6 (**a**) Confocal laser endomicroscopy; (**b**) Moray micro forceps. (Copyright of Springer and US Endoscopy)

new devices and technologies presented above will help us get useful information and in which context we should use them, etc. Hopefully, all the questions will be answered with the help of the new endosonographer colleagues who are being properly prepared reading this book.

References

1. Vilmann P, Jacobsen GK, Henriksen FW, et al. Endoscopic ultrasonography with guided fine needle aspiration biopsy in pancreatic disease. Gastrointest Endosc. 1992;38:172–3.
2. Hebert-Magee S, Bae S, Varadarajulu S, et al. The presence of a cytopathologist increases the diagnostic accuracy of endoscopic ultrasound guided fine needle aspiration cytology for pancreatic adenocarcinoma: a meta-analysis. Cytopathology. 2013;24:159–71.
3. Hewitt MJ, McPhail MJ, Possamai L, et al. EUS-guided FNA for diagnosis of solid pancreatic neoplasms: a meta-analysis. Gastrointest Endosc. 2012;75:319–31.
4. Puli SR, Bechtold ML, Buxbaum JL, et al. How good is endoscopic ultrasound-guided fine-needle aspiration in diagnosing the correct etiology for a solid pancreatic mass?: a meta-analysis and systematic review. Pancreas. 2013;42:20–6.
5. Polkowski M, Larghi A, Weynand B, et al. Learning, techniques, and complications of endoscopic ultrasound (EUS)-guided sampling in gastroenterology: European Society of Gastrointestinal Endoscopy (ESGE) Technical Guideline. Endoscopy. 2012;44(2):190–206.
6. Dumonceau JM, Deprez PH, Jenssen C, et al. Indications, results, and clinical impact of endoscopic ultrasound (EUS)-guided sampling in gastroenterology: European Society of Gastrointestinal Endoscopy (ESGE) Clinical Guideline—updated January 2017. Endoscopy. 2017;49(7):695–714.
7. Cazacu IM, Luzuriaga Chavez AA, Saftoiu A, et al. A quarter century of EUS-FNA: progress, milestones, and future directions. Endosc Ultrasound. 2018;7(3):141–60.
8. Veitch AM, Vanbiervliet G, Gershlick AH, et al. Endoscopy in patients on antiplatelet or anticoagulant therapy, including direct oral anticoagulants: British Society of Gastroenterology (BSG) and European Society of Gastrointestinal Endoscopy (ESGE) guidelines. Endoscopy. 2016;48(4):385–402.
9. European Study Group on Cystic Tumours of the Pancreas. European evidence-based guidelines on pancreatic cystic neoplasms. Gut. 2018;67(5):789–804.
10. Chen JY, Ding QY, Lv Y, et al. Slow-pull and different conventional suction techniques in endoscopic ultrasound-guided fine-needle aspiration of pancreatic solid lesions using 22-gauge needles. World J Gastroenterol. 2016;22(39):8790–7.
11. Carr RA, Yip-Schneider MT, Simpson RE, et al. Pancreatic cyst fluid glucose: rapid, inexpensive, and accurate diagnosis of mucinous pancreatic cysts. Surgery. 2018;163(3):600–5.
12. Lee JH, Kim Y, Choi JW, Kim YS. KRAS, GNAS, and RNF43 mutations in intraductal papillary mucinous neoplasm of the pancreas: a meta-analysis. Springerplus. 2016;5:1172.
13. Raman A, Lennon AM. Cyst fluid biomarkers—diagnosis and prediction of malignancy for cystic lesions of the pancreas. Visc Med. 2018;34(3):178–81.

Ancillary Diagnostic Techniques in EUS

27

Anna Cominardi and Pietro Fusaroli

27.1 EUS Elastography

Endoscopic ultrasound (EUS) elastography is a diagnostic imaging technique based on the measurement of tissue elasticity (hardness); it has a fundamental role in the diagnosis and management of biliopancreatic diseases.

It was introduced in the 1990s and now represents an important tool for a correct characterisation of pancreatic lesions and abdominal and mediastinal lymph nodes.

Two different elastography techniques have been developed and are still part of daily clinical practice: strain and shear wave [1].

The former is a qualitative method based on the evaluation of tissue response to an external or internal force (strain is usually generated by manual compression or cardiovascular pulsation), based on the principle that stiffer tissue is less deformed under compression than softer tissue. Subsequently, tissue deformations within a region of interest (ROI) are compared with each other, and the resultant strains are visualised on the B-mode image as different colours, which demonstrate the different stiffness of the ROI. This technique cannot evaluate the quantity of tissue stiffness, but it can help in identifying malignant lesions because they appear harder than the adjacent tissue.

In brief, strain technique analyses tissue stiffness by a colour-based qualitative and semi-quantitative method: it translates, by assigning a different colour to different grades of tissue deformation after compression, the different elasticity values to a colour scale from dark blue to cyan, green, yellow and red. This colour scale overlays the conventional greyscale EUS image. The red-green-blue colour map describes stiffer areas as blue and the softer ones as green or red [2] (Figs. 27.1 and 27.2).

Another qualitative method is a five-step score method based on the description of the main pattern of the lesion, which can be described as homogenously hard, heterogeneously hard, mixed, heterogeneously soft or homogeneously soft [3].

Qualitative methods can be performed by using both radial and linear echoendoscopes. The pressure generated by the probe and its variations created by vessels pulsation are usually enough to obtain accurate images. It is usually accepted that the target lesion should represent 25–50% of the ROI [4] and the ROI should consist in 50% of lesion and 50% of surrounding tissue [5].

The semi-quantitative method is achieved in two different ways: by strain histograms or strain ratio analysis. The strain histogram, which expresses on X-axis elasticity value and on Y-axis number of pixels, might be created by new

A. Cominardi · P. Fusaroli (✉)
University of Bologna, Bologna, Italy
e-mail: pietro.fusaroli@unibo.it

M. Mutignani et al. (eds.), *Endotherapy in Biliopancreatic Diseases: ERCP Meets EUS*,
https://doi.org/10.1007/978-3-030-42569-2_27

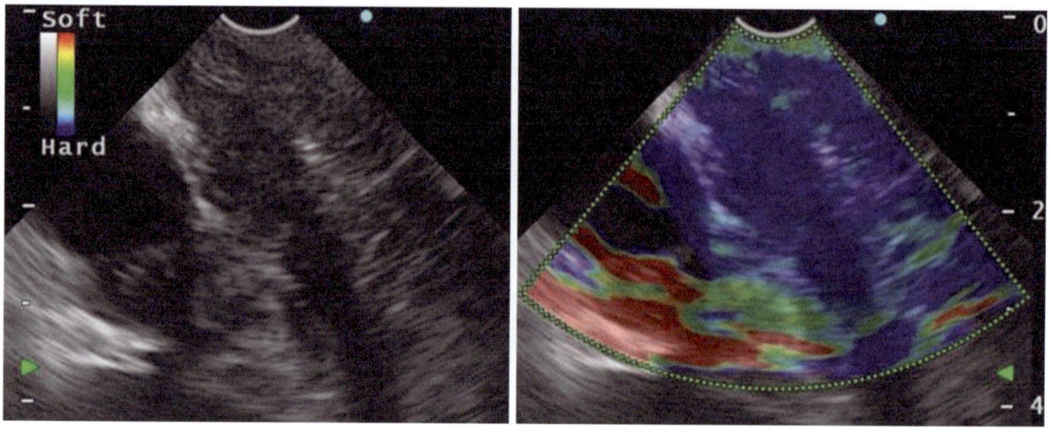

Fig. 27.1 Pancreatic head adenocarcinoma. Comparison between the B-mode image (left) and elastography (right), which shows the blue-coloured malignant lesion. This characteristic is due to the presence of harder tissue in correspondence of the neoplastic area

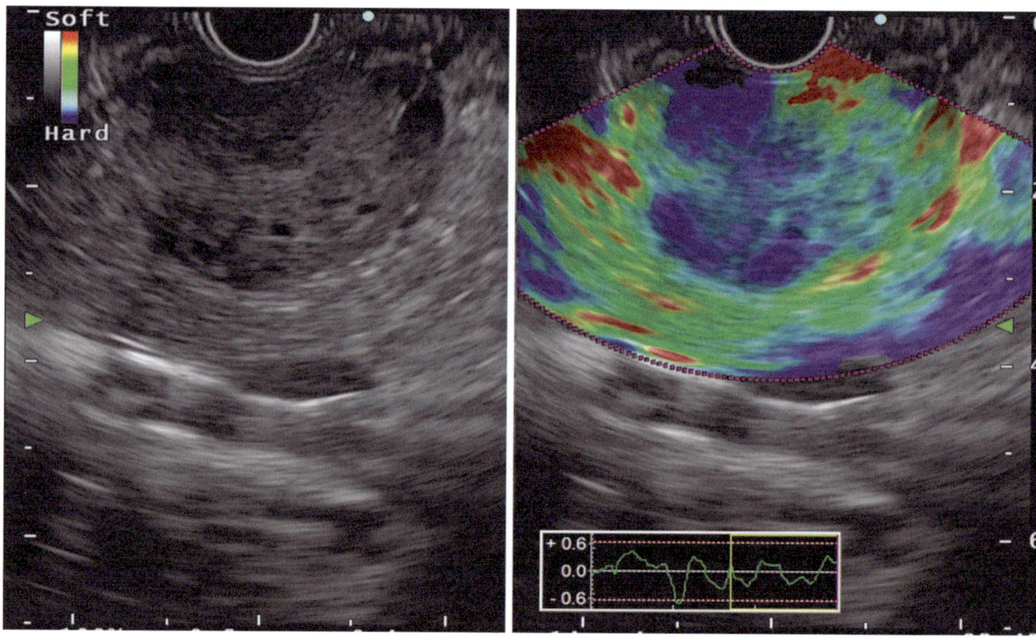

Fig. 27.2 Neuroendocrine tumour (NET) of the pancreas, with a moderate differentiation (G2). Comparison between the B-mode image (left) and elastography (right). This lesion shows a heterogeneous blue/green pattern, representing areas of necrosis inside the tumour

ultrasound machines, and it is a mean value of elasticity strains in a selected region of interest [6]. Alternatively, the strain ratio is the ratio of the mean strain between different ROI [7, 8].

Shear wave elastography has a correlation with tissue elasticity, and it can objectively express tissue hardness by calculating Young's modulus. In this technique, acoustic radiation force impulse is used to excite shear waves. However, as it is not available in EUS, we will not further cover this technique for the purpose of the present chapter.

EUS elastography is intended to perform differential diagnosis throughout different tissue stiffness, just considering that malignant lesions appear harder than benign ones.

EUS elastography can be employed in differential diagnosis of solid pancreatic lesions, lymph nodes and left liver lesions. Pancreatic cysts are seen as an artefact and should not be studied with this technique.

The pancreas is composed of soft tissue, which appears homogenously green at EUS elastography. In the presence of malignancies, this pattern is replaced by stiffer tissue (harder than surrounding pancreatic tissue), which can be visualised as heterogeneous blue lesions. This increased tissue stiffness is due to the presence of fibrosis, necrosis and desmoplasia. Nevertheless, there is no evidence of the existence of a correlation between tumour stiffness and tumour grade.

Giovannini et al. [9] proposed a five score classification for EUS elastography of the pancreas based on the colour patterns of lesions: 1 (green) represents homogenous soft normal pancreatic tissue, 2 (green, yellow and red) shows soft heterogonous fibrotic tissue, and 3, 4 and 5 (mostly blue) scores stand for hard malignant tissue. This classification showed an accuracy of 89.2% and a sensitivity of 92.3% to differentiate benign from malignant pancreatic lesions [10].

EUS elastography allows differentiating pancreatic adenocarcinoma from inflammatory masses and neuroendocrine tumours (sensitivity and specificity 100–96% and 100–88%, respectively) [1]; while carcinomas appear blue, inflammatory masses have mixed colourations (green, yellow and low-intensity blue).

EUS elastography might guide clinical management when EUS-guided tissue sampling is negative or inconclusive, although it cannot be considered a replacement for tissue sampling. Moreover, it might improve the accuracy of fine-needle aspiration/biopsy by helping in the choice of the target area to aspirate.

In patients with high suspicion of malignancies and negative tissue sampling, a combination of EUS elastography and contrast-enhanced colour Doppler ultrasound should be performed in compliance with the fact that malignant lesions appear usually hypovascular on colour Doppler ultrasound and hypo-enhancing on contrast-enhanced ultrasound [11].

In addition, EUS elastography may increase EUS-guided tissue sampling accuracy in nodal staging; it can discriminate from malignant and non-malignant lymph nodes by the qualitative method, because malignant lymph nodes appear harder than benign ones. The latter show homogeneous deformation (yellow-green pattern), while malignant lymph nodes usually have blue hard pattern.

Giovannini et al. [9] showed 100% sensitivity and 50% specificity for this technique in the differential analysis of lymph nodes and a meta-analysis 88 and 85%, respectively [12]. Janssen et al. [13] showed an accuracy up to 86% for malignant lymph nodes and to 88% for benign ones. However, the accuracy of this technique depends on the appropriate selection of the target lymph node to study.

The limitations of EUS elastography are inherent to its subjective nature of an operator-dependent technique (one of its major bias consists on ROI selection by the operator). Furthermore, its depth of penetration is limited, and the strain value might be affected by vessels, bones, cyst presence and an excessive pressure applied by the endosonographer.

27.2 Contrast-Enhanced EUS

Kato et al. first reported the use of contrast agents in EUS for the study of pancreatic masses [14] in 1995; they infused carbon dioxide gas in the superior mesenteric artery through a catheter. This technique had the limitation that can be carried out only during angiography examinations.

The subsequent development of ultrasound contrast agents composed of microbubbles for intravenous use allowed the widespread diffusion of contrast-enhanced EUS.

Ultrasound contrast agents are composed of 2–5 micrometres microbubbles, which are infused through a peripheral vein; when passing under the ultrasonic probe, they backscatter the ultrasound signal and oscillate in response to sound pressure without exiting vessel wall.

First-generation ultrasound contrast agents consisted of microbubbles of air covered by galactose and palmitic acid (Levovist; Bayer Schering Pharma, Berlin, Germany) [15]. However, Levovist needs high acoustic power to oscillate or break its microbubbles; thus it is not suitable for EUS that is equipped with a small transducer, which generates too low signals.

On the other hand, second-generation ultrasound agents are composed of microbubbles of gas (other than air) that oscillated and break under a lower acoustic power [16, 17]. These include SonoVue (Bracco SpA, Milan, Italy), Sonazoid (Daiichi-Sankyo, Tokyo, Japan; GE Healthcare Milwaukee, WI, USA) and Definity (Lantheus Medical Imaging, Billerica, MA, USA) [18].

Contrast-enhanced EUS is represented by CE-power Doppler EUS (CED-EUS) and CE harmonic EUS (CH-EUS).

CED-EUS is based on the principle that ultrasound contrast agent can increase the sensitivity of colour and power Doppler imaging because it can induce phase shift (pseudoDoppler signals), which enhances Doppler signals from vessels [17].

Conversely, CH-EUS is based on its capacity to depict the second harmonic component, which relies on direct visualisation of microbubbles themselves and not of blood flow (as Doppler imaging) [19]. It allows to visualise microvessels as well as parenchymal perfusion and to analyse the vascularisation by the measurement of time-course echogenicity [18]. A recent study showed that overall accuracy for determination of malignancies using CH-EUS was 86%; it increased to 92% when it was combined with EUS elastography [20].

The introduction of CH-EUS has further improved EUS efficacy to characterise pancreatic lesions because it allows an accurate study of vascularisation and it performs high-resolution images of the pancreas (Figs. 27.3, 27.4, and 27.5). CH-EUS can be employed for Tumour,

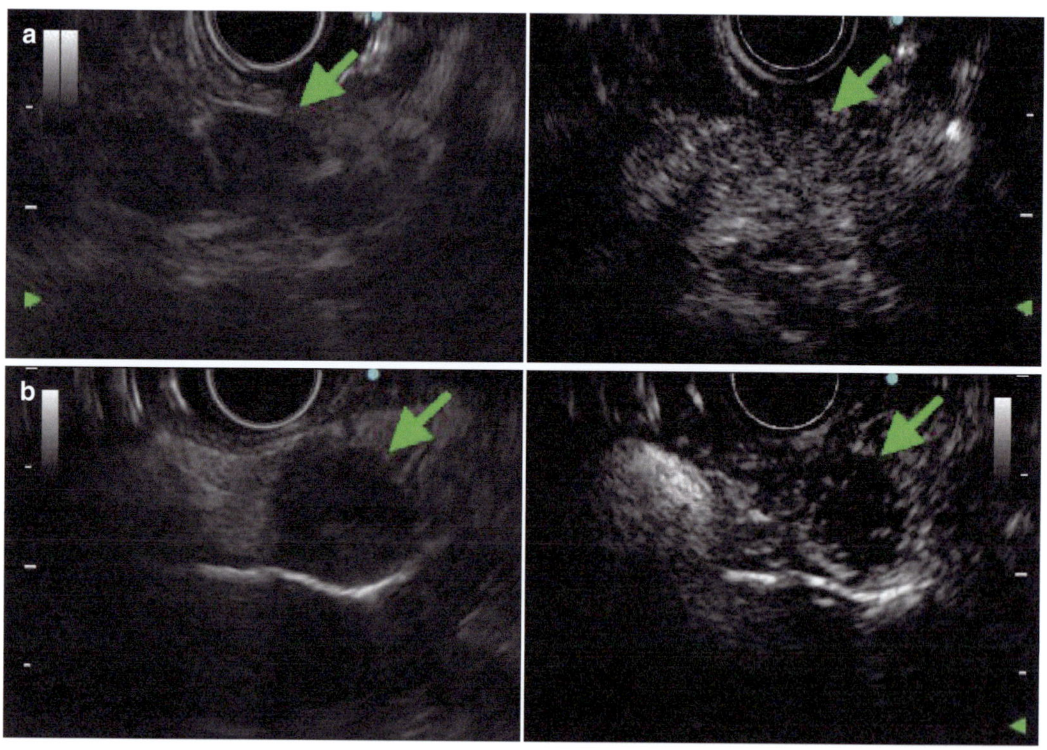

Fig. 27.3 Comparison between a benign and a malignant lymph node. (**a**) B-mode image and CH-EUS image of a benign lymph node (green arrow) which appears homogeneously enhanced. (**b**) B-mode image and CH-EUS image of a hypoenhanced malignant lymph node (green arrow)

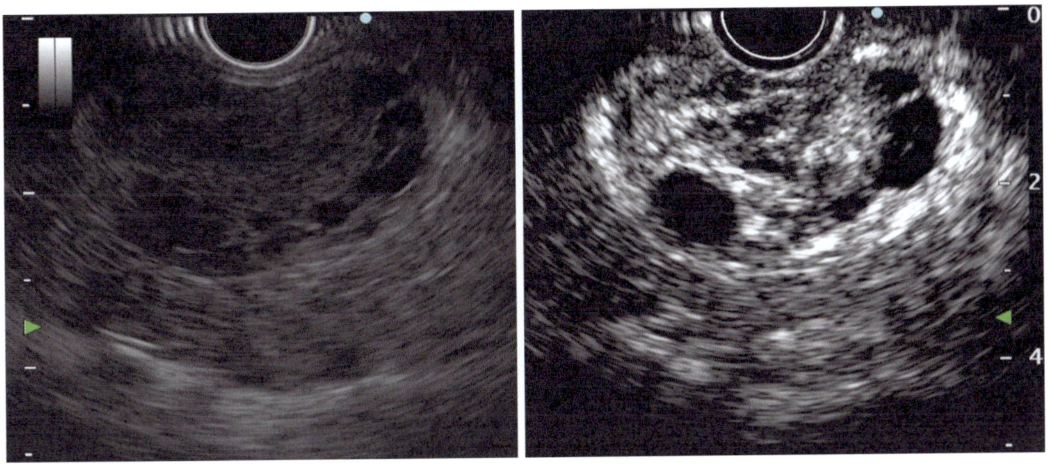

Fig. 27.4 Neuroendocrine tumour (NET) of the pancreas, with moderate differentiation (G2). Comparison between the B-mode (left) and CH-EUS (right), which shows hyperenhanced tumour interspersed with non-enhanced areas corresponding to necrosis

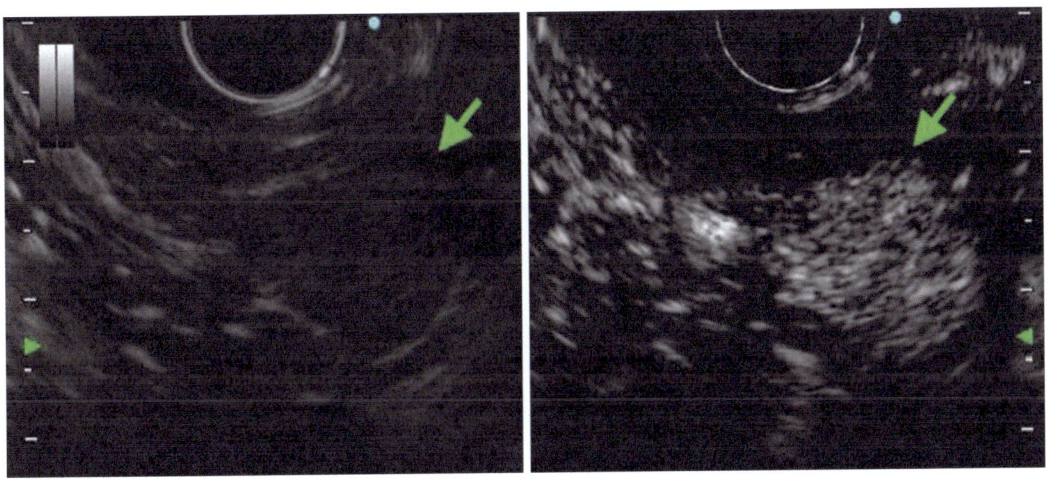

Fig. 27.5 Insulinoma. Comparison between B-mode (left) and CH-EUS (right). The tumour (green arrow) appears homogenously hyperenhanced

Node, Metastasis Cancer (TNM) staging system of pancreatic and biliary carcinomas, and it had been shown that CH-EUS could improve the diagnostic accuracy of preoperative T-staging of pancreatobiliary malignancies [21] (Figs. 27.6 and 27.7). Moreover, the overall accuracy of CH-EUS was higher than accuracy of standard harmonic EUS without contrast enhancement (92% and 69%, respectively) [21].

Pancreatic adenocarcinoma appears as hypoechoic at EUS standard imaging, while it appears hypoenhancing using CH-EUS. A meta-analysis showed that the pooled sensitivity of contrast-enhanced EUS (including both CED-EUS and CH-EUS) for the differential diagnosis of pancreatic adenocarcinomas was 94%, while the specificity was 89%. It also reported hypoenhanced lesions as accurate predictor of carcinomas [22].

Furthermore, CH-EUS sensitivity and specificity (91% and 94%, respectively) for the diagnosis of pancreatic adenocarcinoma were reported to be higher than computed tomography (CT) (71% and 92%, respectively) [23].

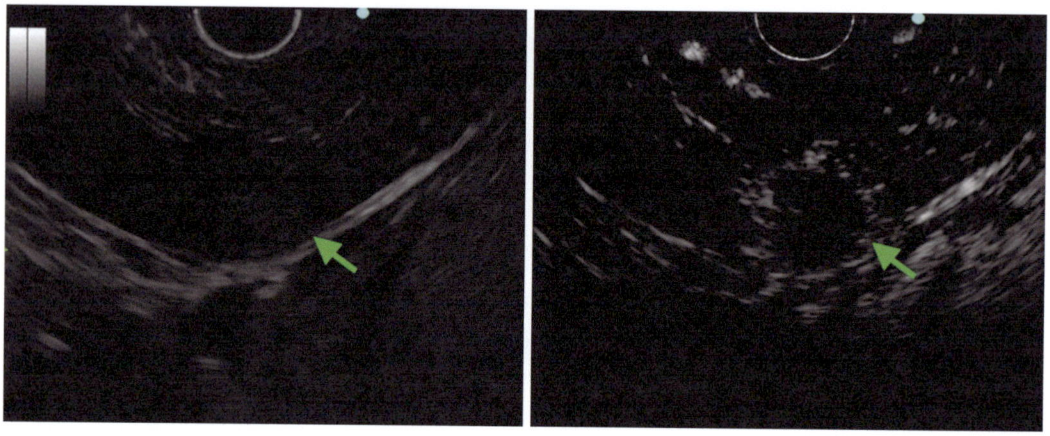

Fig. 27.6 Hepatic metastasis. Comparison between B-mode (left) and CH-EUS hypoenhanced image (on the right) of a hepatic metastasis (green arrow)

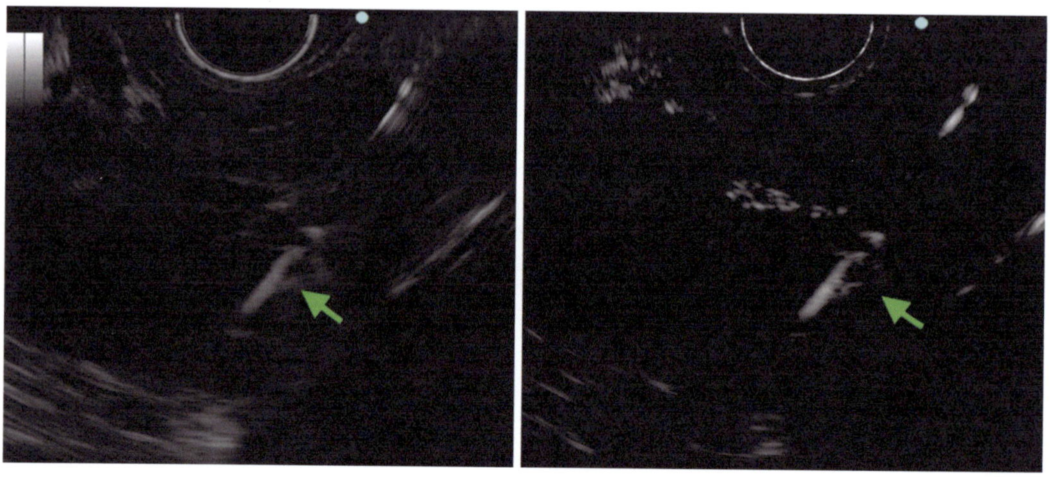

Fig. 27.7 CH-EUS-guided fine-needle aspiration of the previous hepatic metastasis

In particular, CH-EUS demonstrated a greater accuracy for the diagnosis of ductal pancreatic carcinomas ≤2 cm than CT, 89–95% sensitivity and 64–89% specificity for the identification of hypovascularity as a sign of ductal carcinomas [18, 22].

The differentiation between carcinomas, autoimmune pancreatitis and neuroendocrine tumours can also be shown by the elaboration of time-intensity curve during CH-EUS, which reveals the values of maximum intensity, accumulated intensity during observation, intensity reduction rate and the ratio between the uptake inside the mass and the uptake of the surrounding parenchyma [18].

The employment of both EUS elastography and CH-EUS ensures a higher accuracy in the study of biliopancreatic lesions and strengthens the results of fine-needle aspiration biopsy [24, 25] (Fig. 27.8).

The above-mentioned characteristics and its improvements of diagnostic and clinical outcomes make CH-EUS a valid additional tool for the differential diagnosis of biliopancreatic lesions that merits being included in routine use [24].

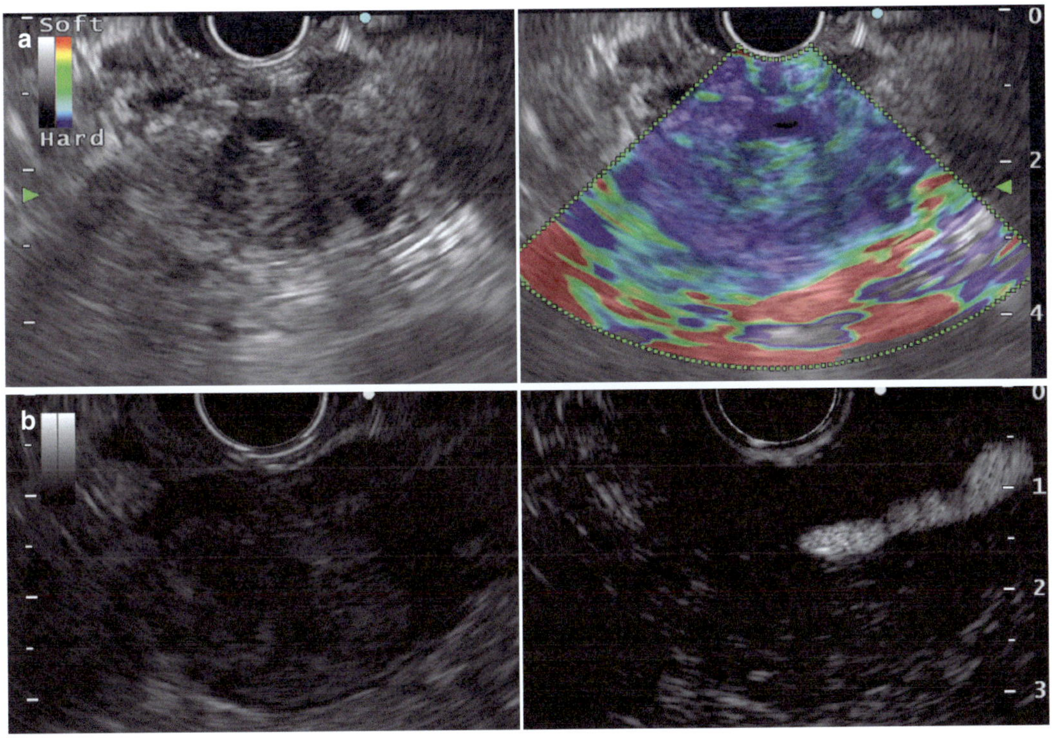

Fig. 27.8 Comparison between elastography (on the top) and CH-EUS (on the bottom) of pancreatic ductal adenocarcinoma. Elastography (**a**) shows a typical neoplastic blue pattern, while in CH-EUS (**b**) the pancreatic adenocarcinoma appears hypo-enhanced

27.3 Endoscopic Ultrasound-Guided Needle-Based Confocal Laser Endomicroscopy

Confocal laser endomicroscopy (CLE) is a contrast-based method, which enables in vivo microscopic imaging during EUS as it allows the visualisation of mucosal layer at a subcellular level of resolution. In other words, it provides in vivo histological images or "virtual biopsies".

The contrast agent is infused intravenously (usually fluorescein) or topically applied through a spray catheter (usually acriflavine), and then, a defined wavelength laser beam (usually blue laser light with a wavelength of 488 nm) is focused towards the target lesion; the recaptured signal is displayed as "optical biopsies" in the horizontal plane [26].

CLE can be performed using dedicated endoscopes (Pentax, Tokyo, Japan, herein termed eCLE) or with probe-based systems (herein termed pCLE) capable of passage through the accessory channel of most endoscopes (Cellvizio, Mauna Kea Technologies, Paris, France) [27]. Moreover, Mauna Kea Technologies (MKT) has developed high-resolution probe for CLE that can pass through the accessory channel of any endoscope [25].

Recently, a novel microprobe that can pass through a 19-gauge EUS-FNA needle has been introduced [28]; thus real-time endomicroscopic information with a needle-based CLE approach (nCLE) can be achieved. Confocal methods allow evaluating pancreatic malignancies and lymph nodes before EUS-guided tissue sampling in order to assess preliminarily the diagnosis of malignancy.

Konda et al. [29] managed a pilot study about the application of needle-based confocal laser endomicroscopy under endosonographic guidance for pancreatic cystic neoplasms; their

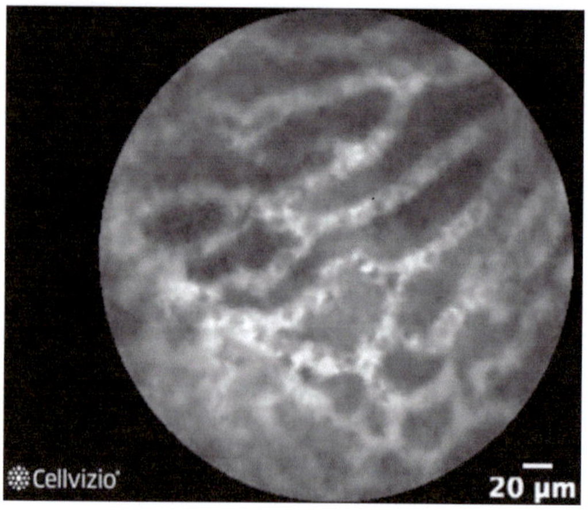

Fig. 27.9 EUS-guided confocal laser endomicroscopy. The regular vessel network is pathognomonic for the diagnosis of serous cystadenoma. (Courtesy of Dr. Bertrand Napoleon, Hospital Mermoz, Lyon, France)

preliminary data showed high nCLE specificity and low sensitivity in detecting this disease, and they suggested that this technique required further evaluation. INSPECT study showed that CLE may increase the detection of pancreatic cystic lesions and aid their management algorithm [30].

This was confirmed by DETECT study, which affirmed that the combination of dual through-the-needle imaging (cystoscopy and nCLE) of pancreatic cysts appears to have strong concordance with the clinical diagnosis of pancreatic cystic lesions (Fig. 27.9) [31].

Since the low negative predictive value of fine-needle aspiration biopsy and the absence of rapid on-site evaluation technique (ROSE) in many institutions, nCLE, in addition of CH-EUS, could be a useful tool for the differential diagnosis of solid pancreatic masses by providing an in vivo cellular assessment, especially since Giovannini et al. [32] in 2016 proposed CLE criteria for the diagnosis of pancreatic adenocarcinoma (dark cell aggregates, irregular vessels with leakages of fluorescein), chronic pancreatitis (residual regular glandular pancreatic structures) and NET (black cell aggregates surrounded by vessels and fibrotic areas).

In conclusion, nCLE has shown to be a valuable supplementary technique for EUS by providing additional information for the study of pancreatic lesions, but its widespread is limited by its cost and learning curve [33].

References

1. Cui XW, Chang JM, Kan QC, Chiorean L, Ignee A, Dietrich CF. Endoscopic ultrasound elastography: current status and future perspectives. World J Gastroenterol. 2015;21(47):13212–24.
2. Dietrich CF, Săftoiu A, Jenssen C. Real time elastography endoscopic ultrasound (RTE-EUS), a comprehensive review. Eur J Radiol. 2014;83(3):405–14.
3. Costache MI, Dumitrescu D, Săftoiu A. Technique of qualitative and semiquantitative EUS elastography in pancreatic examination. Endosc Ultrasound. 2017;6(Suppl 3):S111–4.
4. Havre RF, Elde E, Gilja OH, Odegaard S, Eide GE, Matre K, Nesje LB. Freehand real-time elastography: impact of scanning parameters on image quality and in vitro intra- and interobserver validations. Ultrasound Med Biol. 2008;34(10):1638–50.
5. Hirche TO, Ignee A, Barreiros AP, Schreiber-Dietrich D, Jungblut S, Ott M, Hirche H, Dietrich CF. Indications and limitations of endoscopic ultrasound elastography for evaluation of focal pancreatic lesions. Endoscopy. 2008;40(11):910–7.
6. Săftoiu A, Vilmann P, Gorunescu F, Gheonea DI, Gorunescu M, Ciurea T, Popescu GL, Iordache A, Hassan H, Iordache S. Neural network analysis of dynamic sequences of EUS elastography used for the differential diagnosis of chronic pancreatitis and pancreatic cancer. Gastrointest Endosc. 2008;68(6):1086–94.
7. Schrader H, Wiese M, Ellrichmann M, Belyaev O, Uhl W, Tannapfel A, Schmidt W, Meier J. Diagnostic value of quantitative EUS elastography for malignant pancreatic tumors: relationship with pancreatic fibrosis. Ultraschall Med. 2012;33(7):E196–201.
8. Iglesias-Garcia J, Larino-Noia J, Abdulkader I, Forteza J, Dominguez-Munoz JE. Quantitative endoscopic ultrasound elastography: an accurate method for the differentiation of solid pancreatic masses. Gastroenterology. 2010;139(4):1172–80.
9. Giovannini M, Hookey LC, Bories E, Pesenti C, Monges G, Delpero JR. Endoscopic ultrasound elastography: the first step towards virtual biopsy? Preliminary results in 49 patients. Endoscopy. 2006;38(4):344–8.
10. Giovannini M, Thomas B, Erwan B, Christian P, Fabrice C, Benjamin E, Geneviève M, Paolo A, Pierre D, Robert Y, Walter S, Hanz S, Carl S, Christoph D, Pierre E, Jean-Luc VL, Jacques D, Peter V, Andrian S. Endoscopic ultrasound elastography for evaluation of lymph nodes and pancreatic masses: a multicenter study. World J Gastroenterol. 2009;15(13):1587–93.
11. Sidhu PS, Cantisani V, Dietrich CF, Gilja OH, Saftoiu A, Bartels E, Bertolotto M, Calliada F, Clevert DA,

Cosgrove D, Deganello A, D'Onofrio M, Drudi FM, Freeman S, Harvey C, Jenssen C, Jung EM, Klauser AS, Lassau N, Meloni MF, Leen E, Nicolau C, Nolsoe C, Piscaglia F, Prada F, Prosch H, Adzina M, Savelli L, Weskott HP, Wijkstra H. The EFSUMB guidelines and recommendations for the clinical practice of contrast-enhanced ultrasound (CEUS) in non-hepatic applications: update 2017 (short version). Ultraschall Med. 2018;39(2):154–80.

12. Xu W, Shi J, Zeng X, Li X, Xie WF, Guo J, Lin Y. EUS elastography for the differentiation of benign and malignant lymph nodes: a meta-analysis. Gastrointest Endosc. 2011;74(5):1001–9; quiz 1115.e1–4.
13. Janssen J, Dietrich CF, Will U, Greiner L. Endosonographic elastography in the diagnosis of mediastinal lymph nodes. Endoscopy. 2007;39(11):952–7.
14. Kato T, Tsukamoto Y, Naitoh Y, Hirooka Y, Furukawa T, Hayakawa T. Ultrasonographic and endoscopic ultrasonographic angiography in pancreatic mass lesions. Acta Radiol. 1995;36(4):381–7.
15. Quaia E. Classification and safety of microbubble-based contrast agents. In: Quaia E, editor. Contrast media in ultrasonography. Basic principles and clinical applications. Berlin: Springer; 2005. p. 1–14.
16. Kudo M. Various contrast-enhanced imaging modes after administration of Levovist. In: Kudo M, editor. Contrast harmonic imaging in the diagnosis and treatment of hepatic tumors. Tokyo: Springer; 2003. p. 22–30.
17. Kitano M, Kudo M, Sakamoto H, Nakatani T, Maekawa K, Mizuguchi N, Ito Y, Miki M, Matsui U, von Schrenck T. Preliminary study of contrast-enhanced harmonic endosonography with second-generation contrast agents. J Med Ultrason (2001). 2008;35(1):11 8.
18. Kitano M, Sakamoto H, Kudo M. Contrast-enhanced endoscopic ultrasound. Dig Endosc. 2014;26(Suppl 1):79–85.
19. Kitano M, Sakamoto H, Matsui U, Ito Y, Maekawa K, von Schrenck T, Kudo M. A novel perfusion imaging technique of the pancreas: contrast-enhanced harmonic EUS (with video). Gastrointest Endosc. 2008;67(1):141–50.
20. Iglesias-Garcia J, Lindkvist B, Lariño-Noia J, Abdulkader-Nallib I, Dominguez-Muñoz JE. Differential diagnosis of solid pancreatic masses: contrast-enhanced harmonic (CEH-EUS), quantitative-elastography (QE-EUS), or both? United European Gastroenterol J. 2017;5(2):236–46.
21. Imazu H, Uchiyama Y, Matsunaga K, Ikeda K, Kakutani H, Sasaki Y, Sumiyama K, Ang TL, Omar S, Tajiri H. Contrast-enhanced harmonic EUS with novel ultrasonographic contrast (Sonazoid) in the preoperative T-staging for pancreaticobiliary malignancies. Scand J Gastroenterol. 2010;45(6):732–8.
22. Gong TT, Hu DM, Zhu Q. Contrast-enhanced EUS for differential diagnosis of pancreatic mass lesions: a meta-analysis. Gastrointest Endosc. 2012;76(2):301–9.
23. Kitano M, Kudo M, Yamao K, Takagi T, Sakamoto H, Komaki T, Kamata K, Imai H, Chiba Y, Okada M, Murakami T, Takeyama Y. Characterization of small solid tumors in the pancreas: the value of contrast-enhanced harmonic endoscopic ultrasonography. Am J Gastroenterol. 2012;107(2):303–10.
24. Fusaroli P, Napoleon B, Gincul R, Lefort C, Palazzo L, Palazzo M, Kitano M, Minaga K, Caletti G, Lisotti A. The clinical impact of ultrasound contrast agents in EUS: a systematic review according to the levels of evidence. Gastrointest Endosc. 2016;84(4):587–96.
25. Fusaroli P, Saftoiu A, Dietrich CF. Contrast-enhanced endoscopic ultrasound: why do we need it? A foreword. Endosc Ultrasound. 2016;5(6):349–50.
26. Karstensen JG, Cârþânã T, Constantinescu C, Dumitraşcu S, Kovacevic B, Klausen P, Hassan H, Klausen TW, Bertani H, Bhutani MS, Săftoiu A, Vilmann P. Endoscopic ultrasound guided needle-based confocal laser endomicroscopy in solid pancreatic masses—a prospective validation study. Endosc Int Open. 2018;6(1):E78–85.
27. Giovannini M. Endoscopic ultrasound-guided confocal microscopy: a new tool for the new year? Endosc Ultrasound. 2013;2(1):1–2.
28. Konda VJ, Aslanian HR, Wallace MB, Siddiqui UD, Hart J, Waxman I. First assessment of needle-based confocal laser endomicroscopy during EUS-FNA procedures of the pancreas (with videos). Gastrointest Endosc. 2011;74(5):1049–60.
29. Konda VJ, Meining A, Jamil LH, Giovannini M, Hwang JH, Wallace MB, Chang KJ, Siddiqui UD, Hart J, Lo SK, Saunders MD, Aslanian HR, Wroblewski K, Waxman I. A pilot study of in vivo identification of pancreatic cystic neoplasms with needle-based confocal laser endomicroscopy under endosonographic guidance. Endoscopy. 2013;45(12):1006–13.
30. Konda VJ, Meining A, Jami LH, Giovannini M, Chang KJ, Hwang JH, Wallace MB, Sididiqui UD, Asianian HR, Lo SK, Hart SJ, Waxman I. An international, multi-center trial on needle-based confocal laser endomicroscopy (nCLE): results from the *in vivo* CLE study in the pancreas with endosonography of cystic tumors (INSPECT). Gastroenterology. 2012;142(Suppl):S620.
31. Nakai Y, Iwashita T, Park DH, Samarasena JB, Lee JG, Chang KJ. Diagnosis of pancreatic cysts: EUS-guided, through-the-needle confocal laser-induced endomicroscopy and cystoscopy trial: DETECT study. Gastrointest Endosc. 2015;81(5):1204–14.
32. Giovannini M, Caillol F, Monges G, Poizat F, Lemaistre AI, Pujol B, Lucidarme D, Palazzo L, Napoléon B. Endoscopic ultrasound-guided needle-based confocal laser endomicroscopy in solid pancreatic masses. Endoscopy. 2016;48(10):892–8.
33. Alvarez-Sánchez MV, Napoléon B. New horizons in the endoscopic ultrasonography-based diagnosis of pancreatic cystic lesions. World J Gastroenterol. 2018;24(26):2853–66.

28 EUS-Guided Transenteric Pancreatic Duct Drainage

M. Giovannini

The development of interventional endoscopic ultrasound (EUS) has provided better access to the pancreatic region. Just as pancreatic fluid collections, such as pseudocysts, can be successfully drained from the stomach or duodenum through endoscopic cyst enterostomy or cyst gastrostomy, the same technique could be used to access a dilated pancreatic duct in cases where the duct cannot be drained by conventional ERCP because of complete obstruction.

Main indications of EUS-guided pancreatic duct drainage are stenosis of pancreatico-jejunal or pancreaticogastric anastomosis after Whipple resection, which induce recurrent acute pancreatitis, main pancreatic duct stenosis due to chronic pancreatitis, post-acute pancreatitis, or post-pancreatic trauma after failure of ERCP. The pain associated with chronic pancreatitis (CP) is caused, at least in part, by ductal hypertension. Both surgical and endoscopic treatments can relieve pain by improving ductal drainage. Endoscopic drainage requires transpapillary access to the pancreatic duct during ERCP. EUS-guided pancreaticogastro- or bulbostomy offers an alternative to surgery. Despite the advances in endoscopy, EUS-guided pancreatic duct drainage remains a technically challenging procedure.

M. Giovannini (✉)
Head of Gastroenterology and Endoscopy Department, Paoli-Calmettes Institute, Marseille, France
e-mail: giovanninim@ipc.unicancer.fr

Technical success rates are greater than 70%; however, the average rate of adverse events is nearly 20%, which increases to 55% when stent migration is included. Until recently, a significant difficulty with this technique was the absence of dedicated devices.

28.1 Technical Considerations

By using a linear interventional EUS scope, the dilated MPD was well visualized. EUS-guided pancreatic duct drainage was then performed under combined fluoroscopic and ultrasound guidance, with the tip of the echoendoscope positioned such that the inflated balloon was in the duodenal bulb while the accessory channel remained in the antrum. A 19G needle was inserted transgastrically, or through the bulbus, into the proximal pancreatic duct, and contrast medium was injected. Opacification demonstrated a pancreaticography. A straight or angulated guidewire (0.025 or 0.035 in.) was introduced into the needle; at this time of the procedure, two scenarios are possible.

Option 1: The guidewire passes the stenosis, penetrates the papilla, and travels into the duodenum. A rendezvous technique should be performed by exchanging the EUS scope for a duodenoscope, and "classic" pancreatic endotherapy could be performed. This technique should be the first choice when the anatomy of

M. Mutignani et al. (eds.), *Endotherapy in Biliopancreatic Diseases: ERCP Meets EUS*,
https://doi.org/10.1007/978-3-030-42569-2_28

the patient is intact because the complication rate is very low (Fig. 28.1).

Option 2: The guidewire does not pass the stenosis, or the patient has had a previous surgery (Whipple or gastrectomy). The needle is exchanged over a guidewire (0.025 or 0.035 in.) for a 6.5F or 8F diathermic sheath (Cysto-Gastro set, EndoFlex, Voerde, Germany), which is then used to enlarge the channel between the stomach and the main pancreatic duct. The sheath is introduced using a cutting current. After the exchange over the guidewire (rigid 0.025 or 0.035 in. diameter), a 7F, 7-cm-long pancreaticogastric stent is positioned (Fig. 28.2). This stent will be exchanged for two 7F or one 8.5F stent 1 or 2 months after the first procedure (Fig. 28.3). This technique was first reported in a study on EUS-guided pancreaticogastrostomy by François et al. [1]. Other authors reported different techniques. Although the first steps are similar to the puncture of the main pancreatic duct (pancreatography and guidewire insertion), they [2, 3] used a balloon dilation instead the cystostome as

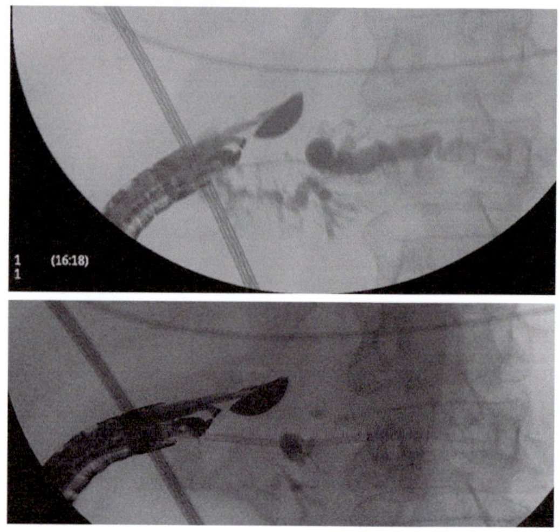

Fig. 28.2 Pancreatico-bulbostomy/chronic pancreatitis with thigh stenosis of the MPD in the head of the pancreas, failure of ERCP

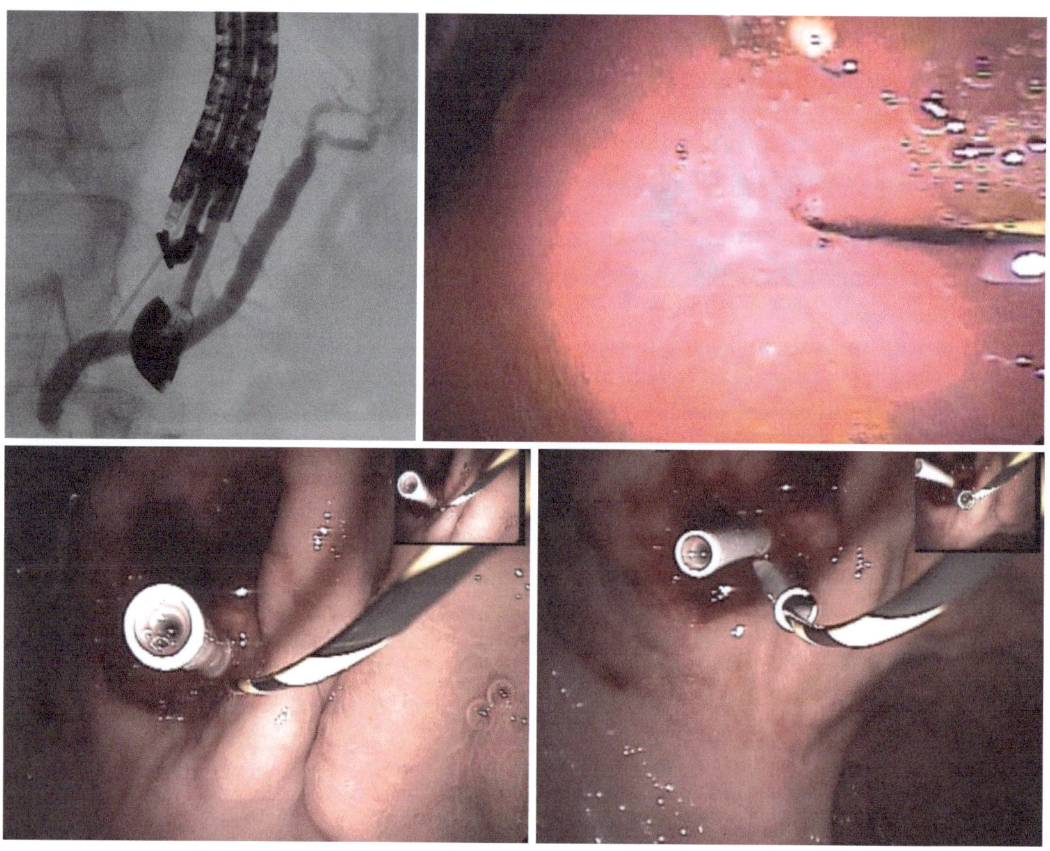

Fig. 28.1 Rendezvous technique on pancreaticogastrostomy/stenosis of a Wirsung gastronomy anastomosis after Whipple resection for benign cystic lesion of the head of the pancreas

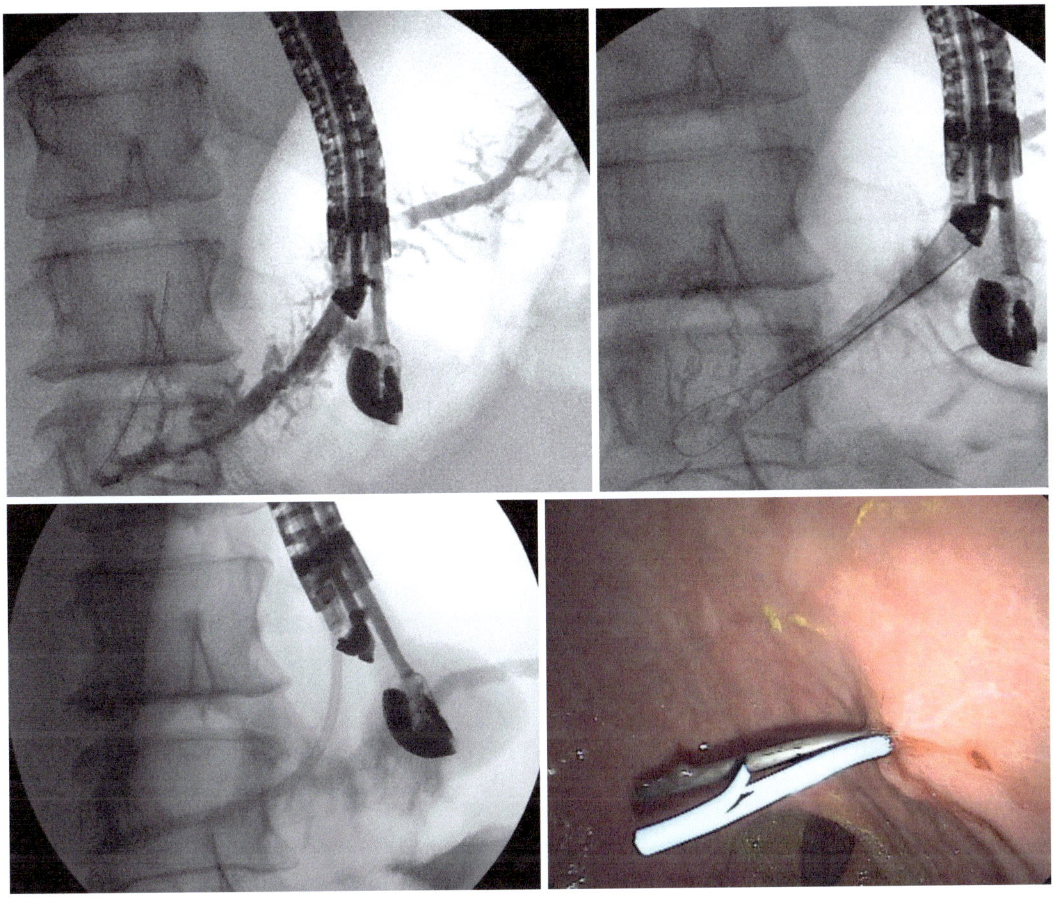

Fig. 28.3 Pancreaticogastrostomy: stenosis of the Wirsung jejunostomy after Whipple surgery for a pancreatic NET of the head of the pancreas

reported in the PRINCEPS study [1] and also in the paper of Tessier et al. [4].

Discussion should be focused on the preventive role of pancreatic juice leakage using the diathermic technique compared to the balloon dilation. In our experience, peripancreatic collection occurred more frequently when a balloon dilation was used compared to a diathermic catheter that prevents the creation of fibrosis around the puncturing tract, causing a leak of pancreatic juice.

The results of the series [2–8] of patients published do not recommend the use of a wider EUS-guided pancreatic duct drainage (Table 28.1), which in any case should be restricted to tertiary centers specializing in biliopancreatic therapy with a pain relief of 70%. However, the complication rate is still high, around 15%, and includes bleeding, pancreatic collection, and perforation. Nevertheless, the possibility of draining the main pancreatic duct into the digestive tract through an endoscopically created fistula, with patency maintained by stent placement, might be interesting as an alternative drainage method without the complication of stent occlusion that is associated with transpapillary drainage.

The first large series of EUS-guided pancreatic duct drainage was published by Tessier et al. [4] on 36 patients. Indications were chronic pancreatitis with complete obstruction (secondary to a tight stenosis, a stone, or main pancreatic duct rupture), inaccessible papilla or impossible cannulation (n = 20), anastomotic stenosis after a Whipple procedure (n = 12), complete main pancreatic duct rupture after acute pancreatitis (AP), or trauma (n = 4). EUS-guided pancreaticogastrostomy or bulbostomy was unsuccessful in three patients; one was lost to follow-up. Major complications occurred in two patients and included one hematoma and one severe acute

Table 28.1 Studies on EUS-guided pancreaticogastrostomy

Authors	Number of Patients	% Success (%)	% Complication (%)	Follow –up (months)
Tessier GIE, 2007	36	70	11	16.5
Kahaleh GIE, 2007	13	92	16	14
Barkay GIE, 2010	21	48	2	13
Ergun Endoscopy, 2011	20	90	10	37
Fuji GIE,2013	45	74	6	32
Will WJG, 2015	94	81.9	8	28
Oh D GIE, 2016	25	100	20	5

pancreatitis. The median follow-up was 14.5 months (range, 4–55 months). Pain relief was complete or partial in 25 patients (69%, intention to treat). Eight patients treated had no improvement of their symptoms (four were subsequently diagnosed with cancer). Stent dysfunction occurred in 20 patients (55%) and required a total of 29 repeat endoscopies.

Fuji et al. [3] reported his experience in 45 patients, where 37 underwent failed ERCP and 29 had surgically altered anatomy. The median follow-up after initial EUS-guided intervention was 23 months. Two patients underwent EUS for stent removal, and EUS-guided pancreatic duct stent placement was attempted in 43 patients. Technical success was achieved in 32/43 (74%) with antegrade (n = 18) or retrograde (n = 14) stent insertion. Serious adverse events occurred in three patients (6%). Patients underwent a median of two (range 1–6) follow-up procedures for revision or removal of stents, without complications. Complete symptom resolution occurred in 24/29 (83%) while stents were in place, with non-dilated ducts in 6 patients. Stents were removed in 23 patients, who were then followed up for an additional median of 32 months; 4 had recurrent symptoms. Among the 11 failed cases, most had persistent symptoms or required surgery.

A larger study was reported by Will et al. [9]. This study enrolled 94 patients who underwent EUS-guided pancreatography and subsequent placement of a drain. In total, 94 patients underwent 111 interventions using one of three different approaches: (1) EUS endoscopic retrograde drainage with a rendezvous technique, (2) EUS-guided drainage of the pancreatic duct, and (3) EUS-guided, internal, anterograde drainage of the pancreatic duct. The technical success rate was 100%, achieving puncture of the pancreatic duct including pancreatography. In patients requiring drainage, the initial drain placement was successful in 47/83 patients (56.6%). Of these, 26 patients underwent transgastric/transbulbar positioning of a stent for retrograde drainage; plastic prostheses were used in 11 and metal stents in 12. A ring drain (anterograde internal drainage) was placed in 3 of these 26 patients due to anastomotic stenosis after a previous surgical intervention. The remaining 21 patients with successful drain placement received transpapillary drains using the rendezvous technique; the majority (n = 19) received plastic prostheses, and only 2 received metal stents (covered self-expanding metal stents). Clinical success, as indicated by reduced or an absence of further pain after the EUS-guided intervention, was achieved in 68/83 patients (81.9%), including several who improved without drainage, but with manipulation of the access route.

In 2015, Fujii-Lau and Levy [10] summarized the current literature on EUS-guided PD drainage, reviewing the published experience of 222 patients. Including both the antegrade and rendezvous techniques, technical success was achieved in 170/222 patients (76.6%). A similar review by Itoi et al. [11] in 2013 reported a technical success rate of >70% in 75 patients using the antegrade technique and a range of success rates from 25 to 100% in 52 patients using the rendezvous technique.

Oh et al. [12] reported in 2016 the use of a pancreatic metallic stent (FCSEMS). Twenty-five consecutive patients with painful obstructive pancreatitis underwent EUS-guided MPD with a FCSEMS after failed ERCP. EUS-guided MPD was successful in all 25 patients (technical success rate, 100%), and symptoms improved in all patients (clinical success rate, 100%). EUS-guided pancreaticogastrostomy ($n = 23$), pancreaticoduodenostomy ($n = 1$), and pancreaticojejunostomy ($n = 1$) were performed. Pain scores improved significantly after FCSEMS placement ($p = 0.001$). Early mild-grade adverse events occurred in five patients (20%), four with self-limited abdominal pain, and one with minor bleeding. No other adverse events related to FCSEMS were observed during the follow-up period, including stent migration, stent clogging, pancreatic sepsis, and stent-induced ductal stricture. Mean stent patency duration was 126.9 days during the mean follow-up period (221.1 days).

Recently, an international, multicenter, retrospective study on the safety and efficacy of EUS-PDI after failed ERP was published [13]. Eighty patients who underwent EUS-guided pancreatic duct drainage at four academic centers in three countries were analyzed. Technical success was achieved in 89% and clinical success in 81% of patients. The success rate in this study was higher than previously reported, which is likely due to increased operator experience and improvements in endoscopic equipment. The transpapillary or trans-anastomotic approaches to stent placement via rendezvous wire access seemed to be the more successful technique, with a trend toward an increased likelihood of complete symptom resolution after adjusting for sex, diagnosis, anatomy, prior failed ERCP, and technical success, but that was not statistically significant. Immediate adverse events (<24 h) occurred in 20% of patients, with 15% experiencing major complications (6 patients with post-ERCP pancreatitis, 4 who developed pancreatic fluid collections, 1 with a main pancreatic duct leak, and 1 with an intestinal perforation. Delayed adverse events (>24 h) occurred in 11% of patients (all of whom also had immediate adverse events—2 pancreatitis, 1 main pancreatic duct leak, and 4 abscesses treated with antibiotics). The method of approach (anterograde vs. rendezvous) was not a predictor of immediate or delayed adverse events, however this could have been due to the small sample size.

While EUS-guided pancreatic duct drainage has been shown to be effective, it appears to be limited by its high rates of complications. However there have been no comparative studies between EUS-guided pancreatic duct drainage and ERCP. A recent international, multicenter, retrospective study [14] was performed to compare these two modalities in terms of technical success, clinical success, and adverse events rates in patients with post-Whipple anatomy. Sixty-six patients underwent 75 procedures (40 EUS-guided pancreatic duct drainage and 35 ERCP). Technical success of EUS-guided pancreatic duct drainage was 92.5% compared with 20% in the ERCP group (odds ratio [OR], 49.3; $p < 0.001$). Clinical success was achieved in 87.5% of EUS-guided pancreatic duct drainage procedures compared with 23.1% in the ERCP group (OR, 23.3; $p < 0.001$). However, adverse events occurred more commonly in the EUS-guided pancreatic duct drainage group (35% vs. 2.9%, $p < 0.001$).

28.2 Clinical Algorithm

ERP should remain a first-line treatment, even in patients with surgically altered anatomy, based on its superior safety profile. This is especially true considering the low case volume of EUS-guided pancreatic duct drainage being performed, even at experienced, expert centers. Regarding the three techniques, the rendezvous technique [7] should be used initially because the complication rate is very low, and EUS-guided pancreatico-bulbostomy is recommended for MPD stenosis in the head of the pancreas because the EUS scope position is stable. EUS-guided pancreaticogastrostomy should be utilized when the patient's anatomy is altered (Whipple or gastrectomy) and mainly in case of stenosis of Wirsung jejunostomy anastomosis. However, this technique is the most difficult with a high prevalence of complications due to the instability of the EUS scope into the stomach [6].

28.3 Conclusion

Considering the major limitations in alternative treatment options after failed ERCP, EUS-guided pancreatic duct drainage has the potential to become standard of care by avoiding more invasive and involved surgical interventions. Therapeutic EUS as pancreaticogastrostomy and EUS-guided biliary drainage currently represents an alternative to surgery or percutaneous biliary drainage when ERCP fails or is impossible due to previous surgery, such as gastrectomy or Whipple resection. Although data has demonstrated that the procedure can be safe and effective, EUS-guided PD drainage remains one of the most technically challenging therapeutic EUS interventions, as evidenced by the multiple considerations on device selection and the risk of severe complications [15]. Therefore, I advocate that this procedure should only be performed in appropriately selected patients by experienced endoscopists trained in both EUS and ERP with well-trained surgical backup available.

References

1. François E, Kahaleh M, Giovannini M, Matos C, Devière J. EUS-guided pancreaticogastrostomy. Gastrointest Endosc. 2002;56(1):128–33.
2. Barkay O, Sheman S, McHenry L, Yoo BM, Fogel EL, Watkins JL, DeWitt J, Al-Haddad MA, Lehman GA. Therapeutic EUS-assisted endoscopic retrograde pancreatography after failed pancreatic duct cannulation at ERCP. Gastrointest Endosc. 2010;7:1166–73.
3. Fujii LL, Topazian MD, Abu Dayyeh BK, Baron TH, Chari ST, Farnell MB, Gleeson FC, Gostout CJ, Kendrick ML, Pearson RK, Petersen BT, Truty MJ, Vege SS, Levy MJ. EUS-guided pancreatic duct intervention: outcomes of a single tertiary-care referral center experience. Gastrointest Endosc. 2013;78(6):854–64.
4. Tessier G, Bories E, Arvanitakis M, Hittelet A, Pesenti C, Le Moine O, Giovannini M, Devière J. US-guided pancreatogastrostomy and pancreatobulbostomy for the treatment of pain in patients with pancreatic ductal dilatation inaccessible for transpapillary endoscopic therapy. Gastrointest Endosc. 2007;65(2):233–41.
5. Kahaleh M, Hernandez AJ, Tokar J, Adams RB, Shami VM, Yeaton P. EUS-guided pancreaticogastrostomy: analysis of its efficacy to drain inaccessible pancreatic ducts. Gastrointest Endosc. 2007;65(2):224–30.
6. Kurihara T, Itoi T, Sofuni A, Itokawa F, Moriyasu F. Endoscopic ultrasonography-guided pancreatic duct drainage after failed endoscopic retrograde cholangiopancreatography in patients with malignant and benign pancreatic duct obstructions. Dig Endosc. 2013;25(Suppl 2):109–16.
7. Takikawa T, Kanno A, Masamune A, Hamada S, Nakano E, Miura S, Ariga H, Unno J, Kume K, Kikuta K, Hirota M, Yoshida H, Katayose Y, Unno M, Shimosegawa T. Pancreatic duct drainage using EUS-guided rendezvous technique for stenotic pancreaticojejunostomy. World J Gastroenterol. 2013;19(31):5182–6.
8. Ergun M, Aouattah T, Gillain C, Gigot JF, Hubert C, Deprez PH. Endoscopic ultrasound-guided transluminal drainage of pancreatic duct obstruction: long-term outcome. Endoscopy. 2011;43:518–25.
9. Will U, Reichel A, Fueldner F, Meyer F. Endoscopic ultrasonography-guided drainage for patients with symptomatic obstruction and enlargement of the pancreatic duct. World J Gastroenterol. 2015;21(46):13140–51.
10. Fujii-Lau LL, Levy MJ. Endoscopic ultrasound-guided pancreatic duct drainage. J Hepatobiliary Pancreat Sci. 2015;22:51–7.
11. Itoi T, Kasuya K, Sofuni A, et al. Endoscopic ultrasonography-guided pancreatic duct access: techniques and literature review of pancreatography, transmural drainage and rendezvous techniques. Dig Endosc. 2013;25:241–52.
12. Oh D, Park DH, Cho MK, et al. Feasibility and safety of a fully covered self-expandable metal stent with antimigration properties for EUS-guided pancreatic duct drainage: early and midterm outcomes (with video). Gastrointest Endosc. 2016;83:366–73.
13. Tyberg A, Sharaiha RZ, Kedia P, et al. EUS-guided pancreatic drainage for pancreatic strictures after failed ERCP: a multicenter international collaborative study. Gastrointest Endosc. 2017;85:164–9.
14. Chen YI, Levy MJ, Moreels TG, et al. An international multicenter study comparing EUS-guided pancreatic duct drainage with enteroscopy-assisted endoscopic retrograde pancreatography after Whipple surgery. Gastrointest Endosc. 2017;85:170–7.
15. Giovannini M. Endoscopic ultrasound-guided pancreatic duct drainage: ready for the prime time? Endosc Ultrasound. 2017;6(5):281–4.

29 EUS-Assisted Ablation Techniques

Silvia Carrara and Milena Di Leo

29.1 Introduction

Endoscopic ultrasound (EUS) is a very fascinating technique that allows the complete exploration of structures adjacent to gastrointestinal lumen with a unique ability to reach the pancreatic parenchyma in a very minimally invasive real-time way. The technique was introduced in the early 1980s after animal and human studies [1], as a diagnostic modality. After that, the advent of the curved linear array echoendoscopes added operative features to EUS. Thanks to the longitudinal plane scanning, similar to that of the transabdominal ultrasound, it is possible to follow under real-time view a needle or any other kind of accessories coming out from the working channel of the echoendoscope. This concept was at the basis of the born of the operative EUS: if you can reach a lesion or an anatomical structure with a needle, you can also bring a device inside it, like a stent, a probe or drugs, exploring new horizons of the therapeutic EUS.

S. Carrara (✉) · M. Di Leo
Digestive Endoscopy Unit, Division of Gastroenterology, Humanitas Clinical and Research Center, Milan, Italy
e-mail: silvia.carrara@humanitas.it; milena.di_leo@humanitas.it

Interventional EUS is increasingly used to treat pancreatic and biliary diseases. Coeliac plexus neurolysis, drainage of pancreatic fluid collections, obstructive malignant biliary drainage after failed ERCP, gallbladder drainage in high-risk surgical candidates, enterostomies, EUS-ERCP rendezvous and haemostatic treatments are the most explored uses of operative EUS [2–5]. This expanding role has been possible because new accessories completely dedicated to EUS have been recently developed, and most of them can be placed with solely endosonographic control, even without fluoroscopic imaging [6].

EUS is also used for fiducial placement to target precise stereotactic body radiotherapy in gastrointestinal malignancies, such as oesophageal/gastro-oesophageal junction cancer, pancreatic cancer and rectal cancer [7, 8].

Therapeutic EUS could be applied to treat pancreatic disease such as pancreatic cystic lesions, neuroendocrine tumours (NET) and pancreatic adenocarcinoma [9].

The ideal effect of an ablative technique should be to homogeneously destroy the entire tumour in a wide enough area to cover the target lesion and with "surgical margins" (0.5–1 cm) without damaging the surrounding tissues. This belief, of course, is extremely optimistic, because the complete destruction of a tumour, especially the pancreatic cancer, with only one technique is overly hopeful. In order to reach the best possible

M. Mutignani et al. (eds.), *Endotherapy in Biliopancreatic Diseases: ERCP Meets EUS*, https://doi.org/10.1007/978-3-030-42569-2_29

outcome, the ablation techniques should be combined with other therapies.

Different ablative techniques have been proposed under EUS guidance, and they could be divided in two groups according to the mechanism of action. One group includes techniques acting directly on the lesion (direct mode), as monopolar or bipolar radiofrequency ablation (RFA), cryothermablation (HTP), photodynamic therapy (PDT), neodymium-doped yttrium aluminium garnet (Nd: YAG) laser ablation and ethanol injection. The second group encloses modality acting with an effect that is mediated by a series of events, such as the delivery of antitumoural drugs, local immunotherapy with cytoimplant and injection of modified viruses [9–11].

This chapter will present the indications and technical features of the most important ablative techniques and the future perspectives.

29.2 Indications

29.2.1 Pancreatic Adenocarcinoma

Pancreatic ductal adenocarcinoma (PDAC) is the fourth leading cause of cancer-related death in the USA, with a growing up incidence [12, 13]. Despite the progressive improvement of diagnostic methods and therapies, survival rate has not been substantially improved during the past 30 years, with a 5-year survival rate of 7.7%, for all stages combined [12]. At the time of diagnosis, about 40% of patients have a locally advanced tumour in which resection is not feasible because of local invasion [14]. An autopsy series identified 30% of patients with pancreatic cancer who died because of locally destructive disease, without evidence of distant progression.

According to National Comprehensive Cancer Network (NCCN) Guidelines [15], PDAC is defined as unresectable when it is locally advanced according to vascular involvement and there is absence of metastasis. The NCCN Guidelines underline the difference between borderline resectable PDAC and locally advanced unresectable PDAC. The second one shows at least one of the following characters: (1) arterial involvement: a contact with superior mesenteric artery or coeliac artery >180° or a contact with first jejunal superior mesenteric artery branch or, for body and tail PDAC, tumour contact with the coeliac artery and aortic involvement and (2) venous contact, unreconstructible superior mesenteric vein/portal vein due to tumour involvement or occlusion (by tumour or bland thrombus) or for head/uncinate process PDAC, a contact with most proximal draining jejunal branch into superior mesenteric vein.

In the presence of one of these characteristics, surgery becomes ineffective and may be dangerous for the patient. Moreover, the surgeon's decision on PDAC resectability has to be based not only on anatomic criteria but also on the biological behaviour of PDAC, since knowledge is growing on the genomic pattern of cancer invasion and metastases.

EUS plays an important role in the diagnosis and staging of PDAC. In locally advanced PDAC, EUS has also been proposed as a therapeutic technique in a multimodality approach where the gastroenterologist joins the oncology team in the treatment of the patients. This context, with patients enrolled in clinical trials approved by ethics committee, could be the ideal setting for a local treatment as EUS-guided ablation in addition to standard oncological treatments. Clinical guidelines, such as those of the Italian Association of Medical Oncology (AIOM) [16], formulated specific statements on local ablative treatment of pancreatic cancer (under EUS guidance, transabdominal ultrasound guidance or during open surgery), and they concluded that this kind of treatments should be performed only in specialized centres and in patients enrolled in clinical trials.

29.2.2 Pancreatic Neuroendocrine Tumours

Pancreatic neuroendocrine tumours (PNETs) are rare pancreatic neoplasms, accounting for less than 3% of pancreatic masses [17, 18]. In the last two decades, the incidence of PNET of all sizes has increased [19]. In particular, the incidence of PNETs smaller than 2 cm has remarkably increased, and the small size does not preclude malignant behaviour [20]. They can be classified according to their features: (1) hormone production (functioning/non-functioning), (2) clinical setting (sporadic/inherited syndromes) and (3) Ki-67 labelling index (three types of grading).

The treatment strategy for PNETs depends on some characteristics of the tumours, in particular the staging, the grading and the production of hormones with hormone-related syndromes. There is a wide heterogeneity in the biological behaviour of PNETs; therefore their therapeutic management includes conservative follow-up and surgery, but also systemic therapy (somatostatin analogues, chemotherapy, peptide receptor radionuclide therapy).

EUS could be used in the different steps of diagnostic and therapeutic workup of PNETs. It has a diagnostic role and its specificity is very high in functional PNETs, like insulinoma, when conventional imaging fails to localize the lesion [21, 22]. EUS-guided biopsy is helpful to confirm diagnosis giving cytological and/or histological samples, and at the same time, it is an accurate method for the grading of pNETs based on Ki-67 labelling index evaluation [23, 24]. Moreover, EUS-guided fine-needle injection can be used to tattoo small pancreatic lesions with India ink to make easier the intraoperative identification during surgery [25].

Small functioning PNETs should be a possible application of EUS-guided ablative techniques as ethanol injection or RFA [26, 27]. In particular, ENETS guidelines [28] suggested the use of endoscopic or percutaneous ablative therapy in patients with resectable insulinoma non-fit for surgery, although surgical approach remains the standard cure.

29.2.3 Pancreatic Cystic Lesions

Pancreatic cysts are incidentally discovered in up to 15% of patients undergoing cross-sectional imaging studies [29]. Mucinous cystic neoplasms carry variable malignant potential [30]. EUS and EUS-guided biopsy is one of the tools in diagnostic flow chart of pancreatic cystic lesions to classify the cyst, to collect cystic fluid and to evaluate worrisome features [31–33].

The incidence of mucinous cysts and their malignancy increase with age. In the setting of elderly patients with malignant cystic lesions unfit for surgery, the EUS-guided ablation may be an optional therapeutic tool. The revised Fukuoka guidelines [32] identified as possible candidate for EUS-guided ablation with ethanol or ethanol followed by paclitaxel patients with unilocular/oligolocular cysts more than 2 cm large and without communication with the main pancreatic duct. These patients generally had refused surgery or were high-risk surgical candidates. At the same time, the guidelines underlined some concerning issues about this procedure, such as complications, standardization of technical aspects and post-operative surveillance. Moreover, in IPMN patients, pancreatic adenocarcinoma could also occur in sites other than cystic lesions [34]. So, the authors stated that further studies are needed, in particular about techniques, materials, long-term outcomes and adequacy of this procedure, and concluded that "At present, EUS-guided ablation cannot be recommended for patients with BD-IPMN outside of a closely monitored research protocol" [32].

29.2.4 Extra-Pancreatic Indications

EUS-guided ablative techniques could also be applied to extra-pancreatic diseases, in particular in the liver, following the idea that if it is possible to puncture a mass with a needle, it would also be possible to insert a device to ablate it. Few case reports described EUS-guided ablation of hepatocellular carcinoma using different ablative techniques [35–37]. One retrospective case series described EUS guidance and percutaneous ethanol lavage therapy for huge hepatic cysts [38].

Other studies reported EUS-guided alcohol ablation of metastatic pelvic lymph nodes [39] and of left adrenal gland metastasis [40].

29.3 Ablative Techniques

The present paragraph will examine the EUS-guided ablative techniques with most data in human studies.

According to the mechanism of action, EUS-guided ablative techniques could be categorized as direct mode techniques and indirect mode techniques. The direct mode techniques act through a locoregional effect, while, in the indirect modes, the antitumoural effect is mediated by a series of events such as the delivery of antitumoural drugs, local immunotherapy with cyto-implant and injection of modified viruses [9–11]. The direct ablation mode not only effectively kills the tumoural cells (as a first direct way) but also acts in an indirect way, by releasing tumour antigens that can provoke an immune response and stimulate the inflammatory response.

Surrounding to the area of necrosis destroyed by local injury, a peripheral zone with a sublethal injury appears. In this area, oxidative stress and inflammation lead to an indirect antitumoural systemic effects.

The histological appearance of an ablated tissue presents different areas that can be easily recognized: (1) a central zone of coagulative necrosis with amorphous material and cellular debris; (2) a surrounding peripheral zone with a sublethal injury that attracts inflammatory cells, with granulation tissue and new blood vessels; and (3) a healthy, surrounding, non-ablated zone.

The advantages of loco-regional ablative techniques, compared to surgical approach, are lower rates of morbidity, less collateral damages to surrounding tissues, shorter hospital stay and overall lower costs. Table 29.1 summarizes the main human studies with hybrid probe and RFA.

29.3.1 Radiofrequency Ablation

29.3.1.1 Mechanism of Action

The radiofrequency ablation (RFA) direct effect is based on high local temperatures, generated by high-frequency alternating current, that induce coagulative necrosis of the tissue with an irreversible cellular damage [41]. Besides thermal damage, RFA seems to act also with an indirect immune-modulative effect.

The hyperthermal damage created by the delivery of high energies results in a destruction of the tumour microenvironment, loss of cell membrane integrity and subcellular injuries, especially in cancer cells that are more heat-sensitive when compared to normal tissue [42, 43].

The volume of necrotic tissue is correlated to temperature and to application time. To produce irreversible cell damage, it takes 4–5 min at 50–55 °C. At temperatures between 60 and 100 °C, there is immediate tissue coagulation. Above 100 °C, tissues vaporize. Therefore, temperatures between 50 and 100 °C are ideal for RFA, while higher temperatures are less effective because of tissue vaporization and carbonization [41] that increase tissue impedance [43] and reduce the tissue electrical conduction.

RFA can be applied percutaneously, intra-operatively or endoscopically. In the latter, two methods are currently available: ERCP-guided and EUS-guided ablation. The two endoscopic techniques have different aims. The ERCP-guided RFA is used for malignant biliary obstruction, and it has a palliative intent in cases of cholangiocarcinoma [44]. Otherwise, EUS-guided RFA has been proposed as a curative method for pancreatic lesions as PDAC, PNETs or pancreatic cystic neoplasms, in a multimodality approach or as a single treatment in case of patients unfit for any other therapy.

RFA has been widely used in the treatment of different kinds of solid tumours (hepatocellular carcinoma, renal cancer, etc.), but its application in the treatment of pancreatic lesions has always been regarded with reluctance by clinicians, for the fear of adverse events in such a thermo-sensitive organ like the pancreas and for the fear of injury to adjacent structures (e.g. the GI tract, major vessels and biliary ducts) [39]. The first RFA experiences during open surgery reported high rates of morbidity and mortality, but they helped the clinicians to understand that the iatrogenic injuries might be limited by applying some technical precautions, such as the reduction of the ablation temperature (<90 °C), the maintenance of a safety margin from major vessels or

Table 29.1 Clinical studies regarding pancreatic EUS-guided thermal ablative therapies (RFA and cryothermablation)

First author (year) [ref num]	Number of patients	Type of ablation (device)	Mean time of application in seconds (range)	Indications	Complications	Outcome
Arcidiacono et al. (2012) [73]	22	Cryothermal ablation (CryoTherm probe, ERBE)	107 ± 86	PDAC III stage	Transient abdominal pain and serum amylase level increase ($n = 3$); minor duodenal bleeding ($n = 1$); jaundice ($n = 2$; 1 with haemobilia and anaemia); duodenal stricture ($n = 1$); cystic fluid collection ($n = 1$)	100% decrease of neoplasia volume (6/6 patients); median survival time 6 months (range 1–12 m)
Wang et al. (2013) [53]	3	Radiofrequency ablation (22G Habib)	120	PDAC III stage	No	13.94% mean reduction in tumour size 46.53% mean reduction in CA19-9 levels
Rossi et al. (2014) [54]	1	Radiofrequency ablation (22G Habib)	360	PNET	No	Complete ablation and clinical response (no recurrence)
Pai et al. (2015) [55]	8	Radiofrequency ablation (19G Habib)	(range 90–120)	MCN ($n = 4$); IPMN ($n = 1$); microcystic adenoma ($n = 1$); PNET ($n = 2$)	Mild abdominal pain ($n = 2$)	33.3% complete resolution of cyst 48.4% reduction of cyst size 100% modified vascularization and presence of central necrosis in PNETs
Armellini et al. (2015) [56]	1	Radiofrequency ablation (18G STARmed)	NR	PNET	No	Complete ablation and clinical response (no recurrence)
Waung et al. (2016) [57]	1	Radiofrequency ablation (Habib)	100 (range 90–120)	Insulinoma	No	Complete ablation and clinical response (no recurrence)
Lakhtakia et al. (2016) [58]	3	Radiofrequency ablation (19G STARmed)	10–15	Insulinoma	No	100% complete clinical response; 33.3% morphologic complete response
Song et al. (2016) [59]	6	Radiofrequency ablation (18G STARmed)	10–15	PDAC III stage ($n = 4$); PDAC IV stage ($n = 2$)	Mild abdominal pain ($n = 2$)	16.7% necrosis with air bubbles in the ablation site

(continued)

Table 29.1 (continued)

First author (year) [ref num]	Number of patients	Type of ablation (device)	Mean time of application in seconds (range)	Indications	Complications	Outcome
Goyal et al. (2017) [60]	5	Radiofrequency ablation (22G Habib)	120	PNET ($n = 1$); MCN ($n = 2$); PDAC III stage ($n = 2$)	No	100% complete clinical response in PNET
Bas-Cutrina et al. (2017) [61]	1	Radiofrequency ablation (22G Habib)	120	PNET	No	Complete ablation and clinical response (no recurrence)
Feng et al. (2017) [62]	1	Radiofrequency ablation (Habib) + lauromacrogol 1% injection	360	SCA	No	Complete ablation and clinical response (no recurrence)
Malikowski et al. (2017) [64]	4	Radiofrequency ablation (Habib)	120	Metastasis from kidney ($n = 2$) and from melanoma ($n = 1$); PNET ($n = 1$)	No	25% complete morphological response; 25% partial morphological response; 25% no presence of morphological response (25% imaging not performed)
Choi et al. (2018) [27]	10	Radiofrequency ablation (22G Habib)	780 (range 600–900)	PNET ($n = 7$); SPN ($n = 2$); Insulinoma ($n = 1$)	Abdominal pain ($n = 1$); pancreatitis ($n = 1$)	70% complete morphological response; 30% partial morphological response
Crino' et al. (2018) [63]	9	Radiofrequency ablation (18G STARmed)	58 (range 15–95)	PDAC III stage ($n = 8$); renal metastasis ($n = 1$)	Mild abdominal pain ($n = 3$); asymptomatic serum amylase and lipase level increase ($n = 1$)	Ablation of 30% tumour mass
Scopelliti et al. (2018) [65]	10	Radiofrequency ablation (18G STARmed)	2149 (range 140–18,000)	PDAC III stage	Mild abdominal pain ($n = 2$); ascites ($n = 2$); peripancreatic oedema ($n = 2$); asymptomatic serum amylase level increase ($n = 2$)	100% intratumour ablation

MCN mucinous cystadenoma, *IPMN* intrapancreatic papillary mucinous neoplasm, *PNET* pancreatic neuroendocrine tumour, *PDAC* pancreatic ductal adenocarcinoma, *NR* not reported, *SPN* solid pseudopapillary neoplasm, *SCA* serous cyst adenoma from the duodenum (which can also be irrigated by cold saline) and the use of a step-up approach in case of large lesions [45–48]. Due to the retroperitoneal position of the pancreas, EUS-guided RFA could be the better choice when compared to transabdominal or surgical approach because EUS is able to guide a real-time procedure into a deeply located target such as the pancreas which is difficult to visualize and to reach by a percutaneous approach. However, the complex anatomy of surrounding structures and the need for development of EUS-specific RFA probes make the procedure more challenging than expected [49].

Two different kinds of RFA technology are currently available: monopolar and bipolar. The second one ensures a better control, because energy delivering is confined between the two electrodes with potentially less injury to the surrounding tissues, but with the trade-off of less efficiency overall [50].

Three ablation devices specifically designed for EUS are currently available:

1. The EUS-RFA System (STARmed, Goyang, South Korea) consists of a 18G needle with a monopolar RFA electrode and a VIVA RF generator (STARmed, Korea). The active electrode tips are manufactured with various lengths: 0.5 cm, 1 cm, 1.5 cm and 2 cm. The device is perfused internally with circulating chilled saline solution that cools the system during the ablation (Fig. 29.1).
2. The Habib EUS-RFA monopolar probe (EMcision Ltd., London, UK) is a 1 Fr wire (0.33 mm), with a working length of 190 cm, that can be connected to RITA (RITA Medical Systems Inc., Fremont, CA). The catheter is passed through a 19 G standard EUS needle (Fig. 29.2).
3. The HybridTherm bipolar flexible probe (ERBE Elektromedizin, Tübingen, Germany) is a 14G probe that combines bipolar RFA with cryotechnology. It has an external protective tube with a diameter of 3.2 mm (an endoscope with a working channel diameter of at least 3). 7 mm is recommended. It is used in conjunction with the VIO 300 D electrosurgical unit and with the ERBECRYO 3 cryosurgical unit (Fig. 29.3).

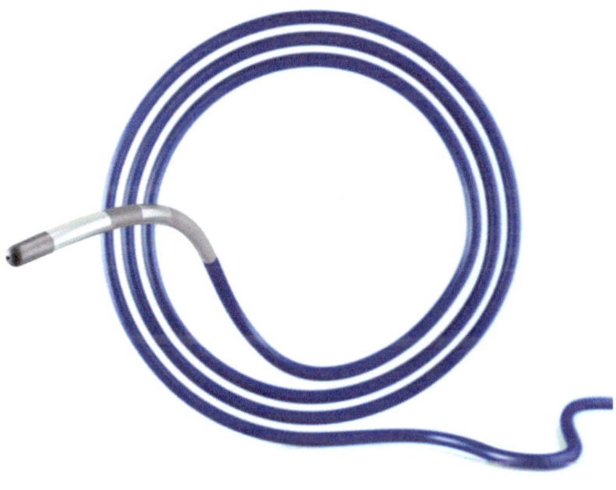

Fig. 29.2 Habib EUS monopolar RFA probe. (EMcision Ltd., London, UK, marketed by Boston Scientific. Photograph owned by Boston Scientific)

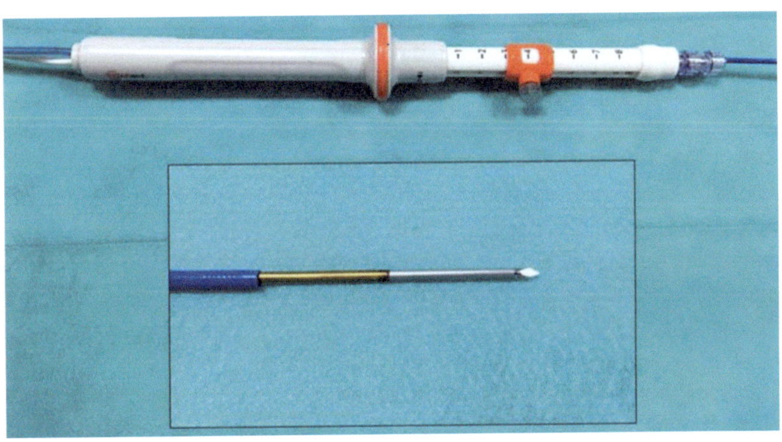

Fig. 29.1 The EUSRA system. (STARmed, Goyang, South Korea. Photograph owned by STARmed)

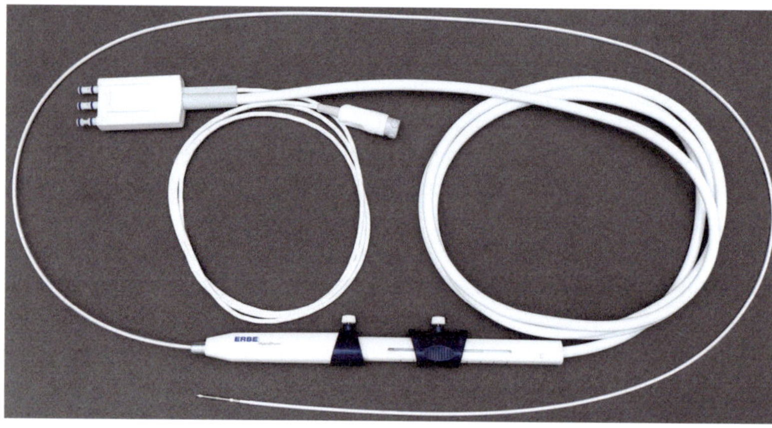

Fig. 29.3 HybridTherm bipolar flexible probe. (ERBE Elektromedizin, Tübingen, Germany. Photograph owned by ERBE)

29.3.1.2 Clinical Data

The first application of RFA in normal porcine pancreas was described by Goldberg in 1999 [51]. A modified 19-gauge Vilmann-type needle (GIP/Medi-Globe, Grassau, Germany) was used to treat 13 pigs. No major complications were observed (one focal pancreatitis, three gastric burns). This first study demonstrated the feasibility and safety of the EUS-guided RFA in porcine pancreas, and it was followed by other similar animal studies with other types of RFA probes; from the umbrella-shaped monopolar electrode used by Varadarajulu et al. in the porcine liver [52] to the new Habib EUS-RFA catheter through the needle (EMcision, London, UK) and 18G EUS-RA RF electrode (STARmed, Goyang, Korea), very similar to EUS biopsy needle. These latter two probes were used also in clinical trials in patients with pancreatic lesions.

Nowadays, 14 studies described RFA [27, 53–65] application to human disease, 9 of them using Habib probes. A total of 63 patients were treated using RFA: 19 with PNETs, 29 with PDAC, 11 with cystic neoplasms and 4 with pancreatic metastasis from other organs. Only one major event (a pancreatitis) was reported. However, further studies are needed to improve the technique, to understand the clinical application and to prevent/treat adverse events.

The EUS-guided RFA could be used in different areas and in multiple sessions in order to have a better control of ablated area.

Wang et al. [53] used EUS-guided RFA through a 22 G needle to treat patients with stage III pancreatic cancers. The current was delivered at 10–15 W for 2 min, and multiple ablations were performed when needed, according to the size of tumour. The authors reported a mean reduction in tumour size of 13.94% and a significant reduction in CA19-9, without any complications.

Song et al. [59] performed RFA in six patients with unresectable pancreatic cancer. They used the EUSRA 18G electrode with a length of 10 mm, applied for 10 s to deliver 20–50 W ablation power. Depending on tumour size, the procedure was repeated to sufficiently cover the tumour.

The procedure was successfully performed in 100% of the patients without major complications.

Crino et al. [63] used the EUSRA 18G electrode needle to treat seven patients with locally advanced pancreatic cancer and one patient with renal cancer metastasis to the pancreas. A 5 or 10 mm exposed tip was chosen according to the size of the tumour. All procedures were started with a preset radiofrequency power of 30 W, and the application time ranged from 15 to 95 s. EUS-RFA was feasible in the patients and an ablated area inside the tumour was achieved in all treated patients. No major complications were observed. Three patients experienced mild abdominal pain after the procedure, which was managed conservatively with anti-inflammatory drugs.

RFA has also been described to treat pancreatic cystic neoplasms and neuroendocrine tumours (Fig. 29.4).

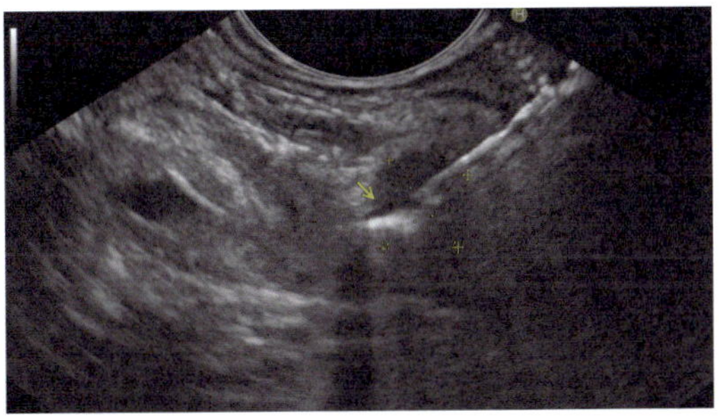

Fig. 29.4 The application of EUSRA in a small neuroendocrine tumour (size <1 cm). The probe is well recognizable as a hyperechoic line inside the mass. A hyperechoic area slowly spread from the electrode tip and is clearly visualized at EUS scan. (Courtesy of Dr. Stefano Francesco Crinò)

Pai et al. [55] performed a multicentre, pilot safety and feasibility study describing RFA in six patients with cystic lesions (four mucinous cysts, one intraductal papillary mucinous neoplasm and one microcystic adenoma) and two patients with neuroendocrine tumours. The ablation was performed with a 1.2-mm Habib EUS-RFA catheter placed through a 19-G or a 22-G fine needle. EUS-RFA was successfully completed in 100% of cases, with a complete resolution in 2/6 patients and a 50% size reduction in 3/6 patients with pancreatic cystic neoplasms. PNETs showed a change in vascularity with central necrosis after EUS-RFA. No major complications occurred.

A few case reports have been described with successful RFA of symptomatic insulinomas in patients unfit for surgery. In some cases, the patients underwent consecutive ablative treatment with complete control of hypoglycaemic symptoms [55–58].

29.3.2 Cryothermablation

29.3.2.1 Mechanism of Action

The HybridTherm bipolar flexible probe has been developed by ERBE (Elektromedizin, Tübingen, Germany), and it combines a radiofrequency ablation with the cooling effect of a cryogenic gas such as CO_2 [66].

The idea to develop a bipolar probe was sustained by the fact that bipolar systems ablate with less collateral thermal damage than monopolar systems but with the trade-off of less efficiency overall [67, 68]. This is one of the reasons at the basis of the association of the cryotechnology to the RFA: to increase the effects of tissue destruction and to overcome the disadvantages of less efficacy.

Moreover, the procedure maintains the systemic response described for RFA that it can hypothetically have therapeutic effect on distant metastasis, as showed in mouse with colon cancer [69] and mice with mammary adenocarcinoma [70, 71].

The probe is similar to a 14G needle and it is easily recognizable under EUS guidance as a hyperechoic line.

Regarding pancreatic application, the first animal study performed on pigs [72] demonstrated the feasibility and safety of the EUS application of this technology, with a good risk profile with no mortality and one major complication (7%). In this study, two procedural aims were showed: the complications were related to the dose and the ablated area was correlated to the duration of application. Furthermore, histological evaluation was performed and described a sharp demarcation between the ablated area and the surrounding pancreatic parenchyma with an inflammatory wall (granulation tissue with fibroblastic reaction, new blood vessels and a remarkable number of lymphocytes and polymorphonucleated neutrophil granulocytes) between the necrotic central area and the peripheral zone.

29.3.2.2 Clinical Data

One preliminary prospective human study [73] was performed enrolling consecutive patients with locally advanced pancreatic adenocarcinoma with no response after standard chemoradiotherapy and with no distant metastasis. The pilot study enrolled 22 patients, but the procedure was performed in 16 of them because in the remaining 6 the probe could not be advanced into the lesion for local tissue stiffness. The study confirmed the previous results in porcine model, in particular the feasibility of the procedure and the good risk profile. One limitation was the ability of the imaging techniques to distinguish the ablated area from inflammation and

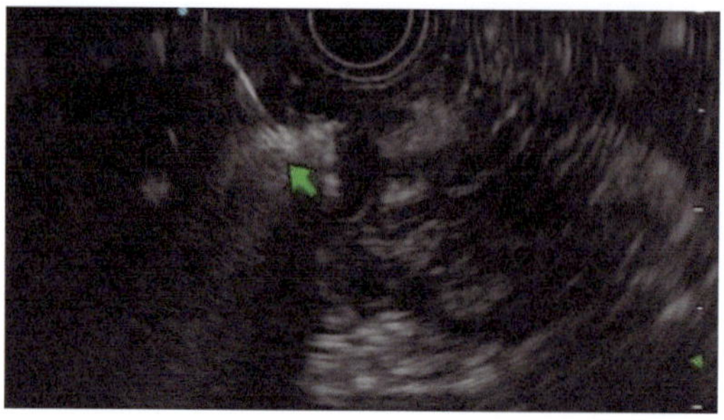

Fig. 29.5 The application of the HybridTherm probe in a patient with locally advanced pancreatic adenocarcinoma. The probe is visible as a hyperechoic line inside the tumour. During the ablation EUS shows generation of bubbles, most likely representing the steam phase during the heating of biological tissue

oedema. A CT scan was performed in all patients, but only in 6 of 16 it was possible to clearly define the tumour margins after ablation. So, other techniques such as MRI and contrast-enhanced EUS should be investigated for this purpose.

Two prospective studies are ongoing [ClinicalTrials.gov Identifier: NCT02336672 and NCT03649035], and they aim to evaluate the clinical efficacy of the procedure in local advance pancreatic adenocarcinoma (Fig. 29.5).

29.3.3 Photodynamic Treatment

29.3.3.1 Mechanism of Action

Photodynamic therapy (PDT) produces tissue necrosis using a light with specific appropriate wavelength that modifies a noncytotoxic photosensitizing agent administrated intravenously in a cytotoxic substance. When photosensitizer is activated, it interacts with oxygen to form reactive oxygen species producing cell apoptosis. It is a well-established treatment for unresectable cholangiocarcinoma [74].

Theoretically, due to its well-structured vascularization, the pancreatic parenchyma has an intense uptake of the photosensitizing agent, and it could be a good target for PDT. The application of PDT for treatment of pancreatic neoplasms was first attempted into a porcine model [75–77]. These studies concluded that EUS-guided PDT could be performed into pancreatic tail with low risk. However, the stiffness of the laser-light catheter, caused by the quartz optic fibre, limited the access to the head of the pancreas [77].

29.3.3.2 Clinical Data

One study [78] evaluated photodynamic therapy performed under EUS guidance, in four neoplastic patients: one pancreatic adenocarcinoma of the pancreatic tail and three with hepato-biliary tumour (two in the caudate lobe of the liver, one in the far distal bile duct). Patients received intravenous chlorin e6 derivative, Photolon (Belmedpreparaty, Minsk, Republic of Belarus), a second-generation photosensitizer with short half-life to minimize side effects. Photodynamic ablation was performed using a novel flexible laser-light catheter (PhotoGlow, South Yarmouth, Massachusetts, USA), which overcomes the stiffness of the previous probes. The laser probe has a quartz core with a diameter of 0.39 mm, polymer coating and cylindrical diffuser tip 1–2 cm long and is compatible with a 19-gauge EUS needle. A Luer Lock on the proximal hub of the FNA needle is used to attach the needle to the probe to avoid probe movements during the procedure. The study results reported no significant procedure-related adverse events and a stable tumour burden after a median follow-up of 5 months.

29.3.4 Neodymium-Doped Yttrium Aluminium Garnet Laser Ablation

29.3.4.1 Mechanism of Action

Laser ablation with neodymium-doped yttrium aluminium garnet (Nd:YAG) produces a necrosis of tissue using a light. The monochromatic light has a specific wavelength that interacts with tissue by three phenomena: scattering, reflection and absorption [79]. The latter one is the most relevant because it is converted into heat and at the end produces cell death. The damage is dependent on both temperature and exposure time [80], but it is also influenced by light wavelength, laser settings (laser power, laser energy and treatment time), physical properties of the tissue and the emission characteristics of the optical applicator [79].

Nd:YAG laser ablation was described for hepatocellular carcinoma, liver metastases, colorectal cancer and others [79].

Application of Nd:YAG ablation to pancreatic parenchyma was firstly attempted into animal model. In 2010, Di Matteo et al. [81] evaluated the procedure in vivo, performing the ablation into normal pancreatic parenchyma of eight pigs, with a good feasibility and no major complications. The same authors, in 2013, performed an ex vivo study [82] on porcine pancreatic tissue, in order to establish the best laser setting of Nd:YAG lasers for pancreatic tissue ablation.

29.3.4.2 Clinical Data

The group of Di Matteo [83] reported the first case in which Nd:YAG laser treatment was applied to human pancreas. They treated a recurrent pancreatic NET in a patient who refused pancreatectomy. The patient was successfully treated with Nd:YAG laser ablation under EUS guidance and she had no recurrence at 1-year follow-up.

Recently, nine patients with stage IIb-III pancreatic adenocarcinoma were treated with Nd:YAG laser ablation under EUS guidance [84] by the same group. Di Matteo used a 1064-nm wavelength laser (Echolaser; Elesta s. r. l, Florence, Italy) with the insertion of a 300-mm optical fibre (Elesta s. r. l.) through a 22-gauge needle and different power settings. The fibre was clearly visible in the target lesion during the procedure, and the presence of a hyperechoic area progressively surrounding the tip of the fibre did not hamper the visualization of the needle (Fig. 29.6).

The procedure was completed in all patients and no adverse events were reported. Di Matteo and colleagues concluded that EUS-guided laser ablation was feasible, with a good profile risk for the treatment of pancreatic cancer.

29.3.5 Ethanol Injection

29.3.5.1 Mechanism of Action

Alcohol produces coagulative necrosis by causing cell membrane lysis, protein denaturation and vascular occlusion [85].

The advantages of ethanol are the low cost, the easy availability and the rapid ablative mechanism.

Percutaneous ethanol injection ablation is routinely used for the treatment of solid and cystic neoplasms in a variety of anatomic locations, as thyroid, kidney, liver and adrenal gland [86].

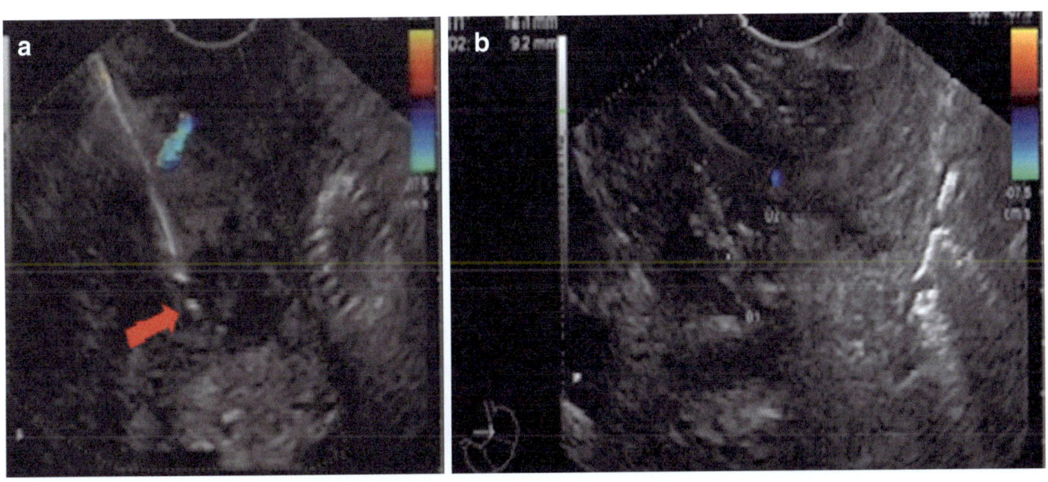

Fig. 29.6 Nd:YAG laser ablation under EUS guidance. (**a**) The hyperechoic spot visible at 5 mm from the tip of the needle inside the tumour (red arrow). (**b**) At the end of the procedure, EUS showed a hyperechoic area along the path of the probe surrounded by non-homogeneous tissue with hyperechoic spots. (Courtesy of Dr. Francesco Di Matteo)

In EUS, the ethanol injection is applied for EUS-guided coeliac plexus neurolysis to relieve pain in pancreatic cancer patients [87].

29.3.5.2 Clinical Data

Nowadays, EUS-guided ethanol injection has been used in case series for the treatment of pancreatic cystic neoplasms and pancreatic neuroendocrine tumours.

The mostly studied application is the ablation of pancreatic cystic neoplasms. Different studies concluded for a high success rate with an achieved cyst resolution in 33–78.6% of patients [88–95]. A recent meta-analysis and systemic review [96] reported that the pooled proportion of patients with complete cyst resolution was 56.20% (95% CI = 48.16–64.08) and partial cyst resolution was 23.72% (95% CI = 17.24–30.89) after EUS-guided ethanol ablation. The pooled percentage of more frequent post-procedure complications was abdominal pain in 6.51% (95% CI = 3.12–11.04) and pancreatitis in 3.90% (95% CI = 1.39–7.60). However, the technique is not standardized, and different alcohol solutions with or without another chemotherapeutic agent were used.

The EUS-guided ethanol ablation for the treatment of pancreatic adenocarcinoma was reported in one study [97]. The authors' aim was to compare the pain control, survival outcomes and safety profile of the combined approach of endoscopic ultrasound-guided tumour ethanol ablation combined with coeliac plexus neurolysis versus coeliac plexus neurolysis alone in patients affected by not resectable pancreatic adenocarcinoma. No severe treatment-related adverse events were reported, and the authors concluded that the combined treatment achieved better pain relief than coeliac plexus neurolysis alone. They reported also a higher median survival in patients with stage III treated with combining approach.

The last application of EUS-guided alcohol ablation for pancreatic disease is the ablation of pancreatic neuroendocrine tumours. Several case reports and case series are currently available regarding this topic [27, 98–114]. Overall 42 patients were treated with alcohol ablation under EUS guidance: 29 insulinomas, 1 gastrinoma and 12 non-functioning pNETs. Clinical remission rate ranged from 75 to 100%, while morphological complete remission rate varied from 61.5 to 100%. The procedure is feasible and easy. The most used needle calibre is the 22G, preferred to a 19G with less manoeuvrability and to 20G CPN needle with more difficult ethanol injection control for its multiple side holes [49]. The most frequent complication is acute mild pancreatitis. Other reported complications are abdominal pain, haemorrhage, infection and pancreatic duct injury.

Collectively, the preliminary studies suggest that ethanol ablation is relatively safe and feasible for clinical use in human pancreas. Therefore, EUS-guided ablation of pancreatic solid and cystic tumours via ethanol injection is a minimally and safely invasive technique that can be proposed for patients who refuse or are not eligible for surgery [85].

29.3.6 Chemotherapy Injection

29.3.6.1 Mechanism of Action

The technique is similar to EUS-guided alcohol ablation while different antitumoural agents are injected into pancreatic cancer aimed to cause either local or systemic biologic response. Some clinical studies were performed; however their value is hampered by small sample size and lack of control group.

29.3.6.2 Clinical Data

Chemotherapy

EUS-guided intratumoural injection of chemotherapy drugs aims to increase local drug concentration avoiding the rising of systemic side effects. Pancreatic adenocarcinoma is theoretically a very good candidate for the procedure because it has a prominent desmoplastic response that can cause an inadequate penetration of chemotherapy in tumour cell.

Levy and colleagues [115] have recently published a prospective study aimed to evaluated EUS injection of gemcitabine in terms of toxicity and ability to downstage neoplasia and increase overall survival in patients affected by unresectable pancreatic adenocarcinoma. A total of 36 patients were enrolled and followed up for 5 years (or until death). The procedure was safe and no adverse events were reported. Twenty percent of patients with stage III PDAC ($n = 4$) had a downstaging and underwent an R0 resection. Median overall survival was 10.4 months.

Cytoimplant

One phase I study [116] evaluated feasibility and safety of allogeneic mixed lymphocyte culture (cytoimplant) delivered by a single EUS-guided fine-needle injection (FNI) in eight patients with unresectable pancreatic carcinoma. Patients did not experience procedure-related complications neither systemic toxicities. Median survival was 13.2 months, and two patients had a partial response (>50% reduction in tumour size measured on imaging) and one a minor response (<50%).

The subsequent randomized multicentre phase II/III study was aimed to evaluate conventional chemotherapy versus cytoimplant injection. The trial was prematurely terminated because the survival and tumour response rates were inferior in the group treated with cytoimplant [11].

Dendritic Cells (DCs)

Currently, four pilot trials [117–120] reported feasibility, safety and clinical response of intratumoural EUS-guided injection of dendritic cells in pancreatic neoplasia of patients affected by unresectable disease. Dendritic cell could help to develop an acquired immune response against neoplastic cell, because they are antigen-presenting cells, generating specific T-cell immunity.

The first study [118] enrolled seven patients and demonstrated that dendritic cell injections were well tolerated without clinical toxicity. It also reported a median survival of 9.9 months with one complete response (complete regression of all lesions lasting at least 1 month) and three partial remissions (>50% decrease of lesions lasting more than 1 month).

The second study [117] enrolled five patients that received intravenous and EUS-guided injection of OK-432-pulsed DCs into a tumour, followed by intravenous infusion of lymphokine-activated killer cells stimulated with anti-CD3 monoclonal antibody. The treatment was safe, and no serious treatment-related adverse events were reported. Moreover, one patient had a partial remission, and two had long stable disease after 6 months of follow-up.

In a third study, Endo et al. [120] determined the feasibility and safety of preoperative EUS-guided injection of immature DC with OK-432 in 9 patients affected by resectable pancreatic adenocarcinoma, compared with 15 patients who underwent surgery without injection. OK-432 (Picibanil) is a lyophilized mixture of group A *Streptococcus pyogenes* with antineoplastic activity. The study results confirmed the safety of DC injection, without increased post-operative complications, but no significant differences in overall survival were reached.

The fourth one [119] added an intravenous adoptive activated T lymphocyte and gemcitabine in 15 enrolled patients. The median overall survival and progression-free survival of 15 patients were 12.0 months and 5.5 months, respectively. A total of 33 adverse events were recorded, in particular grade 3 adverse events occurred in four patients. However, two of them were more likely related to the gemcitabine administrated.

Adenovirus ONYX-015

It is a modified virus with deletion in the E1B gene. This modification leads a preferentially virus replication into neoplastic cell, causing cell death. It was injected in 21 patients with unresectable pancreatic adenocarcinoma in one phase I/II trial [121], plus intravenous gemcitabine. The results showed two patients with partial regressions of the injected tumour, two with minor responses and six with stable disease. As adverse event, the study reported two patients with sepsis and two patients with duodenal perforations.

Tumour Necrosis Factor Alpha (TNF-α)

One phase I/II study [122] evaluated TNFerade Biologic (AdGVEGR.TNF.11D), a replication-deficient adenoviral vector that expresses TNF-α inducible after chemotherapy and radiation. The virus was injected in 50 patients using EUS (27 patients) or percutaneous guidance. They reported 1 case with complete response, 3 patients with partial responses and 12 patients with stable disease, with an overall median survival of 297 days. Three patients experienced dose-limiting toxicities, with pancreatitis and cholangitis.

Unfortunately, the subsequent phase III study [123] concluded that TNFerade was safe but did not increase the survival in patients with LAPC. They randomized 304 patients to receive standard of care alone (90 patients) or standard of care alone plus TNFerade (187 patients), with a median survival of 10.0 months for both groups and a median progression-free survival of 8.6 months and 7.0 months, respectively. Moreover, the group treated with TNFerade had more side effects than the other arm.

BC-819

Hanna et al. published a phase I/II trial [124] study about safety, tolerability, pharmacokinetics and preliminary efficacy of BC-819, a DNA plasmid, administered intratumourally in nine subjects with unresectable non-metastatic pancreatic cancer. No adverse events were recorded. In two subjects, pancreatic tumours were downstaged and became surgically resectable, and in three subjects a partial response was described.

29.4 Future Perspectives

EUS-guided ablation techniques have a very promising rationale: they are aimed to achieve destruction of pancreatic masses using a minimal invasive and real-time imaging modality. They would be an alternative for surgery in patients unfit for surgery or a method for tumour downstaging prior to resection in a context of multimodality approach to pancreatic tumours.

Currently, for pancreatic cysts and PNETs, the technique could be proposed for patients who refuse or are unfit for surgery after a multidisciplinary consultation in a tertiary-level centre.

For pancreatic adenocarcinoma, next to local purpose, EUS-guided ablative techniques aim also to evoke a systemic response, stimulating the patient's immune response against the neoplastic cells. This aspect is crucial for the control of metastatic cells that are an early event in the natural history of PDAC.

Data available show that EUS-guided ablative techniques are feasible and safe.

However, open questions need to be clarified. First of all, advantage in terms of increasing survival and/or quality of life is missing. Secondly, real clinical indications into a multidisciplinary approach should be elucidated. Large multicentre clinical trials with careful patient selection are mandatory to establish a standardized protocol for EUS-guided ablative therapies in pancreatic diseases. The research should also clarify human systemic effects of local ablation, focusing on immunological system that could add another dowel in the complex mechanisms of pancreatic adenocarcinoma.

References

1. DiMagno EP, DiMagno MJ. Endoscopic ultrasonography: from the origins to routine EUS. Dig Dis Sci. 2016;61(2):342–53.
2. Teoh AYB, Dhir V, Kida M, Yasuda I, Jin ZD, Seo DW, et al. Consensus guidelines on the optimal management in interventional EUS procedures: results from the Asian EUS group RAND/UCLA expert panel. Gut. 2018;67(7):1209–28.
3. Law R, Baron TH. Endoscopic ultrasound-guided gallbladder drainage. Gastrointest Endosc Clin N Am. 2018;28(2):187–95.
4. Siddiqui UD, Levy MJ. EUS-guided transluminal interventions. Gastroenterology. 2018;154(7):1911–24.
5. Artifon ELA, Marson FP, Khan MA. Endoscopic ultrasonography-guided hemostasis techniques. Gastrointest Endosc Clin N Am. 2017;27(4):741–7.
6. Anderloni A, Attili F, Carrara S, Galasso D, Di Leo M, Costamagna G, et al. Intra-channel stent release technique for fluoroless endoscopic ultrasound-guided lumen-apposing metal stent placement: changing the paradigm. Endosc Int Open. 2017;5(1):E25–E9.
7. Dhadham GC, Hoffe S, Harris CL, Klapman JB. Endoscopic ultrasound-guided fiducial marker placement for image-guided radiation therapy without fluoroscopy: safety and technical feasibility. Endosc Int Open. 2016;4(3):E378–82.
8. Carrara S, Di Leo M, Zerbi A. The golden compass to the depths. Gastroenterology. 2016;151(5):e7–8.
9. Signoretti M, Valente R, Repici A, Delle Fave G, Capurso G, Carrara S. Endoscopy-guided ablation of pancreatic lesions: technical possibilities

and clinical outlook. World J Gastrointest Endosc. 2017;9(2):41–54.
10. Dabizzi E, Arcidiacono PG. EUS-guided solid pancreatic tumor ablation. Endosc Ultrasound. 2017;6(Suppl 3):S90–S4.
11. Kaplan J, Khalid A, Cosgrove N, Soomro A, Mazhar SM, Siddiqui AA. Endoscopic ultrasound-fine needle injection for oncological therapy. World J Gastrointest Oncol. 2015;7(12):466–72.
12. Siegel RL, Miller KD, Jemal A. Cancer statistics, 2018. CA Cancer J Clin. 2018;68(1):7–30.
13. Rahib L, Smith BD, Aizenberg R, Rosenzweig AB, Fleshman JM, Matrisian LM. Projecting cancer incidence and deaths to 2030: the unexpected burden of thyroid, liver, and pancreas cancers in the United States. Cancer Res. 2014;74(11):2913–21.
14. Iacobuzio-Donahue CA, Fu B, Yachida S, Luo M, Abe H, Henderson CM, et al. DPC4 gene status of the primary carcinoma correlates with patterns of failure in patients with pancreatic cancer. J Clin Oncol. 2009;27(11):1806–13.
15. Tempero MA, Malafa MP, Al-Hawary M, Asbun H, Bain A, Behrman SW, et al. Pancreatic adenocarcinoma, version 2.2017, NCCN clinical practice guidelines in oncology. J Natl Compr Cancer Netw. 2017;15(8):1028–61.
16. Linee Guida AIOM (Associazione italiana oncologia medica) Guidelines for exocrine pancreatic cancer. 2017.
17. Halfdanarson TR, Rabe KG, Rubin J, Petersen GM. Pancreatic neuroendocrine tumors (PNETs): incidence, prognosis and recent trend toward improved survival. Ann Oncol. 2008;19(10):1727–33.
18. Yao JC, Eisner MP, Leary C, Dagohoy C, Phan A, Rashid A, et al. Population-based study of islet cell carcinoma. Ann Surg Oncol. 2007;14(12):3492–500.
19. Lawrence B, Gustafsson BI, Chan A, Svejda B, Kidd M, Modlin IM. The epidemiology of gastroenteropancreatic neuroendocrine tumors. Endocrinol Metab Clin N Am. 2011;40(1):1–18, vii.
20. Kuo EJ, Salem RR. Population-level analysis of pancreatic neuroendocrine tumors 2 cm or less in size. Ann Surg Oncol. 2013;20(9):2815–21.
21. Anderson MA, Carpenter S, Thompson NW, Nostrant TT, Elta GH, Scheiman JM. Endoscopic ultrasound is highly accurate and directs management in patients with neuroendocrine tumors of the pancreas. Am J Gastroenterol. 2000;95(9):2271–7.
22. Ardengh JC, Rosenbaum P, Ganc AJ, Goldenberg A, Lobo EJ, Malheiros CA, et al. Role of EUS in the preoperative localization of insulinomas compared with spiral CT. Gastrointest Endosc. 2000;51(5):552–5.
23. Farrell JM, Pang JC, Kim GE, Tabatabai ZL. Pancreatic neuroendocrine tumors: accurate grading with Ki-67 index on fine-needle aspiration specimens using the WHO 2010/ENETS criteria. Cancer Cytopathol. 2014;122(10):770–8.
24. Weynand B, Borbath I, Bernard V, Sempoux C, Gigot JF, Hubert C, et al. Pancreatic neuroendocrine tumour grading on endoscopic ultrasound-guided fine needle aspiration: high reproducibility and inter-observer agreement of the Ki-67 labelling index. Cytopathology. 2014;25(6):389–95.
25. Lennon AM, Newman N, Makary MA, Edil BH, Shin EJ, Khashab MA, et al. EUS-guided tattooing before laparoscopic distal pancreatic resection (with video). Gastrointest Endosc. 2010;72(5):1089–94.
26. Lakhtakia S. Therapy of pancreatic neuroendocrine tumors: fine needle intervention including ethanol and radiofrequency ablation. Clin Endosc. 2017;50(6):546–51.
27. Choi JH, Seo DW, Song TJ, Park DH, Lee SS, Lee SK, et al. Endoscopic ultrasound-guided radiofrequency ablation for management of benign solid pancreatic tumors. Endoscopy. 2018;50(11):1099–104.
28. Falconi M, Eriksson B, Kaltsas G, Bartsch DK, Capdevila J, Caplin M, et al. ENETS consensus guidelines update for the management of patients with functional pancreatic neuroendocrine tumors and non-functional pancreatic neuroendocrine tumors. Neuroendocrinology. 2016;103(2):153–71.
29. Lee KS, Sekhar A, Rofsky NM, Pedrosa I. Prevalence of incidental pancreatic cysts in the adult population on MR imaging. Am J Gastroenterol. 2010;105(9):2079–84.
30. Karoumpalis I, Christodoulou DK. Cystic lesions of the pancreas. Ann Gastroenterol. 2016;29(2):155–61.
31. Tanaka M, Fernandez-del Castillo C, Adsay V, Chari S, Falconi M, Jang JY, et al. International consensus guidelines 2012 for the management of IPMN and MCN of the pancreas. Pancreatology. 2012;12(3):183–97.
32. Tanaka M, Fernandez-Del Castillo C, Kamisawa T, Jang JY, Levy P, Ohtsuka T, et al. Revisions of international consensus Fukuoka guidelines for the management of IPMN of the pancreas. Pancreatology. 2017;17(5):738–53.
33. European Study Group on Cystic Tumours of the Pancreas. European evidence-based guidelines on pancreatic cystic neoplasms. Gut. 2018;67(5):789–804.
34. Sawai Y, Yamao K, Bhatia V, Chiba T, Mizuno N, Sawaki A, et al. Development of pancreatic cancers during long-term follow-up of side-branch intraductal papillary mucinous neoplasms. Endoscopy. 2010;42(12):1077–84.
35. Armellini E, Leutner M, Stradella D, Ballare M, Occhipinti P. EUS-guided radiofrequency ablation: an option for the extrapancreatic region. Endosc Ultrasound. 2018;7(4):282–3.
36. Di Matteo F, Grasso R, Pacella CM, Martino M, Pandolfi M, Rea R, et al. EUS-guided Nd:YAG laser ablation of a hepatocellular carcinoma in the caudate lobe. Gastrointest Endosc. 2011;73(3):632–6.
37. Nakaji S, Hirata N, Iwaki K, Shiratori T, Kobayashi M, Inase M. Endoscopic ultrasound (EUS)-guided ethanol injection for hepatocellular carcinoma difficult to treat with percutaneous local treatment. Endoscopy. 2012;44(Suppl 2 UCTN):E380.
38. Lee S, Seo DW, Paik WH, Park DH, Lee SS, Lee SK, et al. Ethanol lavage of huge hepatic cysts by

using EUS guidance and a percutaneous approach. Gastrointest Endosc. 2014;80(6):1014–21.
39. DeWitt J, Mohamadnejad M. EUS-guided alcohol ablation of metastatic pelvic lymph nodes after endoscopic resection of polypoid rectal cancer: the need for long-term surveillance. Gastrointest Endosc. 2011;74(2):446–7.
40. Artifon EL, Lucon AM, Sakai P, Gerhardt R, Srougi M, Takagaki T, et al. EUS-guided alcohol ablation of left adrenal metastasis from non-small-cell lung carcinoma. Gastrointest Endosc. 2007;66(6):1201–5.
41. Paiella S, Salvia R, Ramera M, Girelli R, Frigerio I, Giardino A, et al. Local ablative strategies for ductal pancreatic cancer (radiofrequency ablation, irreversible electroporation): a review. Gastroenterol Res Pract. 2016;2016:4508376.
42. Haen SP, Pereira PL, Salih HR, Rammensee HG, Gouttefangeas C. More than just tumor destruction: immunomodulation by thermal ablation of cancer. Clin Dev Immunol. 2011;2011:160250.
43. Chu KF, Dupuy DE. Thermal ablation of tumours: biological mechanisms and advances in therapy. Nat Rev Cancer. 2014;14(3):199–208.
44. Laquiere A, Boustiere C, Leblanc S, Penaranda G, Desilets E, Prat F. Safety and feasibility of endoscopic biliary radiofrequency ablation treatment of extrahepatic cholangiocarcinoma. Surg Endosc. 2016;30(3):1242–8.
45. Girelli R, Frigerio I, Giardino A, Regi P, Gobbo S, Malleo G, et al. Results of 100 pancreatic radiofrequency ablations in the context of a multimodal strategy for stage III ductal adenocarcinoma. Langenbeck's Arch Surg. 2013;398(1):63–9.
46. Wu Y, Tang Z, Fang H, Gao S, Chen J, Wang Y, et al. High operative risk of cool-tip radiofrequency ablation for unresectable pancreatic head cancer. J Surg Oncol. 2006;94(5):392–5.
47. Spiliotis JD, Datsis AC, Michalopoulos NV, Kekelos SP, Vaxevanidou A, Rogdakis AG, et al. Radiofrequency ablation combined with palliative surgery may prolong survival of patients with advanced cancer of the pancreas. Langenbeck's Arch Surg. 2007;392(1):55–60.
48. Spiliotis JD, Datsis AC, Michalopoulos NV, Kekelos SP, Vaxevanidou A, Rogdakis AG, et al. High operative risk of cool-tip radiofrequency ablation for unresectable pancreatic head cancer. J Surg Oncol. 2007;96(1):89–90.
49. Paik WH, Seo DW. Echoendoscopic ablative therapy for solid pancreatic tumors. J Dig Dis. 2017;18(3):135–42.
50. Yoon WJ, Brugge WR. Endoscopic ultrasonography-guided tumor ablation. Gastrointest Endosc Clin N Am. 2012;22(2):359–69, xi.
51. Goldberg SN, Mallery S, Gazelle GS, Brugge WR. EUS-guided radiofrequency ablation in the pancreas: results in a porcine model. Gastrointest Endosc. 1999;50(3):392–401.
52. Varadarajulu S, Jhala NC, Drelichman ER. EUS-guided radiofrequency ablation with a prototype electrode array system in an animal model (with video). Gastrointest Endosc. 2009;70(2):372–6.
53. Wang D, Jin Z, Lei W, Leung JW, Li Z. Mo1524 endoscopic ultrasound guided radiofrequency ablation for the treatment of advanced pancreatic carcinoma. Gastrointest Endosc. 2013;77(5 Suppl):AB414.
54. Rossi S, Viera FT, Ghittoni G, Cobianchi L, Rosa LL, Siciliani L, et al. Radiofrequency ablation of pancreatic neuroendocrine tumors: a pilot study of feasibility, efficacy, and safety. Pancreas. 2014;43(6):938–45.
55. Pai M, Habib N, Senturk H, Lakhtakia S, Reddy N, Cicinnati VR, et al. Endoscopic ultrasound guided radiofrequency ablation, for pancreatic cystic neoplasms and neuroendocrine tumors. World J Gastrointest Surg. 2015;7(4):52–9.
56. Armellini E, Crino SF, Ballare M, Occhipinti P. Endoscopic ultrasound-guided radiofrequency ablation of a pancreatic neuroendocrine tumor. Endoscopy. 2015;47(Suppl 1 UCTN):E600–1.
57. Waung JA, Todd JF, Keane MG, Pereira SP. Successful management of a sporadic pancreatic insulinoma by endoscopic ultrasound-guided radiofrequency ablation. Endoscopy. 2016;48(Suppl 1):E144–5.
58. Lakhtakia S, Ramchandani M, Galasso D, Gupta R, Venugopal S, Kalpala R, et al. EUS-guided radiofrequency ablation for management of pancreatic insulinoma by using a novel needle electrode (with videos). Gastrointest Endosc. 2016;83(1):234–9.
59. Song TJ, Seo DW, Lakhtakia S, Reddy N, Oh DW, Park DH, et al. Initial experience of EUS-guided radiofrequency ablation of unresectable pancreatic cancer. Gastrointest Endosc. 2016;83(2):440–3.
60. Goyal D, Cen P, Wray CJ, Rowe J, Guha S, Singhal S, et al. 1111 Feasibility, safety, and efficacy of endoscopic ultrasound (EUS) guided radiofrequency ablation (RFA) of the pancreatic lesions: single center us experience. Gastrointest Endosc. 2017;85(5):AB144.
61. Bas-Cutrina F, Bargallo D, Gornals JB. Small pancreatic insulinoma: successful endoscopic ultrasound-guided radiofrequency ablation in a single session using a 22-G fine needle. Dig Endosc. 2017;29(5):636–8.
62. Feng X, Linghu E, Chai N, Li H. New treatment of the pancreatic cystic neoplasm: endoscopic ultrasonography-guided radiofrequency ablation combined with lauromacrogol ablation. Turk J Gastroenterol. 2018;29(1):99–102.
63. Crino SF, D'Onofrio M, Bernardoni L, Frulloni L, Iannelli M, Malleo G, et al. EUS-guided radiofrequency ablation (EUS-RFA) of solid pancreatic neoplasm using an 18-gauge needle electrode: feasibility, safety, and technical success. J Gastrointestin Liver Dis. 2018;27(1):67–72.
64. Malikowski T, Gleeson FC, Block M, Chari ST, Abu Dayyeh BK, Kendrick ML, et al. Mo1268 endoscopic ultrasound guided radiofrequency ablation

(EUS-RFA): initial assessment of safety and efficacy. Gastrointest Endosc. 2017;85(5 Suppl):AB484.
65. Scopelliti F, Pea A, Conigliaro R, Butturini G, Frigerio I, Regi P, et al. Technique, safety, and feasibility of EUS-guided radiofrequency ablation in unresectable pancreatic cancer. Surg Endosc. 2018;32(9):4022–8.
66. Hines-Peralta A, Hollander CY, Solazzo S, Horkan C, Liu ZJ, Goldberg SN. Hybrid radiofrequency and cryoablation device: preliminary results in an animal model. J Vasc Interv Radiol. 2004;15(10):1111–20.
67. Van Goethem BE, Rosenveldt KW, Kirpensteijn J. Monopolar versus bipolar electrocoagulation in canine laparoscopic ovariectomy: a non-randomized, prospective, clinical trial. Vet Surg. 2003;32(5):464–70.
68. Lee JM, Han JK, Choi SH, Kim SH, Lee JY, Shin KS, et al. Comparison of renal ablation with monopolar radiofrequency and hypertonic-saline-augmented bipolar radiofrequency: in vitro and in vivo experimental studies. AJR Am J Roentgenol. 2005;184(3):897–905.
69. Joosten JJ, van Muijen GN, Wobbes T, Ruers TJ. Cryosurgery of tumor tissue causes endotoxin tolerance through an inflammatory response. Anticancer Res. 2003;23(1A):427–32.
70. Sabel MS, Arora A, Su G, Chang AE. Adoptive immunotherapy of breast cancer with lymph node cells primed by cryoablation of the primary tumor. Cryobiology. 2006;53(3):360–6.
71. Zhu J, Zhang Y, Zhang A, He K, Liu P, Xu LX. Cryo-thermal therapy elicits potent anti-tumor immunity by inducing extracellular Hsp70-dependent MDSC differentiation. Sci Rep. 2016;6:27136.
72. Carrara S, Arcidiacono PG, Albarello L, Addis A, Enderle MD, Boemo C, et al. Endoscopic ultrasound-guided application of a new internally gas-cooled radiofrequency ablation probe in the liver and spleen of an animal model: a preliminary study. Endoscopy. 2008;40(9):759–63.
73. Arcidiacono PG, Carrara S, Reni M, Petrone MC, Cappio S, Balzano G, et al. Feasibility and safety of EUS-guided cryothermal ablation in patients with locally advanced pancreatic cancer. Gastrointest Endosc. 2012;76(6):1142–51.
74. Park DH, Lee SS, Park SE, Lee JL, Choi JH, Choi HJ, et al. Randomised phase II trial of photodynamic therapy plus oral fluoropyrimidine, S-1, versus photodynamic therapy alone for unresectable hilar cholangiocarcinoma. Eur J Cancer. 2014;50(7):1259–68.
75. Ayaru L, Wittmann J, Macrobert AJ, Novelli M, Bown SG, Pereira SP. Photodynamic therapy using verteporfin photosensitization in the pancreas and surrounding tissues in the Syrian golden hamster. Pancreatology. 2007;7(1):20–7.
76. Chan WM, Lam DS, Lai TY, Liu DT, Li KK, Yao Y, et al. Photodynamic therapy with verteporfin for symptomatic polypoidal choroidal vasculopathy: one-year results of a prospective case series. Ophthalmology. 2004;111(8):1576–84.
77. Yusuf TE, Matthes K, Brugge WR. EUS-guided photodynamic therapy with verteporfin for ablation of normal pancreatic tissue: a pilot study in a porcine model (with video). Gastrointest Endosc. 2008;67(6):957–61.
78. Choi JH, Oh D, Lee JH, Park JH, Kim KP, Lee SS, et al. Initial human experience of endoscopic ultrasound-guided photodynamic therapy with a novel photosensitizer and a flexible laser-light catheter. Endoscopy. 2015;47(11):1035–8.
79. Schena E, Saccomandi P, Fong Y. Laser ablation for cancer: past, present and future. J Funct Biomater. 2017;8(2).
80. Stafford RJ, Fuentes D, Elliott AA, Weinberg JS, Ahrar K. Laser-induced thermal therapy for tumor ablation. Crit Rev Biomed Eng. 2010;38(1):79–100.
81. Di Matteo F, Martino M, Rea R, Pandolfi M, Rabitti C, Masselli GM, et al. EUS-guided Nd:YAG laser ablation of normal pancreatic tissue: a pilot study in a pig model. Gastrointest Endosc. 2010;72(2):358–63.
82. Di Matteo F, Martino M, Rea R, Pandolfi M, Panzera F, Stigliano E, et al. US-guided application of Nd:YAG laser in porcine pancreatic tissue: an ex vivo study and numerical simulation. Gastrointest Endosc. 2013;78(5):750–5.
83. Di Matteo F, Picconi F, Martino M, Pandolfi M, Pacella CM, Schena E, et al. Endoscopic ultrasound-guided Nd:YAG laser ablation of recurrent pancreatic neuroendocrine tumor: a promising revolution? Endoscopy. 2014;46(Suppl 1 UCTN):E380–1.
84. Di Matteo FM, Saccomandi P, Martino M, Pandolfi M, Pizzicannella M, Balassone V, et al. Feasibility of EUS-guided Nd:YAG laser ablation of unresectable pancreatic adenocarcinoma. Gastrointest Endosc. 2018;88(1):168–74.e1.
85. Zhang WY, Li ZS, Jin ZD. Endoscopic ultrasound-guided ethanol ablation therapy for tumors. World J Gastroenterol. 2013;19(22):3397–403.
86. Gelczer RK, Charboneau JW, Hussain S, Brown DL. Complications of percutaneous ethanol ablation. J Ultrasound Med. 1998;17(8):531–3.
87. Wyse JM, Battat R, Sun S, Saftoiu A, Siddiqui AA, Leong AT, et al. Practice guidelines for endoscopic ultrasound-guided celiac plexus neurolysis. Endosc Ultrasound. 2017;6(6):369–75.
88. DeWitt J, McGreevy K, Schmidt CM, Brugge WR. EUS-guided ethanol versus saline solution lavage for pancreatic cysts: a randomized, double-blind study. Gastrointest Endosc. 2009;70(4):710–23.
89. DiMaio CJ, DeWitt JM, Brugge WR. Ablation of pancreatic cystic lesions: the use of multiple endoscopic ultrasound-guided ethanol lavage sessions. Pancreas. 2011;40(5):664–8.
90. Gan SI, Thompson CC, Lauwers GY, Bounds BC, Brugge WR. Ethanol lavage of pancreatic cystic lesions: initial pilot study. Gastrointest Endosc. 2005;61(6):746–52.
91. Moyer MT, Dye CE, Sharzehi S, Ancrile B, Mathew A, McGarrity TJ, et al. Is alcohol required for effective pancreatic cyst ablation? The prospective ran-

domized CHARM trial pilot study. Endosc Int Open. 2016;4(5):E603–7.

92. Oh HC, Seo DW, Kim SC, Yu E, Kim K, Moon SH, et al. Septated cystic tumors of the pancreas: is it possible to treat them by endoscopic ultrasonography-guided intervention? Scand J Gastroenterol. 2009;44(2):242–7.
93. Oh HC, Seo DW, Lee TY, Kim JY, Lee SS, Lee SK, et al. New treatment for cystic tumors of the pancreas: EUS-guided ethanol lavage with paclitaxel injection. Gastrointest Endosc. 2008;67(4):636–42.
94. Oh HC, Seo DW, Song TJ, Moon SH, Park DH, Soo Lee S, et al. Endoscopic ultrasonography-guided ethanol lavage with paclitaxel injection treats patients with pancreatic cysts. Gastroenterology. 2011;140(1):172–9.
95. Park JK, Song BJ, Ryu JK, Paik WH, Park JM, Kim J, et al. Clinical outcomes of endoscopic ultrasonography-guided pancreatic cyst ablation. Pancreas. 2016;45(6):889–94.
96. Kandula M, Moole H, Cashman M, Volmar FH, Bechtold ML, Puli SR. Success of endoscopic ultrasound-guided ethanol ablation of pancreatic cysts: a meta-analysis and systematic review. Indian J Gastroenterol. 2015;34(3):193–9.
97. Facciorusso A, Di Maso M, Serviddio G, Larghi A, Costamagna G, Muscatiello N. Echoendoscopic ethanol ablation of tumor combined with celiac plexus neurolysis in patients with pancreatic adenocarcinoma. J Gastroenterol Hepatol. 2017;32(2):439–45.
98. Bor R, Farkas K, Balint A, Molnar T, Nagy F, Valkusz Z, et al. Endoscopic ultrasound-guided ethanol ablation: an alternative option for the treatment of pancreatic insulinoma. Orv Hetil. 2014;155(41):1647–51.
99. Burghardt K, Kaemmerer D, Michael A, Aschenbach R, Muller UA, Kloos C, et al. Successful endoscopic ultrasound-guided ethanol ablation of a symptomatic sporadic insulinoma in a patient with severe comorbidities not suitable for pancreatic surgery. Diabetes Metab. 2018;44(1):84–6.
100. Dabkowski K, Gajewska P, Walter K, Londzin-Olesik M, Bialek A, Andrysiak-Mammos E, et al. Successful EUS-guided ethanol ablation of insulinoma, four-year follow-up. Case report and literature review. Endokrynol Pol. 2017;68(4):472–9.
101. Deprez PH, Claessens A, Borbath I, Gigot JF, Maiter D. Successful endoscopic ultrasound-guided ethanol ablation of a sporadic insulinoma. Acta Gastroenterol Belg. 2008;71(3):333–7.
102. Jurgensen C, Schuppan D, Neser F, Ernstberger J, Junghans U, Stolzel U. EUS-guided alcohol ablation of an insulinoma. Gastrointest Endosc. 2006;63(7):1059–62.
103. Lee MJ, Jung CH, Jang JE, Hwang JY, Park DH, Park TS, et al. Successful endoscopic ultrasound-guided ethanol ablation of multiple insulinomas accompanied with multiple endocrine neoplasia type 1. Intern Med J. 2013;43(8):948–50.
104. Levy MJ, Thompson GB, Topazian MD, Callstrom MR, Grant CS, Vella A. US-guided ethanol ablation of insulinomas: a new treatment option. Gastrointest Endosc. 2012;75(1):200–6.
105. Luo Y, Li J, Yang A, Yang H, Li F. 68Ga-Exendin-4 PET/CT in evaluation of endoscopic ultrasound-guided ethanol ablation of an insulinoma. Clin Nucl Med. 2017;42(4):310–1.
106. Muscatiello N, Salcuni A, Macarini L, Cignarelli M, Prencipe S, di Maso M, et al. Treatment of a pancreatic endocrine tumor by ethanol injection guided by endoscopic ultrasound. Endoscopy. 2008;40(Suppl 2):E258–9.
107. Paik WH, Seo DW, Dhir V, Wang HP. Safety and efficacy of EUS-guided ethanol ablation for treating small solid pancreatic neoplasm. Medicine (Baltimore). 2016;95(4):e2538.
108. Park DH, Choi JH, Oh D, Lee SS, Seo DW, Lee SK, et al. Endoscopic ultrasonography-guided ethanol ablation for small pancreatic neuroendocrine tumors: results of a pilot study. Clin Endosc. 2015;48(2):158–64.
109. Qin SY, Lu XP, Jiang HX. EUS-guided ethanol ablation of insulinomas: case series and literature review. Medicine (Baltimore). 2014;93(14):e85.
110. Schnack C, Hansen CO, Beck-Nielsen H, Mortensen PM. [Treatment of insulinomas with alcoholic ablation]. Ugeskr Laeger. 2012;174(8):501–2.
111. Teoh AY, Chong CC, Chan AW, Lau JY. EUS-guided alcohol injection of pancreatic neuroendocrine tumor. Gastrointest Endosc. 2015;82(1):167.
112. Trikudanathan G, Mallery SJ, Amateau SK. Successful endoscopic ultrasound-guided alcohol ablation of sporadic insulinoma using three-dimensional targeting (with video). Clin Endosc. 2016;49(4):399–401.
113. Vleggaar FP, Bij de Vaate EA, Valk GD, Leguit RJ, Siersema PD. Endoscopic ultrasound-guided ethanol ablation of a symptomatic sporadic insulinoma. Endoscopy. 2011;43(Suppl 2 UCTN):E328–9.
114. Yang D, Inabnet WB III, Sarpel U, DiMaio CJ. EUS-guided ethanol ablation of symptomatic pancreatic insulinomas. Gastrointest Endosc. 2015;82(6):1127.
115. Levy MJ, Alberts SR, Bamlet WR, Burch PA, Farnell MB, Gleeson FC, et al. EUS-guided fine-needle injection of gemcitabine for locally advanced and metastatic pancreatic cancer. Gastrointest Endosc. 2017;86(1):161–9.
116. Chang KJ, Nguyen PT, Thompson JA, Kurosaki TT, Casey LR, Leung EC, et al. Phase I clinical trial of allogeneic mixed lymphocyte culture (cytoimplant) delivered by endoscopic ultrasound-guided fine-needle injection in patients with advanced pancreatic carcinoma. Cancer. 2000;88(6):1325–35.
117. Hirooka Y, Itoh A, Kawashima H, Hara K, Nonogaki K, Kasugai T, et al. A combination therapy of gemcitabine with immunotherapy for patients with inoperable locally advanced pancreatic cancer. Pancreas. 2009;38(3):e69–74.
118. Irisawa A, Takagi T, Kanazawa M, Ogata T, Sato Y, Takenoshita S, et al. Endoscopic ultrasound-guided fine-needle injection of immature dendritic cells

into advanced pancreatic cancer refractory to gemcitabine: a pilot study. Pancreas. 2007;35(2):189–90.

119. Hirooka Y, Kawashima H, Ohno E, Ishikawa T, Kamigaki T, Goto S, et al. Comprehensive immunotherapy combined with intratumoral injection of zoledronate-pulsed dendritic cells, intravenous adoptive activated T lymphocyte and gemcitabine in unresectable locally advanced pancreatic carcinoma: a phase I/II trial. Oncotarget. 2018;9(2):2838–47.

120. Endo H, Saito T, Kenjo A, Hoshino M, Terashima M, Sato T, et al. Phase I trial of preoperative intratumoral injection of immature dendritic cells and OK-432 for resectable pancreatic cancer patients. J Hepatobiliary Pancreat Sci. 2012;19(4):465–75.

121. Hecht JR, Bedford R, Abbruzzese JL, Lahoti S, Reid TR, Soetikno RM, et al. A phase I/II trial of intratumoral endoscopic ultrasound injection of ONYX-015 with intravenous gemcitabine in unresectable pancreatic carcinoma. Clin Cancer Res. 2003;9(2):555–61.

122. Hecht JR, Farrell JJ, Senzer N, Nemunaitis J, Rosemurgy A, Chung T, et al. EUS or percutaneously guided intratumoral TNFerade biologic with 5-fluorouracil and radiotherapy for first-line treatment of locally advanced pancreatic cancer: a phase I/II study. Gastrointest Endosc. 2012;75(2):332–8.

123. Herman JM, Wild AT, Wang H, Tran PT, Chang KJ, Taylor GE, et al. Randomized phase III multi-institutional study of TNFerade biologic with fluorouracil and radiotherapy for locally advanced pancreatic cancer: final results. J Clin Oncol. 2013;31(7):886–94.

124. Hanna N, Ohana P, Konikoff FM, Leichtmann G, Hubert A, Appelbaum L, et al. Phase 1/2a, dose-escalation, safety, pharmacokinetic and preliminary efficacy study of intratumoral administration of BC-819 in patients with unresectable pancreatic cancer. Cancer Gene Ther. 2012;19(6):374–81.

Intraductal US

30

Claudio Giovanni De Angelis, Ludovica Venezia, and Pablo Cortegoso Valdivia

30.1 Introduction

Intraductal ultrasound (IDUS) is a 360° examination of the pancreatobiliary ducts using a thin-caliber ultrasonic probe, yielding real-time, high-quality, cross-sectional images due to the use of high-frequency ultrasound, during endoscopic retrograde cholangiopancreatography (ERCP) (Fig. 30.1). It allows detailed, high-resolution examination of the extrahepatic bile duct (BD), the main intrahepatic BDs, the main pancreatic duct (MPD), their contents, and periductal structures.

The high-frequency (12–20 MHz) US miniprobes can be passed through the operative channel of the duodenoscope directly into the bile or pancreatic duct. Small caliber (6–8 F), flexibility, and excellent image quality produced by these catheters make them ideal for imaging a narrow ductal cavity, the walls, and the neighboring structures allowing for the evaluation of various biliopancreatic disorders.

IDUS operates at higher frequencies than standard EUS, leading to higher image resolution, optimized by the tubular anatomy of the pancreatic and BDs, filled of fluid and slightly larger in diameter than the probe itself. IDUS is often better than EUS in evaluating the distal biliary system and surrounding structures (such as the right hepatic artery, the portal vein, and the hepatoduodenal ligament); but due to its limited depth of penetration (15–20 mm), image quality is very high within about 2-cm range of radius and cannot be useful for the examination of more distant tissues (e.g., distant lymph nodes and the proximal intrahepatic BDs).

The main limitations of IDUS include costs, limited durability of the probe, limited penetration depth, and difficulty in evaluating intrahepatic ducts. IDUS, either biliary or pancreatic, entails a low complication rate, including acute pancreatitis, such as for ERCP.

30.2 Technical Consideration

Since IDUS catheter has to be placed in the pancreatobiliary duct system, ductal cannulation is a prerequisite, and introduction of the miniprobe into the bile or pancreatic duct can be achieved by guidewire assistance (Fig. 30.2). The over-the-wire model has enabled insertion of the probe into the BD via the papilla without endoscopic sphincterotomy (EST) or balloon dilation. The outer diameter of the miniprobe (range 2.0–3.1 mm) is designed to be inserted via the working channel of a standard endoscope with a diameter of 3.2 mm; the option to use a guidewire allows the insertion of the mini-

C. G. De Angelis (✉) · L. Venezia
P. Cortegoso Valdivia
Gastroenterology Unit, AOU Città della Salute e della Scienza, Molinette Hospital, Turin, Italy

M. Mutignani et al. (eds.), *Endotherapy in Biliopancreatic Diseases: ERCP Meets EUS*,
https://doi.org/10.1007/978-3-030-42569-2_30

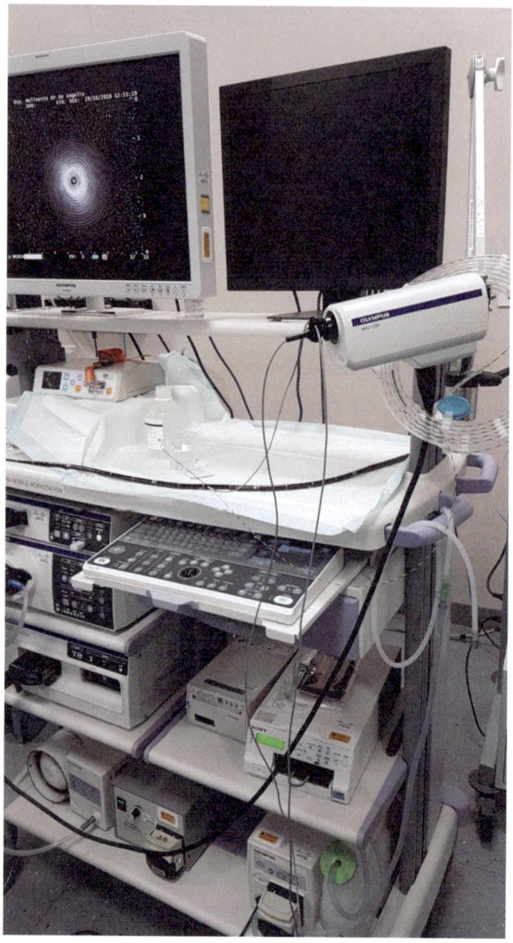

Fig. 30.1 IDUS miniprobe with guidewire, probe-driving unit, endoscopic ultrasonic observation unit

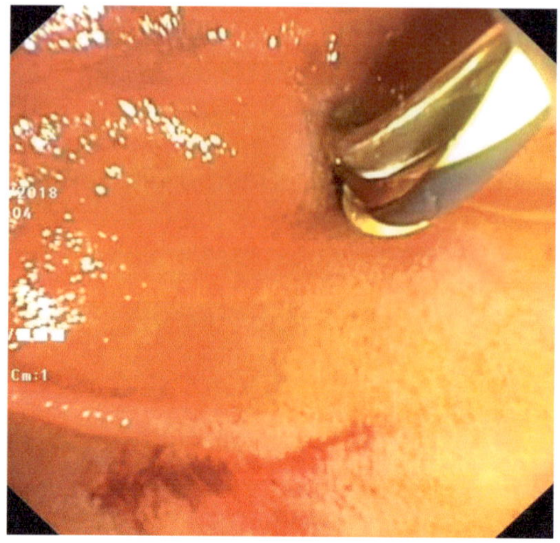

Fig. 30.2 Guidewired 20 MH miniprobe entering a small papilla with EST

probe into even tight strictures. Once the probe has been inserted into the target duct, positioning of the probe and location of scanning are grossly confirmed with the landmarks on the IDUS image. Fluoroscopy can also be used as an aid in localizing the position of the US transducer. EST is required in less than 20% of cases (almost never with a wire-guided probe). Image quality can be compromised in dilated duct due to the difficulty of maintaining the miniprobe in the center of the duct.

The probe can perform a 360° mechanical radial and/or a linear/helical scanning, perpendicular to the direction of insertion, with a frequency of 12–20 MHz. Some types of probes allow for the dual plane reconstruction (DPR) that is the acquisition of a helical ultrasound scan, displaying simultaneously linear as well as radial images and permitting in post-processing a fascinating 3-D reconstruction of the image.

Pneumobilia is a common finding after EST or balloon sphincteroplasty and is an obstacle for IDUS to provide accurate cross-sectional imaging of the biliary system, increasing the possibility of residual CBD stones after stone extraction. Flushing the BD with normal saline through an ERCP catheter placed alongside the probe can remove intraductal air bubbles and enables to perform IDUS simultaneously [1].

30.3 Normal Endosonographic Imaging

Due to its high frequency, the probe only allows visualization of the ductal wall and the immediate periductal vicinity (up to about 15–20 mm). IDUS cannot depict all the intrahepatic BDs due to its limited range of penetration. The normal BD appears as either two or three layers, similar to that seen during standard EUS. Three layers (outer echogenic layer, middle hypoechoic layer, inner echogenic layer) could be visualized in the wall of both the normal extrahepatic BD (Fig. 30.3) and the normal MPD; in addition the pancreatic parenchyma showed a fine reticular pattern [2, 3].

The normal BD wall is 0.31–0.79 mm thick, with smooth inner and outer surfaces and homogeneous internal echoes. When visualized as a

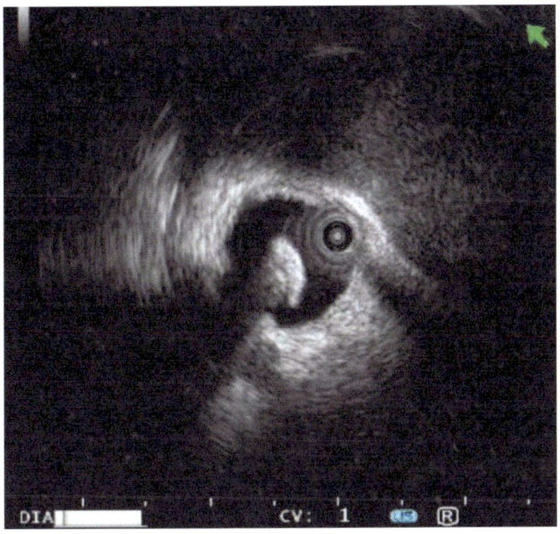

Fig. 30.3 Slightly dilated BD with normal three-layered wall and a stone with acoustic shadowing

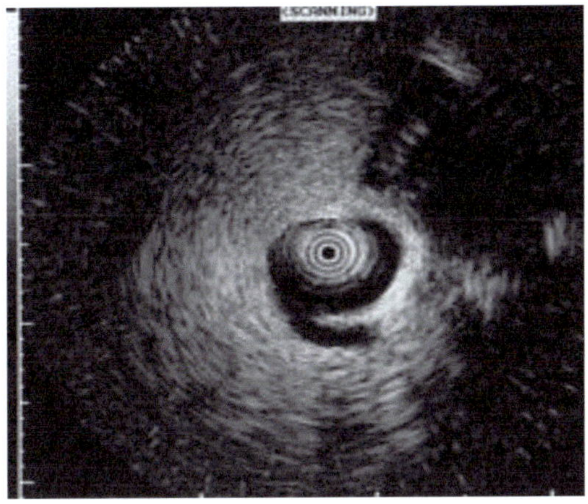

Fig. 30.4 Miniprobe in a dilated MPD with single-layered hyperechoic normal wall and a slightly dilated small branch duct

two-layer structure, an internal hypoechoic layer is seen which represents the mucosa, muscularis propria (fibromuscular layer), and fibrous layer of the subserosa. Occasionally, an interface echo is visualized between the bile and the inner hypoechoic layer. An outer hyperechoic layer represents the adipose layer of the subserosa, the serosa, and the interface echo between the serosa and surrounding organs. A third inner hyperechoic layer, representing an interface, will occasionally be identified. It may not be possible to differentiate the fibromuscular layer from the perimuscular connective tissue in some patients in whom they appear as a single hypoechoic layer.

The endosonographic appearance of the MPD wall varies from a single hyperechoic layer (Figs. 30.4 and 30.5) to three layers. When three layers are present, the inner and outer layers are hyperechoic, with an intervening hypoechoic layer [2].

30.4 Biliary Tree: Indications

30.4.1 Choledocholithiasis

IDUS presents a high diagnostic yield for BD stones. In a prospective comparative study, the sensitivities of magnetic resonance cholangiopancreatography (MRCP), ERCP, and IDUS for identifying choledocholithiasis were 80.0%, 90.0%, and 95.0%, respectively. IDUS can differentiate stones (echogenic foci with acoustic shadowing) (Figs. 30.3 and 30.5) from air bubbles (echoic foci with reverberation artifacts) (Fig. 30.6) and biliary sludge (echogenic foci without acoustic shadowing), enabling visualization of small BD stones or sludge missed on cholangiogram and MRCP [2, 4]. Therefore, it has been considered more effective than ERCP, abdominal CT, and MRI in the diagnosis of CBD stones. Especially, when a bile duct is 12 mm in diameter or greater, IDUS is recommended to detect or deny the presence of stones smaller than 8 mm in diameter.

IDUS can be used to verify stone clearance after supposedly complete stone extraction at ERCP. In a study of 70 examinations, IDUS revealed persistent stones in 40% of patients supposed to be stone-free [5]; another study with 188 patients with supposedly complete stone removal demonstrated less recurrence of stones in the group with IDUS after ERCP than in the group without IDUS (3.4% vs. 13.2%) [6].

IDUS can be also applied to suspected Mirizzi syndrome due to its high sensitivity in detecting a high echoic focus with acoustic shadowing outside of and just next to the common hepatic duct. When compared with EUS, IDUS and EUS are

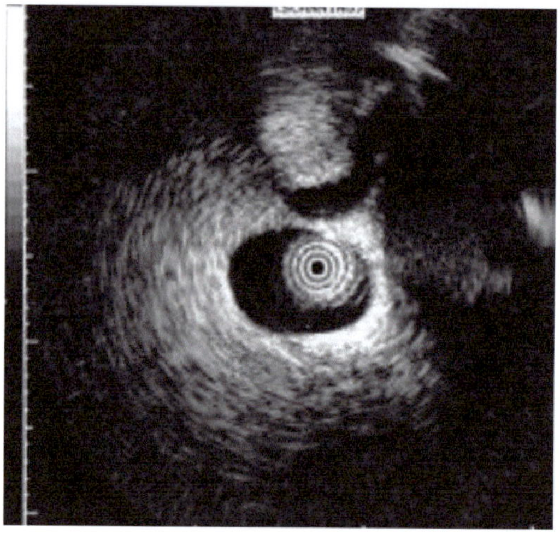

Fig. 30.5 Miniprobe in the MPD with single-layered hyperechoic normal wall and a small stone in the distal CBD

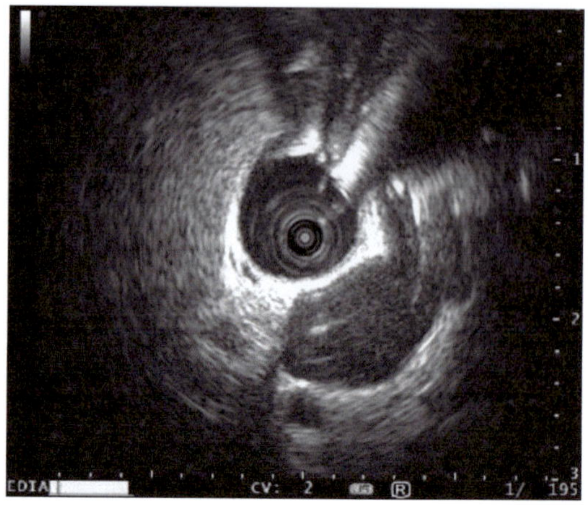

Fig. 30.6 Dilated CBD with normal wall and air bubbles (echoic foci with reverberation artifacts)

both sensitive and accurate for diagnosis of biliary stones and sludge. While EUS is less invasive and is mainly used in order to avoid useless ERCP, IDUS is used during ERCP with all the associated risks and complications.

30.4.2 Bile Duct Strictures

IDUS can help in differentiating malignant from benign biliary strictures, providing high-resolution cross-sectional images of the BD. Many studies demonstrate that IDUS is more accurate than EUS, transpapillary biopsy, or brush cytology for identification of biliary malignancy. Compared with ERCP-guided tissue sampling, IDUS showed significantly better sensitivity (87.5% vs. 62.5%, $P = 0.05$), specificity (90.6% vs. 53.1%, $P < 0.001$), and accuracy (90% vs. 55%, $P < 0.001$) in diagnosing malignancy [4, 7, 8].

Preservation of the normal-layered sonographic appearance of the BD, homogeneous echo-rich masses with smooth margins, and absence of a mass lesion were considered diagnostic of a benign lesion. Some authors describe IDUS image of a benign stricture as a lesion that was hyperechoic and symmetric with intermediate echogenicity (Fig. 30.7) [9].

Features suggestive of malignancy are eccentric wall thickening with an irregular surface (Fig. 30.8), disruption of the normal three-layer sonographic appearance, a papillary surface, a hypoechoic mass with irregular margins, heterogeneous echo-poor areas, and hypoechoic sessile mass with signs of adjacent tissue invasion. Other signs are presence of suspicious lymph nodes (enlarged, hypoechoic, round, and smooth bordered) and evidence of vascular invasion. In addition, measurement of duct wall thickness at the stricture site by IDUS also appeared helpful to predict malignancy: a BD wall thickness of 7 mm or less at the stricture site without extrinsic compression had a 100% negative predictive value for excluding malignancy, while a BD wall thickness >7 mm without extrinsic compression had a positive predictive value of 100% in diagnosing malignancy [3, 10].

IDUS can also be applied to help direct tissue acquisition: with fluoroscopy-guided forceps biopsy or brush cytology after identification of the location of suspected lesion by IDUS or placing IDUS probe alongside biopsy forceps in the bile duct to direct biopsy [11, 12]. In suspected malignant biliary stricture, higher diagnostic yield has been obtained by IDUS-guided transpapillary biopsy compared to the fluoroscopically guided [11]. The sensitivity for diagnosis of malignancy seems to improve with a

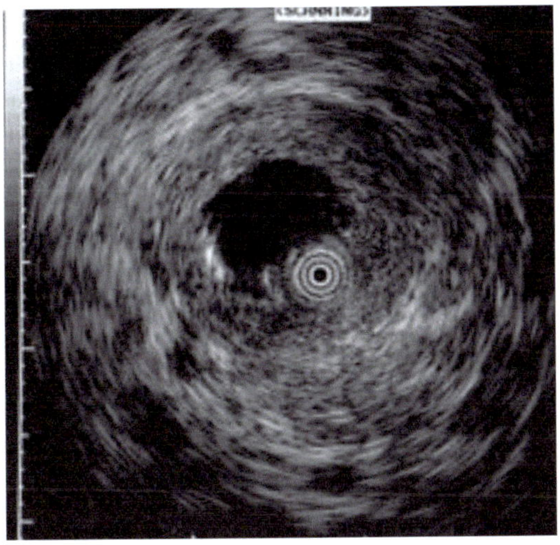

Fig. 30.7 Symmetric concentric echogenic thickening of the CBD wall: benign inflammatory stenosis

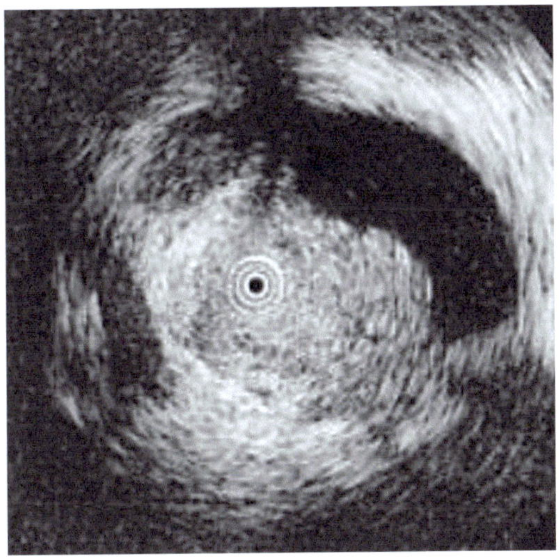

Fig. 30.8 Eccentric mass protruding in the dilated CBD few cm under the hepatic hilum: small cholangiocarcinoma

combination of IDUS and other techniques for tissue acquisition.

30.4.3 Staging of Malignancy

In BD carcinomas IDUS detects early lesions, determines the longitudinal tumor extent, and identifies tumor extension into adjacent organs and major blood vessels with a diagnostic accuracy of nearly 100% [13]. An accurate evaluation of the extent of spread and the necessary margin of resection is important for planning surgery. IDUS can improve the accuracy of local tumor staging, identifying tumor invasion into the pancreatic parenchyma, portal vein, and right hepatic artery. T staging is carried out based on the correlation of the tumor echo and layer structure of the BD wall.

IDUS cannot reliably distinguish T1 from T2 tumors because the miniprobe is not able to depict the fibromuscular layer and the fibrous layer of the subserosa separately. However, it is possible to diagnose invasion of the adipose layer of the subserosa or the serosa of the BD wall, components of the hepatoduodenal ligament such as the portal vein and the right/proper hepatic artery and pancreatic parenchyma. Cumulative accuracy of IDUS in T staging is reported to be 77.7%. Another study showed accuracy rate between 71 and 84% in staging T3 to T1 biliary tumors [14]. IDUS is more accurate than EUS for T staging of hilar and extrahepatic BD carcinoma but has low accuracy in N staging due to limited ultrasound penetration depth outside of the hepatoduodenal ligament, prohibiting its use for M staging.

IDUS plays a role in the evaluation of BD wall thickening. It cannot reliably distinguish tumor spread from inflammation; however, ultrasound criteria may assist in making this distinction. A commonly used feature is based upon the observation that inflammation typically causes symmetrical wall thickening (Fig. 30.7), in contrast to cancer infiltration, which typically causes asymmetrical wall thickening (Fig. 30.8). BD stents, frequently required in patients with biliary obstruction, may also lead to BD wall thickening and overestimation of longitudinal tumor extension. As a result, IDUS should be performed prior to or within a few days of biliary decompression [15].

A limitation is represented by previous history of BD surgery: in this case IDUS is not reliable in differentiating between surgical changes and BD cancer.

30.4.4 Evaluation of Idiopathic Acute or Recurrent Pancreatitis

IDUS can be useful in the detection of suspicious BD stones in idiopathic acute pancreatitis and in the prevention of recurrence of acute biliary pancreatitis, thanks to its ability to detect small CBD stones (Figs. 30.2 and 30.4). EUS is currently recommended before ERCP to detect possible CBD stones or sludge, but when cholangiogram fails to detect CBD stones, especially when a spontaneous stone passage is suspected, IDUS can be helpful. As already told, IDUS can be used to confirm BD clearance right after stone extraction, reducing the recurrence rate of acute biliary pancreatitis, while this can be a difficult task for EUS, mainly due to the interference by air bubbles in the BD (Fig. 30.5) after EST or balloon dilation of the papilla. Pneumobilia can be a problem for diagnosis of residual BD stones also for IDUS, but some tricks can be helpful in this case, normal saline injection in the BD by means of an ERCP catheter inserted alongside the miniprobe to eliminate the air bubbles or a balloon-sheated catheter IDUS probe [1, 16].

30.4.5 Gallbladder Lesions

There are very small series in which IDUS has been claimed useful in evaluating the relatively rare cystic duct cancer, gallbladder cancer [14, 17–19].

30.4.5.1 Ampulla

The significance of IDUS in the assessment of neoplasms of the papilla of Vater is increasing with the widespread performance of endoscopic papillectomy. The clinical problem is to accurately stage ampullomas in order to choose the right treatment. Standard EUS cannot distinguish an adenoma from a T1 carcinoma. Furthermore not all T1 ampullomas are the same: T1 ampullary adenocarcinomas limited to the sphincter of Oddi (d0 in the Japanese classification) carry almost no risk of lymph node metastases, while T1 adenocarcinomas that invade the sphincter (d1) carry a risk of 20–30% of nodal metastases. IDUS accurately visualizes the anatomy of the papilla and is the only procedure that reliably differentiates the sphincter of Oddi's muscle from the rest of the papilla. Oddi's muscle is visualized as a thin (less than 1 mm) hypoechoic layer that surrounds the BD and the MPD. The pancreatic parenchyma shows a fine reticular pattern. Inferior vena cava and lymph nodes at the posterior pancreatic head can also be seen. IDUS enables assessment of intraductal tumor extension along the bile/pancreatic duct terminals beyond the duodenal wall resulting superior to EUS in staging polypoid tumors of the major papilla: early cancer with infiltration limited to Oddi's muscle can be evaluated accurately [9]. Limitations include difficulty in the evaluation of invasion of the pancreas. IDUS can be useful for diagnosing and assessing the size and extent of papillary tumors and for evaluation of surgical resection vs. endoscopic papillectomy. Indeed IDUS is able to identify very small lesions, undetected by previous imaging. Echo attenuation due to the high frequency of miniprobe explains the lower accuracy in advanced stage tumors.

30.4.5.2 Pancreas

IDUS provides a high-resolution imaging of the pancreatic structures: the MPD is usually visualized as a single hyperechoic band, surrounded by the reticular pattern of the normal pancreatic parenchyma (Figs. 30.4 and 30.5) [2].

Limitations in the use of IDUS for the study of the pancreas are the absence of tissue sampling and that the MPD is usually tortuous with a narrow lumen, making the insertion of the probe in the body and tail not always possible; furthermore, its low penetration depth prevents an accurate staging of pancreatic cancer [7].

Nowadays the main indication for IDUS in pancreatic disorders is the preoperative assessment of the extension of intraductal papillary mucinous neoplasms (IPMNs), in order to guide the extent of the surgical resection. The fact that the MPD tends to be dilated because of the hypersecretion of mucin, in IPMNs, makes the use of IDUS easier. In IPMNs a papillary mass is usually visualized, with irregular thickening of the wall of the duct [20].

In some old series pancreatic IDUS has been proposed to distinguish between benign and malignant strictures of the MPD, to detect small pancreatic cancer, to differentiate benign from malignant IPMNs, to determine the nature of cystic lesions, and occasionally to demonstrate communication between the cyst and the MPD and mural nodules undetected by other diagnostic modalities [2, 7, 21, 22].

In a randomized prospective study evaluating 40 patients that underwent surgical resection, IDUS was more accurate in the preoperative evaluation of tumor extent compared to other standard imaging modalities (85% vs. 50%) [20]. In another retrospective study, IDUS evaluated the lateral spreading of branch-duct IPMNs (detection of papillary protrusions in the MPD) in 24 patients before surgery, with a sensitivity, specificity, and accuracy of 92%, 91%, and 92%, respectively; this study also highlighted that the lateral spreading was associated with a dilation of the MPD ≥6 mm [23]. Nevertheless, the necessity of cannulation of the MPD and the absence of tissue/fluid sampling make EUS (not IDUS) the recommended technique by the most recent guidelines in the management of IPMNs [24].

The differentiation of benign and malignant IPMNs was evaluated in a study from Hara et al., comparing the technique to EUS, peroral pancreatoscopy (POPS), and computed tomography: although IDUS had the highest accuracy, a further differential diagnosis between carcinoma in situ and invasive carcinoma was considered impossible [21].

Few old reports from the 1990s evaluated the usefulness of IDUS in patients with chronic pancreatitis or with EUS-negative neuroendocrine tumors, but no further studies have been reported recently [9, 25].

30.5 Other Nonconventional Indications

30.5.1 Primary Sclerosing Cholangitis, IgG-4-Related Cholangitis

IgG4-related sclerosing cholangitis (IgG4-SC) shows various cholangiographic features similar to those of pancreatic cancer, primary SC (PSC), and cholangiocarcinoma. Findings that support IgG4-SC against cholangiocarcinoma are circular-symmetric wall thickening, smooth outer and inner margin, homogeneous internal echo in the stricture, and preservation of the three layers (so-called high-low-high pattern) at the stenotic area [26]. In most cases wall thickness spreads continuously from the intrapancreatic BD to the upper BD, and the BD wall is thicker than 0.8 mm in the non-stenotic area [27]. Findings in favor of cholangiocarcinoma are eccentric wall thickening, disruption of the bile duct wall layers, irregular luminal surface (Fig. 30.8), and a hypoechoic mass with irregular margins [26].

In patients with PSC, all layers of the BD are inflamed and the BD epithelium is severely damaged. IDUS can show specific findings such as disappearance of three layers in the stricture with irregular inner margin and diverticulum-like outpouching. Heterogeneous internal echo, a circular-asymmetric wall thickness, and unclear outer margin are observed on IDUS more frequent in PSC than in IgG4-SC [28].

30.5.2 Directed Endoscopic Biliary Procedures

In order to prevent ERCP complications (e.g., contrast injection-related ascending cholangitis, post-ERCP pancreatitis), recent studies evaluated the usefulness of IDUS instead of radiocontrast cholangiogram: in determining the length of plastic stents (measuring insertion length of the probe between major papilla and the lesions) and in stone removal (with IDUS confirming existence and clearance of stones) [12, 29, 30].

30.5.3 Portal Hypertensive Biliopathy

Portal hypertensive biliopathy is a BD wall abnormality secondary to portal hypertension; compression of periductal or intraductal varices is a rare cause of CBD stricture that can be recognized by IDUS. Biliary varices typically present with multiple, hypoechoic structures in the duct wall or surrounding the bile duct [31, 32].

30.6 Conclusions

IDUS is a relatively safe and sensitive diagnostic tool for various biliopancreatic diseases. Many of the proposed indications for IDUS have not yet been established, but promising roles for this technique could be the differential diagnosis of biliary and MPD strictures of unknown origin, mainly without associated masses on other imaging modalities and the staging of ampullomas, mainly the differentiation between d0 and d1 carcinomas that have clear impact on the therapeutic decision. Staging of biliary malignancies, differential diagnosis between benign and malignant IPMNs, IDUS-guided target biopsies, the possibility to confirm spontaneous stone passage during ERCP and to establish a clean duct after stone extraction, and some IDUS-directed therapeutic biliary procedures in selected cases replacing radiocontrast cholangiograms are all appealing possible applications of this technique, but they warrant further evaluation mainly in comparison with competing modalities such as EUS ± FNA, peroral cholangioscopy and pancreatoscopy with microforceps biopsy, and intraductal probe-based confocal laser endomicroscopy (pCLE). In biliary stenoses of indeterminate nature without mass, after failed normal diagnostic ERCP techniques, we propose an all-in-one approach, with IDUS followed by peroral cholangioscopy with pCLE and then biopsies under direct visualization with microforceps. ERCP forceps biopsies and brushing can of course be repeated in the same session.

References

1. Varadarajulu S. A modified technique to overcome the limitations of intraductal ultrasound for diagnosis of common bile duct stones. Endoscopy. 2008;40(Suppl 2):E152.
2. Bruno M, De Angelis C. IDUS and EDUS. In: De Angelis C, Bocus P, editors. IEC atlas of endoscopic ultrasound. Turin: Ed. Minerva Medica; 2013. p. 141–5.
3. Krishna NB, Saripalli S, Safdar R, Agarwal B. Intraductal US in evaluation of biliary strictures without a mass lesion on CT scan or magnetic resonance imaging: significance of focal wall thickening and extrinsic compression at the stricture site. Gastrointest Endosc. 2007;66(1):90–6.
4. Sun B, Hu B. The role of intraductal ultrasonography in pancreatobiliary diseases. Endosc Ultrasound. 2016;5(5):291–9.
5. Ang TL, Teo EK, Fock KM, Lyn Tan JY. Are there roles for intraductal US and saline solution irrigation in ensuring complete clearance of common bile duct stones? Gastrointest Endosc. 2009;69(7):1276–81.
6. Tsuchiya S, Tsuyuguchi T, Sakai Y, Sugiyama H, Miyagawa K, Fukuda Y, et al. Clinical utility of intraductal US to decrease early recurrence rate of common bile duct stones after endoscopic papillotomy. J Gastroenterol Hepatol. 2008;23(10):1590–5.
7. Tringali A, Lemmers A, Meves V, Terheggen G, Pohl J, Manfredi G, et al. Intraductal biliopancreatic imaging: European Society of Gastrointestinal Endoscopy (ESGE) technology review. Endoscopy. 2015;47(8):739–53.
8. Venezia L, Cortegoso Valdivia P, Rizza S, Bruno M, De Angelis C. Intraductal ultrasound for second-level evaluation of biliary and ampullary stenoses: experience from the Turin Center. Endoscopy. 2018;50(04):S43. https://doi.org/10.1055/s-0038-1637154.
9. Fujita N, Noda Y, Kobayashi G, Ito K, Horaguchi J, Koshita S, et al. Intraductal ultrasonography (IDUS) for the diagnosis of biliopancreatic diseases. Best Pract Res Clin Gastroenterol. 2009;23(5):729–42.
10. Chen L, Lu Y, Wu J-C, Bie L, Xia L, Gong B. Diagnostic utility of endoscopic retrograde cholangiography/intraductal ultrasound (ERC/IDUS) in distinguishing malignant from benign bile duct obstruction. Dig Dis Sci. 2016;61(2):610–7.
11. Moon JH, Choi HJ, Kim HK, Kwon KW, Cheon YK, Cho YD, et al. The usefulness of IDUS-guided transpapillary bile duct biopsy for the diagnosis of malignant biliary strictures. Gastrointest Endosc. 2008;67(5):AB208.
12. Lim S-U, Park C-H, Kee W-J, Lee J-H, Rew S-J, Park S-Y, et al. Intraductal ultrasonography without radiocontrast cholangiogram in patients with extrahepatic biliary disease. Gut Liver. 2015;9(4):540–6.
13. Tamada K, Ido K, Ueno N, Kimura K, Ichiyama M, Tomiyama T. Preoperative staging of extrahepatic bile duct cancer with intraductal ultrasonography. Am J Gastroenterol. 1995;90(2):239–46.
14. Meister T, Heinzow HS, Woestmeyer C, Lenz P, Menzel J, Kucharzik T, et al. Intraductal ultrasound substantiates diagnostics of bile duct strictures of uncertain etiology. World J Gastroenterol. 2013;19(6):874–81.
15. Tamada K, Nagai H, Yasuda Y, Tomiyama T, Ohashi A, Wada S, et al. Transpapillary intraductal US prior to biliary drainage in the assessment of longitudinal spread of extrahepatic bile duct carcinoma. Gastrointest Endosc. 2001;53(3):300–7.
16. Kim H-N, Park C-H, Cho E-A, Rew S-J, Park I-H, Lim S-U, et al. Role of balloon-sheathed intraductal

ultrasonography for patients with extensive pneumobilia. Gut Liver. 2015;9(4):561–5.
17. Obana T, Fujita N, Noda Y, Kobayashi G, Ito K, Sugawara T, et al. Endoscopic biliary imaging and clinicopathological features of cystic duct cancer. J Gastroenterol. 2008;43(2):171–8.
18. Matsubara S, Arizumi T, Togawa O, Sasaki T, Yamamoto N, Nakai Y, et al. Endoscopic transpapillary approach to the gallbladder for diagnosing gallbladder cancer. Can J Gastroenterol. 2007;21(12):809–13.
19. Wehrmann T, Riphaus A, Martchenko K, Kokabpick S, Pauka H, Stergiou N, et al. Intraductal ultrasonography in the diagnosis of Mirizzi syndrome. Endoscopy. 2006;38(7):717–22.
20. Cheon YK, Cho YD, Jeon SR, Moon JH, Jeong SW, Hur KY, et al. Pancreatic resection guided by preoperative intraductal ultrasonography for intraductal papillary mucinous neoplasm. Am J Gastroenterol. 2010;105(9):1963–9.
21. Hara T, Yamaguchi T, Ishihara T, Tsuyuguchi T, Kondo F, Kato K, et al. Diagnosis and patient management of intraductal papillary-mucinous tumor of the pancreas by using peroral pancreatoscopy and intraductal ultrasonography. Gastroenterology. 2002;122(1):34–43.
22. Cellier C, Cuillerier E, Palazzo L, Rickaert F, Flejou JF, Napoleon B, et al. Intraductal papillary and mucinous tumors of the pancreas: accuracy of preoperative computed tomography, endoscopic retrograde pancreatography and endoscopic ultrasonography, and long-term outcome in a large surgical series. Gastrointest Endosc. 1998;47(1):42–9.
23. Kobayashi G, Fujita N, Noda Y, Ito K, Horaguchi J, Obana T, et al. Lateral spread along the main pancreatic duct in branch-duct intraductal papillary-mucinous neoplasms of the pancreas: usefulness of intraductal ultrasonography for its evaluation. Dig Endosc. 2011;23(1):62–8.
24. Elta GH, Enestvedt BK, Sauer BG, Marie Lennon A. ACG clinical guideline: diagnosis and management of pancreatic cysts. Am J Gastroenterol. 2018;113(4):464–79.
25. Menzel J, Domschke W. Intraductal ultrasonography may localize islet cell tumours negative on endoscopic ultrasound. Scand J Gastroenterol. 1998;33(1):109–12.
26. Kamisawa T, Zen Y, Nakazawa T, Okazaki K. Advances in IgG4-related pancreatobiliary diseases. Lancet Gastroenterol Hepatol. 2018;3(8):575–85.
27. Nakazawa T, Naitoh I, Hayashi K. Usefulness of intraductal ultrasonography in the diagnosis of cholangiocarcinoma and IgG4-related sclerosing cholangitis. Clin Endosc. 2012;45(3):331.
28. Naitoh I, Nakazawa T, Hayashi K, Miyabe K, Shimizu S, Kondo H, et al. Comparison of intraductal ultrasonography findings between primary sclerosing cholangitis and IgG4-related sclerosing cholangitis. J Gastroenterol Hepatol. 2015;30(6):1104–9.
29. Lee J-M, Park C-H, Rew S-J, Kim H-N, Lee H-J, Park I-H, et al. Intraductal ultrasonography-directed endoscopic retrograde biliary drainage without fluoroscopy. Endoscopy. 2014;46(Suppl 1 UCTN):E495.
30. Park S-Y, Park C-H, Lim S-U, Cho E-A, Lee D-H, Jun C-H, et al. Intraductal US-directed management of bile duct stones without radiocontrast cholangiography. Gastrointest Endosc. 2015;82(5):939–43.
31. Takagi T, Irisawa A, Shibukawa G, Hikichi T, Obara K, Ohira H. Intraductal ultrasonographic anatomy of biliary varices in patients with portal hypertension. Endosc Ultrasound. 2015;4(1):44–51.
32. Ramchandani M, Nageshwar Reddy D, Lakhtakia S, Gupta R, Tandan M, Rao GV. Role of single-operator per-oral cholangioscopy and intraductal US in assessment of portal biliopathy (with videos). Gastrointest Endosc. 2014;79(6):1015–9.

Part IV

Complications: Prevention, Diagnosis and Management

31 Post-ERCP Acute Pancreatitis

Bernd Kronenberger

31.1 Acute Post-ERCP Pancreatitis

Acute pancreatitis after ERCP (post-ERCP pancreatitis, PEP) occurs in 3–10% of patients [1, 2]. Most patients have a mild or moderate self-limiting course of pancreatitis mainly characterized by abdominal pain radiating to the back lasting for 2–3 or 4–10 days, respectively [3]. Development of hemorrhagic pancreatitis, phlegmon, pseudocyst, or infection indicates severe PEP [4, 5]. Severe PEP may progress to organ failure [1].

31.2 Diagnosis

The diagnosis of PEP relies on the clinical picture, laboratory abnormalities following ERCP, and typical signs of pancreatitis in transabdominal ultrasound (US), computed tomography (CT), or magnetic resonance imaging (MRI). In a consensus conference, PEP was defined as clinical pancreatitis with amylase at least three times the upper limit of normal (ULN) at more than 24 h after the procedure, requiring hospital admission or a prolongation of planned admission [3]. The Atlanta classification for acute pancreatitis may also be used for defining PEP; however, the classification was not primarily developed to define PEP [1, 2]. The Atlanta classification uses three criteria: (1) abdominal pain consistent with acute pancreatitis (acute onset of a persistent, severe, epigastric pain often radiating to the back), (2) serum lipase or amylase activity at least three times the ULN, and (3) characteristic findings of acute pancreatitis on contrast-enhanced CT, MRT, or US. PEP is present when two of the three criteria are fulfilled [1, 2]. Both classifications can be used; however, the classifications were shown to have a poor correlation with each other [2].

The severity of PEP depends on the presence or absence of organ failure and of local or systemic complications. Both classifications use different criteria for the definition of mild, moderate, and severe PEP. The criteria are listed in Table 31.1.

31.3 Pathogenesis of PEP

PEP is a local and systemic inflammatory reaction due to pancreatic damage following manipulation at the papilla and the pancreatic duct. Mechanic and hydrostatic injury are regarded as major factors contributing to edema and sphincter spasm [5, 6]. Obstacle to the flow of pancreatic fluid and direct epithelial and acinar damage may cause a cascade of events leading to activation of pancre-

B. Kronenberger (✉)
Department of Internal Medicine, Gastroenterology, Hepatology, Diabetology, Herz-Jesu-Hospital, Fulda, Germany
e-mail: bernd.kronenberger@email.de

M. Mutignani et al. (eds.), *Endotherapy in Biliopancreatic Diseases: ERCP Meets EUS*,
https://doi.org/10.1007/978-3-030-42569-2_31

Table 31.1 Classification of post-ERCP pancreatitis

Consensus classification (Cotton et al. [3])	Atlanta classification [4]
Mild	
(a) Clinical pancreatitis *And* (b) Amylase at least three times ULN at more than 24 h after the procedure *And* (c) Requiring admission or prolongation of planned admission to 2–3 days	Two of the following: (a) Pain consistent with acute pancreatitis (b) Amylase or lipase >3 times ULN (c) Characteristic findings *And* No organ dysfunction or other adverse events
Moderate	
Pancreatitis requiring hospitalization of 4–10 days	(a) Transient organ failure <48 h *Or* (b) Local or systemic adverse events without persistent organ failure
Severe	
(a) Hospitalization for more than 10 days *Or* (b) Development of hemorrhagic pancreatitis, phlegmon, pseudocyst, or infection *Or* (c) Need of percutaneous drainage or surgery	(a) Persistent single or multiple organ failure >48 h Or (b) Present or persistent systemic inflammatory response syndrome (SIRS)

atic proteolytic enzymes, autodigestion, and release of inflammatory cytokines [5–7]. Contrast material itself in the pancreatic duct is an independent factor that can cause epithelial and acinar damage [5, 6]. Infections are also discussed in the pathogenesis of PEP [5].

31.4 Risk Factors

Risk factors for PEP were intensively studied. Several patient-related risk factors for PEP were identified including prior PEP, female sex, previous recurrent pancreatitis, suspected sphincter Oddi dysfunction, and normal serum bilirubin levels [5, 6]. Chronic pancreatitis has been demonstrated to be protective against PEP [5]. Patients with biliary strictures have a higher risk for post-ERCP pancreatitis than patients with common bile duct stones (6.8% vs. 3.8%) [6]. Procedure-related risk factors are cannulation time ≥5–10 min, repetitive guidewire cannulation, pancreatic injection, precut, pancreatic sphincterotomy, and endoscopic papillary large-balloon dilatation of an intact sphincter [5, 6].

Precut is usually performed in cases of difficult biliary cannulation. Controversy exists whether precut as a procedure itself or the difficult biliary cannulation is the major cause of PEP. Early precut was shown to have a lower risk of PEP than several attempts with the standard technique indicating that prolonged papillary manipulation and not precut is the major risk factor for PEP [2].

31.5 Prevention

31.5.1 Patient Selection

The most effective measure to reduce procedure-related complications is to avoid unnecessary interventions. Due to the availability of less-invasive alternatives for diagnosis or biliopancreatic diseases such as MRI/MRCP and endoscopic ultrasound (EUS), ERCP should not be performed for diagnostic purposes. Especially in patients with common bile duct stones, a thorough evaluation before ERCP should be performed. The diagnostic algorithms and measures are described in the respective chapter.

31.5.2 Pharmacological Prophylaxis

Pancreatitis is mainly caused by an inflammatory response. Attenuation of the inflammatory reaction by nonsteroidal anti-inflammatory drugs may prevent PEP. Studies with conflicting results were published [8]; however, meta-analyses showed that rectal indomethacin or diclofenac administered before or after ERCP reduces the risk for PEP compared to placebo [9]. Therefore, routine pre-ERCP rectal administration of 100 mg indomethacin or diclofenac can be recommended to reduce the risk of post-ERCP pancreatitis in all patients without contraindications [2, 9–11].

31.5.3 Periprocedural Fluid Replacement

Dehydration, hypotonic circulation, and shock support systemic inflammatory reactions and organ dysfunction such as pancreatitis. Therefore, fluid replacement with isotonic crystalloid solutions may prevent development of periprocedural pancreatitis. It has been shown that early replacement of complete electrolyte infusion before, during, and after ERCP reduces the rate of PEP [12, 13].

31.5.4 Guidewire Cannulation

Long cannulation time, several attempts for cannulation, precut, and injection of contrast material increase the risk for PEP. The guidewire cannulation technique reduces PEP, achieves higher rates of cannulation of the desired duct, and reduces the need for precut sphincterotomy [1, 2]. Thus, guidewire cannulation should be the standard approach to the naïve papilla.

31.5.5 Cannulation Attempts and Precut

To reduce trauma by manipulation of the papilla, the number of cannulation attempts should be as low as possible [2]. The risk of PEP seems to be lower in patients receiving early precut than in those with several attempts with the standard technique [2]. In patients with a bile duct dilated down to the papilla, needle-knife fistulotomy seems to be associated with a lower PEP risk than conventional precut and transpancreatic sphincterotomy [2].

31.5.6 Pancreatic Duct Stents

Placement of pancreatic stents to reduce the risk for PEP is well supported by randomized-controlled studies and meta-analyses [1, 2]. Therefore, placement of small prophylactic pancreatic stents e.g. 5-French over a guidewire in the pancreatic duct is strongly recommended in patients with high risk for post-ERCP pancreatitis [1, 2, 11]. Pancreatic stents should remain for at least 12–24 h and be removed not later than 3–5 days [1, 2, 11].

31.6 Management

Management of PEP depends on the severity of pancreatitis [14]. In mild to moderate cases, fluid replacement and pain management are sufficient. In severe cases with hemodynamic instability, systemic reactions, and organ failure, intensive care management is necessary. Most important is sufficient fluid replacement and the preservation of hemodynamics. Antibiotic treatment is only necessary if cholangitis or infectious complications have occurred. Severe acute pancreatitis with necrosis in the pancreatic parenchyma or surrounding fat tissue may require percutaneous drainage, transgastric stenting, and endoscopic or surgical necrosectomy [15].

References

1. Chandrasekhara V, Khashab MA, Muthusamy VR, Acosta RD, Agrawal D, Bruining DH, et al. Adverse events associated with ERCP. Gastrointest Endosc. 2017;85(1):32–47. [cited 2018 Apr 28]. http://www.ncbi.nlm.nih.gov/pubmed/27546389.
2. Dumonceau J-M, Andriulli A, Elmunzer B, Mariani A, Meister T, Deviere J, et al. Prophylaxis of post-ERCP pancreatitis: European Society of Gastrointestinal Endoscopy (ESGE) guideline—updated June 2014. Endoscopy. 2014;46(9):799–815. [cited 2018 Apr 29]. http://www.ncbi.nlm.nih.gov/pubmed/25148137.
3. Cotton PB, Lehman G, Vennes J, Geenen JE, Russell RC, Meyers WC, et al. Endoscopic sphincterotomy complications and their management: an attempt at consensus. Gastrointest Endosc. 1991;37(3):383–93. [cited 2018 Apr 29]. http://www.ncbi.nlm.nih.gov/pubmed/2070995.
4. Banks PA, Bollen TL, Dervenis C, Gooszen HG, Johnson CD, Sarr MG, et al. Classification of acute pancreatitis—2012: revision of the Atlanta classification and definitions by international consensus. Gut. 2013;62(1):102–11. [cited 2018 Apr 29]. http://gut.bmj.com/lookup/doi/10.1136/gutjnl-2012-302779.
5. Tryliskyy Y, Bryce G. Post-ERCP pancreatitis: pathophysiology, early identification and risk stratification. Adv Clin Exp Med. 2018;27(1):149–54.

[cited 2018 Apr 29]. http://www.ncbi.nlm.nih.gov/pubmed/29521055.
6. Zheng L, Wang X, Tao Q, Liang S, Wang B, Luo H, et al. Different pattern of risk factors for post-ERCP pancreatitis in patients with biliary stricture. Scand J Gastroenterol. 2018;53(5):604–10. [cited 2018 Apr 7]. http://www.ncbi.nlm.nih.gov/pubmed/29117728.
7. European Association for the Study of the Liver (EASL). EASL clinical practice guidelines on the prevention, diagnosis and treatment of gallstones. J Hepatol. 2016;65(1):146–81.
8. Ishiwatari H, Urata T, Yasuda I, Matsusaki S, Hisai H, Kawakami H, et al. No benefit of oral diclofenac on post-endoscopic retrograde cholangiopancreatography pancreatitis. Dig Dis Sci. 2016;61(11):3292–301. 22 [cited 2018 Apr 12]. http://link.springer.com/10.1007/s10620-016-4251-x.
9. Yu L-M, Zhao K-J, Lu B. Use of NSAIDs via the rectal route for the prevention of pancreatitis after ERCP in all-risk patients: an updated meta-analysis. Gastroenterol Res Pract. 2018;2018:1027530. [cited 2018 Apr 29]. http://www.ncbi.nlm.nih.gov/pubmed/29576766.
10. Garg R, Mohan BP, Krishnamoorthi R, Rustagi T. Pre-endoscopic retrograde cholangiopancreatography (ERCP) administration of rectal indomethacin in unselected patients to reduce post-ERCP pancreatitis: a systematic review and meta-analysis. Indian J Gastroenterol. 2018;37(2):120–6. [cited 2018 Apr 29]. http://www.ncbi.nlm.nih.gov/pubmed/29619673.
11. Lammert F, Neubrand M, Bittner R, Feussner H, Greiner L, Hagenmüller F, et al. S3-Leitlinie der Deutschen Gesellschaft für Verdauungs- und Stoffwechselkrankheiten und der Deutschen Gesellschaft für Viszeralchirurgie zur Diagnostik und Behandlung von Gallensteinen. Z Gastroenterol. 2007;45(9):971–1001. [cited 2018 Apr 22]. http://www.ncbi.nlm.nih.gov/pubmed/17874360.
12. Choi J-H, Kim HJ, Lee BU, Kim TH, Song IH. Vigorous periprocedural hydration with lactated ringer's solution reduces the risk of pancreatitis after retrograde cholangiopancreatography in hospitalized patients. Clin Gastroenterol Hepatol. 2017;15(1):86–92.e1. [cited 2018 Apr 29]. http://www.ncbi.nlm.nih.gov/pubmed/27311618.
13. Mok SRS, Ho HC, Shah P, Patel M, Gaughan JP, Elfant AB. Lactated ringer's solution in combination with rectal indomethacin for prevention of post-ERCP pancreatitis and readmission: a prospective randomized, double-blinded, placebo-controlled trial. Gastrointest Endosc. 2017;85(5):1005–13. [cited 2018 Apr 29]. http://www.ncbi.nlm.nih.gov/pubmed/27816497.
14. Tenner S, Baillie J, DeWitt J, Vege SS, American College of Gastroenterology. American College of Gastroenterology guideline: management of acute pancreatitis. Am J Gastroenterol. 2013;108(9):1400–15. [cited 2018 Mar 29]. http://www.ncbi.nlm.nih.gov/pubmed/23896955.
15. Isayama H, Nakai Y, Rerknimitr R, Khor C, Lau J, Wang H-P, et al. Asian consensus statements on endoscopic management of walled-off necrosis Part 1: epidemiology, diagnosis, and treatment. J Gastroenterol Hepatol. 2016;31(9):1546–54. [cited 2018 Apr 29]. http://www.ncbi.nlm.nih.gov/pubmed/27044023.

Bleeding 32

Stefanos M. Dokas

32.1 ERCP-Related Bleeding

Endoscopic sphincterotomy is an endoscopic procedure with high hemorrhagic risk (Table 32.1). Bleeding during endoscopic sphincterotomy is not uncommon. Usually this is a transient phenomenon which stops spontaneously within a few minutes without any specific treatment. This is not considered an adverse event and has no impact on scheduled treatment. Clinically significant bleeding occurs whenever excessive blood impairs the delivery of scheduled treatment or manifests as melena, hematemesis, or hypovolemic shock, thus requiring admission with or without transfusions or prolongation of hospital stay or further interventions such as endoscopic hemostasis, angiographic embolization, and surgery. The incidence of significant bleeding after biliary sphincterotomy is less than 2% [1–3] although this figure was estimated a bit higher in the early days of ERCP [4]. The bleeding-related mortality rate is around 3.5% (CI 1.08–6.00) [1].

The severity of post-sphincterotomy bleeding is graded as mild, moderate, severe, and fatal (Table 32.2) according to the drop of hemoglobin, the need for transfusion, and/or further interventions. Delayed bleeding may occur anywhere between hours up to 7 or even 10 days postoperatively.

Table 32.1 Risk stratification of endoscopic procedures based on the risk of haemorrhage [16]

High risk	Low risk
Endoscopic polypectomy ERCP with sphincterotomy Sphincterotomy + large balloon papillary dilatation Ampullectomy Endoscopic mucosal resection or endoscopic submucosal dissection Endoscopic dilatation of strictures in the upper or lower GI tract Endoscopic therapy of varices Percutaneous endoscopic gastrostomy EUS with FNA Esophageal, enteral, or colonic stenting	Diagnostic procedures ± biopsy Biliary or pancreatic stenting Device-assisted enteroscopy without polypectomy

Endoscopic ampullectomy carries a high bleeding risk. Post-ampullectomy bleeding has been reported to range between 2 and 30% [5]. Bleeding during or after ampullectomy is managed the same way as post-sphincterotomy bleeding.

32.2 EUS-Related Bleeding

Bleeding may complicate EUS interventions. Fine needle aspiration and treatment of pancreatic fluid collections are the procedures most frequently asso-

S. M. Dokas (✉)
Endoscopy Department, St. Luke's Private Hospital, Thessaloniki, Greece
e-mail: altair@med.auth.gr

M. Mutignani et al. (eds.), *Endotherapy in Biliopancreatic Diseases: ERCP Meets EUS*,
https://doi.org/10.1007/978-3-030-42569-2_32

Table 32.2 Bleeding severity after endoscopic sphincterotomy [4] and further adapted from [50]

Mild	Moderate	Severe	Fatal
Clinical (i.e., not just endoscopic) evidence of bleeding Hemoglobin drop <3 g, without need for transfusion	Transfusion (4 units or less), no angiographic intervention or surgery	Transfusion 5 units or more or intervention (angiographic or surgical)	Death

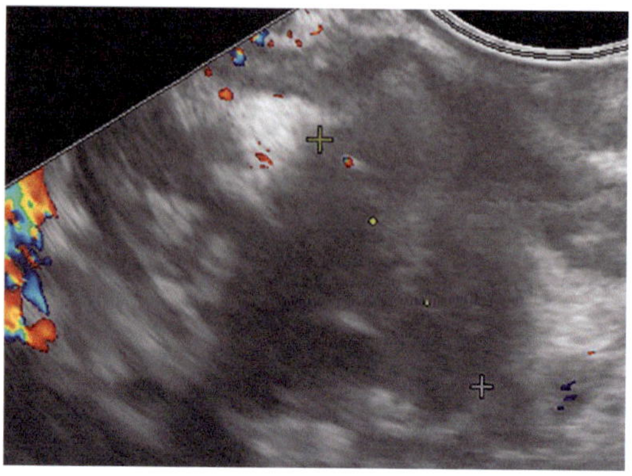

Fig. 32.1 Bleeding after EUS-FNA (Kindly granted by M. Mutignani)

ciated with hemorrhage. Intraprocedural bleeding may be observed in as much as 4% of cases, but it is usually mild and no intervention is needed. Bleeding may be evident as a small rim of fluid or a stable duodenal wall hematoma (Fig. 32.1) [6]. Extraluminal bleeding is rare and may complicate 1.3% of EUS-FNA procedures [7] or up to 6% of EUS-FNA of pancreatic cystic lesions [8]. Compression of the bleeding site with the echoendoscope for a few minutes usually is enough to stop the bleeding. On the other hand, EUS-FNA for solid lesions seems safer in terms of hemorrhage [9].

Hemorrhage during or after EUS-guided treatment of peripancreatic fluid collections, mainly walled-off necrosis, is not uncommon and can be massive [10, 11]. Bleeding may occur during the puncture [12] or later as a result of metal stent-induced vessel erosion [10]. A recent study suggested that placing a double pigtail stent through the lumen-apposing stent (LAMS) inserted for the treatment of peripancreatic fluid collection yielded significantly less adverse events; bleeding was the most frequent adverse event [13]. Most bleeding cases are due to eroded pseudoaneurysms arising either from the splenic or the gastroduodenal artery. Bleeding from the rim of the puncture may be controlled with dilating balloon tamponade or with LAMS placement. Delayed bleeding may be controlled endoscopically through the LAMS or by means of interventional radiology [14].

32.3 Risk Factors - Preventive Measures

Risk factors definitely associated with increased bleeding incidence include coagulopathy, thrombocytopenia, acute cholangitis, initiation of anticoagulants less than 3 days after ERCP, bleeding during ERCP, and operator with low case volume. Liver cirrhosis, renal insufficiency/dialysis, periampullary diverticula, dilated common bile duct (CBD), and needle-knife sphincterotomy are potentially associated with increased bleeding risk. On the other hand, the use of aspirin or nonsteroidal anti-inflammatory drugs (NSAIDs), a wide sphincterotomy, extension of a previous sphincterotomy, and the presence of ampullary tumor do not increase the bleeding risk (Table 32.3).

It is now clear that there is no increased risk of hemorrhage after sphincterotomy in patients receiving aspirin or nonsteroidal anti-inflammatory drugs (NSAIDs) [15]. It is not necessary to hold aspirin in order to perform endoscopic sphincterotomy or EUS-FNA. Ampullectomy, on the contrary, has a very high bleeding risk, and individual patient parameters should be taken into account before deciding whether to discontinue aspirin or not. The risk of hemorrhage in patients treated with clopidogrel and other thienopyridine agents is unclear, although current guidelines both from the ESGE and the ASGE clearly suggest that antiplatelets other than aspirin should be discontinued for 5–7 days prior to

Table 32.3 Risk factors for hemorrhage after sphincterotomy [51]

Definite	Maybe	No
Coagulopathy	Cirrhosis	Aspirin or NSAIDs use
Anticoagulation <3 days after ES	Dilated CBD	Ampullary tumor
Cholangitis before ERCP	CBD stone	Longer sphincterotomy
Bleeding during ES	Periampullary diverticulum	Extension of prior ES
Low ERCP case volume	Precut sphincterotomy	

the procedure [16, 17]. On the other hand, a recent nationwide Japanese study which included 61,000 patients concluded that endoscopic sphincterotomy is safe in patients receiving *any single antiplatelet drug* [18].

In case of dual antiplatelet therapy, consultation from the attending physician should be solicited. Usually, aspirin is continued and the second antiplatelet agent is held depending on thrombotic risk. Thrombotic risk is very high whenever both agents are stopped [19]. Sphincterotomy or other high-risk endoscopic procedure can be performed 5–7 days after discontinuation of clopidogrel or equivalent agent. Whenever the thrombotic risk is high, or in emergencies, balloon sphincteroplasty following a small sphincterotomy or biliary stenting without sphincterotomy to relieve obstruction are valid alternatives [20–22].

In patients with thrombocytopenia, sphincterotomy may be performed after platelet transfusion with a goal of platelet count above 50,000/mm^3. Coagulopathy from cirrhosis or other causes may be reversed with the use of fresh frozen plasma (FFP) and/or vitamin K in an emergency setting. Patients on hemodialysis are on particularly high risk of post-sphincterotomy bleeding [15]. Improving platelet function with 1-desamino-8d-arginine vasopressin (DDAVP) or estrogens and correction of anemia may help reduce bleeding risk in this particular group of patients.

Vitamin K antagonists, such as warfarin, should be stopped approximately 5 days prior to the procedure. Bridging therapy with low molecular weight heparin can be performed when indicated. For emergencies, three options exist for warfarin reversal: the use of prothrombinase complex concentrate, FFP transfusion, and vitamin K administration. Four-factor prothrombinase complex concentrate delivers coagulation factors II, IX, X, and VII and can reverse the anticoagulation from vitamin K antagonists immediately. Fresh frozen plasma transfusion rapidly restores missing coagulation factors. Transfusion of six units of FFP is usually enough to achieve adequate coagulation. Vitamin K increases the liver production of factors II, VII, XI, and X. Sufficient factor VII levels can be reached 6 h after intravenously administered vitamin K (2 mg). Orally administered vitamin K (5 mg) restores factor VII levels after 12 h [23, 24]. In any case, INR monitoring during pharmacologic manipulations with target ≤1.5 ensures adequate coagulation. Reinitiating warfarin with the usual dose at the night of the procedure is suggested by current guidelines from both ESGE and ASGE [16, 17].

Unfractionated heparin may be reversed with protamine sulphate for emergencies; otherwise, for elective cases, bridging with low molecular weight heparin can be performed.

Direct oral anticoagulants were initially introduced in 2009 and include the direct thrombin inhibitor dabigatran and the direct factor Xa inhibitors rivaroxaban, apixaban, and edoxaban. Dabigatran is metabolized and excreted from the kidneys. Discontinuation for 2–3 days is usually enough in patients with normal renal function. An antidote for dabigatran (idarucizumab) is available and can be used in case of life-threatening bleeding. Rivaroxaban, apixaban, and edoxaban have to be discontinued for 1–2 days before the procedure. Reinitiating direct oral anticoagulants is advised whenever adequate hemostasis is ensured.

The use of blended current from automated current delivery generators has been shown to reduce the risk of immediate but not delayed bleeding [20, 25, 26]. Uncontrolled or "zipper cut" may be prevented using the ENDOCUT mode [27]. Directing the cut at the arc between

11 and 1 o'clock, where the density of vessels is low, reduces bleeding risk besides preventing perforations [28]. Bleeding during the intervention usually stops, but it is also a predisposing factor for delayed bleeding. If even minor bleeding or oozing persists by the end of the procedure, endoscopic hemostasis better be performed before terminating the procedure.

32.4 Management

Intraprocedural bleeding is often encountered during ERCP. This is usually minor hemorrhage which stops spontaneously. The first thing to do when bleeding starts during sphincterotomy is to apply coagulating current via the sphincterotome wire at the top of the sphincterotomy and to continue cutting up to desired length, especially if the bleeding seems of arterial origin [29]. If bleeding persists or impairs the visibility and inhibits treatment, further measures must be taken to arrest hemorrhage. The simplest and easiest method to achieve hemostasis is injecting diluted epinephrine with the usual concentration (1:10,000) at the edges and the apex of the sphincterotomy (Fig. 32.2a–c). A few milliliters of injected solution will usually stop the bleeding. The effectiveness of injected epinephrine is very high, between 96 and 100% [30, 31]. Care must be taken so that epinephrine is not injected into the pancreas. The aim is to create a submucosal bleb. The use of standard sclerotherapy needles through the duodenoscope may present with some difficulties. For a smooth injection procedure, the needle is first advanced to the edge of the sheath. The sheath is passed over the elevator with the elevator relaxed. When the sheath exits the working channel, the needle is pushed forward. Then the elevator can be raised to target the bleeding spot. It is best to maintain the sheath outside the working channel with the needle protruding while injecting to various sites. If the needle is withdrawn into the sheath, readvancing may be difficult, or may damage the needle. This is due to sheath kinking from the elevator. A spring sheath stainless steel needle may overcome such difficulties when injecting through the duodenoscope.

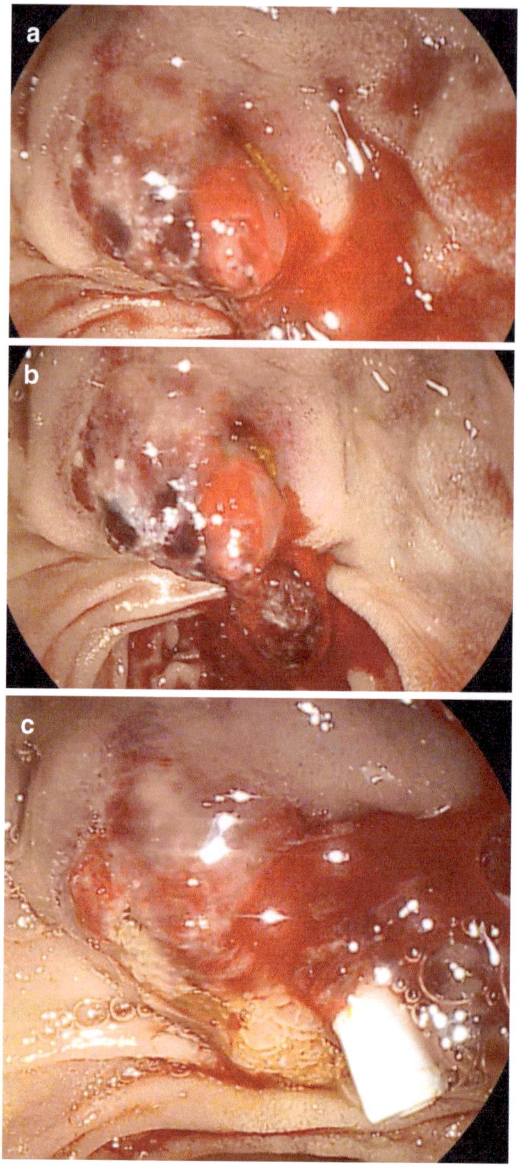

Fig. 32.2 (**a**) Late bleeding after EBS. (**b**) Late bleeding after EBS. (**c**) Prophylactic biliary stent insertion after adrenaline injection. (Kindly granted by M. Mutignani)

Alternative hemostatic methods include tamponade of the bleeding site with a stone retrieval balloon. The balloon is inserted into the bile duct and withdrawn while fully inflated without exiting the duct so as to compress the tissue between the balloon and the tip of the endoscope. This compression is maintained for 3–5 min. Treatment may be complemented with other hemostatic methods for a more permanent result.

If bleeding persists, coaptive monopolar or bipolar coagulation can be applied [32, 33]. When coagulation is applied, care should be taken so that the pancreatic orifice is protected and spared. The use of coagulating probes with injection ability is a good choice when bleeding is blocking the view, and a fast hemostasis is necessary. Coagulating current may be applied through the tip of a polypectomy snare [34], through the tip of a closed Dormia basket via an electrosurgical pencil [29] or with the use of coagulating forceps [35]. Coaptive coagulation is also highly recommended for active arterial bleeding during ampullectomy [36]. Argon plasma coagulation (APC) has been used to treat successfully two cases of post-sphincterotomy bleeding more than 10 years ago [37].

Endoclips can also be used to treat post-sphincterotomy bleeding (Figs. 32.3a, b and 32.4a, b). Their deployment is challenging through the duodenoscope. Failed attempts are to be expected often [38, 39]. A recent study

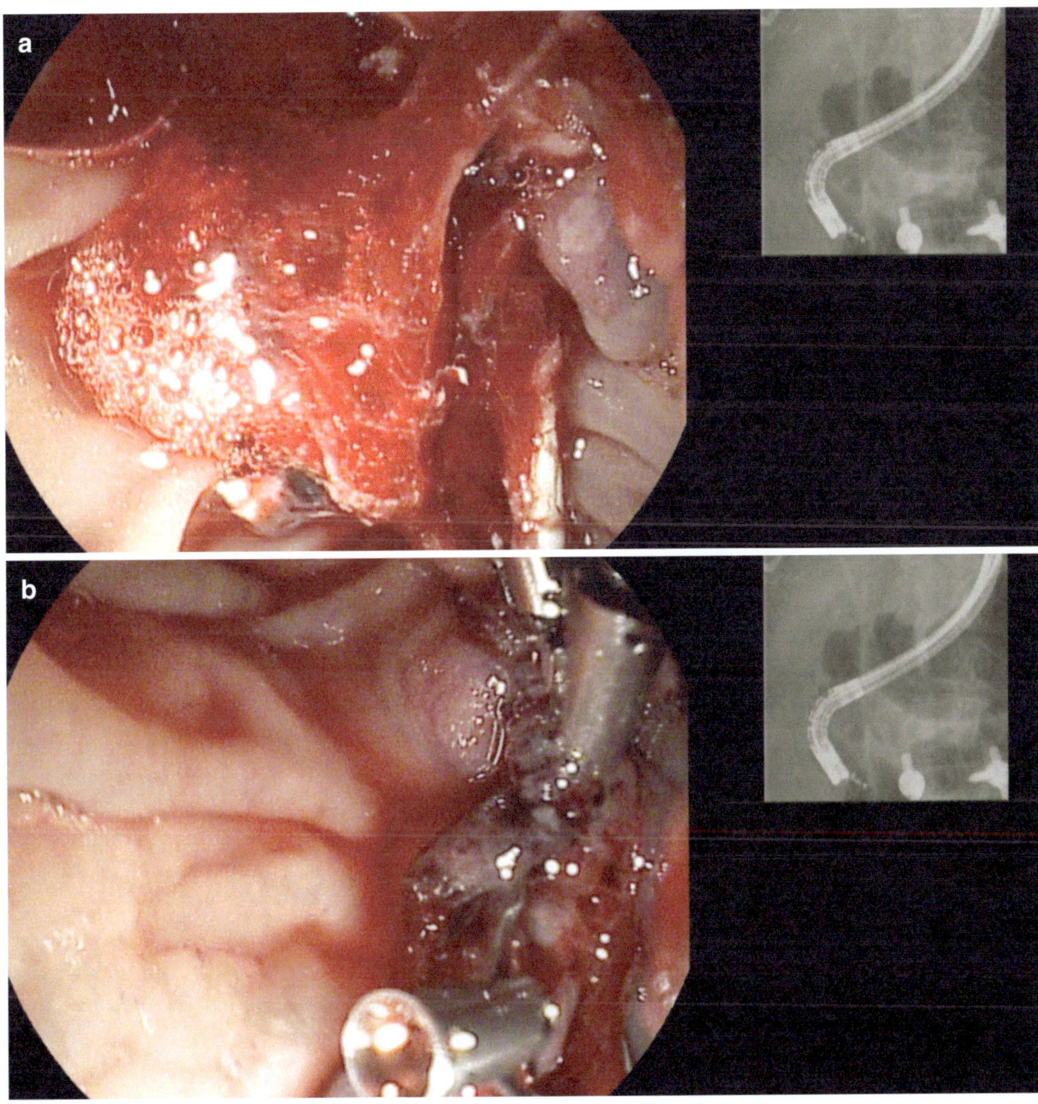

Fig. 32.3 (**a**) Acute bleeding after Endoscopic Sphincterotomy. (**b**) Clipping successfully controlled the bleeding. (Kindly granted by M. Mutignani)

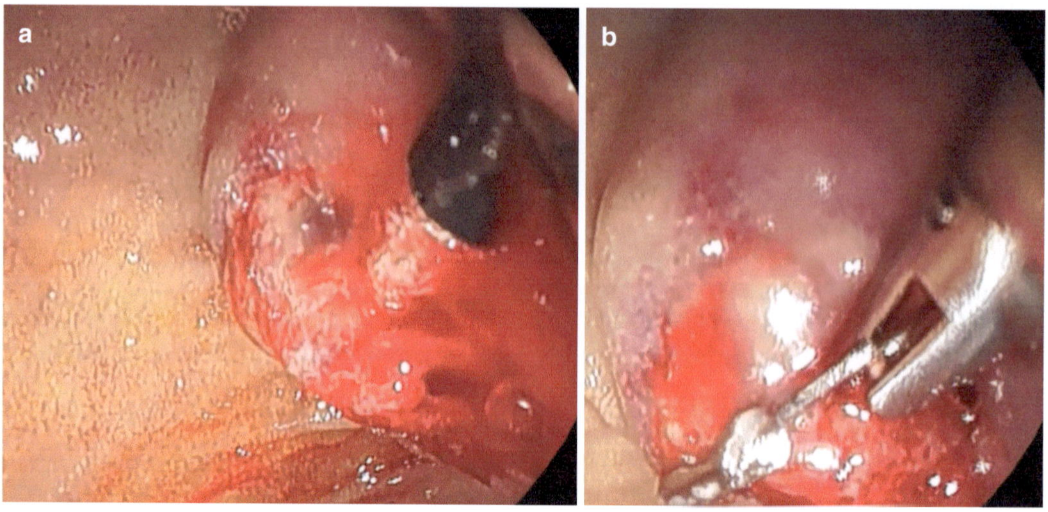

Fig. 32.4 (**a**) Bleeding during needle knife papillotomy. (**b**) Clispping to control hemorrhage. (Kindly granted by M. Mutignani)

reported 100% control of post-sphincterotomy bleeding with endoclips deployed through a forward-viewing gastroscope equipped with a transparent hood [40].

Fully covered self-expanding metal stents (FCSEMS) have also been used to treat post-biliary sphincterotomy bleeding. The deployment of a metal stent exerts a tamponade effect. The promising results from the first case series [41, 42] were confirmed by a larger retrospective cohort which included 23 patients treated with FCSEMS [43]. In all cases, bleeding stopped after the insertion of the FCSEMS. The stents were retrieved early (within 8 days) in one study [41] and later, between 8 and 12 weeks, in other studies [42, 43]. In order to avoid difficulties during removal, it seems reasonable to opt for early stent removal.

Hemostatic powder spray (TC-325; Cook Medical Inc., Winston-Salem, NC) is an inorganic powder which achieves hemostasis by adhering to the bleeding site and promotes thrombus formation by concentrating and activating platelets and coagulation factors [44]. This substance is sprayed via a dedicated catheter onto the bleeding site. It has been used to treat post-sphincterotomy bleeding, and a few case reports have been published [45, 46]. The treatment was successful in all published cases. Bile duct occlusion from a blood clot was reported in one case [47], but this may potentially complicate any case of post-sphincterotomy bleeding.

The medical treatment of post-sphincterotomy bleeding is the same with upper gastrointestinal bleeding. It includes close monitoring, fluid replenishment, and hemodynamic support, correction of coagulopathy, and plasma and blood transfusion if needed.

There is no consensus on the type of endoscopic therapy used to treat post-sphincterotomy bleeding. Operator preference and familiarity with various hemostatic methods are definitely a major factor. The use of dual endoscopic treatment such as epinephrine plus coagulation or clipping, like in the treatment of peptic ulcer bleeding, seems reasonable, especially when brisk bleeding is encountered. Repeat endoscopy is usually offered in the case of recurrent bleeding. Alternative hemostatic methods should be applied during repeat endoscopy.

If repeated endotherapy is not successful, angiographic embolization can occlude the bleeding vessel efficiently in most cases [48], although literature data are scarce. Surgery is indicated for refractory cases. The incidence of surgical treatment of post-sphincterotomy hemorrhage is very low, below 0.1% [49].

It is important never to lose access to the bile duct. Maintaining a guidewire deeply into the bile duct during hemostasis is strongly advised.

Massive bleeding may result in intraductal clot formation which in turn may obstruct the bile duct. Maintaining ductal patency, preferably with a nasobiliary catheter, is wise, especially if there is fear of recurrent bleeding.

To summarize, keeping calm, maintaining ductal access/patency, and hemostasis either with adrenaline injection, coagulation with various methods, tamponade (balloon/FCSEMS), clipping, or hemostatic powder spray are the steps to follow for a successful endoscopic management.

32.5 Conclusion

Bleeding may be immediate or delayed after endoscopic sphincterotomy or therapeutic EUS. Patient- and operator-dependent risk factors contribute to the occurrence of bleeding. Proper patient preparation and endoscopic technique are key factors to minimize bleeding risk. Numerous endoscopic hemostatic methods are available in order to achieve durable hemostasis, but the optimal endoscopic hemostatic technique is not yet defined. Newer hemostatic modalities have enriched the armamentarium of the modern endoscopist.

References

1. Andriulli A, Loperfido S, Napolitano G, Niro G, Valvano MR, Spirito F, et al. Incidence rates of post-ERCP complications: a systematic survey of prospective studies. Am J Gastroenterol. 2007;102(8):1781–8. https://doi.org/10.1111/j.1572-0241.2007.01279.x. AJG1279 [pii].
2. Williams EJ, Taylor S, Fairclough P, Hamlyn A, Logan RF, Martin D, et al. Risk factors for complication following ERCP; results of a large-scale, prospective multicenter study. Endoscopy. 2007;39(9):793–801. https://doi.org/10.1055/s-2007-966723.
3. Freeman ML, Nelson DB, Sherman S, Haber GB, Herman ME, Dorsher PJ, et al. Complications of endoscopic biliary sphincterotomy. N Engl J Med. 1996;335(13):909–18. https://doi.org/10.1056/NEJM199609263351301.
4. Cotton PB, Lehman G, Vennes J, Geenen JE, Russell RC, Meyers WC, et al. Endoscopic sphincterotomy complications and their management: an attempt at consensus. Gastrointest Endosc. 1991;37(3):383–93. S0016-5107(91)70740-2 [pii].
5. Ito K, Fujita N, Noda Y. Endoscopic diagnosis and treatment of ampullary neoplasm (with video). Dig Endosc. 2011;23(2):113–7. https://doi.org/10.1111/j.1443-1661.2010.01101.x.
6. Voss M, Hammel P, Molas G, Palazzo L, Dancour A, O'Toole D, et al. Value of endoscopic ultrasound guided fine needle aspiration biopsy in the diagnosis of solid pancreatic masses. Gut. 2000;46(2):244–9.
7. Affi A, Vazquez-Sequeiros E, Norton ID, Clain JE, Wiersema MJ. Acute extraluminal hemorrhage associated with EUS-guided fine needle aspiration: frequency and clinical significance. Gastrointest Endosc. 2001;53(2):221–5. S0016-5107(01)70372-0 [pii].
8. Varadarajulu S, Eloubeidi MA. Frequency and significance of acute intracystic hemorrhage during EUS-FNA of cystic lesions of the pancreas. Gastrointest Endosc. 2004;60(4):631–5. S0016-5107(04)01891-7 [pii].
9. Eloubeidi MA, Tamhane A, Varadarajulu S, Wilcox CM. Frequency of major complications after EUS-guided FNA of solid pancreatic masses: a prospective evaluation. Gastrointest Endosc. 2006;63(4):622–9. https://doi.org/10.1016/j.gie.2005.05.024. S0016-5107(05)02108-5 [pii].
10. Bang JY, Hasan M, Navaneethan U, Hawes R, Varadarajulu S. Lumen-apposing metal stents (LAMS) for pancreatic fluid collection (PFC) drainage: may not be business as usual. Gut. 2017;66(12):2054–6. https://doi.org/10.1136/gutjnl-2016-312812. gutjnl-2016-312812 [pii].
11. Stecher SS, Simon P, Friesecke S, Glitsch A, Kuhn JP, Lerch MM, et al. Delayed severe bleeding complications after treatment of pancreatic fluid collections with lumen-apposing metal stents. Gut. 2017;66(10):1871–2. https://doi.org/10.1136/gutjnl-2016-313562. gutjnl-2016-313562 [pii].
12. Mejia Perez LK, Brahmbhatt B, Gomez V. Massive bleeding after EUS-guided walled-off necrosis drainage. VideoGIE. 2018;3(1):13–4. https://doi.org/10.1016/j.vgie.2017.09.014. S2468-4481(17)30211-4 [pii].
13. Puga M, Consiglieri CF, Busquets J, Pallares N, Secanella L, Pelaez N, et al. Safety of lumen-apposing stent with or without coaxial plastic stent for endoscopic ultrasound-guided drainage of pancreatic fluid collections: a retrospective study. Endoscopy. 2018;50(10):1022–6. https://doi.org/10.1055/a-0582-9127.
14. Jiang TA, Xie LT. Algorithm for the multidisciplinary management of hemorrhage in EUS-guided drainage for pancreatic fluid collections. World J Clin Cases. 2018;6(10):308–21. https://doi.org/10.12998/wjcc.v6.i10.308.
15. Nelson DB, Freeman ML. Major hemorrhage from endoscopic sphincterotomy: risk factor analysis. J Clin Gastroenterol. 1994;19(4):283–7.
16. Veitch AM, Vanbiervliet G, Gershlick AH, Boustiere C, Baglin TP, Smith LA, et al. Endoscopy in patients on antiplatelet or anticoagulant therapy, including direct oral anticoagulants: British Society of

Gastroenterology (BSG) and European Society of Gastrointestinal Endoscopy (ESGE) guidelines. Gut. 2016;65(3):374–89. https://doi.org/10.1136/gutjnl-2015-311110. gutjnl-2015-311110 [pii].

17. Acosta RD, Abraham NS, Chandrasekhara V, Chathadi KV, Early DS, Eloubeidi MA, et al. The management of antithrombotic agents for patients undergoing GI endoscopy. Gastrointest Endosc. 2016;83(1):3–16. https://doi.org/10.1016/j.gie.2015.09.035. S0016-5107(15)02950-8 [pii].
18. Hamada T, Yasunaga H, Nakai Y, Isayama H, Matsui H, Horiguchi H, et al. Bleeding after endoscopic sphincterotomy or papillary balloon dilation among users of antithrombotic agents. Endoscopy. 2015;47(11):997–1004. https://doi.org/10.1055/s-0034-1392408.
19. Eisenberg MJ, Richard PR, Libersan D, Filion KB. Safety of short-term discontinuation of antiplatelet therapy in patients with drug-eluting stents. Circulation. 2009;119(12):1634–42. https://doi.org/10.1161/CIRCULATIONAHA.108.813667. CIRCULATIONAHA.108.813667 [pii].
20. Freeman ML. Complications of endoscopic retrograde cholangiopancreatography: avoidance and management. Gastrointest Endosc Clin N Am. 2012;22(3):567–86. https://doi.org/10.1016/j.giec.2012.05.001. S1052-5157(12)00026-8 [pii].
21. Chung JW, Chung JB. Endoscopic papillary balloon dilation for removal of choledocholithiasis: indications, advantages, complications, and long-term follow-up results. Gut Liver. 2011;5(1):1–14. https://doi.org/10.5009/gnl.2011.5.1.1.
22. Baron TH, Harewood GC. Endoscopic balloon dilation of the biliary sphincter compared to endoscopic biliary sphincterotomy for removal of common bile duct stones during ERCP: a metaanalysis of randomized, controlled trials. Am J Gastroenterol. 2004;99(8):1455–60. https://doi.org/10.1111/j.1572-0241.2004.30151.x. AJG30151 [pii].
23. Hunt BJ, Levi M. Urgent reversal of vitamin K antagonists. BMJ. 2018;360:j5424. https://doi.org/10.1136/bmj.j5424.
24. Tran HA, Chunilal SD, Harper PL, Tran H, Wood EM, Gallus AS. An update of consensus guidelines for warfarin reversal. Med J Aust. 2013;198(4):198–9. https://doi.org/10.5694/mja12.10614.
25. Balmadrid B, Kozarek R. Prevention and management of adverse events of endoscopic retrograde cholangiopancreatography. Gastrointest Endosc Clin N Am. 2013;23(2):385–403. https://doi.org/10.1016/j.giec.2012.12.007. S1052-5157(12)00170-5 [pii].
26. Perini RF, Sadurski R, Cotton PB, Patel RS, Hawes RH, Cunningham JT. Post-sphincterotomy bleeding after the introduction of microprocessor-controlled electrosurgery: does the new technology make the difference? Gastrointest Endosc. 2005;61(1):53–7. S0016-5107(04)02454-X [pii].
27. Norton ID, Petersen BT, Bosco J, Nelson DB, Meier PB, Baron TH, et al. A randomized trial of endoscopic biliary sphincterotomy using pure-cut versus combined cut and coagulation waveforms. Clin Gastroenterol Hepatol. 2005;3(10):1029–33. S1542-3565(05)00528-8 [pii].
28. Mirjalili SA, Stringer MD. The arterial supply of the major duodenal papilla and its relevance to endoscopic sphincterotomy. Endoscopy. 2011;43(4):307–11. https://doi.org/10.1055/s-0030-1256229.
29. Costamagna G. What to do when the papilla bleeds after endoscopic sphincterotomy. Endoscopy. 1998;30(1):40–2. https://doi.org/10.1055/s-2007-993727.
30. Leung JW, Chan FK, Sung JJ, Chung SC. Endoscopic sphincterotomy-induced hemorrhage: a study of risk factors and the role of epinephrine injection. Gastrointest Endosc. 1995;42(6):550–4. https://doi.org/10.1016/S0016-5107(95)70009-9. S0016-5107(95)70009-9 [pii].
31. Wilcox CM, Canakis J, Monkemuller KE, Bondora AW, Geels W. Patterns of bleeding after endoscopic sphincterotomy, the subsequent risk of bleeding, and the role of epinephrine injection. Am J Gastroenterol. 2004;99(2):244–8.
32. Sherman S, Hawes RH, Nisi R, Lehman GA. Endoscopic sphincterotomy-induced hemorrhage: treatment with multipolar electrocoagulation. Gastrointest Endosc. 1992;38(2):123–6. S0016-5107(92)70375-7 [pii].
33. Kuran S, Parlak E, Oguz D, Cicek B, Disibeyaz S, Sahin B. Endoscopic sphincterotomy-induced hemorrhage: treatment with heat probe. Gastrointest Endosc. 2006;63(3):506–11. https://doi.org/10.1016/j.gie.2005.09.039. S0016-5107(05)02942-1 [pii].
34. Katsinelos P, Kountouras J, Chatzimavroudis G, Zavos C, Fasoulas K, Katsinelos T, et al. Endoscopic hemostasis using monopolar coagulation for postendoscopic sphincterotomy bleeding refractory to injection treatment. Surg Laparosc Endosc Percutan Tech. 2010;20(2):84–8. https://doi.org/10.1097/SLE.0b013e3181d76ace. 00129689-201004000-00006 [pii].
35. Dubravcsik Z, Hritz I, Fejes R, Szepes A, Madácsy L. Endoscopic therapy of refractory post-papillotomy bleeding with electrocautery forceps coagulation method combined with prophylactic pancreatic stenting. Video J Encycl GI Endosc. 2014;1(3):628–31. https://doi.org/10.1016/j.vjgien.2013.06.002.
36. Bassan M, Bourke M. Endoscopic ampullectomy: a practical guide. J Interv Gastroenterol. 2012;2(1):23–30. https://doi.org/10.4161/jig.20131. 2154-1280-2-1-9 [pii].
37. Oviedo JA, Barrison A, Lichtenstein DR. Endoscopic argon plasma coagulation for refractory postsphincterotomy bleeding: report of two cases. Gastrointest Endosc. 2003;58(1):148–51. https://doi.org/10.1067/mge.2003.320. S0016510703014871 [pii].
38. Baron TH, Norton ID, Herman L. Endoscopic hemoclip placement for post-sphincterotomy bleeding. Gastrointest Endosc. 2000;52(5):662. https://doi.org/10.1067/mge.2000.108621. S0016-5107(00)00334-5 [pii].

39. Lin LF, Siauw CP, Ho KS, Tung JN. Hemoclip treatment for post-endoscopic sphincterotomy bleeding. J Chin Med Assoc. 2004;67(10):496–9.
40. Chon IIK, Kim TH. Endoclip therapy of post-sphincterotomy bleeding using a transparent cap-fitted forward-viewing gastroscope. Surg Endosc. 2017;31(7):2783–8. https://doi.org/10.1007/s00464-016-5287-x. 10.1007/s00464-016-5287-x [pii].
41. Itoi T, Ijima M, Kobatake T, Kurihara E, Watanuki Y, Okuno N. Hemostasis by using a fully covered self-expandable biliary metal stent for massive bleeding during EUS-guided cystogastrostomy. Gastrointest Endosc. 2014;80(4):726–7. https://doi.org/10.1016/j.gie.2013.12.028. S0016-5107(13)02711-9 [pii].
42. Shah JN, Marson F, Binmoeller KF. Temporary self-expandable metal stent placement for treatment of post-sphincterotomy bleeding. Gastrointest Endosc. 2010;72(6):1274–8. https://doi.org/10.1016/j.gie.2010.08.012. S0016-5107(10)01968-1 [pii].
43. Cochrane J, Schlepp G. Comparing endoscopic intervention against fully covered self-expanding metal stent placement for post-endoscopic sphincterotomy bleed (CEASE Study). Endosc Int Open. 2016;4(12):E1261–4. https://doi.org/10.1055/s-0042-118227.
44. Aslanian HR, Laine L. Hemostatic powder spray for GI bleeding. Gastrointest Endosc. 2013;77(3):508–10. https://doi.org/10.1016/j.gie.2012.11.034. S0016-5107(12)02986-0 [pii].
45. Appleby VJ, Hutchinson JM, Beckett CJ, Moreea S. Use of the haemostatic agent TC-325 in the treatment of bleeding secondary to endoscopic retrograde cholangiopancreatography sphincterotomy. QJM. 2015;108(1):79–80. https://doi.org/10.1093/qjmed/hcu135. hcu135 [pii].
46. Baracat FI, Tranquillini CV, Brunaldi VO, Baracat R, de Moura EGH. Hemostatic powder: a new ally in the management of postsphincterotomy bleeding. VideoGIE. 2017;2(11):303–4. https://doi.org/10.1016/j.vgie.2017.07.002. S2468-4481(17)30139-X [pii].
47. Moosavi S, Chen YI, Barkun AN. TC-325 application leading to transient obstruction of a post-sphincterotomy biliary orifice. Endoscopy. 2013;45(Suppl 2 UCTN):E130. https://doi.org/10.1055/s-0032-1326370.
48. Dunne R, McCarthy E, Joyce E, McEniff N, Guiney M, Ryan JM, et al. Post-endoscopic biliary sphincterotomy bleeding: an interventional radiology approach. Acta Radiol. 2013;54(10):1159–64. https://doi.org/10.1177/0284185113491567. 0284185113491567 [pii].
49. Christensen M, Matzen P, Schulze S, Rosenberg J. Complications of ERCP: a prospective study. Gastrointest Endosc. 2004;60(5):721–31. S0016-5107(04)02169-8 [pii].
50. Cotton PB, Eisen GM, Aabakken L, Baron TH, Hutter MM, Jacobson BC, et al. A lexicon for endoscopic adverse events: report of an ASGE workshop. Gastrointest Endosc. 2010;71(3):446–54. https://doi.org/10.1016/j.gie.2009.10.027. S0016-5107(09)02613-3 [pii].
51. Freeman ML. Adverse outcomes of ERCP. Gastrointest Endosc. 2002;56(6 Suppl):S273–82. https://doi.org/10.1067/mge.2002.129028. S0016-5107(02)70025-4 [pii].

ERCP-Related Perforations

33

Alberto Tringali, Marcello Cintolo, and Massimiliano Mutignani

Abbreviations

ABX	Antibiotics
BS	Biliary stent
C	Conservative treatment
CBD	Common bile duct
CR	Case report
CS	Case series
CT	Computed tomography
E	Endoscopy
EBL	Endoscopic band ligation
ERCP	Endoscopic retrograde cholangio-pancreatography
FCSEMS	Fully covered self-expandable metal stent
IV	Intravenous
NBD	Naso-biliary drainage
NBM	Nil-by-mouth
NDT	Naso-duodenal tube
NGT	Nasogastric tube
NNR	Number not reported
NR	Not reported
OTSC	Over-the-scope clip
PBS	Plastic biliary stent
PCD	Percutaneous drainage (surgical)
PTC	Percutaneous transhepatic cholangiography
R	Retrospective
S	Surgery
TTSC	Through-the-scope clip

A. Tringali (✉)
Endoscopy Unit, ASST Grande Ospedale Metropolitano Niguarda, Milan, Italy

ULSS 2 Marca Trevigiana, Conegliano Hospital, Conegliano, Italy
e-mail: alberto.tringali@ospedaleniguarda.it

M. Cintolo · M. Mutignani
Endoscopy Unit, ASST Grande Ospedale Metropolitano Niguarda, Milan, Italy
e-mail: marcello.cintolo@ospedaleniguarda.it; massimiliano.mutignani@ospedaleniguarda.it

33.1 Epidemiology and Types of Perforation

In the last decades endoscopic retrograde cholangiopancreatography (ERCP) has evolved from diagnostic to a therapeutic procedure, leading to a higher risk of adverse events, morbidity, and mortality. The most common adverse events related to ERCP are post-ERCP pancreatitis (3–10%), cholangitis (0.5–3%), bleeding (0.3–2%), and perforation [1].

Overall perforation rate during ERCP varies among the different series, ranging between 0.08 and 2.2% [2, 3], with a pooled median incidence of one perforation each almost 200 procedures (0.47%).

M. Mutignani et al. (eds.), *Endotherapy in Biliopancreatic Diseases: ERCP Meets EUS*,
https://doi.org/10.1007/978-3-030-42569-2_33

ERCP-related perforations are usually divided into four groups according to Stapfer's classification [4]. This classification is based on anatomical criteria (Fig. 33.1): type 1 perforations (15–17%) include all injuries of the duodenal wall, type 2 perforations are the most common (60–65%) and are localized in the periampullary region, and type 3 perforations (13–20%) include biliary ductal injuries and leaks [5].

A rare case of Stapfer's type 3 perforation is the injury of the glissonian capsule, with the risk to cause subcapsular hematoma [6, 7] and/or abscesses [8, 9]; mortality rate of this adverse event is near to 10% of patients and is crucial to recognize it promptly. Some case reports also reported gaseous embolisms [10].

Finally, types 4 are not properly considered perforations, because includes all cases in which after ERCP is possible to detect retroperitoneal free air at the abdomen CT scan. However, many studies demonstrated that the presence of retroperitoneal air after sphincterotomy, in absence of clinical and biochemical signs of alarm, should be considered of no clinical significance [11].

Howard et al. proposed another classification, less used, categorizing perforations into three groups on the basis of the type of injury: guidewire's perforation of the duct (group I), periampullary perforation (group II), and duodenal perforation remote from the papilla (group III) [12].

33.2 Mechanisms of Perforation and Risk Factors

Type 1 perforations are usually caused by direct damage of the scope, type 2 perforations are commonly due to sphincterotomy, precut, or papillary balloon dilation. Type 3 perforations are caused by guidewires or other devices used during ERCP, such as Dormia's basket to retrieve biliary stones or balloon dilation in case of biliary stricture [5]. The subglissonian injuries are mainly due to the peripheral intrahepatic damage by using long guidewires [13].

Many published data analyzed predictive factors for an increased risk of ERCP-related perforation [14, 15]; in a multivariate analysis, Cotton et al. found that only the presence of surgically altered anatomy (Billroth II gastrectomy, Roux-en-Y diversion, and Whipple procedure) is signifi-

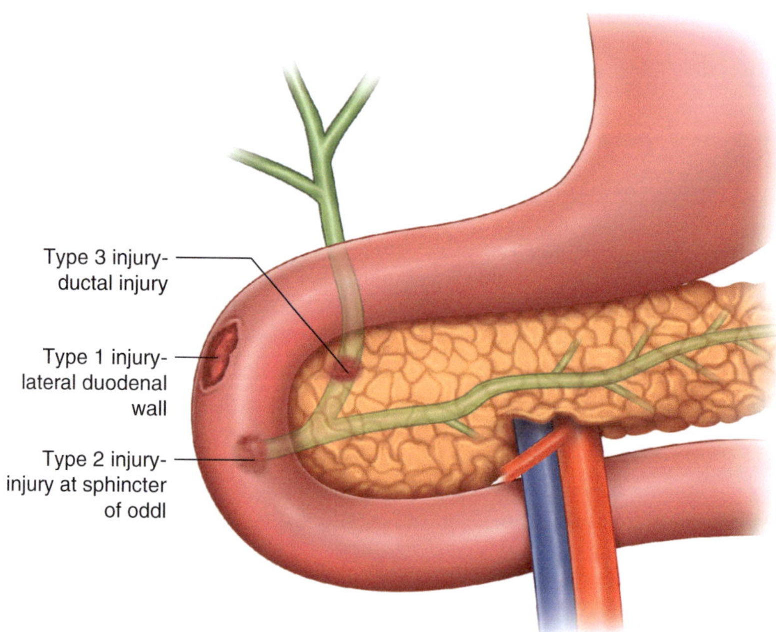

Fig. 33.1 Classification of ERCP-related perforations according to Stapfer et al.

cantly correlated to risk of type 1 perforation [16]. Enns et al. showed that greater age, biliary balloon dilation, precut, sphincterotomy, and a longer duration of the procedure are all associated with a high risk of type 1 and 2 perforations [17]. The presence of a periampullary diverticula is usually considered a possible risk factor for ERCP-related complication and perforation; nevertheless a recent meta-analysis including 16 studies for a total of 2794 patients concluded that the presence of a periampullary diverticula is not related to an increased risk of complication during ERCP [18].

A detail of risk factors according to the different types of perforation are summarized in the following table.

Risk factors for perforation
Type 1
Greater age
Altered anatomy (e.g., gastrectomy, pancreaticoduodenectomy)
Duodenal strictures
Periampullary diverticula
Longer duration of the procedure
Type 2
Greater age
Sphincterotomy
Precut
Oddi dysfunction
Dilated common bile duct
Periampullary diverticula
Longer duration of the procedure
Endoscopic papillary balloon dilation
Type 3
Dilation of biliary stricture
Guidewires

33.3 Diagnosis

The immediate recognition of an ERCP-related perforation is the key point to achieve a better outcome. Perforation during the procedure could be immediately suspected by endoscopy, in case of an evident mucosal breach, or by fluoroscopy, in case of onset of free peritoneal or retroperitoneal air and/or extravasation of contrast medium (Fig. 33.2a, b). The availability of high-quality radiological images and the development of a good experience in interpreting the radiologic findings are highly recommended. The execution of an abdomen CT scan without contrast medium can confirm or exclude the perforation, sometimes detecting the exact site of the leak and showing the presence of abdominal free air and/or fluid collections (Fig. 33.3a, b); the presence of peritoneal or retroperitoneal fluid collections at the CT scan could be an indication to urgent surgery. Among patients who do not need surgery, in absence of clinical and biochemical signs of infection, it could be useful to repeat a CT scan 3–5 days later, to check the reduction of the abdominal collections.

The diagnosis of subglissonian injury could be suspected during the procedure at the fluoroscopy, if the guidewire's tip seems to be deep in the peripheral ducts or even beyond the liver's profile. The onset of fever, anemia, and/or abdominal pain in the post-procedural period should be considered as alarm sign, and an abdominal CT scan with contrast is strongly suggested to exclude this adverse event.

Sometimes, diagnosis of perforation is delayed and can be suspected few hours after the procedures for the onset of clinical signs and symptoms, such us abdominal pain, peritoneal irritation, and fever.

An important role for the diagnosis and monitoring of the clinical course is played by biochemical tests: leukocytosis and increased CRP levels are almost always present and usually reach a peak in second-third day after the procedure [19]. Moreover, levels of lactate and procalcitonin are accurate markers of clinical severity, especially in case of presence of abdominal fluid collections and infection [20]. A rapid deterioration of clinical condition, a concomitant hypovolemia, tachycardia, and worsening of liver and renal functions denote the onset of septic shock with poor prognosis.

Differential diagnosis with cholangitis is sometimes challenging, although the increase of aminotransferase, conjugated bilirubin, and cholestasis index should orient the physician toward the diagnosis of post-ERCP cholangitis. Post-ERCP pancreatitis is characterized usually by typical pain with the increased levels of amylase and lipase three times normal [21], although also

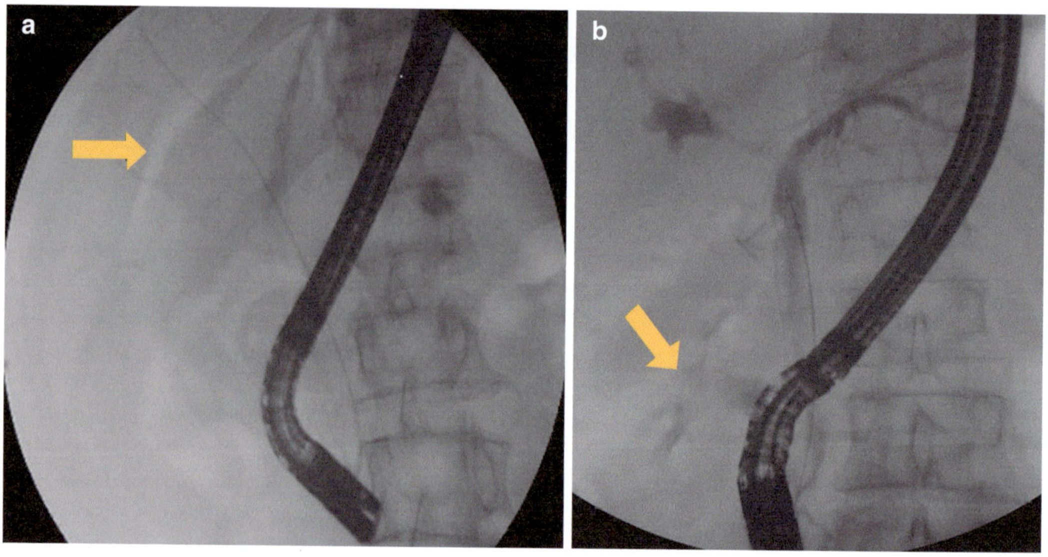

Fig. 33.2 (**a** and **b**) Free air (**a**) and extravasation of medium contrast (**b**) at the fluoroscopy

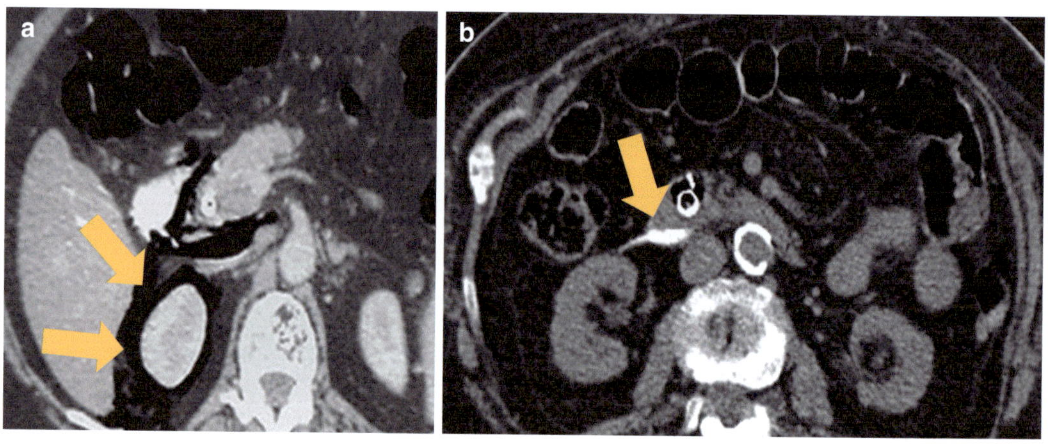

Fig. 33.3 (**a** and **b**) Presence of pararenal free air (**a**) and retroperitoneal extravasation of medium contrast (**b**) at the abdominal CT scan

in case of type 1 perforation, with outflow of pancreatic juice into the peritoneal space, an increase of amylase and lipase could be observed. In these cases, only the abdominal CT scan could orient toward a correct diagnosis.

33.4 Prevention

An enteral self-expandable metal stent could be previously placed, in case of malignant duodenal stricture, to permit a safe and easier procedure, avoiding the wall lateral stress caused by the passage of the scope. In case of surgically altered anatomy, the learning curve and the experience are crucial [22], for this reason these patients should be referred to a tertiary center. A pediatric colonoscope should allow to reach the ampullary region using frontal view and with good standard of safety [23]. In surgically altered anatomy, especially in Billroth II reconstruction, the use of the fluoroscopy to follow the progression of the scope into the bowel and to assess the correct anatomy is recommended [24].

Generally, the use of precut is associated with high risk of perforation [25]; thus its application should be carefully considered; in case of difficult common bile duct (CBD) cannulation,

EUS-guided or percutaneous rendezvous is strongly suggested, in relation to the expertise of the center. In case of repeated cannulation of pancreatic duct, a trans-pancreatic papillary septotomy is a valid and safer option to guarantee a cutting plan to accede to CBD [26]. To avoid subglissonian injuries, a careful use of the guidewires, especially the longer ones, is strongly recommended.

33.5 Therapy

33.5.1 Type 1 Perforations

33.5.1.1 Endoscopy

Duodenal lateral perforation, occurring in about 0.18% of the procedures, is one of the most threatening complications during ERCP and is usually caused by the tip of the scope during the shortening maneuver. It consists of a full-thickness laceration with the immediate flowing out of gastrointestinal fluids into the peritoneal cavity, although the duodenal perforation is not always easy to detect because of lateral view of duodenoscope [27].

A timely diagnosis and therapy are paramount; in fact an immediate recognition of the mucosal wound or the onset of free air on imaging allows to try an early closure by endoscopy or an urgent surgical intervention [28].

The simply conservative approach, which consists of a wait-and-see attitude, antibiotic therapy, and supportive measures, with no surgery or endoscopic treatment, in case of radiologic confirmation of perforation with extravasation of fluids, should be strongly discouraged because of the low success rate and high mortality, reaching a 50% of cases in some small series [3].

Nowadays, several endoscopic devices are available to attempt the endoscopic closure of mucosal leaks. Most of the published data, although limited by the presence of only some case reports and short case series, showed promising technical and clinical results of endotherapy in this setting, without need for surgery and mortality [29].

In the event of perforation, we suggest using a frontal-view endoscope with large operative channel, to place a guidewire in the peritoneal cavity, which serves as guide to localize the perforation site and to make easier the OTSC placement (Fig. 33.4a, b). Furthermore, we suggest, in case that the procedure has been carried out in air, to switch to CO_2 insufflation to reduce the risk of complications.

After verifying the effectiveness of the endoscopic closure, by intraluminal injection of hydrosoluble contrast medium, the placement of a nose-jejunal tube is strongly suggested for the subsequent enteral nutrition distally to the perforation site. A wide review of the literature about surgical, endoscopic, and conservative treatment in type I perforations is synthesized in Table 33.1.

Here are the most used endoscopic devices:

- Through-the-Scope (TTS) Clips: the use of these devices changes according to the size and the shape of the leak. For small leaks, it could be necessary to place some endoclips in order to bring the edges of the breach together [29], while for the greater leaks, it could be

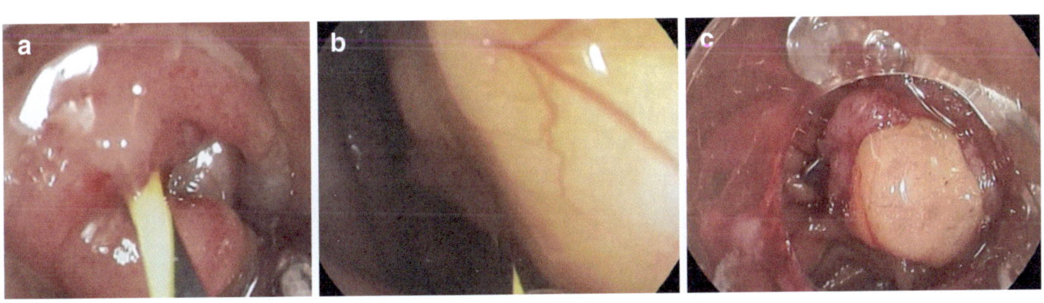

Fig. 33.4 (**a**, **b**, and **c**) Guidewire inserted into the duodenal perforation (**a**). An intraperitoneal view by facing the scope through the duodenal leak (**b**). Closure of the leak by the placement of an OTSC, with omentum trapped among the teeth of the clip (**c**)

Table 33.1 Baseline characteristics and outcomes of type 1 perforations

Author, year	N. type 1 perf	Study type	Number of ERCP	Number of pts with ERCP perforation	Age (years) Median (range)	Endoscopic treatment (system used)	Endoscopic success rate	Conservative treatment	Conservative success rate	Surgical treatment	Surgical success rate	Mortality	LoS
Stapfer [4], 2000	5	R	1413	14 (1%)	59.5 ± 8.2	0/5	–	1/5	0/1 (0%)	4/5	3/4 (75%)	2/5 (40%) 1C,1S	66.6 ± 72.4
Preetha [36], 2003	6	R	4030	18 (0.45%)	73.9 ± 8.0	0/6	–	0/6	–	6/6	4/6 (66%)	2/6 (33%) 2 S	17.8 ± 13.1
Avgerinos [27], 2009	9	R	4358	15 (0.34%)	64.3 ± 12.5	0/9	–	0/9	–	9/9	9/9 (100%)	0/9 (0%)	16.1 ± 6.4
Palanivelu [42], 2008	1	CR	NR	NR	60 (–)	0/1	–	0/1	–	1/1	1/1 (100%)	0/1 (0%)	9
Kim [43], 2009	10	R	2247	20 (0.89%)	69.1 ± 3.5	0/10	–	4/10	4/4(100%)	6/10	5/6 (87.5%)	1/10 (10%) 1 S	C = 13 ± 9.8 S = 33 ± 23.2
Nakagawa [30], 2010	1	CR	NR	NR	88 (–)	1/1 (endoclip + endoloop)	1/1 (100%)	0/1	–	0/1	–	0/1 (0%)	NR
Lee [29], 2010	4	CS	NR	NR	71.1 ± 4.2	4/4 (endoclip)	4/4 (100%)	0/4	–	0/4	–	0/4 (0%)	14.7 ± 7.1
Polydorou [37], 2011	7	R	9880	44 (0.4%)	74.5 ± 9.2	0/7	–	1/7	1/1 (100%)	6/7	4/6 (66%)	2 (29%) 2 S	29.5 ± 28.7
Kim [44], 2011	4	R	7638	20 (0.16%)	71.8 ± 1.7	1/4 (endoclip)	1/1 (100%)	0/4	–	3/4	3/3 (100%)	0/4 (0%)	23.0 ± 11.2
Ercan [38], 2012	17	R	9209	52 (0.56%)	59.7 ± 15.2	0/17	–	0/17	–	17/17	9/17 (53%)	8/17 (47%) 8 S	11.1 ± 4.0
Kim [45], 2012	13	R	11,048	68 (0.61%)	NR	NR	–	NR	–	NR	–	4/13 (30%) poor outcome	NNR

Rabie [46], 2013	3	R	597	10 (1.67%)	NR	0/3	–	0/3	–	3/3	2/3 (66%)	1/3 (33%) 1 S	NNR
Li Y [47], 2014	1	CR	NR	NR	77 (–)	1/1 (EBL)	1/1 (100%)	0/1	–	0/1	–	0/1 (0%)	NNR
Armas Ojeda [48], 2015	3	R	1923	15 (0.78%)	61.6 ± 15.5	0/3	–	0/3	–	3/3	2/3 (66%)	1/3 (33%) 1 S	25.3 ± 18.8
Yang [49], 2015	1	CR	NR	NR	70 (–)	1/1 (fibrin sealant)	1/1 (100%)	0/1	–	0/1	–	0/1 (0%)	14
Kumbhari [3], 2016	7	R	NR	76 (–)	NR	0/7	–	2/7	1/2 (50%)	5/7	5/5 (100%)	1/7 (14.2%) 1 C	10.1 ± 7.2
Angsuwatc-harakon [31], 2016	4	CS	NR	NR	56.1 ± 7.7	4/4 (OTSC)	4/4 (100%)	0/4	–	0/4	–	0/4 (0%)	9.2 ± 4.8
Overall	96	–	52.343	352 (0.67%)	68.4 ± 8.3	12/83	12/12 (100%)	8/83	6/8	63/83	47/63 (74%)	18/83 (21%) 16 S 2 C	20.9 ± 14.7

used as a mixed technique: by using a double-channel scope, two or more clips are placed on the edges of the breach, clipping at the same time the snare of an endoloop; at the end of the procedure, endoloop is closed and the edges of the wound are brought together [30].

- Over-the-Scope (OTS) Clips: this type of clip has to be mounted over the distal part of the scope and consists of a plastic cap with a large, super elastic, biocompatible Nitinol clip which, once released, compresses the tissue between its teeth (Fig. 33.4c). The role of the cap is to facilitate the suction of the tissues, including omentum, before releasing the clip [31]. Several types of forceps are available in order to bring the flaps of the leak together, during the suction; in some cases, the twin grasper forceps are very useful to approach two distant flaps, being able to staple separately two different flaps of mucosa.
- Apollo OverStitch®: a recent OTS device developed to permit endoscopic suturing in order to guarantee a safe and firm fistula closure [32]. This device, used also for bariatric surgery applications [33], has been employed in particular to solve postsurgical and endoscopic complications, although it needs expertise and training (Fig. 33.5).

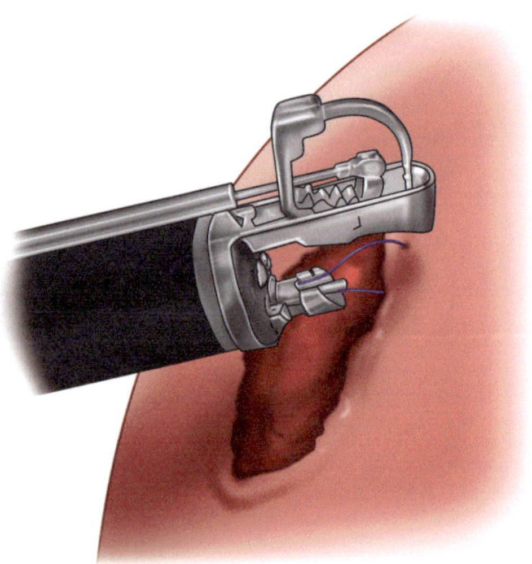

Fig. 33.5 Apollo OverStitch®

- Fibrin glue and other sealants: these substances are used, alone or mainly in association with other techniques, to permit the closure of abdominal fistulas and leaks; however, their use in literature is episodic and the results in terms of long-term follow-up and outcomes are missing [34].
- Another option, if endoscopic closure of the perforation fails, could be the "triple stenting technique" that is based on the placement of a large diameter fully covered SEMS (20–24 mm) through the scope in the duodenum with enough length to cover the perforation site. The first step is to perform a cholangiopancreatography with sphincterotomy to facilitate the localization of the biliopancreatic orifice at a later stage. After the placement of the enteral stent with trans-stent duodenoscope it is possible, by using a straight guidewire, to cannulate CBD and pancreatic duct to allow the placement, through the mesh, of a FCSEMS of 8–10 mm in diameter and 4–6 cm long in the CBD and a 7–8.5 Fr × 5–7 cm long plastic stent, in the pancreatic duct [35] (Fig. 33.6). Usually it is necessary to dilate the mesh of the enteral FCSEMS with a balloon to facilitate the stent placement. This procedure allows to close the perforation site and divert the pancreatic and biliary juice into the cover SEMS avoiding the fluid collected in the peritoneum. The stents were usually left in place for a period of 4–8 weeks.

In addition to endoscopic treatment, i.v. (intravenous) broad-spectrum antibiotic therapy should be started, together with i.v. PPI, parenteral nutrition, and other supportive cares.

33.5.1.2 Surgery

Until a few years ago, the unique therapeutic option consisted of urgent surgery; also in case of timely intervention, clinical outcomes in this setting remain poor, with a long hospital stay and high morbidity and mortality [36]. Some recent studies reported high mortality rate associated with surgery, ranging in some series between 29 and 47% [37, 38]. Surgical treatments consist of a primary surgical repair of the duodenal wall and peritoneal toilette (with or without the place-

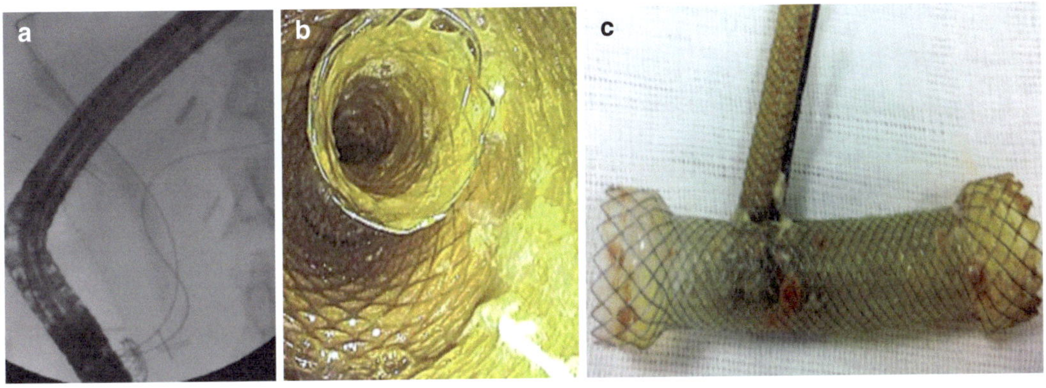

Fig. 33.6 Use of triple stenting for duodenal wall perforation: placement of the stents, seen at the fluoroscopy (**a**); biliary stent through the mash of the enteral stent, seen at the endoscopy (**b**). The stents' complex, after removal (**c**) [35]

Table 33.2 Comparison of outcomes of type 1 perforations

Type of treatment	N (%)	Clinical success	Mortality	LoS (days)
Surgery	63/83 (76%)	47/63 (74.6%)	16/63 (25.4%)	–
Endoscopy	12/83 (14.4%)	12/12 (100%)	0 (0%)	–
Conservative	8/83 (9.6%)	2/8 (25%)	2 (25%)	–
Overall	–	61/83 (73.4%)	18/83 (21.6%)	20.9 ± 14.7

ment of surgical drainages and T-tube), while other authors described the necessity to perform a gastrojejunostomy with pyloric exclusion to divert the gastroduodenal fluids from the perforated tract [4].

In this type of perforation, surgeons should not be focused on the detection of the perforation site because it is often difficult to localize.

Immediate surgery is mandatory in case of endoscopic failure; in fact a delay in surgery could dramatically affect the short- and long-term outcomes, with higher morbidity and mortality, that could reach almost 50% of cases [27, 38].

Comparison of outcomes according to the treatment is obtained analyzing data from the studies collected in the review in Table 33.1 and is reported in Table 33.2.

33.5.2 Type 2 and 3 Perforations

Periampullary perforations (type 2) occur in 0.25% of ERCPs, involve generally the papilla and the retroperitoneal space, and are mainly caused by sphincterotomy, precut, or endoscopic papillary balloon dilation, rarely by guidewire or other devices. In this setting the need for surgery is 21% of cases with an overall mortality of 9.4% of cases. Among patients requiring surgery, mortality rises to 38%.

Ductal perforations (type 3) occur in about 0.07% of ERCPs and are mainly generated by guidewires, pneumatic or mechanical dilation of the CBD, stent retrieval, and some other procedure, like the placement of a biliary stent or the use of Dormia's basket for stone removal. Surgery for type 3 perforation is required in 14% of cases, with a mortality rate lower than 1%.

A large review of the literature regarding type 2 and 3 is synthesized in Table 33.3.

33.5.2.1 Conservative Treatment

These conditions are often treated conservatively, by the placement of nasogastric tube; administration of intravenous fluids; proton pump inhibitors; antibiotics, in some case somatostatin, especially in the past; and nil-by-mouth regimen, although sometimes this approach resulted in the need for percutaneous drainage and delay of surgery with higher risk of mortality, as reported in Table 33.3.

Table 33.3 Baseline characteristics and outcomes of type 2–3 and 4 perforations

First author, year	Type of studies	Perfor type	N type 2–3 perfor	N. of pts. with ERCP	N. of pts. with ERCP-related perforation	Age (years) mean ± SD	Altered anatomy	Diagnosis Immediate	Endoscopic treatment (system used)	FCSEMS removal days	Endoscopic AE	Conservative treatment	Surgery	Time of surgery <24 h	Success rate	Mortality	LOS Days mean ± SD
Loperfido [50], 1998	P	2	12	3356	28 (0.83%)	NR	NR	NR	0/12	–	–	6/12	6/12	NR	NR	1/12	NR
Howard [12], 1999	R	2 3	22 14	6040	40 (0.66%)	57 ± 12 53 ± 13	NR	20/22 14/14	18/22 11/14 (PBS, NBD)	–	8/18 3/ 11	3/22 3/14 NGT, NDT	1/22 0/14	0/1	S = 0/1 C = 6/6 E = 27/29	1/22 (1 S) 0/14	8.5 ± 7 3.5 ± 3
Stapfer [4], 2000	R	2 3	6 3	1413	14 (0.99%)	41 ± 10.5 47.6 ± 7.2	NR	5/6 3/3	0/6 0/3	–	–	5/6 2/3	1/6 1/3	2/2	C = 5/7 S = 2/2	0/6 0/3	46.4 ± 25.5 14 ± 4
Enns [17], 2002	R	2 3	13 14	9314	33 (0.35%)	NR NR	NR	10/13 9/14	5/13 PBS (2/13 PTCS) 4/14 PBS	–	NR	6/13 7/14 (ABX, NBM)	2/13 1/14	NR	C = 13/13 E = 9/9 S = 3/3	0/13 0/14	6.5 ± 2.7 7.5 ± 3.2
Preetha [36], 2003	R	2 3 4	7 4 1	4030	18 (0.44%)	58 ± 19.2 55 ± 9.2	NR	1/7 1/4	0/7 0/4	–	–	0/7 0/4	7/7 4/4	1/7 2/4	S = 10/11	1/7 (1 S) 0/4	29.7 ± 6.5 10 ± 1.2
Christensen [51], 2004	P	2	12	1177	13 (1.1%)	73	0/12	12/12	0/12	–	–	12/12 (ABX, NBM)	0/12	NR	C = 9/12	1/12 (1 C)	NR
Kayhan [52], 2004	CS	2	15	3124	17 (0.54%)	NR	NR	15/15	0/15	–	–	6/15	9/15	NR	NR	NR	NR
Wu [53], 2006	R	2 3	11 7	6620	30 (0.45%)	60 ± 17 66 ± 18	NR	4/11 7/7	2/11 BS 1/7 BS (2/7 PTCS)	NR	NR	5/11 6/7 (ABX, NBM)	4/11 0/7	NR	C = 9/11 S = 2/4 E = 3/3	4/11 (2 C, 2 S) 0/7	26.5 ± 25.8 4.4 ± 2.1
Sarli [54], 2007	R	2	18	NR	18	58.9 ± 13.5	NR	4/18	0/18	–	–	13/18	5/18	NR	S = 4/5 C = 12/13	0/18	12.6 ± 2.7
Assalia [55], 2007	P cs	2 3	17 2	3104	20 (0.64%)	63.8 mean	NR	16/17 2/2	3/17 (BPS, NBD) 0/2	NR	NR	14/17 2/2	0/17 0/2	NR	C = 14/16 E = 3/3	1/18 (1C) 0/2	6.2 ± 2.3
Fatima [56], 2007	R	2 3	19 36	12,427	75 (0.6%)	NR NR	NR	NR	0/19 0/36	–	–	13/19 31/36	6/19 5/36	NR	C = 42/44 S = 8/11	5/19 (1C, 4S) 0/36	
Knudson [57], 2008	R	2 3	11 7	4919	32 (0.65%)	NR	4/18	NR	0/18	–	–	6/11 5/7	5/11 2/7	NNR	C = 11/11 S = 7/7	0/11 0/7	9 ± 5 7 ± 3 C 12 ± 6 S

continued

Mao [58], 2008	R cs	2 3	8 1	2432	9 (0.37%)	58	NR	3/9	0/9	–	–	5/8 1/1	3/9 0/1	NR	C = 6/6 S = 2/3	0/8 0/1	S = 12.6 ± 4 C = 50 ± 13.2
Avgerinos [27], 2009	R	2 4	3 1	4358	15 (0.34%)	83.3 ± 2.7	NR	0/3	0/3	–	–	1/3 (NBM, ABX)	2/3	NR	C = 0/1 S = 2/2	1/3 (1C)	26 ± 0.5
Kim [43], 2009	R	2 3	9 1	2247	18 (0.8%)	NR	NR	3/9 1/1	0/9 0/1	–	–	8/9 1/1	1/9 0/1	NR	C = 9/9 S = 1/1	0/9 0/1	NR
Morgan [15], 2009	R	2	12	12,817	24 (0.18%)	53	0/12	3/12	0/12	–	–	12/12 (NBM)	0/12	NR	C = 12/12	0/12	9
Vezakis [59], 2011 CR	CR	2	1	NR	1	61	0/1	1/1	1/1 (FCSEMS+ NBD)	–	0/1	1/1	0/1	NR	E = 1/1	0/1	60
Jeon [60], 2011	CR	2	1	NR	1	82	0/1	0/1	1/1 (FCSEMS rescue)	–	0/1	1/1	0/1	NR	E = 1/1	0/1	16
Dubecz [2], 2012	R Cs	2 3 4	3 1 4	12,232	11 (0.08%)	77.3 ± 13 62	0/3 0/1	3/3 0/1	0/4	–	–	3/3 0/1	0/3 1/1	NR	C = 1/3 S = 1/1	2/3 (2C) 0/1	20.5 ± 4.2
Kwon [61], 2012	R	2	32	8381	53 (0.63%)	65 ± 2.2	NR	21/32	0/32	–	6/32	31/32	1/32	NR	C = 30/31 S = 1/1	1/32 (1C)	19.3 ± 2.2
Park [62], 2012	CR	2	1	–	1	–	–	0/1	1/1 (FCSEMS rescue)	10	0/1	0/1	0/1	–	E = 1/1	0/1	23
Alfieri [41], 2013	R	2 3 4	15 1 8	14,618	30 (0.2%)	55.3 ± 11.7	NR	NR	0/16	–	NR	6/15 (PCD, NBM) 1/1	9/15 0/1	NR	C = 7/7 S = 6/9	1/15 (1S) 0/1	48.6 ± 19.7 15
Miller [63], 2013	R	2 3 4	11 5 5	1638	26 (1.5%)	67.3 ± 16	NR	9/12 5/5	1/11 (FCSEMS) 0/5	NR	NR	8/11 (PCD) 5/5	2/11 0/5	NR	S = 2/2 C = 0/8 E = 1/1	6/11 (6C) 0/5	NR
Polydorou [37], 2013	R	2 3 4	30 5 2	9880	44 (0.44%)	63 ± 14.2	NR	29/30 5/5	3/30 (FCSEMS)	–	NR	27/30 (NBM, PCD)	0/30 0/5	.	C = 23/27 E = 3/3	0/30 0/5	NR
Canena [64], 2013	R	2	4	NR	4	48.9 ± 11.7	NR	0/4	4/4 (rescue FCSEMS)	29,5 (21–30)	0/4	0/4	0/4	–	E = 4/4	0/4	9.6 ± 1.2

Table 33.3 (continued)

First author, year	Type of studies	Perfor type	N type 2–3 perfor	N. of pts. with ERCP	N. of pts. with ERCP-related perforation	Age (years) mean ± SD	Altered anatomy	Diagnosis Immediate	Endoscopic treatment (system used)	FCSEMS removal days	Endoscopic AE	Conservative treatment	Surgery	Time of surgery <24 h	Success rate	Mortality	LOS Days mean ± SD
Rabie [46], 2013	R	2 3 4	1 3 3	597	10 (1.67%)	57.4 ± 16.5	NR	NR	0/1 0/3	–	–	1/1 3/3 (ABX, NBM)	0/1 0/3	–	C = 4/4	0/4	NR
Jin [65], 2013	R	2 3	36 6	22,988	58 (0.25%)	NNR	NNR	NNR	NNR	NR	NR	NNR	NNR	NNR	NR	NNR	NR
Koc [66], 2014	R	2 3 4	17 9 2	2972	28 (0.94%)	51.1 ± 12.5 56.6 ± 8.7	NR	2/17 0/9	0/17 0/9	–	–	11/17 7/9	6/17 2/9	NR	C = 12/18 S = 6/8	1/17 (1C) 1/9 (1S)	10.7 ± 3.7 10.4 ± 1
Armas Ojeda [48], 2015	R	2	12	1923	15 (0.78%)	67.7 ± 15.7	NR	8/12	0/12	–	–	7/12	5/12	5/5	C = 1/7 S = 4/5	2/12 (2C)	22.7 ± 8
Kumbhari [3], 2016	R	2 3 4	54 9 6	3331	76 (2.28%)	51.3 ± 15.8	5 BII, 7 diverticula, 3 Roux	6/61	1/49 (FCSEMS)	NR	NR	49/54	4/49	NR	NR	1/54	9.5 ± 3.7
Odemis [67], 2016	R	2	20	7471	25 (0.33%)	49 ± 19.2	5/20 diverticula	NR	10/20 (FCSEMS)	NR	6/20	10/20 (NBD, NBM, ABX)	0/20	NR	C = 9/10 E = 10/10	1/20 (1C)	19.5 ± 8.7
Trikudanath [68], 2018	R	2	15	4860	15 (0.3%)	61.7 ± 19	1 Roux, 5 diverticula	15/15	15/15 (FCSEMS)	30.5 (14–45)	0/15	0/16	0/15	NR	E = 15/15	0/15	3.6 ± 2.5
Tringali [19], 2018	R	2	16	7298	16 (0.21%)	66.9 ± 11.5	0/16	15/16	16/16 (FCSEMS)	43 (2–105)	2/16	0/16	0/16	NR	E = 16/16	0/16	11.3 ± 4.2
34 studies		2 3 4	474 128 32	176,317	828 (0.47%) 474/634 (74.7%) 128/634 (20.3%) 32/634 (5%)	Type 2: 61.2 ± 10.0 Type 3: 58.1 ± 5.6	31/163	Type 2: 210/356 Type 3: 50/75	97/530	34(±6.3)–30 (29–43)	–	234/379 44/103	Type 2: 89/423 Type 3: 16/113	14/24	S = 69/117 C = 248/276 E = 91/93	Type 2: 32/427 11/32 S 19/32 C 2/32 U 0/32 E Type 3: 1/110 1/1 = C	Type 2: 20.3 ± 14.9 Type 3: 13.3 ± 11.4

Therapy of subglissonian injuries is essentially conservative, if the patient is hemodynamically stable: i.v. fluids, antibiotics, and careful clinical observation are mandatory; embolization and surgery should be considered only for those patients who are unstable. A percutaneous drainage of the hematoma or the abscess could be also performed [39].

33.5.2.2 Endoscopy

In this case, an immediate recognition of the leak or the onset of retroperitoneal air (Fig. 33.2a, b) is diagnostic for perforation. To make the diagnosis during the same procedure allows to perform an early treatment placing a fully covered self-expandable metal stent (FCSEMS) into the CBD.

European guidelines suggested performing abdominal CT scan to confirm the initial suspect of type 2 perforations.

The role of the FCSEMS in type 2 perforations is to compress the edge of the sphincterotomy, virtually closing the breach and avoiding the outflow of bile and secretions in the retroperitoneum (Fig. 33.7).

According to ESGE guidelines, the management of the type 2 perforations suspected during ERCP is essentially conservative; in case of no contrast medium extravasation, only supportive measures should be considered, while in case of extravasation, a biliary stenting could be placed; nevertheless it is not specified what type of stent is recommended to be used.

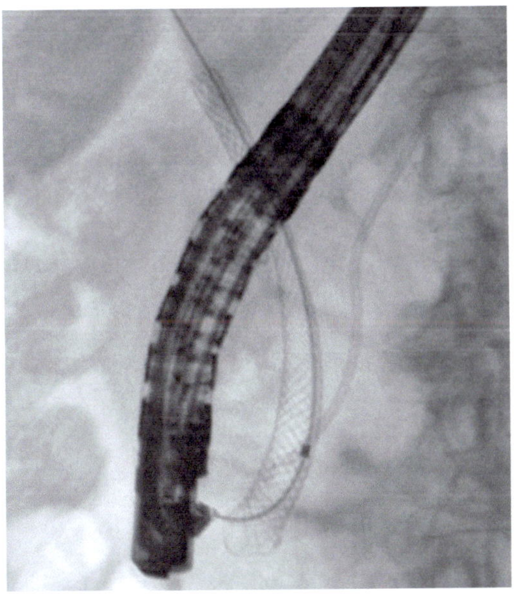

Fig. 33.7 FCSEMS placed into CBD

Endoscopic treatment could be considered on a case-by-case basis if the presence of contrast medium extravasation is evident on imaging, in order to drain the biliary tree; surgery is suggested in case of a great abdominal collection of medium contrast or signs of toxicity [40].

ASGE guidelines conversely highlighted the need to place immediately a FCSEMS, whereas feasible, if an intra-procedural diagnosis of perforation is made [1]. Although conservative management in type 2 and 3 perforations is generally considered appropriate, recent studies underline the importance of immediate FCSEMS placement; even if a delayed diagnosis is made, then the placement of a fully covered metal stent seems to guarantee a good outcome, avoiding further outflows of duodenal fluids into the retroperitoneum. Immediate treatment with FCSEMS for Stapfer 2 and 3 perforations seems to be associated with earlier postoperative feeding and shorter hospital stay [19]. Stent's removal could be considered usually 1 month after the placement.

Technique of SEMS placement: consists of placement of guidewire of 0.035 in. in the common bile duct and inserts over the wire with the rapid exchange system a trans-papillary FCSEMS of 10 mm in diameter, 4 or 6 cm in length (see Chap. 19 for technique details).

In type 3 perforations, placement of a FCSEMS could directly cover the leak of the duct, but most of its function is to change intraductal pressure in favor of the outflow of bile into the duodenal lumen.

In case of type 3 perforation due to a large papillary balloon dilation (≥10 mm), we suggest the placement of two FCSEMS side by side, to perfectly cover the perforation site.

33.5.2.3 Surgery

The presence of peritonitis makes the surgical option mandatory, according to European guidelines (ESGE).

Table 33.4 Comparison of outcomes of type 2 perforations

Type of treatment	N (%)	Clinical success	Mortality	LoS (days)
Surgery	89/423 (21%)	69/117 (58.9%)	11/80 (13.7%)	–
Endoscopy	97/530 (18.3%)	91/93 (97.8%)	0/81 (0%)	–
Conservative	234/379 (61.7%)	248/276 (89.8%)	21/264 (7.9%)	–
Overall	–	408/486 (83.9%)	32/425 (7.5%)	20.3 ± 14.9

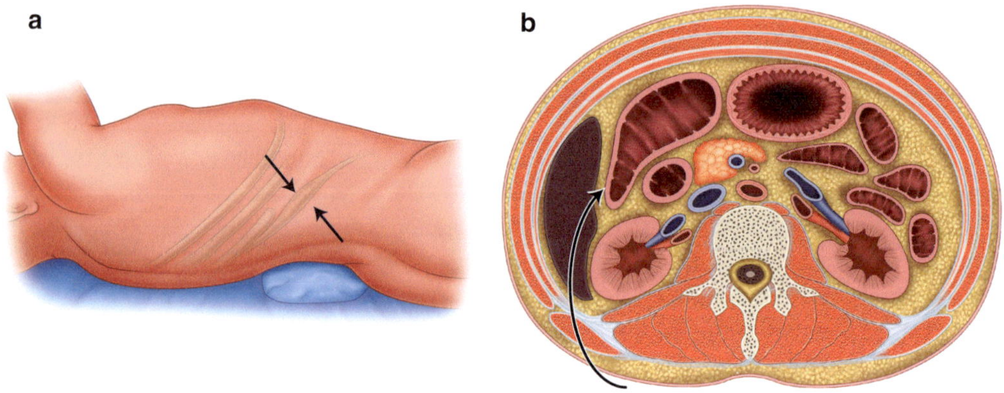

Fig. 33.8 Oblique lumbotomy

A primary repair is feasible if the exact site of the leak is identified. In some cases, when the leak is larger and repairing is not possible, it could be necessary to perform a choledochojejunostomy or a hepaticojejunostomy, with or without gastrojejunostomy and pyloric exclusion.

Surgery in type 2 and 3 perforations should be considered for more severe cases, as clinical outcomes seem to be scanty and mortality higher, if compared with endoscopic management (in Table 33.4 are analyzed data from the reviews collected in Table 33.3).

In all cases of retroperitoneal collection, an oblique lumbotomy could be performed combined with 12th rib resection and extended anteriorly, if necessary [41]. This access allows a good exposure and debridement of the prerenal and retrorenal spaces, reaching the duodenum when necessary (Fig. 33.8).

33.5.3 Type 4 Perforations

This pathological entity should not be treated and is managed only by clinical observation; biochemical tests could confirm the benignity of this condition.

33.6 Summary

1. Timing in diagnosis of perforation is crucial to guarantee an immediate endoscopic treatment or an early surgical intervention.
2. Symptoms, biochemical markers, and imaging are accurate for guiding therapy.
3. Endoscopic treatment depends on type of Stapfer perforations.
4. Treatment of type 1 perforations is based on surgery, although an endoscopic closure with OTSC placement or other technique including triple stenting, followed by medical treatment, could be attempted.
5. Type 2 and 3 perforations are basically based on immediate placement of FCSEMS, unlike the previous suggestion, that allows early refeeding and reduces hospitalization with benefit for the patients and cost saving.
6. Surgery is indicated in case of onset of sign of peritoneal irritation or all retroperitoneal col-

lections and depends on leak size and clinical and imaging sign of infected collection that needs to perform an oblique lumbotomy.

References

1. ASGE Standards of Practice Committee, Chandrasekhara V, Khashab MA, Muthusamy VR, Acosta RD, Agrawal D, Bruining DH, Eloubeidi MA, Fanelli RD, Faulx AL, Gurudu SR, Kothari S, Lightdale JR, Qumseya BJ, Shaukat A, Wang A, Wani SB, Yang J, DeWitt JM. Adverse events associated with ERCP. Gastrointest Endosc. 2017;85(1):32–47. https://doi.org/10.1016/j.gie.2016.06.051. Epub 2016 Aug 18.
2. Dubecz A, Ottmann J, Schweigert M, Stadlhuber RJ, Feith M, Wiessner V, Muschweck H, Stein HJ. Management of ERCP-related small bowel perforations: the pivotal role of physical investigation. Can J Surg. 2012;55(2):99–104. https://doi.org/10.1503/cjs.027110.
3. Kumbhari V, Sinha A, Reddy A, Afghani E, Cotsalas D, Patel YA, Storm AC, Khashab MA, Kalloo AN, Singh VK. Algorithm for the management of ERCP-related perforations. Gastrointest Endosc. 2016;83(5):934–43. https://doi.org/10.1016/j.gie.2015.09.039.
4. Stapfer M, Selby RR, Stain SC, Katkhouda N, Parekh D, Jabbour N, Garry D. Management of duodenal perforation after endoscopic retrograde cholangiopancreatography and sphincterotomy. Ann Surg. 2000;232(2):191–8.
5. Cirocchi R, Kelly MD, Griffiths EA, Tabola R, Sartelli M, Carlini L, Ghersi S, Di Saverio S. A systematic review of the management and outcome of ERCP related duodenal perforations using a standardized classification system. Surgeon. 2017;15(6):379–87. https://doi.org/10.1016/j.surge.2017.05.004.
6. Horn TL, Peña LR. Subcapsular hepatic hematoma after ERCP: case report and review. Gastrointest Endosc. 2004;59:594–6.
7. Chi KD, Waxman I. Subcapsular hepatic hematoma after guide wire injury during ERCP. Endoscopy. 2004;36:1019–21.
8. Sharma A, Mukewar S, Mara KC, Dierkhising RA, Kamath PS, Cummins N. Epidemiologic factors, clinical presentation, causes, and outcomes of liver abscess: a 35-year Olmsted County Study. Mayo Clin Proc Innov Qual Outcomes. 2018;2(1):16–25.
9. Oliveira Ferreira A, Tato Marinho R, Velosa J. Infected hepatic hematoma 10 days after ERCP. Endoscopy. 2013;45(Suppl 2 UCTN):E402–3. https://doi.org/10.1055/s-0033-1344865.
10. Voigt P, Schob S, Gottschling S, Kahn T, Surov A. Systemic air embolism after endoscopy without vessel injury—a summary of reported cases. J Neurol Sci. 2017;376:93–6.
11. Genzlinger JL, McPhee MS, Fisher JK, Jacob KM, Helzberg JH. Significance of retroperitoneal air after endoscopic retrograde cholangiopancreatography with sphincterotomy. Am J Gastroenterol. 1999;94:1267–70.
12. Howard TJ, Tan T, Lehman GA, Sherman S, Madura JA, Fogel E, Swack ML, Kopecky KK. Classification and management of perforations complicating endoscopic sphincterotomy. Surgery. 1999;126(4):658–63; discussion 664–5.
13. Zizzo M, Lanaia A, Barbieri I, Zaghi C, Bonilauri S. Subcapsular hepatic hematoma after endoscopic retrograde cholangiopancreatography: a case report and review of literature. Medicine (Baltimore). 2015;94(26):e1041. https://doi.org/10.1097/MD.0000000000001041.
14. Wilkinson ML, Engelman J, Hanson P. Intestinal perforation after ERCP in Billroth II partial gastrectomy. Gastrointest Endosc. 1994;40(3):389.
15. Morgan KA, Fontenot BB, Ruddy JM, Mickey S, Adams DB. Endoscopic retrograde cholangiopancreatography gut perforations: when to wait! When to operate! Am Surg. 2009;75(6):477.
16. Cotton PB, Garrow DA, Gallagher J, Romagnuolo J. Risk factors for complications after ERCP: a multivariate analysis of 11,497 procedures over 12 years. Gastrointest Endosc. 2009;70(1):80–8. https://doi.org/10.1016/j.gie.2008.10.039.
17. Enns R, Eloubeidi MA, Mergener K, Jowell PS, Branch MS, Pappas TM, Baillie J. ERCP-related perforations: risk factors and management. Endoscopy. 2002;34(4):293–8.
18. Jayaraj M, Mohan BP, Dhindsa BS, Mashiana HS, Radhakrishnan G, Dhir V, Trindade AJ, Adler DG. Periampullary diverticula and ERCP outcomes: a systematic review and meta-analysis. Dig Dis Sci. 2019;64(5):1364–76. https://doi.org/10.1007/s10620-018-5314-y.
19. Tringali A, Pizzicanella M, Andrisani G, Cintolo M, Hassan C, Adler D, Dioscoridi L, Pandolfi M, Mutignani M, Di Matteo F. Temporary FC-SEMS for type II ERCP-related perforations: a case series from two referral centers and review of the literature. Scand J Gastroenterol. 2018;53(6):760–7. https://doi.org/10.1080/00365521.2018.1458894.
20. Novotny AR, Emmanuel K, Hueser N, Knebel C, Kriner M, Ulm K, Bartels H, Siewert JR, Holzmann B. Procalcitonin ratio indicates successful surgical treatment of abdominal sepsis. Surgery. 2009;145(1):20–6. https://doi.org/10.1016/j.surg.2008.08.009.
21. Cotton PB, Eisen GM, Aabakken L, Baron TH, Hutter MM, Jacobson BC, Mergener K, Nemcek A Jr, Petersen BT, Petrini JL, Pike IM, Rabeneck L, Romagnuolo J, Vargo JJ. A lexicon for endoscopic adverse events: report of an ASGE workshop. Gastrointest Endosc. 2010;71(3):446–54. https://doi.org/10.1016/j.gie.2009.10.027.
22. Bove V, Tringali A, Familiari P, Gigante G, Boškoski I, Perri V, Mutignani M, Costamagna G. ERCP in

patients with prior Billroth II gastrectomy: report of 30 years' experience. Endoscopy. 2015;47(7):611–6. https://doi.org/10.1055/s-0034-1391567.

23. Nakaji S, Hirata N, Yamauchi K, Shiratori T, Kobayashi M, Fujii H, Ishii E. Endoscopic retrograde cholangiopancreatography using a cap-assisted highly flexible colonoscope in patients with Roux-en-Y anastomosis. Endoscopy. 2014;46(6):529–32. https://doi.org/10.1055/s-0034-1365516.
24. ASGE Technology Committee, Enestvedt BK, Kothari S, Pannala R, Yang J, Fujii-Lau LL, Hwang JH, Konda V, Manfredi M, Maple JT, Murad FM, Woods KL, Banerjee S. Devices and techniques for ERCP in the surgically altered GI tract. Gastrointest Endosc. 2016;83(6):1061–75. https://doi.org/10.1016/j.gie.2016.03.018.
25. Artifon EL, Paulo S, Cardillo GZ, Ishioka S. Suprapapillary needle puncture for common bile duct access: laboratory profile. Arq Gastroenterol. 2006;43(4):299–304.
26. Kapetanos D, Kokozidis G, Christodoulou D, Mistakidis K, Dimakopoulos K, Katodritou E, Kitis G, Tsianos EV. Case series of transpancreatic septotomy as precutting technique for difficult bile duct cannulation. Endoscopy. 2007;39(9):802–6.
27. Avgerinos DV, Llaguna OH, Lo AY, Voli J, Leitman IM. Management of endoscopic retrograde cholangiopancreatography: related duodenal perforations. Surg Endosc. 2009;23(4):833–8. https://doi.org/10.1007/s00464-008-0157-9.
28. Bill JG, Smith Z, Brancheck J, Elsner J, Hobbs P, Lang GD, Early DS, Das K, Hollander T, Doyle MBM, Fields RC, Hawkins WG, Strasberg SM, Hammill C, Chapman WC, Edmundowicz S, Mullady DK, Kushnir VM. The importance of early recognition in management of ERCP-related perforations. Surg Endosc. 2018;32(12):4841–9. https://doi.org/10.1007/s00464-018-6235-8.
29. Lee TH, Bang BW, Jeong JI, Kim HG, Jeong S, Park SM, Lee DH, Park SH, Kim SJ. Primary endoscopic approximation suture under cap-assisted endoscopy of an ERCP-induced duodenal perforation. World J Gastroenterol. 2010;16(18):2305–10.
30. Nakagawa Y, Nagai T, Soma W, Okawara H, Nakashima H, Tasaki T, Hisamatu A, Hashinaga M, Murakami K, Fujioka T. Endoscopic closure of a large ERCP-related lateral duodenal perforation by using endoloops and endoclips. Gastrointest Endosc. 2010;72(1):216–7. https://doi.org/10.1016/j.gie.2009.10.040.
31. Angsuwatcharakon P, Prueksapanich P, Kongkam P, Rattanachu-Ek T, Sottisuporn J, Rerknimitr R. Efficacy of the Ovesco clip for closure of endoscope related perforations. Diagn Ther Endosc. 2016;2016:9371878. https://doi.org/10.1155/2016/9371878.
32. Chon SH, Toex U, Plum PS, Fuchs C, Kleinert R, Bruns C, Goeser T. Successful closure of a gastropulmonary fistula after esophagectomy using the Apollo Overstitch and endoscopic vacuum therapy. Endoscopy. 2018;50(7):E149–50. https://doi.org/10.1055/a-0592-6384.
33. Sartoretto A, Sui Z, Hill C, Dunlap M, Rivera AR, Khashab MA, Kalloo AN, Fayad L, Cheskin LJ, Marinos G, Wilson E, Kumbhari V. Endoscopic sleeve gastroplasty (ESG) is a reproducible and effective endoscopic bariatric therapy suitable for widespread clinical adoption: a Large, International Multicenter Study. Obes Surg. 2018;28(7):1812–21. https://doi.org/10.1007/s11695-018-3135-x.
34. Sakaguchi Y, Tsuji Y, Yamamichi N, Fujishiro M, Koike K. Successful closure of a large perforation during colorectal endoscopic submucosal dissection by application of polyglycolic acid sheets and fibrin glue. Gastrointest Endosc. 2016;84(2):374–5. https://doi.org/10.1016/j.gie.2016.03.787.
35. Mutignani M, Dioscoridi L, Dokas S, Aseni P, Carnevali P, Forti E, Manta R, Sica M, Tringali A, Pugliese F. Endoscopic multiple metal stenting for the treatment of enteral leaks near the biliary orifice: a novel effective rescue procedure. World J Gastrointest Endosc. 2016;8(15):533–40. https://doi.org/10.4253/wjge.v8.i15.533.
36. Preetha M, Chung YF, Chan WH, Ong HS, Chow PK, Wong WK, Ooi LL, Soo KC. Surgical management of endoscopic retrograde cholangiopancreatography-related perforations. ANZ J Surg. 2003;73(12):1011–4.
37. Polydorou A, Vezakis A, Fragulidis G, Katsarelias D, Vagianos C, Polymeneas G. A tailored approach to the management of perforations following endoscopic retrograde cholangiopancreatography and sphincterotomy. J Gastrointest Surg. 2011;15(12):2211–7. https://doi.org/10.1007/s11605-011-1723-3.
38. Ercan M, Bostanci EB, Dalgic T, Karaman K, Ozogul YB, Ozer I, Ulas M, Parlak E, Akoglu M. Surgical outcome of patients with perforation after endoscopic retrograde cholangiopancreatography. J Laparoendosc Adv Surg Tech A. 2012;22(4):371–7. https://doi.org/10.1089/lap.2011.0392.
39. Imperatore N, Micheletto G, Manes G, Redaelli DG, Reitano E, de Nucci G. Systematic review: features, diagnosis, management and prognosis of hepatic hematoma, a rare complication of ERCP. Dig Liver Dis. 2018;50(10):997–1003. https://doi.org/10.1016/j.dld.2018.07.010. Epub 2018 Jul 20.
40. Paspatis GA, Dumonceau JM, Barthet M, Meisner S, Repici A, Saunders BP, Vezakis A, Gonzalez JM, Turino SY, Tsiamoulos ZP, Fockens P, Hassan C. Diagnosis and management of iatrogenic endoscopic perforations: European Society of Gastrointestinal Endoscopy (ESGE) position statement. Endoscopy. 2014;46(8):693–711. https://doi.org/10.1055/s-0034-1377531. Epub 2014 Jul 21.
41. Alfieri S, Rosa F, Cina C, Tortorelli AP, Tringali A, Perri V, Costamagna G, Doglietto GB. Management of duodenopancreato-biliary perforations after ERCP: outcomes from an Italian tertiary referral center. Surg Endosc. 2013;27:2005–12.
42. Palanivelu C, Jategaonkar PA, Rangarajan M, Anand NV, Senthilnathan P. Laparoscopic management of a retroperitoneal duodenal perforation following ERCP for periampullary cancer. JSLS. 2008;12(4):399–402.

43. Kim JH, Yoo BM, Kim JH, Kim MW, Kim WH. Management of ERCP-related perforations: outcomes of single institution in Korea. J Gastrointest Surg. 2009;13(4):728–34. https://doi.org/10.1007/s11605-008-0786-2. Epub 2009 Jan 6.
44. Kim BS, Kim IG, Ryu BY, et al. Management of endoscopic retrograde cholangiopancreatography-related perforations. J Korean Surg Soc. 2011;81:195–204.
45. Kim J, Lee SH, Paik WH, Song BJ, Hwang JH, Ryu JK, Kim YT, Yoon YB. Clinical outcomes of patients who experienced perforation associated with endoscopic retrograde cholangiopancreatography. Surg Endosc. 2012;26(11):3293–300. https://doi.org/10.1007/s00464-012-2343-z.
46. Rabie ME, Mir NH, Al Skaini MS, El Hakeem I, Hadad A, Ageely H, Shaban AN, Obaid M, Hummadi AM. Operative and non-operative management of endoscopic retrograde cholangiopancreatography-associated duodenal injuries. Ann R Coll Surg Engl. 2013;95(4):285–90. https://doi.org/10.1308/003588413X13511609958578.
47. Li Y, Han Z, Zhang W, Wang X, Li A, Xu Y, Zhou D, Wan T, Zhong J, Mi W, Liu S. Successful closure of lateral duodenal perforation by endoscopic band ligation after endoscopic clipping failure. Am J Gastroenterol. 2014;109(2):293–5. https://doi.org/10.1038/ajg.2013.415.
48. Armas Ojeda MD, Ojeda Marrero V, Roque Castellano C, Cabrera Marrero JC, Mathías Gutierrez Mdel P, Ceballos Santos D, Marchena Gómez J. [Duodenal perforations after endoscopic retrograde cholangiopancreatography]. Cir Esp. 2015;93(6):403–10. https://doi.org/10.1016/j.ciresp.2015.01.004.
49. Yang HY, Chen JH. Endoscopic fibrin sealant closure of duodenal perforation after endoscopic retrograde cholangiopancreatography. World J Gastroenterol. 2015;21(45):12976–80. https://doi.org/10.3748/wjg.v21.i45.12976.
50. Loperfido S, Angelini G, Benedetti G, Chilovi F, Costan F, De Berardinis F, De Bernardin M, Ederle A, Fina P, Fratton A. Major early complications from diagnostic and therapeutic ERCP: a prospective multicenter study. Gastrointest Endosc. 1998;48(1):1–10.
51. Christensen M, Matzen P, Schulze S, Rosenberg J. Complications of ERCP: a prospective study. Gastrointest Endosc. 2004;60(5):721–31.
52. Kayhan B, Akdoğan M, Sahin B. ERCP subsequent to retroperitoneal perforation caused by endoscopic sphincterotomy. Gastrointest Endosc. 2004;60(5):833–5.
53. WuHM,DixonE,MayGR,SutherlandFR.Management of perforation after endoscopic retrograde cholangiopancreatography (ERCP): a population-based review. HPB (Oxford). 2006;8(5):393–9. https://doi.org/10.1080/13651820600700617.
54. Sarli L, Porrini C, Costi R, Regina G, Violi V, Ferro M, Roncoroni L. Operative treatment of periampullary retroperitoneal perforation complicating endoscopic sphincterotomy. Surgery. 2007;142(1):26–32.
55. Assalia A, Suissa A, Ilivitzki A, Mahajna A, Yassin K, Hashmonai M, Krausz MM. Validity of clinical criteria in the management of endoscopic retrograde cholangiopancreatography related duodenal perforations. Arch Surg. 2007;142(11):1059–64.
56. Fatima J, Baron TH, Topazian MD, Houghton SG, Iqbal CW, Ott BJ, Farley DR, Farnell MB, Sarr M. Pancreaticobiliary and duodenal perforations after periampullary endoscopic procedures: diagnosis and management. Arch Surg. 2007;142(5):448–54; discussion 454–5.
57. Knudson K, Raeburn CD, McIntyre RC Jr, Shah RJ, Chen YK, Brown WR, Stiegmann G. Management of duodenal and pancreaticobiliary perforations associated with periampullary endoscopic procedures. Am J Surg. 2008;196(6):975–81; discussion 981–2. https://doi.org/10.1016/j.amjsurg.2008.07.045.
58. Mao Z, Zhu Q, Wu W, Wang M, Li J, Lu A, Sun Y, Zheng M. Duodenal perforations after endoscopic retrograde cholangiopancreatography: experience and management. J Laparoendosc Adv Surg Tech A. 2008;18(5):691–5. https://doi.org/10.1089/lap.2008.0020.
59. Vezakis A, Fragulidis G, Nastos C, Yiallourou A, Polydorou A, Voros D. Closure of a persistent sphincterotomy-related duodenal perforation by placement of a covered self-expandable metallic biliary stent. World J Gastroenterol. 2011;17(40):4539–41. https://doi.org/10.3748/wjg.v17.i40.4539.
60. Jeon HJ, Han JH, Park S, Youn S, Chae H, Yoon S. Endoscopic sphincterotomy-related perforation in the common bile duct successfully treated by placement of a covered metal stent. Endoscopy. 2011;43(Suppl 2 UCTN):E295–6. https://doi.org/10.1055/s-0030-1256464.
61. Kwon W, Jang JY, Ryu JK, Kim YT, Yoon YB, Kang MJ, Kim SW. Proposal of an endoscopic retrograde cholangiopancreatography-related perforation management guideline based on perforation type. J Korean Surg Soc. 2012;83(4):218–26. https://doi.org/10.4174/jkss.2012.83.4.218.
62. Park WY, Cho KB, Kim ES, Park KS. A case of ampullary perforation treated with a temporally covered metal stent. Clin Endosc. 2012;45(2):177–80. https://doi.org/10.5946/ce.2012.45.2.177.
63. Miller R, Zbar A, Klein Y, Buyeviz V, Melzer E, Mosenkis BN, Mavor E. Perforations following endoscopic retrograde cholangiopancreatography: a single institution experience and surgical recommendations. Am J Surg. 2013;206(2):180–6. https://doi.org/10.1016/j.amjsurg.2012.07.050.
64. Canena J, Liberato M, Horta D, Romão C, Coutinho A. Short-term stenting using fully covered self-expandable metal stents for treatment of refractory biliary leaks, postsphincterotomy bleeding, and perforations. Surg Endosc. 2013;27(1):313–24. https://doi.org/10.1007/s00464-012-2368-3.
65. Jin YJ, Jeong S, Kim JH, Hwang JC, Yoo BM, Moon JH, Park SH, Kim HG, Lee DK, Jeon YS, Lee DH. Clinical course and proposed treatment strategy for ERCP-related duodenal perforation: a multicenter analysis. Endoscopy. 2013;45(10):806–12. https://doi.org/10.1055/s-0033-1344230.

66. Koc B, Bircan HY, Adas G, Kemik O, Akcakaya A, Yavuz A, Karahan S. Complications following endoscopic retrograde cholangiopancreatography: minimal invasive surgical recommendations. PLoS One. 2014;9(11):e113073. https://doi.org/10.1371/journal.pone.0113073. eCollection 2014.
67. Odemis B, Oztas E, Kuzu UB, Parlak E, Disibeyaz S, Torun S, Kayacetin E. Can a fully covered self-expandable metallic stent be used temporarily for the management of duodenal retroperitoneal perforation during ERCP as a part of conservative therapy? Surg Laparosc Endosc Percutan Tech. 2016;26(1):e9–e17. https://doi.org/10.1097/SLE.0000000000000240.
68. Trikudanathan G, Hoversten P, Arain MA, Attam R, Freeman ML, Amateau SK. The use of fully-covered self-expanding metallic stents for intra-procedural management of post-sphincterotomy perforations: a single-center study (with video). Endosc Int Open. 2018;6(1):E73–7. https://doi.org/10.1055/s-0043-121884.

34 Miscellany Complications of ERCP

Zito Francesco Paolo, Germani Ugo, D' Alessandro Alessandra, Zullo Angelo, and Raffaele Manta

34.1 Infectious Adverse Events

Asymptomatic and transient bacteremia is common after both diagnostic and therapeutic ERCP, as well as other invasive procedures, being reported in 3–27% of patients. However, it is generally not relevant and antibiotic prophylaxis is not routinely recommended after ERCP [1, 2]. Endoscopy-related transmission of infections may occur when contaminated equipment is used, mainly during therapeutic procedures, with microorganisms diffusing into the bloodstream. Several studies have reported a high incidence of infections caused by multidrug-resistant (MDR) organisms in patients performing ERCPs, so that reprocessing procedures for duodenoscopes have been recently reviewed [3–5]. Therefore, these recommendations need to be accurately followed in clinical practice for prevention of infections. Cholangitis is the most common infectious adverse event associated with ERCP, but other infections may occur, including cholecystitis, cholangitic abscess, and endocarditis [4, 6].

Z. F. Paolo · D'. A. Alessandra
Digestive Endoscopy Unit, Pineta Grande Hospital, Caserta, Italy

G. Ugo · R. Manta
(*)
Digestive Endoscopy Unit, University Hospital of Perugia, Perugia, Italy

Z. Angelo
Gastroenterology and Digestive Endoscopy Unit of Nuovo Regina Margherita Hospital, Rome, Italy

34.1.1 Cholangitis

According to updated ESGE guidelines, acute cholangitis is considered one of the most important indications to emergency ERCP. However, cholangitis itself is a potential complication of ERCP, frequently occurring after the endoscopic procedure in up to 0.5–3% of patients [7–9]. On the other hand, delayed post-ERCP cholangitis is less frequent and typically occurs as a consequence of biliary stent—both plastic and metallic—occlusion in patients requiring long-term biliary drainage. From a clinical point of view, iatrogenic cholangitis is similar to other acute cholangitis, with classical symptomatic triad characterized by shivering fever, jaundice, and abdominal pain (Charcot triad), while hypotension or mental confusion occurs only in the most severe and life-threatening cases. According to the Tokyo Guidelines, acute cholangitis can be diagnosed when one item for each of the following criteria is fulfilled: evidence of systemic inflammation (fever or elevated white cell blood count), cholestasis (elevated bilirubin or transaminases), biliary dilation, or evidence of an etiology (stones, stricture, etc.) on imaging [2, 6].

M. Mutignani et al. (eds.), *Endotherapy in Biliopancreatic Diseases: ERCP Meets EUS*,
https://doi.org/10.1007/978-3-030-42569-2_34

Several factors may increase the risk for post-ERCP acute cholangitis, including either clinical or endoscopic-related parameters. Patients with incomplete biliary drainage, such as those with hilar cholangiocarcinoma, primary sclerosing cholangitis, or widespread metastatic liver disease, and those after liver transplantation are at increased risk. Similarly, the combination of ERCP with percutaneous biliary drainage or stenting of malignant biliary stricture may favor the onset of this complication. For these reasons, current guidelines strongly recommend proper opacification and complete drainage of intra- and extrahepatic bile ducts as mainstay of each ERCP in order to reduce the risk of post-procedural cholangitis. Moreover, an appropriate noninvasive imaging evaluation (MRCP or CT scan) may create a preoperative "road map" resulting in useful indication for the operator. Indeed, a previous assessment of biliary system may avoid excessive intraductal injection of contrast during cholangioscopy. Moreover, the endoscopist may schedule the proper therapeutic strategy, regarding the technique of cannulation, the number and the type stents needed, as well as other specific equipment. Besides biliary strictures, incomplete stone extraction or retained fragment after lithotripsy may increase the incidence of acute post-ERCP cholangitis up to 10%, as reported by Chang et al. [10]. For this reason, whenever imperfect biliary clearance is suspected and stone fragment may still be inside the common bile duct (up to 30% after lithotripsy), a biliary stent should be left in place, and endoscopic papillary large balloon dilation (EPLBD) should be performed aiming to facilitate the extraction of large bile stones. It has been reported that EPLBD is associated with a lower risk of cholangitis compared to mechanical lithotripsy (0% vs 13.3%, respectively) with similar results in terms of biliary stone clearance (98% vs 91%, respectively). However, data of another randomized trial failed to confirm these results [4–6, 9].

Current guidelines discourage the routine antibiotic therapy before ERCP and recommend antibiotic prophylaxis only in those patients with liver transplantation or biliary diseases associated with high risk of incomplete biliary drainage (i.e., primary sclerosing cholangitis, hilar stricture). Antibiotics specific for enteric gram-negative bacteria and enterococci should be preferred, and therapy should be continued after the procedure when biliary drainage is incomplete [2, 5].

Up to 13% of patients who underwent biliary stenting may experience cholangitis as delayed adverse event when the stent occlusion occurs prior the scheduled removal or exchange. It has been found that only biliary stenting increases the risk of cholangitis, while pancreatic duct stenting is not associated with such complication. Stent, both plastic and metallic, may occlude because of several reasons, such as stone fragment, biliary sludge, tumor or tissue overgrowth, food material, or stent migration.

Although many factors may play a role, the presence of cancer and placement of multiple biliary stents were found to be the main risk factors for post-ERCP delayed cholangitis. Patients with inoperable pancreatic cancer or cholangiocarcinoma usually require long-term biliary stenting as palliative treatment, and the risk of cholangitis, due to stent occlusion, is directly related to the length of patient survival [4]. In detail, up to 40–60% of patients develop cholangitis within 1 year from metallic stent placement, generally due to neoplastic ingrowth. However, self-expandable metal stents (SEMSs) are associated with lower occlusion rate, less therapeutic failure, lower number of procedure, and lower incidence of cholangitis when compared to plastic stents [6–8]. On the other hand, plastic stents are easy to remove and replace (every 3 months) and are less expensive. Based on these observations, the choice of the most appropriate stent (plastic vs metal) is very important to reduce the risk of this complication. The choice should be based on several aspects, such as the etiology and location of the stricture, the outcome of previous treatment, the skill of operator, and survival expectance [7].

34.1.2 Cholecystitis

Post-ERCP cholecystitis is a very uncommon complication (up to 0.5% of patients) presenting with fever, abdominal pain, leukocytosis, and positive Murphy's sign. The clinical diagnosis should be confirmed by imaging technique, since symptomatic pattern is very similar to that of cholangitis and misdiagnosis may occur [3].

Although no clear predictors of post-ERCP cholecystitis have been identified, gallbladder contamination with nonsterile contrast or cystic duct obstruction due to metallic stent placement may be potential risk factors. Indeed, deployment of fully covered metal stents at level of cystic duct orifice may increase the incidence of this complication up to 12%, and the risk further increased when the cystic duct is partially involved by the neoplastic stricture [7]. Whether uncovered metallic or plastic stents may reduce such a complication still remains controversial. However, the use of uncovered metal stent for the palliation of malignant biliary stricture involving the distal part of the biliary system is generally suggested, since the opened mesh of the stent does not obstruct the cystic duct [2, 9, 10].

Therapeutic management of post-ERCP cholecystitis should include wide-spectrum antibiotics, preferably specific against gram-negative organisms, as first-line therapy, while cholecystectomy should be considered only for cholecystitis unresponsive to medical treatment. Moreover, in patients unfit for surgery because of severe comorbidities or inoperable biliary strictures, EUS-guided cholecystic drainage from the stomach or duodenum could be a valid option. Finally, if the patient develops post-ERCP cholecystitis after a covered metal stent placecment, stent removal and replacement with uncovered stent could be considered [11–15].

34.1.3 Duodenoscope-Related Infections

An increased incidence of infections with MDR organisms associated with duodenoscope use has been recently highlighted. Differently from other endoscope-transmitted bacterial infections, where contamination is usually associated with breaches of standard reprocessing protocol, the use of duodenoscopes is associated with an increased risk due to presence of difficult-to-clean parts of the instrument (i.e., elevator and its own cable, the cable channel itself, and nearby areas) [16–18]. In fact, a contamination by carbapenem-resistant Enterobacteriaceae in nearly 2% of duodenoscopes and several cases of post-ERCP *Pseudomonas* and *Klebsiella* infections have been described despite a regularly performed reprocessing of instrument. On the contrary, no viral, fungal, or parasitic infection has been reported in association with the use of duodenoscopes [2, 7, 19–23].

Each endoscope with an elevator channel, both duodenoscopes and linear-array echoendoscopes, requires high effective reprocessing, according to current guidelines (ESGE-ESGENA 2018) [18]. Moreover, according to FDA, further measures should be applied, including microbial assessment every month or following 60 procedures. In case of confirmed contamination or when endoscopes are used in patients with known MDR infection, opportune measures of disinfection need to be accurately followed. In case of transmission of a MDR infection, blood sample culture should be performed in order to choose the most appropriate therapy [5, 24, 25].

34.2 Hepatic Hematoma

Hepatic hematoma (HH) is a rare, but potentially severe adverse event following ERCP caused by an injury to the intrahepatic biliary ducts or vessels. In most cases this complication occurs as parenchymatous damage during a deep cannulation with the guidewire [3, 7, 10]. In patients with choledocholithiasis, HH may occur also due to intrahepatic injury related to the traction applied with the balloon during stone extraction. HH is predominantly found in the right hepatic lobe (95.1%) and rarely in the left or in both lobes. A recent systematic review of all published cases estimated an overall incidence of 0.15%. However, the real incidence may be underestimated since this complication may develop without symptoms [4].

Clinical presentation usually includes acute onset of abdominal pain within 48 h after the procedure, while anemia, hypotension, and fever are less common symptoms, and they may suggest a more severe condition. When HH is suspected, an imaging exam such as abdominal ultrasonography, CT scan, or magnetic resonance should be performed to confirm the diagnosis and rule out other complications with similar clinical presentation [26–29]. Laboratory tests are not specific for HH, although a decrease in the hemoglobin level may occur.

Therapeutic management should be tailored according to the general conditions of the patient, and multidisciplinary approach is mandatory [2, 4, 30]. In hemodynamically stable patients with a limited and noncompressive hematomas, a conservative management with intravenous fluids and broad-spectrum prophylactic antibiotics is recommended. On the other hand, surgical or minimally invasive radiological approach should be reserved in case of general condition deterioration, hemodynamically instability, or presence of hepatic abscess unresponsive to medical therapy. Outcome depends on the clinical presentation and need for invasive therapies. A sudden rupture represents a life-threatening complication with high risk of mortality due to hypovolemic shock [3, 31].

34.3 Hepatic Abscess

Hepatic abscess is a very rare but life-threatening complication of ERCP with high risk of mortality. It is defined as a capsulated, suppurative collection within the liver parenchyma which may be infected by several types of microorganisms such as bacteria, fungi, or parasites [2]. The common risk factors for pyogenic liver abscess (PLA) are underlying biliary tract abnormalities, age >50 years, malignancy, diabetes, and interventional biliary or hepatic procedures. Indeed, endoscopic sphincterotomy (ES) creates a connection between intestinal lumen and biliary tree facilitating the spread to the liver of bowel microbes and, in particular conditions, the formation of liver abscess [13, 32, 33]. A recent cohort study from Taiwan compared the risk for pyogenic liver abscess (PLA) in patients undergoing ERCP with or without endoscopic sphincterotomy followed up for 5 years. Interestingly, the overall incidence of PLA was significantly higher when ES was performed (4.20 vs 0.94 per 1000 person-years) with an adjusted hazard ratio of 4.50 (95% CI 3.38–6.58). Although higher in the first year, the risk remained significantly increased over the next 4–5 years of follow-up [4, 7].

The most common presenting symptoms of liver abscess are fever and right-upper abdominal pain, nausea, and vomiting, while jaundice is very rare. Blood examinations usually reveal neutrophilic leukocytosis, abnormal liver tests, low serum albumin, and, infrequently, clotting impairment. Although diagnostic in half cases, blood cultures should be performed when a PLA is suspected. Abdominal CT scan and ultrasound are the main diagnostic tools, allowing drainage of the lesion as well. MRI has a very high sensitivity for small abscess, but it is not recommended as first diagnostic examination [34, 35].

Broad-spectrum antibiotic therapy is the mainstay of treatment and should be started empirically when the diagnosis of liver abscess is suspected. Antibiotic therapy could be tailored following a successful bacterial culture. Such therapy is successful in the majority of patients with liver abscesses <3 cm in diameter [36]. Abscess drainage is another therapeutic approach whose timing should be evaluated on response to previous antibiotic therapies or general condition of the patient [37]. Urgent drainage is needed only when hemodynamic instability with shock or multi-organ dysfunction occurs [38]. According to its size, location, and complexity, PLA can be drained with needle aspiration (most commonly under radiographic guidance), placement of an indwelling catheter (most commonly under radiographic guidance), open or laparoscopic surgical drainage, surgical resection of the abscess, or endoscopic drainage [39–42].

34.4 Stent-Related Complication

Placement of biliary stent adverse events is usually associated with the deployment of metallic metal stent. Early complications are rare and include hemorrhage, pancreatitis, stent misplacement, perforation, and injury to the CBD or main pancreatic duct [2, 3]. On the other hand, chronic stent-related complications are more common and include stent obstruction (25–35% of patients), migration (up to 6% of subjects), and infections such as cholangitis, liver abscess, or sepsis. Displacement of stents may occur proximally into the biliary tree, typically in patients with malignant stenosis, or distally into the gut with the risk of bowel perforation [14]. Jaundice, cholangitis, pancreatitis, or perforation may develop as consequence of stent migration, requiring stent removal. Several techniques of extraction have been described, including the use of specific stent retrieval devices, forceps, snares, or balloons. Pancreatic duct stenting may rarely cause ductal irregularity, side branch dilation, and stricture formation, mimicking radiological features associated with chronic pancreatitis [21, 23].

34.5 Splenic Injury

Splenic injury is a very rare and potentially life-threatening complication of ERCP, including subcapsular hematoma, peri-splenic hematoma, laceration, rupture, avulsion of splenic vessels, or avulsion of spleen from the capsule. The incidence of this complication is unknown, and a recent systematic review described data of 24 cases [43, 44]. Although etiology remains unclear, it has been hypothesized that traction applied on the spleen, during the procedure, may induce damage and consequent spleen infraction. For this reason, patients with abdominal adhesions due to previous major abdominal surgery or subjects with calcification and fibrosis of splenocolic and gastrosplenic ligaments, due to chronic pancreatitis, may be at high risk for splenic injury during ERCP [2–4]. However, the technique used during the ERCP may itself predispose to this adverse event due to pressure and the torsion of the instrument on the greater curvature and, consequently on the splenic hilum, during access to duodenum or papilla cannulation.

Patients with splenic injury usually complain of abdominal pain immediately after the procedure, and, in case of severe splenic damage, hemodynamic instability and acute anemia may occur. As for other post-ERCP complications characterized by severe abdominal pain, diagnosis of splenic injury should be confirmed with a radiological exam such as abdominal ultrasonography or CT scan [43].

The therapeutic management should be tailored on the severity of splenic damage and may include a conservative approach, angiographic embolization of splenic artery, or splenectomy in case of hemodynamic instability.

34.6 Cardiopulmonary Adverse Events

Cardiopulmonary adverse events occurring during ERCP are usually related to procedural sedation/anesthesia and include hypoxia, hypotension, cardiac dysrhythmia, and aspiration. If transient hypoxia and hypotension are excluded, the incidence of clinically relevant cardiopulmonary complication ranges from 0.07% up to 2.4%, but the risk increases in elderly and debilitated patients. In the last years, along with the increase in complexity of endoscopic procedures, the use of sedation changed [1, 5, 31, 45]. In fact, ERCP, as well as other advanced endoscopic procedures, requires longer and deeper sedation than ambulatory endoscopy. Therefore, the presence of an anesthesiologist in the endoscopic room is usually recommended. Moreover, a proper pre-procedural examination should be always performed to assess the anesthesiological risk, and the endoscopic room for ERCPs needs to be properly equipped for emergency (i.e., ventilator system, intubation equipment, defibrillator). Several systematic reviews have reported that, unless of severe comorbidities, ERCP can be performed safely without intubation in the majority of patients, even in case of propofol-based anesthesia. In randomized trials, patients undergoing ERCP with propofol sedation had similar mortality rate or incidence of serious cardiopulmonary adverse events compared to traditional medications. On the contrary, propofol-based anesthesia was associated with shorter recovery times and better sedation with higher level of amnesia [6, 8, 10].

34.6.1 Air Embolism

Air embolism is a very rare but potentially fatal complication of ERCP. The incidence is unknown because it is a very uncommon adverse event, only 26 cases being reported in the literature. Air embolism may occur when traumatic injury or inflammation of the bile ducts, contrast administration, insufflation, rubbing of the endoscope, and ERCP accessories allow the passage of air directly into the vascular system. Patients with past history of surgery, previous extraction of large bile stones, or placement of metal stents, as well as those undergoing cholangioscopy or endoscopic necrosectomy, are at increased risk for this complication. However, use of CO_2 insufflation during ERCPs and the use of water for the distension of biliary ducts during cholangioscopy reduce the risk [46].

Unexpected onset of severe hypotension and hypoxia or sudden impairment of neurological status, during or immediately after the endoscopic procedure, typically occur in case of systemic air embolism. Whenever such complication is suspected, the endoscopic procedure must be immediately stopped in order to allow rapid endotracheal intubation and ventilation [3, 5]. Then, the patient should be positioned in the Trendelenburg and left lateral decubitus to reduce the amount of air arriving to the brain. Once hemodynamically stable, a total body CT scan and a transthoracic echocardiogram should be performed to confirm the diagnosis of systemic air embolism [47, 48].

References

1. Miyatani H, et al. Post-ERCP biliary complications in patients with biliary type sphincter of Oddi dysfunction. Sci Rep. 2018;8(1):9951. https://doi.org/10.1038/s41598-018-28309-w.
2. Freeman ML, et al. Complications of endoscopic biliary sphincterotomy. N Engl J Med. 1996;335(13):909–18. https://doi.org/10.1056/NEJM199609263351301.
3. Kahaleh M, Freeman M. Prevention and management of post-endoscopic retrograde cholangiopancreatography complications. Clin Endosc. 2012;45(3):305–12. https://doi.org/10.5946/ce.2012.45.3.305.
4. Chandrasekhara V, et al. Adverse events associated with ERCP. Gastrointest Endosc. 2017;85(1):32–47. https://doi.org/10.1016/j.gie.2016.06.051.
5. Kwon CI, et al. Unusual complications related to endoscopic retrograde cholangiopancreatography and its endoscopic treatment. Clin Endosc. 2013;46(3):251–9. https://doi.org/10.5946/ce.2013.46.3.251.
6. Guda ML, Nalini FL. Overview of ERCP complications: prevention and management. ERCP and EUS. Springer Science; 2015. https://doi.org/10.1007/978-1-4939-2320-5_3.
7. ASGE Quality Assurance in Endoscopy Committee, Calderwood AH, et al. ASGE guideline for infection control during GI endoscopy. Gastrointest Endosc. 2018;87(5):1167–79. https://doi.org/10.1016/j.gie.2017.12.009.
8. Vila JJ, et al. Post-endoscopic retrograde cholangiopancreatography complications: how can they be avoided? World J Gastrointest Endosc. 2012;4(6):241–6. https://doi.org/10.4253/wjge.v4.i6.241.
9. Petersen BT, et al. Infection using ERCP endoscopes. Gastroenterology. 2016;151(1):46–50. https://doi.org/10.1053/j.gastro.2016.05.040.
10. Cheng CL, et al. Risk factors for post-ERCP pancreatitis: a prospective multicenter study. Am J Gastroenterol. 2006;101:139–47.
11. Vandervoort J, et al. Risk factors for complic-ations after performance of ERCP. Gastrointest Endosc. 2002;56:652–6.
12. Masci E, et al. Complications of diagnostic and therapeutic ERCP: a prospective multicenter study. Am J Gastroenterol. 2001;96:417–23.
13. Wang P, et al. Risk factors for ERCP-related complications: a prospective multicenter study. Am J Gastroenterol. 2009;104:31–40.
14. Katsinelos P, et al. Risk factors for therapeutic ERCP-related complications: an analysis of 2,715 cases performed by a single endoscopist. Ann Gastroenterol. 2014;27:65–72.
15. Du M, et al. Post-ERCP infection and its epidemiological and clinical characteristics in a large Chinese tertiary hospital: a 4-year surveillance study. Antimicrob Resist Infect Control. 2017;6:131. https://doi.org/10.1186/s13756-017-0290-0.
16. Talukdar R. Complications of ERCP. Best Pract Res Clin Gastroenterol. 2016;30(5):793–805. https://doi.org/10.1016/j.bpg.2016.10.007.
17. Beilenhoff U, et al. Prevention of multidrug-resistant infections from contaminated duodenoscopes: position statement of the European Society of Gastrointestinal Endoscopy (ESGE) and European Society of Gastroenterology Nurses and Associates (ESGENA). Endoscopy. 2017;49(11):1098–106. https://doi.org/10.1055/s-0043-120523.
18. Kwak MS, et al. Risk factors of post- endoscopic retrograde cholangiopancreatography bacteremia. Gut Liver. 2013;7(2):228–33. https://doi.org/10.5009/gnl.2013.7.2.228.
19. Kim MH, et al. The impact of gallbladder status on biliary complications after the endoscopic removal of choledocholithiasis. Dig Dis Sci. 2016;61(4):1165–71. https://doi.org/10.1007/s10620-015-3915-2.
20. Smith ZL, et al. Transmission of carbapenem-resistant Enterobacteriaceae during ERCP: time to revisit the

current reprocessing guidelines. Gastrointest Endosc. 2015;81(4):1041–5. https://doi.org/10.1016/j.gie.2014.11.006.
21. Alfa MJ, et al. A survey of reprocessing methods, residual viable bioburden, and soil levels in patient-ready endoscopic retrograde cholangiopancreatography duodenoscopes used in Canadian centers. Infect Control Hosp Epidemiol. 2002;23:198–206.
22. Kola A, et al. An outbreak of carbapenem-resistant OXA-48—producing Klebsiella pneumonia associated to duodenoscopy. Antimicrob Resist Infect Control. 2015;4:8. https://doi.org/10.1186/s13756-015-0049-4.
23. Wendorf KA, et al. Endoscopic retrograde cholangiopancreatography-associated AmpC Escherichia coli outbreak. Infect Control Hosp Epidemiol. 2015;36:634–42.
24. Robertson P, et al. Transmission of Salmonella enteritidis after endoscopic retrograde cholangiopancreatography because of inadequate endoscope decontamination. Am J Infect Control. 2017;45(4):440–2. https://doi.org/10.1016/j.ajic.2016.11.024.
25. Chen M, et al. Risk factor analysis of post-ERCP cholangitis: a single-center experience. Hepatobiliary Pancreat Dis Int. 2018;17(1):55–8. https://doi.org/10.1016/j.hbpd.2018.01.002.
26. Freeman ML. Complications of endoscopic retrograde cholangiopancreatography: avoidance and management. Gastrointest Endosc Clin North Am. 2012;22:567–86.
27. Kostrzewska M, et al. Complications of endoscopic retrograde cholangio-pancreatography (ERCP) and their risk factors. Adv Med Sci. 2011;56:6–12.
28. Hanau LH, Steigbigel NH. Acute (ascending) cholangitis. Infect Dis Clin North Am. 2000;14:521–46.
29. Tierney J, et al. Predictive risk factors associated with cholangitis following ERCP. Surg Endosc. 2018;32(2):799–804. https://doi.org/10.1007/s00464-017-5746-z.
30. Buxbaum JL, et al. Inoperable pancreatic cancer patients who have prolonged survival exhibit an increased risk of cholangitis. JOP. 2011;12(4):377–83.
31. Pola S, et al. Long-term risk of cholangitis in patients with metal stents for malignant biliary obstruction. Dig Dis Sci. 2012;57(10):2693–6.
32. Glomsaker T, et al. Patterns and predictive factors of complications after endoscopic retrograde cholangiopancreatography. Br J Surg. 2013;100:373–80.
33. Agostoni M, et al. Adverse events during monitored anesthesia care for GI endoscopy: an 8-year experience. Gastrointest Endosc. 2011;74:266–75.
34. Zappa MA, Aiolfi A, Antonini I, Musolino CD, Porta A. Subcapsular hepatic haematoma of the right lobe following endoscopic retrograde cholangiopancreatography: case report and literature review. World J Gastroenterol. 2016;22(17):4411–5. https://doi.org/10.3748/wjg.v22.i17.4411.
35. Imperatore N, et al. Systematic review: features, diagnosis, management and prognosis of hepatic hematoma, a rare complication of ERCP. Dig Liver Dis. 2018;50(10):997–1003. https://doi.org/10.1016/j.dld.2018.07.010.
36. Ortega Deballon P, et al. Liver hematoma following endoscopic retrograde cholangiopancreatography (ERCP). Surg Endosc. 2000;14:767.
37. Horn TL, Pena LR. Subcapsular hepatic hematoma after ERCP: case report and review. Gastrointest Endosc. 2004;59:594–6.
38. Chi KD, Waxman I. Subcapsular hepatic hematoma after guide wire injury during endoscopic retrograde cholangiopancreatography: management and review. Endoscopy. 2004;36:1019–21.
39. Liu L, et al. Pyogenic liver abscess: a retrospective study of 105 cases in an emergency department from East China. J Emerg Med. 2017;52(4):409–16. https://doi.org/10.1016/j.jemermed.2016.09.026.
40. Kalaitzakis E. All-cause mortality after ERCP. Endoscopy. 2016;48(11):987–94. https://doi.org/10.1055/s-0042-111319.
41. Lardiere-Deguelte S, et al. Hepatic abscess: diagnosis and management. J Visc Surg. 2015;152(4):231–43. https://doi.org/10.1016/j.jviscsurg.2015.01.013.
42. Peng YC, et al. Risk of pyogenic liver abscess and endoscopic sphincterotomy: a population-based cohort study. BMJ Open. 2018;8(3):e018818. https://doi.org/10.1136/bmjopen-2017-018818.
43. Oliveira-Cunha M, et al. Late complications after endoscopic sphincterotomy. Surg Laparosc Endosc Percutan Tech. 2016;26(1):1–5. https://doi.org/10.1097/SLE.0000000000000226.
44. Pamudurthy V, et al. Etiologies and risks of splenic decapsulation after endoscopic retrograde cholangiopancreatography: case report and literature review. Endosc Int Open. 2018;6(3):E271–3. https://doi.org/10.1055/s-0043-125145.
45. Chawla S, Willingham FF. Cardiopulmonary complications of endoscopic retrograde cholangiopancreatography. Tech Gastrointest Endosc. 2014;16:144–9.
46. Sharma VK, et al. A national study of cardiopulmonary unplanned events after GI endoscopy. Gastrointest Endosc. 2007;66:27–34.
47. El Hajj II, et al. Life threatening hemobilia after endoscopic retrograde cholangiopancreatography (ERCP). Dig Liver Dis. 2017;49(12):1336–7. https://doi.org/10.1016/j.dld.2017.09.001.
48. Fujii L, et al. Successful nonsurgical treatment of pneumomediastinum, pneumothorax, pneumoperitoneum, pneumoretroperitoneum, and subcutaneous emphysema following ERCP. Gastroenterol Res Pract. 2010;2010:289135. https://doi.org/10.1155/2010/289135.

EUS Complications

35

Ilaria Tarantino and Michele Amata

35.1 Introduction

In recent years, endoscopic ultrasound (EUS) has established itself as a complete and innovative technology in the endoscopy. In the diagnostic and, more recently, the operative setting, EUS has permitted a high accuracy in GI cancer staging, with its own mini-invasive approach, even if this technique remains skill- demanding. This chapter focuses on the adverse events (AEs) associated with the main applications of EUS: diagnostic, EUS fine-needle aspiration (FNA), and EUS fine-needle injection procedures.

35.2 Complications of Diagnostic EUS

Historically, EUS started as a diagnostic procedure for the diagnosis of GI diseases and was performed mainly with radial echoendoscopes. Today, diagnostic EUS is currently being performed with either radial or linear echoendoscope (Fig. 35.1). EUS is a safe and efficient procedure in expert hands, but it shares the risks and adverse effects of the other endoscopic procedures, such as cardiovascular events, unwelcome effects of conscious and deeper sedation, and allergic reactions to medications.

Though rare, the main complications in diagnostic EUS are perforation, bleeding, and infections. The incidence of GI perforation ranged from 0 to 0.4% in prospective series. Perforation is probably more common with upper gastrointestinal (UGI) EUS than with EGD, even if there is scant evidence in the literature [1]. This risk is mostly secondary to the echoendoscope design, which combines oblique or side-viewing optics with a relatively long rigid tip that extends well beyond the optical lens. In fact, the currently available echoendoscopes, both radial and linear, have an ultrasound (US) transducer located at the tip, making the distal part of the scope less flexible and stiffer than standard ones. In addition, the EUS optical lens have an oblique viewing and is located 1–2 cm proximally from the tip. In such way, the echoendoscope insertion and advancement of the instruments, especially across the bends, are semi-blind maneuvers, and the risk of perforation can increase, especially in areas of angulation (oropharynx or apex of duodenal bulb), stenosis (esophageal cancer), or a blind lumen (pharyngeal or esophageal diverticula). This complication is more common in the early phase of EUS training or when skilled endosonographers use new equipment with different designs and lengths of the tip [2].

I. Tarantino (✉) · M. Amata
Endoscopy Service, Department of Diagnostic and Therapeutic Services, Istituto Mediterraneo per i Trapianti e Terapie ad alta specializzazione (IRCCS-ISMETT), Palermo, Italy
e-mail: itarantino@ismett.edu

M. Mutignani et al. (eds.), *Endotherapy in Biliopancreatic Diseases: ERCP Meets EUS*,
https://doi.org/10.1007/978-3-030-42569-2_35

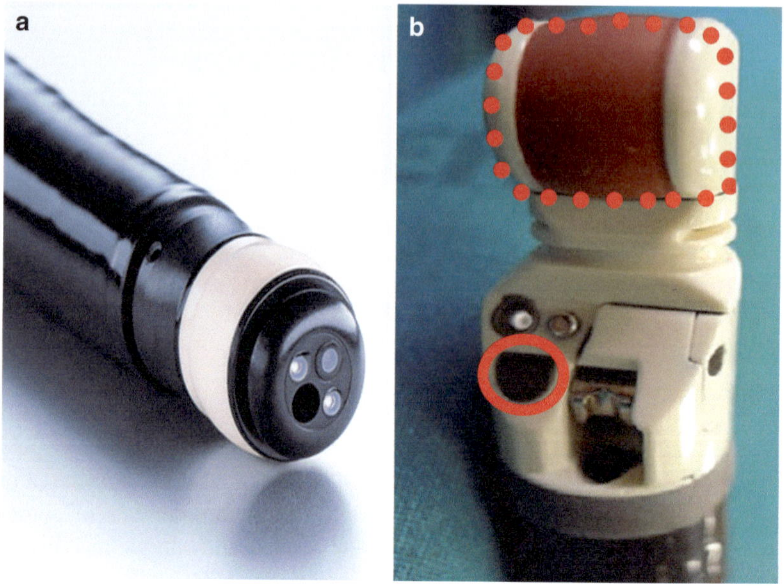

Fig. 35.1 Focus on the tip of a radial (**a**) and linear (**b**) echoendoscope. Red circular line, optical lens with oblique or side view; red dashed line, US transducer

Esophageal intubation with the echoendoscope is a partially blind maneuver, and cervical perforation is an extremely rare collateral effect as evaluated in a prospective large series study [3]. In a US survey with 43,852 cases, the incidence of perforation was 0.03% (16 patients, with 1 death) [4]. An accurate anamnesis for the detection of potential risk factors, like older age (>65 years), history of difficult intubation, cervical spine kyphosis, and swallowing disease, may help to recognize high-risk patients and help in reducing the incidence.

Esophageal cancer and esophageal strictures are both associated with increased incidence of esophageal perforation. Approximately 15–40% of esophageal cancer cases are stenosing tumor, and the stricture often restricts the passage of the scopes, limiting the EUS staging assessment. Some authors have proposed the dilatation of the lumen, increasing the accuracy of EUS for T and N staging for traversable versus non-traversable tumors (81% vs. 28% and 86% vs. 72%, respectively) [5]. In the other hands, dilation of the stricture carries high risk of perforation in up to one out of four cases [6], even if distant lymphadenopathy (M1a tumor staging) is only possibly diagnosed in 10–40% of patients who require this technique [7]. Though past studies have reported different perforation rates (higher than 24%) following esophageal dilation, more recent studies have found this practice to be safe thanks to the technology innovations in stiffness and caliber size of endoscopes and operator consciousness of the AEs in hazardous hydropneumatic dilatation. For patients with circumferential stenosis, judicious stepwise dilation is undertaken to a maximum of 15 mm, even more if a sequential 1-mm stepwise bougienage is applied [7]. Dilation has allowed immediate passage of the echoendoscope beyond the tumor in 75–85% of cases, but extreme caution is necessary also when a simple semi-circumferential infiltration is present. Alternative modalities are also known, such as choosing mini-probes, thinner and softer but with limited US depth penetration [8], and the EBUS device, which is much more flexible and slim (6.9 mm in diameter), providing a complete staging evaluation and allowing FNA sampling of celiac nodes or liver lesions [9].

35.3 Complications of EUS-FNA

FNA is the most common EUS intervention performed to obtain tissue from solid masses and nodes or to aspirate liquid from cystic lesions. The EUS-FNA morbidity has a range between 0 and 2.5% in prospective series, with 0.04%

incidence of death (1 case reported in 2486 patients) [10]. The main frequent complications are infection, bleeding, and acute pancreatitis. Moreover, a needle with a larger caliber does not seem to be associated with a higher complication risk. As described in two randomized control trials (RCTs) comparing needles of different sizes (22G vs. 25G and 19G vs. 25G), the authors did not find significant differences in complications [11, 12]. In another study, the number of needle passes was not associated with increased risk of complications [13]. On the other hand, operator experience may play a role as an important risk factor because, as shown in the literature, the highest frequencies of complications were observed in the first phase of training or in the early period of endoscopic experience [14].

35.3.1 Infection

The infection rate after EUS-FNA, including FNA of rectal and perirectal lesions, is generally low, with a similar incidence compared to upper GI endoscopy or diagnostic EUS. The bacteremia following EUS-FNA in rare cases develops as clinical illness or septic status. According to the latest guidelines, prophylactic antibiotics are not recommended for EUS-FNA in solid lesions or lymph nodes, also for the prevention of infective endocarditis in the patients with cardiac risk factors. Indeed, sepsis has been reported after EUS-FNA of cystic lesions (pancreatic or mediastinal ones), and, in fact, prophylactic infusion of antibiotics is mandatory in these cases. Wiersema et al. reported a significantly higher incidence of complications for EUS-FNA of pancreatic fluid collections than for pancreatic solid lesions (3/22 [14%] vs. 2/452 [0.5%], respectively; $P < 0.001$) [15]. In the studies evaluated for the latest ESGE guidelines, the antibiotic prophylaxis was administered before EUS-FNA of pancreatic fluid collections, but nevertheless the overall morbidity remained higher than for solid masses (5/210 [2.4%] vs. 10/1386 [0.7%], respectively) [10]. Therefore, the cystic character of the lesion is considered a risk factor for complications, both of infection and bleeding.

35.3.2 Pancreatitis

Pancreatitis can occur after EUS-FNA of both solid and pancreatic cystic lesions (PCL), with a low incidence (range of 0.26% in a large multicenter study and 2% in a prospective small study) [10]. Iatrogenic pancreatitis following EUS-FNA is generally mild and self-limiting, but severe scenarios with fatal complications have been reported [16]. The median time of hospitalization for pancreatitis treatment is 3 days (range 1–21 days). The injury of normal intervening parenchyma of the pancreas during EUS-FNA or the damage of pancreatic ducts develops local complications, with activation of an inflammatory process. Limiting the number of needle passes in order to minimize the amount of "normal" pancreatic parenchyma that must be traversed and avoiding the pancreatic duct during EUS-FNA procedures are all safe tricks that all operators must use in their practice [6]. A known history of recent pancreatitis, size tumors ≤20 mm in diameter, and puncture of a benign pancreatic lesion, especially pancreatic neuroendocrine tumors (PNET), are factors that may predispose to post-EUS-FNA pancreatitis of solid lesions, but a significant relationship has still not been shown [17].

35.3.3 Hemorrhage

Clinically significant bleeding has been reported, though it is a very rare condition, with an incidence between 0 and 0.5% as reported in large prospective series [18]. Significant hemorrhage can be manifest if a large vessel is punctured or in cases of bleeding disorder. Indeed, self-limited intra-procedural bleeding with no clinical consequence is much more common. The risk of bleeding is related mainly to the performance and quality of FNA and may generate an extraluminal (expanding echo-poor region adjacent to the sampled lesion) or an intra-cystic bleeding (hyperechoic area increasing in size, inside the cyst). This last condition is much more frequent and has a rate of 6% of self-limited bleeding. The management of these conditions consists in halting other needle passages, observed by EUS, and infusing a dose of antibiotics (β-lactam antibiotic preferably) to prevent a subsequent infection [6, 10, 19]. For an extra-luminal hemorrhage following EUS-FNA, one study specifically evaluated 277 patients over a 13-month period, with evidence of a 1.3% rate. These complications occurred just in three patients, during the aspiration of a pancreatic islet cell mass, a peritumoral lymph node in a patient with esophageal cancer, and a PCL. In all cases, the hemorrhage was seen with US, and mechanical pressure was gently applied with the endoscope to tamponade the hemorrhage [20]. Indeed, in the literature there are few rare cases of intra-procedural bleeding that required luminal intervention, such as adrenaline injection and hemostatic clips [10], and just one fatal case secondary to a massive bleed after EUS-FNA [21]. EUS-FNA should be avoided in patients taking oral anticoagulants [22] according to recent guidelines on endoscopy and antiplatelet agents [23]. EUS-FNA of solid masses can be performed in patients taking aspirin or NSAIDS, but not in patients taking thienopyridines (e.g., clopidogrel). EUS-FNA of cystic lesions should not be performed in patients taking any kind of antiplatelet agents [24]. Thromboembolic risk and its relative risk-to-benefit ratio must at all times be considered if a change or interruption in the antithrombotic therapy is strictly necessary for the performance of EUS-FNA [6]. EUS-through-the-needle biopsy (EUS-TTNB) has been recently introduced for the tissue acquisition in PCLs. The micro-forceps was specifically designed to be used through a 19-gauge needle after EUS-guided puncture of PCL with a high diagnostic yield and lower AEs. In a recent retrospective multicenter study, Barresi et al. had showed a 16% of AEs, 3/56 patients experienced abdominal pain, and 7/56 developed intra-cystic hemorrhage. Intra-cystic hemorrhage was defined as an active bleeding inside the cyst as a spurting vessel enhanced by color Doppler or a cystic lesion that progressively increases in size after evacuation, with change in morphological aspect from anechoic to hyperechoic PCL (Fig. 35.2), in both cases the bleeding spontaneously stopped [25].

35.3.4 Tumor Seeding

The seeding of tumorous cells along the needle tract is less frequent, but is a serious complication that can impair patient survival. A retrospective study suggests that peritoneal carcinomatosis, correlated with pancreatic cancer, may occur more frequently after abdominal percutaneous (ranges from 0.003 to 0.009%) compared to EUS-guided FNA [26]. Since this first report of tumor dissemination after diagnostic EUS-FNA of pancreatic tumors, needle tract seeding has been reported in 15 cases, of which 80% (12/15 cases) of the total of the tumors were located in the body or tail of the pancreas. In fact, the preferred location of tumor seeding was the posterior gastric wall (12/15) and the gastroesophageal junction (3/15). Indeed, there are no reports of tumor seed-

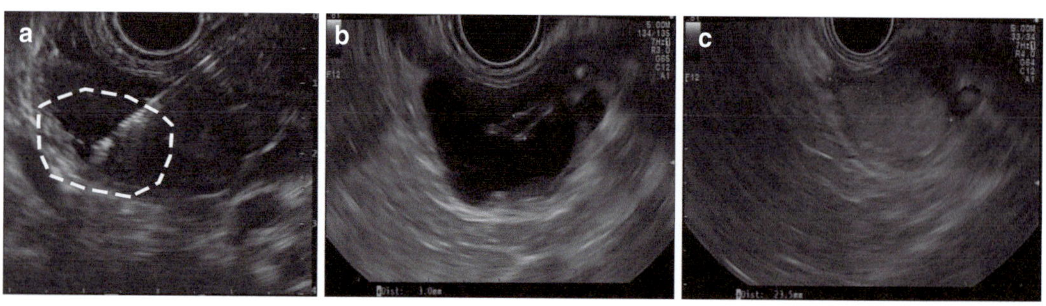

Fig. 35.2 Endoscopic ultrasound-through-the-needle biopsy for the sampling of a PCL. (**a**) EUS view of the biopsy forceps with opened blades (white dashed line). Intra-cystic bleeding after TTNB: initial phase (**b**) and complete morphological change of the cyst with typical hyperechoic aspect (**c**)

ing following EUS-FNA of the pancreatic head tumors, which can be explained by the fact that the needle tract site is resected together with the lesions (duodenocefalopancreasectomy). Endosonographers need to bear in mind the possibility of needle tract seeding when performing EUS-FNA for resectable tumors located in the pancreatic body or tail [27]. Moreover, the risk of needle tract seeding can be reduced by performing EUS-FNA only when the results obtained are useful for management and therapeutic decision-making, as described by Fujii [28]. Needle tract seeding following EUS-FNA can be avoided by setting the needle tract line within the surgical resection margins, if technically possible. Furthermore, follow-up of the needle puncture sites by performing endoscopy and imaging modalities for early detection of needle tract seeding can help to guarantee a radical cure. However, further prospective studies with larger cohorts are necessary to estimate the real risk of needle tract seeding following EUS-FNA [27].

35.3.5 Bile Peritonitis

Though rare, bile peritonitis can occur after the puncture of the gallbladder and\or obstructed bile ducts, with an increased risk if the operator hits the target on the bile rather than a gallbladder mass. In fact, EUS-FNA of solid gallbladder masses has been reported as safe in one small case series [29]. If biliary puncture occurs, antibiotics should be administered to patients who do not have biliary obstruction. Bile duct peritonitis frequently requires surgery. A case of bile peritonitis requiring laparotomy following EUS-FNA of a pancreatic head mass with biliary obstruction, who had inadvertent perforation of distal common bile duct, has been reported [30].

35.4 Complications of EUS Fine-Needle Injection Procedures

EUS can be used to perform celiac plexus block (CPB) or celiac plexus neurolysis (CPN) in order to achieve analgesia in chronic pancreatitis or pancreatic cancer pain. The technique needs the direct injection of corticosteroids (in blockade) or absolute alcohol (in neurolysis) plus a local anesthetic into the celiac plexus using a EUS-FNA needle. The common AEs are transient diarrhea (4–15%) due to unintentionally local injury of mesenteric plexus, transient orthostatic hypotension (1%), temporary increase of pain (9%), and abscess development [31]. In order to reduce the incidence of orthostasis, adequate intravenous hydration before and after the procedure must be adopted. Hofman et al. reported a large case series (189 CPB and 31 CPN) with one case of asymptomatic hypotension after neurolysis, one case of retroperitoneal abscess, and two cases of severe self-limited post-procedural pain after CPB [32]. The CPN AEs with EUS-guided and percutaneous approach are almost similar in incidence to hemorrhage [33]. Even though it has been postulated that the EUS anterior access would avoid the rare but devastating AEs of spinal cord infarction associated with the posterior percutaneous approach, Fujii and colleagues have described bilateral lower extremity paralysis after EUS-guided CPN by the involvement of the anterior spinal artery after alcohol injection [34]. The most frightening complication after CPN is death, which may be due to thrombosis or necrosis, with associated perforation of the celiac artery and aorta, leading to end-stage organ ischemia. There are few published case reports on this fatal event secondary to EUS-FNA injection procedures [35, 36].

35.5 Complications of Pancreatic Fluid Collection Drainage

According to the Atlanta classification [37], walled-off pancreatic necrosis (WOPN) and pseudocyst (PC) are encapsulated pancreatic fluid collections (PFCs), respectively, with or without solid necrotic debris inside, which can be located within the pancreatic parenchyma or in peri-pancreatic space, and develop after an episode of acute pancreatitis or pancreatic trauma. Traditionally, the drainage of PFCs was accomplished by surgical or percutaneous methods. Subsequently, EUS-guided cystogastroduodenostomy with double pigtail plastic stent placement emerged as an effective nonsurgical or radiological treatment for PFCs, but with a lower success rate for WOPN treatment [38]. Recently, new dedicated lumen-apposing metal stents (LAMS) with antimigratory properties have been used for EUS drainage of PFCs [39]. These LAMS are specifically designed to create an anastomosis between the cyst cavity and the gut lumen, allowing an easy access of the collection to perform repeated sessions of direct endoscopic necrosectomy (DEN). The simplicity of the procedure plays a key role in terms of safety and efficacy, with a technical success greater than 90% and treatment success varying between 70 and 90% according to the specific characteristics of the drained PFC [40]. The EUS drainage procedure of PFCs is reasonably safe in experienced hands. However, post-procedural complications have been reported and include perforation, bleeding, buried stent, migration, and maldeployment of the stent. Prospective, randomized trials have conclusively proven that the technical outcomes and safety profile of EUS are superior to conventional endoscopy for transmural drainage of pancreatic PCs in terms of lower hemorrhage and perforation [41]. In fact, the EUS approach is able to identify vascular structures by using Doppler and helps to assess maturity of PFCs by the clear evaluation of the wall thickness and the selection of the thinnest point of entrance, even in non-bulging collections. Despite these clear advantages, perforation and bleeding are the most frequent complications, as evidenced in several studies [42, 43]. The frequency of these complications can vary according to the type of PFCs, the concurrent infective process, and procedural techniques: the approximate incidence rate is around 10% (mainly bleeding and perforation). Sadik et al. reported a 94% success rate with a 5% complication rate in simple PCs vs. 80% success rate and 30% complication rate in infected ones [44]. Similar results have been reported by Varadarajulu et al. [45]. According to this evidence, while EUS-guided drainage is still effective and safe, infected PCs are more difficult to treat, with higher complication rates [6].

35.5.1 Perforation

Perforation has been reported as a complication in several studies and may be more common when uncinate lesions are drained [42, 43, 46]. Varadarajuluet al. reported perforation in two patients requiring surgery in a group of 148 patients undergoing EUS-guided drainage of PFCs with double pigtails [47]. In these studies, the electrocautery used for transmural puncture caused the majority of perforations. Another risk factor is the use of non-coaxial needle knife to create the fistula (the tangential direction of the needle force can dissect the GI wall) and the balloon dilatation catheter with a very large caliber. The adoption of a coaxial over-the-wire cystotome can help to avoid this adverse invent, such as the use of a graded dilation technique without the use of electrocautery [6]. However, most perforations are generally small, and conservative measures are sufficient, especially if CO_2 has been used as gas for insufflations and if the nasogastric drainage and intravenous antibiotics were promptly chosen. Initial enteral nutrition has been shown to decrease systemic infections, the need for surgical intervention, and mortality compared with parenteral nutrition. As shown in a recent Asian-Pacific consensus statement, the majority of perforations after WOPN drainage and DEN (71.4%, 20/28) could be treated conservatively, with efficacy [48]. The rest of non-responders require immediate surgical rescue therapy.

35.5.2 Bleeding

While EUS-Doppler allows for the recognition and avoidance of the interposing blood vessels in the site of puncture (entry point) or inside the novel cavity, bleeding can occur during or after EUS-guided drainage, with a median reported incidence rate of 18% [49]. In fact, following the initial tamponaded action by the mechanical compression inside the cavity, some small vessels can start to bleed when the PFCs become empty, especially if the liquid component is prominent. Moreover, use of the needle knife adds a risk of hemorrhage from the entry point, even with wire guidance [6]. The number of available published studies evaluating EUS-guided drainage of PFCs with LAMS and their own AEs is scant, and mostly contradictory, and with short follow-up. Initially, Bang et al. reported 10 AEs in 31 patients (8/10 within the first 5 months): two cases with buried LAMS in the gastric wall, three cases of bleeding from the stent entry site, and three cases of stent-induced biliary stricture. All three patients presented with severe GI bleeding required admission to the intensive care unit and blood transfusions after 3- (1\3) and 5-week (2\3) stent placement. Computed tomography angiography showed a new pseudoaneurysm in all three patients, which were promptly managed by interventional-radiology-guidance coil embolization [50]. The authors, however, considered few pathophysiological theories. Plastic stents gravitate toward the GI lumen after resolution of PFC; indeed LAMS remain fixed in place, with the resultant friction against regional vasculature surrounding the necrotic cavity, causing bleeding. Once the PFC resolves, it is the immobility of the LAMS that increases the risk of bleeding, occlusion, or deeply burial in the gastric wall layers. To prevent stent-related adverse effects, the authors suggest a follow-up with CT at 3–4 weeks in order to evaluate PFC resolution and to schedule LAMS removal [51], which must not exceed 4 weeks according to ESGE guidelines [52]. Recently, Zeissig et al. conducted the largest multicenter cohort of LAMS interventions for PFCs, confirming the efficacy and safety of LAMS for the drainage of PFCs and demonstrating a low rate of hemorrhage [53]. In 219 patients, the German authors recorded just 6 (3%) bleeding events, of which none was fatal (2/6 required interventional radiology embolization, 1/6 treated by LAMS removal, 1/6 resolved by administration of prothrombin complex concentrate, 2/6 required no interventions) [53]. Though the LAMS were removed after a median time of 71 days (IQR 32–97 days), the authors reported only a minor percentage of delayed bleeding events, in contradiction to Stecher et al., in which the total and delayed bleeding rate was, respectively, 17.4% (8/46 patients) and 11% (5/46 patients) [54]. In our opinion, CT scan and LAMS removal can be scheduled sooner if the PFCs contain much more liquid than necrotic components or if the clinical scenario rapidly changes, with acute abdominal pain, organ failure, sepsis, and other signs of local complications. We also believe that a daily and frequent check-up of the clinical conditions may be the correct strategy to manage the correct timing and follow-up. However, further prospective studies are needed to compare double pigtail stents with LAMS in patients with pancreatic PCs or WON. Endoscopic methods described to control bleeding after drainage include dilute epinephrine injection, balloon tamponade, through-the-scope endo-clips, electrosurgical hemostatic forceps (EHF), placement of large diameter, fully covered self-expandable metal stent (FC-SEMS), or hemostatic powder [6]. Placing a large caliber FC-SEMS, if bleeding is noted during the drainage procedure, helps to control this, thanks to its intrinsic characteristics (cover, tensile strength, and ability to self-expand). In all cases of suspected hemorrhage, the physician should consider pseudoaneurysm as a source of the bleeding, which can be confirmed with dynamic contrast-enhanced CT [48]. In cases of uncontrolled bleeding, urgent angiographic embolization or surgical exploration is required. In all cases, a multidisciplinary approach involving skilled interventional endoscopists, radiologists, and surgeons is mandatory to manage cases of severe bleeding [6].

35.5.3 Buried LAMS

Buried LAMS refers to the situation in which GI mucosa grows over the flanged end of the LAMS and may be secondary to its tight apposition between the enteric and PFC lumen. Bang et al. [51] reported an incidence of buried LAMS syndrome of 17% (2/12 patients), and the question of its management has been described in several other case reports [55–57]. In addition, some authors have proposed that placing the stent across the gastric antrum (rather than the gastric body) may increase the risk of buried LAMS because of the significantly stronger motility of the gastric antrum [58]. The use of a snare or forceps may be sufficient, but in inconvenient cases, the dilation of the stent with a direct capture of the internal flange may facilitate removal [59].

35.5.4 Stent Migration

The migration of plastic stent inside the PFCs is more likely if the site of puncture is in the esophagus or at the gastric cardia or if the endoscopic visualization during the deployment is challenging. Gradual withdrawal combined with torqueing movements of the echoendoscope is a crucial maneuver to reduce this kind of complication. The risk of internal migration is higher with the use of short-length devices, even with FC-SEMS or plastic pigtail stent. This condition can possibly be managed by a quick checkup of the procedure and if the guidewire is still in situ [60]. Otherwise, the fistula track has to be re-dilated with a balloon, and successively the internally migrated stent must be retrieved from the cavity by use of a foreign body forceps [61]. LAMS migration rates have been reported in few case reports and at approximately 19% [59]. Migration can occur either in the cyst cavity or back in the gut lumen, such as the stomach [62] or in the colon [63]. This condition can occur immediately or spontaneously after a few weeks of stent placement or also due to subsequent manipulation of the stent during endoscopic debridement procedures. In order to stabilize the LAMS architecture, some endoscopists have opted to place a double pigtail stent through the LAMS, but it is unknown whether this approach can help to reduce the risk of LAMS migration. If stent migration is recognized during routine imaging or endoscopy, endoscopic removal of the stent should be urgently executed. In the case of migration into the upper-GI lumen, direct retrieval is done as soon as possible. Indeed, further distal migration of the stent can be managed operatively with a deep enteroscopy or conservatively with serial abdominal X-rays to confirm passage, with prompt surgical management if bowel obstruction occurs [64].

35.5.5 Maldeployment

Proper LAMS placement requires the correct deployment and expansion of the proximal (outward, deployed second) and the distal (inward, deployed first) flares. Maldeployment consists in a technical impossibility of complete and safe release of both flanges of the stent. This condition is rare, but severe AEs in cases of EUS-guided drainage of PFCs with LAMS can occur when there is decreased space in the GI lumen secondary to a large extra-luminal cavity that may compress the echoendoscope, making it hard to reach a stable position. In addition, the necrotic component inside the PFCs, especially if in a large quantity, can impede the complete release of the distal flare inside the new cavity due to the steady friction and robust compression of solid necrosis, leaving insufficient space for the full opening of the stent. In addition, image quality and accuracy of ultrasound can be limited and disturbed by the necrotic tissue. These conditions can hinder the operator in recognizing the structures or the correct entry point and can lead to AEs such as inward deployment. In case of technical difficulties, a preventive placement of a guidewire through the LAMS catheter allows a safe access for PFC, for the deployment of a second LAMS and\or FC-SEMS [65]. In the same way, Lera et al. described a rescue procedure with SEMS-in-LAMS technique, after LAMS misplacement [66]. Indeed, outward LAMS migration occurs most frequently when the intervening distance between the stent and the targets is greater than 15 mm [67].

35.5.6 Direct Endoscopic Necrosectomy (DEN)

Symptomatic infected WOPN is a well-recognized, life-threatening complication that historically has been managed by surgical debridement, which is associated with high rates of AEs (34–95%), death (11–39%), and long-term pancreatic insufficiency [68]. As an alternative to open necrosectomy, less invasive techniques have been used to drain WOPN, such as percutaneous drainage but still with numerous

AEs such as catheter occlusion, secondary infections, and fistula formation [69]. After ineffective plastic stent (insufficient drainage due to its easy occlusion by necrotic debris) and FC-SEMS (stent migration and bleeding complications) placement, LAMS has become the favored modality to allow multiple sessions of DEN, with an increase in the survival rate [70, 71]. DEN is a minimally invasive technique for performing debridement of the cyst cavity, with success rates of 75–91%, superior to the surgical approach [72]. DEN consists in the insertion of a therapeutic gastroscope inside the cavity through the stent in order to remove all the necrotic debris using non-dedicated devices such as a stone-retrieval basket (Fig. 35.3). The use of CO_2 reduces the risk of air embolism, which is a rare, severe, and potentially lethal complication when air insufflation is adopted during DEN. Air embolism has been reported [73], with an incidence of 0.9–2% [52], and must be promptly recognized if cardiovascular and/or respiratory symptoms suddenly

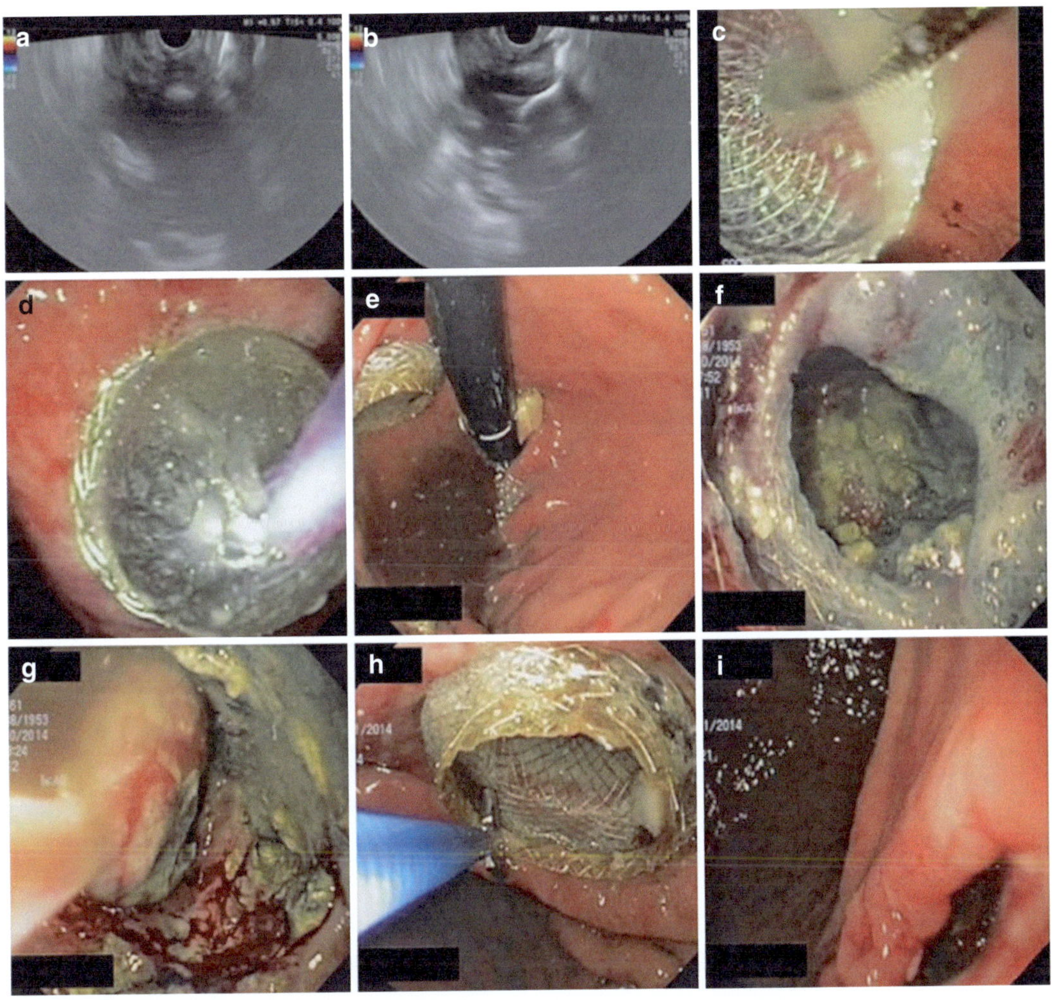

Fig. 35.3 EUS-guided drainage with LAMS and necrosectomy in an infected WOPN. (**a**) EUS view of the WOPN. (**b**) Distal flange of the stent opened inside the cavity. (**c**) Endoscopic view of the proximal flange of the stent. (**d**) Balloon dilation of the LAMS. (**e**) Proximal flange of the LAMS in the gastric cavity. (**f**) Necrotic tissue inside the WOPN. (**g**) Endoscopic visualization of internal part of the collection: retrieval of necrosis fragment with a standard stone-retrieval basket. (**h**) LAMS removal with a biopsy forceps. (**i**) Endoscopic visualization of the cystogastrostomy immediately following the stent removal

develop [74]. The overall complication rate is 36% [52]: the most frequent complications of DEN are bleeding (18%) from larger vessels at its base and perforation (4%). As shown in an Asian consensus on endoscopic management of WOPN, the morbidity and mortality rates were 27.3% (173/633) and 4.4% (28/633), respectively [75]. The reported bleeding rate was 12.6% (80/633), which can occur during both balloon dilation of the GI tract fistula and necrosectomy. In cases of occasional evidence of crossing blood vessel inside the cavity, the use of EHF has been successfully applied to prevent a major bleeding by clipping and transaction (Fig. 35.4) [76]. Perforation (4.4%; 28/633) was the second most frequent complication, and air embolism was observed in just five patients (0.8%; 5/633) [75].

35.6 Complications of EUS-Guided Biliary Drainage

EUS-guided pancreaticobiliary access is a relatively new technique to access and drain obstructed biliary and pancreatic ducts via EUS-guided needle puncture through the gastric or duodenal wall. The technique was developed as a salvage therapy, an alternative to percutaneous or surgical approach, when conventional ERCP fails, and can be secondary to altered anatomy or

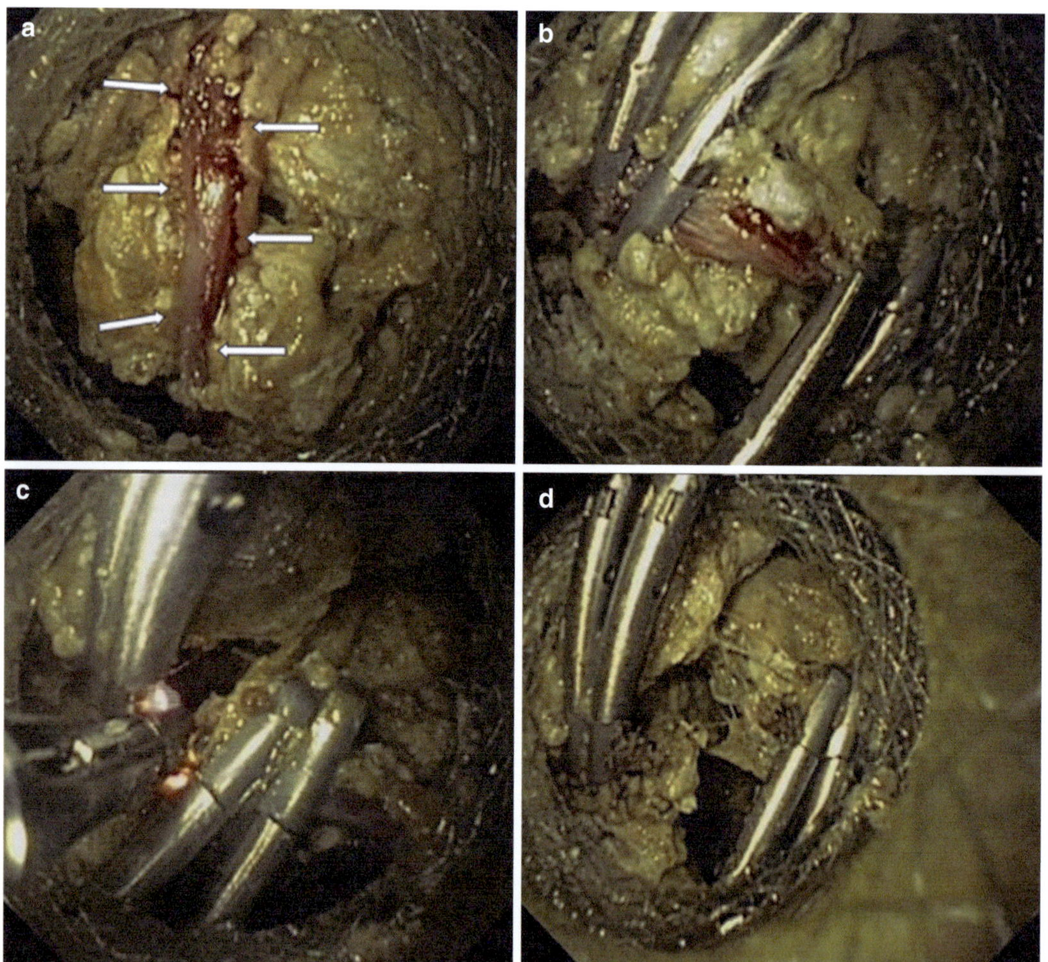

Fig. 35.4 (**a**) Crossing blood vessel at high risk of bleeding (arrows) next to the edge of the distal flange of the LAMS. (**b**) Clips positioned at the ends of the vessel. (**c**) Coagulation of the vessel between clips with a monopolar forceps. (**d**) Blood vessel after transection

in the presence of locally advanced pancreatico-biliary cancer. Diagnostic cholangiography was first reported by Wiersema et al. by EUS-guided puncture of the bile duct, in 1996 [77]. Later, Giovannini et al. described the first EUS-guided biliary drainage (EUS-BD), in 2001 [78]. EUS-guided biliary drainage procedures include EUS-guided choledochoduodenostomy (EUS-CDS) and EUS-guided hepatico-gastrostomy (EUS-HGS). EUS-BD has achieved high technical and clinical success rates (more than 90%) at high-volume centers [6]. On the other hand, these procedures are associated with significant risks of leakage and infection [79]. In fact, the adverse events for EUS-BD have been reported at a range of 3.4–38.6%, with an average adverse event rate of 17–18.9% [80]. As a described risk factor for adverse events, the operator should avoid [81], as much as technically possible, the use of a needle knife when creating the fistula tract to the bile duct. The complications associated with EUS-guided biliary interventions are related to many factors: the route of entry into the biliary system (trans-gastric via hepatic route or transduodenal via CBD), type of devices used, stage or extent of disease, and experience of the operator [80]. The usual complications include bile leak and bile peritonitis (3%); bleeding (2.7%); cholangitis due to the incomplete or unsuccessful drainage of the obstructed biliary system, which may require antibiotic prophylaxis and re-intervention such as alternative endoscopic procedures or PTBD; stent migration or maldeployment; pneumoperitoneum (managed conservatively with antibiotic and continuous nasogastric drainage); and perforation. In this last case, and if the procedure is unsuccessful, the transmural defect can be closed with endoscopic placement of mechanical clips or with over-the-scope clips [6, 80].

35.6.1 Bile Leak

Bile leak occurs when bile liquid from the obstructed high-pressure system is drained off into the potential space between the GI and bile duct wall, manifesting either as biloma (localized bile collection) or bile peritonitis. It is more common with the use of small caliber plastic stents or uncovered SEMS. Indeed, FC-SEMS result in a lower incidence [6]. Kawakubo et al. reported that bile leakage was more frequently observed in patients who underwent plastic stent placement (11%) than in those receiving covered metal stents (4%) [82]. Similarly, Khashab et al. conducted an international multicenter study on EUS-HGS compared with EUS-CDS and found that AEs were significantly more common in the plastic stent population than the metallic one (43% vs. 13%) [83]. For LAMS application, bile leak has been described in just a few case series [51]. The specific design and architecture of the LAMS may partially explain the lower complication rates. Most bile leakages are self-limiting and improve with conservative management.

35.6.2 Stent Migration and Maldeployment

In the published literature, internal stent migration in the peritoneal cavity associated with perforations has been reported as a rare AE, but with possible fatal evolution [84–86]. Usually, the liver and stomach are non-adherent, and there is a potential loss of space between the two organs that may favor migration. In fact, FC-SEMS can potentially migrate into the liver or peritoneal cavity, especially if the protruding luminal part of the stent is short. This complication is more common with EUS-HGS, which results in many more types of complications than EUS-CDS [6]. The use of a long SEMS with bare inner part (for anchoring within liver and avoiding blockage of draining biliary side branches), leaving longer segment (5 cm) in the gastric end of HGS, and placing antimigratory features on the stent are methods to prevent internal migration. Most complications with EUS-BD are associated with the initial/beginner training. Therefore, experts recommend mentor's supervision during at least the first 20 cases [87] because lower technical success rates and higher complication rates are clearly reported during the first 20 EUS-BD procedures [88]. In addition, a French experience showed that there is a significant learning curve, directly related to the total number of AEs [89]. The recent introduction of LAMS has reduced such complications [90], even if there are a few case reports of maldeployment resolved with the precautionary use of a guidewire through the LAMS catheter (Fig. 35.5) [91].

35.7 Complication of EUS-Guided Gallbladder Drainage

EUS-guided gallbladder drainage (EUS-GBD) has recently emerged as an alternative approach to percutaneous cholecystostomy in high-risk patients with acute cholecystitis [92]. In fact, EUS-GBD has been clearly found to be superior in terms of technical\clinical success and lower AEs compared to percutaneous cholecystostomy (19 [32.2%] vs. 44 [74.6%]) [93]. The radiological approach has reported a maximum of 25% of AEs, such as intrahepatic hemorrhage, pneumothorax, and biliary peritonitis. Anatomically, the gallbladder is often (but not always) in proximity to the gastric antrum or the duodenal bulb, a distance that makes technically possible a safe and feasible EUS-guided access [94]. Older approaches, using double pigtail stents and FC-SEMS, are still in use but with lower frequency due to the recent application of LAMS. In addition, plastic stents or FC-SEMS can migrate into the gallbladder or into the peritoneum [95]. LAMS have decreased the risk of bile leak because its shape and architecture seal the gap between the GI lumen and the gallbladder wall, promoting lumen apposition. The high technical and clinical success of EUS-GBD with LAMS has been reported [96], but with inhomogeneous data on AE rates. Initially, in a multicenter prospective study, AEs (LAMS obstruction, stent-related or procedure-related) were observed in 50% of patients, with an overall mortality of 23% [97]. Anderloni et al. found lower AE rate (10%) and mortality (10%) in a retrospective tertiary-care center study [98]. Moreover, a multicenter (seven tertiary care referral centers) retrospective study showed 10.7% of AEs and 9.3% of 30-day mortality in high-risk surgical patients with acute cholecystitis who underwent EUS-GBD with LAMS [99]. There are a few anatomical factors that can limit the feasibility of EUS-GD. The tissue's thickness between the gallbladder and the duodenum or stomach, the gallbladder's distensibility, and the presence of a contracted or fibrotic gallbladder are all factors that the operators must take in consideration in order to avoid such tragic outcomes. The most frequently described AEs following EUS-GB are abdominal pain, bile leak with peritonitis, perforation, bleeding that requires blood product transfusion or different kinds of interventions, maldeployment, and the buried syndrome. Teoh et al. reported a fatal maldeployment that was not detected during the procedure [93]. It is extremely important that the endoscopist knows all the possible complications, recognizes any adverse events promptly, and manages them accordingly. Ligresti et al. reported a buried LAMS following EUS-BG successfully managed with a LAMS-in-LAMS technique (Fig. 35.6) [100].

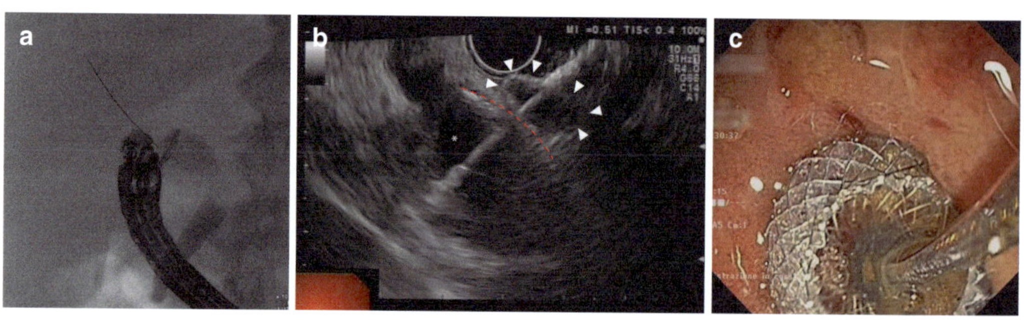

Fig. 35.5 (**a**) Fluoroscopic view of the maldeployed distal flange of the stent inside the common bile duct (CBD). (**b**) Endoscopic ultrasound view of the distal flange of the stent (arrowheads) fully released outside of the common bile duct (CBD wall: red dashed line). (**c**) Endoscopic view of choledochoduodenostomy showing proximal flange of the stent released and correctly in place in the duodenal bulb

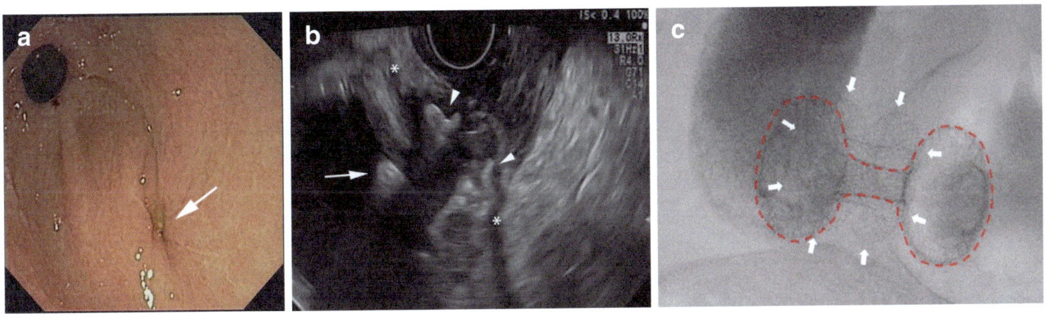

Fig. 35.6 Buried LAMS in the gastric antrum. (**a**) Endoscopic view with a 2-mm fistulous orifice (arrow). (**b**) EUS view showing the proximal flange (arrowheads) within the gastric wall; a clearly visible hypoechoic gastric muscular layer (∗) and the distal flange in place in the gallbladder (arrow). (**c**) LAMS-in-LAMS technique: the second (red dashed line) and first LAMS (arrows) in coaxial direction

References

1. Cotton PB, Eisen GM, Aabakken L, Baron TH, Hutter MM, Jacobson BC, Mergener K, Nemcek A Jr, Petersen BT, Petrini JL, Pike IM, Rabeneck L, Romagnuolo J, Vargo JJ. A lexicon for endoscopic adverse events: report of an ASGE workshop. Gastrointest Endosc. 2010;71(3):446–54.
2. Gonsalves WI, Pruthi RK, Patnaik MM. The new oral anticoagulants in clinical practice. Mayo Clin Proc. 2013;88(5):495–511.
3. Eloubeidi MA, Tamhane A, Lopes TL, Morgan DE, Cerfolio RJ. Cervical esophageal perforations at the time of endoscopic ultrasound: a prospective evaluation of frequency, outcomes, and patient management. Am J Gastroenterol. 2009;104(1):53–6.
4. Das A, Sivak M, Chak A. Cervical esophageal perforation during EUS: a national survey. Gastrointest Endosc. 2001;53(6):599–602. [cited 2016 Jul 13].
5. Wallace MB, Hawes RH, Sahai AV, Van Velse A, Hoffman BJ. Dilation of malignant esophageal stenosis to allow EUS guided fine-needle aspiration: safety and effect on patient management. Gastrointest Endosc. 2000;51(3):309–13.
6. Lakthakia S. Complications of diagnostic and therapeutic endoscopic ultrasound. Best Pract Res Clin Gastroenterol. 2016;30(5):807–23. https://doi.org/10.1016/j.bpg.2016.10.008. Epub 2016 Oct 28. Review. PubMed PMID: 27931638.
7. Pfau PR, Ginsberg GG, Lew RJ, Faigel DO, Smith DB, Kochman ML. Esophageal dilation for endosonographic evaluation of malignant esophageal strictures is safe and effective. Am J Gastroenterol. 2000;95(10):2813–5.
8. Mennigen R, Tuebergen D, Koehler G, Sauerland C, Senninger N, Bruewer M. Endoscopic ultrasound and conventional probe and miniprobe in preoperative staging of esophageal cancer. J Gastrointest Surg. 2008;12(2):256–62.
9. Liberman M, Hanna N, Duranceau A, Thiffault V, Ferraro P. Endobronchial ultrasonography added to endoscopic ultrasonography improves staging in esophageal cancer. Ann Thorac Surg. 2013;96(1):232–8.
10. Polkowski M, Larghi A, Weynand B, Boustière C, Giovannini M, Pujol B, Dumonceau J-M. Learning, techniques, and complications of endoscopic ultrasound (EUS)-guided sampling in gastroenterology: European society of Gastrointestinal Endoscopy (ESGE) technical guidelines. Endoscopy. 2012;44(2):190–205.
11. Siddiqui UD, Rossi F, Rosenthal LS, Padda MS, Murali-Dharan V, Aslanian HR. EUS-guided FNA of solid pancreatic masses: a prospective, randomized trial comparing 22-gauge and 25-gauge needles. Gastrointest Endosc. 2009;70:1093–7.
12. Song TJ, Kim JH, Lee SS, Eum JB, Moon SH, Park DY, Seo DW, Lee SK, Jang SJ, Yun SC, Kim MH. The prospective randomized, controlled trial of endoscopic ultrasound-guided fine-needle aspiration using 22G and 19G aspiration needles for solid pancreatic or peripancreatic masses. Am J Gastroenterol. 2010;105:1739–45.
13. O'Toole D, Palazzo L, Arotçarena R, et al. Assessment of complications of EUS-guided fine-needle aspiration. Gastrointest Endosc. 2001;53:470–4.
14. Thomas T, Kaye PV, Ragunath K, Dancour A, Aubert A, Hammel P, Amaris J, Ruszniewski P. Efficacy, safety, and predictive factors for a positive yield of EUS-guided Trucut biopsy: a large tertiary referral center experience. Am J Gastroenterol. 2009;104:584–91.
15. Wiersema MJ, Vilmann P, Giovannini M, Chang KJ, Wiersema LM. Endosonography-guided fine-needle aspiration biopsy: diagnostic accuracy and complication assessment. Gastroenterology. 1997;112:1087–95.
16. Eloubeidi MA, Gress FG, Savides TJ, Wiersema MJ, Kochman ML, Ahmad NA, Ginsberg GG, Erickson

RA, Dewitt J, Van Dam J, Nickl NJ, Levy MJ, Clain JE, Chak A, Sivak MV Jr, Wong R, Isenberg G, Scheiman JM, Bounds B, Kimmey MB, Saunders MD, Chang KJ, Sharma A, Nguyen P, Lee JG, Edmundowicz SA, Early D, Azar R, Etemad B, Chen YK, Waxman I, Shami V, Catalano MF, Wilcox CM. Acute pancreatitis after EUS guided FNA of solid pancreatic masses: a pooled analysis from EUS centers in the United States. Gastrointest Endosc. 2004;60:385–9.
17. Katanuma A, Maguchi H, Yane K, Hashigo S, Kin T, Kaneko M, Kato S, Kato R, Harada R, Osanai M, Takahashi K, Nojima M. Factors predictive of adverse events associated with endoscopic ultrasound-guided fine needle aspiration of pancreatic solid lesions. Dig Dis Sci. 2013;58(7):2093–9.
18. Eloubeidi MA, Tamhane A, Varadarajulu S, Wilcox CM. Frequency of major complications after EUS-guided FNA of solid pancreatic masses: a prospective evaluation. Gastrointest Endosc. 2006;63:622–9.
19. Varadarajulu S, Eloubeidi MA. Frequency and significance of acute intracystic hemorrhage during EUS-FNA of cystic lesions of the pancreas. Gastrointest Endosc. 2004;60(4):631–5.
20. ASGE Standards of Practice Committee, Early DS, Acosta RD, Chandrasekhara V, et al. Adverse events associated with EUS and EUS with FNA. Gastrointest Endosc. 2013;77(6):839–43. https://doi.org/10.1016/j.gie.2013.02.018.
21. Mortensen MB, Fristrup C, Holm FS, Pless T, Durup J, Ainsworth AP, Nielsen HO, Hovendal C. Prospective evaluation of patient tolerability, satisfaction with patient information, and complications in endoscopic ultrasonography. Endoscopy. 2005;37(2):146–53.
22. ASGE Standards of Practice Committee, Anderson MA, Ben-Menachem T, Gan SI, Appalaneni V, Banerjee S, Cash BD, et al. Management of antithrombotic agents for endoscopic procedures. Gastrointest Endosc. 2009;70(6):1060–70.
23. Committee ASGE Standards of Practice. The management of antithrombotic agents for patients undergoing GI endoscopy. Gastrointest Endosc. 2016;83(3):678.
24. Boustiere C, Veitch A, Vanbiervliet G, Bulois P, Deprez P, Laquiere A, et al. European Society of Gastrointestinal Endoscopy. Endoscopy and antiplatelet agents. European society of gastrointestinal endoscopy (ESGE) guideline. Endoscopy. 2011;43(5):445–58.
25. Barresi L, Crinò SF, Fabbri C, Attili F, Poley JW, Carrara S, Tarantino I, Bernardoni L, Giovanelli S, Di Leo M, Manfrin E, Tacelli M, Bruno MJ, Traina M, Larghi A. Endoscopic ultrasound-through-the-needle biopsy in pancreatic cystic lesions: a multicenter study. Dig Endosc. 2018;30(6):760–70. https://doi.org/10.1111/den.13197. Epub 2018 Jul 5.
26. Jenssen C, Alvarez-Sánchez MV, Napoléon B, Faiss S. Diagnostic endoscopic ultrasonography: assessment of safety and prevention of complications. World J Gastroenterol. 2012;18:4659–76.
27. Minaga K, Takenaka M, Katanuma A, Kitano M, Yamashita Y, Kamata K, Yamao K, Watanabe T, Maguchi H, Kudo M. Needle tract seeding: an overlooked rare complication of endoscopic ultrasound-guided fine-needle aspiration. Oncology. 2017;93(Suppl 1):107–12.
28. Fujii LL, Levy MJ. Basic techniques in endoscopic ultrasound-guided fine needle aspiration for solid lesions: adverse events and avoiding them. Endosc Ultrasound. 2014;3:35–45.
29. Jacobson BC, Pitman MB, Brugge WR. EUS-guided FNA for the diagnosis of gallbladder masses. Gastrointest Endosc. 2003;57(2):251–4.
30. Chen HY, Lee CH, Hsieh CH. Bile peritonitis after EUS-guided fine-needle aspiration. Gastrointest Endosc. 2002;56:594–6.
31. Gress F, Schmitt C, Sherman S, Ciaccia D, Ikenberry S, Lehman G. Endoscopic ultrasound-guided celiac plexus block for managing abdominal pain associated with chronic pancreatitis: a prospective single center experience. AmJ Gastroenterol. 2001;96:409–16.
32. Hoffman BJ. EUS-guided celiac plexus block/neurolysis. Gastrointest Endosc. 2002;56(4 Suppl):S26–8.
33. ASGE Standards of Practice Committee. Adverse events associated with EUS and EUS with FNA. Gastrointest Endosc. 2013;77(6):839–43.
34. Fujii L, Clain JE, Morris JM, et al. Anterior spinal cord infarction with permanent paralysis following endoscopic ultrasound celiac plexus neurolysis. Endoscopy. 2012;44(Suppl 2):E265–6.
35. Gimeno-Garcia AZ, Ekwassuef A, Paquin SC, Sahai AV. Fatal complication after endoscopic ultrasound-guided celiac plexus neurolysis. Endoscopy. 2012;44:E267.
36. Loeve US, Mortensen MB. Lethal necrosis and perforation of the stomach and the aorta after multiple EUS-guided celiac plexus neurolysis procedures in a patient with chronic pancreatitis. Gastrointest Endosc. 2013;77(1):151–2.
37. Pancreatitis Across Nations Clinical Research and Education Alliance (PANCREA), Dellinger EP, Forsmark CE, Layer P, et al. Determinant-based classification of acute pancreatitis severity: an international multidisciplinary consultation. Ann Surg. 2012;256:875–80.
38. Seewald S, Ang TL, Kida M, et al. EUS 2008 Working Group document: evaluation of EUS-guided drainage of pancreatic-fluid collections (with video). Gastrointest Endosc. 2009;69:S13–21.
39. Shah RJ, Shah JN, Waxman I, Kowalski TE, Sanchez-Yague A, Nieto J, Brauer BC, Gaidhane M, Kahaleh M. Safety and efficacy of endoscopic ultrasound-guided drainage of pancreatic fluid collections with lumen-apposing covered self-expanding metal stents. Clin Gastroenterol Hepatol. 2014;13:747–52.
40. Varadarajulu S, Tamhane A, Blakely J. Graded dilation technique for EUS-guided drainage of peripancreatic fluid collections: an assessment of outcomes

and complications and technical proficiency (with video). Gastrointest Endosc. 2008;68(4):656–66.
41. Varadarajulu S, Christein JD, Tamhane A, Drelichman ER, Wilcox CM. Prospective randomized trial comparing EUS and EGD for transmural drainage of pancreatic pseudocysts (with videos). Gastrointest Endosc. 2008;68(6):1102–11.
42. Giovannini M, Pesenti C, Rolland AL, Moutardier V, Delpero JR. Endoscopic ultrasound-guided drainage of pancreatic pseudocysts or pancreatic abscesses using a therapeutic echo endoscope. Endoscopy. 2001;33(6):473–7.
43. Antillon MR, Shah RJ, Stiegmann G, Chen YK. Single-step EUS-guided transmural drainage of simple and complicated pancreatic pseudocysts. Gastrointest Endosc. 2006;63(6):797–803.
44. Sadik R, Kalaitzakis E, Thune A, Hansen J, Jonson C. EUS-guided drainage is more successful in pancreatic pseudocysts compared with abscesses. World J Gastroenterol. 2011;17(4):499–505.
45. Varadarajulu S, Bang JY, Phadnis MA, Christein JD, Wilcox CM. Endoscopic transmural drainage of peripancreatic fluid collections: outcomes and predictors of treatment success in 211 consecutive patients. J Gastrointest Surg. 2011;15(11):2080–8.
46. Will U, Wegener C, Graf K-I, Wanzar I, Manger T, Meyer F. Differential treatment and early outcome in the interventional endoscopic management of pancreatic pseudocysts in 27 patients. World J Gastroenterol. 2006;12(26):4175–8.
47. Varadarajulu S, Christein JD, Wilcox CM. Frequency of complications during EUS-guided drainage of pancreatic fluid collections in 148 consecutive patients. J Gastroenterol Hepatol. 2011;26(10):1504–8.
48. Isayama H, Nakai Y, Rerknimitr R, et al. Asian consensus statements on endoscopic management of walled-off necrosis Part 1: epidemiology, diagnosis, and treatment. J Gastroenterol Hepatol. 2016;31(9):1546–54. https://doi.org/10.1111/jgh.13394. Review. PubMed PMI.
49. Van Brunschot S, Fockens P, Bakker OJ, Besselink MG, Voermans RP, Poley JW, Gooszen HG, Bruno M, van Santvoort HC. Endoscopic transluminal necrosectomy in necrotizing pancreatitis: a systematic review. Surg Endosc. 2014;28(5):1425–38.
50. Bang JY, Navaneethan U, Hasan MK, Sutton B, Hawes R, Varadarajulu S. Non-superiority of lumen-apposing metal stents over plastic stents for drainage of walled-off necrosis in a randomised trial. Gut. Published Online First: 01 June 2018. https://doi.org/10.1136/gutjnl-2017-315335.
51. Bang JY, Hasan M, Navaneethan U, Hawes R, Varadarajulu S. Lumen-apposing metal stents (LAMS) for pancreatic fluid collection (PFC) drainage: may not be business as usual. Gut. 2017;66(12):2054–6. https://doi.org/10.1136/gutjnl-2016-312812. Epub 2016 Aug 31.
52. Arvanitakis M, Dumonceau JM, Albert J, Badaoui A, Bali MA, Barthet M, Besselink M, Deviere J, Oliveira Ferreira A, Gyökeres T, Hritz I, Hucl T, Milashka M, Papanikolaou IS, Poley JW, Seewald S, Vanbiervliet G, van Lienden K, van Santvoort H, Voermans R, Delhaye M, van Hooft J. Endoscopic management of acute necrotizing pancreatitis: European Society of Gastrointestinal Endoscopy (ESGE) evidence-based multidisciplinary guidelines. Endoscopy. 2018;50(5):524–46. https://doi.org/10.1055/a-05.
53. Zeissig S, Sulk S, Brueckner S, Matthes K, Hohmann M, Reichel S, Ellrichmann M, Arlt A, Will U, Hampe J. Severe bleeding is a rare event in patients receiving lumen-apposing metal stents for the drainage of pancreatic fluid collections. Gut. Published Online First: 20 April 2018. https://doi.org/10.1136/gutjnl-2018-316581.
54. Stecher SS, Simon P, Friesecke S, Glitsch A, Kühn JP, Lerch MM, Mayerle J. Delayed severe bleeding complications after treatment of pancreatic fluid collections with lumen-apposing metal stents. Gut. 2017;66:1871–2.
55. Fabbri C, Luigiano C, Marsico M, Cennamo V. A rare adverse event resulting from the use of a lumen-apposing metal stent for drainage of a pancreatic fluid collection: "the buried stent". Gastrointest Endosc. 2015;82:585–7. https://doi.org/10.1016/j.gie.2015.04.035. [PMID: 26279357].
56. Rodrigues-Pinto E, Grimm IS, Baron TH. Removal of buried gastroduodenal stents after drainage of pancreatic fluid collections: silence of the LAMS (with video). Gastrointest Endosc. 2016;83:853–4. https://doi.org/10.1016/j.gie.2015.11.017. [PMID: 26975290].
57. Sanchez-Ocana R, Peñas-Herrero I, Santos-Santamarta F, de la Serna-Higuera C, Perez-Miranda M. EUS-guided removal of a buried lumen-apposing metal stent caused by delayed inward migration after cyst-gastrostomy. Gastrointest Endosc. 2017;86(1):229.
58. Irani S, Kozarek RA. The Buried Lumen Apposing Metal Stent (LAMS): is this a stent problem, a location problem or both. A case series. Gastrointest Endosc. 2016;83:AB186–7.
59. DeSimone ML, Asombang AW, Berzin TM. Lumen apposing metal stents for pancreatic fluid collections: Recognition and management of complications. World J Gastrointest Endosc. 2017;9(9):456–63.
60. Lakhtakia S, Basha J, Nabi Z, Ramchandani M, Reddy DN. Salvaging a malpositioned fully covered self-expanding metal stent for pancreatic fluid collection drainage. Endoscopy. 2016;48:2015–6.
61. Wang GX, Liu X, Wang S, Ge N, Guo JT, Liu W, Sun SY. Stent displacement in endoscopic pancreatic pseudocyst drainage and endoscopic management. World J Gastroenterol. 2015;21(7):2249–53.
62. Itoi T, Binmoeller KF, Shah J, Sofuni A, Itokawa F, Kurihara T, Tsuchiya T, Ishii K, Tsuji S, Ikeuchi N, Moriyasu F. Clinical evaluation of a novel lumen-apposing metal stent for endosonography-guided pancreatic pseudocyst and gallbladder drainage (with videos). Gastrointest Endosc. 2012;75(4):870–6.

63. Mahmood SK, Kaimakliotis P. Migration of a lumen-apposing metal stent into the colon. ACG Case Rep J. 2018;5:e14. https://doi.org/10.14309/crj.2018.14. Published 2018 Feb 14.
64. Razzak A, Larsen M, Irani S, Gan SI, Ross A. Small-bowel obstruction due to a migrated lumen-apposing metal stent. Gastrointest Endosc. 2016;84:867–9.
65. Azeem N, Freeman ML, Amateau SK. Immediate retrieval of a maldeployed lumen-apposing metal stent from a walled-off cavity. Endoscopy. 2018;50(03):E76–7. https://doi.org/10.1055/s-0043-124759.
66. Lera ME, Matuguma SE, Madruga-Neto AC, Brunaldi VO, Minata MK, Guedes HG, de Moura EGH. Self-expandable metal stent in lumen-apposing metal stent (the SEMS-in-LAMS procedure): a simple salvage procedure after LAMS misplacement. Endoscopy. 2019;51(4):E77–8. https://doi.org/10.1055/a-0820-1456.
67. Amateau SK, Freeman ML. Avoidance, recognition, and management of complications associated with lumen-apposing metal stents. Gastrointest Endosc Clin N Am. 2018;28(2):219–31. https://doi.org/10.1016/j.giec.2017.11.009. Epub 2018 Feb 4. Review. PubMed PMID: 2951.
68. Howard TJ, Patel JB, Zyromski N, Sandrasegaran K, Yu J, Nakeeb A, Pitt HA, Lillemoe KD. Declining morbidity and mortality rates in the surgical management of pancreatic necrosis. J Gastrointest Surg. 2007;11:43–9.
69. Neff R. Pancreatic pseudocysts and fluid collections: percutaneous approaches. Surg Clin North Am. 2001;81:399–403.
70. Tarantino I, Ligresti D, Tuzzolino F, Barresi L, Curcio G, Granata A, Traina M. Clinical impact of EUS treatment of walled-off pancreatic necrosis. Endosc Int Open. 2017;5(8):E784–91. https://doi.org/10.1055/s-0043-112494. Epub 2017 Aug 7.
71. Carbajo López AY, Brunie Vegas FJ, García-Alonso FJ, Cimavilla Román M, Torres Yuste R, Simón PG, de la Serna-Higuera C, Fernández Pérez GC, Pérez-Miranda M. Retrospective cohort study comparing endoscopic ultrasound-guided and percutaneous drainage of upper abdominal abscesses. Dig Endosc. 2019;31(4):431–8. https://doi.org/10.1111/den.13342.
72. Bakker OJ, van Santvoort HC, van Brunschot S, Geskus RB, Besselink MG, Bollen TL, van Eijck CH, Fockens P, Hazebroek EJ, Nijmeijer RM, Poley JW, van Ramshorst B, Vleggaar FP, Boermeester MA, Gooszen HG, Weusten BL, Timmer R, Dutch Pancreatitis Study Group. Endoscopic transgastric vs surgical necrosectomy for infected necrotizing pancreatitis. JAMA. 2012;307:1053–61.
73. Yasuda I, Nakashima M, Iwai T, Isayama H, Itoi T, Hisai H, Inoue H, Kato H, Kanno A, Kubota K, Irisawa A, Igarashi H, Okabe Y, Kitano M, Kawakami H, Hayashi T, Mukai T, Sata N, Kida M, Shimosegawa T. Japanese multicenter experience of endoscopic necrosectomy for infected walled-off pancreatic necrosis: the JENIPaN study. Endoscopy. 2013;45(8):627–34.
74. Kumar N, Conwell DL, Thompson CC. Direct endoscopic necrosectomy versus step-up approach for walled-off pancreatic necrosis: comparison of clinical outcome and health care utilization. Pancreas. 2014;43(8):1334–9.
75. Isayama H, Nakai Y, Rerknimitr R, Khor C, Lau J, Wang HP, Seo DW, Ratanachu-Ek T, Lakhtakia S, Ang TL, Ryozawa S, Hayashi T, Kawakami H, Yamamoto N, Iwashita T, Itokawa F, Kuwatani M, Kitano M, Hanada K, Kogure H, Hamada T, Ponnudurai R, Moon JH, Itoi T, Yasuda I, Irisawa A, Maetani I. The Asian consensus statements on endoscopic management of walled-off necrosis Part 1: epidemiology, diagnosis and treatment. Gastroenterol Hepatol. 2016;31(9):1546–54.
76. Tarantino I, Ligresti D, Barresi L, Granata A, Traina M. Clipping and transection of a crossing blood vessel during transgastric endoscopic necrosectomy. Gastrointest Endosc. 2016;83(4):833–4. https://doi.org/10.1016/j.gie.2015.10.028. Epub 2015 Oct 30.
77. Wiersema MJ, Sandusky D, Carr R, Wiersema LM, Erdel WC, Frederick PK. Endosonography-guided cholangiopancreatography. Gastrointest Endosc. 1996;43(2 Part 1):102–6.
78. Giovannini M, Moutardier V, Pesenti C, Bories E, Lelong B, Delpero JR. Endoscopic ultrasound-guided bilioduodenal anastomosis: a new technique for biliary drainage. Endoscopy. 2001;33:898–900.
79. Jang JW, Lee SS, Park DH, Seo DW, Lee SK, Kim MH. Feasibility and safety of EUS-guided transgastric/transduodenal gallbladder drainage with single-step placement of a modified covered self-expandable metal stent in patients unsuitable for cholecystectomy. Gastrointest Endosc. 2011;74(1):176–81. https://doi.org/10.1016/j.gie.2011.03.1120.
80. Baars JE, Kaffes AJ, Saxena P. EUS-guided biliary drainage: a comprehensive review of the literature. Endosc Ultrasound. 2018;7(1):4–9. https://doi.org/10.4103/eus.eus_105_17.
81. Park DH, Jang JW, Lee SS, Seo DW, Lee SK, Kim MH. EUS-guided biliary drainage with transluminal stenting after failed ERCP: predictors of adverse events and long-term results. Gastrointest Endosc. 2011;74(6):1276–84.
82. Kawakubo K, Isayama H, Kato H, Itoi T, Kawakami H, Hanada K, Ishiwatari H, Yasuda I, Kawamoto H, Itokawa F, Kuwatani M, Iiboshi T, Hayashi T, Doi S, Nakai Y. Multicenter retrospective study of endoscopic ultrasound guided biliary drainage for malignant biliary obstruction in Japan. J Hepatobiliary Pancreat Sci. 2014;21(5):328–43.
83. Khashab MA, Messallam AA, Penas I, Nakai Y, Modayil RJ, De la Serna C, Hara K, El Zein M, Stavropoulos SN, Perez-Miranda M, Kumbhari V, Ngamruengphong S, Dhir VK, Park DH. International multicenter comparative trial of transluminal EUS guided biliary drainage via

hepatogastrostomy vs. choledochoduodenostomy approaches. Endosc Int Open. 2016;4:E175–81.
84. Minaga K, Kitano M, Yamashita Y, Nakatani Y, Kudo M. Stent migration into the abdominal cavity after EUS guided hepaticogastrostomy. Gastrointest Endosc. 2017;85:263–4.
85. Okuno N, Hara K, Mizuno N, Susumu H, Imao H, Kenji Y. Stent migration into the peritoneal cavity following endoscopic ultrasound-guided hepaticogastrostomy. Endoscopy. 2015;47:E311.
86. Martins FP, Rossini LGB, Ferrari AP. Migration of a covered metallic stent following endoscopic ultrasound-guided hepaticogastrostomy: fatal complication. Endoscopy. 2010;42(Suppl. 2):126–7.
87. Hara K, Yamao K, Mizuno N, Hijioka S, Imaoka H, Tajika M, Tanaka T, Ishihara M, Okuno N, Hieda N, Yoshida T, Niwa Y. Endoscopic ultrasonography-guided biliary drainage: who, when, which, and how? World J Gastroenterol. 2016;22:1297–303.
88. Vila JJ, Pérez-Miranda M, Vazquez-Sequeiros E, Abadia MA, Pérez-Millán A, González-Huix F, Gornals J, Iglesias-Garcia J, De la Serna C, Aparicio JR, Subtil JC, Alvarez A, de la Morena F, García-Cano J, Casi MA, Lancho A, Barturen A, Rodríguez-Gómez SJ, Repiso A, Juzgado D, Igea F, Fernandez-Urien I, González-Martin JA, Armengol-Miró JR. Initial experience with EUS-guided cholangiopancreatography for biliary and pancreatic duct drainage: a Spanish national survey. Gastrointest Endosc. 2012;76:1133–41.
89. Poincloux L, Rouquette O, Buc E, Privat J, Pezet D, Dapoigny M, Bommelaer G, Abergel A. Endoscopic ultrasound-guided biliary drainage after failed ERCP: cumulative experience of 101 procedures at a single center. Endoscopy. 2015;47:794–801.
90. Mussetto A, Fugazza A, Fuccio L, Triossi O, Repici A, Anderloni A. Current uses and outcomes of lumen-apposing metal stents. Ann Gastroenterol. 2018;31(5):535–40.
91. Ligresti D, Amata M, Granata A, Cipolletta F, Barresi L, Traina M, Tarantino I. Salvage procedure following lumen-apposing metal stent maldeployment during endoscopic ultrasound-guided biliary drainage. Endoscopy. 2018;50(7):E190–1. https://doi.org/10.1055/a-0605-3198. Epub 2018 Jun 12.
92. Anderloni A, Buda A, Vieceli F, Khashab MA, Hassan C, Repici A. Endoscopic ultrasound-guided transmural stenting for gallbladder drainage in high-risk patients with acute cholecystitis: a systematic review and pooled analysis. Surg Endosc. 2016;30(12):5200–8.
93. Teoh AYB, Serna C, Penas I, Chong CCN, Perez-Miranda M, Ng EKW, Lau JYW. Endoscopic ultrasound-guided gallbladder drainage reduces adverse events compared with percutaneous cholecystostomy in patients who are unfit for cholecystectomy. Endoscopy. 2017;49(2):130–8.
94. Irani S, Baron TH, Grimm IS, Khashab MA. EUS-guided gallbladder drainage with a lumen-apposing metal. Gastrointest Endosc. 2015;82(6):1110–5. https://doi.org/10.1016/j.gie.2015.05.045. Epub 2015 Jul 2.
95. Choi JH, Lee SS, Choi JH, Park DH, Seo DW, Lee SK, Kim MH. Long-term outcomes after endoscopic ultrasonography-guided gallbladder drainage for acute cholecystitis. Endoscopy. 2014;46:656–61.
96. Peñas-Herrero I, de la Serna-Higuera C, Perez-Miranda M. Endoscopic ultrasoundguided gallbladder drainage for the management of acute cholecystitis (with video). J Hepatobiliary Pancreat Sci. 2015;22:35–43.
97. Walter D, Teoh AY, Itoi T, Pérez-Miranda M, Larghi A, Sanchez-Yague A, Siersema PD, Vleggaar FP. EUS-guided gall bladder drainage with a lumen-apposing metal stent: a prospective long-term evaluation. Gut. 2016;65:6–8.
98. Anderloni A, Leo MD, Carrara S, Fugazza A, Maselli R, Buda A, Amato A, Auriemma F, Repici A. Endoscopic ultrasound-guided transmural drainage by cautery-tipped lumen-apposing metal stent: exploring the possible indications. Ann Gastroenterol. 2018;31(6):735–41.
99. Dollhopf M, Larghi A, Will U, Rimbaş M, Anderloni A, Sanchez-Yague A, Teoh AYB, Kunda R. EUS-guided gallbladder drainage in patients with acute cholecystitis and high surgical risk using an electrocautery-enhanced lumen-apposing metal stent device. Gastrointest Endosc. 2017;86(4):636–43. https://doi.org/10.1016/j.gie.2017.02.027. Epub 2017 Mar 1.
100. Ligresti D, Cipolletta F, Amata M, Cimavilla M, Traina M, Tarantino I. Buried lumen-apposing metal stent (LAMS) following endoscopic ultrasound-guided gallbladder drainage: the LAMS-in-LAMS rescue treatment. Endoscopy. 2018;50(8):822–3.

Part V

Biliopancreatic Diseases: Clinical Results

Common Bile Duct Stones

36

Bernd Kronenberger

36.1 Introduction

Common bile duct stones (CBDS) are the most common cause of benign biliary obstruction requiring endoscopic treatment [1–3]. Sequelae of biliary obstruction by CBDS are pain, jaundice, biliary pancreatitis, and cholangitis [1–4]. Complications of CBDS may progress to severe and life-threatening disease [4].

The clinical picture of CBDS disease is heterogeneous. CBDS may appear as single or multiple calculi causing a varying degree of cholestasis [5]. The size of CBDS ranges from small barely visible microconcrements (microlithiasis) to large stones in the order of centimeters [5, 6]. CBDS smaller than the diameter of the bile duct migrate in the bile duct, and if they do not cause biliary obstruction, they may be asymptomatic and difficult to detect [5, 7]. Clinically relevant problems usually occur when stones get stuck and cholestasis develops. Small stones are more likely to cause distal obstruction and larger stones proximal obstruction [1].

Stone extraction is required in patients with symptomatic CBDS and may be an emergency in those patients with biliary obstruction and with complications [3]. Several methods for stone extraction exist including endoscopic, radiologic, and surgical approaches. Endoscopic retrograde cholangiopancreatography (ERCP) is less invasive than radiologic or surgical methods and therefore usually chosen as first-line treatment for stone extraction [1, 3]. Nevertheless, ERCP bears the risk for severe procedure-associated complications such as pancreatitis, bleeding, cholangitis, and perforation. To reduce complications, unnecessary ERCPs should be avoided, and ERCP should only be performed for therapeutic stone extraction [4]. Making the decision to treat CBDS can be a challenge when direct detection of CBDS is not possible. Guidelines suggest a stepwise diagnostic approach to evaluate the probability for symptomatic CBDS [1, 3, 4, 8, 9]. Diagnostic approaches and risk-based management options for CBDS are described in the following chapter.

36.2 Etiology and Risk Factors

Bile stones develop when substances in the bile reach their limit of solubility and form microcrystals [10]. Sludge is the result when microcrystals get stuck in the bile mucus [10]. Over time, microcrystals grow and form large or multiple stones [10].

According to their origin, CBDS can be classified into primary and secondary stones [1, 4]. Primary stones form de novo in the intra- or

B. Kronenberger (✉)
Department of Internal Medicine, Gastroenterology, Hepatology, Diabetology, Herz-Jesu-Hospital, Fulda, Germany
e-mail: bernd.kronenberger@email.de

M. Mutignani et al. (eds.), *Endotherapy in Biliopancreatic Diseases: ERCP Meets EUS*,
https://doi.org/10.1007/978-3-030-42569-2_36

extrahepatic bile ducts, while secondary CBDS occur by migration from the gallbladder [4]. Most CBDS are secondary stones that are found in 3–12% of patients with stones in the gallbladder [4, 5, 11]. Conversely, 95% of patients with CBDS have stones in the gallbladder [1–4]. Predisposing conditions for primary stones are biliary infections and reduced bile flow in dilated bile ducts [12].

White to yellowish cholesterol stones and black pigment stones account for 90–95% of secondary CBDS [12]. Black pigmented stones show an association with comorbidities affecting bilirubin and calcium homeostasis such as hematologic or hemolytic disorders, liver cirrhosis, Crohn's disease, and primary hyperparathyroidism [12, 13]. In contrast to cholesterol and black pigment stones, brown pigment stones are the major source of primary stones [14]. Predisposing factors are dilated bile ducts including Caroli's disease and anaerobic infections [15]. Brown pigment stones are also associated with juxtapapillary diverticula [12, 14].

Drugs may also cause cholelithiasis. Ceftriaxone is known to cause reversible biliary stones/sludge which is called pseudolithiasis [16]. Biliary pseudolithiasis is usually asymptomatic and disappears spontaneously after discontinuing the drug; some patients develop biliary obstruction and need endoscopic treatment [16].

36.3 Clinical Spectrum of Common Bile Duct Stones

36.3.1 Symptomatic Bile Duct Stones with Cholestasis

Most patents with CBDS develop symptoms [1, 17]. The typical clinical presentation is acute pain in the right upper abdominal quadrant or the epigastrium [1, 4]. The duration varies between minutes and several hours. The pain is caused by distention of the bile duct. Pain can be missing in elderly patients [1]. Depending on the time and extent of obstruction, jaundice may develop. Fever and suspicious inflammation parameters indicate cholangitis which may require urgent treatment.

Stones impacted in the sphincter of Oddi or spontaneous stone passage may cause biliary pancreatitis [1]. Acute biliary pancreatitis is observed in 4–8% of patients with gallbladder stones.

36.3.2 Symptomatic Bile Stones Without Cholestasis

Depending on the size, mobility, and location, common bile duct stones may cause intermittent symptoms without cholestasis. Passage of the stones into the duodenum or backward into the distended duct may relieve the pain [1].

36.3.3 Asymptomatic Bile Duct Stones

Bile duct stones are occasionally found in asymptomatic patients [17–20]. As most asymptomatic common bile duct stones are not recognized, the natural history of asymptomatic stones is not well characterized. Overall, it seems that the natural history of asymptomatic common bile duct stones is more benign than that of symptomatic stones [1]. CBDS in asymptomatic patients are usually of moderate size [21]. Asymptomatic stones are most frequently found in patients with dilated bile ducts following cholecystectomy and in patients with Caroli's syndrome [15]. Especially, elderly patients may be asymptomatic carriers of CBDS. The risk of complications such as obstruction and cholangitis is increased [18]. Follow-up studies with patients after cholecystectomy indicate that only 5–12% of patients with common bile duct stones are asymptomatic [1, 7, 17, 19]. In a large retrospective analysis including 3828 patients with CBDS, CBDS associated complications occurred in 25.3% of patients when no measures for stone extraction were performed. The risk was significantly lower (12.5%) when stone extraction was performed [21]. Therefore, asymptomatic stones can be treated to prevent complications [1, 9]. On the other hand, asymptomatic patients were shown to have a higher risk of post-ERCP pancreatitis than symptomatic patients (12.5% vs. 3.9%) [20].

36.3.4 Recurrent Common Bile Duct Stones

The highest risk factor for recurrent CBDS is calculus gallbladder. Therefore, calculus gallbladder should be removed to reduce the risk of recurrent biliary complications.

Patients after Endoscopic sphinterotomy (EST) and cholecystectomy are at risk for CBDS recurrence. Recurrence was reported to occur in up to 18.5% patients [22] within 6 months to 15 years after initial treatment [23]. Factors associated with recurrence are the number of CBD stones (≥2), CBD stone diameter (≥10 mm), stone composition, stone consistency, CBD diameter (≥15 mm), bile duct dilatation pattern, sharp bile duct angulation (<145°), balloon dilatation, large balloon (>12 mm) dilatation, endoscopic mechanical lithotripsy, endoscopic sphincterotomy, and endoscopic papillary balloon dilatation, stricture of the major papilla post EST to 2–5 mm, and the presence of the ampulla within or on the edge of a duodenal diverticulum [22, 23].

36.3.5 Acute Cholecystitis and Common Bile Duct Stones

Cholangitis due to CBDS and cholecystitis are both associated with an inflammatory response and alteration of liver enzymes. Diagnosis of CBDS in patients with acute cholecystitis may be difficult. The reported prevalence of CBDS in patients with acute cholangitis shows a large variation between 0.92 and 16.5% [24]. Score predictors for choledocholithiasis showed a poor performance when acute cholecystitis is present. Suspicion of common bile duct stones by transabdominal ultrasound, total bilirubin >4 mg/dL, CBD dilatation >6 mm on Transabdominal ultrasound (US), abnormal liver test results, and biliary pancreatitis were all not predictive for bile duct stones in patients with acute cholecystitis [24]. Because CBDS associated cholangitis requires preoperative ERCP, endoscopic ultrasound (EUS) is advisable in patients with acute cholecystitis and suspicion of common bile duct stones.

36.3.6 Mirizzi Syndrome

Multiple impacted gallstones or a single large impacted gallstone in Hartmann's pouch of the gallbladder may cause obstruction of the hepatic or choledochyl duct. This form of external bile duct compression is referred to as Mirizzi syndrome [10]. Mirizzi syndrome is a rare condition that occurs in 0.1% of patients with gallstones [10]. The condition is difficult to diagnose as the symptoms are similar to cholecystitis or bile obstruction by CBDS. The true incidence of Mirizzi syndrome may be underdiagnosed preoperatively. The syndrome should be considered when patients are symptomatic for biliary obstruction, but a clear reason cannot be detected [10].

36.4 Diagnosis of Common Bile Duct Stones

The management of common bile duct stones depends on the extent and severity of symptoms, cholestasis, and complications. When CBDS are clinically suspected, laboratory analysis of liver and cholestasis parameters, parameters for inflammation, and transabdominal ultrasound should be promptly performed.

36.4.1 Laboratory Evaluation

The predictive value of abnormal liver biochemical parameters for CBDS is limited as there are several factors that influence increase of liver biochemical parameters other than common bile duct stones. Alanine aminotransferase (ALT) and aspartate aminotransferase (AST) are released from damaged hepatocytes, while gamma-glutamyl transferase (GGT), alkaline phosphatase (AP), and bilirubin increase following damage to the biliary system. Therefore, concomitant liver or bile duct diseases must be considered. Furthermore, the release of biochemical liver parameters follows different kinetic pattern after damage. The liver enzymes AST and ALT usually rise early after biliary obstruction, while AP, GGT, and bilirubin levels gradually rise if obstruction persists.

In a series of more than 1000 patients undergoing laparoscopic cholecystectomy, the negative predictive value of completely normal liver biochemical parameters was 94.7–97.7%, whereas the positive predictive value of any abnormal liver biochemical test results was only 15% [25, 26]. Thus, liver biochemical parameters have the most utility in excluding common bile duct stones [26].

Increased C-reactive protein (CRP) levels and/or elevated leukocyte levels with left shift indicate infectious complications and/or pancreatitis [1]. Procalcitonin elevation is helpful for the diagnosis of sepsis. Amylase and lipase are important predictors of early pancreatic damage.

36.4.2 Transabdominal Ultrasound

When CBDS are suspected, abdominal ultrasound should be the first imaging method. CBDS typically present as hyperechoic structures with dorsal shadowing. While bile stones in the gallbladder can be visualized with high sensitivity and specificity, intraductal stones are more difficult to identify. Transabdominal ultrasound achieves a sensitivity of 22–55% for detecting CBDS in patients with stones in the gallbladder [26].

The Vaterian papilla is difficult to evaluate by use of transabdominal ultrasound. Therefore, prepapillary concrements can frequently only be detected by indirect signs such as dilatation of the common bile duct and/or dilatation of the intrahepatic biliary branches. The normal bile duct diameter is 3–6 mm [26]. Biliary dilatation to a diameter greater than 7–8 mm in patients with gallbladder indicates biliary obstruction [26].

Gallbladder stones also have a predictive value for choledocholithiasis. It was shown that multiple small bile stones of less than 5 mm have a higher risk to migrate into the bile duct system than lager stones [26].

36.4.3 Endoscopic Ultrasound

Endoscopic ultrasound (EUS) is a minimally invasive procedure with a procedural risk that is similar to that of gastroscopy. A major advantage is the lack of radiation and the availability to the endoscopist. EUS allows evaluation of the bile duct and the gallbladder. Complete visualization of the extrahepatic duct system can be achieved in up to 96% of patients [27, 28]. Due to the proximity of the transducer to the papilla, EUS allows visualization of the distal bile duct entering the papilla making EUS the procedure of choice for evaluation of small stones impacted in the papilla [29]. With high frequencies in the order of 7.5–12 MHz, the resolution is less than 1 mm [27]. EUS achieves a sensitivity and specificity of 95% and 97%, respectively, [28]; however, bile duct obstruction in the hilum or in right hepatic duct may be overlooked. EUS may be difficult in patients with gastrectomy.

EUS can be performed with a linear or a radial echo endoscope. In the hands of experienced endoscopists, the diagnostic accuracy of linear or radial scanner is not different [27]. Small stones, biliary sludge, and microlithiasis can be detected. Larger stones usually appear as hyper-echoic foci with strong acoustic shadowing, while sludge produces low amplitude echoes without shadowing. Positioning the echo endoscope in the apex of the duodenal bulb allows evaluation of the common bile duct, the pancreatic duct, and the portal vein [27]. Withdrawal and counterclockwise torque leads to visualization of the bile duct toward the hilum, while insertion of the scope and clockwise torque leads to the distal bile duct and the papilla [27]. Positioning the transducer perpendicular to the papilla allows visualization of the distal bile duct entering the papilla. Detection of CBDS is difficult in patients with calcifications in the pancreas and duodenal diverticula and air within the bile duct.

36.4.4 Magnetic Resonance Imaging (MRI/MRCP)

The sensitivity and specificity of MRI/magnetic resonance cholangiopancreatography (MRCP) for CBDS are 93% and 96%, respectively [28]. The accuracy for CBDS is similar for MRI/MRCP and EUS [28]. Patients with negative MRI/MRCP or EUS do not need further invasive tests, unless symptoms persist. The choice between magnetic resonance tomography (MRT) and EUS depends on availability and experience. MRT may have an advantage over EUS in detection of hilar or intrahepatic stones and in detection and localization of neoplasia, while EUS may be better for detection of small papillary calculi [30].

36.4.5 Computed Tomography (CT)

CT has a sensitivity for common bile duct stones of 66.7% in patients with acute biliary pancreatitis [30]. The overall accuracy of MRI/MRCP in detecting choledocholithiasis was higher than that of CT (93.3% vs. 66.7%) [30].

36.4.6 Endoscopic Retrograde Cholangiopancreatography (ERCP)

With a sensitivity and specificity of 96% and 99%, respectively, ERCP shows an excellent diagnostic performance for detection of CBDS which is superior compared with other conventional diagnostic tests including transabdominal ultrasound, CT, MRT, common bile duct diameter, and liver biochemical parameter [25]. Due to the procedural complication risk, ERCP is not justified for diagnostic purposes unless alternatives are available.

36.5 Indication for Treatment of Common Bile Duct Stones

CBDS can cause several health problems including pain, jaundice, cholangitis, and acute pancreatitis [3, 4]. Extraction of CBDS in patients with symptomatic obstruction of the bile duct relieves the symptoms and reduces the risk for development of complications. Therefore, patients with symptomatic CBDS should receive stone extraction.

Several methods for stone extraction differing in invasiveness and complexity are available [3]. ERCP is the most convenient and least invasive method and performed as first-line treatment in most patients [1, 4]. However, ERCP shows complication and mortality rates in the order of 0.8–11.1% and 0.1–3.3%, respectively [1, 4, 31]. Therefore, ERCP is only justified when CBDS can be confirmed or are very likely the cause for the complaints of the patient. As diagnosis of CBDS can be difficult in oligosymptomatic patients, a stepwise diagnostic algorithm is necessary to avoid unnecessary and potentially harmful stone extraction procedures [18].

Diagnostic evaluation of patients with suspected CBDS should start with analysis of liver function tests and transabdominal ultrasound [1, 3, 26]. The strongest predictor for common bile duct stones is ultrasonographic evidence of a bile duct stone [1, 3, 26]. Patients with confirmed CBDS can be directly referred to stone extraction and need no further diagnostic evaluation especially when these patients are symptomatic [1, 3, 26]. On the other hand, patients with normal liver function tests have a very low likelihood for CBDS and need no further evaluation of the CBD [1, 3, 26].

Diagnosis of CBDS can be a challenge when stones are not detectable by transabdominal ultrasound. Several indirect predictive factors for CBDS have been described. The criteria mostly refer to patients with known gallbladder stones as most studies were performed in series of patients with indication for cholecystectomy. Except visualization of the stone, no single parameter is sufficient for strong prediction of symptomatic choledocholithiasis [26]. Guidelines recommend a risk stratification according to clinical signs, laboratory abnormalities, and abdominal ultrasound features [1, 3, 4, 9, 26]. Criteria for the probability of CBDS in patients with choledocholithiasis are listed in Table 36.1. The criteria vary slightly between the guidelines, and the scores have not been fully evaluated [1, 3, 4, 26].

The guidelines agree in the recommendation that patients with a high probability for CBDS should receive treatment with preoperative ERCP [4]. Patients with intermediate risk should receive further imaging diagnosis by EUS or MRCP depending on availability [4]. Preoperative ERCP should be performed when CBDS can be detected [4]. Patients without evidence of CBDS in EUS or MRCP or patients with a low probability can be ruled out and should not receive preoperative ERCP [4]. However, it must be considered that small stones may migrate in the CBD and that some patients assigned to CBDS low risk may develop severe complications in the long term [32].

Table 36.1 Probability of CBD in patients with symptomatic cholelithiasis

High > 50%	
CBD stone transabdominal US	DGVS, ASGE, EASL, BSG
Signs of ascending cholangitis	DGVS, ASGE, EASL, BSG
Bilirubin > 4 mg/dL	ASGE
CBD > 7 mm + abnormal bilirubin + abnormal GGT, AP, ALT, or AST	DGVS
CDB > 6 mm + abnormal bilirubin >1.8 mg/dL	ASGE
Pain, CBD dilatation, jaundice in patients with history of gallstones	BSG
Low < 5%	
CBD ≤ 7 mm	DGVS
Normal liver biochemical parameters	DGVS, ASGE, EASL
Absence of a preceding clinical predictor such as cholangitis or biliary pancreatitis	DGVS, ASGE

36.5.1 CBDS in Elderly Patients

The risk for gallstones increases with age, and CBDS are common in the elderly population. Most patients older than 80 years have concomitant diseases (73%) and are treated with antithrombotic drugs (25%) [33]. Therefore, safety concerns about ERCP in the elderly population have been raised. Recent studies comparing success and complication rates of ERCP between patients older or younger than 80–85 years showed no significant age-related differences in technical success and failure rates of ERCP [33–35]. The most common complication was post-ERCP pancreatitis. Thus, ERCP can be effectively and safely performed in elderly patients despite concomitant diseases.

36.6 Extraction Techniques

36.6.1 ERCP

ERCP with endoscopic sphincterotomy and subsequent removal of stones is a well-established treatment for CBDS and performed in many centers as first-line approach to CBDS. CBDS removal by ERCP has a success rate of more than 90% [4, 33–35]. In patients with altered anatomy (e.g., previous Roux-en-Y anastomosis, bariatric surgery), standard ERCP is less promising. In these cases, percutaneous or endoscopic balloon endoscopy-assisted treatment of bile duct stones should be considered [1].

36.6.1.1 Cannulation of the Papilla

After placement of the duodenoscope in the duodenum and identification of the papilla, the procedure starts with the cannulation of the bile duct orifice with the standard catheter or a standard sphincterotome. The rate of successful cannulation is around 95% [36] with lower rates when ERCP is performed for the first time (92%) [36].

After successful cannulation, the catheter is advanced into the common bile duct over a guided wire. To visualize the stones, fluoroscopy is performed. The stones become visible by a filling defect [5]. Fluoroscopy is usually performed from the proximal to the distal bile duct. It should be only performed when the wire is clearly located in the bile duct. Fluoroscopy of the pancreatic duct should be avoided due to the high risk of pancreatitis.

Small papillary office is a factor related to difficult biliary cannulation [18, 37]. Especially in asymptomatic patients with common bile duct stones, the rate of difficult deep cannulation was shown to be significantly higher than in symptomatic patients [18]. In asymptomatic patients, small papillary orifice might be more often than in symptomatic patients because of low bile duct pressure [18]. Difficult cannulation leading to edema of the papilla with consecutive impairment of pancreatic juice flow, activation of autodigestion, and inflammation can explain why post-ERCP pancreatitis occurs more likely in asymptomatic patients [18].

36.6.1.2 Endoscopic Sphincterotomy

Once a stone is confirmed, endoscopic sphincterotomy should be performed. This is usually achieved by a wire-guided sphincterotome. The size of the sphincterotomy depends on the size of the stones. It should be done as small as possible and as large as necessary to remove the stones.

Endoscopic sphincterotomy is associated with immediate complications such as bleeding (clinically relevant 0.8–15%), sepsis (1.2%), pancreatitis (2–3.5%), and perforation (1.2–1.8%) [37, 38]. Long-term adverse events such as Oddi dysfunction also have to be considered [37, 38].

Recurrent common bile duct stone formation occurs in 4–24% of patients following initial ERCP with endoscopic sphincterotomy. In patients with recurrent or retained bile duct stones after previous sphincterotomy, extension of a previous sphincterotomy can be safely done. Vezakis et al. showed that the complication rate of extension sphincterotomy is lower than after first-time sphincterotomy (0.8% vs. 5.3%) [38]. The most common complication was hemorrhage which was also less frequent following extension endoscopic sphincterotomy (20% vs. 29%) [38].

36.6.1.3 Pre-cut Sphincterotomy and Fistulotomy

If direct introduction of the papilla is not successful, pre-cut papillotomy with a needle knife or a pre-cut sphincterotome over the pancreatic duct can be performed. It must be considered that pre-cut is associated with an increased risk of duodenal perforation, bleeding, and the development of pancreatic fistula compared with conventional sphincterotomy [37]. Pre-cut papillotomy with a needle knife in patients with acute severe cholangitis and impacted common bile duct stones was associated with a 100% success rate and a complication rate of 4% (hemorrhage, pancreatitis) [39].

Papillary fistulotomy is another approach for secondary biliary access. Papillary fistulotomy is performed by an incision on the mucosa above the papillary office by using a needle-knife catheter. The cut is made in distal to proximal direction, aiming at the papillary apex [40]. The fistula can be cannulated into the bile duct with a guidewire and sphincterotome, and it can be enlarged by cutting the sphincter.

In a small recently published randomized trial comparing fistulotomy and conventional cannulation for treatment of CBDS, complication and success rates (perforation and pancreatitis) were 2% and 100% for papillary fistulotomy and 13.7% and 75% for conventional cannulation [40]. Thus, papillary fistulotomy appears safe and effective and should be evaluated in larger trials.

36.6.1.4 Large Balloon Dilatation of the Papilla

Endoscopic sphincterotomy is associated with complications including hemorrhage, retroperitoneal perforation, cholangitis, pancreatitis, and recurrent common bile duct stones [41]. Therefore, alternative approaches with lower bleeding risk are needed in special patient populations. Endoscopic balloon dilatation of the sphincter of Oddi represents an alternative procedure to remove common bile duct stones [41]. However, balloon dilatation is not recommended as first-line approach as it was reported to have a higher risk for complications than EST (17.9% vs. 3.3%) [42]. A recent meta-analysis showed that endoscopic sphincterotomy plus large balloon dilatation causes fewer overall complications than endoscopic sphincterotomy alone (OR, 0.53) [43]. Endoscopic sphincterotomy plus large balloon dilatation was more effective than endoscopic sphincterotomy alone especially for removal of large stones >15 mm [43]. Maruta et al. investigated long-term complications in patients after endoscopic sphincterotomy vs. large balloon dilatation due to common bile duct stones [44]. The estimated 1–3-year late complication rates were 5–15% and not associated with the type of intervention [44].

36.6.2 Stone Extraction

36.6.2.1 Stone Extraction Balloon

Stone extraction by balloon catheter is a technique which is suited for extraction of smaller CBDS and intrahepatic stones. Larger stones can be impacted in the papilla by the balloon technique. Balloons can also be used for diagnostic purposes to localize stones or strictures. The balloon can be used to bring calculi in position for other stone extraction techniques.

The stone extraction balloon is mounted at the end of a plastic catheter. For stone extraction, the catheter is introduced in the distal bile duct, and a hydrophilic guidewire is placed in the desired bile duct. Then, the deflated balloon catheter is advanced over the guidewire so that the balloon is placed behind the stone. When the balloon is in the right position, it can be inflated by injecting air from the outer end of the catheter. The balloon diameter should be adapted to the diameter of the bile duct. In the next step, the balloon can be pulled down though the papilla with the calculi. As the diameter of the bile ducts may change, it can be necessary to adapt the size of the balloon. Several attempts may be necessary as the stone gets frequently lost when the balloon is pulled down.

36.6.2.2 Stone Extraction Basket

The standard technique of capturing a stone is to use a four-wire basket and advance it upstream of the stone [45]. When the catheter with the enclosed basket is behind the stone, the basket is opened slowly while pulling back the catheter. The basket can be moved up and down to capture the stone. Once the stone has been drawn, the basket can be closed and pulled back to extract the stone. This should be done carefully because if the stone is grasped too tightly, it may break into several fragments.

There are several maneuvers to remove the stone from the papilla [45]. The first is to pull back the basket catheter through the scope. This technique is promising when the stone is not too large and the spincteromy is large enough. The second is to release the up-angle of the scope and to push the scope forward. The third is to turn the scope clockwise. Manipulation at the papilla is associated with the risk of lacerating the papilla and injuring bile duct and pancreas. The risk is greatest when the scope is removed with the basket. This maneuver should be avoided.

If patients have multiple stones, it is necessary to insert the extraction device repeatedly to capture and remove the stones. It is important that distal stones are captured first as capture of proximal stones can lead to impaction of the basket.

If extraction of small stones with the four-wire basket is not successful, it can be switched to a balloon extraction catheter. An alternate approach may be an eight-wire basket which is shaped like a net and is superior to the four-wire basket in the extraction of small stones [45].

Large stones, especially those larger than 15 mm, carry the risk of basket impaction. This usually happens if the stone diameter exceeds the lumen of the papilla. Then the stone cannot be extracted in total, and lithotripsy must be performed. Not every basket is suited for lithotripsy. Therefore, if larger stones are found in fluoroscopy, a special reinforced basket suited for lithotripsy should be chosen.

36.6.2.3 Mechanical Lithotripsy

Bile duct stones greater than 10 mm have a decreased incidence of successful endoscopic extraction and often require lithotripsy. The standard procedure for large bile duct stones is mechanical lithotripsy. Sufficient endoscopic sphincterotomy and/or large balloon dilatation is required.

Mechanical lithotripsy requires a special device consisting of a reinforced stone extraction basket in a metal outer sheath. For lithotripsy, the stone is caught by the basket first. Then, the metal sheath is advanced until the trapped stone in the basket breaks. The procedure must be done carefully to avoid damage of the common bile duct. After fragmentation of the stone, the fragments can be extracted using standard techniques with basket or balloon.

Emergency lithotripsy is necessary when a stone has been trapped by a standard basket and both cannot be removed though the papilla. Then the handle of the basket is cut off and the endoscope is removed. A flexible metal sheath is then carefully advanced over the remaining cable under fluoroscopic control until it reaches the basket with the stone. When placing the metal sheath, it is important not to apply too much force on the papilla and to place the metal sheath so that the basket with stone and metal sheath are in a straight line. Then the metal sheath can be further advanced with a special crushing device fixed at the outer end until the stone breaks.

36.6.3 Prophylactic Saline Irrigation of the Bile Duct to Reduce the Rate of Residual Common Bile Duct Stones

Recurrent cholangitis due to residual common bile duct stone occurs frequently even after endoscopic stone removal. Preventive saline irrigation in the bile duct after endoscopic removal of CBDS could decrease residual CBDS. A randomized trial showed that the incidences of residual CBDS were 6.8% in patients after preventive saline irrigation and 22.7% in the control group [46]. The study indicates that routine saline irrigation after endoscopic stone removal may be effective and safe to reduce residual common bile duct stones [46].

36.6.3.1 Stent Placement

Complex biliary stones often cannot be completely extracted in a single session [47]. To reduce the time of procedure and to reduce disease-associated complications, it can be of use to split the ERCP. Saito et al. compared ERCP-related complications between single- and two-stage endoscopic stone removal [48]. There was a trend to lower complication rates after two-stage ERCP than after single-stage ERCP (7.4% vs. 13.2%) [48].

Temporary stent placement can be performed before a repeat attempt [49]. The stent ensures bile flow, leads to mechanic destruction of the stone, and is prophylactic for bleeding. Usually, plastic non-self-expandable stents are used. However, the volume of biliary drainage with these stents may be insufficient. Therefore, multiple stents may be necessary. Covered self-expandable stents are larger and have been shown to be effective and safe for treatment of complex bile stones [47, 49]. Cost-effectiveness of these stents should be considered.

36.6.3.2 Intraductal Lithotripsy

Intraductal lithotripsy techniques are electrohydraulic lithotripsy (EHL) and laser lithotripsy [50, 51]. Both techniques are second-line techniques. The most common indication is large impacted stones or stones behind a stricture. With advanced techniques, clearance can be obtained in 99% of patients; however, multiple sessions and combinations of different approaches may be necessary [51].

EHL is performed with a coaxial bipolar lithotripsy probe that is placed in the bile duct nearby the stone. The probe is connected with a charge unit. Discharging produces sparks which generate in aqueous medium high-frequency hydraulic pressure waves which in turn lead to fragmentation of the stone. Continuous irrigation of saline is necessary during the procedure. Accidental application of the shock waves to the bile duct wall may lead to perforation. Therefore, the procedure should be performed by using centering balloons or if available by direct cholangioscopy.

In laser lithotripsy, a pulsed laser is used to induce high power density shock waves for fragmentation of the stone. The technique can be applied peroral under fluoroscopic or cholangioscopic guidance or by transhepatic approach.

36.6.4 Cholangioscopy with Lithotripsy

If standard mechanical lithotripsy fails, cholangioscopy guided lithotripsy is an adjunct [50–56]. The difficulty of cholangioscopy is the access to the bile duct. Peroral cholangioscopy (POCS) can be performed by introducing an ultrathin videoendoscope in the bile duct [57]. The maneuver is difficult to perform and limited by the flexibility of the scope and the diameter of the bile duct. Another approach is mother-baby cholangioscopy which is performed with a miniaturized baby single-use endoscope that is advanced through the working channel of the duodenoscope like a standard catheter [52]. The baby endoscope has four-way steerability. Through the working channel, laser or electrohydraulic lithotripsy can be performed. Costs, fragility, and a small working channel are limitations of this technique. A large endoscopic sphincterotomy is the prerequisite for introduction of the cholangioscope. Cholangioscopy is difficult to perform in patients with surgically altered anatomy, a periampullary diverticulum, or a sigmoid-shaped common bile duct [50].

A major advantage of cholangioscopy is that guided lithotripsy is possible and strictures can be evaluated [55]. The success rate for complete bile duct stone removal is 91–95% [52, 53]. However, repeated procedures may be necessary to achieve final stone clearance [52]. Cholangitis is the most common complication of cholangioscopy which can be reduced by antibiotic prophylaxis [52].

Peroral transluminal cholangioscopy is a novel and advanced technique in which cholangioscopy is performed through a fistula between the intrahepatic bile duct and the stomach or intestine [50]. In a pilot study, electrohydraulic lithotripsy by ERC guided cholangioscopy or by peroral transluminal cholangioscopy demonstrated a complete stone extraction rate of 98% [50]. Cholangitis and pancreatitis occurred in 14% of treated patients [50].

36.6.5 Extracorporeal Shock Wave Lithotripsy (ESWL)

ESWL utilizes electrohydraulic or electromagnetic energy generated outside the body to fragment gallstones. ESWL is usually performed under US or fluoroscopic guidance. For fluoroscopic identification and targeting of the gallstones, insertion of a nasobiliary drain is required. In general, patients are sedated and receive antibiotic prophylaxis for the treatment.

Successful clearance can be achieved in 60–90% of patients [58].

36.6.6 Percutaneous Transhepatic Cholangiography (PTC)

In case of severe cholestasis and frustrating endoscopy, PTC can be performed as an alternative [59]. Complications of PTCD (bleeding, pneumothorax, perforation) are more frequent than complications from ERCP. Small calculi can be pushed forward through the papilla [45]. As this maneuver may damage the papilla, balloon dilatation should be performed before stone extraction [60]. Larger stones require lithotripsy. If extraction is not possible, placement of a drainage can be performed [61]. The drainage restores the bile flow and may lead to fragmentation of the stone. Stone extraction can be successful in a second attempt. The percutaneous route can also be used to introduce a thin videoendoscope to perform cholangioscopy with Laser-based lithotripsy or electrohydraulic lithitripsy [62].

36.6.6.1 Cholecysto-Choledocholithiasis

The currently most widespread method for treatment of cholecysto-choledocholithiasis is a two-step approach by performing an ERCP first and a laparoscopic cholecystectomy later [31]. Surgical bile duct revision is an alternative therapy for common bile duct stones when endoscopic procedures including cholangioscopy fail [52]. Progress in laparoscopic surgery made it possible to treat cholecysto-choledocholithiasis by a single-stage approach with similar efficacy, mortality, and morbidity to a double-stage procedure [31, 63]. The single-stage approach has not been standardized and presents various technical options with varying degrees of complexity from the technological and manual standpoint [31]. A complete clearance of the bile duct via laparoscopic approach in a single session can be obtained by trans-cystic laparoscopic bile duct clearance, laparoscopic common bile duct exploration, or rendezvous intraoperative endoscopic retrograde cholangiography [31]. Trans-cystic treatment is the simplest approach. However, this method is limited in case of large stones or papillary stenosis [31]. A recent meta-analysis including 13 studies with overall 1757 patients indicated that laparoscopic common bile duct exploration and laparoscopic cholecystectomy were superior to preoperative endoscopic sphincterotomy and cholecystectomy with respect to CBDS clearance (94% vs. 90%) and perioperative complications (7.6% vs. 12.0%) [64]. Laparoscopic common bile duct exploration and rendezvous intraoperative endoscopic retrograde cholangiography are more time consuming and are technically more difficult. The rendezvous approach requires the presence of the endoscopist. Subsequent studies should indicate the predictive parameters in order to choose the best option for a truly personalized surgery [31].

References

1. European association for the study of the liver (EASL). Electronic address: easloffice@easloffice.eu. EASL Clinical Practice Guidelines on the prevention, diagnosis and treatment of gallstones. J Hepatol. 2016;65(1):146–81. https://doi.org/10.1016/j.jhep.2016.03.005.
2. Farthing M, Roberts SE, Samuel DG, Williams JG, Thorne K, Morrison-Rees S, et al. Survey of digestive health across Europe: final report. Part 1: the burden of gastrointestinal diseases and the organisation and delivery of gastroenterology services across Europe. United Eur Gastroenterol J [Internet]. 2014 Dec 13 [cited 2018 Apr 9];2(6):539–43. Available from: http://journals.sagepub.com/doi/10.1177/2050640614554154.
3. Williams E, Beckingham I, El Sayed G, Gurusamy K, Sturgess R, Webster G, et al. Updated guideline on the management of common bile duct stones (CBDS). Gut [Internet]. 2017 May [cited 2018 Apr 12];66(5):765–82. Available from: http://www.ncbi.nlm.nih.gov/pubmed/28122906.
4. Kuzu UB, Ödemiş B, Dişibeyaz S, Parlak E, Öztaş E, Saygılı F, et al. Management of suspected common bile duct stone: diagnostic yield of current guidelines. HPB (Oxford) [Internet]. 2017 Feb [cited 2018 Apr 22];19(2):126–32. Available from: http://linkinghub.elsevier.com/retrieve/pii/S1365182X16319724.
5. Collins C, Maguire D, Ireland A, Fitzgerald E, O'Sullivan GC. A prospective study of common bile duct calculi in patients undergoing laparoscopic cholecystectomy: natural history of choledocholithiasis revisited. Ann Surg [Internet]. 2004 Jan [cited 2018 Apr 22];239(1):28–33. Available from: https://insights.ovid.com/crossref?an=00000658-200401000-00005.
6. Choi CS, Ku YJ, Yoon DY, Yun EJ, Seo YL, Lim KJ, et al. Harmonic ultrasonography for the detection of microlithiasis in the gallbladder. Ultrasonography [Internet]. 2014 Jun 28 [cited 2018 Apr 22];33(4):275–82. Available from: http://www.ncbi.nlm.nih.gov/pubmed/25060185.
7. Frossard JL, Hadengue A, Amouyal G, Choury A, Marty O, Giostra E, et al. Choledocholithiasis: a prospective study of spontaneous common bile duct stone migration. Gastrointest Endosc [Internet]. 2000 Feb [cited 2018 Apr 22];51(2):175–9. Available from: http://www.ncbi.nlm.nih.gov/pubmed/10650260.
8. Ramchandani M, Pal P, Reddy DN. Endoscopic management of acute cholangitis as a result of common bile duct stones. Dig Endosc [Internet]. 2017 Apr [cited 2018 Apr 28];29:78–87. Available from: http://www.ncbi.nlm.nih.gov/pubmed/28425658.
9. Lammert F, Neubrand M, Bittner R, Feussner H, Greiner L, Hagenmüller F, et al. S3-Leitlinie der Deutschen Gesellschaft für Verdauungs- und Stoffwechselkrankheiten und der Deutschen Gesellschaft für Viszeralchirurgie zur Diagnostik und Behandlung von Gallensteinen. Z Gastroenterol [Internet]. 2007 Sep [cited 2018 Apr 22];45(9):971–1001. Available from: http://www.ncbi.nlm.nih.gov/pubmed/17874360.
10. Jones MW, Ferguson T. Gallbladder, Mirizzi Syndrome [Internet]. StatPearls. StatPearls Publishing; 2018 [cited 2018 Mar 25]. Available from: http://www.ncbi.nlm.nih.gov/pubmed/29494098.
11. Koo KP, Traverso LW. Do preoperative indicators predict the presence of common bile duct stones during laparoscopic cholecystectomy? Am J Surg [Internet]. 1996 May [cited 2018 Apr 22];171(5):495–9. Available from: http://www.ncbi.nlm.nih.gov/pubmed/8651393.
12. Wittenburg H. Pathogenesis of gallstones. Der Gastroenterol. 2018;13:6–14.
13. Chen C-H, Lin C-L, Kao C-H. Association between inflammatory bowel disease and cholelithiasis: a nationwide population-based cohort study. Int J Environ Res Public Health [Internet]. 2018 Mar 14 [cited 2018 Mar 24];15(3):513. Available from: http://www.ncbi.nlm.nih.gov/pubmed/29538289.
14. Sandstad O, Osnes T, Skar V, Urdal P, Osnes M. Common bile duct stones are mainly brown and associated with duodenal diverticula. Gut [Internet]. 1994 Oct [cited 2018 Apr 21];35(10):1464–7. Available from: http://www.ncbi.nlm.nih.gov/pubmed/7959206.
15. Mabrut J-Y, Kianmanesh R, Nuzzo G, Castaing D, Boudjema K, Létoublon C, et al. Surgical management of congenital intrahepatic bile duct dilatation, Caroli's disease and syndrome. Ann Surg [Internet]. 2013 Nov [cited 2018 May 5];258(5):713–21. Available from: http://content.wkhealth.com/linkback/openurl?sid=WKPTLP:landingpage&an=00000658-201311000-00008.

16. Doi Y, Takii Y, Ito H, Jingu N, To K, Kimura S, et al. Usefulness of endoscopic managements in patients with ceftriaxone-induced pseudolithiasis causing biliary obstruction. Case Rep Med [Internet]. 2017 [cited 2018 Mar 30];2017:1–5. Available from: http://www.ncbi.nlm.nih.gov/pubmed/29230246.
17. Caddy GR, Kirby J, Kirk SJ, Allen MJ, Moorehead RJ, Tham TC. Natural history of asymptomatic bile duct stones at time of cholecystectomy. Ulster Med J [Internet]. 2005 Sep [cited 2018 Apr 22];74(2):108–12. Available from: http://www.ncbi.nlm.nih.gov/pubmed/16235763.
18. Saito H, Kakuma T, Kadono Y, Urata A, Kamikawa K, Imamura H, et al. Increased risk and severity of ERCP-related complications associated with asymptomatic common bile duct stones. Endosc Int Open [Internet]. 2017 Sep 5 [cited 2018 Mar 31];5(9):E809–17. Available from: http://www.ncbi.nlm.nih.gov/pubmed/28879226.
19. Rosseland AR, Glomsaker TB. Asymptomatic common bile duct stones. Eur J Gastroenterol Hepatol [Internet]. 2000 Nov [cited 2018 Apr 22];12(11):1171–3. Available from: http://www.ncbi.nlm.nih.gov/pubmed/11111771.
20. Kim SB, Kim KH, Kim TN. Comparison of outcomes and complications of endoscopic common bile duct stone removal between asymptomatic and symptomatic patients. Dig Dis Sci [Internet]. 2016 Apr 20 [cited 2018 May 6];61(4):1172–7. Available from: http://www.ncbi.nlm.nih.gov/pubmed/26589817.
21. Möller M, Gustafsson U, Rasmussen F, Persson G, Thorell A. Natural course vs interventions to clear common bile duct stones: data from the Swedish Registry for Gallstone Surgery and Endoscopic Retrograde Cholangiopancreatography (GallRiks). JAMA Surg [Internet]. 2014 Oct 1 [cited 2018 May 6];149(10):1008–13. Available from: http://archsurg.jamanetwork.com/article.aspx?doi=10.1001/jamasurg.2014.249.
22. Yoo ES, Yoo BM, Kim JH, Hwang JC, Yang MJ, Lee KM, et al. Evaluation of risk factors for recurrent primary common bile duct stone in patients with cholecystectomy. Scand J Gastroenterol [Internet]. 2018 Feb 19 [cited 2018 Mar 25];1–5. Available from: http://www.ncbi.nlm.nih.gov/pubmed/29457922.
23. Nzenza TC, Al-Habbal Y, Guerra GR, Manolas S, Yong T, McQuillan T. Recurrent common bile duct stones as a late complication of endoscopic sphincterotomy. BMC Gastroenterol [Internet]. 2018 Dec 15 [cited 2018 Mar 24];18(1):39. Available from: http://www.ncbi.nlm.nih.gov/pubmed/29544453.
24. Gouveia C, Loureiro R, Ferreira R, Oliveira Ferreira A, Santos AA, Santos MPC, et al. Performance of the choledocholithiasis diagnostic score in patients with acute cholecystitis. GE - Port J Gastroenterol [Internet]. 2018 Jan [cited 2018 Mar 25];25(1):24–9. Available from: http://www.ncbi.nlm.nih.gov/pubmed/29457047.
25. Yang M-H, Chen T-H, Wang S-E, Tsai Y-F, Su C-H, Wu C-W, et al. Biochemical predictors for absence of common bile duct stones in patients undergoing laparoscopic cholecystectomy. Surg Endosc. 2008;22(7):1620–4.
26. Maple JT, Ben-Menachem T, Anderson MA, Appalaneni V, Banerjee S, Cash BD, et al. The role of endoscopy in the evaluation of suspected choledocholithiasis. Gastrointest Endosc [Internet]. 2010 Jan [cited 2018 Apr 12];71(1):1–9. Available from: http://www.ncbi.nlm.nih.gov/pubmed/20105473.
27. Aljebreen A. Role of endoscopic ultrasound in common bile duct stones. Saudi J Gastroenterol [Internet]. 2007 [cited 2018 Apr 28];13(1):11. Available from: http://www.ncbi.nlm.nih.gov/pubmed/19858606.
28. Giljaca V, Gurusamy KS, Takwoingi Y, Higgie D, Poropat G, Štimac D, et al. Endoscopic ultrasound versus magnetic resonance cholangiopancreatography for common bile duct stones [Internet]. Vol. 2015, Cochrane Database Syst Rev. 2015 [cited 2018 Apr 28]. p. CD011549. Available from: http://www.ncbi.nlm.nih.gov/pubmed/25719224.
29. Vaynshtein J, Sabbag G, Pinsk I, Rahmani I, Reshef A. Predictors for choledocholitiasis in patients undergoing endoscopic ultrasound. Scand J Gastroenterol [Internet]. 2018 Mar 4 [cited 2018 Mar 25];53(3):335–9. Available from: http://www.ncbi.nlm.nih.gov/pubmed/29421933.
30. Lee S-L, Kim H-K, Choi H-H, Jeon B-S, Kim T-H, Choi J-M, et al. Diagnostic value of magnetic resonance cholangiopancreatography to detect bile duct stones in acute biliary pancreatitis. Pancreatology [Internet]. 2018 Jan [cited 2018 Mar 29];18(1):22–8. Available from: http://www.ncbi.nlm.nih.gov/pubmed/29246689.
31. Bove A, Di Renzo RM, Palone G, Testa DC, Malerba V, Bongarzoni G. Single-stage procedure for the treatment of cholecysto-choledocolithiasis: a surgical procedures review. Ther Clin Risk Manag [Internet]. 2018 Feb [cited 2018 Mar 25];Volume 14:305–12. Available from: http://www.ncbi.nlm.nih.gov/pubmed/29503549.
32. Akashi T, Tachibana Y, Matsuo S, Gibo J. Worsening of acute cholangitis caused by a bile duct stone after hospitalization: a case series. Gastroenterol Res [Internet]. 2018 Feb [cited 2018 Mar 24];11(1):58–61. Available from: http://www.ncbi.nlm.nih.gov/pubmed/29511408.
33. Yang J, Li W, Si X, Zhang J, Cao Y. Efficacy and safety of therapeutic ERCP in the elderly. Surg Laparosc Endosc Percutan Tech [Internet]. 2018 Jan 18 [cited 2018 Mar 29];1. Available from: http://www.ncbi.nlm.nih.gov/pubmed/29252934.
34. Yıldırım AE, Öztürk ZA, Konduk BT, Balkan A, Edizer B, Gulsen MT, et al. The safety and efficacy of ERCP in octogenarians: a comparison of two geriatric age cohorts. Acta Gastroenterol Belg [Internet]. [cited 2018 Mar 24];80(2):263–70. Available from: http://www.ncbi.nlm.nih.gov/pubmed/29560692.
35. Iida T, Kaneto H, Wagatsuma K, Sasaki H, Naganawa Y, Nakagaki S, et al. Efficacy and safety of endoscopic procedures for common bile duct stones in patients aged 85 years or older: a retrospective study. Pagnini C, editor. PLoS One [Internet]. 2018 Jan 3

[cited 2018 Mar 29];13(1):e0190665. Available from: http://www.ncbi.nlm.nih.gov/pubmed/29298346.
36. Al-Mansour MR, Fung EC, Jones EL, Zayan NE, Wetzel TD, Martin del Campo SE, et al. Surgeon-performed endoscopic retrograde cholangiopancreatography. Outcomes of 2392 procedures at two tertiary care centers. Surg Endosc [Internet]. 2017 Dec 22 [cited 2018 Mar 29]. Available from: http://www.ncbi.nlm.nih.gov/pubmed/29273876.
37. Barthet M, Lesavre N, Desjeux A, Gasmi M, Berthezene P, Berdah S, et al. Complications of endoscopic sphincterotomy: results from a Single Tertiary Referral Center. Endoscopy [Internet]. 2002 Dec [cited 2018 Mar 31];34(12):991–7. Available from: http://www.ncbi.nlm.nih.gov/pubmed/12471544.
38. Vezakis A, Polydorou A, Kontis E, Pantiora E, Papanikolaou IS, Fragulidis G. Safety and efficacy of extending a previous endoscopic sphincterotomy for the treatment of retained or recurrent common bile duct stones. Ann Gastroenterol [Internet]. 2017 [cited 2018 Mar 29];31(1):109–14. Available from: http://www.ncbi.nlm.nih.gov/pubmed/29333075.
39. Zheng M, Liu X, Li N, Li W-Z. Emergency endoscopic needle-knife precut papillotomy in acute severe cholangitis resulting from impacted common bile duct stones at duodenal papilla. Dig Liver Dis [Internet]. 2018 Mar [cited 2018 Mar 29];50(3):267–70. Available from: http://www.ncbi.nlm.nih.gov/pubmed/29361439.
40. Furuya CK, Sakai P, Marinho FRT, Otoch JP, Cheng S, Prudencio LL, et al. Papillary fistulotomy *vs* conventional cannulation for endoscopic biliary access: a prospective randomized trial. World J Gastroenterol [Internet]. 2018 Apr 28 [cited 2018 May 5];24(16):1803–11. Available from: http://www.wjgnet.com/1007-9327/full/v24/i16/1803.htm.
41. Tsai T-J, Lin C-K, Lai K-H, Chan H-H, Wang E-M, Tsai W-L, et al. Does preserved sphincter of Oddi function prevent common bile duct stones recurrence in patients after endoscopic papillary balloon dilation? J Chinese Med Assoc [Internet]. 2018 Apr [cited 2018 Mar 25];81(4):311–5. Available from: http://www.ncbi.nlm.nih.gov/pubmed/29499900.
42. Disario JA, Freeman ML, Bjorkman DJ, Macmathuna P, Petersen BT, Jaffe PE, et al. Endoscopic balloon dilation compared with sphincterotomy for extraction of bile duct stones. Gastroenterology [Internet]. 2004 Nov [cited 2018 Mar 25];127(5):1291–9. Available from: http://www.ncbi.nlm.nih.gov/pubmed/15520997.
43. Yang X-M, Hu B. Endoscopic sphincterotomy plus large-balloon dilation vs endoscopic sphincterotomy for choledocholithiasis: A meta-analysis. World J Gastroenterol [Internet]. 2013 Dec 28 [cited 2018 Apr 13];19(48):9453. Available from: http://www.ncbi.nlm.nih.gov/pubmed/24409076.
44. Maruta A, Iwashita T, Uemura S, Yoshida K, Iwata K, Mukai T, et al. Comparison of late adverse events after endoscopic sphincterotomy versus endoscopic papillary large balloon dilation for common bile duct stones: a propensity score-based cohort analysis. Dig Endosc [Internet]. 2018 Feb 27 [cited 2018 Mar 29]. Available from: http://www.ncbi.nlm.nih.gov/pubmed/29399885.
45. Yasuda I. Novel retrieval basket for small bile duct stones. Dig Endosc [Internet]. 2015 Sep [cited 2018 Apr 12];27(6):712–712. Available from: http://doi.wiley.com/10.1111/den.12496.
46. Ahn D-W, Lee SH, Paik WH, Song BJ, Park JM, Kim J, et al. Effects of saline irrigation of the bile duct to reduce the rate of residual common bile duct stones: a multicenter, prospective, randomized study. Am J Gastroenterol [Internet]. 2018 Apr 27 [cited 2018 Apr 7];113(4):548–55. Available from: http://www.ncbi.nlm.nih.gov/pubmed/29610513.
47. García-Cano J, Reyes-Guevara AK, Martínez-Pérez T, Valiente-González L, Martínez-Fernández R, Viñuelas-Chicano M, et al. Fully covered self-expanding metal stents in the management of difficult common bile duct stones. Rev Esp Enferm Dig [Internet]. 2013 Jan [cited 2018 Apr 8];105(1):7–12. Available from: http://www.ncbi.nlm.nih.gov/pubmed/23548005.
48. Saito H, Kadono Y, Kamikawa K, Urata A, Imamura H, Matsushita I, et al. The incidence of complications in single-stage endoscopic stone removal for patients with common bile duct stones: a propensity score analysis. Intern Med [Internet]. 2018 Feb 15 [cited 2018 Mar 31];57(4):469–77. Available from: http://www.ncbi.nlm.nih.gov/pubmed/29151506.
49. Cerefice M, Sauer B, Javaid M, Smith LA, Gosain S, Argo CK, et al. Complex biliary stones: treatment with removable self-expandable metal stents: a new approach (with videos). Gastrointest Endosc [Internet]. 2011 Sep [cited 2018 Apr 8];74(3):520–6. Available from: http://www.ncbi.nlm.nih.gov/pubmed/21872710.
50. Kamiyama R, Ogura T, Okuda A, Miyano A, Nishioka N, Imanishi M, et al. Electrohydraulic lithotripsy for difficult bile duct stones under endoscopic retrograde cholangiopancreatography and peroral transluminal cholangioscopy guidance. Gut Liver [Internet]. 2018 Feb 8 [cited 2018 Mar 25]. Available from: http://www.ncbi.nlm.nih.gov/pubmed/29409310.
51. Brown NG, Camilo J, Nordstrom E, Yen RD, Fukami N, Brauer BC, et al. Advanced ERCP techniques for the extraction of complex biliary stones: a single referral center's 12-year experience. Scand J Gastroenterol [Internet]. 2018 Apr 12 [cited 2018 May 6];1–6. Available from: http://www.ncbi.nlm.nih.gov/pubmed/29644909.
52. Turowski F, Hügle U, Dormann A, Bechtler M, Jakobs R, Gottschalk U, et al. Diagnostic and therapeutic single-operator cholangiopancreatoscopy with SpyGlassDS™: results of a multicenter retrospective cohort study. Surg Endosc [Internet]. 2018 Mar 12 [cited 2018 Mar 24]. Available from: http://www.ncbi.nlm.nih.gov/pubmed/29532224.
53. Brewer Gutierrez OI, Bekkali NLH, Raijman I, Sturgess R, Sejpal D V., Aridi HD, et al. Efficacy and safety of digital single-operator cholangioscopy for difficult biliary stones. Clin Gastroenterol Hepatol [Internet]. 2017 Oct 24 [cited 2018 Mar

31]. Available from: http://www.ncbi.nlm.nih.gov/pubmed/29074446.

54. Buxbaum J, Sahakian A, Ko C, Jayaram P, Lane C, Yu CY, et al. Randomized trial of cholangioscopy-guided laser lithotripsy versus conventional therapy for large bile duct stones (with videos). Gastrointest Endosc [Internet]. 2018 Apr [cited 2018 Apr 12];87(4):1050–60. Available from: http://linkinghub.elsevier.com/retrieve/pii/S0016510717322034.
55. Deprez P, Garces Duran R, Moreels T, Furneri G, Demma F, Verbeke L, et al. The economic impact of using single-operator cholangioscopy for the treatment of difficult bile duct stones and diagnosis of indeterminate bile duct strictures. Endoscopy [Internet]. 2018 Feb 24 [cited 2018 Mar 31];50(2):109–18. Available from: http://www.ncbi.nlm.nih.gov/pubmed/29172216.
56. Ghersi S, Fuccio L, Bassi M, Fabbri C, Cennamo V. Current status of peroral cholangioscopy in biliary tract diseases. World J Gastrointest Endosc [Internet]. 2015 May 16 [cited 2018 Apr 29];7(5):510. Available from: http://www.ncbi.nlm.nih.gov/pubmed/25992189.
57. Okugawa T, Tsuyuguchi T, K C S, Ando T, Ishihara T, Yamaguchi T, et al. Peroral cholangioscopic treatment of hepatolithiasis: Long-term results. Gastrointest Endosc [Internet]. 2002 Sep [cited 2018 Apr 29];56(3):366–71. Available from: http://www.ncbi.nlm.nih.gov/pubmed/12196774.
58. Ellis RD, Jenkins AP, Thompson RP, Ede RJ. Clearance of refractory bile duct stones with extracorporeal shockwave lithotripsy. Gut [Internet]. 2000 Nov [cited 2018 Apr 29];47(5):728–31. Available from: http://www.ncbi.nlm.nih.gov/pubmed/11034593.
59. Clouse ME, Stokes KR, Lee RG, Falchuk KR. Bile duct stones: percutaneous transhepatic removal. Radiology [Internet]. 1986 Aug [cited 2018 May 6];160(2):525–9. Available from: http://www.ncbi.nlm.nih.gov/pubmed/3726136.
60. Nagashima I, Takada T, Shiratori M, Inaba T, Okinaga K. Percutaneous transhepatic papillary balloon dilation as a therapeutic option for choledocholithiasis. J Hepatobiliary Pancreat Surg [Internet]. 2004 Aug [cited 2018 May 6];11(4):252–4. Available from: http://link.springer.com/10.1007/s00534-003-0851-x.
61. Peng Y-C, Chow W-K. Alternative percutaneous approach for endoscopic inaccessible common bile duct stones. Hepatogastroenterology [Internet]. [cited 2018 May 6];58(107–108):705–8. Available from: http://www.ncbi.nlm.nih.gov/pubmed/21830373.
62. Weigand K, Kandulski A, Zuber-Jerger I, Mueller M, Goessmann H. Cholangioscopy-guided electrohydraulic lithotripsy of large bile duct stones through a percutaneous access device. Endoscopy [Internet]. 2018 Feb 16 [cited 2018 May 6];50(5):E111–2. Available from: http://www.ncbi.nlm.nih.gov/pubmed/29452436.
63. Liu Z, Zhang L, Liu Y, Gu Y, Sun T. Efficiency and safety of one-step procedure combined laparoscopic cholecystectomy and eretrograde cholangiopancreatography for treatment of cholecysto-choledocholithiasis: a randomized controlled trial. Am Surg [Internet]. 2017 Nov 1 [cited 2018 Mar 31];83(11):1263–7. Available from: http://www.ncbi.nlm.nih.gov/pubmed/29183529.
64. Pan L, Chen M, Ji L, Zheng L, Yan P, Fang J, et al. The safety and efficacy of laparoscopic common bile duct exploration combined with cholecystectomy for the management of cholecysto-choledocholithiasis. Ann Surg [Internet]. 2018 Mar 12 [cited 2018 Mar 24];1. Available from: http://www.ncbi.nlm.nih.gov/pubmed/29533266.

Intrahepatic Stones

37

Bernd Kronenberger

37.1 Introduction

Hepatolithiasis is defined as the presence of biliary stones proximal to the confluence of the left and/or right hepatic ducts [1]. Intrahepatic stones may long be asymptomatic. Symptoms occur in association with complications. The most common symptoms are abdominal pain, colics, jaundice, and fever. The main risk factors for hepatolithiasis are cholestasis, infections (by bacteria or intrahepatic parasites), and anatomic abnormalities of the bile duct [1]. Anastomotic strictures, sclerosing cholangitis, congenital choledochal cysts, and Caroli's disease support hepatolithiasis [1, 2]. The characteristic features of hepatolithiasis such as stones, inflammation, and strictures influence each other and aggravate the disease [1]. The prognosis is determined by acute and chronic complications. Ascending infections are the most frequent acute complication. Chronic complications include secondary biliary cirrhosis, segmental or lobar atrophy, liver abscess, and cholangiocarcinoma [1, 3, 4]. Endoscopic treatments involve percutaneous transhepatic cholangioscopic lithotripsy, peroral cholangioscopy, and endoscopic retrograde cholangiopancreatography (ERCP) [1, 3–6]. The surgical treatment includes hepatic resection, reconstruction of bile duct stricture, and liver transplantation [1].

B. Kronenberger (✉)
Department of Internal Medicine, Gastroenterology, Hepatology, Diabetology, Herz-Jesu-Hospital, Fulda, Germany
e-mail: bernd.kronenberger@email.de

37.2 Diagnosis

Transabdominal ultrasound should be the first diagnostic approach in case of suspecting hepatolithiasis. It can identify bile ducts that are obstructed by calcified and non-calcified intrahepatic bile stones. If stones are not visible by transabdominal ultrasound, and to visualize the whole of the biliary tree, magnetic resonance cholangiopancreatography (MRCP) should be the next step. MRCP achieves a sensitivity of 97% for hepatolithiasis and can reliably detect bile duct strictures as well as lesions proximal to the obstruction and outside of the bile ducts [3]. In computed tomography (CT), dilated ducts and strictures and liver abscesses can be demonstrated, while stones are often not directly visible [3]. ERCP is invasive and shows an inferior sensitivity (59%) for the detection of intrahepatic stones [3]. Endoscopic ultrasound can also be used to detect intrahepatic stones [5]. Intrahepatic bile duct stones frequently cause difficulties in diagnosing concomitant cholangiocarcinomas. As hepatolithiasis frequently occurs in association with stones in the gallbladder and with common bile duct stones, similar diagnostic evaluations as for common bile duct stones should be performed.

M. Mutignani et al. (eds.), *Endotherapy in Biliopancreatic Diseases: ERCP Meets EUS*,
https://doi.org/10.1007/978-3-030-42569-2_37

37.3 Treatment

Symptomatic patients and patients with complications have a strong indication for treatment. In asymptomatic patients, watchful waiting may be more appropriate [3]. The primary treatment focus is restoration of bile drainage. Stones should be removed and strictures dilated [4]. The access to intrahepatic stones is more difficult than that to common bile duct stones and may require a multidisciplinary approach.

37.3.1 ERCP

ERCP can only be successful if the bile duct is not completely occluded by bile stones or by strictures. As the sensitivity for detection of hepatolithiasis is limited by ERCP, previous localization of the affected bile ducts by means of imaging is necessary. After endoscopic sphincterotomy, a hydrophilic guidewire should be inserted into the desired duct behind the stone under fluoroscopic control. Then, a balloon catheter or a basket can be maneuvered behind the stone, and if this procedure is successful, the stone can be extracted. However, frustrating attempts to extract the stone may cause further impaction of the stone and deterioration of the patient's condition. If strictures are detected, dilatation should be performed. Stenting may be considered to prevent restenosis.

37.3.2 Cholangioscopy

Peroral cholangioscopy can be performed either by mother-baby technique with a baby cholangioscope that is advanced through the working channel of the duodenoscope (mother-baby Peroral cholangioscopy (POC)) or via direct retrograde videocholangioscopy by insertion of a small-diameter endoscope (5–6 mm) directly into the bile duct (direct retrograde video-cholangioscopy) [7]. Peroral cholangioscopy (POC) offers several options for stone extraction under endoscopy guidance. Small stones can be mobilized by irrigation and suction. Manipulation with forceps or baskets may also be useful to extract stones. Large stones may be destructed by laser or electrohydraulic therapy. The major problem with this technique is to achieve a sufficient stability in advancement of the cholangioscope. POC lithotripsy of hepatolithiasis showed a success rate of 64% [8].

If the transpapillary route is not successful, percutaneous transhepatic cholangioscopy can be performed. However, prerequisite of this technique is percutaneous drainage of the affected bile duct. For percutaneous cholangioscopic lithotripsy, complete stone removal rates of 80–85% have been reported [3]. Postoperative cholangioscopy via the T-tube sinus tract is an option for patients with hepatolithiasis after cholecystectomy with high success rates in the order of 60–90% [4].

37.3.3 Endoscopic Ultrasound-Guided Drainage

Difficult to access bile ducts can be punctured with a fine-needle-aspiration needle from the upper gastrointestinal tract under EUS guidance [9]. Through the needle, a guidewire can be placed in the duodenum, and biliary cannulation can be attempted. EUS-guided puncture of the bile duct can be performed from the duodenal bulb. The left intrahepatic bile ducts are accessible from the stomach. Success rates in the order of 80–95% and adverse events in the order of 15% were reported for this procedure [9].

37.3.4 Extracorporeal Shock Wave Lithotripsy (ESWL)

Bile duct stones which cannot be removed endoscopically can be fragmented by ESWL. The method was shown to be applicable in patients with intrahepatic stones [6]. The method should be combined with other stone extraction procedures such as ERCP.

37.3.5 Surgical Treatment

Hepatectomy is the most invasive approach for treatment of hepatolithiasis. The advantage of hepatectomy is that stones and lesions are removed simultaneously. Surgical resection should be considered in severe, refractory cases with unilateral diseased hepatic lobes or segments with atrophy, fibrosis, cirrhosis, or refractory cholangitis [4, 10]. Hepatectomy is not suitable in patients with bilateral and diffuse intrahepatic stone disease. Stone clearance rates higher than 80% and fewer recurrence rates compared with endoscopic modalities can be achieved [3]. Intraoperative exploration of the bile ducts during hepatectomy can be applied to identify and remove further stones [10].

References

1. Ran X, Yin B, Ma B. Four Major factors contributing to intrahepatic stones. Gastroenterol Res Pract. [Internet]. 2017 [cited 2018 Apr 29];2017:1–5. Available from: http://www.ncbi.nlm.nih.gov/pubmed/28163717.
2. Mabrut J-Y, Kianmanesh R, Nuzzo G, Castaing D, Boudjema K, Létoublon C, et al. Surgical management of congenital intrahepatic bile duct dilatation, Caroli's disease and syndrome. Ann Surg. [Internet]. 2013 [cited 2018 May 5];258:713–21. Available from: http://content.wkhealth.com/linkback/openurl?sid=WKPTLP:landingpage&an=00000658-201311000-00008.
3. European association for the study of the liver (EASL). Electronic address: easloffice@easloffice.eu. EASL Clinical Practice Guidelines on the prevention, diagnosis and treatment of gallstones. J Hepatol. 2016;65(1):146–81. https://doi.org/10.1016/j.jhep.2016.03.005.
4. Wen X, Wang T, Huang Z, Zhang H, Zhang B, Tang L, et al. Step-by-step strategy in the management of residual hepatolithiasis using post-operative cholangioscopy. Therap Adv Gastroenterol. [Internet]. 2017 [cited 2018 Mar 31];10:853–64. Available from: http://www.ncbi.nlm.nih.gov/pubmed/29147136.
5. Puspok A, Lomoschitz F, Dejaco C, Hejna M, Sautner T, Gangl A. Endoscopic ultrasound guided therapy of benign and malignant biliary obstruction: a case series. Am J Gastroenterol. [Internet]. 2005 [cited 2018 May 6];100:1743–7. Available from: http://www.ncbi.nlm.nih.gov/pubmed/16086710.
6. Ellis RD, Jenkins AP, Thompson RP, Ede RJ. Clearance of refractory bile duct stones with extracorporeal shockwave lithotripsy. Gut [Internet]. 2000 [cited 2018 Apr 29];47:728–31. Available from: http://www.ncbi.nlm.nih.gov/pubmed/11034593.
7. Ghersi S, Fuccio L, Bassi M, Fabbri C, Cennamo V. Current status of peroral cholangioscopy in biliary tract diseases. World J Gastrointest Endosc. [Internet]. 2015 [cited 2018 Apr 29];7:510. Available from: http://www.ncbi.nlm.nih.gov/pubmed/25992189.
8. Okugawa T, Tsuyuguchi T, K C S, Ando T, Ishihara T, Yamaguchi T, et al. Peroral cholangioscopic treatment of hepatolithiasis: long-term results. Gastrointest Endosc. [Internet]. 2002 [cited 2018 Apr 29];56:366–71. Available from: http://www.ncbi.nlm.nih.gov/pubmed/12196774.
9. Iwashita T, Yasuda I, Mukai T, Iwata K, Ando N, Doi S, et al. EUS-guided rendezvous for difficult biliary cannulation using a standardized algorithm: a multicenter prospective pilot study (with videos). Gastrointest Endosc. [Internet]. 2016 [cited 2018 May 6];83:394–400. Available from: http://www.ncbi.nlm.nih.gov/pubmed/26089103
10. Zhou Y, Zha W-Z, Wu X-D, Fan R-G, Zhang B, Xu Y-H, et al. Biliary exploration via the left hepatic duct orifice versus the common bile duct in left-sided hepatolithiasis patients with a history of biliary tract surgery. Medicine (Baltimore). [Internet]. 2018 [cited 2018 Mar 24];97:e9643. Available from: http://insights.ovid.com/crossref?an=00005792-201801190-00034.

38 Acute Cholangitis

Bernd Kronenberger

38.1 Introduction

Acute cholangitis is a severe complication of biliary obstruction. The most common cause of cholangitis is common bile duct stones (CBDS); less common causes are benign biliary strictures and neoplasms. Cholangitis is a potentially life-threatening condition when it progresses to sepsis and multiple organ failure [1]. For optimal management, early diagnosis and immediate treatment with antibiotics and biliary drainage are mandatory [1, 2].

38.2 Symptoms

Cholangitis must be suspected in patients with biliary obstruction and symptoms of infection. The typical clinical presentation is abdominal pain, fever, and jaundice (Charcot's triad). Fever is present in most patients with cholangitis (90%), while jaundice is observed in 60–70% only [1]. Abdominal pain may be the single symptom; however, it may also be missing. Furthermore, abdominal pain is not specific for cholangitis because pain is also a typical symptom of cholecystitis. Especially in elderly or in immunocompromised patients, typical clinical criteria may be missing.

38.3 Diagnosis of Cholangitis

The Charcot's triad has a strong specificity (95.9%) but poor sensitivity (26.4%) for cholangitis. Thus, the presence of Charcot's triad strongly suggests acute cholangitis; however, if the criteria are not fulfilled, cholangitis cannot be ruled out [1, 3]. Therefore, additional criteria are necessary.

The diagnosis of cholangitis relies on the presence of infection/inflammation on the one hand and biliary obstruction on the other hand. The evaluation of patients with suspected cholangitis starts with a profound clinical examination with focus on assessment of the level of consciousness, of yellowing of the conjunctiva, and of abdominal pain [4]. Vital signs such as blood pressure, heart rate, and body temperature must be determined [4].

Laboratory parameters for infection/inflammation such as leukocyte count, CRP, and/or procalcitonin should be determined as well as liver function parameters such as alanine aminotransferase (ALT), aspartate aminotransferase (AST), gamma-glutamyl transferase (GGT), alkaline phosphatase (ALP), and bilirubin [4]. Furthermore, a transabdominal ultrasound should be performed. If the diagnosis is unclear, com-

B. Kronenberger (✉)
Department of Internal Medicine, Gastroenterology, Hepatology, Diabetology, Herz-Jesu-Hospital, Fulda, Germany
e-mail: bernd.kronenberger@email.de

M. Mutignani et al. (eds.), *Endotherapy in Biliopancreatic Diseases: ERCP Meets EUS*, https://doi.org/10.1007/978-3-030-42569-2_38

puted tomography (CT) or magnetic resonance imaging (MRI)/magnetic resonance cholangiopancreatography (MRCP) should be considered. The performance of the different diagnostic approaches for CBDS and cholestasis is described in detail in the respective chapter.

A risk stratification for the probability of cholangitis can be performed according to the Tokyo guidelines (TG18/13). The guidelines report a diagnostic algorithm including clinical signs and laboratory and imaging criteria for infection and cholestasis to predict acute cholangitis (Table 38.1) [1]. Validation of the TG18/13 criteria showed a high sensitivity (87.6%) and specificity (77.7%) for acute cholangitis [1]. The algorithm can be used for risk stratification and management of acute cholangitis [3].

If acute cholangitis is suspected but criteria are not fulfilled, a diagnostic reassessment every 6–12 h should be performed until a diagnosis is reached [5].

38.4 Initial Management

First-line treatment includes general supportive measures including adequate intravenous hydration and empiric antibiotic treatment [4]. The need for biliary drainage depends on severity of cholangitis. Assessment of the severity of cholangitis is also described in the Tokyo guidelines. The stratification mainly depends on signs of sepsis with organ dysfunction (Table 38.2) [1].

Table 38.1 TG18/TG13 diagnostic criteria for acute cholangitis

A. Systemic inflammation	
A-1	Fever >38 °C and/or shaking chills
A-2	Laboratory data: evidence of inflammatory response
	WBC count <4000 or >10,000/μL or CRP ≥ 1 mg/dL
B. Cholestasis	
B-1	Jaundice (bilirubin ≥2 mg/dL)
B-2	Laboratory data: abnormal liver function tests (ALT, AST, GGT, ALP > 1.5XSTD)
C. Imaging	
C-1	Biliary dilatation
C-2	Evidence of the etiology on imaging (stricture, stone, stent, etc.)

Modified according to [1]

Suspected diagnosis: one item in A plus one item in either B or C

Definite diagnosis: one item in A, one item in B, and one item in C

38.4.1 Grade III (Severe Acute Cholangitis)

Severe acute cholangitis is defined as cholangitis with sepsis induced-organ failure. Grade III cholangitis is present when any one of the following criteria is met: cardiovascular dysfunction, neurological dysfunction, respiratory dysfunction, renal dysfunction, or hematological dysfunction [4]. Grade III cholangitis is a life-threatening condition which requires immediate appropriate respiratory and circulatory management. Tracheal intubation and artificial ventilation and catecholamines may be necessary. Antibiotic treatment is urgent. Biliary drainage is urgent and should be performed as soon as possible after the patient's condition has been improved by initial treatment [4]. If the patient is not stable for endoscopic retrograde cholangiopancreatography (ERCP), per-

Table 38.2 Severity assessment criteria for acute cholangitis

Grade III (severe) acute cholangitis (at least one condition)
Cardiovascular dysfunction: hypotension requiring dopamine ≥5 μg/kg per min or any dose of norepinephrine
Neurological dysfunction: disturbance of consciousness
Respiratory dysfunction: PaO_2/FiO_2 ratio <300
Renal dysfunction: PT-INR >1.5
Hematological dysfunction: platelet count <100,000/mm^3
Grade II (moderate) acute cholangitis (at least two conditions)
Abnormal WBC count (>12,000/mm^3, <4000/mm^3)
High fever (≥29 °C)
Age (≥75 years)
Hyperbilirubinemia (total bilirubin ≥5 mg/dL)
Hypoalbuminemia (<STD × 0.73)
Grade I (mild) acute cholangitis
Not grade II or grade III

Modified according to [1]

cutaneous transhepatic biliary drainage could be performed as an alternative in some cases [4].

38.4.2 Grade II (Moderate Acute Cholangitis)

Moderate cholangitis is present if at least two of the following criteria are fulfilled: WBC ≥12,000 or <4000, temperature ≥39 °C, age ≥75 years, total bilirubin ≥5 mg/dL, or albumin <lower limit of normal (× 0.73). Moderate acute cholangitis requires early biliary drainage.

38.4.3 Grade I (Mild Acute Cholangitis)

Patients with mild cholangitis do not meet the criteria for grade II and III cholangitis. Empiric antibiotic treatment and general supportive care are sufficient. Most patients do not require biliary drainage [4]. Biliary drainage should be considered in patients who do not respond to initial therapy [4].

38.5 Antimicrobial Therapy [6]

Antibiotic treatment is the mainstay of treatment for patients with cholangitis. A large spectrum of bacteria including gram-negative (*Escherichia coli*, *Klebsiella* spp., *Pseudomonas* spp., *Enterobacter* spp., *Acinetobacter* spp., *Citrobacter* spp.), gram-positive microorganisms (*Enterococcus* spp., *Streptococcus* spp., *Staphylococcus* spp.) and anaerobes can be found in the bile [6, 7]. Blood cultures should be obtained before starting antibiotic treatment [6]. At the beginning of any procedure, bile cultures should be performed [6]. Bile cultures are more often positive than blood culture and frequently reveal a polymicrobial content [7]. Antibiotics for empiric therapy should be chosen according to the local resistance patterns and the severity of the cholangitis. Due to the polymicrobial content of infected bile, broad-spectrum antibiotics covering aerobic gram-negative and anaerobic bacteria should be chosen at initial therapy. Antibiotic treatment should be adapted when results from bile and blood cultures are available [7]. For grade III acute cholangitis, agents with anti-pseudomonal activity are recommended as empirical therapy [6]. Once the source of infection is controlled, antimicrobial therapy should be maintained for 4–7 days [6].

38.6 Biliary Decompression

As described in the previous chapter about common bile duct stones (CBDS), several methods for biliary decompression exist. ERCP is less invasive than surgical methods and percutaneous drainage and comes along with a better outcome [8]. Therefore, ERCP should be the first choice for treatment of biliary obstruction in patients with cholangitis [8]. Empiric antibiotic treatment should start before endoscopy, and stabilization of the patients, especially those with severe cholangitis, is mandatory. Patients with severe grade III cholangitis should receive intervention within 12 h if they are stable. The greatest benefit from early biliary decompression within 24 h seems to have patients with moderate grade II cholangitis because decompression may stop progression to grade III cholangitis [6].

The primary goal of endoscopic treatment of cholangitis is biliary decompression which can be achieved by biliary stenting or nasobiliary drainage with equal efficacy [8]. To reduce the risk of bleeding, endoscopic sphincterotomy can also be avoided [8]. If CBDS are present, removal can be performed in a single session if the extraction is uncomplicated and patients are in a hemodynamic stable condition. In patients with severe cholangitis or in patients with difficult stones, removal should be performed in a second session after drainage [8]. If treatment by ERCP is not possible, percutaneous transhepatic drainage and endoscopic ultrasonography-guided drainage are alternative options [8]. Those treatment options are described in the respective chapter.

References

1. Ramchandani M, Pal P, Reddy DN. Endoscopic management of acute cholangitis as a result of common bile duct stones. Dig Endosc. [Internet]. 2017 [cited 2018 Apr 28];29:78–87. Available from: http://www.ncbi.nlm.nih.gov/pubmed/28425658.
2. Karvellas CJ, Abraldes JG, Zepeda-Gomez S, Moffat DC, Mirzanejad Y, Vazquez-Grande G, et al. The impact of delayed biliary decompression and antimicrobial therapy in 260 patients with cholangitis-associated septic shock. Aliment Pharmacol Ther. [Internet]. 2016 [cited 2018 Apr 28];44:755–66. Available from: http://doi.wiley.com/10.1111/apt.13764.
3. Kiriyama S, Kozaka K, Takada T, Strasberg SM, Pitt HA, Gabata T, et al. Tokyo Guidelines 2018: diagnostic criteria and severity grading of acute cholangitis (with videos). J Hepatobiliary Pancreat Sci. [Internet]. 2018 [cited 2018 Apr 28];25:17–30. Available from: http://www.ncbi.nlm.nih.gov/pubmed/29032610.
4. Miura F, Okamoto K, Takada T, Strasberg SM, Asbun HJ, Pitt HA, et al. Tokyo Guidelines 2018: initial management of acute biliary infection and flowchart for acute cholangitis. J Hepatobiliary Pancreat Sci. [Internet]. 2018 [cited 2018 Apr 28];25:31–40. Available from: http://www.ncbi.nlm.nih.gov/pubmed/28941329.
5. Mayumi T, Okamoto K, Takada T, Strasberg SM, Solomkin JS, Schlossberg D, et al. Tokyo Guidelines 2018: management bundles for acute cholangitis and cholecystitis. J Hepatobiliary Pancreat Sci. [Internet]. 2018 [cited 2018 Apr 28];25:96–100. Available from: http://www.ncbi.nlm.nih.gov/pubmed/29090868.
6. Gomi H, Solomkin JS, Schlossberg D, Okamoto K, Takada T, Strasberg SM, et al. Tokyo Guidelines 2018: antimicrobial therapy for acute cholangitis and cholecystitis. J Hepatobiliary Pancreat Sci. [Internet]. 2018 [cited 2018 Apr 28];25:3–16. Available from: http://www.ncbi.nlm.nih.gov/pubmed/29090866.
7. European Association for the Study of the Liver (EASL). Electronic address: easloffice@easloffice.eu. EASL clinical practice guidelines on the prevention, diagnosis and treatment of gallstones. J Hepatol. 2016;65(1):146–81. https://doi.org/10.1016/j.jhep.2016.03.005.
8. Mukai S, Itoi T, Baron TH, Takada T, Strasberg SM, Pitt HA, et al. Indications and techniques of biliary drainage for acute cholangitis in updated Tokyo Guidelines 2018. J Hepatobiliary Pancreat Sci. [Internet]. 2017 [cited 2018 Apr 28];24:537–549. Available from: http://www.ncbi.nlm.nih.gov/pubmed/28834389.

Papillectomy: Clinical Results

39

Alberto Mariani

Adenoma is the most common benign ampullary lesion and clinically most important because of its potential to undergo malignant transformation to ampullary cancer. Adenocarcinoma is the most common malignant ampullary lesion, the others mainly being neuroendocrine carcinoma, signet ring cell carcinoma, and some metastatic neoplasms, such as melanoma and lymphoma. While the standard treatment of ampullary carcinoid tumor and high-grade neuroendocrine carcinoma is surgery, that of an ampullary adenoma is more and more frequently endoscopy, also because of its early and increased detection by routine screening endoscopic procedures and advanced imaging modalities.

The goal of endoscopic papillectomy (EP) is to achieve complete resection of ampullary neoplasms. The complete resection is the only method of ascertaining that an ampullary adenoma does not harbor undetected foci of carcinoma. To reach this goal, a careful selection of patients in referral centers with expertise in endoscopic retrograde cholangiopancreatography (ERCP) is a crucial issue. No specific guidelines about the management of EP are available.

A. Mariani (✉)
Pancreato-Biliary Endoscopy and Endosonography Division, Pancreas Translational and Clinical Research Center, San Raffaele Scientific Institute IRCCS, Vita Salute San Raffaele University, Milan, Italy
e-mail: mariani.alberto@hsr.it

39.1 Indications

Standardized indications for EP are not yet well established [1–4].

- EP is considered as the procedure of choice for the curative treatment of ampullary adenoma without evidence of intraductal involvement. Endoscopic characteristics of a benign lesion generally include well-defined and not friable margins, absence of ulcerations, and soft consistency.
- EP may be considered as a curative treatment in case of ampullary adenoma with high-grade intraepithelial dysplasia or well-differentiated in situ tumor (Tis).
- EP may be indicated in patients with intramucosal cancer (T1 cancer confined to mucosa) and/or intraductal involvement who are unfit for surgery or refuse surgery, making it clear that radical surgery is the only curative treatment for these patients.

39.2 Contraindications

- Absolute contraindications to EP are metastases, invasive cancer beyond the mucosa (increased risk of metastatic lymph nodes), and intraductal extension ≥1 cm [5, 6].
- Relative contraindications are tumor size ≥4 cm, T1 cancer confined to mucosa,

M. Mutignani et al. (eds.), *Endotherapy in Biliopancreatic Diseases: ERCP Meets EUS*,
https://doi.org/10.1007/978-3-030-42569-2_39

intraductal extension <1 cm, poor patient compliance to follow-up, and no ERCP expertise.

Preoperative assessment of tumor depth (T staging) by using abdominal endoscopic ultrasound (EUS) and/or computed tomography (CT) is needed to decide between endoscopic and surgical resection.

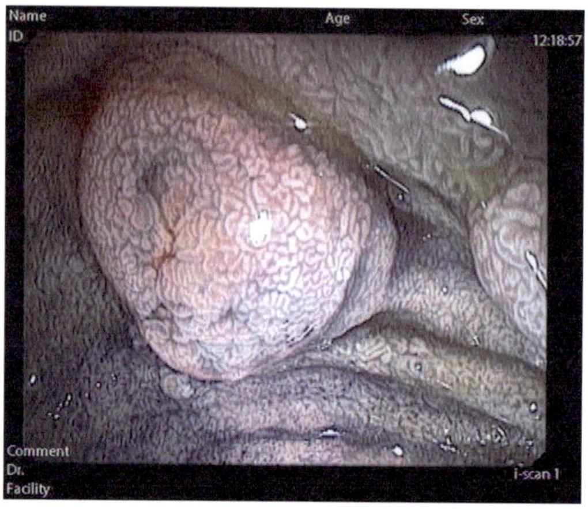

Fig. 39.1 Endoscopic images showing lesions at the papilla in patients previously evaluated by using abdominal CT and EUS to provide indication for endoscopic papillectomy (EP)—adenoma with low-grade dysplasia for which EP was a curative treatment. At the time of EP, the histological examination of the resected tissue showed no signs of carcinoma and negative resection margins

Figures 39.1, 39.2, 39.3, and 39.4 show endoscopic images of some papillary lesions with their indication for EP.

39.3 Clinical Results

Most of the published studies evaluating the results of EP for the treatment of papillary tumors are referred to retrospective small and single center series [4]. In Table 39.1, the results of prospective and the largest retrospective published series are reported [3, 6–13]. Overall success rate is 85%, ranging from 73 to 100%. Overall recurrence rate of ampullary adenoma is equal to 14%, ranging from 5.4 to 29.8%. The wide range of the reported success depends on the heterogeneity in study design, inclusion criteria, techniques, and, not least, the definition of success. Some authors define success at the time of first treatment in presence of a complete excision of the lesion on visual inspection; others define success as the absence of recurrence on follow-up. Anyway it may be difficult to assess whether the tumor has been completely removed or not, because of possible coagulation artifacts at its lateral margins or of difficulties to detect its intraductal ingrowth. This is a reason for an appropriate surveillance endoscopy. When the ampullary adenoma is a part of familial adenomatous polyposis (FAP),

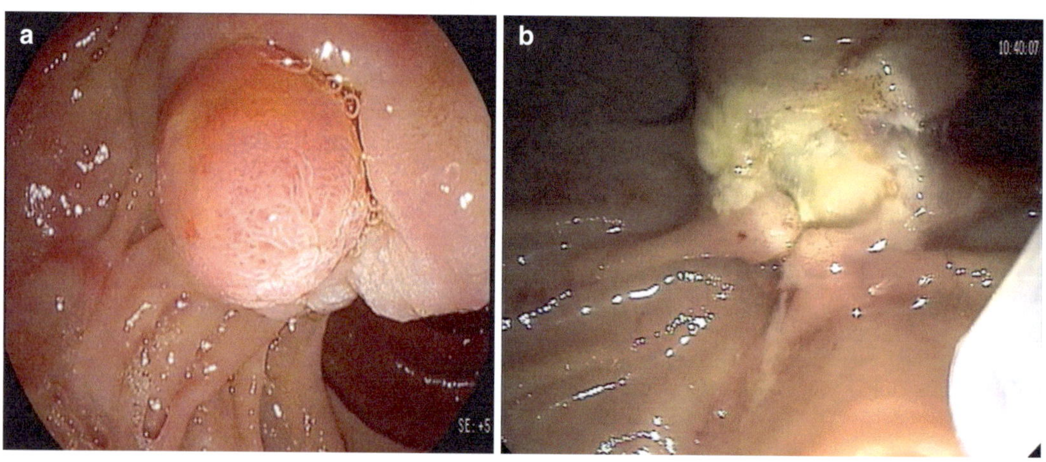

Fig. 39.2 Endoscopic images showing lesions at the papilla in patients previously evaluated by using abdominal CT and EUS to provide indication for endoscopic papillectomy (EP)—(**a**) Adenoma with high-grade dysplasia; (**b**) papillectomy which was a curative treatment: at 5 years of follow-up, no residual tumor was detected

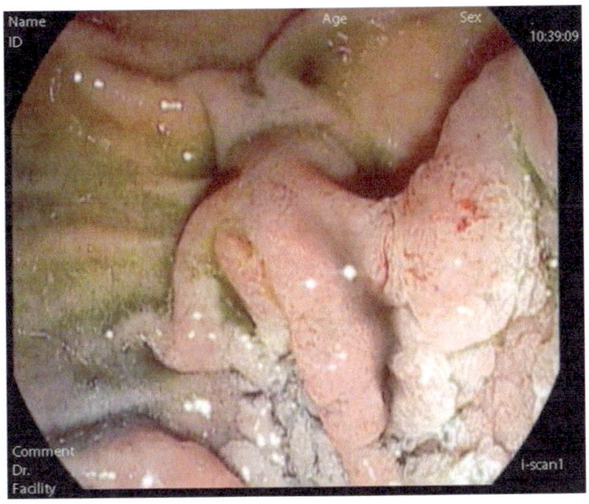

Fig. 39.3 Endoscopic images showing lesions at the papilla in patients previously evaluated by using abdominal CT and EUS to provide indication for endoscopic papillectomy (EP)—adenoma with low-grade dysplasia associated with a large laterally spreading tumor of the second portion of the duodenum cured by EP and piecemeal mucosectomy, respectively

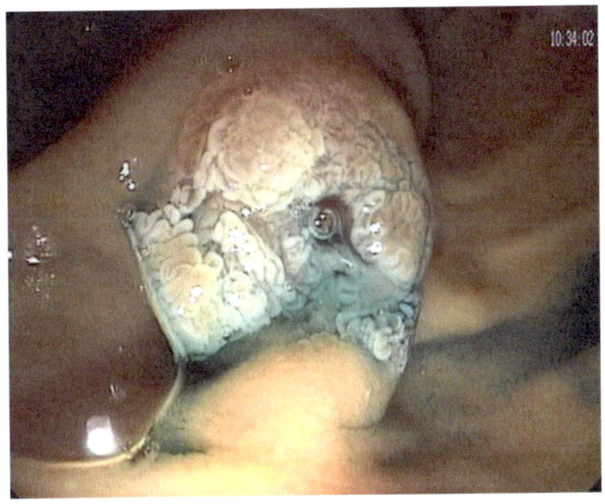

Fig. 39.4 Endoscopic images showing lesions at the papilla in patients previously evaluated by using abdominal CT and EUS to provide indication for endoscopic papillectomy (EP)—intramucosal cancer for which EP was performed in a patient who was unfit for surgery

the indication for EP remains controversial because the complete excision of the tumor may not eliminate the risk of recurrence; therefore, some authors suggest the simple endoscopic surveillance with biopsies only. Such an approach has the advantage of avoiding the risks of EP but the limitations of underestimating foci of high-grade dysplasia or carcinoma.

In a recent retrospective monocenter series [13], 110 consecutive patients underwent EP between 2000 and 2017 and were followed-up for a mean of 31.6 months (range 1–108) scheduling endoscopic re-evaluation at 1, 3, 6, and 12 months after EP for the first year and yearly for the following 5 years. Indications were dysplasia in 57.2% of cases, focal or intramucosal adenocarcinoma in 37.4%, and neuroendocrine tumor in 5.4%. 77.3% of these patients were submitted to en bloc resection and 22.7% to piecemeal resection. Complications were observed in 22 patients (20% of cases): delayed bleeding in 19 (17.3%) and retroperitoneal perforation in three (2.7%), all of which were successfully treated by surgical or percutaneous drainage. Forty-seven patients (42.7%) had residual (29.8%) or recurrent (20.2%) adenomas successfully retreated by endoscopy in 43 and surgery in four.

There are some factors that affect the success rate. Predictors of long-term success on multivariate analysis include patient age >48 years, lesion size ≤24 mm, male sex, and absence of polyposis syndrome [7]. Absence of dilated ducts may predict clinical success [9]; the presence of intraductal adenoma growth may predict clinical failure and greater need for surgery [6]. Failure to achieve a cleavage plane with submucosal injection has been shown as the strongest predictor of malignancy [8]. Risk factors for recurrence include high-grade dysplasia and, also if not fully demonstrated, larger lesion size (>24 mm) [9, 14] which are more likely to be incompletely excised at the initial endoscopic procedure. Pancreatobiliary histologic subtype is an adverse prognostic factor [15].

39.4 Results in Relation to EP Techniques

En bloc resection ought to be the preferable EP technique compared to piecemeal because it may provide a complete tissue sample with clear margins for precise histopathologic evaluation and in a shorter procedure time. Piecemeal resection is usually limited to larger and more sessile lesions which are theoretically at higher risk of incom-

Table 39.1 Outcome of papillectomy in prospective or large sample size retrospective studies

References	Design	No. of patients	FAP %	Success %	Recurrence %	Need for surgery %	Follow-up mean months (range)
Catalano et al. [7]	Retrospective Multicenter	103	31	83	10	16	36 (12–78)
Kahaleh et al. [8]	Prospective Single center?	56	[a]	86	nr	[a]	[a]
Bohnacker et al. [6]	Prospective Single center	106	5	73	15	9	40 (22–174)
Irani et al. [9]	Retrospective Single center	102	22	84	8	16	32 (2–68)[b]; 48 (3–88)[c]
Salmi et al. [3]	Prospective Single center	61	10	82	8.8	8.2	36
Onkendy et al. [10]	Retrospective Single center[d]	130	42	[a]	29	7	52
Napoleon et al. [11]	Prospective Multicenter	93	21	81	5.4	5.4	33 (1–36)
Kang et al. [12]	Retrospective Multicenter	104	[a]	89.4	6.7	7.7	44.2 (6–90)
Valerij et al. [13]	Retrospective Single center[e]	110	25	100	29.8	11	31.6 (1–108)
Klein et al. [18]	Retrospective Single center	125	11.2	97.6	17 (at first surveillance)	6.4	29 (18–48)[f]
Total		990					
Mean				86.2	14.4	9.6	38
Range				73–100	5.4–29.8	5.4–16	1–174

[a]Not reported
[b]Sporadic
[c]FAP (familial adenomatous polyposis)
[d]Comparison of endoscopy and surgery
[e]Abstract
[f]Median and interquartile range

plete resection and consequently higher recurrences. In the only published comparative series [16], 81 patients with ampullary adenomas and 44 with laterally spreading lesions of the papilla of Vater (LSL-P) were resected endoscopically over 9 years. LSL-P had comparable outcomes to standard papillectomy (similar recurrence at first surveillance: 16.4% vs. 17.9%), despite higher rates of intra-procedural and delayed bleeding (Table 39.2). At the first follow-up evaluation, histologically proven recurrence was associated with piecemeal resection (P = 0.02) and number of resected specimens (P = 0.02) but not with lesion size.

Whether or not submucosal injection of a diluted epinephrine solution should be used to lift ampullary tumors during endoscopic snare papillectomy is unclear. In a prospective multicenter study, 50 patients with biopsy-proven papillary adenomas were randomized to undergo either simple snare papillectomy (SSP) or submucosal injection papillectomy (SIP) using 1:10,000 diluted epinephrine [17]. Complete resection rates in the SSP and SIP groups were 80.8% (21/26) and 50.0% (12/24), respectively (P = 0.02). However, rates of tumor persistence at 1 month (15.4% vs. 8.3%, P = 0.62), recurrence at 12 months (12.0% vs. 9.5%, P = 0.58), and adverse events, such as bleeding (42.3% vs. 45.8%, P = 0.80), were similar. According to these results, SSP may be a simpler and primarily recommendable technique.

Table 39.2 Complications of papillectomy

References	Design	Patients no.	Overall %	Pancreatitis %	Bleeding %	Perforation %	Papillary stenosis %	Cholangitis %	Mortality %
Catalano et al. [7]	Retrospective Multicenter	103	10	5	2	0	3	0	0
Kahaleh et al. [8]	Prospective Single center?	56	13	7	4	0	2	0	2
Bohnacker et al. [6]	Prospective Single-center	106	19	6	13	0	–	0	0
Irani et al. [9]	Retrospective Single-center	102	21	10	5	2	1	3	0
Salmi et al. [3]	Prospective Single center	61	18	10	5	3	–	–	0
Onkendy et al. [10]	Retrospective Single center	130	29	14.6	13	0.7	–	0	0
Napoleon et al. [11]	Prospective Multicenter	93	35	20	10	3.6	1.8	7	0.9
Kang et al. [12]	Retrospective Multicenter	104	32	15.4	17.3	7.7	–	–	1.9
Valerij et al. [13]	Retrospective Single center	110	20	0	17.3	2.7	–	–	0
Klein et al. [18]	Retrospective Single center	125	–	7.6 vs. 7.1[a]	50 vs. 24.7[a,b] 25 vs. 12.3[a,c]	0.8	–	–	0
Total		990							
Mean			21.9	9.5	9.6	2	0.9	1.1	0.5
Range			10–35	0–15.4	2–17.3	0–7.7	1–3	0–7	0–2

[a]Laterally spreading lesions vs. conventional ampullary adenomas
[b]Immediate bleeding
[c]Delayed bleeding

39.5 Adverse Events

Adverse events reported in prospective and large retrospective series are shown in Table 39.2. According to these series, the overall adverse events rate is about 22%, ranging from 10 to 35%. The mortality rate is very low, averaging 0.4% (range from 0 to 2%). The most frequent adverse events are bleeding and pancreatitis. Underlying malignancy and lateral extension have been reported as possible risk factors for bleeding and perforation, respectively [9]. Immediate bleeding can be stopped by epinephrine injection, electrocautery, or clip placement, while delayed bleeding may require blood transfusion. The release of clips through a duodenoscope is technically challenging and requires the correct use of the elevator for a proper positioning. Caution has to be given to the site of clips' release, avoiding the occlusion of the biliary and/or pancreatic orifice.

The overall rate of pancreatitis is about 10% so that EP can be considered a high-risk procedure for such a complication, despite most cases being mild. It is difficult to establish whether pancreatitis results from resection, the electrocautery setting, or intraprocedural manipulations, including sphincterotomy, stenting, and potential additional ablation. As shown in Table 39.3, from most of the studies, rates of pancreatitis were lower in patients with pancreatic stent in place than in those without. It is useful to mention that the presence of pancreas divisum makes the prophylactic pancreatic stent placement unnecessary.

In the only randomized, controlled trial that evaluated the protective effect of pancreatic stents, placed immediately after EP without pancreatic sphincterotomy [18], the rate of pancreatitis was significantly lower in the stent group (0 vs. 33 %, $P = 0.02$). However, the positive results of this study could be limited by the fact that a single additional pancreatitis in the stent group would have significantly modified the effectiveness of the stenting. In a French large prospective multicenter study [11], the effectiveness of pro-

Table 39.3 Rates of pancreatitis according to the placement of pancreatic stent in patients undergoing papillectomy

References	Design	Patients no.	Pancreatitis no. (%)	Pancreatic stent %	No pancreatic stent %	*P* value
Catalano et al. [7]	Retrospective Multicenter	103	5 (5)	3	17	ns
Kahaleh et al. [8]	Prospective Single center	56	4 (7)	75	2	ns
Bohnacker et al. [6]	Prospective Single center	106	13 (6)	11	14	ns
Irani et al. [9]	Retrospective Single center	102	10 (10)	10	13	ns
Salmi et al. [3]	Prospective Single center	61	6 (10)	3	20	<0.05
Onkendy et al. [10]	Retrospective Single center[a]	130	19 (14.6)	63	6	[b]
Napoleon et al. [11]	Prospective Multicenter	93	22 (20)	14	25	=0.046
Kang et al. [12]	Retrospective Multicenter	104	16 (15.4)	20	9.1	ns
Valerij et al. [13]	Retrospective Single center[c]	110	0	[b]	[b]	[b]
Klein et al. [18]	Retrospective Single center	125	9 (7.2)	6.6	13.3	ns
Total		990				
Mean			104 (10.5)			
Range %			0–15.4			

ns not significant
[a]Comparison of endoscopy and surgery
[b]Not reported
[c]Abstract

phylactic pancreatic stenting after EP was confirmed by a significantly lower rate of acute pancreatitis in the stent group (14% vs. 25%). The duration of pancreatic stenting ranges from 24 h to 3 months [4]: a short stent duration (from 1 to 3 days) minimizes stent-induced ductal changes. Both the 5-F stent and the 3-F stent have similar spontaneous passage at 2 weeks; however, the former has the advantage of an easier and faster placement [19].

Although further data is needed, the use of prophylactic pancreatic stenting after EP should be suggested to reduce the incidence of post-procedural pancreatitis and papillary stenosis as well [20]. Whether rectal nonsteroidal anti-inflammatory drugs (NSAIDs) alone or in addition to pancreatic stenting has a better prophylactic effect is still to be evaluated.

However, when immediately at the end of papillectomy the pancreatic orifice remains well visible, the placement of a pancreatic stent may be avoided. Similar considerations can be given for the prevention or reduction of the risk of papillary stenosis which is a late complication of EP. Some investigators advocate routinely placing pancreatic stent [6, 7, 9, 21], but others suggest its selected use only in cases of delayed pancreatic drainage after EP [8, 22]. Similarly, a systematic use of prophylactic biliary stenting to reduce the risk of cholangitis and of biliary stricture is usually considered unnecessary, except in cases of suspected inadequate biliary drainage (sphincterotomy plus stenting) [20]. Some experts also perform biliary stent placement when there is a concern for microperforation after resection.

Figures 39.5, 39.6, and 39.7 show the endoscopic view of hemostatic treatments of post-EP bleeding.

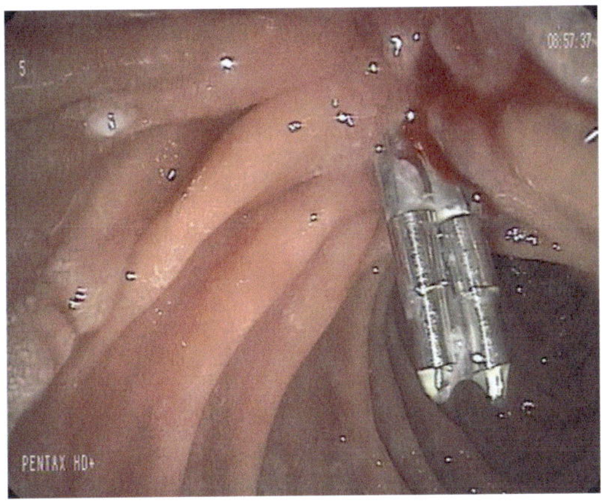

Fig. 39.5 Treatment of post-EP bleeding—after en bloc resection, two hemoclips were applied for bleeding control

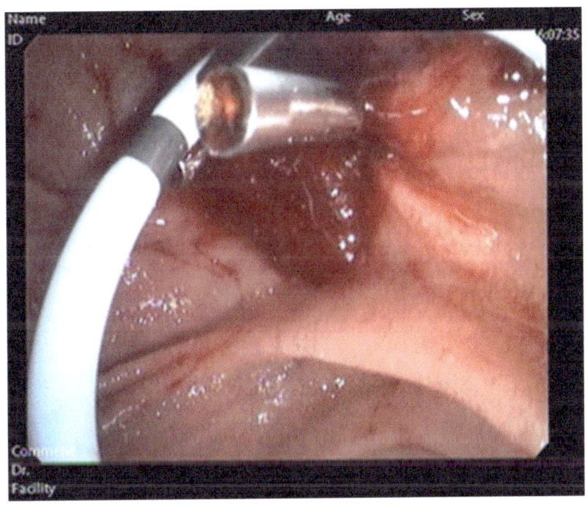

Fig. 39.6 Treatment of post-EP bleeding—hemostasis after placement of one hemoclip in a patient with bleeding the day after EP and with prophylactic pancreatic stent in place

39.6 Surveillance for Residual or Recurrent Neoplastic Tissue

It is not always possible to establish the difference between residual and recurrent neoplastic tissue. The detection of a worse histology in a short follow-up period is, for example, more suspicious for residual than recurrent tumor. The optimal strategy for post-EP surveillance is unknown. The surveillance intervals are not standardized and can be related to the degree of dysplasia, estimate of resection completeness, and evidence of intraductal involvement. Some authors suggest a first endoscopic re-evaluation at 1–6 months after the index procedure followed by intervals of 3–12 months during at least 2 years [20]. Endoscopic surveillance program is needed to ensure complete tissue removal and to assess for disease recurrence. As reported in

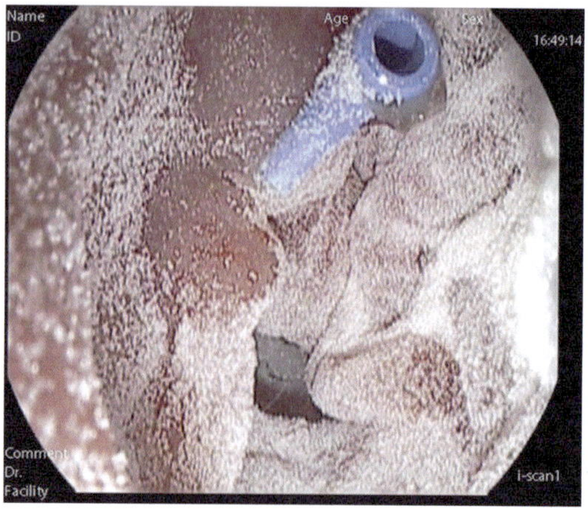

Fig. 39.7 Treatment of post-EP bleeding—hemostasis by spraying with inorganic Hemospray powder (Cook Medical) just after the placement of a prophylactic pancreatic stent

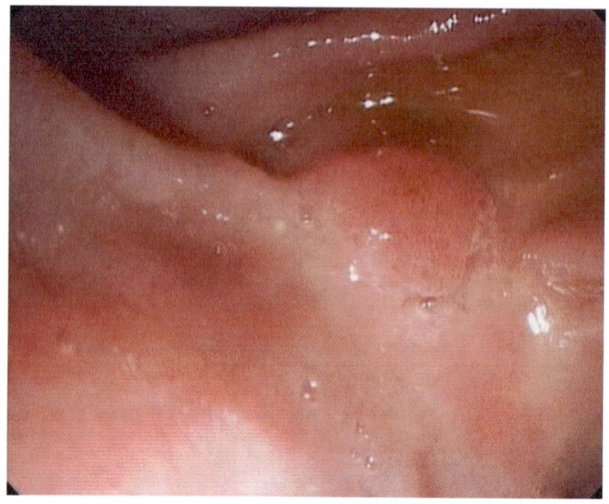

Fig. 39.9 Endoscopic findings of papillary area during follow-up—recurrent adenomatous tissue at the top of the scar area

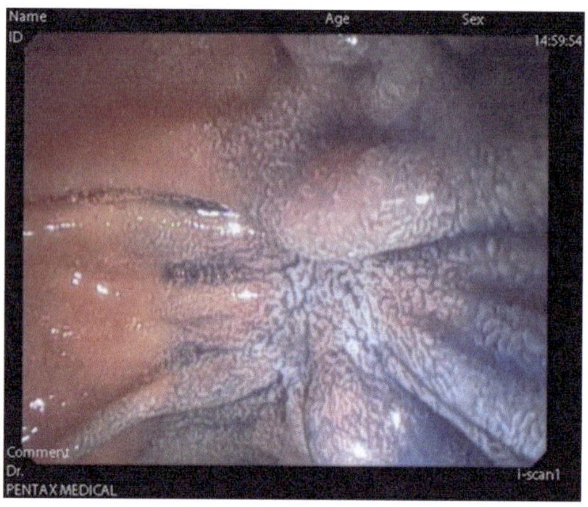

Fig. 39.8 Endoscopic findings of papillary area during follow-up—endoscopic view revealing no residual tumor at 2 years after EP

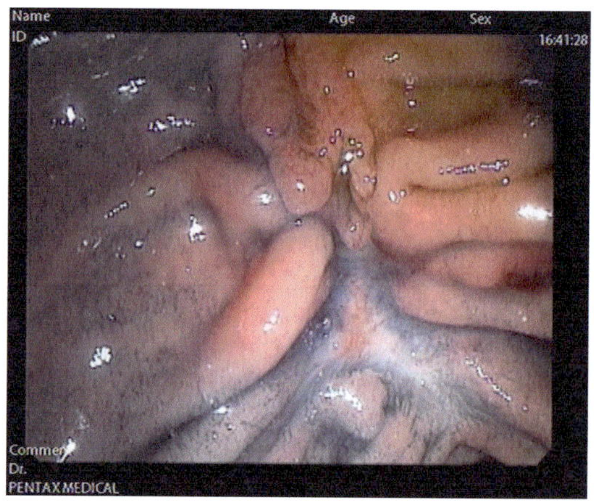

Fig. 39.10 Endoscopic findings of papillary area during follow-up—recurrent adenomatous tissue at the top of the scar area

ASGE guidelines on the role of endoscopy in ampullary and duodenal adenomas [20], some authors recommend a post-resection surveillance strategy for sporadic (non-FAP) ampullary polyps similar to that used for patients with colon polyps treated with piecemeal resection.

As shown in Table 39.1, recurrence rates after EP range from 5.4 to 29.8%.

In Figs. 39.8, 39.9, 39.10, and 39.11, endoscopic images of surveillance after EP are shown.

39.7 Treatment of Residual or Recurrent Endobiliary Neoplastic Tissue

Considering surgical risks, local endobiliary treatment, such as intraductal radiofrequency ablation (ID-RFA), can play a role in the management of residual or recurrent endobiliary neoplastic tissue after EP. In patients with short intrabiliary extension of ampullary adenomas,

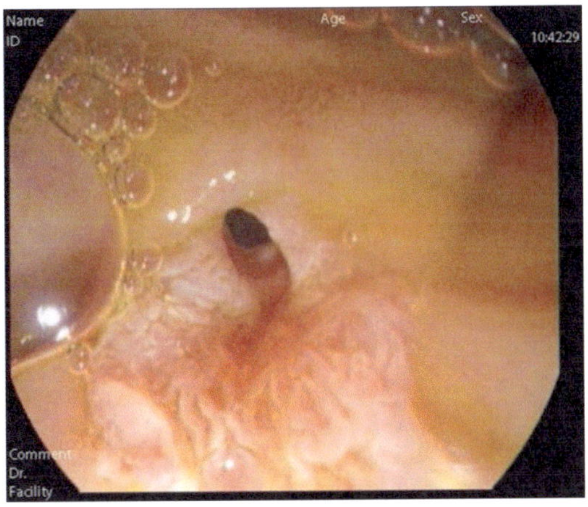

Fig. 39.11 Endoscopic findings of papillary area during follow-up—recurrent adenomatous tissue at the lower area of the biliary orifice

ID-RFA can be an effective alternative therapeutic option to pancreaticoduodenectomy, which generally remains the standard of care. ID-RFA is simpler and easier to use than photodynamic therapy or argon plasma coagulation, but definitive studies establishing its benefit are lacking.

In a recent study [23], 20 patients with histologically proven endobiliary adenoma remnant (15 low-grade and five high-grade dysplasia with ductal extent <20 mm) after EP for ampullary tumor were enrolled in a prospective multicenter study to evaluate the efficacy and safety of ID-RFA. All patients underwent one successful ID-RFA session (Habib Endo HPB 8F bipolar wire-guide catheter; setting: 10 W, effect 8, 30 s) followed by biliary stent placement and, in five of them (25%), by pancreatic stent too. The rates of residual adenoma were 15% and 30% at 6 and 12 months, respectively. At 12 months, the success rate of RFA was equal to 70%, and only two patients (10%) were referred for surgery: one with adenocarcinoma on endobiliary biopsies at 6 months and the other with suspected carcinoma that had low-grade dysplasia at histology instead. Eight patients (40%) experienced at least one adverse event: three mild pancreatitis (medical treatment), one melena (red blood transfusion), one cholangitis (medical treatment), and three mild biliary strictures (dilation and fully covered self-expanding metal stent [SEMS], placement). No major adverse events occurred. Treatment failure at 12 months (=dysplasia recurrence) was higher in patients with high-grade dysplasia than in those with low grade dysplasia (67% vs. 7%; $P = 0.014$).

Although no patients developed an invasive carcinoma on pathologic analysis, authors underlined the need for a close follow-up in all patients undergoing ID-RFA treatment. Adenomas may grow slowly, and residual intraductal adenoma might be missed for long periods of time. In their method, authors scheduled ERCP and EUS at 6 and 12 months with systematic endobiliary biopsy sampling and brush cytology.

The optimal electrosurgical generator settings and duration of biliary ID-RFA treatment are unknown. It is not clear if multiple ID-RFA sessions and/or higher settings are more effective, especially in patients with negative predictors of ID-RFA success, those with endobiliary adenoma remnant with high-grade dysplasia. Against a high efficacy, ID-RFA treatment may be affected by high rates of biliary strictures and pancreatitis, as observed in a retrospective series by Rustagi et al. [24]. Seventeen patients underwent a mean of 2.6 treatment sessions, with applications longer than 60 s, sometimes with multiple treatment applications during each ERCP. Seven patients had additional treatments (thermal probes, argon plasma coagulation, and/or photodynamic therapy). ID-RFA alone was effective in 100% of cases, but 36% developed a biliary stricture. Other studies also reported post-RFA infectious adverse events, such as cholecystitis and periduodenal abscess [25, 26].

Some authors [26, 27] to decrease complications, suggest to not perform EP and biliary ID-RFA during the same treatment session. They perform intraductal RFA 6–12 weeks later EP by allowing the papillectomy site to heal.

After RFA treatment, a biliary stent placement is recommended, but it is unclear whether fully covered SEMS offer an advantage over plastic stents. Concerning the pancreatic stenting, with the limitations of the small sample size, the study of Camus showed a trend toward less post-procedure pancreatitis when pancreatic duct stents were used. The effects of intraductal biliary RFA by means of a newly designed temperature controlled RFA catheter (ELRA® STARmed, Seoul, Korea) are under evaluation.

39.8 Ablative Therapies

Argon plasma coagulation (APC) is a monopolar electrosurgical procedure that may be used as additional treatment during EP for thermal ablation of residual adenoma and/or hemostasis after snare resection [9]. It may be better not to systematically use APC, as we carry out repeated snaring to resect all visible remnant tumors first, rather than ablating all residual tumors with APC. In fact, electrocautery effect during snaring can burn residual tumors and make APC ablation unnecessary. The efficacy of APC on the recurrence of the disease is not clear because the available data is not enough to draw conclusions.

Short- and long-term adverse events of additional APC ablation during EP for ampullary adenoma were analyzed in a recent comparative retrospective study on 109 patients with potentially resectable biopsy-proven ampullary adenoma (41 patients in EP+APC group and 41 EP-only group, after propensity score matching) [28]. APC ablation (forced APC mode, effect 2, and maximal watts 40) was selectively done at the discretion of the endoscopist for the prevention of post-procedural bleeding, the control of possible immediate bleeding, or ablation of suspected microscopic remnant tumor. Bleeding rates were significantly lower in the EP+APC group than in the EP group (7.3% vs. 31.7%, odds ratio = 0.180, $P < 0.01$). There were no significant differences in other procedure-related early adverse events, such as pancreatitis (12.2% vs. 19.5%, $P = 0.365$), cholangitis (2.4% vs. 9.8%, $P = 0.198$), and perforation (2.4% vs. 2.4%, $P = 1.000$). During the follow-up period (mean 904 ± 868 days), papillary stricture (9.8% vs. 4.9%, $P = 0.405$) and recurrence rates (24.4% vs. 24.4%, $P = 0.797$) were not significantly different between the two groups. Authors concluded that APC ablation may provide benefit in preventing bleeding events during EP without increasing the likelihood of pancreatitis when using a prophylactic pancreatic stent that is placed before APC.

Figures 39.12 and 39.13 show the endoscopic view of the treatment of residual and recurrent adenoma, respectively.

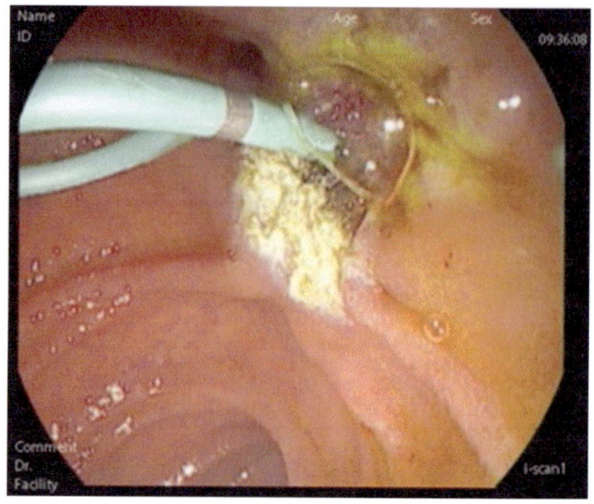

Fig. 39.12 Treatment of residual or recurrent adenoma—Argon plasma coagulation for the thermal ablation of residual adenoma just after the placement of a prophylactic pancreatic stent

39.9 Comparison of EP and Surgery

Randomized controlled studies comparing EP to surgery (surgical ampullectomy or pancreaticoduodenectomy) are lacking. Pancreaticoduodenectomy (PD) is associated with higher cure rates and lower recurrence rates rather than EP but has the disadvantage of a longer hospital stay (mean, 3 weeks) and high morbidity (15–63%) with a mortality from 0 to 13% [29].

These results have been confirmed in the largest series comparing EP and surgery for the resection of benign adenomas [10]. One hundred eighty patients were treated either with EP ($n = 130$) or surgical resection ($n = 50$, including ampullectomy or PD). EP was associated with fewer complications compared to surgery (29% vs. 58%, $P < 0.001$) but a fivefold higher recurrence rate ($P = 0.006$). The need for two or more endoscopic resections to achieve a complete tumor removal was associated with 13-fold greater risk of recurrence ($p < 0.001$). However, when comparing patients who underwent local resections only, there was no difference in the recurrence rate between endoscopic resection and ampullectomy (32% vs. 33%; $P = 0.49$). Ampullectomy is associated with a lower morbidity and mortality than PD (from 14 to 27% and from 0 to 4%, respectively) but with higher

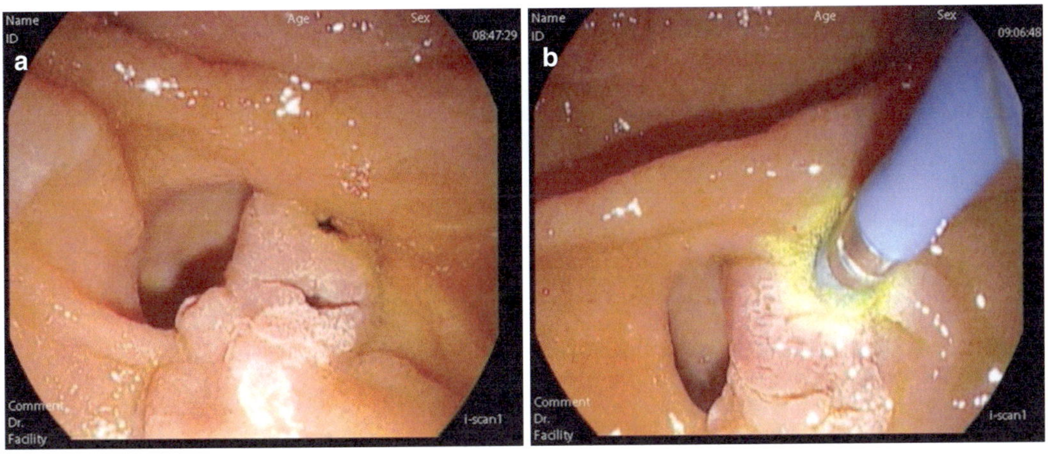

Fig. 39.13 Treatment of residual or recurrent adenoma—(**a**) Recurrent adenomatous tissue associated with a short (5 mm) intraductal biliary involvement; (**b**) intraductal radiofrequency ablation by using a temperature-controlled ELSA STARmed catheter

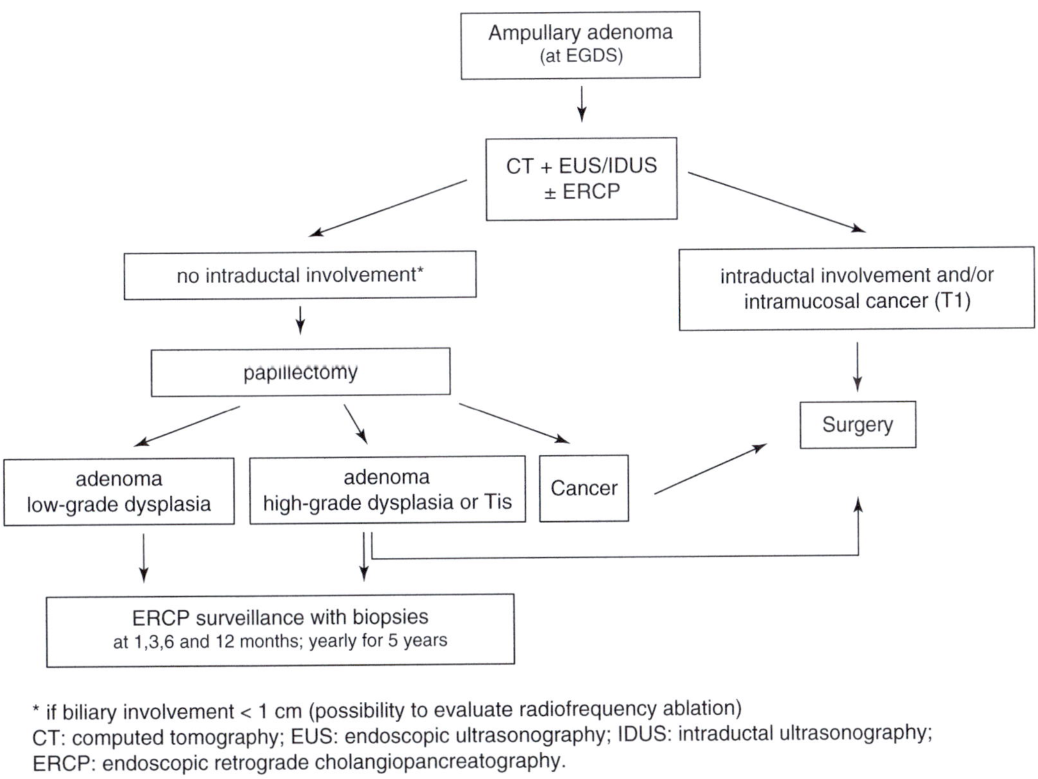

Fig. 39.14 Proposed algorithm for the management of ampullary adenoma

recurrence rates (from 17 to 32%) for which an accurate endoscopic surveillance is needed. The main limitation of ampullectomy is the lack of lymphadenectomy, as lymph node involvement has been frequently observed in apparently low-risk carcinoma [29].

A proposed algorithm for the management of ampullary adenoma is shown in Fig. 39.14.

References

1. El Hajj II, Coté GA. Endoscopic diagnosis and management of ampullary lesions. Gastrointest Endosc Clin N Am. 2013;23:95–109.
2. Petrone G, Ricci R, Familiari P, Inzani F, Matsuoka M, Mutignani M, Delle Fave G, Costamagna G, Rindi G. Endoscopic snare papillectomy: a possible radical treatment for a subgroup of T1 ampullary adenocarcinomas. Endoscopy. 2013;45:401–4.
3. Salmi S, Ezzedine S, Vitton V, Ménard C, Gonzales JM, Desjeux A, Grimaud JC, Barthet M. Can papillary carcinomas be treated by endoscopic ampullectomy? Surg Endosc. 2012;26(4):920–5.
4. Kim H-K, Lo SK. Endoscopic approach to the patients with benign or malignant ampullary lesions. Gastrointest Endosc Clin N Am. 2013;23:347–83.
5. Seewald S, Omar S, Soehendra N. Endoscopic resection of tumors of the ampulla of Vater: how far up and how deep down can we go? Gastrointest Endosc. 2006;63:789–91.
6. Bohnacker S, Seitz U, Nguyen D, et al. Endoscopic resection of benign tumors of the duodenal papilla without and with intraductal growth. Gastrointest Endosc. 2005;62:551–60.
7. Catalano MF, Linder JD, Chak A, et al. Endoscopic management of adenoma of the major duodenal papilla. Gastrointest Endosc. 2004;59:225–32.
8. Kahaleh M, Shami VM, Brock A, et al. Factors predictive of malignancy and endoscopic resectability in ampullary neoplasia. Am J Gastroenterol. 2004;99:2335–9.
9. Irani S, Arai A, Ayub K, et al. Papillectomy for ampullary neoplasm: results of a single referral center over a 10-year period. Gastrointest Endosc. 2009;70:923–32.
10. Onkendi EO, Naik ND, Rosedahl JK, Harmsen SW, Gostout CJ, Baron TH, Sarr MG, Que FG. Adenomas of the ampulla of Vater: a comparison of outcomes of operative and endoscopic resections. J Gastrointest Surg. 2014;18:1588–96.
11. Napoleon B, Gincul R, Ponchon T, et al. Endoscopic papillectomy for early ampullary tumors: long-term results from a large multicentre prospective study. Endoscopy. 2014;46:127–34.
12. Kang SH, Kim KH, Kim TN, et al. Therapeutic outcomes of endoscopic papillectomy for ampullary neoplasms: retrospective analysis of a multicenter study. BMC Gastroenterol. 2017;17:69–76.
13. Valerij G, Tringali A, Bove V, Landi R, Barbaro F, Boskoski I, Familiari P, Perri V, Costamagna G. Endoscopic papillectomy: long-term results in 110 consecutive patients. Endoscopy. 2018;50(4):S68–9.
14. Kim JH, Han JH, Yoo BM, et al. Is endoscopic papillectomy safe for ampullary adenomas with high-grade dysplasia? Ann Surg Oncol. 2009;16:2547–54.
15. Adsay V, Ohike N, Tajiri T, et al. Ampullary region carcinomas. Definition and site specific classification with delineation of four clinicopathologically and prognostically distinct subsets in an analysis of 249 cases. Am J Surg Pathol. 2012;36:1592–608.
16. Hyun JJ, Lee TH, Park JS, et al. Prospective multicenter study of submucosal injection to improve endoscopic snare papillectomy for ampullary adenoma. Gastrointest Endosc. 2017;85:746–55.
17. Harewood GC, Pochron NL, Gostout CJ. Prospective, randomized, controlled trial of prophylactic pancreatic stent placement for endoscopic snare excision of the duodenal ampulla. Gastrointest Endosc. 2005;62:367–70.
18. Klein A, Qi Z, Bahin FF, et al. Outcomes after endoscopic resection of large laterally spreading lesions of the papilla and conventional ampullary adenomas are equivalent. Endoscopy. 2018;50:972–83.
19. Zolotarevsky E, Fehmi SM, Anderson MA, et al. Prophylactic 5-Fr pancreatic duct stents are superior to 3-Fr stents: a randomized controlled trial. Endoscopy. 2011;43:325–30.
20. Chathadi KV, Khashab MA, Acosta RD, et al. The role of endoscopy in ampullary and duodenal adenomas Prepared by: Asge Standards of Practice Committee. Gastrointest Endosc. 2015;82(5):773–81.
21. Cheng CL, Sherman S, Fogel EL, et al. Endoscopic snare papillectomy for tumors of the duodenal papillae. Gastrointest Endosc. 2004;60:757–64.
22. Patel R, Davitte J, Varadarajulu S, et al. Endoscopic resection of ampullary adenomas: complications and outcomes. Dig Dis Sci. 2011;56:3235–40.
23. Camus M, Napoléon B, Vienne A, Marc LR, Leblanc S, Barret M, Chaussade S, Robin F, Kaddour N, Prat F. Efficacy and safety of endobiliary radiofrequency ablation for the eradication of residual neoplasia after endoscopic papillectomy: a multicenter prospective study. Gastrointest Endosc. 2018;88:511–8.
24. Rustagi T, Irani S, Reddy DN, Abu Dayyeh BK, Baron TH, Gostout CJ, Levy MJ, Martin J, Petersen BT, Ross A, Topazian MD. Radiofrequency ablation for intraductal extension of ampullary neoplasms. Gastrointest Endosc. 2017;86(1):170–6.
25. Mensah ET, Martin J, Topazian M. Radiofrequency ablation for biliary malignancies. Curr Opin Gastroenterol. 2016;32:238–43.
26. McCarty TR, Rustagi T. New indications for endoscopic radiofrequency ablation. Clin Gastroenterol Hepatol. 2018;16(7):1007–101.
27. Chandrasekhara V, Topazian M. Biliary radiofrequency ablation: burning issues. Gastrointest Endosc. 2018;88(3):519–20.
28. Nam K, Song TJ, Kim RE, Cho DH, Cho M, Oh O, Hyun Park D, Soo Lee S, Seo DW, Lee SK, Kim MH, Baek S. Usefulness of argon plasma coagulation ablation subsequent to endoscopic snare papillectomy for ampullary adenoma. Dig Endosc. 2018;30:485–92.
29. Panzeri F, Crippa S, Castelli P, Aleotti F, Pucci A, Partelli S, Zamboni G, Falconi M. Management of ampullary neoplasms: a tailored approach between endoscopy and surgery. World J Gastroenterol. 2015;21(26):7970–87.

Endoscopic Management in Malignant Biliary Strictures: Tips and Tricks

40

Alberto Tringali

40.1 Tips and Tricks for Malignant Biliary Strictures

Massimiliano Mutignani

- **Preliminary Tests**. Preprocedural evaluation is crucial: surgical resectability and histological diagnosis should be defined before ERCP.
- **Adequate Equipment**. Dedicated equipment has to be preliminarily available: hydrophilic guidewires from different brands, different stiffness, and diameters must be prepared. Every guidewire has a different behavior in relationship with the type of stricture. Moreover, different tips can be useful in different situations (as explained in Fig. 40.1). Adequate guidewires improve the chance of complete drainage in these settings.
- **Preliminary Dilation**. Dilation is an important step before stenting. In tight strictures, mechanical dilation can be used as well as hydropneumatic dilation: my recommendation is not to exceed in strictures' dilations, especially using hydropneumatic dilation, to avoid iatrogenic perforations (as explained in Fig. 40.2). In the most challenging and hard strictures, dilation can be performed using Sohendra's screw or cystoenterostome over-the-wire, in tertiary referral centers (Fig. 40.3).
- **Stents' Length: Never Too Long**. Stents' length is important: the proximal edge of the biliary stent should be left not too long into the biliary duct because, according to biochemical laws, a foreign body in the bile flow creates a nucleation point and can lead to bile ducts' secondary obstructions. That is why the proximal edge should be just above the stricture (as you can see in Fig. 40.4), but never too long proximally to the stricture. A too long stent, especially in hilar tumors, causes also reparative and hyperplastic reactions that can contribute to secondary obstructions.
- **Preoperative Drainage**. Preoperative drainage can be performed both by plastic and metal stenting. Plastic stenting is not always the best choice because of the morphology of the biliary tree. If it is necessary according to the anatomical situation, the plastic stent can be placed backward after adequate modification in tertiary referral centers (as you can see in Fig. 40.5). Furthermore, many studies demonstrated that metal stenting is better if neoadjuvant chemotherapy is needed.
- **Hilar Tumors**. A challenging case is represented by the endoscopic drainage of hilar tumors. The discussion present in the international literature on unilateral vs. bilateral is questionable and, in my opinion, not useful in clinical practice. On the other hand, the most important difference is between complete and incomplete drainage. Whatever we introduce

A. Tringali (✉)
Endoscopy Unit, ASST Grande Ospedale Metropolitano Niguarda, Milan, Italy
e-mail: alberto.tringali@ospedaleniguarda.it

M. Mutignani et al. (eds.), *Endotherapy in Biliopancreatic Diseases: ERCP Meets EUS*,
https://doi.org/10.1007/978-3-030-42569-2_40

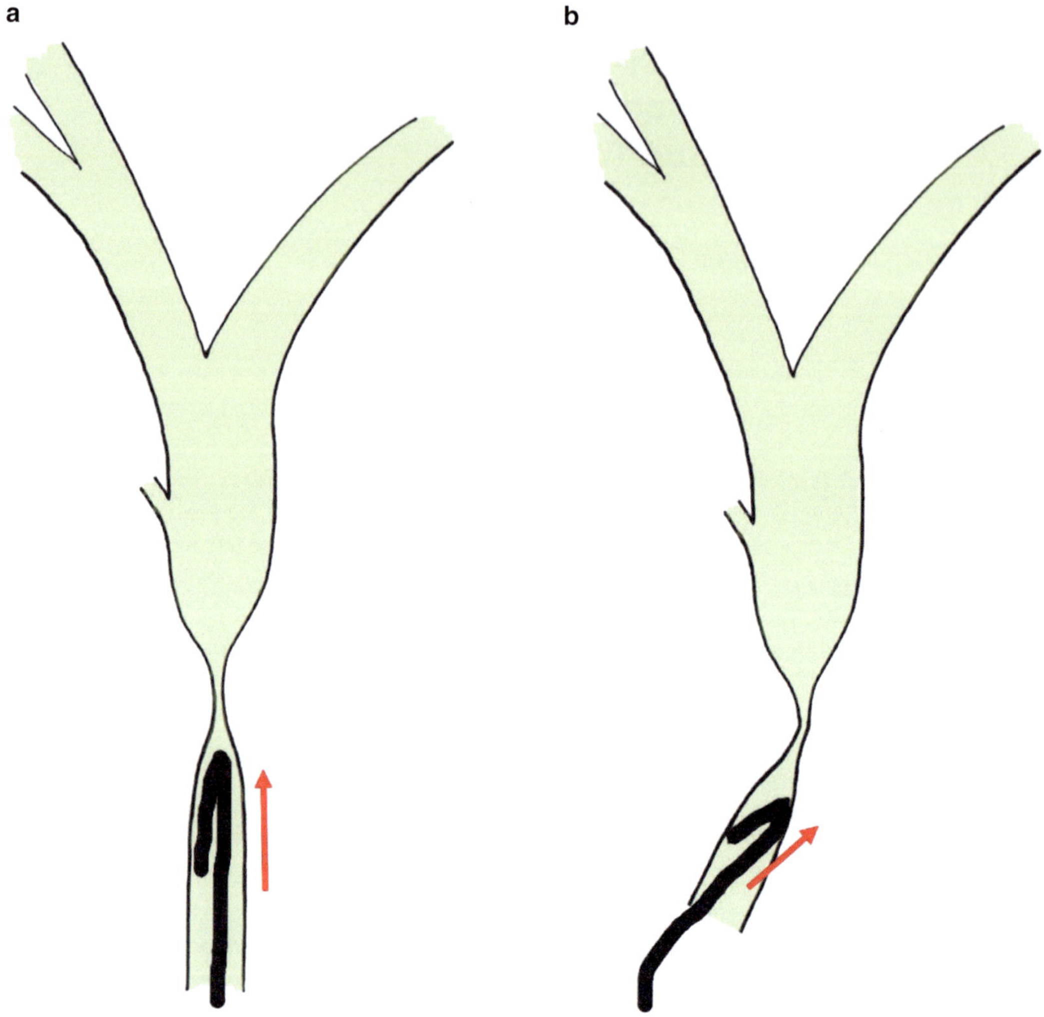

Fig. 40.1 The same guidewire can act differently in different strictures: (**a**) Pushing the loop of the guidewire, it will overpass the stricture because of linear force application. (**b**) If the stenosis is angled, the loop of the guidewire will not be able to overpass the stricture because of only side force application

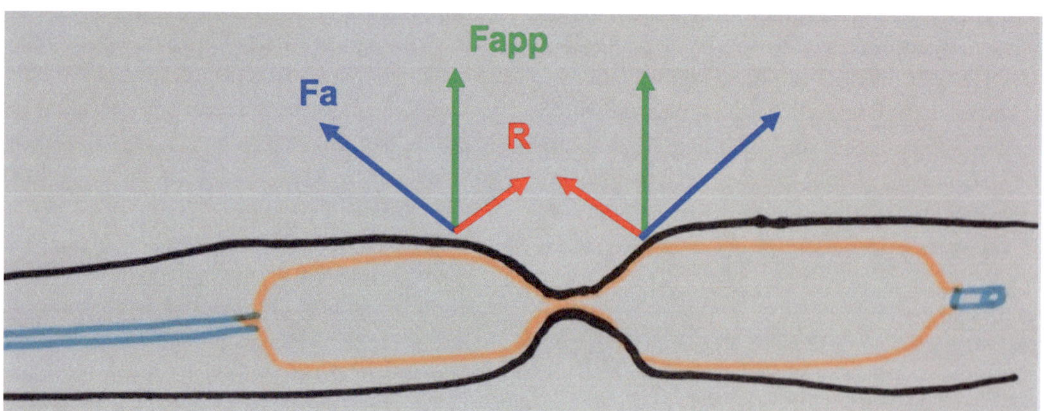

Fig. 40.2 Force application during hydropneumatic dilation is not homogeneous and can lead to perforations. *Fa* active force, *Fapp* applicative force, *R* resistance

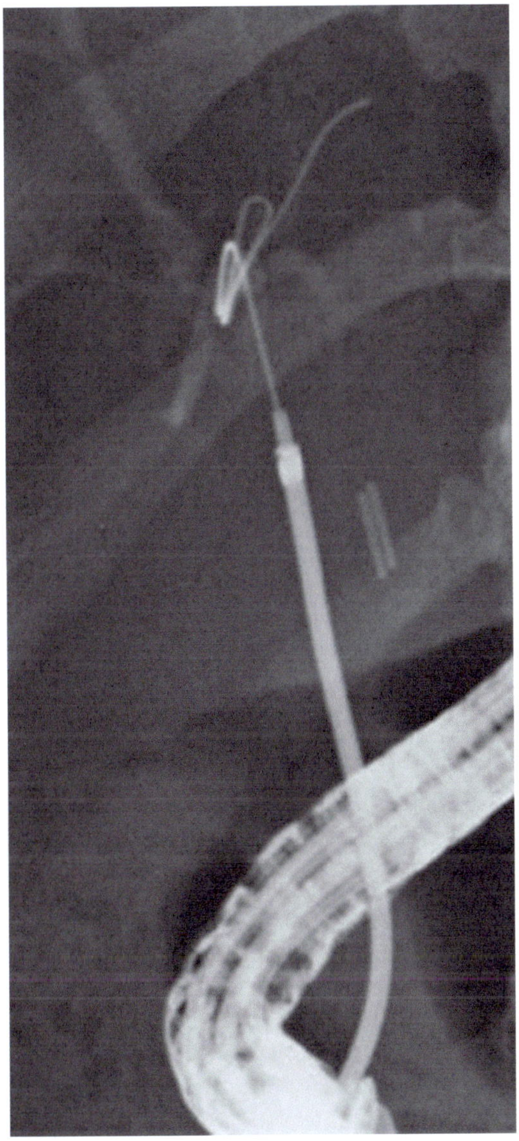

Fig. 40.3 Sohendra screw used to overpass tight malignant strictures

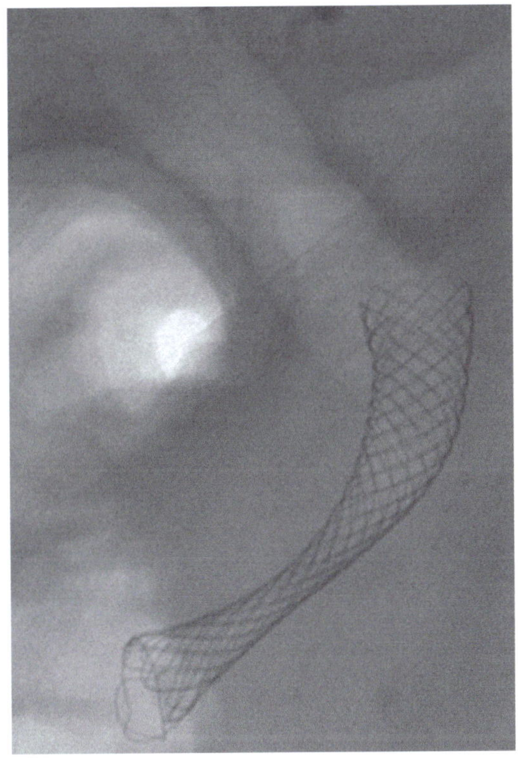

Fig. 40.4 Proximal edge of the stent is placed just above the stricture

into the biliary tree (i.e., contrast medium, guidewires, air) would contaminate the bile and can lead to cholangitis and severe sepsis. That is why preprocedural CT scan and/or cholangioMRI are mandatory before the procedure to obtain a complete mapping of the biliary tree and to define the type and site of stricture. This mapping is important to perform endoscopic drainage using a "blind technique": the guidewire is pushing into the bile duct that we previously decided to drain (on the basis of preprocedural mapping) without contrast injection. If the guidewire was accidentally placed in another duct, I recommend leaving it in place and to stent also that duct.

40.2 Distal Malignant Biliary Stricture (DMBO)

Common causes of distal malignant biliary obstruction include pancreatic carcinoma, cholangiocarcinoma, ampullary cancer, and metastatic lymphadenopathy of metastatic lesions [1, 2].

The mechanisms of malignant biliary obstruction by these tumors are direct tumor infiltration, extrinsic compression, adjacent inflammation, desmoplastic reaction, or a combination of these factors [3].

Malignant biliary obstruction can present with jaundice due to intrahepatic biliary dilation

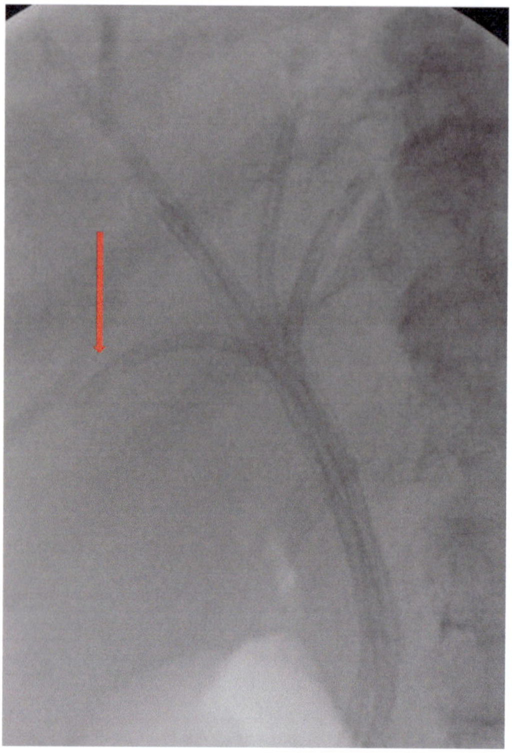

Fig. 40.5 Backward placement of biliary plastic stent (red arrow) to adapt to stricture morphology and to obtain more stability

(Fig. 40.6) and requires palliative drainages if it is unresectable. Restoration of biliary flow, together with relief of jaundice and pruritus, is the primary goal in the palliation of malignant biliary obstruction, and it also prevents biliary obstruction-related complications such as cholangitis, coagulopathy, malabsorption, and hepatocellular dysfunction [2, 4].

Drainage can be approached in three ways: surgical bypass (e.g., hepaticojejunostomy or choledochojejunostomy), percutaneous transhepatic biliary drainage, and endoscopic stenting by endoscopic retrograde cholangiopancreatography (ERCP) or EUS-guided [1, 4].

40.2.1 Surgery Versus Endoscopic Approach

Tip: Endoscopic approach has same clinical success and is the most cost-effective than surgery.

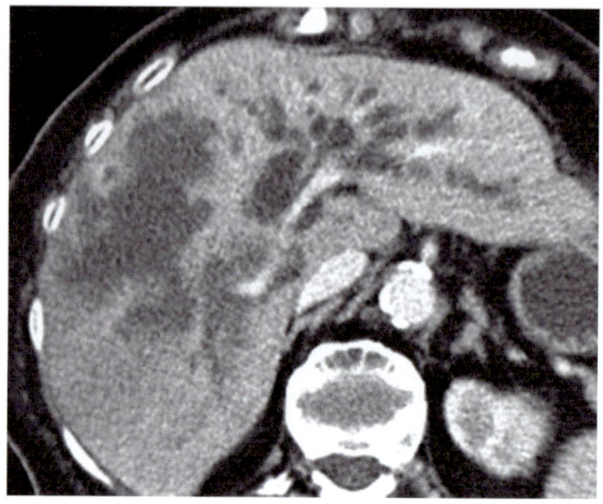

Fig. 40.6 Intrahepatic biliary duct dilation due to Klatskin tumor

Comparison of primary biliary stenting and surgical bilio-digestive anastomosis for malignant biliary obstruction has been performed in three meta-analyses [5–7]; the two most recent ones included five identical randomized controlled trials (RCTs) (379 patients), of which four used ERCP and one the percutaneous approach to insert mostly plastic stents (self-expandable metal stents (SEMSs) were used in 15 patients only); two RCTs were added compared with the older meta-analysis [5, 6].

In the two recent meta-analyses, procedure-related complications were more frequent with surgery vs. biliary stenting as well as 30-day mortality (16.3% vs. 9.6% as stated by de Lima et al. [6]; incorrectly calculated by Glazer et al. [5]); short-term success rates were similar with both techniques, but recurrent biliary obstruction was less frequent after surgical bypass vs. stenting. Of note, the single RCT (30 patients) that used SEMSs found no difference between endoscopy and surgery in terms of late-onset complications and patient readmission [8].

A meta-analysis of endoscopic and surgical bypass outcomes in malignant distal biliary obstruction showed the same technical and therapeutic success for endoscopic stenting as for surgical drainage procedures, with similar quality of life and overall survival but with a reduced risk of complications, albeit with an increased risk of recurrent biliary obstruction for endoscopic stenting [9–11].

More treatment sessions are needed after endoscopic stenting than after surgical bypass, but endoscopic stenting still continues to be the most cost-effective approach [8]. Percutaneous transhepatic biliary drainage is associated with considerable morbidity, patient discomfort, and the need for repeated intervention [10].

Endoscopic biliary stenting is presently the standard of care for the palliation of distal malignant biliary obstruction [1, 9, 10]. It provides effective palliation and may offer lower morbidity and mortality, shorter hospital stay, and diminished overall cost when compared with surgical or radiological approaches [1].

Quality of life was assessed in two RCTs; one of these reported better results for endoscopic stenting [12], while the other one reported similar results for both drainage approaches. The total duration of hospital stay, including patient readmissions, was shorter for biliary stenting vs. surgery in all of the five RCTs. Costs were analyzed in a single RCT: total costs (including readmissions) with endoscopic SEMS placement were approximately half those of surgery (4271 ± 2411 vs. 8321 ± 1821 USD) [8]. A similar difference has been reported in a large multicenter retrospective study that included 622 patients [13].

40.2.2 Is the ERCP the First Choice Compared to EUS-BD?

Tip: *Yes. ERCP is still the first choice reserving EUS-BD when ERCP fails.*

Endoscopic ultrasound-guided biliary drainage (EUS-BD) has been more recently employed and is rapidly gaining acceptance: four meta-analyses (16–42 studies including 5–12 prospective ones; for a total of 528–1192 patients) reported that EUS-BD was clinically successful in 87–94% of cases with adverse events reported in 16–29% [14–17].

EUS-BD has mostly been used in malignant conditions (87% of biliary obstructions in a meta-analysis that included 1186 patients) [15]. EUS-BD had a higher functional success rate in malignant vs. benign conditions in the single meta-analysis that analyzed that outcome, although technical success rates were similar [17].

This technique has mostly been used following failed ERCP although it has been used in pilot trials as a first-line option [12, 18].

A systematic review and meta-analysis [19] showed that with adequate endoscopy expertise, EUS-BD could show similar efficacy (technical and clinical success) and safety (total adverse events RR 0.68 95%CI 0.31–1.48) when compared with ERCP BD for primary palliation of distal MBOP and exhibits several clinical advantages (lower rates of pancreatitis; stent dysfunction, and tumor ingrowth and overgrowth).

A small prospective clinical study including 18 patients showed that EUS-BD is safe and effective as a first-line BD therapy with success rates of 94% and a complication rate of 11% [12].

A multicenter retrospective study comparing ERCP-BD with EUS-BD suggested that both techniques were equally effective [20].

> *ESGE recommends restricting the use of EUS-guided biliary drainage to cases where biliary drainage using standard ERCP techniques has failed.*

EUS-BD might therefore be a good primary alternative in patients with an expected difficult cannulation due to altered anatomy or malignant obstruction. Future randomized studies are needed to further explore this indication of EUS-BD as primary drainage.

Future Development: Moreover, the EUS-BD with antegrade stenting method has the advantage that the entire procedure can be carried out through an endoscopically created temporary fistula between the upper intestine and the intrahepatic bile ducts, without the need for the scope to reach the biliary orifice.

A recently published pilot study showed that EUS-BD with antegrade stenting is also feasible and safe in patients with an altered anatomy [21]. In a small cohort of 20 patients with an altered anatomy, a Japanese group demonstrated a 95% technical and clinical success rate of EUS-guided antegrade stenting.

In addition, EUS-BD can be used as an alternative to precut sphincterotomy. A recent retrospective study showed that the ERCP failure rate decreases when EUS-BD is available [22]. The success for EUS-BD (95.1%, 95% CI, 89.7–100) was significantly higher than for precut (75.3%, 95% CI, 68.2–82.4), $P < 0.001$, which supports the role for EUS-BD as an alternative to precut after failed cannulation.

40.2.3 How to Treat Patients in Case of ERCP Failure?

Tips: A repeated attempt at ERCP is suggested. Anyway in case of second failure or patients with complex postsurgical anatomy (including BII gastrectomy), we strongly suggest to refer to a specialized center.

EUS-BD is a preferred approach in case of ERCP failure but in expert hands and tertiary center.

Nine studies [23–31] analyzed the role of repeated attempt at ERCP showing that repeat ERCP was successful in 82% of cases especially if ERCP was repeated after 2 or 4 days after the first attempt. The explanation suggested includes better visualization of the opening of the bile duct because of decreased edema and availability of device (e.g., hydrophilic guidewire, referral to expert endoscopist at the same institution or high volume center).

Endoscopic ultrasound-guided biliary drainage can be an effective alternative for percutaneous transhepatic biliary drainage after failed endoscopic retrograde cholangiopancreatography (ERCP) [32].

ERCP fails in 5–10% of cases due to inaccessible papilla or inability to cannulate the papilla [33]. Reasons for ERCP failure include altered anatomy, ampullary distortion, periampullary diverticulum, gastric outlet obstruction, or duodenal stents in situ. Conventionally, percutaneous transhepatic biliary drainage (PTBD) has been performed when ERCP fails. However, PTBD is associated with high adverse event rates that are seen in up to 33% and include bleeding, bile leak, dislocation of the external catheter, recurrent infection, and acute cholangitis. Catheter-related morbidity from the external drainage is well known and may also worsen the patient's quality of life [34].

EUS-BD has emerged as a welcome alternative to PTBD or surgery when ERCP fails. EUS-BD was first described by Giovannini et al. [35]. Over the last decade, a wealth of data has surfaced demonstrating efficacy and safety of this technique. EUS-BD has several advantages. First, it is minimally invasive and can be performed directly after a failed ERCP in the same session by the same proceduralist. Second, drainage of both the intrahepatic and extrahepatic bile ducts may be achieved. Third, it is minimally invasive with minimal or no procedural pain. Fourth, as opposed to PTBD, there is no external drain that can dislocate or that limits patient's daily activities. In addition, a short hospital stay (similar to ERCP) is expected, and the reported adverse event rate is far lower than for PTBD [36–38].

40.2.4 EUS-BD: Intrahepatic (HGS) Versus Extrahepatic (CDS) Approach. Which Is the Best?

Tips: Overall data show that EUS-guided hepaticogastrostomy (EUS-HGS) and EUS-guided choledochoduodenostomy (EUS-CDS) are equally effective and safe. However, there is limited data available in favor of EUS-CDS with regard to safety.

Several studies have investigated the intrahepatic approach vs. the extrahepatic approach showing different results. A large retrospective study, including 245 patients, revealed a similar success rate for the both approach [39, 40].

However, the intrahepatic approach was associated with higher postprocedural pain, longer procedure time, and longer hospital admissions [39].

The latter was confirmed by a retrospective analysis of 65 patients which showed that the intrahepatic approach was associated with more complications and three patients in whom the intrahepatic approach was used died after the procedure [41]. However, the success rate was the same for all techniques, and there was neither significant difference in complication rates among transluminal and transpapillary stent placements nor between direct and rendezvous stenting. This was confirmed in a prospective, international, multicenter study looking at the efficacy and safety of EUS-BD in which an extrahepatic approach was significantly associated with decreased procedure time, length of hospital stay, and risk of moderate adverse events [42].

A retrospective study of 39 patients with obstructive jaundice caused by lower biliary obstruction and duodenal obstruction due to malignant tumors showed that EUS-HGS was associated with longer stent patency than EUS-CDS [43]. Moreover, CDS was the only risk factor associated with adverse events related to EUS-BD, in particular, reflux cholangitis (odds ratio, 10.28; 95% confidence interval [CI], 1.686–62.733; $p = 0.012$). In a single-center prospective study, Artifon *et al.* randomized 49 patients with unresectable distal malignant biliary obstruction and failed ERCP to either HGS or CDS [44]. Both methods yielded similar technical success rates, safety, and procedure time (48 min). Moreover, a quality-of-life assessment revealed that no specific drainage route was superior. There was a minor trend in favor of HGS with regard to clinical success. However, this was not statistically significant.

A systematic review showed no significant difference between transduodenal and transgastric approaches for EUS-BD with regard to efficacy and safety. [17], while another meta-analysis [15] showed that adverse events were less frequent with the extrahepatic vs. intrahepatic route (OR, 0.40; 95% CI, 0.18–0.87; $p = 0.022$).

A recent meta-analysis including 572 patients, assessing EUS guided CDS [45], showed that the pooled rate of adverse events was 0.136 (95% CI, 0.097–0.188; $p = 0.01$) and pooled rates were 4.2% for cholangitis, 4.1% for bleeding, 3.7% for bile leakage, and 2.9% for perforation. On subgroup analysis, the pooled rate of adverse events with the use of lumen-apposing metal stent (LAMS) was 9.3% (95% CI 4.8–17.3%), while the rate of adverse events such as cholangitis, bleeding, and bile leakage was 13.4%. According to a recent meta-analysis of 686 patients, assessing the role of endoscopic ultrasound guided-hepaticogastrostomy, overall clinical success and technical success were 84% (95% CI 80–88%) and 96% (95% CI 93–98%), respectively, but the success rate was only 65% in non-expert hands; the rate of adverse events was relatively high (29%), including bile leakage, stent migration, bleeding, and peritonitis.

Finally, the last meta-analysis published by Hedjoudjie et al. including 17 studies for a total of 686 patients showed that the overall clinical and technical success rates were 84% (95% CI 80–88) and 96% (95% CI 93–98), respectively, for HGS and 87% and 95%, respectively, for CDS and reported adverse event rates were significantly higher for HGS (29%) compared to CDS (20%). Compared to HGS, the pooled odds ratio for the complication rate of CGDS was 2.10 (95% CI, 1.25–3.24) ($p = 0.0042$).

EUS-guided CDS is indicated for obstruction in the middle and lower bile duct due to pancreaticobiliary malignancy in case of ERCP failure but is contraindicated in patients with surgically altered anatomy (e.g., Roux-en-Y anastomosis or tumor invasion-associated duodenal obstruction). In such cases, EUS-guided hepaticogastrostomy may be indicated because the access route is the stomach and in case of inaccessible papilla due to duodenal obstruction caused by tumor. Furthermore, in case of contraindication to PTBD due to the development of ascites, HGS could be useful; however, if massive ascites is present, EUS-HGS could not be used for preventing formation of gastrohepatic fistula.

40.2.5 EUS-BD Versus PTBD After Failed ERCP: The Winner Is

Tip: EUS-BD should be preferred because of lower adverse events, lower cost, and lower reintervention rates and it is more cost-effective.

As mentioned earlier, PTBD is associated with substantial morbidity [34]. There is only limited prospective, randomized data available evaluating the efficacy and safety of EUS-BD in comparison with PTBD. Artifon et al. were the first to compare the efficacy and safety of CDS *vs.* PTBD in a small prospective randomized study including 25 patients [46]. They concluded both methods had equal technical success, clinical success, and adverse event profile. Giovannini et al. started another prospective multicenter study comparing EUS-BD with PTBD and randomized 41 patients [36]. They excluded patients with right-sided bile duct stenosis. Interim analysis showed a complication rate of 60% in the PTBD group *vs.* 35% in the EUS-BD group, and recruitment in the PTBD arm was consequently ceased thereafter. A retrospective study including 73 patients with failed ERCP showed that although technical success rate was higher in the PTBD group, clinical success was equivalent [37]. However, PTBD was associated with higher adverse event rate and higher costs. In a recent meta-analysis, there was no difference in technical success between EUS-BD and PTBD, but EUS-BD was associated with better clinical success and fewer postprocedural adverse events [38]. Importantly, EUS-BD was associated with lower reintervention rates and was more cost-effective [38].

Another meta-analysis that compared PTBD with EUS-BD after failed ERCP has been published by Baniya et al. [47] (three RCTs and three retrospective; total, 312 patients) and found that clinical success was similar with both techniques (OR 1.48, 95% CI 0.46–4.79) but fewer adverse events in the EUS-BD group (0.34, 95% CI 0.20–0.59); severe adverse events accounted for this difference, and the reintervention rates and costs were lower with EUS-BD.

40.2.5.1 When Percutaneous Biliary Drainage Should Be Used?

Tip: We suggest to use PTBD in patients who fail ERCP in case of absence of EUS experts or in case with altered anatomy.

Percutaneous transhepatic biliary drainage is most often used when endoscopic biliary stenting has failed [10]. Endoscopic ultrasound-guided biliary drainage can be an effective alternative for percutaneous transhepatic biliary drainage after failed endoscopic retrograde cholangiopancreatography (ERCP) [32]. Surgical bypass is usually reserved for unsuccessful or unfeasible endoscopic/percutaneous drainage [9].

40.2.6 Do We Need to Perform ES Before SEMS Placement?

TIps: There is no increased rate of post-ERCP acute pancreatitis (PEP) in patients when a stent is placed without sphincterotomy, but study has some statistical flaws. We suggest to perform a small sphincterotomy that allows the stent to be placed easily and not increase the risk of perforation.

Endoscopic sphincterotomy (ES) before stent placement in patients with distal malignant biliary obstruction is still a controversial issue. Some authors suggested that ES before stent deployment has a protective role in avoiding the risk of post-ERCP pancreatitis, but this approach is not currently evidence based. We found four RCTs [48–51] and six observational studies [52–57] that showed there is no increased rate of PEP in the ES group compared to non endoscopic sphincterotomy before stent placement in patients with distal malignant biliary obstruction; therefore, ES is not mandatory in patients with distal malignant biliary obstruction because it is associated with higher rate of adverse events. However, due to the small number of patients, the study heterogeneity, and missing relevant data in the trials included, more RCTs are required before a firm recommendation could be made, and a subgroup analysis should be performed taking into account tumor type (pancreatic cancer vs. distal cholangiocarcinoma) to distinguish the rate of PEP.

European Society of Gastrointestinal Endoscopy (ESGE) suggests against routine endoscopic biliary sphincterotomy before the insertion of a single plastic stent or an uncovered /partially covered SEMS.

40.2.7 Is There a Greater Risk of Cholecystitis After Placing an FCSEMS?

Tip: There is no increased risk of cholecystitis after placing a fully covered self-expanding metal stent (FCSEMS).

Anyway we suggest to follow simple recommendations:

(a) *Check the stent position with the cystic duct insertion and adjust stent position.*
(b) *Place a stent in the gallbladder in case of tumor infiltration.*

A major concern of the endoscopist is the risk of cholecystitis in case of placing an FCSEMS in a patient with distant malignant stricture (DMS). The risk is due to malignant infiltration of the cystic duct and the presence of gallbladder stone [58].

In a recent meta-analysis of our group that was published, we found no statistically significant difference in the rate of cholecystitis in patients with DMS when an FC SEMS was placed [59].

We found that a careful visualization of the insertion of cystic duct to consider the need for the correct placement of FCSEMS could prevent the risk of cholecystitis as well as the fluoroscopic evidence of cystic duct involvement from tumor that could increase the risk of cholecystitis. We also suggest to avoid overinjecting the cystic duct and gallbladder to prevent chemical irritation in a patient without an adequate gallbladder drainage and the presence of stone.

40.2.8 Treatment of Malignant Bilioduodenal Obstruction (Type II GOO); Is It Always Possible to Place a Stent?

Tip: Place a duodenal uncovered SEMS (USEMS) before and in the same day or 2 days after placing a biliary covered SEMS (CSEMS) through the mesh of duodenal uncovered SEMS.

The management of type II bilioduodenal strictures may be challenging due to the involvement of the papilla as well as technical problems in getting a good scope position relative to the papilla. For the same reason, technical success is lower with type II strictures than with type I and III strictures [60–62].

With respect to the approach for biliary drainage, the recommendation made above to prefer biliary stenting over surgical bypass is even stronger in the setting of malignant duodenal obstruction, as life expectancy of patients who present both duodenal and biliary stricture is short: in a retrospective study (81 patients with bilioduodenal stenting), median survival was 73 days [63]; even in patients with a "good" prognosis identified by a higher World Health Organization (WHO) score, another study reported a median survival of 139 days [64].

Although the procedure may be technically difficult, success rates of 86–100% have been reported by experts in a prospective study, with lower success rates reported in cases where the duodenal stricture involves the papilla [60]. The technique and sequence of biliary and duodenal stenting according to different clinical scenarios are detailed in the ESGE Technical Review [65]. In the case of failed duodenal or biliary stenting, other interventions (e.g., PTBD, EUS-BD restricted to research settings) should be considered [66, 67].

ESGE suggests endoscopic insertion of a biliary SEMS and an uncovered duodenal SEMS in patients with both biliary and duodenal malignant obstructions.

40.2.9 Which Stent: Plastic Versus Metal?

Tip: Metal stents are preferred over plastic stents

The main drawbacks of plastic stents is their propensity to occlude leading to recurrent symptoms of biliary obstruction within 3–4 months. The main lesson learned from the limitation of plastic stent is that larger is better.

The USEMS were developed to expand the stent diameter and reduce the risk of stent occlusion.

A systematic review and meta-analysis of seven trials have proved that SEMS are superior to plastic because of less risk of stent occlusion at 6 months, lower risk of recurrent biliary obstruction, and finally their cost-effectiveness in patients surviving more than 6 months [68–71]. Initial higher cost of SEMS is balanced by a decreased need for reintervention if survival >4 months [72].

Five meta-analyses have compared SEMSs with plastic stents for the endoscopic drainage of distal malignant biliary obstruction [73–77].

Compared with plastic stents, SEMSs are associated with a longer patient survival, a lower risk of stent dysfunction/cholangitis, and fewer reinterventions. Costs associated with palliation of malignant biliary obstruction with SEMSs vs. plastic stents have been compared in a meta-analysis (eight RCTs, 311 patients with hilar or extrahepatic malignant biliary obstruction) and in a more recent RCT (18 centers, 219 patients with extrahepatic malignant biliary obstruction) [68, 77]. No significant differences in costs were reported in these studies, and the more recent RCT showed total costs were also similar for plastic stents vs. SEMSs in patients with a short survival duration (≤3 months) or those with metastatic disease [68]. A follow-up study (140 patients) of that RCT showed that health-related quality of life, both general and disease specific, was better over time with SEMSs vs. plastic stents [78].

40.2.10 ESGE Recommends SEMS Insertion for Palliative Drainage of Malignant Extrahepatic Biliary Obstruction

40.2.10.1 Which Metal Stent Should Be Used: *USEMS Versus PCSEMS Versus CSEMS? A Battle of Superiority?*

Tip: New CSEMS are preferred because of greater stent survival and need for reintervention.

The limit of USEMS is due to the tumor ingrowth as cause of recurrent biliary obstruction. Uncovered metal stents are superior to plastic stents in terms of patency. However, tissue ingrowth and stent dysfunction are common through their bare wire mesh. Covered metal stents have been developed to overcome tissue ingrowth and prolong stent patency but are associated with higher migration rate. Currently available covered metal stents differ according to their structure, stent and covering material, and mechanical properties (radial and axial force). The "battle of superiority" between covered and uncovered metal stents continues with contrasting results in recent studies. The choice of covered or uncovered metal stents should be individualized to the needs of each patient [79]. Recent developments in covered metal stents include different antimigration designs, covering membrane thickness (50–60 μm) to prevent tumor ingrowth, antireflux properties for preventing stent occlusion and cholangitis due to duodenobiliary reflux (pilot study), and drug-eluting capabilities.

The mechanical properties of SEMS also play an important role in migration. A SEMS with low axial force (AF) and high radial force (RF) is less likely to migrate. Isayama et al. compared the results between different covered SEMS and correlated them with their mechanical properties. CSEMS with the maximum AF had the highest migration rates [80].

Seven meta-analyses have compared covered and uncovered SEMS [81–87]; the covered SEMSs used in the original studies included partially covered SEMSs (PCSEMSs) and FCSEMSs. No differences in the proportions of patients with stent dysfunction, overall complications, or patient survival were reported, except for stent dysfunction in two meta-analyses [85, 86].

Covered SEMSs were associated with a lower risk of tumor ingrowth but a higher risk of stent migration, tumor overgrowth, and sludge formation. With respect to concerns about cholecystitis following covered SEMS placement [88], the four meta-analyses that reported this outcome found no increased risk of cholecystitis after insertion of covered vs. uncovered SEMS [81, 82, 84, 86].

Of note, measures taken in some studies to prevent this complication have included placement of the stent covering below the level of the cystic duct implantation in patients with an intact gallbladder [89] and the use of covered SEMS with transmural drainage holes [90]. Finally, nitinol stents have replaced stainless steel stents as they perform better (Fig. 40.7) [91, 92].

Specific SEMS designs have been investigated:

- *Antireflux covered SEMSs* were compared with SEMSs without an antireflux valve (an uncovered SEMS and a covered SEMS) in two RCTs [93, 94]. Both RCTs reported a similar efficacy in decreasing bilirubin serum levels and a longer patency of antireflux vs.

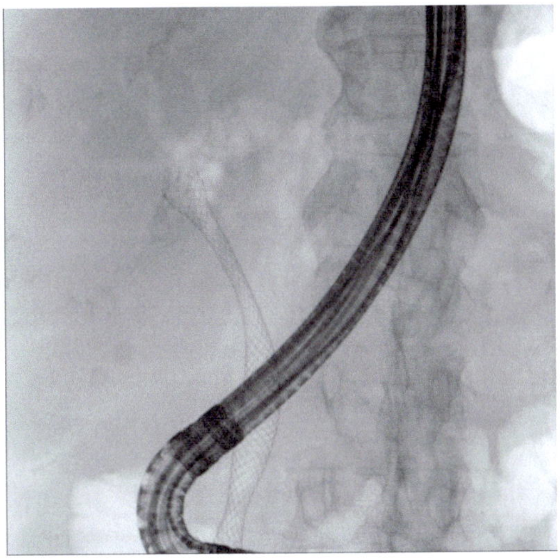

Fig. 40.7 Endotherapy of type I cholangiocarcinoma according to Bismuth-Corlette classification by a single fully covered metal stent

conventional SEMS. This is consistent with the finding that duodenal-biliary reflux is independently associated with biliary stone recurrence [95]. It appears promising for preventing stent occlusion and cholangitis due to duodenobiliary reflux.

- *Antimigration systems,* including flared ends and anchoring flaps, have been tested with covered SEMSs [96, 97]. Anchoring flaps have yielded promising results in patients with benign strictures [97], but no study has compared identical stent designs with or without an antimigration system, precluding definitive conclusions. Stent models combining antireflux and antimigration systems have been tested in pilot trials [98].
- *A radioactive stent,* inserted percutaneously, provided longer patient survival than a similar, nonradioactive, stent in an RCT that included 23 patients with malignant biliary obstruction [99]. Another RCT (55 patients) that used a radioactive strand inserted between the stent and the biliary wall also reported prolonged patient survival [100].
- *Paclitaxel-eluting stents* provided no advantage compared with standard SEMSs in an RCT (72 patients) [101]. The concept of drug-eluting stents (DES) originated from intervention cardiology. The chemotherapeutic agents (paclitaxel or gemcitabine) used in DES have cytotoxic, anti-inflammatory, and antiproliferative properties.
- *Biodegradable stents: the advantages of these stents include elimination of the need for stent removal, reduced proliferation, and impregnation with antitumor agents.*

A recent systematic review and meta-analysis [102] including 11 RCTs with a total of 1272 patients concluded that there was a risk reduction of about 32% for both stent failure and patient mortality with covered SEMS, but this difference was not significant. Migration and sludge rates were higher with covered SEMS, whereas tumor ingrowth was more likely with uncovered SEMS. However, stent migration and sludge formation were much more common with covered SEMS (odds ratio [OR], 5.11; 95% CI, 1.84–14.17; OR, 2.46; 95% CI, 1.37–4.43). The use of covered SEMS was associated with a lower rate of tumor ingrowth (OR, 0.21; 95% CI, 0.09–0.50) but a higher rate of tumor overgrowth (OR, 2.00; 95% CI, 1.15–3.48) compared with uncovered stents. The rates of procedure-related adverse events were similar in both groups.

Unfortunately, stent characteristics have never been evaluated systematically, and the RCTs available for statistical analysis used covered SEMS without the recent technical improvements developed to overcome the limitations of the covering membranes. In particular, the only rational conclusion about the higher rate of tumor overgrowth in the covered SEMS group is that the covering membrane did not inhibit tumor overgrowth.

We speculate that the type of covering membrane, technical characteristics of the covered SEMS, such as the axial and radial force of the stents, and the antimigration system might play significant roles. Most of the covered stents in the RCTs were characterized by inefficient covering membrane or unfavorable axial or radial force, which may have influenced the comparison between covered and uncovered SEMS. Thus, the current statistical analysis may prompt many physicians to continue to place uncovered SEMS. However, we suggest that on the basis of a stent failure rate reduction of 32% favoring covered SEMS, these stents should be considered as the first option until new, better designed RCTs are published.

Finally the comparison, in a stratified analysis, between the CSEMS, PCSEMS, and USEMS did not find substantial differences when compared with the overall estimates.

40.2.11 How to Drain DMBO of Unconfirmed Etiology

In large series, 5–10% of patients operated for pancreatic cancer prove to have benign disease at surgery [103]. Uncovered SEMSs are known to have poor long-term patency in benign disease [104]. These stents are difficult or impossible to remove, and although a new "stent-in-stent" technique has been successfully used to remove uncovered SEMSs mistakenly inserted in patients with a benign disease [105, 106], this technique is laborious and adverse events are frequent [107].

40.2.12 Preoperative Biliary Drainage (PBD) in DMBO

Among ten unique meta-analyses that assessed the potential benefit of PBD in patients with a distal biliary obstruction, none found differences in terms of mortality, and with respect to morbidity, nine found it to be similar [108–116] with vs. without PBD; a single study reported a lower morbidity (serious adverse events) with vs. without PBD [117]. Although the meta-analyses were limited by the characteristics of the original studies, including selection bias, the use of the percutaneous or the endoscopic route for PBD, and the inclusion in some studies of patients with proximal biliary obstruction, they represent the best available evidence.

Of note, two retrospective studies that compared PBD and no PBD in a total of 170 patients reported an independent association between endoscopic PBD and shorter patient survival [118, 119].

Apart from well-accepted indications for PBD such as cholangitis, severe jaundice was suggested to be an adequate indication: a recent, mostly retrospective, study (1200 patients) found that a total serum bilirubin ≥ 300 µmol/L was associated with a high risk of severe postoperative complications [120].

Of note, patients with a total serum bilirubin ≥ 250 µmol/L were excluded from the largest RCT of PBD vs. no PBD [121].

On the other hand, a retrospective matched case–control study (152 patients) suggested that even in patients with relatively severe jaundice (bilirubin ≥ 15 mg/dL [256 µmol/L]) classified as grade 2 on the American Society of Anesthesiologists (ASA) scale, PBD presented no advantage [122]. Thus, the validity of severe jaundice as an indication for PBD remains unclear.

ESGE recommends against routine preoperative biliary drainage in patients with malignant biliary obstruction; preoperative biliary drainage should be reserved for patients with cholangitis, severe symptomatic jaundice (e.g., intense pruritus), or delayed surgery, or before neoadjuvant chemotherapy in jaundice patients.

ESGE recommends the endoscopic placement of a 10-mm-diameter self-expandable metal stent (SEMS) for preoperative biliary drainage of extrahepatic malignant biliary obstruction.

40.2.12.1 Which Route of PBD Is Preferred? PTBD Versus ERCP

If a decision is made to proceed with PBD in patients with malignant distal biliary obstruction who are undergoing curative resection, the endoscopic route is preferred over the percutaneous route because data from three retrospective series with long-term follow-up that compared the two approaches (total, 1213 patients) showed longer patient survival and less frequent peritoneal/liver recurrence in the endoscopic groups [123–125].

40.2.12.2 Which Stent Should Be Placed in Case of PBD?

With respect to the use of plastic stents vs. self-expandable metal stents (SEMSs) for PBD, a meta-analysis (four retrospective cohorts and one prospective cohort; total, 704 patients) found that SEMSs were associated with a lower rate of endoscopic reintervention (3.4% vs. 14.8%) and no difference in overall surgical morbidity or mortality [126]. The interval between biliary drainage and surgery was not reported, but we calculated that neoadjuvant therapy, an indicator of long PBD duration, was performed in 337 (48%) patients.

In a more recent multicenter RCT (86 patients) comparing plastic stents and fully covered SEMSs (FCSEMSs), there were similar outcomes including need for reintervention, surgery-related adverse events, and mortality, but the interval between biliary drainage and surgery was only 13 days [127].

In the setting of neoadjuvant therapy, an RCT (54 patients) found that use of FCSEMSs resulted in a longer stent patency duration and fewer days of delay in neoadjuvant therapy compared with plastic stents and uncovered SEMSs; total costs associated with PBD were similar for all stent models [128]. Similarly, two retrospective studies (total, 72 patients) found that, compared with SEMSs, plastic stents were associated with more complications; one of the studies also analyzed the delay in neoadjuvant therapy and costs: with SEMSs, the delay was shorter and the total costs were similar [129, 130]. The type of SEMS was stated in one study only (FCSEMS) [130]. FCSEMSs also present the advantage of being removable if surgical resection is finally not performed. Finally, SEMSs do not compromise R0 resection or increase the risk of local unresectability according to a retrospective analysis of 593 patients [131], but the presence of a biliary plastic stent or SEMS prolongs operative duration [122, 131].

Clinical Pearls for Adequate Stenting Using Metallic Stent in Distal Malignant Biliary Obstruction

1. Insertion of a SEMS with a 10-mm diameter is recommended when patient life expectancy is longer than 4 months. When the stent is occluded, the second stent should be a CSEMS if
2. the first metal stent is an uncovered model.
3. Good SEMSs have a high radial force and a low axial force.
4. Remember that the removal of an uncovered metal stent is extremely difficult after embedding.
5. The desired location of the stent is from 1 to 2 cm above the proximal end of the stricture to 1 cm below the papilla.
6. Biliary sphincterotomy may not be necessary for insertion of a SEMS.
7. Some delivery systems of the SEMS have a function for recapturing during deployment.

40.2.13 Proximal Malignant Biliary Stricture (Hilar) (HMBO)

40.2.13.1 Introduction

The malignant hilar stricture poses a difficult management challenge to the endoscopist with complex and varied endoscopic techniques for diagnosis and treatment (Fig. 40.8).

The etiology of hilar stricture can be benign or malignant, with malignant strictures being primary tumors (cholangiocarcinoma), local extension of other tumors (gallbladder cancer, hepatocellular carcinoma), and rarely lymph node metastasis (breast, colon, stomach, ovaries, lymphoma, and melanoma) with cholangiocarcinoma being the most common [132].

Biliary papillomatosis (BP) is a rare disease characterized by multiple papillary adenomas of

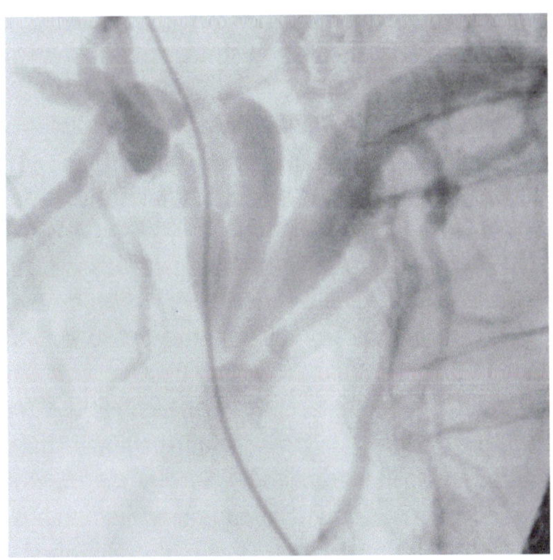

Fig. 40.8 Fluoroscopic image of hilar cholangiocarcinoma. The anterior and posterior right ducts are divided by the neoplasm

variable distribution and extent in the extrahepatic and/or intrahepatic biliary tree, manifesting as recurrent abdominal pain, jaundice, and cholangitis [133]. BP is a new entity with a high malignant potential in papillary adenocarcinoma [133] causing hilar stricture that should be remembered in the differential diagnosis.

40.2.13.2 Diagnosis

1. *How Do You Perform Diagnosis of Malignant Hilar Stricture?*

Tips: Imaging raise the suspicion of tumor and allow staging and guide treatment.

Brushing and biopsy failed to give a diagnosis in 30–40%v of cases. There is a need to always perform EUS-FNA.

In case of doubt, perform cholangioscopy with targeted biopsy.

The diagnostic imperative when encountering a hilar stricture, be it from the clinical presentation or an imaging study, is to determine malignant vs. benign etiology and to determine potential surgical respectability [132]. This is easier said than done. However, even in patients with elevated plasma bilirubin/alkaline phosphatase, elevated carcinoembryonic antigen (CEA)/carbohydrate antigen (CA) 19.9 levels, suspicious imaging findings, and direct cholangiographic findings showing an irregular hilar stricture, up to 20% can have benign disease at the time of surgical resection [134].

Cross-sectional imaging (computed tomography (CT) scan and magnetic resonance imaging (MRI)) may raise the suspicion of malignant stricture but can only guide endoscopic evaluation for respectability and treatment and should always be performed before the treatment.

There are multiple endoscopic techniques for tissue acquisition in a suspected malignant hilar stricture, which are generally done at the time of endoscopic retrograde cholangiopancreatography. These include brush cytology, intraductal biopsies, endoluminal fine needle aspiration (FNA), and targeted biopsies through direct cholangioscopy.

In a recent systematic review and a meta-analysis, the pooled sensitivity of brushing for the diagnosis of malignant biliary strictures was 45% with a high specificity of 99% [135, 136].

The sensitivity reported for intraductal biopsies ranges between 43 and 81% with a very high specificity (97–100%) [136–138].

A multimodal approach combining the two techniques could potentially be more effective. Weber et al. found that the combination of brush and biopsies yielded a sensitivity of 60.3%, a minor increase from either technique individually [139].

In a meta-analysis of nine studies comparing the two techniques, the combination of two modalities modestly increased the sensitivity to 59%, again higher than either technique alone [135, 136].

Endoluminal FNA has been reported to have a sensitivity of 38%, but when the three techniques were combined (brush, biopsy, FNA), sensitivity rose to 73% [137]; endoscopic ultrasound with FNA has been shown to have a sensitivity of 77% in proximal biliary strictures, which had negative brush cytology results; however, the negative predictive value is too low to exclude malignancy following a negative biopsy [140] and can be associated with a disease dissemination [141].

The Asia-Pacific Working Group on Hepatobiliary Disorders recommends at least a combination of two techniques for all suspicious strictures [142].

The role of peroral cholangioscopy in the diagnosis of biliary strictures is evolving with the new Spyglass System because direct visualization of the biliary system is allowed as well as targeted biopsies with mini forceps through the cholangioscope [143], but its availability is limited due to cost in tertiary care centers. It has been shown that visual interpretation alone was successful in differentiating malignant vs. benign in 89% of patients with biopsies successful in 82% of patients who had inconclusive ERCP evaluation [144].

Visual characteristics of malignancy included visible mass, dilated tortuous vessels, papillary or villous projections, and intraductal nodules. In a recent meta-analysis of peroral cholangioscopy with biopsies of indeterminate biliary strictures, the pooled sensitivity and specificity to detect cholangiocarcinoma were 66% and 97%, respectively [143]. When compared to brushing and intraductal biopsies, mini forceps biopsy provided significantly better sensitivity and overall accuracy (76.5%) [145].

The role of fluorescence in situ hybridization (FISH) and digital image analysis (DIA) is currently limited with low sensitivity (34%); the role of probe-based confocal laser endomicroscopy (pCLE) using the Cholangioflex probe during ERCP is promising with a described sensitivity of 98% in single prospective study [146]. The limit of this technique is that the results are operator dependent result and low agreement between observer.

40.2.13.3 Treatment

Tip: The goal of endoscopic treatment remains adequate biliary drainage to improve the quality of life and prolong survival by increasing the stent patency time without increasing the incidence of adverse events.

Given that 70–90% of patients presenting with malignant biliary obstruction have unresectable disease with poor overall prognosis, the ultimate goal of therapy is palliation with relief of biliary obstruction.

Over the last 20 years, endoscopic decompression has emerged as the preferred treatment option with lower complication rates, lower morbidity, lower overall cost, and shorter hospitalization [11].

Specifically, endoscopic stenting of hilar cholangiocarcinoma can offer relief of biliary obstruction and alleviate symptoms of pain, intractable pruritus, and cholangitis [147].

Approximately 55–60% of the liver volume is excreted through the right hepatic duct, 30–35% through the left hepatic duct, and 10% from the caudate lobe.

Previously, it had been recommended that at least 25% of the total liver volume be diverted for adequate biliary drainage in patients with biliary obstruction [148]. However, recently, ≥50% drainage of the total liver volume has been proposed [142, 149]. Drainage of ≥50% of the total liver volume was associated with prolonged survival than was drainage of <50% [149].

While biliary stenting does not improve overall mortality, photodynamic therapy (PDT) is an emerging endoscopic treatment modality that offers the possibility of remodeling the tumor mass and may actually improve survival in patients with non-resectable cholangiocarcinoma [150, 151]. Endoscopic modalities for therapeutic management of malignant hilar strictures are summarized in Table 40.1

Table 40.1 Endoscopic modalities for treatment of HMBO

Endoscopic retrograde cholangiopancreatography (ERCP) with stenting
– Plastic stent
– Self-expanding metal stent (straight, side-by-side, or Y-shaped)
Endoscopic ultrasound-guided biliary drainage
Hepaticogastrostomy
Photodynamic therapy
Radiofrequency ablation

40.2.13.4 Endoscopic Versus Percutaneous Approach

Percutaneous transhepatic biliary drainage (PTBD) may be superior to endoscopic drainage in patients with advanced HMBO because it has greater technical feasibility and makes reaching the lobar section of the bile duct easier. The technical success rate for PTBD was higher, stent patency was longer, and the complication rate was similar to that of the endoscopic approach [152–154].

Lee et al. [153] showed that the median stent patency was longest in internal stenting via PTBD (180 days) followed by endoscopic retrograde biliary drainage (ERBD) (120 days) and external PTBD (59 days) ($p = 0.02$ for internal stenting via PTBD *vs.* ERBD, $p < 0.01$ for ERBD *vs.* external PTBD, $p < 0.01$ for internal stenting via PTBD *vs.* external PTBD). Paik et al. [154] revealed that successful biliary decompression in patients with advanced type III or IV hilar cholangiocarcinoma (HCCA) was significantly higher with the percutaneous self-expandable metal stents (SEMS) than with the endoscopic SEMS group (92.7% *vs.* 77.3%, respectively, $p = 0.049$) with similar complication rates.

Jang et al. [152] also reported that technical success rate was higher in the PTBD group (100%) than in the endoscopic group (72.4%) without statistical differences in clinical success, stent patency, patient survival, and complication rate. However, the technical feasibility of, and durability after, reintervention showed marked differences because of limitations of retrospective studies.

A meta-analysis and systematic review, including seven retrospective studies and two RCTS for a total of 546 patients, concluded that PTBD was superior to endoscopic drainage in patients with advanced (Bismuth type III–IV) unresectable hilar malignancy (OR, 2.53; 95% CI, 1.57–4.08) [155].

Overall adverse events and 30-day mortality were similar for both approaches. Bismuth types I and II MHS were not included in the meta-analysis because ERCP was believed to represent the optimal approach for palliative drainage of such strictures. Of note, drainage of Bismuth type I MHS is technically similar to that of extrahepatic biliary strictures. The value of this meta-analysis is limited by the fact that most data were retrospective, including three noncomparative studies. With respect to quality of life, it improves with both approaches [156, 157], but an RCT (54 patients) suggested that some health parameters improve more with PTBD vs. ERCP [156, 157].

In the 2013 Asia Pacific Consensus, the percutaneous approach was preferred over the endoscopic approach for bilateral or multisectoral drainage >50% of the total liver volume in patients with high-grade hilar stricture (Bismuth type II to IV) [142].

However, the disadvantages of PTBD are inconvenient to the patient, reduce the quality of life, and result in loss of bile through the external drainage tube. Frequent dislodgement of the PTBD tube or infection is also problematic.

Furthermore, from the technical point of view, PTBD is difficult if the intrahepatic bile duct (IHD) is not fully dilated, or if there are multiple liver metastases, ascites, or blood clots, while an endoscopic approach may be more patient-friendly than a percutaneous approach in terms of convenience and quality of life.

Recent studies of SEMS placed under endoscopic guidance reported higher technical feasibility and clinical success, and good stent patency, without an increased incidence of complications [158–170].

ESGE suggests palliative drainage of malignant hilar strictures by means of ERCP for Bismuth types I and II, and PTBD or a combination of PTBD and ERCP for Bismuth types III and IV, to be modulated according to local expertise.

In summary, the initial percutaneous approach might be preferred, especially in advanced HMBO, judging from the literature. However, recent endoscopic reports revealed higher technical and clinical feasibility in advanced HMBO because of the technical advances and development of stents and accessories. Endoscopic palliation is now preferred and recommended as a primary intervention in usual setting.

40.2.13.5 Is the Drainage of Advanced Hilar Stricture for All?

A meta-analysis (13 studies, 59,437 ERCPs) showed that ERCP success is more frequent when it is performed by high volume vs. low volume endoscopists (OR, 1.6; 95% CI, 1.2–2.1) and in high volume vs. low volume hospitals (OR, 2.0; 95% CI, 1.6–2.5), while adverse events are less frequent when ERCP is performed by high volume endoscopists [171].

ESGE recommends performing drainage of malignant hilar stricture in high volume centers with a multidisciplinary hepatobiliary team.

40.2.14 Endoscopic Stenting

40.2.14.1 Should We Perform ES Before Stent Placement? Yes. We Should Do

The role of routine ES before stenting is still controversial, and no clear guidelines exist to govern its use. Additionally, ES is also an independent risk factor for complications such as pancreatitis, bleeding, and perforation, with a reported complication rate of approximately 10%. Bilateral stent placements for Bismuth type II to IV hilar cholangiocarcinoma are also very complicated and result in increased endoscopic manipulations [172]. The higher incidence of post-ERCP complications in patients who had two SEMSs (bilateral stents) placed could be related to these reasons. In these situations, limited ES before stenting could be an effective strategy for facilitating more complex stenting procedures [173]. Limited ES may allow for easier stent placement and reduce resistance to biliary instrumentation. Additionally, proximal bile duct strictures may contribute to a fulcrum effect resulting in medial displacement of the distal stent and, consequently, stent-related compression of the pancreatic duct [174]. Limited ES might prevent the risk of pancreatitis by reducing stent-related pancreatic duct obstruction.

With regard to endoscopic stenting, there are two main considerations: plastic vs. metal stent and unilateral vs. bilateral stenting of the hepatic ducts [175, 176].

Regardless of the type of stent used or the segments drained, drainage of adequate liver volume (>30%) is needed to relieve jaundice [148].

In fact, in a recent retrospective study of 107 patients, the main factor determining effective drainage (decrease in serum bilirubin by 50% at day 30) and longer survival was a decrease in liver volume by >50% following stenting of malignant hilar strictures [148]. Procedural complications for stenting in general can include occlusion (tissue overgrowth, ingrowth, debris), migration, and infection (cholangitis, cholecystitis) [176].

SEMS can be either uncovered or covered with material to prevent tumor overgrowth, though uncovered ones are preferred in strictures at the hilum as to not occlude drainage from the contralateral biliary system or the cystic duct [176].

40.2.14.2 Which Stent for Hilar Malignant Stricture? Plastic Versus Metal

Both plastic stents (PS) and SEMS have been used for malignant hilar strictures, with recent prospective studies comparing the two methods ranging between 60 and 100 patients [177–179]. Although PS are less expensive than SEMS, the duration of their patency is low, typically about 3 months [180, 181].

In contrast, SEMSs are patent for much longer, around 6–12 months [177, 181, 182].

In a recent pooled meta-analysis comparing SEMS and PS for malignant hilar obstruction, SEMS had a lower 30-day occlusion rate, lower long-term occlusion rate, higher rate of successful stent insertion, lower rate of therapeutic failure, and lower rate of cholangitis [76]. Given this, SEMSs are overall more cost-effective when compared to PS in malignant hilar obstruction [183]. Therefore, two consensus statements from separate groups in Asia prefer metallic stenting when palliating malignant hilar strictures, particularly in patients with a predicted survival of longer than 3 months and Bismuth II–IV HCCA lesions [142, 184].

SEMSs have several advantages over plastic stents. The open wire mesh of metal stents does not occlude the side branches of the IHDs or the cystic duct. The larger diameter of metal stents prolongs their patency. Furthermore, when stricture is severe, plastic stent insertion may be more difficult.

In summary, based on reported comparative studies, SEMSs are primarily preferred for adequate palliation of HMBO to prolong stent patency and reduce the reintervention rate without increasing the rate of adverse events. In patients with HMBO who are expected to survive for at least 3 months, SEMSs are preferred to plastic stent.

40.2.14.3 Do We Need to Perform Unilateral or Bilateral Drainage?

There is still some debate as to whether unilateral stenting should be performed vs. bilateral stenting in malignant hilar obstruction. In one randomized controlled trial of 157 patients in Italy, unilateral drainage had a higher rate of successful stent insertion, lower rate of complications, and lower rate of early cholangitis, with no difference in mortality, in an intention-to-treat analysis [185].

Vienne et al. analyzed factors predictive of drainage effectiveness during endoscopic stenting for HMBO [149].

Therefore, bilateral or multi-sectoral stenting to achieve drainage of ≥50% of the total liver volume may be required for favorable clinical efficacy in patients with high-grade hilar stricture (Bismuth type II to IV) [142].

In a pooled meta-analysis of seven studies comprising a total of 574 patients, there was no statistically significant difference in occlusion rate, therapeutic failure, cholangitis, and mortality between unilateral and bilateral stenting [76]. Bilateral stenting may be needed if both ductular systems become contaminated with contrast injection, in which case parallel stents can be placed side by side or a newly available Y-shaped stent can be deployed with reasonable success [166].

40.2.14.4 Complete Versus Incomplete Drainage

The concept of unilateral and bilateral biliary drainage should then be revised according to the anatomy of the hilar stricture and be replaced by the terms "complete" (all liver segments drained) and "incomplete" biliary drainage [186].

Only "complete" drainage of the biliary tree would thus protect from septic complications, at least theoretically. Here is the point: while "monolateral" stenting in type ≥II MHS means always "incomplete" drainage, "bilateral" stenting with two prostheses provides "complete" drainage in type II, but "incomplete" drainage in types III and IV. It is therefore improper to compare "monolateral" to "bilateral" stenting in type III and IV MHS because they will provide an incomplete drainage in both circumstances.

In fact, if a single stent cannot drain >50% of the estimated total liver volume in patients with HMBO, bilateral or multisegmental drainage should be considered. Furthermore, we always should keep in mind that if we inject contrast agents, we potentially could contaminate all liver segments as we must drain all!

Two recent meta-analyses [76, 187] compared unilateral and bilateral drainage of MHS obtaining similar results in terms of jaundice palliation, complications, and 30-day mortality. Some authors suggest preferring unilateral drainage due to the higher technical success [76, 188]. Many studies, included in the meta-analyses, enrolled also patients with Bismuth-Corlette type I MHS, where one stent can drain all the liver, while other used two stents to drain Bismuth-Corlette type III or IV MHS obtaining an incomplete drainage leaving opacified and undrained biliary ducts theoretically, even in Bismuth-Corlette type III strictures, only one stent placed in one of the right sectoral ducts (each one drains approximately 30% of the hepatic parenchyma) or in the left hepatic duct (40%) should be enough to palliate symptoms if the drained parenchyma is not atrophic. However, currently, drainage of at least 50% of the parenchyma is recommended because it has been shown to be more effective [149, 173, 189, 190].

40.2.14.5 How Do You Drain?

Endoscopists should plan their drainage strategy based on CT or magnetic resonance cholangiopancreatography findings, with selective wire-guided cannulation of the desired side and placement of a single SEMS to drain at least 30–50% of the total liver volume [148, 149, 175, 191]. Hintze and colleagues reported a high successful drainage (86%) and a low post-ERCP cholangitis (6%) in 35 patients with type III and IV malignant hilar obstruction who underwent MRCP-guided unilateral stenting with minimal contrast injection above the stricture [192].

40.2.14.6 How to Perform Biliary Drainage?

Endoscopist should revised all CT scan and MRI and perform biliary drainage without using contrast agents to avoid to contaminate all biliary tree causing a high risk of cholangitis and sepsis that could be impossible to drain leading patients to high risk of death. Therefore, we use a guidewire cannulation after analyzing MRI and planning to drain one, two, or three ducts according to the imaging study. After performing ES, we place the guidewire in the desired duct and start opening the first stent that should be placed just above the stricture. To do that, we open the stent and we retrieved the stent under fluoroscopic control identifying the stricture just below the proximal flange.

40.2.14.7 Is There a Role of CSEMS in the Hilar Tumor?

The USEMS limit is due to tumor ingrowth as cause of recurrent biliary obstruction (RBO).

Other cause of RBO for USEMS is that the excessive length of the SEMS causes hyperplastic reaction or de novo development of sludge and stone closing the side branch and as a result the occlusion of SEMS determining the difficulties to reintervention that is often troublesome.

Similarly to other scenario, the use of CSEMS could avoid the tumor ingrowth. Unfortunately, the presence of ducts (lateral or secondary) and the risk of closing leading to cholangitis have limited the use of CSEMS in this setting. Early or delayed septic complications developing in the obstructed biliary ducts are a major issue when dealing with palliative treatment of complex MHS.

First of all, we should determine if the CSEMS is applicable for all patients, for any situations, and by any endoscopists.

From my point of view, the applicability depends on patient anatomy and operator expertise. It is more easy to apply in the left duct because the side branch arises more distally compared to the right branch allowing the placement of CSEMS. Unfortunately, few data are available with the fully covered design, but the risk of cholangitis due to side branch occlusion is the major concern.

The study by Kitamura et al. [193] inserted a 6-mm partially covered SEMS (side by side) showing a lower time to RBO compared to other studies and that the RBO is shorter in case of advanced or complex tumor (bismuth 3–4)/9 days compared to more simple stricture (Bismuth 1–2).

However, Inoue et al. *[194]* reported technical and clinical success rates for FCSEMS of >90% with an incidence of liver abscess of 7%.

Yoshida et al. [195] described similar technical and clinical feasibility, but mean stent patency was only 95 days.

It seems that CSEMS do not show a significant difference in patency compared to plastic stents, and further large prospective comparative trials are needed to assess the role of CSEMS.

Tips: Therefore, insertion of covered SEMS in patients with hilar malignant stricture is not generally recommended. ESGE recommends uncovered SEMSs for palliative drainage of malignant hilar obstruction. Of note, if a decision for palliation has not been taken, plastic stents are recommended because removal of uncovered SEMSs is usually not possible [152], and it sometimes could be useful to place more than one SEMS in case of small caliber of common bile duct (caliber the duct!)

40.2.15 Stent in Stent (SIS) Versus Side by Side (SBS): Which Is the Best Technique?

Tip: We suggest to use SBS as easier reintervention in case of stent occlusion.

The "side-by-side" and "stent-in-stent" positioning of multiple SEMSs have been found equivalent in a meta-analysis (four studies, 158 patients) with respect to the rates of successful stent placement, successful drainage, early and late complications, and stent occlusions and adverse event rate [196].

The choice of the technique thus seems to be at the discretion of the endoscopist, with the "side-by-side" and "stent-in-stent" techniques more frequently used in Western and Asian countries, respectively. The appropriate methods should be select based on the technical difficulty, degree of bile duct dilations, and level of operator's experience. The insertion of side-by-side SEMSs has become easier with the availability of small-diameter delivery catheters that can be passed simultaneously in a standard therapeutic channel duodenoscope and permit simultaneous SEMS deployment [197].

Different precautions should be taken with each technique (e.g., with the "side-by-side" technique, the SEMSs should cross the papilla or their lower extremities should be positioned at the same level in the CBD to facilitate further stent access).

40.2.15.1 How to Treat Stent Dysfunction?

The diagnosis of stent dysfunction has not been standardized; it is usually based on the combination of clinical criteria and liver function tests, complemented with transabdominal ultrasound in some cases. Examples of definitions of stent dysfunction used in RCTs are a decline in bilirubin <20% following stent insertion (failed biliary drainage), development of cholangitis, jaundice, or a flu-like syndrome, and cholestasis [198]. More recent RCTs have mostly used para-clinical tests, as in the study by Schmidt et al. who defined stent dysfunction as the presence of two of the three following criteria:

(a) Ultrasound showing new dilatation of intrahepatic or extrahepatic bile ducts
(b) Bilirubin ≥ 2 mg/dL (34.2 μmol/L) with an increase ≥1 mg/dL (17.1 μmol/L) compared to the value after initial successful drainage, or elevation of alkaline phosphatases/gamma-glutamyl transferase to more than twice the upper limit of normal values with an increase of at least 30 U/L
(c) Signs of cholangitis (fever and leukocyte count >10,000/μL or C-reactive protein (CRP) > 20 mg/dL) [199]

A meta-analysis (seven retrospective studies, 314 patients) found no difference in stent reocclusion when plastic stents vs. SEMSs were used to treat occluded SEMSs in patients with a malignant biliary obstruction (relative risk, 1.24; 95% CI, 0.92–1.67) [200].

In a more recent RCT, 48 patients with a malignant biliary obstruction who developed stent dysfunction were randomized to insertion of a plastic stent, uncovered SEMS, or PCSEMS [68]. Of these, 11 patients (23%) again developed stent dysfunction, eight in the plastic stent group, one in the uncovered SEMS group, and two in the PCSEMS group, with mean functional durations of 170 days, 367 days, and 326 days, respectively (plastic stent vs. SEMS; $p = 0.026$). No differences in overall costs were found between secondarily placed SEMSs or plastic stents. Another RCT (43 patients with a nonfunctioning uncovered SEMS in a malignant distal biliary obstruction) found no difference in time to stent occlusion between covered and uncovered SEMS (112 vs. 181 days, respectively; $P > 0.05$) [201].

Dysfunction of plastic stents is treated by stent removal, cleaning of ductal debris, and SEMS insertion, unless the diagnosis is not yet clear or patient life expectancy is very limited.

In the case of SEMS occlusion, cleaning of ductal debris with a balloon is suggested, followed by cholangiographic assessment of the degree of tissue ingrowth/overgrowth and subsequent insertion of an inner plastic stent or SEMS [202]; a retrospective study (52 patients) reported a longer patency (131 days vs. 47 days) with SEMSs vs. plastic stents [203]. Radiofrequency ablation might be an alternative option although data are sparse and comparison with insertion of a plastic stent has been reported in only one retrospective study [204].

ESGE suggests that in a patient with a DMBO and a nonfunctioning stent, a plastic stent should be replaced by a SEMS and, in the case of a SEMS, a plastic stent or a new SMS should be inserted within the original SEMS.

40.2.15.2 Preoperative Biliary Drainage (PBD): Is There a Role

Two systematic reviews (11 studies, 711 patients, and nine studies, 892 patients) reported that preoperative biliary drainage of hilar cholangiocarcinoma was associated with a higher postoperative morbidity rate, in particular because of infections, and no significant difference in postoperative mortality [205, 206].

However, many authors have suggested that in specific situations (e.g., cholangitis, predicted future liver remnant volume of ≤30% following surgery), preoperative drainage could be indicated [207].

These situations have been associated with a high risk of postoperative liver failure and may thus benefit from portal vein embolization and drainage limited to the future liver remnant segments [208].

ESGE suggests against routine preoperative biliary drainage in patients with malignant hilar obstruction. The indication and route for preoperative biliary drainage should be decided by a multidisciplinary team based on patient characteristics and institutional experience.

40.2.15.3 How to Perform PBD?

With respect to the choice between the endoscopic and percutaneous approaches for preoperative biliary drainage, two meta-analyses (four retrospective studies, 433 patients, and three retrospective studies, 265 patients) reported a similar [209] or higher [210] procedure-related morbidity for ERCP vs. PTBD.

On the other hand, a large, more recent, retrospective study (280 patients) found that major postoperative morbidity was more frequent after PTBD vs. ERCP for drainage of MHS [211].

A single meta-analysis analyzed long-term survival; it was shorter following PTBD vs. ERCP (30% vs. 46% at 5 years) [209].

A similarly shorter patient survival following PTBD vs. ERCP was reported in three large retrospective studies (793 patients) not included in the meta-analyses [212–214].

Peritoneal metastasis was more frequent following PTBD vs. ERCP; it may be associated with the duration of PTBD (60 days or more) and the presence of multiple PTBD catheters [215].

A similar association between preoperative PTBD and shorter survival has not been found in a Western bicentric study (245 patients) with a different use of PTBD catheters [216].

40.2.15.4 Which Stent Should Be Used for PBD?

If endoscopic preoperative drainage of MHS is performed, plastic stents or nasobiliary drains are preferred [217]; although less comfortable for the patient, nasobiliary drains are preferred in particular by Japanese authors because of the lower incidence of cholangitis due to tube occlusion [218]. The use of SEMSs for preoperative drainage of MHS is discouraged because of the paucity of the literature [219] and the risk of precluding curative surgery.

40.2.15.5 Which Length? Is the Length Important?

There are no studies that assess this relevant point. We must remember that placing a long USEMS in case of HMBO is one of the causes of stent occlusion due to development of hyperplastic reaction of lateral duct and sludge and stone formation.

40.2.15.6 Is There a Role of Drug-Eluting SEMS?

Drug-eluting SEMSs have been designed in an attempt to improve SEMS to prevent tumor ingrowth and stent occlusion.

An early multicenter prospective study using a paclitaxel-eluting stent did not show improved performance compared to conventional USEMS, though other stents are currently in development [220].

Antireflux stents have been developed to limit duodenal contents into the bile ducts and stent occlusion [221].

Initial experience with antireflux SEMS has yielded conflicting results; one study showed long-term patency possibly exceeding conventional SEMS, while a smaller study showed a disappointing rate of early occlusion [222]. Further studies are needed to demonstrate the efficacy of antireflux and drug-eluting SEMS to determine their role in maintaining long-term patency.

40.2.15.7 Endoscopic Adjuvant Treatment of Biliary Obstruction: Advance Beyond the SEMS

Patients with cholangiocarcinoma and pancreatic cancer continue to have poor prognosis when surgery is not an option. Meta-analysis has not shown a significant improvement with standard chemoradiation regimens for biliary malignancies [223] likely due to a late presentation and aggressive nature on presentation. However, two endoscopic therapies aimed at providing local control of biliary malignancy have shown some promise in early studies to improve stent function, quality of life, and overall survival in patients with advanced, unresectable disease.

The use of photodynamic therapy (PDT) has been studied for palliation of unresectable cholangiocarcinoma.

An RCT of PDT when compared to biliary stenting alone showed a dramatic increase in survival time from 98 days to 493 days [151]. Another RCT also showed a median survival increased from 210 days to 630 days [224].

Retrospective data also support increase of survival and quality of life when PDT is used in addition to biliary stents as well as chemotherapy [225, 226].

Several studies have demonstrated the ability of PDT to locally control tumor, improve stent patency and quality of life, and even improve survival in patients with unresectable cholangiocarcinoma [151, 224, 227–231].

Three meta-analyses confirmed that palliative treatment of cholangiocarcinoma with PDT is associated with improved biliary drainage, better quality of life, and increased survival, though all noted that the overall quality of evidence is low, with few randomized trials and low number of patients [232–234]. Side effects from phototherapy are mainly related to photosensitivity. The high cost of PDT may be a factor preventing its widespread use for local control of unresectable cholangiocarcinoma.

40.2.15.8 Radiofrequency Ablation

Radiofrequency ablation (RFA), compared to PDT, offers low cost and is technically simple to perform inducing ablative necrosis and can be used to palliate biliary malignancies by using a bipolar probe placed at the site of obstruction [230].

RFA can be performed through a percutaneous route or via catheter inserted via ERCP creating a coagulative necrosis of the intraductal tumor mass. Plastic stent is applied when future ablation is planned, while SEMS may be used when a single session is planned.

The risk of adverse events is low but includes hemobilia and biliary fistula.

The literature supporting RFA for biliary malignancies is not as robust as that for PDT, consisting mostly of retrospective series [235].

A retrospective comparison by Strand et al. [236] compared results in 48 patients (16 RFA, 32 PDT) which demonstrated similar median survival (9.6 months in RFA, 7.5 months in PDT). Future studies will be required to determine the optimal techniques for RFA, as well as the patient populations who are most likely to benefit.

European studies have also investigated the use of RFA therapy to treat occlusion of SEMS without the need for additional stent placement [237].

An open label prospective pilot study demonstrated successful RFA of the biliary system in 21 of 22 patients, but only six had cholangiocarcinoma [238].

References

1. Cipolletta L, Rotondano G, Marmo R, et al. Endoscopic palliation of malignant obstructive jaundice: an evidence-based review. Dig Liver Dis. 2007;39:375–88.
2. Stern N, Sturgess R. Endoscopic therapy in the management of malignant biliary obstruction. Eur J Surg Oncol. 2008;34:313–7.
3. Irisawa A, Katanuma A, Itoi T. Otaru consensus on biliary stenting for unresectable distal malignant biliary obstruction. Dig Endosc. 2013;25(Suppl 2):52–7.
4. Wassef W, Syed I. Designer stents: are we there yet? Gastrointest Endosc. 2007;66:804–8.
5. Glazer ES, Hornbrook MC, Krouse RS. A meta-analysis of randomized trials: immediate stent placement vs. surgical bypass in the palliative management of malignant biliary obstruction. J Pain Symptom Manage. 2014;47:307–14.
6. de Lima SLA, Bustamante FAC, de Moura EGH, et al. Endoscopic palliative treatment versus surgical bypass in malignant low bile duct obstruction: a systematic review and meta-analysis. Int J Hepatobiliary Pancreat Dis. 2015;5:35–46.
7. Taylor MC, McLeod RS, Langer B. Biliary stenting versus bypass surgery for the palliation of malignant distal bile duct obstruction: a meta-analysis. Liver Transpl. 2000;6:302–8.
8. Artifon EL, Sakai P, Cunha JE, et al. Surgery or endoscopy for palliation of biliary obstruction due to metastatic pancreatic cancer. Am J Gastroenterol. 2006;101:2031–7.
9. Jaganmohan S, Lee JH. Self-expandable metal stents in malignant biliary obstruction. Expert Rev Gastroenterol Hepatol. 2012;6:105–14.
10. Lee JH. Self-expandable metal stents for malignant distal biliary strictures. Gastrointest Endosc Clin N Am. 2011;21:463–80, viii–ix.
11. Moss AC, Morris E, Leyden J, et al. Malignant distal biliary obstruction: a systematic review and meta-analysis of endoscopic and surgical bypass results. Cancer Treat Rev. 2007;33:213–21.
12. Hara K, Yamao K, Hijioka S, et al. Prospective clinical study of endoscopic ultrasound-guided choledochoduodenostomy with direct metallic stent placement using a forward-viewing echoendoscope. Endoscopy. 2013;45:392–6.
13. Bliss LA, Eskander MF, Kent TS, et al. Early surgical bypass versus endoscopic stent placement in pancreatic cancer. HPB (Oxford). 2016;18:671–7.
14. Fabbri C, Luigiano C, Lisotti A, et al. Endoscopic ultrasound-guided treatments: are we getting evidence based – a systematic review. World J Gastroenterol. 2014;20:8424–48.
15. Khan MA, Akbar A, Baron TH, et al. Endoscopic ultrasound-guided biliary drainage: a systematic review and meta-analysis. Dig Dis Sci. 2016;61:684–703.

16. Moole H, Bechtold ML, Forcione D, et al. A meta-analysis and systematic review: success of endoscopic ultrasound guided biliary stenting in patients with inoperable malignant biliary strictures and a failed ERCP. Medicine. 2017;96:e5154.
17. Wang K, Zhu J, Xing L, et al. Assessment of efficacy and safety of EUS-guided biliary drainage: a systematic review. Gastrointest Endosc. 2016;83:1218–27.
18. Kawakubo K, Kawakami H, Kuwatani M, et al. Endoscopic ultrasound guided choledochoduodenostomy vs transpapillary stenting for distal biliary obstruction. Endoscopy. 2016;48:164–9.
19. Jin Z, Wei Y, Lin H, et al. Endoscopic ultrasound-guided versus endoscopic retrograde cholangiopancreatography-guided biliary drainage for primary treatment of distal malignant biliary obstruction: A systematic review and meta-analysis. Dig Endosc. 2020;32(1):16–26.
20. Dhir V, Itoi T, Khashab MA, et al. Multicenter comparative evaluation of endoscopic placement of expandable metal stents for malignant distal common bile duct obstruction by ERCP or EUS-guided approach. Gastrointest Endosc. 2015;81:913–23.
21. Iwashita T, Yasuda I, Mukai T, et al. Endoscopic ultrasound-guided antegrade biliary stenting for unresectable malignant biliary obstruction in patients with surgically altered anatomy: Single-center prospective pilot study. Dig Endosc. 2017;29:362–8.
22. Lee A, Aditi A, Bhat YM, et al. Endoscopic ultrasound-guided biliary access versus precut papillotomy in patients with failed biliary cannulation: a retrospective study. Endoscopy. 2017;49:146–53.
23. Church NI, Seward EW, Pereira SP, et al. Success of repeat ERCP following initial therapeutic failure. Gastrointest Endosc. 2006;63:AB293.
24. Colan-Hernandez J, Aldana A, Concepción M, et al. Optimal timing for a second ERCP after failure of initial biliary cannulation following precut sphincterotomy: an analysis of experience at two tertiary centers. Surg Endosc. 2017;31:125.
25. Donnellan F, Enns R, Kim E, et al. Outcome of repeat ERCP after initial failed use of a needle knife for biliary access. Dig Dis Sci. 2012;57:1069–71.
26. Hisai H, Okagawa Y, Wada H, et al. Outcome of repeat ERCP after biliary cannulation failure following needle knife sphincterotomy. Gastrointest Endosc. 2013;77:AB291.
27. Kevans D, Zeb F, Donnellan F, et al. Failed biliary access following needle knife fistulotomy: is repeat interval ERCP worthwhile? Scand J Gastroenterol. 2010;45:1238–41.
28. Kim J, Ryu JK, Ahn D-W, et al. Results of repeat endoscopic retrograde cholangiopancreatography after initial biliary cannulation failure following needle-knife sphincterotomy. J Gastroenterol Hepatol. 2012;27:516–20.
29. Pavlides M, Barnabas A, Fernandopulle N, et al. Repeat endoscopic retrograde cholangiopancreaticography after failed initial precut sphincterotomy for biliary cannulation. World J Gastroenterol. 2014;20:13153–8.
30. Ramirez FC, Dennert B, Sanowski RA. Success of repeat ERCP by the same endoscopist. Gastrointest Endosc. 1999;49:58–61.
31. Swan MP, Bourke MJ, Williams SJ, et al. Failed biliary cannulation: clinical and technical outcomes after tertiary referral endoscopic retrograde cholangiopancreatography. World J Gastroenterol. 2011;17(45):4993–8.
32. Park do H, Jang JW, Lee SS, et al. EUS-guided biliary drainage with transluminal stenting after failed ERCP: predictors of adverse events and long-term results. Gastrointest Endosc. 2011;74: 1276–84.
33. Enochsson L, Swahn F, Arnelo U, et al. Nationwide, population-based data from 11,074 ERCP procedures from the Swedish Registry for Gallstone Surgery and ERCP. Gastrointest Endosc. 2010;72:1175–84.e1-3.
34. Nennstiel S, Weber A, Frick G, et al. Drainage-related complications in percutaneous transhepatic biliary drainage: an analysis over 10 years. J Clin Gastroenterol. 2015;49:764–70.
35. Giovannini M, Moutardier V, Pesenti C, et al. Endoscopic ultrasound-guided bilioduodenal anastomosis: a new technique for biliary drainage. Endoscopy. 2001;33:898–900.
36. Giovannini M. Multicenter randomized phase II study: Percutaneous biliary drainage vs. EUS guided biliary drainage: results of interim analysis. Gastrointest Endosc. 2015;81:AB171.
37. Khashab MA, Valeshabad AK, Afghani E, et al. A comparative evaluation of EUS-guided biliary drainage and percutaneous drainage in patients with distal malignant biliary obstruction and failed ERCP. Dig Dis Sci. 2015;60:557–65.
38. Sharaiha RZ, Khan MA, Kamal F, et al. Efficacy and safety of EUS-guided biliary drainage in comparison with percutaneous biliary drainage when ERCP fails: a systematic review and meta-analysis. Gastrointest Endosc. 2017;85:904–14.
39. Dhir V, Bhandari S, Bapat M, et al. Comparison of transhepatic and extrahepatic routes for EUS-guided rendezvous procedure for distal CBD obstruction. United European Gastroenterol J. 2013;1:103–8.
40. Gupta K, Perez-Miranda M, Kahaleh M, et al. Endoscopic ultrasound-assisted bile duct access and drainage: multicenter, long-term analysis of approach, outcomes, and complications of a technique in evolution. J Clin Gastroenterol. 2014;48:80–7.
41. Dhir V, Artifon EL, Gupta K, et al. Multicenter study on endoscopic ultrasound-guided expandable biliary metal stent placement: choice of access route, direction of stent insertion, and drainage route. Dig Endosc. 2014;26:430–5.
42. Khashab MA, Van der Merwe S, Kunda R, et al. Prospective international multicenter study on endoscopic ultrasound-guided biliary drainage for patients with malignant distal biliary obstruction after failed endoscopic retrograde cholangiopancreatography. Endosc Int Open. 2016;4:E487–96.

43. Ogura T, Chiba Y, Masuda D, et al. Comparison of the clinical impact of endoscopic ultrasound-guided choledochoduodenostomy and hepaticogastrostomy for bile duct obstruction with duodenal obstruction. Endoscopy. 2016;48:156–63.
44. Artifon EL, Marson FP, Gaidhane M, et al. Hepaticogastrostomy or choledochoduodenostomy for distal malignant biliary obstruction after failed ERCP: is there any difference? Gastrointest Endosc. 2015;81:950–9.
45. Mohan BO, Shakhatreh M, Garg R, et al. Efficacy and safety of endoscopic ultrasound-guided choledoduodenostomy: a systematic review and meta-analysis. J Clin Gastroenterol. 2019;53:243–50.
46. Artifon EL, Aparicio D, Paione JB, et al. Biliary drainage in patients with unresectable, malignant obstruction where ERCP fails: endoscopic ultrasonography-guided choledochoduodenostomy versus percutaneous drainage. J Clin Gastroenterol. 2012;46:768–74.
47. Baniya R, Upadhaya S, Amdal S, et al. Endoscopic ultrasound-guided biliary drainage versus percutaneous transhepatic biliary drainage after failed ERCP: a meta-analysis. Clin Exp Gastroenterol. 2017;10:67–74.
48. Artifon ELA, Sakai P, IShioka S, et al. Endoscopic sphincterotomy before deployment of covered metal stent is associated with greater complication rate: a prospective randomized controlled trial. J Clin Gastroenterol. 2008;42(7):815–9.
49. Giorgio PD, Luca LD. Comparison of treatment outcomes between biliary plastic stent placements with and without endoscopic sphincterotomy for inoperable malignant common bile duct obstruction. World J Gastroenterol. 2004;10:1212–121.
50. Hayashi T, Kawakami H, Osanai M, et al. No benefit of endoscopic sphincterotomy before biliary placement of self-expandable metal stents for unresectable pancreatic cancer. Clin Gastroenterol Hepatol. 2015;13(6):1151–8.
51. Zhou H, Li L, Zhu S, et al. Endoscopic sphincterotomy associated cholangitis in patients receiving proximal biliary self-expanding metal stent. Hepatobiliary Pancreat Dis Int. 2012;11(6): 643–9.
52. Banerjee N, Hiloden K, Baron TH, et al. Endoscopic sphincterotomy is not required for transpapillary SEMS placement for biliary obstruction. Dig Dis Sci. 2011;56(2):591–5.
53. Kawakubo K, Isayama H, Nakai Y, et al. Risk factors for pancreatitis following transpapillary self-expandable metal stent placement. Surg Endosc. 2012;26:771–6.
54. Margulies C, Siqueira ES, Silverman WB, Lin XS, Martin JA, Rabinovitz M, Slivka A. The effect of endoscopic sphincterotomy on acute and chronic complications of biliary endoprostheses. Gastrointest Endosc. 1999;49:716–9.
55. Nakahara K, Okuse C, Suetani K, et al. Covered metal stenting for malignant lower biliary stricture with pancreatic duct obstruction: is endoscopic sphincterotomy needed? Gastroenterol Res Pract. 2013;2013:375613.
56. Shimizu I, Naitoh T, Nakazawa T, et al. Predictive factors for pancreatitis and cholecystitis in endoscopic covered metal stenting for distal malignant biliary obstruction. J Gastroenterol Hepatol. 2013;28(1):68–72.
57. Wilcox CM, Kim H, Ramesh J, et al. Biliary sphincterotomy is not required for bile duct stent placement. Dig Endosc. 2014;26(1):87–92.
58. Suk KT, Kim HS, Kim JW, et al. Risk factors for cholecystitis after metal stent placement in malignant biliary obstruction. Gastrointest Endosc. 2006;64(4):522–9.
59. Tringali A, Hassan C, Rota M, et al. Covered vs. uncovered self-expandable metal stents for malignant distal biliary strictures: a systematic review and meta-analysis. Endoscopy. 2018;50(6):631–41.
60. Mutignani M, Tringali A, Shah SG, et al. Combined endoscopic stent insertion in malignant biliary and duodenal obstruction. Endoscopy. 2007;39:440–7.
61. Staub J, Siddiqui A, Taylor LJ, Loren D, Kowalski T, Adler DG. ERCP performed through previously placed duodenal stents: a multicenter retrospective study of outcomes and adverse events. Gastrointest Endosc. 2018;87(6):1499–504.
62. Yao JF, Zhang L, Wu H. Analysis of high risk factors for endoscopic retrograde cholangiopancreatography biliary metallic stenting after malignant duodenal stricture SEMS implantation. J Biol Regul Homeost Agents. 2016;30:743–8.
63. Matsumoto K, Kato H, Tsutsumi K, et al. Long-term outcomes and risk factors of biliary stent dysfunction after endoscopic double stenting for malignant biliary and duodenal obstructions. Dig Endosc. 2017;29:617–25.
64. Jeurnink SM, Steyerberg EW, Vleggaar FP, et al. Predictors of survival in patients with malignant gastric outlet obstruction: a patient-oriented decision approach for palliative treatment. Dig Liver Dis. 2011;43:548–52.
65. Dumonceau JM, Heresbach D, Deviere J, et al. Biliary stents: models and methods for endoscopic stenting. Endoscopy. 2011;43:617–26.
66. Canena J, Coimbra J, Carvalho D, et al. Endoscopic bilio-duodenal bypass: outcomes of primary and revision efficacy of combined metallic stents in malignant duodenal and biliary obstructions. Dig Dis Sci. 2014;59:2779–89.
67. Khashab MA, Valeshabad AK, Leung W, et al. Multicenter experience with performance of ERCP in patients with an indwelling duodenal stent. Endoscopy. 2014;46:252–5.
68. Walter D, van Boeckel PGA, Groenen MJ, et al. Cost efficacy of metal stents for palliation of extrahepatic bile duct obstruction in a randomized controlled trial. Gastroenterology. 2015;149:130–8.
69. Moss AC, Morris E, Leyden J, et al. Do the benefits of metal stents justify the costs? A systematic

review and meta-analysis of trials comparing endoscopic stents for malignant biliary obstruction. Eur J Gastroenterol Hepatol. 2007;19(12):1119–24.

70. Yeoh KG, Zimmerman MJ, Cunningham JT, et al. Comparative costs of metal versus plastic biliary stent strategies for malignant obstructive jaundice by decision analysis. Gastrointest Endosc. 1999; 49(4 Pt 1):466–71.
71. Mohankumar D, Garner H, Ruff K, et al. Characterization of right wrist posture during simulated colonoscopy: an application of kinematic analysis to the study of endoscopic maneuvers. Gastrointest Endosc. 2014;79(3):480–9.
72. Soderlund C, Linder S. Covered metal versus plastic stents for malignant common bile duct stenosis: a prospective, randomized, controlled trial. Gastrointest Endosc. 2006;63(7):986–95.
73. Almadi MA, Barkun A, Martel M. Plastic vs. self-expandable metal stents for palliation in malignant biliary obstruction: a series of meta-analyses. Am J Gastroenterol. 2017;112:260–73.
74. Hong WD, Chen XW, Wu WZ, et al. Metal versus plastic stents for malignant biliary obstruction: an update meta-analysis. Clin Res Hepatol Gastroenterol. 2013;37:496–500.
75. Moole H, Jaeger A, Cashman M, et al. Are self-expandable metal stents superior to plastic stents in palliating malignant distal biliary strictures? A meta-analysis and systematic review. Med J Armed Forces India. 2017;73:42–8.
76. Sawas T, Al Halabi S, Parsi MA, et al. Self-expandable metal stents versus plastic stents for malignant biliary obstruction: a meta-analysis. Gastrointest Endosc. 2015;82:256–267.e7.
77. Zorron PL, de Moura EG, Bernardo WM, et al. Endoscopic stenting for inoperable malignant biliary obstruction: a systematic review and meta-analysis. World J Gastroenterol. 2015;21:13374–85.
78. Walter D, van Boeckel PGA, Groenen MJM, et al. Higher quality of life after metal stent placement compared with plastic stent placement for malignant extrahepatic bile duct obstruction: a randomized controlled trial. Eur J Gastroenterol Hepatol. 2017;29:231–7.
79. Tringali A, Mutignani M, Adler DG. Fully covered self-expandable metal stents versus uncovered self-expandable metal stents in patients with distal malignant biliary stricture: Is this the right question? Gastrointest Endosc. 2019;89(4):897–8.
80. Isayama H, Nakai Y, Kawakubo K, et al. Covered metallic stenting for malignant distal biliary obstruction: clinical results according to stent type. J Hepatobiliary Pancreat Sci. 2011;18(5):673–47.
81. Alastal Y, Hammad T, Khan AM, et al. Risk of post-ERCP pancreatitis with the placement of covered versus uncovered self-expandable biliary metal stents: systematic review and meta-analysis. JOP. 2015;16:452–8.
82. Almadi MA, Barkun AN, Martel M. No benefit of covered vs uncovered self-expandable metal stents in patients with malignant distal biliary obstruction: a meta-analysis. Clin Gastroenterol Hepatol. 2013;11:27–37.e21.
83. Chen M-Y, Lin J-W, Zhu H-P, et al. Covered stents versus uncovered stents for unresectable malignant biliary strictures: a meta-analysis. Biomed Res Int. 2016;2016:6408067.
84. Li J, Li T, Sun P, et al. Covered versus uncovered self-expandable metal stents for managing malignant distal biliary obstruction: a meta-analysis. PLoS One. 2016;11:e0149066.
85. Moole H, Bechtold ML, Cashman M, et al. Covered versus uncovered self-expandable metal stents for malignant biliary strictures: a meta-analysis and systematic review. Indian J Gastroenterol. 2016;35:323–30.
86. Saleem A, Leggett CL, Murad MH, et al. Meta-analysis of randomized trials comparing the patency of covered and uncovered self-expandable metal stents for palliation of distal malignant bile duct obstruction. Gastrointest Endosc. 2011;74:321–327.e321–3.
87. Yang Z, Wu Q, Wang F, et al. A systematic review and meta-analysis of randomized trials and prospective studies comparing covered and bare self-expandable metal stents for the treatment of malignant obstruction in the digestive tract. Int J Med Sci. 2013;10:825–83.
88. Fumex F, Coumaros D, Napoleon B, et al. Similar performance but higher cholecystitis rate with covered biliary stents: results from a prospective multicenter evaluation. Endoscopy. 2006;38:787–92.
89. Isayama H, Komatsu Y, Tsujino T, et al. A prospective randomised study of "covered" versus "uncovered" diamond stents for the management of distal malignant biliary obstruction. Gut. 2004;53:729–34.
90. Krokidis M, Fanelli F, Orgera G, et al. Percutaneous treatment of malignant jaundice due to extrahepatic cholangiocarcinoma: covered Viabil stent versus uncovered Wallstents. Cardiovasc Intervent Radiol. 2010;33:97–106.
91. Isayama H, Mukai T, Itoi T, et al. Comparison of partially covered nitinol stents with partially covered stainless stents as a historical control in a multicenter study of distal malignant biliary obstruction: the WATCH study. Gastrointest Endosc. 2012;76:84–92.
92. Soderlund C, Linder S, Bergenzaun PE, et al. Nitinol versus steel partially covered self-expandable metal stent for malignant distal biliary obstruction: a randomized trial. Endoscopy. 2014;46:941–8.
93. Hu B, Wang TT, Wu J, et al. Antireflux stents to reduce the risk of cholangitis in patients with malignant biliary strictures: a randomized trial. Endoscopy. 2014;46:120–6.
94. Lee YN, Moon JH, Choi HJ, et al. Effectiveness of a newly designed antireflux valve metal stent to reduce duodenobiliary reflux in patients with unresectable distal malignant biliary obstruction: a randomized,

controlled pilot study (with videos). Gastrointest Endosc. 2016;83:404–12.
95. Zhang R, Luo H, Pan Y, et al. Rate of duodenal-biliary reflux increases in patients with recurrent common bile duct stones: evidence from barium meal examination. Gastrointest Endosc. 2015;82:660–5.
96. Minaga K, Kitano M, Imai H, et al. Evaluation of anti-migration properties of biliary covered self-expandable metal stents. World J Gastroenterol. 2016;22:6917–9.
97. Park do H, Lee SS, Lee TH, et al. Anchoring flap versus flared end, fully covered self-expandable metal stents to prevent migration in patients with benign biliary strictures: a multicenter, prospective, comparative pilot study (with videos). Gastrointest Endosc. 2011;73:64–70.
98. Hamada T, Isayama H, Nakai Y, et al. Antireflux metal stent with an antimigration system for distal malignant biliary obstruction: a feasibility pilot study. Surg Laparosc Endosc Percutan Tech. 2015;25:212–7.
99. Zhu H-D, Guo J-H, Zhu G-Y, et al. A novel biliary stent loaded with (125)I seeds in patients with malignant biliary obstruction: preliminary results versus a conventional biliary stent. J Hepatol. 2012;56:1104–11.
100. Hasimu A, Gu J-P, Ji W-Z, et al. Comparative study of percutaneous transhepatic biliary stent placement with or without iodine-125 seeds for treating patients with malignant biliary obstruction. J Vasc Intervent Radiol. 2017;28:583–93.
101. Jang SI, Lee SJ, Jeong S, et al. Efficacy of a multiplex paclitaxel emission stent using a Pluronic® mixture membrane versus a covered metal stent in malignant biliary obstruction: a prospective randomized comparative study. Gut Liver. 2017;11:567–73.
102. Tringali A, Hassan C, Rota M, et al. Correction: covered vs. uncovered self-expandable metal stents for malignant distal biliary strictures: a systematic review and metaanalysis. Endoscopy. 2018;50(6):C5.
103. Wolfson D, Barkin JS, Chari ST, et al. Management of pancreatic masses. Pancreas. 2005;31:203–17.
104. Siriwardana HP, Siriwardena AK. Systematic appraisal of the role of metallic endobiliary stents in the treatment of benign bile duct stricture. Ann Surg. 2005;242:10–9.
105. Arias Dachary FJ, Chioccioli C, Deprez PH. Application of the "covered- stent-in-uncovered-stent" technique for easy and safe removal of embedded biliary uncovered SEMS with tissue ingrowth. Endoscopy. 2010;42(Suppl 2):E304–5.
106. Tan DM, Lillemoe KD, Fogel EL. A new technique for endoscopic removal of uncovered biliary self-expandable metal stents: stent-in-stent technique with a fully covered biliary stent. Gastrointest Endosc. 2012;75:923–5.
107. Tringali A, Blero D, Boskoski I, et al. Difficult removal of fully covered self expandable metal stents (SEMS) for benign biliary strictures: the "SEMS in SEMS" technique. Dig Liver Dis. 2014;46:568–71.
108. Cabral V, Zhou J. Preoperative biliary drainage for pancreatic head carcinoma: a systematic review and meta-analysis. Biomed Lett. 2015;1:81–7.
109. Chen Y, Ou G, Lian G, et al. Effect of preoperative biliary drainage on complications following pancreatoduodenectomy: a meta-analysis. Medicine. 2015;94:e1199.
110. Fang Y, Gurusamy KS, Wang Q, et al. Meta-analysis of randomized clinical trials on safety and efficacy of biliary drainage before surgery for obstructive jaundice. Br J Surg. 2013;100:1589–96.
111. Qiu Y-D, Bai J-L, Xu F-G, et al. Effect of preoperative biliary drainage on malignant obstructive jaundice: a meta-analysis. World J Gastroenterol. 2011;17:391–6.
112. Saleh MMA, Nørregaard P, Jørgensen HL, et al. Preoperative endoscopic stent placement before pancreaticoduodenectomy: a meta-analysis of the effect on morbidity and mortality. Gastrointest Endosc. 2002;56:529–34.
113. Scheufele F, Schorn S, Demir IE, et al. Preoperative biliary stenting versus operation first in jaundiced patients due to malignant lesions in the pancreatic head: a meta-analysis of current literature. Surgery. 2017;161:939–50.
114. Sewnath ME, Karsten TM, Prins MH, et al. A meta-analysis on the efficacy of preoperative biliary drainage for tumors causing obstructive jaundice. Ann Surg. 2002;236:17–27.
115. Sun C, Yan G, Li Z, et al. A meta-analysis of the effect of preoperative biliary stenting on patients with obstructive jaundice. Medicine. 2014;93:e189.
116. Velanovich V, Kheibek T, Khan M. Relationship of postoperative complications from preoperative biliary stents after pancreaticoduodenectomy. A new cohort analysis and meta-analysis of modern studies. JOP. 2009;10:24–9.
117. Moole H, Bechtold M, Puli SR. Efficacy of preoperative biliary drainage in malignant obstructive jaundice: a meta-analysis and systematic review. World J Surg Oncol. 2016;14:182.
118. Barauskas G, Urbonas K, Smailyte G, et al. Preoperative endoscopic biliary drainage may negatively impact survival following pancreatoduodenectomy for ampullary cancer. Dig Surg. 2016;33:462–9.
119. Furukawa K, Shiba H, Shirai Y, et al. Negative impact of preoperative endoscopic biliary drainage on prognosis of pancreatic ductal adenocarcinoma after pancreaticoduodenectomy. Anticancer Res. 2015;35:5079–83.
120. Sauvanet A, Boher JM, Paye F, et al. Severe jaundice increases early severe morbidity and decreases long-term survival after pancreaticoduodenectomy for pancreatic adenocarcinoma. J Am Coll Surg. 2015;221:380–9.
121. van der Gaag NA, Rauws EA, van Eijck CH, et al. Preoperative biliary drainage for cancer of the head of the pancreas. N Engl J Med. 2010;362:129–37.

122. Arkadopoulos N, Kyriazi MA, Papanikolaou IS, et al. Preoperative biliary drainage of severely jaundiced patients increases morbidity of pancreaticoduodenectomy: results of a case-control study. World J Surg. 2014;38:2967–72.
123. Miura F, Sano K, Wada K, et al. Prognostic impact of type of preoperative biliary drainage in patients with distal cholangiocarcinoma. Am J Surg. 2017;214:256–61.
124. Strom TJ, Klapman JB, Springett GM, et al. Comparative long-term outcomes of upfront resected pancreatic cancer after preoperative biliary drainage. Surg Endosc. 2015;29:3273–81.
125. Uemura K, Murakami Y, Satoi S, et al. Impact of preoperative biliary drainage on long-term survival in resected pancreatic ductal adenocarcinoma: a multicenter observational study. Ann Surg Oncol. 2015;22(Suppl. 3):1238–46.
126. Crippa S, Cirocchi R, Partelli S, et al. Systematic review and meta-analysis of metal versus plastic stents for preoperative biliary drainage in resectable periampullary or pancreatic head tumors. Eur J Surg Oncol. 2016;42:1278–85.
127. Song TJ, Lee JH, Lee SS, et al. Metal versus plastic stents for drainage of malignant biliary obstruction before primary surgical resection. Gastrointest Endosc. 2016;84:814–21.
128. Gardner TB, Spangler CC, Byanova KL, et al. Cost-effectiveness and clinical efficacy of biliary stents in patients undergoing neoadjuvant therapy for pancreatic adenocarcinoma in a randomized controlled trial. Gastrointest Endosc. 2016;84:460–6.
129. Adams MA, Anderson MA, Myles JD, et al. Self-expanding metal stents (SEMS) provide superior outcomes compared to plastic stents for pancreatic cancer patients undergoing neoadjuvant therapy. J Gastrointest Oncol. 2012;3:309–13.
130. Tsuboi T, Sasaki T, Serikawa M, et al. Preoperative biliary drainage in cases of borderline resectable pancreatic cancer treated with neoadjuvant chemotherapy and surgery. Gastroenterol Res Pract. 2016;2016:7968201.
131. Cavell LK, Allen PJ, Vinoya C, et al. Biliary self-expandable metal stents do not adversely affect pancreaticoduodenectomy. Am J Gastroenterol. 2013;108:1168–73.
132. Larghi A, Tringali A, Lecca PG. Management of hilar biliary strictures. Am J Gastroenterol. 2008;103:458–73.
133. Lee SS, Kim MH, Lee SK, et al. Clinicopathologic review of 58 patients with biliary papillomatosis. Cancer. 2004;100:783–93.
134. Koea J, Holden A, CahuK MJ. Differential diagnosis of stenosing lesions at the hepatic hilus. World J. Surg. 2004;28:466–70.
135. de Bellis M, Sherman S, Fogel EL. Tissue sampling at ERCP in suspected malignant biliary stricture (part 2). Gastrointest Endosc. 2002;56:383–90.
136. Navaneethan U, Njei B, Lourdusamy V, et al. Comparative cost effectiveness of biliary brush cytology and intraductal biopsy for detection of malignant biliary strictures: a systematic review and meta-analysis. Gastrointest Endosc. 2015;81:168–76.
137. Jailwala J, Fogel EL, Sherman S. Triple tissue sampling at ERCP in malignant biliary obstruction. Gastrointest Endosc. 2000;51:383–90.
138. Ponchon T, Gagnon P, Berger F, et al. Value of endobiliary brush cytology and biopsies for the diagnosis of malignant bile duct stenosis: results of a prospective study. Gastrointest Endosc. 1995;42:565–72.
139. Weber A, von Weyhem C, Fend F, et al. Endoscopic trasnpapillary brush cytology and forceps biopsy in patients with hilar cholangiocarcinoma. World J Gastroenterol. 2008;14:1097–101.
140. De witt J, Misra VL, Leblanc JK, et al. EUS-guided FNA of proximal biliary strictures after negative ERCP brush cytology results. Gastrointest Endosc. 2006;64:325–33.
141. Heimbach JK, Sanchez W, Rosen CB, et al. Trasnperitoneal fine needle aspiration biopsy of hilar cholangiocarcinoma is associated with disease dissemination. HPB. 2011;13:356–60.
142. Rerknimitr R, Angsuwatcarakon P, Ratanachu-ek T, et al. Asian Pacific consensus recommendations for endoscopic and interventional management of hilar cholangiocarcinoma: consensus for hilar cholangiocarcinoma. J Gastroenterol Hepatol. 2013;28:593–607.
143. Navaneethan U, Hasan MK, Lourdusamy V, et al. Single-operator cholangioscopy and targeted biopsies in the diagnosis of indeterminate biliary strictures: a systematic review. Gastrointest Endosc. 2015;82(4):608–14.e2.
144. Ramchandani M, Reddy DN, Gupta R, et al. Role of single operator cholangioscopy and targeted biopsies in the diagnosis of indeterminate biliary lesions: a single center, prospective studies. Gastrointest. Endosc. 2011;74:511–9.
145. Draganov PV, Chauhan S, Wagh MS, et al. Diagnostic accuracy of conventional and cholangioscopy-guided sampling in indeterminate biliary lesions at the time of ERCP: a prospective long-term follow up study. Gastrointest Endosc. 2012;75:437–53.
146. Meining A, Chen YK, Pleskoww D, et al. Direct visualization of indeterminate pancreaticobiliary strictures with probe based confocal laser endomicroscopy: a multicenter experience. Gastrointest Endosc. 2011;74:961–8.
147. Goenka MK, Goenka U. Palliation: Hilar cholangiocarcinoma. World J Hepatol. 2014;6:559–69.
148. Dowsett JF, Vaira D, Hatfield AR, et al. Endoscopic biliary therapy using the combined percutaneous and endoscopic technique. Gastroenterology. 1989;96:1180–6.
149. Vienne A, Hobeika E, Gouya H, et al. Prediction of drainage effectiveness during endoscopic stenting of malignant hilar strictures: the role of liver volume assessment. Gastrointest Endosc. 2010;72:728–35.
150. Berr F, Tannapfel A, Lamesch P, et al. Neoadjuvant photodynamic therapy before curative resec-

tion of proximal bile duct carcinoma. J Hepatol. 2000;32:352–7.
151. Ortner ME, Caca K, Berr F, et al. Successful photodynamic therapy for nonresectable cholangiocarcinoma: a randomized prospective study. Gastroenterology. 2003;125:1355–63.
152. Jang SI, Hwang JH, Lee KH, et al. Percutaneous biliary approach as a successful rescue procedure after failed endoscopic therapy for drainage in advanced hilar tumors. J Gastroenterol Hepatol. 2017;32:932–8.
153. Lee SH, Park JK, Yoon WJ, et al. Optimal biliary drainage for inoperable Klatskin's tumor based on Bismuth type. World J Gastroenterol. 2007;13:3948–55.
154. Paik WH, Park YS, Hwang JH, et al. Palliative treatment with self-expandable metallic stents in patients with advanced type III or IV hilar cholangiocarcinoma: a percutaneous versus endoscopic approach. Gastrointest Endosc. 2009;69:55–62.
155. Moole H, Dharmapuri S, Duvvuri A, et al. Endoscopic versus percutaneous biliary drainage in palliation of advanced malignant hilar obstruction: a meta-analysis and systematic review. Can J Gastroenterol Hepatol. 2016;2016:4726078.
156. Barkay O, Mosler P, Schmitt CM, et al. Effect of endoscopic stenting of malignant bile duct obstruction on quality of life. J Clin Gastroenterol. 2013;47:526–31.
157. Gamanagatti S, Singh T, Sharma R. Unilobar versus bilobar biliary drainage: effect on quality of life and bilirubin level reduction. Indian J Palliat Care. 2016;22:50–62.
158. Cahal P, Baron TH. Expandable metal stents for endoscopic bilateral stent-within-stent placement for malignant hilar biliary obstruction. Gastrointest Endosc. 2010;71:195–9.
159. Dumas R, Demuth N, Buckley M, et al. Endoscopic bilateral metal stent placement for malignant hilar stenoses: identification of optimal technique. Gastrointest Endosc. 2000;51:334–8.
160. Hwang JC, Kim JH, Lim SG, et al. Y-shaped endoscopic bilateral metal stent placement for malignant hilar biliary obstruction: prospective long-term study. Scand J Gastroenterol. 2011;46:326–32.
161. Ishiwatari H, Hayashi T, Ono M, et al. Newly designed plastic stent for endoscopic placement above the sphincter of Oddi in patients with malignant hilar biliary obstruction. Dig Endosc. 2013;25(Suppl 2):94–9.
162. Kato H, Tsutsumi K, Harada R, et al. Endoscopic bilateral deployment of multiple metallic stents for malignant hilar biliary strictures. Dig Endosc. 2013;25(Suppl 2):75–80.
163. Kawamoto H, Tsutsumi K, Fujii M, et al. Endoscopic 3-branched partial stent-in-stent deployment of metallic stents in high-grade malignant hilar biliary stricture (with videos). Gastrointest Endosc. 2007;66:1030–7.
164. Kim JY, Kang DH, Kim HW, et al. Usefulness of slimmer and open-cell-design stents for endoscopic bilateral stenting and endoscopic revision in patients with hilar cholangiocarcinoma (with video). Gastrointest Endosc. 2009;70:1109–15.
165. Kogure H, Isayama H, Nakai Y, et al. Newly designed large cell Niti-S stent for malignant hilar biliary obstruction: a pilot study. Surg Endosc. 2011;25:463–7.
166. Lee JH, Kang DH, Kim JY, et al. Endoscopic bilateral metal stent placement for advanced hilar cholangiocarcinoma: a pilot study of a newly designed Y stent. Gastrointest Endosc. 2007;66:364–9.
167. Lee TH, Moon JH, Kim JH, et al. Primary and revision efficacy of cross-wired metallic stents for endoscopic bilateral stent-in-stent placement in malignant hilar biliary strictures. Endoscopy. 2013;45:106–13.
168. Lee TH, Park do H, Lee SS, et al. Technical feasibility and revision efficacy of the sequential deployment of endoscopic bilateral side-by-side metal stents for malignant hilar biliary strictures: a multicenter prospective study. Dig Dis Sci. 2013;58:547–55.
169. Naitoh I, Hayashi K, Nakazawa T, et al. Side-by-side versus stent-in-stent deployment in bilateral endoscopic metal stenting for malignant hilar biliary obstruction. Dig Dis Sci. 2012;57:3279–85.
170. Park do H, Lee SS, Moon JH, et al. Newly designed stent for endoscopic bilateral stent-in-stent placement of metallic stents in patients with malignant hilar biliary strictures: multicenter prospective feasibility study (with videos). Gastrointest Endosc. 2009;69:1357–60.
171. Keswani RN, Qumseya BJ, O'Dwyer LC, et al. Association between endoscopist and center endoscopic retrograde cholangiopancreatography volume with procedure success and adverse outcomes: a systematic review and meta-analysis. Clin Gastroenterol Hepatol. 2017;15:1866–1875.e3.
172. Itoi T, Sofuni A, Itokawa F, Tonozuka R, Ishii K. Current status and issues regarding biliary stenting in unresectable biliary obstruction. Dig Endosc. 2013;25(Suppl 2):63–70.
173. Dumonceau JM, Tringali A, Blero D, Devière J, Laugiers R, Heresbach D, Costamagna G. Biliary stenting: indications, choice of stents and results: European Society of Gastrointestinal Endoscopy (ESGE) clinical guideline. Endoscopy. 2012;44:277–98.
174. Tarnasky PR, Cunningham JT, Hawes RH, Hoffman BJ, Uflacker R, Vujic I, Cotton PB. Transpapillary stenting of proximal biliary strictures: does biliary sphincterotomy reduce the risk of postprocedure pancreatitis? Gastrointest Endosc. 1997;45:46–51.
175. Kozarek RA. Inflammation and carcinogenesis of the biliary tract: update on endoscopic treatment. Clin Gastroenterol Hepatol. 2009;7:S89–94.
176. Webb K, Saunders M. Endoscopic management of malignant bile duct strictures. Gastrointest Endosc Clin N Am. 2013;23:313.
177. Mukai T, Yasuda I, Nakashima M, et al. Metallic stents are more efficacious than plastic stents in

unresectable malignant hilar biliary strictures: a randomized controlled trial. J Hepatobiliary Pancreat Sci. 2013;20:214–22.
178. Perdue DG, Freeman ML, DiSario JA, et al. Plastic versus self-expanding metallic stents for malignant hilar biliary obstruction: a prospective multicenter observational cohort study. J Clin Gastroenterol. 2008;42:1040.
179. Sangchan A, Kongkasame W, Pugkhem A, et al. Efficacy of metal and plastic stents in unresectable complex hilar cholangiocarcinoma: a randomized controlled trial. Gastrointest Endosc. 2012;76:93–9.
180. Donelli G, Guaglianone E, Di Rosa R, et al. Plastic biliary stent occlusion: factors involved and possible preventive approaches. Clin Med Res. 2007;5:53–60.
181. Raju RP, Jaganmohan SR, Ross WA, et al. Optimum palliation of inoperable hilar cholangiocarcinoma: comparative assessment of the efficacy of plastic and self-expanding metal stents. Dig Dis Sci. 2011;56:1557–64.
182. Cheng JL, Bruno MJ, Bergman JJ, et al. Endoscopic palliation of patients with biliary obstruction caused by nonresectable hilar cholangiocarcinoma: efficacy of self-expandable metallic Wallstents. Gastrointest Endosc. 2002;56:33–9.
183. Sangchan A, Chaiyakunapruk N, Supakankunti S, et al. Cost utility analysis of endoscopic biliary stent in unresectable hilar cholangiocarcinoma: decision analytic modeling approach. Hepatogastroenterology. 2014;61:1175–81.
184. Katanuma A, Irisawa A, Itoi T. Otaru consensus on biliary stenting for unresectable malignant hilar biliary obstruction. Dig Endosc. 2013;25(Suppl 2):58–62.
185. De Palma GD, Galloro G, Siciliano S, et al. Unilateral versus bilateral endoscopic hepatic duct drainage in patients with malignant hilar biliary obstruction: results of a prospective, randomized, and controlled study. Gastrointest Endosc. 2001;53:547–53.
186. Costamagna G, Tringali A. Can we insert a covered stent, partially or not, in case of hilar biliary stenosis? Endosc Int Open. 2017;05:E1218–9.
187. Puli SR, Kalva N, Pamulaparthy SR, et al. Bilateral and unilateral stenting for malignant hilar obstruction: a systematic review and meta-analysis. Indian J Gastroenterol. 2013;32:355–62.
188. Hong W, Sun X, Zhu Q. Endoscopic stenting for malignant hilar biliary obstruction: should it be metal or plastic and unilateral or bilateral? Eur J Gastroenterol Hepatol. 2013;25:1105–12.
189. Bulajic M, Panic N, Radunovic M, et al. Clinical outcome in patients with hilar malignant strictures type II Bismuth-Corlette treated by minimally invasive unilateral versus bilateral endoscopic biliary drainage. Hepat Pancreatic Dis Int. 2012;11: 209–14.
190. Takahashi E, Fukasawa M, Sato T, et al. Biliary drainage strategy of unresectable malignant hilar strictures by computed tomography volumetry. World J Gastroenterol. 2015;21:4946–53.
191. Freeman ML, Overby C. Selective MRCP and CT-targeted drainage of malignant hilar biliary obstruction with self-expanding metallic stents. Gastrointest Endosc. 2003;58:41–9.
192. Hintze R, Abou-Rebyeh H, Adler A, Veltzke-Schlieker W, Felix R, Wiedenmann B. Magnetic resonance cholangiopancreatography-guided unilateral endoscopic stent placement for Klatskin tumors. Gastrointest Endosc. 2001;53:40–6.
193. Kitamura K, Yamamiya A, Ishii Y, et al. Side-by-side partially covered self-expandable metal stent placement for malignant hilar biliary obstruction. Endosc Int Open. 2017;5:1211–7.
194. Inoue T, Okumura F, Naitoh I, et al. Feasibility of the placement of a novel 6-mm diameter threaded fully covered self-expandable metal stent for malignant hilar biliary obstructions (with videos). Gastrointest Endosc. 2016;84:352–7.
195. Yoshida T, Hara K, Imaoka H, et al. Benefits of side-by-side deployment of 6-mm covered self-expandable metal stents for hilar malignant biliary obstructions. J Hepatobiliary Pancreat Sci. 2016;23:548–5.
196. Hong W, Chen S, Zhu Q, et al. Bilateral stenting methods for hilar biliary obstructions. Clinics (Sao Paulo). 2014;69:647–52.
197. Inoue T, Ishii N, Kobayashi Y, et al. Simultaneous versus sequential side-by-side bilateral metal stent placement for malignant hilar biliary obstructions. Dig Dis Sci. 2017;62:2542–9.
198. Davids PH, Groen AK, Rauws EA, et al. Randomised trial of self-expanding metal stents versus polyethylene stents for distal malignant biliary obstruction. Lancet. 1992;340:1488–92.
199. Schmidt A, Riecken B, Rische S, et al. Wing-shaped plastic stents vs self-expandable metal stents for palliative drainage of malignant distal biliary obstruction: a randomized multicenter study. Endoscopy. 2015;47:430–6.
200. Shah T, Desai S, Haque M, et al. Management of occluded metal stents in malignant biliary obstruction: similar outcomes with second metal stents compared to plastic stents. Dig Dis Sci. 2012;57:2765–73.
201. Lee BS, Ryu JK, Jang DK, et al. Reintervention for occluded metal stent in malignant bile duct obstruction: a prospective randomized trial comparing covered and uncovered metal stent. J Gastroenterol Hepatol. 2016;31:1901–7.
202. Fujii M, Kawamoto H, Tsutsumi K, et al. Management of occluded metallic stents in malignant hilar biliary stricture. Hepatogastroenterology. 2013;60:447–51.
203. Inoue T, Naitoh I, Okumura F, et al. Reintervention for stent occlusion after bilateral self-expandable metallic stent placement for malignant hilar biliary obstruction. Dig Endosc. 2016;28(7):731–7.
204. Kadayifci A, Atar M, Forcione DG, et al. Radiofrequency ablation for the management of occluded biliary metal stents. Endoscopy. 2016;48:1096–101.

205. Celotti A, Solaini L, Montori G, et al. Preoperative biliary drainage in hilar cholangiocarcinoma: systematic review and meta-analysis. Eur J Surg Oncol. 2017;43:1628–163.
206. Liu F, Li Y, Wei Y, et al. Preoperative biliary drainage before resection for hilar cholangiocarcinoma: whether or not? A systematic review. Dig Dis Sci. 2011;56:663–72.
207. Wiggers JK, Groot Koerkamp B, Cieslak KP, et al. Postoperative mortality after liver resection for perihilar cholangiocarcinoma: development of a risk score and importance of biliary drainage of the future liver remnant. J Am Coll Surg. 2016;223:321–331.e321.
208. Olthof PB, Wiggers JK, Koerkamp BG, et al. Postoperative liver failure risk score: identifying patients with resectable perihilar cholangiocarcinoma who may benefit from portal vein embolization. J Am Coll Surg. 2017;225:387–94.
209. Hameed A, Pang T, Chiou J, et al. Percutaneous vs. endoscopic pre-operative biliary drainage in hilar cholangiocarcinoma – a systematic review and meta-analysis. HPB (Oxford). 2016;18:400–41.
210. Al Mahjoub A, Menahem B, Fohlen A, et al. Preoperative biliary drainage in patients with resectable perihilar cholangiocarcinoma: is percutaneous transhepatic biliary drainage safer and more effective than endoscopic biliary drainage? A meta-analysis. J Vasc Intervent Radiol: JVIR. 2017;28:576–82.
211. Kishi Y, Shimada K, Nara S, et al. The type of preoperative biliary drainage predicts short-term outcome after major hepatectomy. Langenbecks Arch Surg. 2016;401:503–11.
212. Ebata T, Mizuno T, Yokoyama Y, et al. Surgical resection for Bismuth type IV perihilar cholangiocarcinoma. Br J Surg. 2018;105:829–38.
213. Hirano S, Tanaka E, Tsuchikawa T, et al. Oncological benefit of preoperative endoscopic biliary drainage in patients with hilar cholangiocarcinoma. J Hepatobiliary Pancreat Sci. 2014;21:533–40.
214. Komaya K, Ebata T, Yokoyama Y, et al. Verification of the oncologic inferiority of percutaneous biliary drainage to endoscopic drainage: a propensity score matching analysis of resectable perihilar cholangiocarcinoma. Surgery. 2017;161:394–404.
215. Takahashi Y, Nagino M, Nishio H, et al. Percutaneous transhepatic biliary drainage catheter tract recurrence in cholangiocarcinoma. Br J Surg. 2010;97:1860–6.
216. Wiggers JK, Groot Koerkamp B, Coelen RJ, et al. Percutaneous preoperative biliary drainage for resectable perihilar cholangiocarcinoma: no association with survival and no increase in seeding metastases. Ann Surg Oncol. 2015;22(Suppl 3):S1156–16.
217. Kawashima H, Itoh A, Ohno E, et al. Preoperative endoscopic nasobiliary drainage in 164 consecutive patients with suspected perihilar cholangiocarcinoma: a retrospective study of efficacy and risk factors related to complications. Ann Surg. 2013;257:121–7.
218. Kawakami H, Kuwatani M, Onodera M, et al. Endoscopic nasobiliary drainage is the most suitable preoperative biliary drainage method in the management of patients with hilar cholangiocarcinoma. J Gastroenterol. 2011;46:242–8.
219. Grünhagen DJ, Dunne DFJ, Sturgess RP, et al. Metal stents: a bridge to surgery in hilar cholangiocarcinoma. HPB (Oxford). 2013;15:372–8.
220. Jang SI, Kim JH, You JW, et al. Efficacy of metallic stent covered with a paclitaxel-incorporated membrane versus a covered metal stent for malignant biliary obstruction: a prospective comparative study. Dig Dis Sci. 2013;58:865–71.
221. Misra SP, Dwivedii M, et al. Reflux of duodenal contents and cholangitis in patients undergoing self-expanding metal stent placement. Gastrointest Endosc. 2009;70:317–21.
222. Kim DU, Kwon CI, Kang DH, et al. New antireflux self-expandable metal stent for malignant lower biliary obstruction: in vitro and in vivo preliminary study. Dig Endosc. 2013;25:60–6.
223. Horgan AM, Amir E, Walter T, Knoxx JJ, et al. Adjuvant therapy in the treatment of biliary tract cancer: a systematic review and meta-analysis. J Clin Oncol. 2012;30:1934–40.
224. Zoepf T, Jakobs R, Arnold JC, et al. Palliation of nonresectable bile duct cancer: improved survival after photodynamic therapy. Am J Gastroenterol. 2005;100:2426–30.
225. Hong MJ, Cheon YK, Lee EJ, et al. Long-term outcome of photodynamic therapy with systemic chemotherapy compared to photodynamic therapy alone in patients with advanced hilar cholangiocarcinoma. Gut Liver. 2014;8:318–23.
226. Park do H, Lee SS, Lee JL, et al. Randomized phase II trial of photodynamic therapy plus oral fluoropyrimidine, S-1, versus photodynamic therapy alone for unresectable hilar cholangiocarcinoma. Eur J Cancer. 2014;50:1259–68.
227. Cheon YK, Lee TY, Lee SM. Long-term outcome of photodynamic therapy compared with biliary stenting alone in patients with advanced hilar cholangiocarcinoma. HPB (Oxford). 2012;14:185–93.
228. Hong MJ, Cheon YK, Lee EJ, et al. Long term outcome of photodynamic therapy with systemic chemotherapy compared to photodynamic in patients with advanced hilar cholangiocarcinoma. Gut Liver. 2014;8:318–23.
229. Kahaleh M, Mishra R, Shami VM, et al. Unresectable cholangiocarcinoma: comparison of survival in biliary stenting alone versus stenting with photodynamic therapy. Clin Gastroenterol Hepoatol. 2008;6:290–7.
230. Lee TY, Cheon YK, Shim CS, et al. Photodynamic therapy prolongs metal stent patency in patients with unresectable hilar cholangiocarcinoma. World J Gastroenterol. 2012;18:5589–94.
231. Witzigmann H, Berr F, Ringel U. Surgical and palliative management and outcome in 184 patients with hilar cholangiocarcinoma: palliative photodynamic

therapy plus stenting is comparable to r1/r2 resection. Ann Surg. 2006;244:230–9.
232. Gao F, Bai Y, Ma SR, et al. Systematic review: photodynamic therapy for unresectable cholangiocarcinoma. J Hepatobiliary Pancreat Sci. 2010;17:125–31.
233. Leggettt CL, Gorospe EC, Murad MH, et al. Photodynamic therapy for unresectable cholangiocarcinoma: a comparative effectiveness systematic review and meta-analysis. Photodiagnosis Photodyn Ther. 2012;9:189–95.
234. Lu Y, Liu L, Wu JC, et al. Efficacy and safety of photodynamic therapy for unresectable cholangiocarcinoma: a meta-analysis. Clin Res Hepatol Gatsroenterol. 2015;39(6):718–24.
235. Dolak W, Schreiber F, Scheighofer H, et al. Endoscopic radiofrequency ablation for malignant biliary obstruction: a nationwide retrospective study of 84 consecutive patients. Surg Endosc. 2014;28:854–60.
236. Strand DS, Cosgrove ND, Patrie TJ, et al. ERCP-directed radiofrequency ablation and photodynamic therapy are associated with comparable survival in the treatment of unresectable cholangiocarcinoma. Gastrointest Endosc. 2014;80:794–804.
237. Pai M, VAlek V, Tomas A, Doros A, et al. Percutaneous intraductal radiofrequency ablation for clearance of occluded metal stent in malignant biliary obstruction: feasibility and early results. Cardiovasc Intervent Radiol. 2014;37:235–40.
238. Steel AAW, Postgate AJ, Khorsandi S, et al. Endoscopically applied radiofrequency ablation appears to be safe in the treatment of malignant biliary obstruction. Gastrointest Endosc. 2011;73:149–53.

41 Results of EUS Transmural Biliary Drainage

Raffaele Salerno

41.1 Introduction

Endoscopic retrograde cholangiopancreatography (ERCP) with stent placement is the standard therapeutic modality for the management of benign and malignant biliary obstruction.

In the United States, about 500,000 ERCPs are performed annually with a failure rate of 5–7% [1].

The reasons for failure can be classified in two different categories: in some patients, the papilla is endoscopically accessible, and in others it is not. In the first group, the failure is due to several technical aspects like ampullary pathology, periampullary diverticulum, and ampullary neoplastic infiltration. In the second group, benign (peptic stenosis) or malignant duodenal stenosis or postsurgical anatomy like gastrointestinal bariatric bypass, Roux-en-Y gastric bypass, and Billroth II gastroenterostomy may prevent access to the papilla.

Percutaneous transhepatic biliary drainage (PTBD) is a rescue procedure that is often used when ERCP fails.

According to the literature, the morbidity associated to PTBD can range up to 33% [2], including catheter dislocation, infection, bleeding, biliary leakages, acute cholangitis, and pneumothorax [3]. Endoscopic ultrasonography-guided biliary drainage (EUS-BD) is an alternative to PTBD with advantages of internal drainage and a single session procedure by the same operator without the discomfort of an external catheter.

Wiersema and colleagues showed for the first time in 1996 the feasibility of performing a cholangiogram under endoscopic ultrasonography guidance [4].

The first report of EUS-guided bilio-digestive anastomosis was by Giovanni et al. in 2001 [5], and it was then performed worldwide with reported cumulative technical success and post-procedure adverse events of 90% and 17%, respectively [6].

A recent systematic review and meta-analysis by Sharaiha et al. compared the efficacy and safety of EUS-BD and PTBD [7]. Nine studies [8–16] were included in the final analysis. Of these, three were RCTs [8, 12, 16], and six were retrospective studies [9, 11, 13–15]. All nine studies used metal stents in patients undergoing EUS-BD and were conducted at tertiary centers. One study [12] included benign and malignant etiologies of biliary obstruction, whereas the remaining studies included patients with malignant etiologies only.

EUS-BD and PTBD showed equivalent technical success (OR, 1.78; 95% CI, 0.69–4.59; $I^2 = 22\%$), but EUS-BD was associated with a better clinical success (OR, 0.45; 95% CI, 0.23–0.89; $I^2 = 0\%$), fewer postprocedure adverse events (OR, 0.23; 95% CI, 0.12–0.47; $I^2 = 57\%$),

R. Salerno (✉)
Gastroenterology and Endoscopy Unit ASST Fatebenefratelli Sacco, Milan, Italy
e-mail: raffaele.salerno@asst-fbf-sacco.it

M. Mutignani et al. (eds.), *Endotherapy in Biliopancreatic Diseases: ERCP Meets EUS*,
https://doi.org/10.1007/978-3-030-42569-2_41

and a lower rate of reinterventions (OR, 0.13; 95% CI, 0.07–0.24; $I^2 = 0\%$). No significant differences in hospitalization between EUS-BD and PTBD were found, but EUS-BD was more cost-effective.

41.2 Techniques

Transmural EUS-BD should be performed by an experienced endoscopist with at least 20 cases done under supervision of a tutor [17] and trained in both EUS and ERCP. Skilled staff and carbon dioxide insufflation are mandatory for guidewire manipulation and to reduce the risk of pneumoperitoneum, respectively.

According to the access to the biliary tree, two approaches can be performed: the intrahepatic approach (hepatogastric anastomosis EUS-HPA or antegrade stent placement EUS-AS) and the extrahepatic approach (choledochoduodenostomy EUS-CDS or transgallbladder EUS-GBD).

EUS-guided rendezvous transpapillary drainage will not be discussed in this chapter.

41.2.1 Intrahepatic Approach

This kind of approach is typically preferred in cases where endoscopic access to the papilla is impeded by gastric outlet obstruction or an obstructing proximal duodenal tumor, or in patients with a surgically altered anatomy. Dilatation of intrahepatic ducts is mandatory for the choice of this approach. Cancer infiltration of the gastric wall within the planned path of approach to the bile ducts or massive ascites and coagulopathy are considered as contraindications.

With the tip of the echoendoscope positioned along the small curvature of the stomach, the dilated left hepatic duct (segment III) is correctly visualized. Transgastric needle (19–22 G) insertion into the left hepatic duct and contrast injection clearly show the biliary tree under fluoroscopy (Fig. 41.1). The next step is the exchange of the needle over a guidewire for a 6.5-Fr cystostome used to create by cutting current the fistula between the stomach and the left hepatic duct.

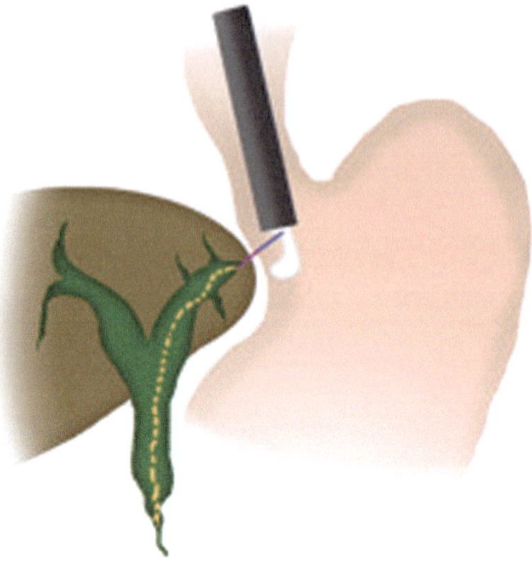

Fig. 41.1 Transhepatic approach

Plastic stent or a self-expandable metal stent (SEMS) is then positioned over the guidewire (hepatico-gastric stent) or advancing a guidewire across the stricture and the papilla to complete an antegrade stent placement (EUS-AS).

This kind of technique is not actually standardized, and there is no scientific evidence to prefer one over the other of different devices. The choice of the needle is still debated. Some operators suggest the 19 G needle because the large diameter reduces the risk of shearing the guidewire coating during manipulation. On the other hand, the 19 G needle can be stiffer and more difficult to handle compared to the 22 G one. Usually, a hydrophilic guidewire is preferred because it makes it easier to cross the strictures. The 0.025-in. guidewire matches with a 22 G needle, and this flexibility may help during the manipulation maneuvers but at the same time can make the stent insertion challenging due to the lack of stiffness and less stable scope position.

The optimal biliary access point and learning curve for technically successful EUS-HGA were evaluated by Oh et al. in 129 consecutive patients who underwent EUS-HGA [18]. Measurements were taken for the intrahepatic bile duct diameter at the point of puncture, the hepatic portion length and bile duct segment for each needle puncture attempt, and procedure times (from initial bile duct puncture to final transmural stenting) in each EUS-HGA session.

In the logistic regression model, intrahepatic bile duct diameter of puncture site ≤5 mm (OR, 3.7; 95% CI, 1.71–8.1; $p < 0.01$) and hepatic portion length >3 cm (OR, 5.7; 95% CI, 2.7–12; $p < 0.01$) were related with low technical success. The learning curve for technical success was evaluated by measuring procedure time and adverse events by using the moving average method and cumulative sum (CUSUM) analysis, respectively. Procedure time and adverse events were shorter after 24 cases and stabilized at 33 cases of EUS-HGA, respectively.

These data suggest that a bile duct diameter >5 mm and hepatic portion length 1 to ≤3 cm on EUS may guide the choice for the optimal site of puncture for successful EUS-HGS and that 33 cases of EUS-HGA are needed to achieve technical proficiency.

A crucial step is the creation of the fistula that can potentially impact on the technical success and on the complications like bile leakage, bilioperitoneum, or perforation. The dilatation of the fistula is mandatory for stent insertion and can be performed by using balloon dilator, stiff gradual catheters, needle knife, and cystostome with cutting current. Advancing of stiff catheter may form tissue resistance creating a gap between the stomach and the liver, with postprocedure bile leak, and balloon dilatation generates radial force as well; that is why some endoscopists prefer a 6.5 Fr cystostome. In a recent meta-analysis of EUS-BD technique, Wang and colleagues reported adverse event rates of 20% (49/249) with needle knife, 20.37 % (44/216) with balloon catheter, and 38.46% (10/26) with cystotome [19].

The type of the stent used depends on the indication (benign vs. malignant), the degree of ductal dilatation, whether the wire could cross the anastomosis, the length of fistula tract, and surgical candidacy of the patient [20]. In the first cases of HGA reported, plastic stents were used with significant postprocedure bile leakage. On the other hand, fully covered self-expandable metal stent (FCSEMS) may cause side bile duct obstruction with cholangitis, and significant stent migration may occur too. To prevent these complications, Giovannini and colleagues used the "stent-in-stent technique" with insertion of two metal stents: a first uncovered metal stent of 8- or 10-cm length placed to prevent migration and the occlusion of side biliary branches and in the second time, a fully covered stent of 6-cm length in the uncovered to prevent the bile leakage. Recently, Song et al. reported no proximal and distal stent migration in any of 27 patients who underwent EUS-BD, using hybrid metal stents (Standard Sci Tech Inc., Seoul, South Korea), which are partially covered self-expandable metal stents (uncovered in the intrahepatic portion and covered in the transmural distal) [21]. Tyberg et al. described an algorithm for EUS-BD based on patient anatomy [20]. In 41 of the 52 patients in study (79%) and in 11 patients (21%), SEMS and plastic stents were respectively inserted following clinical settings like the degree of dilation, the underlying disease, the capability to cross the anastomosis, the length of the fistulous tract, and the potential resectability of the patient. Bigger caliber and longer patency of SEMS make them an appealing option over plastic stents when reintervention for stent exchange is not required.

41.2.2 Extrahepatic Approach

This approach includes the endoscopic ultrasound-guided choledochoduodenostomy (EUS-CDS) and, when feasible, choledochoantrostomy. It is usually used in case of failure of selective cannulation of common bile duct because of ampullary neoplasm or neoplastic infiltration from pancreatic cancer, or when the access to the papilla is prevented by benign (peptic stenosis) or malignant duodenal stenosis. In all these cases, there is no consensus about the choice between the intrahepatic approach and the extrahepatic approach, depending on the endoscopist's discretion and expertise.

More recently, some authors described gallbladder drainage for biliary drainage in patients with distal biliary obstruction and patent cystic duct [22, 23] so that this technique may be literally considered as an extrahepatic approach.

The tip of the echoendoscope is advanced to the duodenal bulb or, when feasible, to the antrum wall, where the dilated common bile duct is closer to the wall. Likewise the technique of extrahepatic approach, the access to the bile duct is achieved with a 19-gauge EUS needle, with subsequent bile aspiration, 0.035-in. guidewire manipulation into the intrahepatic tree, dilatation of the fistula, and stent insertion. Similarly to HGA, stent migration is the main postprocedural complication, so some endoscopists suggest fully covered biliary metal stents with a length of more than 4 cm. On the other hand, using these stents, reintervention can be sometimes difficult, and the distal portion of the stent may cause duodenal trauma and even perforation.

Kawakubo and colleagues compared the clinical efficacy and safety of EUS-CDS versus endoscopic transpapillary stenting (ETS) as first-line treatment in 82 patients with distal malignant biliary obstruction, finding equivalent clinical success rate (EUS-CDS, 96.2%; ETS, 98.2%; $P = 0.54$) and overall adverse event rate (EUS-CDS, 26.9%, ETS, 35.7%; $P = 0.46$) but a shorter mean procedural time with EUS-CDS than with ETS (19.7 vs. 30.2 min; $P < 0.01$) [24]. These data were confirmed in a prospective multicenter study by Nakai et al. [25].

Lumen-apposing metal stents (LAMS) were introduced to drain peripancreatic fluid collections but recently were used for EUS-BD too. The features of this stent are represented by the full silicone covered, wider lumen and bigger flanges to prevent tissue ingrowth, provide fast drainage, reduce the risk of migration with bile leakage, and allow removability. There is now available new cautery-enhanced delivery system (Hot AXIOS device, Boston Scientific) that allows the EUS-BD in one step with no need for prior needle puncture or guidewire insertion and even fluoroscopy too (Fig. 41.2). Bile duct dilatation and a distance of no more than 10 mm are required to avoid stent migration, leakage, and pressure necrosis.

EUS-CDS using a LAMS was proposed as an alternative approach for patients with malignant obstructive jaundice and failed ERCP. Tsuchiya and colleagues evaluated prospectively the long-term outcome (median, 184 days; range, 12–819) in 19 patients who underwent EUS-CDS using a fully covered LAMS with a cautery-enhanced delivery system [26]. Technical success was achieved in all patients and jaundice improvement in 95% of patients (18/19).

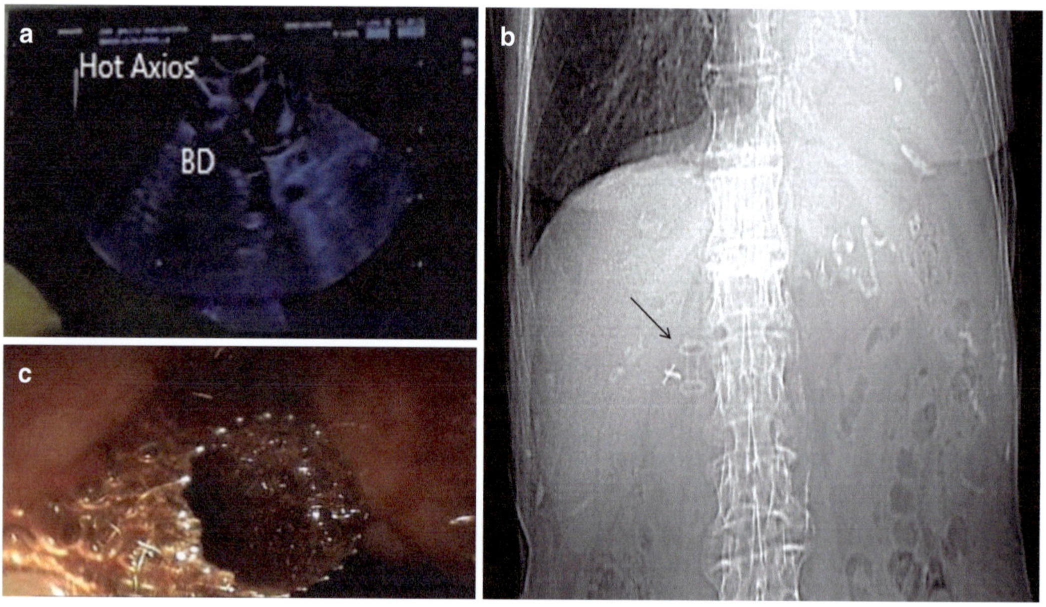

Fig. 41.2 Extrahepatic approach (**a**) Endoscopic ultrasonography-guided choledochoduodenostomy using a LAMS (Hot AXIOS device, Boston Scientific) (**b**) CT-scan view (**c**) Endoscopic view. *BD=bile duct*

No intraprocedural adverse events were recorded, but the postprocedure-related adverse events ratio was 15.8% (3/19; acute cholangitis [n = 2] and fever [n = 1]). Five patients had secondary stent obstruction because of food residue (n = 2), kinking (n = 1), suspected tumor ingrowth (n = 1), and spontaneous dislodgement (n = 1) with reintervention in four of these five patients. The authors supposed the food impaction and the bile duct kinking as a consequence of the small diameter of the LAMS used (6–8 mm diameter could have shorter patency compared to 10 mm diameter) and of the absence of the spontaneous outflow of the bile after decompression, respectively. The efficacy of EUS-CDS using the LAMS was recently confirmed by Anderloni and colleagues in a retrospective analysis in 46 patients [27]. They reported technical and clinical success rate of 93.5% and 97.7%, respectively, but adverse events in five patients (11.6%) with one fatal bleeding 17 days after stent placement, three episodes of stent occlusion (food impaction), and one spontaneous migration (all four requiring reintervention). In spite of these encouraging results, the authors suggested a careful evaluation before using the stent in this clinical setting because of not negligible adverse events.

Recently, EUS-guided gallbladder drainage (EUS-GBD) was reported to be useful for acute cholecystitis in patients unfit for surgery. Jang et al. found that EUS-GBD was comparable to percutaneous transhepatic gallbladder drainage in terms of technical feasibility, efficacy, and safety of the procedures [28].

In a pooled analysis on the efficacy and safety of EUS-GBD with LAMS in nonoperative candidates with acute cholecystitis, Kalva et al. showed that technical success was 93.86% (95% CI = 90.56–96.49) and clinical success was 92.48% (95% CI = 88.9–95.42). Overall complication rate was 18.31% (95% CI = 13.49–23.68), and stent-related complication rate was 8.16% (95% CI = 4.03–14.96) in the pooled percentage of patients [29].

Some authors proposed EUS-GBD in case of failure to treat malignant distal biliary obstruction and patent cystic duct, with encouraging results. Imai and colleagues reported technical success rates and functional success rate in 100 % and 91.7% of cases, respectively, with adverse events in 16.7% of cases in a series of 12 patients with obstructive jaundice due to unresectable malignant distal biliary stricture who underwent EUS-GBD after ERCP failed [22].

41.2.3 Algorithm for EUS-BD Guidance

Artifon and colleagues compared in a prospective randomized trial the outcomes of hepaticogastrostomy and choledochoduodenostomy in 49 patients with distal malignant biliary obstruction [30]. The technical success rate was 96% and 91% with clinical success rate of 91% and 77% and similar procedural time for HPA and CDS, respectively. The overall adverse event rate was 16.3% (20% for the HPA group and 12.5% for the CDS group). These data show no significant differences between the two techniques.

The anatomic site of transmural biliary drainage was evaluated too in a review on 42 studies with 1192 patients by Wang and colleagues [19].

They calculated the cumulative technical success rate (TSR), functional success rate (FSR), and adverse event rate of EUS-BD and the pooled odds ratio of TSR, FSR, and adverse event rate of the transduodenal (TD) approach versus transgastric (TG) approach, finding no significant difference.

Some authors have proposed different algorithms to guide the choice of approach.

Park et al. evaluated an algorithm based on enhanced guidewire manipulation for EUS-BD after failed ERCP in 45 patients, achieving overall technical and functional success rates of 91% (intention to treat, n = 41/45) and 95% (per protocol, n = 39/41), respectively [31].

More recently, some other authors proposed an algorithm for biliary drainage based on patient anatomy (Fig. 41.3) [20].

Patients with a dilated intrahepatic biliary tree (IHBT) on cross-sectional imaging received an intrahepatic (IH) approach, while patients with a nondilated IHBT on cross-sectional imaging underwent an extrahepatic (EH) approach. In case of failure of IH drainage, conversion to an EH approach was proposed.

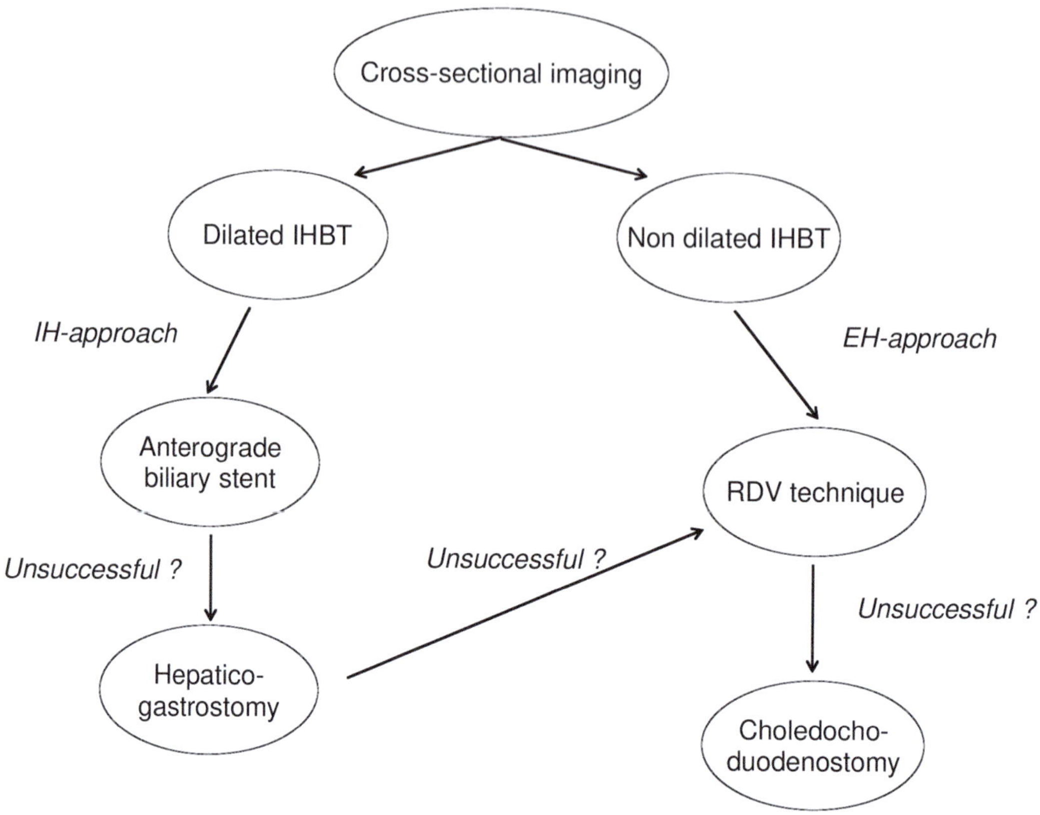

Fig. 41.3 Algorithm for biliary drainage based on patient anatomy proposed by Tyberg and colleagues. *IHBT=intrahepatic biliary tree; IH=intraheaptic; EH=extrahepatic; RDV=rendez-vous*

Following this algorithm, they reported technical success in 50/52 patients (96%) with adverse events in five patients (10%).

41.3 Summary

PTBD is a rescue procedure used in case of failure of ERCP. The technical success rate of PTBD is more than 95% with adverse event overall rates of 33% or higher, including bleeding, infection, dislodgement, bile leak, and tract seeding [3]. Moreover, this technique is uncomfortable to the patient because of the external drainage catheter and is not suitable in case of ascites or multiple liver metastasis. EUS-BD has been an evolving alternative to PTBD with better clinical success (OR, 0.45), fewer adverse events (OR, 0.23), and fewer reinterventions (OR, 0.13) [7]. EUS transmural biliary drainage can be achieved by the puncture of intrahepatic duct in the III segment (*intrahepatic approach*) and the insertion of hepatico-gastric (HGA) stent or advancing a guidewire across the stricture and the papilla to complete an antegrade stent placement (EUS-AS), or by the puncture of common bile duct or the gallbladder (*extrahepatic approach*) with choledochoduodenostomy (CDS) or cholecystoduodenostomy (GBD).

There is no formal consensus on how to choose between intrahepatic approach and extrahepatic approach.

Some proposed algorithms for biliary drainage based on patient anatomy [20] or guidewire manipulation [31], both with encouraging results.

The most crucial step for both approaches is represented by the dilatation of the fistula that potentially can impact on the technical success or failure of the drainage procedure. For this reason, the operators mostly prefer transpapillary (rendezvous) EUS-BD or anterograde technique because of the smaller risk of postprocedure bile leak.

The recent availability of the LAMS improves this field by reducing leakage and the mean procedural time, but it still needs careful evaluation because of potential severe adverse event [27].

In 2011, a consortium involving 40 international experts met to standardize terminology, nomenclature, and indications of EUS-BD, concluding that because of the potential serious adverse events associated with the procedure, EUS-BD should only be performed by endoscopists trained in both EUS and ERCP, performing pancreatico-biliary EUS and FNA, with large ERCP and EUS experience for nearly 4–5 years (at least 200–300 EUS and ERCP each year) with 95–98% success rate for standard ERCP, with a surgical and interventional radiology backup [32].

Therefore, the endoscopist must have mastery of multiple techniques to fully use EUS-BD.

References

1. Cote GA, et al. Association between volume of endoscopic retrograde cholangiopancreatography at an academic medical center and use of pancreatobiliary therapy. Clin Gastroenterol Hepatol. 2012;10:920–4.
2. Nennstiel S, et al. Drainage-related complications in percutaneous transhepatic biliary drainage: an analysis over 10 years. J Clin Gastroenterol. 2015;49:764–70.
3. Yarmohammadi H, et al. Percutaneous biliary interventions and complications in malignant bile duct obstruction. Chin Clin Oncol. 2016;5(5):68.
4. Wiersema MJ, et al. Endosonography-guided cholangiopancreatography. Gastrointest Endosc. 1996;43:102–6.
5. Giovannini M, et al. Endoscopic ultrasound-guided bilioduodenal anastomosis: a new technique for biliary drainage. Endoscopy. 2001;33(10):898–900.
6. Khan MA, et al. Endoscopic ultrasound-guided biliary drainage: a systematic review and meta-analysis. Dig Dis Sci. 2016;61:684–703.
7. Sharaiha RZ, et al. Efficacy and safety of EUS-guided biliary drainage in comparison with percutaneous biliary drainage when ERCP fails: a systematic review and meta-analysis. Gastrointest Endosc. 2017;85:904–14.
8. Artifon EL, et al. Biliary drainage in patients with unresectable, malignant obstruction where ERCP fails: endoscopic ultrasonography-guided choledochoduodenostomy versus percutaneous drainage. J Clin Gastroenterol. 2012;46:768–74.
9. Bapaye A, et al. Comparison of endosonography-guided vs. percutaneous biliary stenting when papilla is inaccessible for ERCP. United Eur Gastroenterol J. 2013;1:285–93.
10. Khashab MA, et al. A comparative evaluation of EUS-guided biliary drainage and percutaneous drainage in patients with distal malignant biliary obstruction and failed ERCP. Dig Dis Sci. 2015;60:557–65.
11. Bill J, et al. A comparison between endoscopic ultrasound guided rendezvous and percutaneous biliary drainage after failed ERCP for malignant biliary obstruction [abstract]. Gastrointest Endosc. 2015;81:AB531.
12. Giovannini M, et al. Multicenter randomized phase II study: percutaneous biliary drainage vs EUS guided biliary drainage: results of the intermediate analysis [abstract]. Gastrointest Endosc. 2015;81:AB174.
13. Sharaiha RZ, et al. Endoscopic ultrasound-guided biliary drainage versus percutaneous transhepatic biliary drainage: predictors of successful outcome in patients who fail endoscopic retrograde cholangiopancreatography. Surg Endosc. 2016;30:5500–5.
14. Torres-Ruiz MF, et al. Biliary drainage in malignant obstruction: a comparative study between EUS-guided vs percutaneous drainage in patients with failed ERCP [abstract]. Gastrointest Endosc. 2016;83:AB356.
15. Sportes A, et al. Comparative trial of EUS-guided hepatico-gastrostomy and percutaneous transhepatic biliary drainage for malignant obstructive jaundice after failed ERCP [abstract]. Gastrointest Endosc. 2016;83:AB522–3.
16. Lee TH, et al. Similar efficacies of endoscopic ultrasound-guided transmural and percutaneous drainage for malignant distal biliary obstruction. Clin Gastroenterol Hepatol. 2016;14:1011–9.
17. Hara K, et al. Endoscopic ultrasonography-guided biliary drainage: who, when, which, and how? World J Gastroenterol. 2016;22:1297–303.
18. Oh D, et al. Optimal biliary access point and learning curve for endoscopic ultrasound-guided hepaticogastrostomy with transmural stenting. Therap Adv Gastroenterol. 2017;10(1):42–53.
19. Wang K, et al. Assessment of efficacy and safety of EUS-guided biliary drainage: a systematic review. Gastrointest Endosc. 2016;83:1218–27.
20. Tyberg A, et al. EUS-guided biliary drainage after failed ERCP: a novel algorithm individualized based on patient anatomy. Gastrointest Endosc. 2016;84(6):941–6.
21. Song TJ, et al. Preliminary report on a new hybrid metal stent for EUS-guided biliary drainage (with videos). Gastrointest Endosc. 2014;80(4):707–11.
22. Imai H, et al. EUS-guided gallbladder drainage for rescue treatment of malignant distal biliary

obstruction after unsuccessful ERCP. Gastrointest Endosc. 2016;84:147–51.
23. Itoi T, et al. Endoscopic ultrasonography-guided cholecystogastrostomy using a lumen-apposing metal stent as an alternative to extrahepatic bile duct drainage in pancreatic cancer with duodenal invasion. Dig Endosc. 2013;25:137–41.
24. Kazumichi K, et al. EUS-guided choledochoduodenostomy for distal biliary obstruction. Endoscopy. 2016;48:164–9.
25. Nakai Y, et al. Prospective multicenter study of primary EUS-guided choledochoduodenostomy using a covered metal stent. Endosc Ultrasound. 2018;8(2):111–7.
26. Tsuchiya T, et al. Long-term outcomes of EUS-guided choledochoduodenostomy using a lumen-apposing metal stent for malignant distal biliary obstruction: a prospective multicenter study. Gastrointest Endosc. 2018;87(4):1138–46.
27. Anderloni A, et al. Single-stage EUS-guided choledochoduodenostomy using a lumen-apposing metal stent for malignant distal biliary obstruction. Gastrointest Endosc. 2019;89(1):69–76.
28. Jang JW, et al. Endoscopic ultrasound-guided transmural and percutaneous transhepatic gallbladder drainage are comparable for acute cholecystitis. Gastroenterology. 2012;142:805–11.
29. Kalva NR, et al. Efficacy and safety of lumen apposing self-expandable metal stents for EUS guided cholecystostomy: a meta-analysis and systematic review. Can J Gastroenterol Hepatol. 2018;2018:7070961.
30. Everson LA, et al. Hepaticogastrostomy or choledochoduodenostomy for distal malignant biliary obstruction after failed ERCP: is there any difference? Gastrointest Endosc. 2015;81:950–9.
31. Park DH, et al. Prospective evaluation of a treatment algorithm with enhanced guidewire manipulation protocol for EUS-guided biliary drainage after failed ERCP (with video). Gastrointest Endosc. 2013;78(1):91–101.
32. Kahaleh M, et al. Endoscopic ultrasonography guided biliary drainage: Summary of consortium meeting, May 7th, 2011, Chicago. World J Gastroenterol. 2013;19(9):1372–9.

Postoperative Biliary Stricture 42

Paolo Cantù and Aurelio Mauro

Abbreviations

ERCP	Endoscopic retrograde cholangiopancreatography
LC	Laparoscopic cholecystectomy
OC	Open cholecystectomy
POBS	Postoperative biliary stricture
SEMS	Self-expandable metal stent

42.1 Epidemiology and Risk Factors

Postoperative biliary strictures (POBS) may develop after any type of biliary surgical procedures. Laparoscopic cholecystectomy (LC) is the most common cause of POBS with a rate that is two to six times higher than open cholecystectomy (OC) [1]. Biliary injuries after cholecystectomy have relevant medical and legal implications as well [2]. In a large LC series involving more than 10,000 patients, the reported rate of biliary injuries ranges from 0.18% to 0.6% [3]. Partial or complete clipping and some thermal injury of the common bile duct (CBD) are the well-known mechanisms leading to stricture. Clipping the cystic duct too close to its implantation may lead to traction of the CBD and to its obstruction as well as in case of non-dilated CBD. This condition is encountered during LC when a countertraction force on the CBD is not applicable during the traction of the cystic duct to be clipped. In up to 30–40% of patients, the stricture is caused by concomitant ischemia secondary to dissection or a thermal injury [4] of the right hepatic artery. The application of clips around the bile duct can compromise its blood supply by damaging the vascular net running in the 3 and 9 o'clock positions of the bile duct [5].

Rare causes of POBS are other abdominal surgeries where the bile ducts are exposed to surgical devices, such as hepatectomy, hepatic and biliary repair after an abdominal trauma, portacaval shunting, pancreatoduodenectomy, gastrectomy (especially for deep duodenal ulcers), and bilateral supradrenalectomy [4, 6].

The risk factors for POBS are summarized according to different factors such as biliary and vascular variant anatomies, severity of local inflammation, and operator expertise.

Anatomic variants of the cystic duct implantation to CBD, which in 20% of patients runs parallel and in 5% posterior to the CBD [7] and as of the hilar bifurcation in up to 20% (Fig. 42.1), may increase the difficulty of the correct identification of Calot's triangle, also known as the cystohepatic triangle, delimited on the upper side by

P. Cantù (✉) · A. Mauro
Gastroenterology and Endoscopy Unit, Fondazione IRCCS Ca' Granda Ospedale Maggiore Policlinico, Department of Pathophysiology and Transplantation, Università degli Studi di Milano, Milan, Italy
e-mail: paolo.cantu@policlinico.mi.it

M. Mutignani et al. (eds.), *Endotherapy in Biliopancreatic Diseases: ERCP Meets EUS*,
https://doi.org/10.1007/978-3-030-42569-2_42

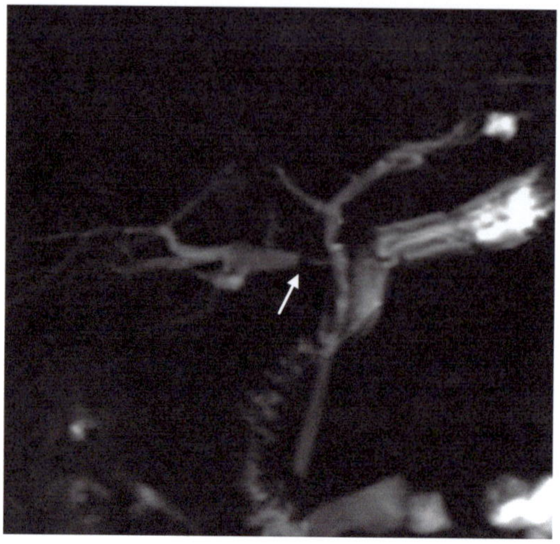

Fig. 42.1 Type E5 Strasberg stricture associated to an aberrant right hepatic duct. Ten days after cholecystectomy, the patients presented with jaundice. He was successfully treated with endoscopic multistenting

the inferior surface of the liver or the cystic artery, the cystic duct laterally, and the CBD medially [5]. Acute inflammation or excess bleeding during LC may also reduce the visibility. In this condition, low levels of expertise and involvement of trainees (i.e., with less than 100 cholecystectomies performed) are additional risk factors for POBS [1, 8, 9]. In difficult conditions, intraoperative cholangiography can be of great help to prevent possible visual perceptual illusion or for intraoperative confirmation of a relevant biliary injury [10]. In patients with any type of biliary injury after cholecystectomy (leak, stricture, and complete transection), it has been shown that proximal injury, repair in the acute phase, and late referral to tertiary centers have worse outcomes [11]. The presence of a bile leak after cholecystectomy is per se a risk factor associated to POBS with a reported incidence from 10 to 70% in selected series [11, 12].

42.2 Classifications

Several systems have been proposed for the classification of iatrogenic bile duct lesions aiming to summarize a large plethora of injury pictures. Such classifications describe injury mechanisms and their preventive strategies but fail to take into account short-term prognostic factors.

Table 42.1 Bismuth's classification of biliary strictures based on available healthy biliary mucosa

Type	Definition
I	Common hepatic or main bile duct stump ≥2 cm
II	Common hepatic duct stump <2 cm
III	Ceiling of the biliary confluence is intact; right and left ductal system s communicate
IV	Ceiling of the confluence is destroyed; bile ducts are separated
V	Type I, II, or III stricture of an isolated right duct

Adapted from Bismuth et al. [13]

The most dated and probably the most used classification system is the one authored by Bismuth [13]. The Bismuth classification was originally designed to guide the surgical reconstruction of the biliary tree based on the available healthy biliary mucosa and is useful for the evaluation of outcomes after repair. Five types of stricture are described (Table 42.1) according to the progressive reduction of the available healthy biliary mucosa, from more than 2 cm of a spared CBD or main bile duct stump (type I) to the complete separation of right and left hepatic ducts (type IV); in type V, there is the involvement of an aberrant right second-order duct with or without concomitant CBD stricture.

The Strasberg classification also includes leak injuries and allows the differentiation as types A to D between small, i.e., bile leakage from the cystic duct or aberrant right branch, and major injuries performed during laparoscopic cholecystectomy. Type E of the Strasberg classification (Fig. 42.2) includes the scenarios of the Bismuth classification. In 1996, Bergman published a very simple classification of injuries after LC, which gives practical information for their treatment. It describes four groups of lesions (types A to D) ranging from minor bile leaks to major bile leaks with or without stricture, isolated biliary stricture, and, finally, a complete biliary transection. Type A and type D lesions are treated endoscopically and surgically, respectively; type B ones may require a combined treatment, whereas endoscopy is the first choice for type C lesions, but surgery may be an option in case of failure [14].

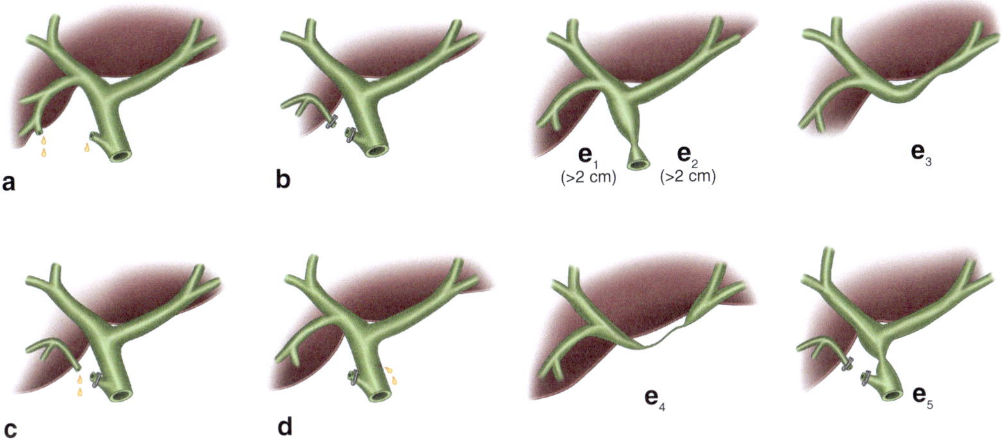

Fig. 42.2 Strasberg classification. In types A, C, and D are depicted the different levels of leakage, whereas the different subtypes E depict the strictures. (Adapted from Chun K, Korean J Hepatobiliary Pancreat Surg. 2014;18:69–72 [16])

The Csendes system provides a detailed classification based on the types of injury with the standard devices used during LC [15].

Other ancillar classifications are the MacMahon classification based on the levels of CBD laceration and the Neuhaus classification, which includes prognostic information about the risk of stricture recurrence [16].

The main criticism of all the aforementioned classification systems concerns the lack of consideration of any additional vascular injury level. Ten to 30% of all patients present with vascular involvement, which is important to detect because of a potentially worse outcome. The Stewart-Way and Hannover classification systems overcome this drawback [10, 17]. The Stewart-Way classification was created taking into account surgery reports and videotapes of biliary injury during cholecystectomy. It describes four types of injury based on their mechanisms (Fig. 42.3). In type I, an incomplete CBD transection can occur secondary to the misidentification of CBD instead of the cystic duct, and the correct identification during early surgery avoids the complete transection of the CBD. Type II injury consists of damage near the CBD secondary to clipping and cautery damage during attempts to control bleeding. Type III injury is the most frequent (60% of cases) and consists in the complete CBD transection followed by the failure of identification during surgery. Type IV injury involves damage of the right hepatic duct or a second-order hepatic duct, associated to injury of the right hepatic artery in 60% of cases. Vascular involvement was less frequent in types I, II, and III than type IV, i.e., 5%, 18%, and 27%, respectively, vs. 60% stated. The Hannover classification is an expansion of the Stewart-Way one, resulting in 21 different subtypes of injury grouped in five main classes, making it difficult to apply in everyday practice.

42.3 Clinical Presentation and Diagnosis

POBS has a variable clinical presentation mainly because of the severity of the iatrogenic stricture. Only 10% of strictures are suspected within the first postoperative week. Its early presentation relates to major injuries such as complete CBD transection with or without associated leakage and ranges from abdominal discomfort to jaundice and cholangitis. Two-thirds of patients with POBS are diagnosed later and within the first 6 months following cholecystectomy. These patients undergo evaluation for paucisymptomatic cholestasis, recurrent cholangitis, and/or intrahepatic stone formation. Secondary biliary cirrhosis may develop [1, 4, 6] in patients with delayed clinical presentation (>6 months) leading to late repair.

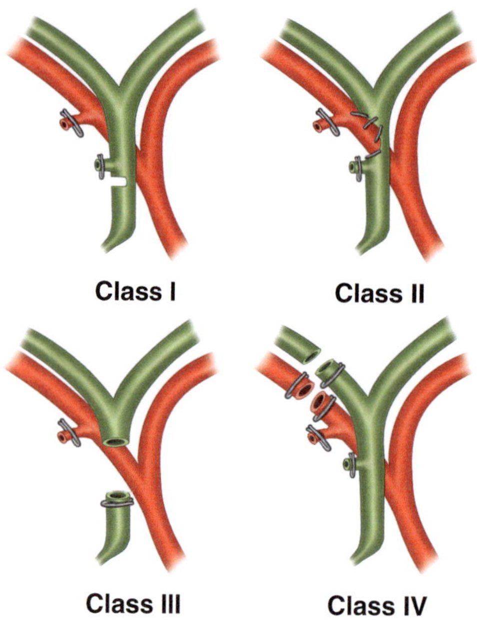

Fig. 42.3 Stewart-Way classification. Both biliary and vascular injuries are depicted. (Adapted from Way LW et al., Ann Surg. 2003;237:460–9 [10])

In the setting of sepsis of biliary origin, the first aim of the first evaluation is to assess complications such as bile collection. The second aim is to assess the type and extent of injury in order to plan the mode and timing of intervention according to the expertise [2] locally available.

Noninvasive imaging tests should also be used accordingly. Abdominal ultrasound evaluates the presence of fluid collection and intrahepatic biliary dilatation. Computed tomography has higher accuracy compared to ultrasound (96% vs. 70%) in detecting any fluid collection and is useful if the latter is equivocal. If bile duct injury is strongly suspected, in aiming to study its location or in case of bile flow from abdominal drain, a cholangiography is indicated [18]. Both direct (endoscopic or percutaneous) and MR cholangiographies are comparable with regard to the detection of any intrahepatic bile duct dilatation and the assessment of the level of injury and presence of associated lithiasis. However, MR cholangiography is noninvasive and facilitates the study of a disconnected biliary duct, otherwise not accessible by endoscopy, and provides additional information on associated fluid collection, secondary portal hypertension, and atrophy of injured liver [19]. The interpretation of cholangiographies and their multidisciplinary discussion are the first step to plan successful treatment. The first step is to assess the integrity of the CBD and to rule out any disconnection of intrahepatic ducts. There is no longer a role for exploratory surgery (laparotomy/re-laparoscopy) or invasive cholangiographies to delineate the biliary anatomy for diagnostic purposes only. The assessment of vascular lesions is of pivotal role especially in the case of a previous repair attempt and in the management of proximal injury, which may be associated with the injury of the right hepatic artery. With the advent of MR cholangiography, hepatobiliary scintigraphy has been progressively underused in the diagnostic work-up of these conditions.

42.4 Endoscopic Therapy

Nowadays, endoscopic therapy is considered the first-line treatment of POBS, thanks to its high success rate and low risk of relevant complications [20]. On the contrary, surgery leads to a considerable risk of perioperative mortality (up to 4%) with morbidity ranging from 9 to 42% [21, 22]. Most published series about endotherapy have consisted of patients presenting with a miscellanea of POBS of different origins, e.g., cholecystectomy, liver transplantation, right or left hepatectomy, etc., thus leading to criticisms in the discussion on results.

Three decades ago, in the endoscopic scenario, balloon dilation and single plastic stenting were put forward, but a high rate of stricture recurrence has occurred [4]. Costamagna and Mutignani et al. [4] suggested the progressive dilation of any tight stricture by means of a progressive number of plastic stents placed side by side across the stricture. Their study involved patients presenting with a biliary stricture after hepatic or biliary surgery (post-cholecystectomy) [4]. Sixty percent of them had Bismuth type I or II biliary strictures, and 40% had more complex type III–V strictures. A median number of 4.1 ± 1.3 endoscopic procedures was needed, and the median duration of therapy was 12.1 ± 5.3 months. Hydrostatic balloon dilation was used only to assist the insertion of the maximal number of stents. No difference was found comparing early (<30 days after surgery) or late (>30 days) strictures in terms of radiological success. Complications occurred in 9% of patients on endoscopic therapy and consisted of cholangitis or mild-moderate pancreatitis. The patients of this series have been followed up on a very long term (median time length of 13 years) [21], and only 11% of them have presented with new-onset biliary obstruction secondary to the recurrence of the stricture. An endoscopic rescue therapy with multi-stenting was proposed again, and success was achieved for all such patients. Multi-stenting with a less aggressive treatment, i.e., by means of a median of only two plastic side-by-side stents to treat patients presenting with a Bismuth type I–II (92% of cases) or type III–V (8%) stricture after cholecystectomy, achieved clinical success in 91% of cases, but with a higher recurrence rate (20%) during the 9.1-year-long follow-up[23]. Moreover, a low rate of success has been recorded by other authors in patients with Bismuth type III–V postoperative strictures compared to type I–II, i.e., 25% vs. 80% [24]. In summary, in order to successfully treat more complex POBS, an aggressive policy is needed. Otherwise, cholangitis in the series of patients who have undergone multi-stenting therapy is relatively low secondary to the soiling alongside the occluded stents. In this setting, death related to sepsis of biliary origin secondary to stent dysfunction was reported [23]. A local registry on patients' recall is required in order to limit the risk of emergency presentation with cholangitis secondary to stents clogging. Patients' compliance should be taken into account at the time of planning endoscopic or surgical options. The optimal timing to definitively remove plastic stents has not been defined by means of controlled studies. According to different authors, the end of endotherapy is defined as ranging from the disappearance of any waste at stricture level or the easy passage of an inflated balloon catheter at the level of the previous stricture to the rapid drainage of the contrast medium above the stricture [4, 23–25].

More recently, multi-stenting has become the reference standard for the first-line treatment of this condition (Figs. 42.4, 42.5 and 42.6), but criticism has risen. The need of multiple procedures and hospitalization contributes to high direct and indirect healthcare provision costs. In recent years, self-expandable metal stents with plastic coverage made of permalume or silicone, at first designed for malignant strictures, have been marketed for benign biliary strictures of different origin, such as chronic pancreatitis and post-orthotopic liver transplantation. In addition to their large diameter up to 10 mm that is achieved through metal meshes after the delivery of the plastic coverage surrounding, the metal meshes allow for removability after 6–12 months, thanks to the absence of in-growth secondary to hyperplastic tissue [26]. The development of a removable metal stent in this area potentially translates into limiting of the endoscopic therapies down to two procedures only, i.e., stent-in and stent-out procedures [27–32], leading to a decrease in healthcare provision costs in comparison to the multi-stenting policy.

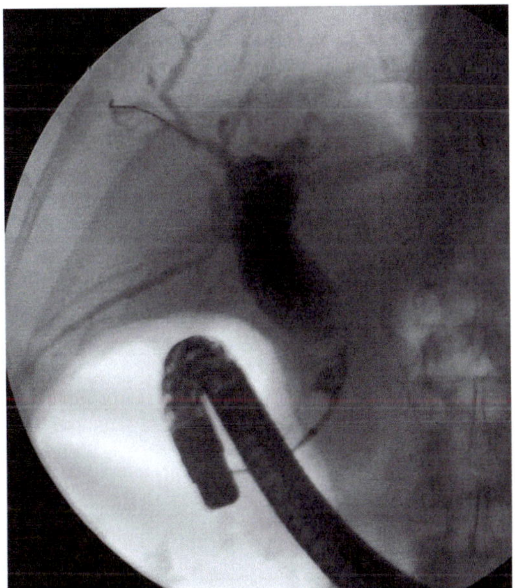

Fig. 42.4 Type 1 Bismuth stricture after cholecystectomy. The distal stricture was tight and angulated; the common bile duct was dilated above the stricture

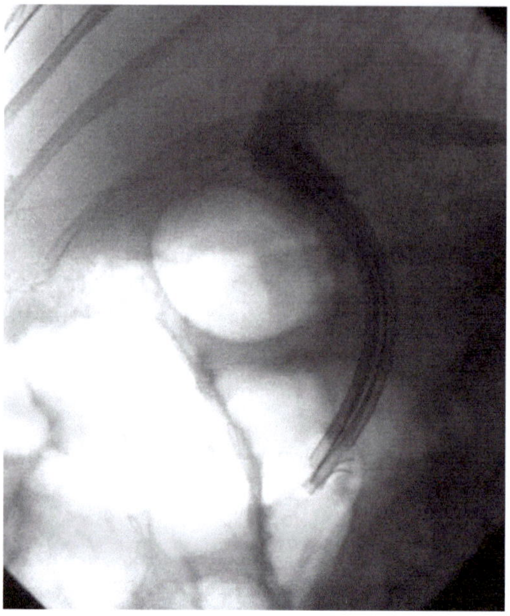

Fig. 42.5 Multiple plastic stenting was proposed to the patient who underwent four ERCPs in a year

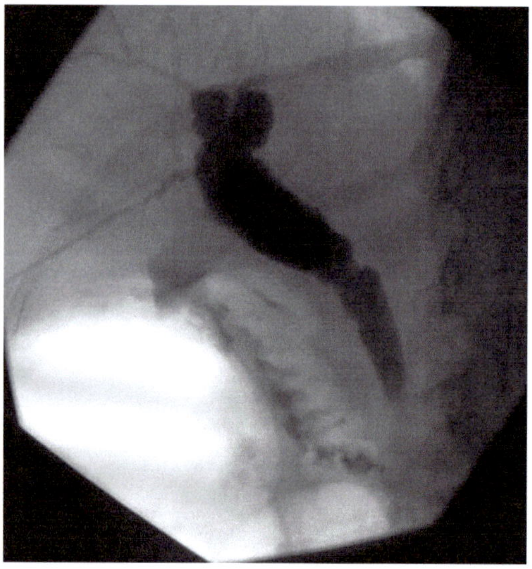

Fig. 42.6 At 1 year, the maximal stenting with five 10 Fr stents was achieved leading to a suboptimal radiological result secondary to a residual waist at the level of the stricture. Otherwise, clinical and laboratory results were maintained at 3 years follow-up

In case of a biliary stricture after cholecystectomy that is more than 2 cm below the hilum, endoscopic treatment by means of a fully covered self-expandable metal stent has been proposed [33], and favorable results have been reported for 72% of patients at 18 months. Waiting for long-term clinical results, the migration is considered the "Achilles' heel" of the use of fully covered SEMS, ranging from 3% to 25% of patients with a benign biliary stricture, including patients with a miscellanea of POBS (Table 42.2). None of the solutions proposed to date in order to reduce the migration risk rate of fully covered SEMSs has been validated by prospective studies; they are the placement of a stent without prior sphincterotomy or with the major portion above the stricture, clipping the stent to the duodenal mucosa, or suspending a short conic-shape stent across the stricture. Distal migration impacts on the success rate, while proximal migration potentially implies difficult removal with standard techniques (rat tooth forceps, snaring) in up to 4% of patients in large series [33]. In difficult scenarios secondary to overgrowth at the level of the distal impaction of the metal meshes, stent-in-stent removal has been proposed [34]. The use of a second covered stent bridging the previous impacted covered one can be of help to treat the overgrowth tissue by compression leading to ischemia of the hyperplastic tissue, thus allowing the disimpaction of the stent and easy removal of both stents [34].

After cholecystectomy, benign strictures rising at the level of the hilum (Fig. 42.7) or proximal to it (Fig. 42.8) can be multiple and bilateral, as associated to a vascular lesion, leading to an acute and chronic ischemia of the biliary ducts. In this condition, endotherapy with multiple bilateral plastic stents is proposed as a first-step approach in tertiary referral centers [4, 23]. After the clogging of the stent, the soiling of bile alongside the stents allows the second-order ducts [35] to drain. Exchange at a 3-month interval is usually planned in this scenario, as well. In case of a biliary stricture involving the hilum, the use of multiple fully covered metal stents has been traditionally contraindicated secondary to the risk of secondary biliary duct occlusion leading to sepsis of biliary origin [22]. A fully covered metal stent with side holes has been designed for this condition and will be available soon in the market. In the setting of benign biliary strictures, randomized controlled trials that aim to compare the use of multiple plastic stents vs. fully covered

Table 42.2 Endoscopic therapies for postoperative stricture

Authors	Year	No. of patients [a]	Study design	Endotherapy	Rx success ITT	Complications	Migration	Recurrence	Follow-up	Rescue TP	Clinical success PP
Costamagna	2001	45	Retro	PM	89%	9%	2%	0%	48 months	–	89%
Bergman	2001	74	Retro	PM	59%	19%	4%	20%	9.1 years	PM-surg	74%
Draganov	2002	16	Retro	PM	80%	<1%	0%	20%	48 months	PM-surg	80%
Kahaleh	2008	3	Retro	PC SEMS	100%	NA	NA	0%	12 months	–	100%
Costamagna	2010	35	Retro	PM	89%	9%	2%	11%	13.7 years	PM	100%
Mangiavillano	2014	11	Prosp	FCSEMS	100%	0%	9%	9%	6 months	Percut	91%
Chaput	2016	14	Prosp	FCSEMS	61%	NA	25%	22%	12 months	PM-FC-surg	61%
Schmidt	2017	4	Prosp	FCSEMS	82%	0%	25%	0%	24 months	PM-FC	82%
Wu	2017	17	Retro	FCSEMS	84%	18%	3%	33%	43 months	NA	84%
				PM	83%	24%	8%	25%	43 months	NA	83%

Retro retrospective, *Prosp* prospective, *PM* plastic multistenting, *PC* partially covered, *FC* fully covered, *SEMS* self-expandable metal stent, *surg* surgery, *percut* percutaneous, *ITT* intention-to-treat analysis, *PP* per-protocol analysis, *NA* not assessed

[a]Chronic pancreatitis and liver transplanted patients were excluded

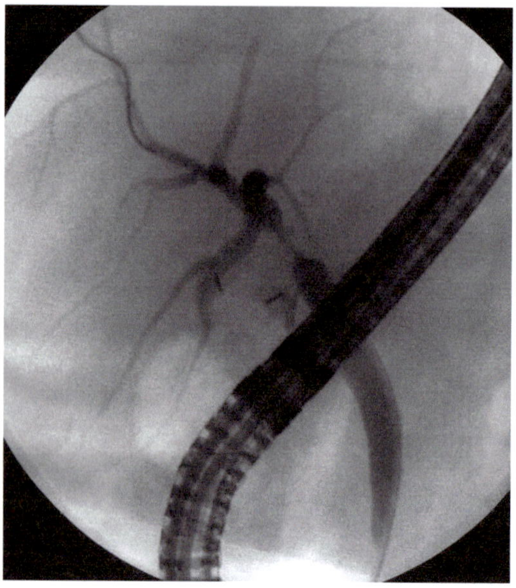

Fig. 42.7 Type 3 Bismuth stricture. The left hepatic duct was not injected with contrast medium because of a complex hilar stricture

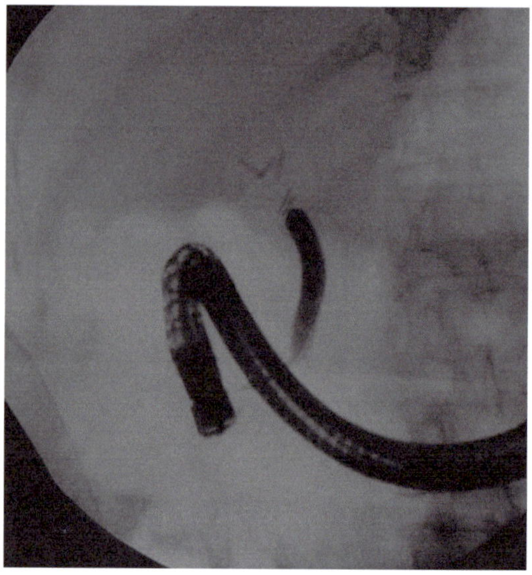

Fig. 42.9 Type E1 Strasberg stricture of the common bile duct by inappropriate clip release and transection of the hepatic duct. Hepatico-jejunal anastomosis was performed 4 days after cholecystectomy

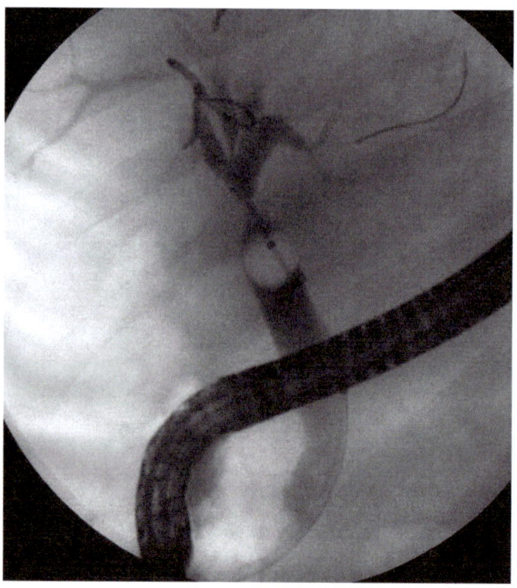

Fig. 42.8 Type 2 Bismuth stricture after cholecystectomy as seen during an occlusive cholangiography

metal stents are welcome: such trials will help to define the best approach on the basis of a cost-effective analysis.

When a leak is associated to a stricture, stenting should aim at dilating the stricture and reducing the pressure gradient of the biliary tree above the stricture and the duodenum. In case of extrahepatic leak, the stent should pass through both the stricture and the leak; in case of intrahepatic leak, the proximal end of the stent should be at the level of the hepatic ducts, and traversing the leak is not usually needed (law of communicating vessels). When a complete transection of the CBD occurs (Fig. 42.9), some authors have suggested an early endoscopic attempt to restore the integrity of the biliary tree by forcing the site of the clipping to access the disconnected proximal CBD. When stenting fails in this condition, hepatico-jejunal anastomosis is to be performed.

To date, the experiences on biologic stents dissolving over time or metal stents eluting drugs against hyperplasia of the tissue are too limited to deserve any discussion in the field of benign biliary strictures.

42.5 Non-endoscopic Therapies

At present, no large randomized control trials have been planned, and no cost analysis is available to compare endoscopic therapies vs. non-endoscopic ones. The higher rates of complications following non-endoscopic treatments limit their application to second-line approaches. The aim of second-line treatments remains that of preventing secondary biliary cirrhosis. Traditionally, in case of any failure of endoscopic drainage, also after referral to a tertiary referral center, percutaneous drainage is attempted in case of dilated intrahepatic biliary ducts. Published results on outcome after the radiological approach are scanty, and the long-term success rate ranges from 75 to 90% [35, 36]. In case of a bilateral postoperative stricture, a bilateral percutaneous drainage should be attempted. Multiple procedures have to be planned in order to progressively dilate the stricture using larger external or internal-external drainages. Complications are consistent with cholangitis, hemobilia, and hepatic hematoma and are usually treated with antibiotics and transfusional support. The level of quality of life for patients with a definitive external drainage is considered a limitation of this approach, and, whenever possible, the endoscopic approach is preferred. Of note in the field of tight and angulated strictures, the percutaneous approach does potentially help any subsequent endoscopic stenting (rendezvous technique).

In the centers of referral for endoscopic therapies, surgery is considered after the failure of endoscopic and percutaneous approaches for the above-mentioned reasons. In non-tertiary endoscopic centers, surgery is considered at the early stages of the management of these conditions. When a biliary lesion is confirmed at an accurate intraoperative evaluation at the time of cholecystectomy and repair is then attempted, a high rate of success is achieved. Little data currently confirms that early surgical repair leads to long-term success [37, 38], especially in case of complicated postoperative biliary lesions with a leak and an associated stricture [39]. On the contrary, late surgical treatment shows a lower rate of success. In case of extrahepatic biliary strictures, the traditional surgery consisted in hepatico-jejunal anastomosis to achieve an optimal drainage above the stricture. Facing with a hilar stricture, biductal hepatico-jejunostomy involving the right and left hepatic ducts should be considered and guided by percutaneous transhepatic cholangiography. Overall long-term success ranges from 70% to 90% at 3–9 years with a stricture complicating in 6–20% of bilio-enteric anastomosis cases. In case of intrahepatic strictures not amenable to radiological drainage or surgical bilio-enteric anastomosis (especially when associated to cholangitis, intrahepatic stones, and segmental hepatic atrophy), resection is the only curative option [40]. The rationale for this approach is that by removing the atrophic parenchyma and performing a bilio-enteric anastomosis, good long-term results can be achieved. Liver resection may prevent biliary malignancy secondary to chronic biliary stasis or recurrent cholangitis. Moreover, the removal of the damaged liver tissue (right or left hepatectomy) with exposure of the biliary tree can contribute to a large anastomosis in non-fibrotic, well-vascularized tissue. Early complications have occurred in 7% to 42% of the series including hepatic or intra-abdominal abscess, empyema, or wound infections [41]. Overall long-term clinical outcomes are optimal or good in more than 90% of cases when an appropriate timing for surgical repair is considered [40]. After unsuccessful endoscopic and non-endoscopic repairs, only a few patients may present with recurrent attacks of cholangitis or chronic cholestasis leading to secondary liver fibrosis, cirrhosis, and portal hypertension. In this setting, liver transplantation should be considered, and a few cases have been reported [42]. In such a subset of patients, the criteria and the timing for liver transplantation have not been defined yet by means of international guidelines, and this option is to be considered as a center-based decision according to the locally available expertise.

References

1. Costamagna G, Shah SK, Tringali A. Current management of postoperative complications and benign biliary strictures. Gastrointest Endosc Clin N Am. 2003;13:635–48, ix.
2. Bharathy KG, Negi SS. Postcholecystectomy bile duct injury and its sequelae: pathogenesis, classi-

fication, and management. Indian J Gastroenterol. 2014;33:201–15.
3. Cai XJ, Ying HN, Yu H, et al. Blunt dissection: a solution to prevent bile duct injury in laparoscopic cholecystectomy. Chin Med J (Engl). 2015;128:3153–7.
4. Costamagna G, Pandolfi M, Mutignani M, et al. Long-term results of endoscopic management of postoperative bile duct strictures with increasing numbers of stents. Gastrointest Endosc. 2001;54:162–8.
5. MacFadyen BV Jr, Vecchio R, Ricardo AE, et al. Bile duct injury after laparoscopic cholecystectomy. The United States experience. Surg Endosc. 1998;12:315–21.
6. Smith MT, Sherman S, Lehman GA. Endoscopic management of benign strictures of the biliary tree. Endoscopy. 1995;27:253–66.
7. Smadja C, Blumgart L. Surgery of the liver and biliary tract; The biliary tract and the anatomy of biliary exposure. Edinburgh: Churchill Livingstone; 1988.
8. Woods MS, Traverso LW, Kozarek RA, et al. Characteristics of biliary tract complications during laparoscopic cholecystectomy: a multi-institutional study. Am J Surg. 1994;167:27–33; discussion 33-4.
9. Andren-Sandberg A, Alinder G, Bengmark S. Accidental lesions of the common bile duct at cholecystectomy. Pre- and perioperative factors of importance. Ann Surg. 1985;201:328–32.
10. Way LW, Stewart L, Gantert W, et al. Causes and prevention of laparoscopic bile duct injuries: analysis of 252 cases from a human factors and cognitive psychology perspective. Ann Surg. 2003;237:460–9.
11. de Reuver PR, Grossmann I, Busch OR, et al. Referral pattern and timing of repair are risk factors for complications after reconstructive surgery for bile duct injury. Ann Surg. 2007;245:763–70.
12. Lokesh HM, Pottakkat B, Prakash A, et al. Risk factors for development of biliary stricture in patients presenting with bile leak after cholecystectomy. Gut Liver. 2013;7:352–6.
13. Bismuth H, Majno PE. Biliary strictures: classification based on the principles of surgical treatment. World J Surg. 2001;25:1241–4.
14. Bergman JJ, van den Brink GR, Rauws EA, et al. Treatment of bile duct lesions after laparoscopic cholecystectomy. Gut. 1996;38:141–7.
15. Csendes A, Navarrete C, Burdiles P, et al. Treatment of common bile duct injuries during laparoscopic cholecystectomy: endoscopic and surgical management. World J Surg. 2001;25:1346–51.
16. Chun K. Recent classifications of the common bile duct injury. Korean J Hepatobiliary Pancreat Surg. 2014;18:69–72.
17. Bektas H, Schrem H, Winny M, et al. Surgical treatment and outcome of iatrogenic bile duct lesions after cholecystectomy and the impact of different clinical classification systems. Br J Surg. 2007;94:1119–27.
18. Lee CM, Stewart L, Way LW. Postcholecystectomy abdominal bile collections. Arch Surg. 2000;135:538–42; discussion 542-4.
19. Chaudhary A, Negi SS, Puri SK, et al. Comparison of magnetic resonance cholangiography and percutaneous transhepatic cholangiography in the evaluation of bile duct strictures after cholecystectomy. Br J Surg. 2002;89:433–6.
20. Dumonceau JM, Tringali A, Blero D, et al. Biliary stenting: indications, choice of stents and results: European Society of Gastrointestinal Endoscopy (ESGE) clinical guideline. Endoscopy. 2012;44:277–98.
21. Costamagna G, Tringali A, Mutignani M, et al. Endotherapy of postoperative biliary strictures with multiple stents: results after more than 10 years of follow-up. Gastrointest Endosc. 2010;72:551–7.
22. Kaino S, Sen-Yo M, Shinoda S, et al. Side-by-side placement of bilateral endoscopic metal stents for the treatment of postoperative biliary stricture. Clin J Gastroenterol. 2017;10:68–72.
23. Bergman JJ, Burgemeister L, Bruno MJ, et al. Long-term follow-up after biliary stent placement for postoperative bile duct stenosis. Gastrointest Endosc. 2001;54:154–61.
24. Draganov P, Hoffman B, Marsh W, et al. Long-term outcome in patients with benign biliary strictures treated endoscopically with multiple stents. Gastrointest Endosc. 2002;55:680–6.
25. Wu J, Zhou DX, Wang TT, et al. A new fully covered self-expandable metal stent for the treatment of postsurgical benign biliary strictures. Dig Dis Sci. 2017;62:2550–7.
26. Mangiavillano B, Manes G, Baron TH, et al. The use of double lasso, fully covered self-expandable metal stents with new "anchoring flap" system in the treatment of benign biliary diseases. Dig Dis Sci. 2014;59:2308–13.
27. Kahaleh M, Behm B, Clarke BW, et al. Temporary placement of covered self-expandable metal stents in benign biliary strictures: a new paradigm? (with video). Gastrointest Endosc. 2008;67:446–54.
28. Cote GA, Slivka A, Tarnasky P, et al. Effect of covered metallic stents compared with plastic stents on benign biliary stricture resolution: a randomized clinical trial. JAMA. 2016;315:1250–7.
29. Mahajan A, Ho H, Sauer B, et al. Temporary placement of fully covered self-expandable metal stents in benign biliary strictures: midterm evaluation (with video). Gastrointest Endosc. 2009;70:303–9.
30. van Boeckel PG, Vleggaar FP, Siersema PD. Plastic or metal stents for benign extrahepatic biliary strictures: a systematic review. BMC Gastroenterol. 2009;9:96.
31. Schmidt A, Pickartz T, Lerch MM, et al. Effective treatment of benign biliary strictures with a removable, fully covered, self-expandable metal stent: a prospective, multicenter European study. United Eur Gastroenterol J. 2017;5:398–407.
32. Chaput U, Vienne A, Audureau E, et al. Temporary placement of fully covered self-expandable metal stents for the treatment of benign biliary strictures. United Eur Gastroenterol J. 2016;4:403–12.

33. Deviere J, Nageshwar Reddy D, Puspok A, et al. Successful management of benign biliary strictures with fully covered self-expanding metal stents. Gastroenterology. 2014;147:385–95; quiz e15.
34. Tringali A, Blero D, Boskoski I, et al. Difficult removal of fully covered self expandable metal stents (SEMS) for benign biliary strictures: the "SEMS in SEMS" technique. Dig Liver Dis. 2014;46:568–71.
35. Singh RR, Singh V. Endoscopic management of hilar biliary strictures. World J Gastrointest Endosc. 2015;7:806–13.
36. Ramos-De la Medina A, Misra S, Leroy AJ, et al. Management of benign biliary strictures by percutaneous interventional radiologic techniques (PIRT). HPB (Oxford). 2008;10:428–32.
37. Huszar O, Kokas B, Matrai P, et al. Meta-analysis of the long term success rate of different interventions in benign biliary strictures. PLoS One. 2017;12:e0169618.
38. Maddah G, Rajabi Mashhadi MT, Parvizi Mashhadi M, et al. Iatrogenic injuries of the extrahepatic biliary system. J Surg Res. 2017;213:215–21.
39. Eum YO, Park JK, Chun J, et al. Non-surgical treatment of post-surgical bile duct injury: clinical implications and outcomes. World J Gastroenterol. 2014;20:6924–31.
40. Barbier L, Souche R, Slim K, et al. Long-term consequences of bile duct injury after cholecystectomy. J Visc Surg. 2014;151:269–79.
41. Pekolj J, Yanzon A, Dietrich A, et al. Major liver resection as definitive treatment in post-cholecystectomy common bile duct injuries. World J Surg. 2015;39:1216–23.
42. Perini MV, Herman P, Montagnini AL, et al. Liver resection for the treatment of post-cholecystectomy biliary stricture with vascular injury. World J Gastroenterol. 2015;21:2102–7.

43 Biliary Complications After Liver Transplantation

Jörg G. Albert

Abbreviations

ABS	Anastomotic biliary stricture
CBD	Common bile duct
CC	Choledocho-choledochostomy
CJ	Choledocho-jejunostomy
cSEMS	(Fully) Covered self-expanding metal stent
ERCP	Endoscopic retrograde cholangio-pancreatography
HAT	Hepatic artery thrombosis
ITBL	Ischemic-type biliary lesion
LDLT	Living donor liver transplantation
MPS	Multiple plastic stents
MRCP	Magnetic resonance cholangiopan-creatography
NAS	Non-anastomotic stricture
NEPS	Non-expanding plastic stent
OLT	Orthotopic liver transplantation
PSC	Primary sclerosing cholangitis
PTCD	Percutaneous transhepatic cholan-giodrainage
SEMS	Self-expanding metal stent
SSC-CIP	Cholangiopathy of the critically ill patient

J. G. Albert (✉)
Abteilung für Gastroenterologie, Hepatologie und Endokrinologie, Robert-Bosch-Krankenhaus, Auerbachstraße, Stuttgart, Germany
e-mail: joerg.albert@rbk.de

43.1 Introduction

Since the first experiences with liver transplantation in the 1960s, this procedure has become a standard treatment for end stage liver disease. Limited by the donor liver supply, the number of orthotopic liver transplants (OLT) has nevertheless continued to increase over time. Although surgical techniques improved constantly and the rate of biliary complications following liver transplantation has been decreasing, they remain a major source of morbidity and mortality for the patient: Biliary complications may occur in a substantial number of patients after orthotopic liver transplantation (OLT) and significantly influence the outcome. Biliary leaks, bile duct strictures, choledocholithiasis, biliary casts, and strictures of the bile duct anastomosis all contribute to symptomatic disease with impact on morbidity and mortality of OLT. T-tube biliary reconstruction, Roux-en-Y anastomosis, ischemia, reperfusion injury, hepatic artery thrombosis (HAT), cytomegalovirus infection, and primary sclerosing cholangitis (PSC) are some of the risk factors in post-liver transplantation biliary complications (Table 43.1). The incidence of biliary complications after liver transplantation ranges from about 5 to 25% (Tables 43.2 and 43.3).

Many of these conditions are successfully treated by endoscopic means today. This reflects the change of treatment approaches that consisted of surgical repair before the 1990s and were

M. Mutignani et al. (eds.), *Endotherapy in Biliopancreatic Diseases: ERCP Meets EUS*,
https://doi.org/10.1007/978-3-030-42569-2_43

interventional with use of ERCP or PTCD in the 1990s, changing to a predominant use of ERCP in the 2000s in most centers [1].

43.2 Considering Surgical Technique Before Starting Endoscopic Treatment

The choice of biliary anastomosis is a major determinant of the risk of biliary complications after OLT. The two most common biliary reconstruction are choledocho-choledochostomy (CC, duct-to-duct anastomosis) and choledocho-jejunostomy (CJ). CC is usually preferred today because of technical ease, preserving of the Sphincter of Oddi, and the easy endoscopic access to the biliary system after surgery. With the Sphincter of Oddi still in place, risk of ascending cholangitis might be less frequent. Adding a T-tube to CC allows measurement of bile output in the early postoperative period and maintains easy access for radiological evaluation of the biliary system. However, T-tubes have been associated with bile leak and cholangitis at the time of their removal and were associated to an increased rate of overall complications (33% vs. 15%), and even survival might be slightly reduced after T-tube placement [2]. Thus, CC (duct-to-duct anastomosis) without T-tube insertion is the surgical technique most frequently performed in OLT today, and it may result in stricture formation in about 20% of cases [3]. The stricture may occur weeks to years after the transplantation. Small size of donor CBD, age of recipient, and biliary leakage are risk factors for biliary stricture, and operative technique seems to contribute [4].

CJ may be preferred in patients with preexisting biliary disease, e.g., primary sclerosing cholangitis, or prior biliary surgery, and in cases of size mismatch between donor and recipient ducts. Compared to CC, CJ adversely affects the ability to perform an endoscopic evaluation of the biliary system after the liver transplantation. Potential complications of CJ include intestinal perforation, stricture, leakage, and bleeding at the jejuno-jejunostomy.

Table 43.1 Examples for etiology of bile duct injury in patients after liver transplantation

Bile duct obstruction	Bile duct stones, biliary casts
	Anastomotic stricture (choledocho-choledochal or bilio/hepato-jejunal anastomosis)
	Recurrence of primary sclerosing cholangitis (PSC)
Infections	Bacterial cholangitis
	Cytomegalovirus infection (CMV)
Ischemia	Ischemic bile duct injury, e.g., non-anastomotic ischemic type like lesions (ITBL)
	Vascular disease: e.g., hepatic artery thrombosis (HAT)
	Cholangiopathy of the critically ill patient (SSC-CIP), long-term ventilator dependence

43.3 Diagnostics Before Interventional Treatment

Ductography (ERCP, PTCD) findings are the gold standard for establishing the diagnosis of biliary complication after liver transplantation. However, non-invasive diagnostics should precede ERCP or PTCD. Ultrasonography and/or MRI + MRCP or

Table 43.2 Incidence of biliary complications after liver transplantation

Author	Year	*n*		Rate of biliary complications	Rate of anastomotic stenosis	Rate of anastomotic leakage	Rate of non-anastomotic stricture
Stratta	1989	226	DDLT	19.1%	8.3%	–	–
Greif	1994	1792	DDLT	12.1%	3.9%	3.2%	0.6%
Chen	2003	766	LDLT	17.8%	10.5%	7.3%	
Suarez	2008	498	HBD vs. NHBD	–	13.9 %(HBD) 12.5% (NHBD)	7.7% (HBD) 4.2 (NHBD)	2.3% (HBD) 25% (NHBD)
Parks	2008	283	LDLT		20.5%		
Marubashi	2009	83	LDLT	8.4%	7.2%	1.2%	–

HBD heart-beating donor, *NHBD* non-heart-beating donor, *DDLT* deceased donor liver transplantation, *LDLT* life donor liver transplantation

Table 43.3 Interventional treatment of anastomotic biliary stricture after OLT

Author	Year	*N*	Concept	Intervention	Number of ERCPs	Mean number/ diameter of stents	Mean duration of stenting [month]	Success of treatment
Morelli	2003	25	Retrospective	Dilation + stents	3 (1–6)	2 (0–7)		80%
Zöpf	2005	72	Retrospective, comparative	Dilation (BD) vs. dilation + stents (BD+S)	4 (1–11)	17 Fr (10–21.5)	4 (1–27)	Immediate: 88%/87%, long-term 38% (BD)/69% (BD + S)
Alazmi	2006	143	Retrospective	Dilation + stents	3.1	14.6 ± 6.8 Fr	4.8 [145 (11–1000) days]	82%
Holt	2007	53	Prospective	Dilation + stents	3	4	11	92% (early); 69% (late)
Pasha	2007	25	Retrospective	Dilation + multiple stents	3.5 (1–9)	5.3	4.6	88% (early); 80% (20/25 late)
Morelli	2008	38	Prospective case series	Dilation + multiple stents	3.4 (2–6)	2.5 (1–6)	3.5 [107 (20–198) days]	87%
Tabibian	2010	69	Retrospective	Dilation + multiple stents	3 (2–7)	8 vs. 3.5 (success vs. failure)	15 (12–60)	94%

CT evaluates the diagnosis of biliary disease in liver transplant patients. An abdominal ultrasound allows for the evaluation of the biliary tree and the corresponding hepatic vasculature. The positive predictive value of abdominal ultrasound is high, but sensitivity for detecting biliary obstruction ranges below 70%. Magnetic resonance cholangiopancreatography (MRCP) provides a high sensitivity in detecting biliary strictures, and MRCP can offer a road map for the endoscopist in planning the intervention [5].

43.4 Stricturing Disease After Liver Transplantation

Biliary stricture should be suspected in any OLT patient who presents with jaundice, fever, abdominal pain, and in patients with asymptomatic biochemical cholestasis [6]. Dilatation of the bile duct system may be observed on imaging studies but is not a prerequisite for the correct diagnosis (!). Histologic findings may be suggestive of biliary obstruction, e.g., pericholangitis or bile duct proliferation.

Anastomotic biliary stricture (ABS) has to be distinguished from non-anastomotic strictures (NAS) that are mainly due to temporary ischemia of the biliary epithelia. NAS are defined as strictures involving the donor hepatic duct proximal to the anastomosis and the right and/or left hepatic duct and/or intrahepatic branches. The latter are ischemic type biliary lesion (ITBL) in most instances. Treatment by ERCP should not be prolonged, but ERCP is rarely an urgent emergency intervention. ERCP with maximal stent placement strategy has become widely accepted and allows a >80% resolution rate of all duct-to-duct ABSs. Recurrence of ABS might again be treated endoscopically, and the need for surgical intervention or retransplantation is a rare event. Thereby, plastic stents are inserted into the bile duct bridging the ABS and the number of stents is increased with every stent exchange session, up to the maximum stent number that is achieved at the size of the donor and/or recipient CBD size. This "stent-exchange-program" (multiple plastic stent, MPS) is lasting for an average of 1 year [7–10].

In NAS and ITBL, treatment has to be highly individualized in each case and is based on NEPS placement and bile duct cast removal as needed. In patients with CJ reconstruction, the initial treatment usually involves drainage insertion and/or hydrostatic balloon dilation by the percutaneous approach (PTCD).

SEMS for endoscopic treatment of duct strictures are increasingly used for the stricture of the choledocho-choledochal anastomosis but rarely ideal for ITBLs that are often proximally located to the anastomosis. Covered self-expanding metal stents (cSEMS) might significantly help to reduce the number of endoscopic interventions to achieve similar efficacy as multiple plastic stents and might become a new treatment standard. However, the optimal duration of cSEMS therapy is not yet clarified and stricture recurrence tends to be higher in the cSEMS treatment groups in some studies [11, 12]. The ideal type of cSEMS has not yet been identified; intra-ductal SEMS can be compared to a SEMS extruding from the papilla; there are SEMS with anti-migration waist, anchoring flaps, fixed-cell structure vs. non-fixed cell structure, and many others. In meta-analysis, fully covered SEMS and MPS had equal ABS resolution and recurrence, although there was a trend toward a higher recurrence rate in FC-SEMS that disappeared when trials with a shorter stent indwelling time were excluding. No difference was found in overall adverse events or migration rate [13, 14].

Recurrence of ABS is observed in up to one in five patients after initial successful endoscopic therapy [15]. The optimal type of endoscopic therapy that would minimize the risk of stricture recurrence is ambiguous, though. A second treatment approach with interventional/endoscopic stenting can be advocated in most patients and will again be successful in up to 80% of these cases [16].

43.5 Bile Duct Leaks

Bile duct leak should be suspected in any patient who develops abdominal pain, fever, or any sign of peritonitis after liver transplantation and might occur after T-tube removal. Bile leaks not related to T-tube removal typically present within the first 30 days after OLT. Some patients, especially those on corticosteroids, may be asymptomatic, with no signs of pain or fever. In such cases, any unexplained elevations in serum bilirubin, fluctuation in immunosuppressive medication levels, or bilious ascites should raise immediate suspicion for a bile leak.

Bile duct leaks are often located at the site of the anastomosis and might be due to ischemia and incomplete healing of the anastomosis. The occurrence of leaks may be associated to surgical technique, ischemia time, and others. For example, intraoperative intraductal trans-anastomotic stenting in duct-to-duct biliary reconstruction seems to result in an increased risk of leak formation. Bile leakage can be classified as early (immediate) or late (within days to weeks). Early leakage is usually detected at the anastomotic site. Late leakage is typically associated with the removal of the T-tube, which is infrequently used in most centers now. ERCP with stenting of the bile duct, sphincterotomy, nasobiliary drainage, or a combination of these techniques has a high rate of success [17].

Severe stricture formation due to a chronic inflammatory reaction may accompany the healing of the leak. Stenting after sphincterotomy to decrease the bile pressure gradient over the papilla is the basic treatment procedure of leaks. It is highly advisable to add stenting up to several months to prevent complications from stricture formation.

Refractory anastomotic bile leaks after liver transplantation are associated with decreased event-free survival. Hepatic artery disease is associated with refractory leaks. Future, large-scale prospective studies may help to define the optimal management of patients at risk for refractory bile leaks.

43.6 Adverse Events from Bile Duct Content

Bile duct stones, sludge, and casts, together called bile duct filling defects, occur in approximately 5–10% of patients after LDLT and after deceased donor OLT and are frequently accompanied by other biliary complications, most commonly biliary strictures. Patients present with abdominal pain, cholestatic liver tests, and cholangitis. The increase of the viscosity of bile or a reduced bile flow can predispose to the formation of sludge and stones. Bile duct mucosal damage due to obstruction, ischemia, or infection can develop bile casts. Patients presenting with biliary stones and sludge will frequently provide an underlying stricture. In addition, medications such as cyclosporine may play a role in bile lithogenicity by inhibiting bile secretion and promoting functional biliary stasis [6]. In liver transplant patients, bile is supersaturated with cholesterol, which is aggravated by T-tube drainage and depletion of the bile acid pool.

Simple stones without other biliary lesions present occur late a a predominant use of ERCP in the 2000s in most centers fter OLT and are treated by stone removal, similarly to non-OLT patients. Bile duct stones secondary to stricture are differed from biliary casts due to ischemic destruction of biliary epithelia, mixed with bilirubin. Addressing the therapy of the stricture together with stone removal is crucial for a successful treatment in these cases. In addition, bile duct sludge formation is frequent in patients that undergo prolonged endoscopic stenting; stent exchange intervals might need to be shortened to minimize symptomatic stone disease and cholangitis in some of these patients.

43.7 Bilioma and Liver Abscess Formation

Bile leak within the liver or abdominal cavity may result in the formation of a biloma that can undergo infection, i.e., abscess formation. A small biloma communicating with the biliary tree may resolve on its own. Larger bilioma and abscess need treatment with antibiotics and percutaneous drainage, and in some cases, placement of a biliary stent in the extrahepatic bile duct is required. In case there is an underlying stricture preventing the evacuation of the bilioma, a transhepatic/trans-bilioma percutaneously placed drainage (trans-bilioma PTCD) may be very helpful [18]. Surgical drainage of a bilioma is a last resort option.

43.8 Summary and Diagnostic Algorithm

Biliary complications are frequently well attributed by interventional treatment approaches and should be swiftly addressed. With the increase of cholestatic enzymes or detection of bile in a surgically placed drain, further diagnostics are warranted that may include Duplex/sonography, MRI/MRCP, CT, and/or ERCP. Anastomotic strictures and leakage are the most frequent postoperative complications in the early course after liver transplantation, and strictures may also occur later after.

Anastomotic strictures are well treated by placing multiple plastic stents or—in the case of appropriate anatomy—cSEMS by ERCP or, alternatively, by PTCD. The prognosis of treatment success is excellent. Ischemic-type biliary lesions (ITBL), i.e., non-anastomotic strictures, should be handled by ERCP likewise, preferring endoscopic balloon dilation over stent insertion of combining both; however, treatment success is lower than in treating ABS. in the case of refractory strictures and/or recurring cholangitis or progressive liver failure, re-transplantation must be considered an alternative treatment.

References

1. Schwartz DA, Petersen BT, Poterucha JJ, Gostout CJ. Gostout. Endoscopic therapy of anastomotic bile duct strictures occurring after liver transplantation. Gastrointest Endosc. 2000;51(2):169–74.
2. Scatton O, Meunier B, Cherqui D, Boillot O, Sauvanet A, Boudjema K, Launois B, Fagniez PL, Belghiti J, Wolff P. Randomized trial of choledochocholedochostomy with or without a T tube in orthotopic liver transplantation. Ann Surg. 2001;233:432–7.
3. Poley JW, Lekkerkerker MN, Metselaar HJ, Kuipers EJ, Bruno MJ. Clinical outcome of progressive stenting in patients with anastomotic strictures after orthotopic liver transplantation. Endoscopy. 2013;45:567–70.

4. Park JB, Kwon CHD, Choi G-S, Chun JM, Jung GO, Kim S-J, Joh J-W, Lee S-K. Prolonged cold ischemic time is a risk factor for biliary strictures in duct-to-duct biliary reconstruction in living donor liver transplantation. Transpl. 2008;86(11):1536–42
5. Kitazono MT, Qayyum A, Yeh BM, Chard PS, Ostroff JW, Coakley FV. Magnetic resonance cholangiography of biliary strictures after liver transplantation: a prospective double-blind study. J Magn Reson Imaging. 2007;25:1168–73.
6. Kochhar G, Parungao JM, Hanouneh IA, Parsi MA. Biliary complications following liver transplantation. World J Gastroenterol. 2013;19(19):2841–6. https://doi.org/10.3748/wjg.v19.i19.2841.
7. Aepli P, St John A, Gupta S, Hourigan LF, Vaughan R, Efthymiou M, Kaffes A. Success and complications of an intra-ductal fully covered self-expanding metal stent (ID-FCSEMS) to treat anastomotic biliary strictures (AS) after orthotopic liver transplantation (OLT). Surg Endosc. 2017;31(4):1558–63 . Epub 2016 Aug 29. https://doi.org/10.1007/s00464-016-5138-9.
8. Coté GA, Slivka A, Tarnasky P, Mullady DK, Elmunzer BJ, Elta G, Fogel E, Lehman G, McHenry L, Romagnuolo J, Menon S, Siddiqui UD, Watkins J, Lynch S, Denski C, Xu H, Sherman S. Effect of covered metallic stents compared with plastic stents on benign biliary stricture resolution: a randomized clinical trial. JAMA. 2016;315(12):1250–7. https://doi.org/10.1001/jama.2016.2619.
9. Phillips MS, Bonatti H, Sauer BG, Smith L, Javaid M, Kahaleh M, Schmitt T. Elevated stricture rate following the use of fully covered self-expandable metal biliary stents for biliary leaks following liver transplantation. Endoscopy. 2011;43(6):512–7 . Epub 2011 May 26. https://doi.org/10.1055/s-0030-1256389.
10. Santosh Kumar KY, Mathew JS, Balakrishnan D, Bharathan VK, Thankamony Amma BSP, Gopalakrishnan U, Narayana Menon R, Dhar P, Vayoth SO, Sudhindran S. Intraductal transanastomotic stenting in duct-to-duct biliary reconstruction after living-donor liver transplantation: a randomized trial. J Am Coll Surg. 2017;225(6):747–54 . Epub 2017 Sep 13. https://doi.org/10.1016/j.jamcollsurg.2017.08.024.
11. Martins FP, De Paulo GA, Contini MLC, Ferrari AP. Metal versus plastic stents for anastomotic biliary strictures after liver transplantation: a randomized controlled trial. Gastrointest Endosc. 2018;87(1):131.e1–131.e13. https://doi.org/10.1016/j.gie.2017.04.013.
12. Tal AO, Finkelmeier F, Filmann N, Kylänpää L, Udd M, Parzanese I, Cantù P, Dechêne A, Penndorf V, Schnitzbauer A, Friedrich-Rust M, Zeuzem S, Albert JG. Multiple plastic stents versus covered metal stent for treatment of anastomotic biliary strictures after liver transplantation: a prospective, randomized, multicenter trial. Gastrointest Endosc. 2017;86(6):1038–45. https://doi.org/10.1016/j.gie.2017.03.009.
13. Tringali A, Tarantino I, Barresi L, Traina M, Bonato G, Cintolo M, Hassan C, Mutignani M, Adler DG. Multiple plastic versus fully covered metal stents for managing post-liver transplantation anastomotic biliary strictures: a meta-analysis of randomized controlled trials. Ann Gastroenterol. 2019;32(4):407–15. Epub 2019 Apr 13. https://doi.org/10.20524/aog.2019.0376.
14. Zeair S, Butkiewicz F, Butkiewicz J, Stasiuk R. Application of fully covered self-expandable metallic stents with and without antimigration waist versus repeated plastic biliary stent placement in management of anastomotic biliary strictures after orthotopic liver transplantation. Ann Transplant. 2017;22:719–24.
15. Alazmi W, Fogel E, Watkins J, McHenry L, Tector J, Fridell J, Mosler P, Sherman S, Lehman G. Recurrence rate of anastomotic biliary strictures in patients who have had previous successful endoscopic therapy for anastomotic narrowing after orthotopic liver transplantation. Endoscopy. 2006:38(6):571–4.
16. Albert JG, Filmann N, Elsner J, Moench C, Trojan J, Bojunga J, Sarrazin C, Friedrich-Rust M, Herrmann E, Bechstein WO, Zeuzem S, Hofmann WP. Long-term follow-up of endoscopic therapy in stenosis of the bilio-biliary anastomosis associated with orthotopic liver transplantation. Liver Transpl. 2013;19(6):586–93. https://doi.org/10.1002/lt.22643.
17. Thuluvath PJ, Pfau PR, Kimmey MB, Ginsberg GG. Biliary complications after liver transplantation: the role of endoscopy. Endoscopy. 2005;37:857–63.
18. Albert J, Finkelmeier F, Friedrich-Rust M, Kronenberger B, Trojan J, Zeuzem S, Sarrazin C. Identifying indications for percutaneous (PTC) vs. endoscopic ultrasound (EUS)- guided "Rendezvous" procedure in biliary obstruction and incomplete endoscopic retrograde cholangiography (ERC). Zeitschrift für Gastroenterologie. 2014:52(10):1157–63

44 Biliary Leaks: Role of ERCP in Post-operative Biliary Complications

Jörg G. Albert

Abbreviations

BDI	Bile duct injury
CT	Computed tomography
CBD	common bile duct
CHD	common hepatic duct
ERC	Endoscopic-retrograde cholangiography
ERCP	Endoscopic retrograde cholangiopancreatography
EUS	Endoscopic ultrasound
HIDA	Hepatobiliary iminodiacetic acid
LHD	left hepatic duct
MRCP	Magnetic resonance cholangiopancreatography
MRI	Magnetic resonance imaging
PTCD	Percutaneous transhepatic cholangiodrainage
RHD	right hepatic duct
US	Percutaneous ultrasound

44.1 Introduction

Iatrogenic bile duct injury (BDI) necessitates ERCP to establish a thorough diagnosis and—in many cases—to offer an effective treatment. Surgical interventions that might lead to BDI include cholecystectomy, liver transplantation, and partial liver resection, but also any other kind of abdominal surgeries may be involved. In the case of BDI, leaks are most common, followed by stricture formation, i.e., from ischemic healing, e.g., at the site of a biliary anastomosis or biliary suture. Secondary complications might be the formation of bile duct stones and casts. Less common is the sump syndrome, defined by reflux of intestinal contents into the surgically altered biliary tree. BDI may successfully be treated by endoscopic means: Therefore, ERCP is indicated in all patients with proven or highly suspected post-operative biliary complication. The treatment plan should be based on an interdisciplinary discussion amongst interventionalists and hepato-biliary surgeons. Other types of bile duct infringement, e.g., from trauma, are very rare and may be treated in analogy to therapy of iatrogenic BDI.

Bile duct injury occurs in about 1% of patients who undergo laparoscopic or open surgery of the gallbladder in benign disease. Thereby, complete dissection of the common bile duct may occur in less than 0.1% and postoperative leak of the biliary system in 0.5–1.5% of cases. The frequency of complications did not significantly change with the replacement of open gallbladder resection by laparoscopic technique. However, the characteristics of lesions shifted to indirect trauma and thermic injury or misplaced clips.

J. G. Albert (✉)
Hepatologie und Endokrinologie, Abteilung für Gastroenterologie, Robert-Bosch-Krankenhaus, Auerbachstraße, Stuttgart, Germany
e-mail: joerg.albert@rbk.de

M. Mutignani et al. (eds.), *Endotherapy in Biliopancreatic Diseases: ERCP Meets EUS*,
https://doi.org/10.1007/978-3-030-42569-2_44

BDI is not only associated with increased medical costs but also an increased mortality rate, which can be as high as 20% in complicated cases. In minor injury the prognosis is good, though.

Patients' presentation in post-operative biliary complications is often non-specific and symptoms may range from pruritus, fatigue, jaundice, and abdominal pain to frank cholangitis and sepsis. Cholestatic liver tests and abdominal ultrasonography can be indicative but sensitivity of ultrasonography might be as low as 60%. Persisting percutaneous drainage of bile-containing fluid from an intraoperatively placed drain, increasing CRP and bilirubin, should cause concern. Magnetic resonance imaging (MRI) together with MR-cholangiopancreatography (MRCP) has taken a central place for the evaluation of the biliary system in these patients. MRI and computed tomography (CT) are applied for visualizing fluid collections such as bilioma and may hint at strictures by revealing prestenotic bile duct dilation. Scintigraphy (e.g., hepatobiliary iminodiacetic acid (HIDA), paraisopropyl iminodiacetic acid (PIPIDA), or diisopropyl iminodiacetic acid (DISIDA)) may detect extravasation of bile flow, and cross-sectional imaging can further highlight the presence of biliary complications such as bilioma and abscess. Endoscopic ultrasound (EUS) of the biliary tract is of particular interest in order to detect intraductal stones or sludge formations. EUS may also help to drain bilioma internally or to access the bile duct system for drainage purposes.

44.2 ERCP in Bile Duct Injury

BDI is either dealt with by ERCP, PTC, or surgical re-intervention; and the selection of the optimal treatment approach is crucial for a successful outcome. Endoscopic therapy is combined with a percutaneous drainage in the case of fluid collections and/or abscess. The treatment principle is based upon reestablishing the physiological bile flow route and to optimize pressure within the bile duct system to provide outflow of fluid to the desired location and to enable healing. The human sphincter of Oddi provides a fairly steady basal pressures with superimposed forceful contractions. The normal sphincter basal pressures range from 10 to 15 mmHg with strong phasic contractions of up to 150 mmHg. ERCP allows for simple sphincterotomy in order to decrease intraductal pressure and to support drainage of the common bile duct system into the duodenum. Moreover, hydrostatic balloon dilation in combination with or without stent placement counteracts stricture formation. Both plastic straight and pigtail stents can be used. Plastic stents are removed or replaced after 2–3 months or preterm when signs of stent occlusion occur. In some suitable cases, placement of a large bore stent, i.e., fully covered self-expandable metal stent, can seal a biliary leak. Fully covered metallic stents can remain in place for a longer period of time but should be removed after 6–9 months in most cases. We chose shorter plastic stent exchange intervals for patients who need immunosuppressive medication and longer intervals when multiple stenting is applied. Recently, we adopted fully covered self-expandable metal stent placement as a valuable alternative to multiple plastic stenting in appropriate situations [1–7].

44.3 Evaluation and Subsequent Treatment of Bile Duct Injury

There have been several classification systems developed to highlight findings in BDI and to assign treatment approaches accordingly. One of the first systematic descriptions of bile duct injury is authored by H. Bismuth in 1982 [8]. This classification illustrates the location of the injury within the biliary tract and might be helpful in assessing prognosis after surgical repair. Bile duct injuries fall into four classes based on the Stewart-Way classification [9] (Fig. 44.1). Class 1 injury occurs when the CBD is mistaken for the cystic duct, but the error is recognized before CBD is divided. Class 2 injuries involve damage to CHD from clips or cautery used too close to the duct. Class 3 injury, maybe the most common type, occurs when CBD is mistaken for the cystic duct. The common duct is transected and a variable portion including the junction of the cystic and common duct is excised or removed. Class 4 BDI involves damage to the

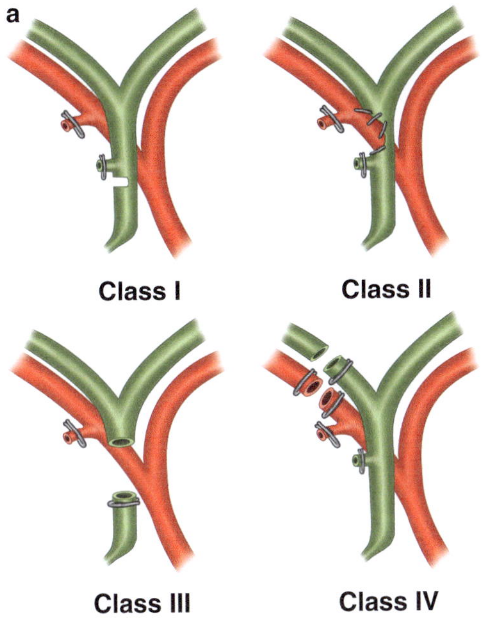

Fig. 44.1 (**a**) Stewart-Way classification of bile duct injury from laparoscopic cholecystectomy. (**b**) Strasberg types of laparoscopic bile duct injuries. Type A lesions are cystic duct leaks or leaks from small ducts in the liver bed. Type B + C injuries almost always involve aberrant right hepatic ducts with Type B denoting occlusion of a RHD and Type C denoting leakage from an RHD. Type D injuries are lateral injuries to major bile ducts. The distances in Type E1 and type E2 indicate the length of common hepatic duct remaining with E1 implying a CHD stump of >2cm, E2 signifying a CHD stump of <2cm, E3 is a hilar stricture/injury with preserved biliary confluence, E4 with involvement of the confluence, and E5 denotes an injury to an aberrant RHD and the CHD

right hepatic duct (RHD), either because this structure is mistaken for the cystic duct or because it is injured during dissection. Thus, the Stewart-Way system originates in the mechanism of the injury and origin of the lesion. Within the last two decades of the twentieth century, minimally invasive endoscopic treatment was replacing surgical repair in many indications, and laparoscopic cholecystectomy ousted open cholecystectomy in most cases. New classifications allowed for acknowledging these developments: The Amsterdam classification contemplates the treatment approach, which is successfully accomplished endoscopically in almost all type A lesions and in almost none of type D. The Strasberg classification was the first to define distinct types of laparoscopic BDI and the Neuhaus (Berlin) or Klempnauer (Hannover surgical group) classification modified Strasberg's parameters to refer to endoscopic vs. surgical treatment approaches (Figs. 44.2 and 44.3; Table 44.1) [10, 11].

In one large series, an overall success rate of 88% was achieved by tailoring percutaneous, endoscopic, and surgical approaches to the types of lesions (Table 44.2) [13]. Strasberg A bile leaks accounted for 45% of the patients with 96% managed successfully by endoscopists. In 289 patients with bile duct injuries (Strasberg B-E), a successful outcome was achieved most often for patients managed by hepatobiliary surgeons (88%) followed by endoscopists (76%) and interventional radiologists (50%) ($P < 0.05$). Overall outcomes were improved in 2004–2010 compared with 1993–2003 (78% vs. 69%). Outcomes were worse in (a) endoscopically managed patients who presented relatively late (2–6 months) and (b) patients who underwent surgery 2–4 weeks after the injury. Surgical management and stenting for 6–12 months remained significant predictors of a successful outcome in a multivariable analysis.

In patients with Roux-en-Y reconstruction, endoscopic treatment—i.e., dilation with or without stent placement—is feasible but more challenging. A conventional side-viewing duodenoscope may be less ideal to reach the bilio-enteric anastomosis. Forward-viewing endoscopes such as a pediatric colonoscope or balloon-assisted endoscopes are more apt for the task. The use of an overtube may help to maintain endoscope position before the papilla.

44.4 Other Post-operative Complications

Sump syndrome is defined by the reflux of intestinal contents into the operated biliary tree, causing recurrent cholangitis, in particular after a side-to-side choledocho-duodenostomy. Since this type of surgical interventions has been abandoned for many years now, sump syndrome is usually found in elderly people with a history of

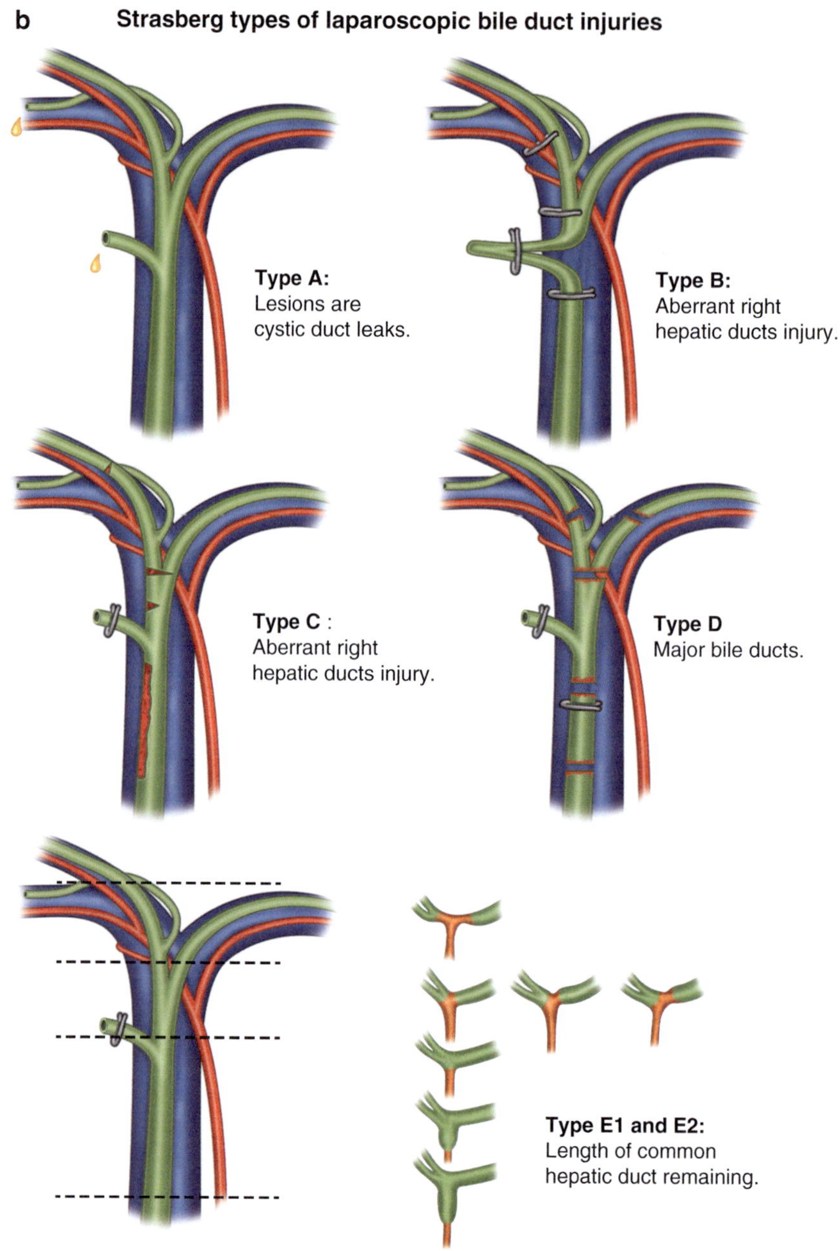

Fig. 44.1 (continued)

biliary surgery. It is characterized by recurrent ascending cholangitis due to food remnants in the poorly drained distal common bile duct. Endoscopic sphincterotomy and distal common bile duct clearance using extraction balloon or dormia basket is usually the treatment of choice.

Bilioma and/or abscess occurring together with a biliary leak may be located intrahepatically, e.g., in concomitant ischemic complications. In these cases, a combined percutaneous-endoscopic drain insertion might be necessary, cp. Chap. 28.

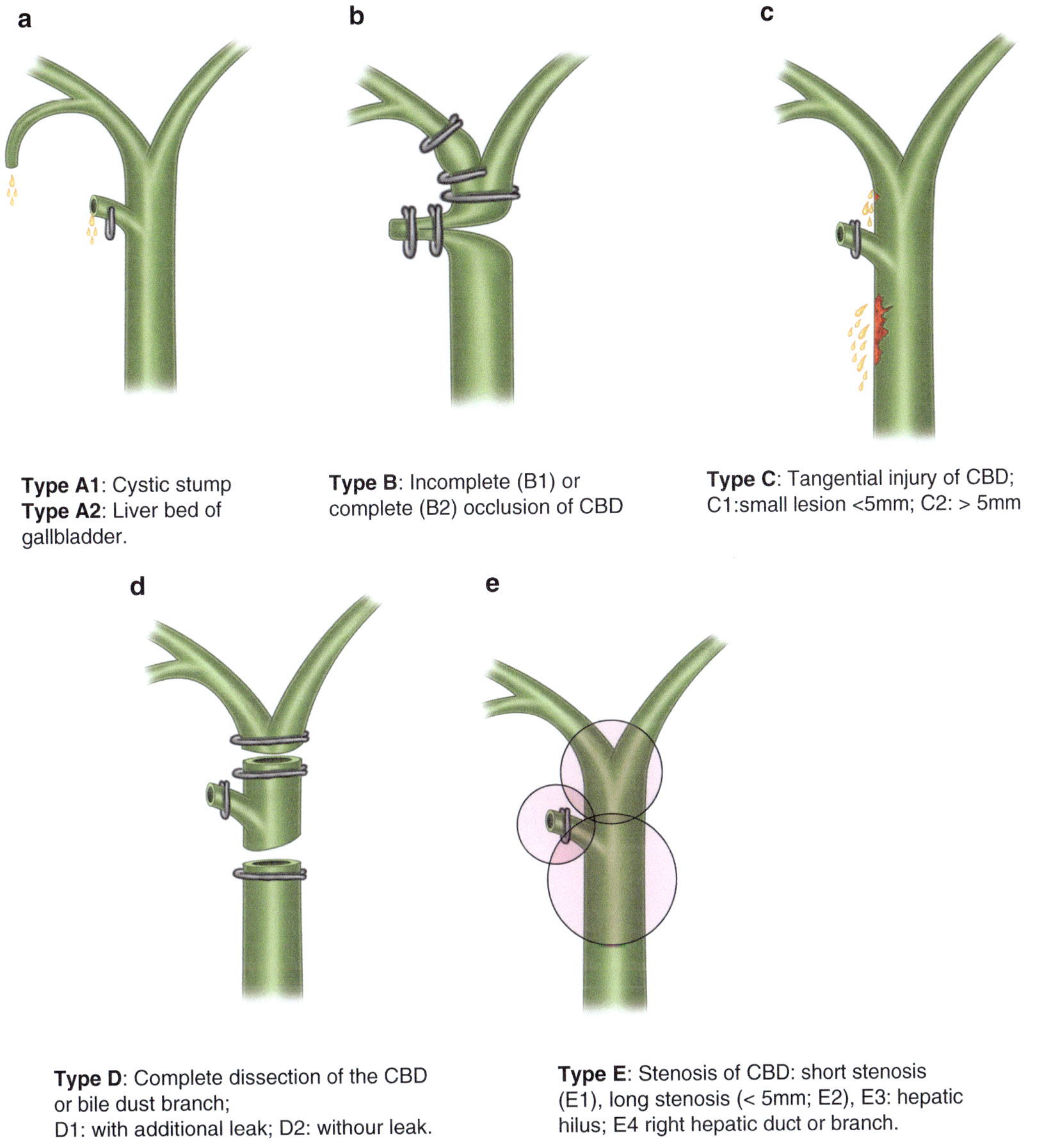

Fig. 44.2 Hannover/Berlin modification of Strasberg classification with direct deduction of treatment (Tx). Type A1: leak from cystic stump, A2: leak from the gallbladder bed. Tx: endoscopic papillotomy ± stent placement. Type B: Incomplete (B1) or complete (B2) occlusion of CBD (mostly misplaced clips). Tx for B1: Endoscopic Tx may be an option; Tx B2: removal of clip. Type C. Tangential injury of the CBD, continuity preserved. C1: small lesion <5 mm; C2: lesion >5 mm. Tx: Endoscopic papillotomy and stenting in small lesions; T-drain or saturation. New option: covered SEMS. Type D: End-to-end anastomosis, hepatojejunostomy. (D1/D2: CBD), D3: at the hepatic bifurcation, D4: above the hepatic bifurcation. Type E: Stenosis of CBD: short stenosis (E1), long stenosis (>5 mm; E2), E3: hepatic hilus; E4 right hepatic duct or branch. Tx options: endoscopic Tx in short stenosis, surgery in longer or complex stenosis

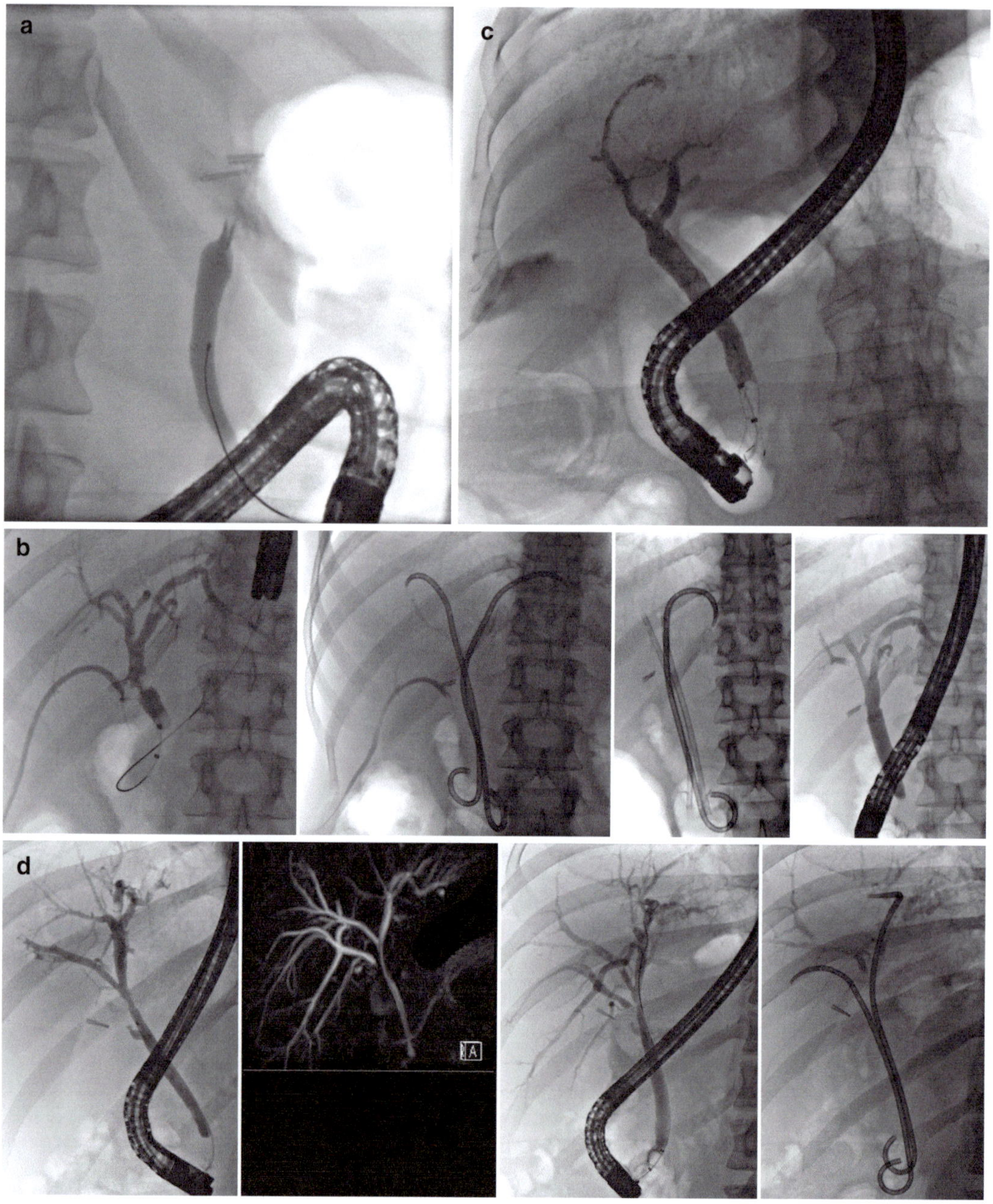

Fig. 44.3 (**a**) Type B2 post-cholecystectomy stricture (Neuhaus). Complete obstruction of CBD by misplaced clips. (**b**) Endoscopic treatment of type B1 stricture. (**c**) Folly covered, self-expanding metal stent for type C lesion. The cSEMS completely covers the lesion. (**d**) Type D lesion with complete closure of a branch of the right hepatic duct. MRCP reveals the missing segment, and endoscopic treatment is thereby realized. (**e**) Subhilar type E stenosis and multistenting with an excellent final outcome. (**f**) Type E stenosis of the distal CBD: almost 3 years after laparoscopic cholecystectomy, occlusion of the lower common bile (CBD) duct occurred in a male patient. Of note, the cystic duct inserts very low into the CBD which might have made surgery more difficult. Fibrosis due to ischemia might have caused the late stricture. Hydrostatic balloon dilation had been performed. An increasing number of plastic stents (multistenting) were used to dilate the stricture permanently

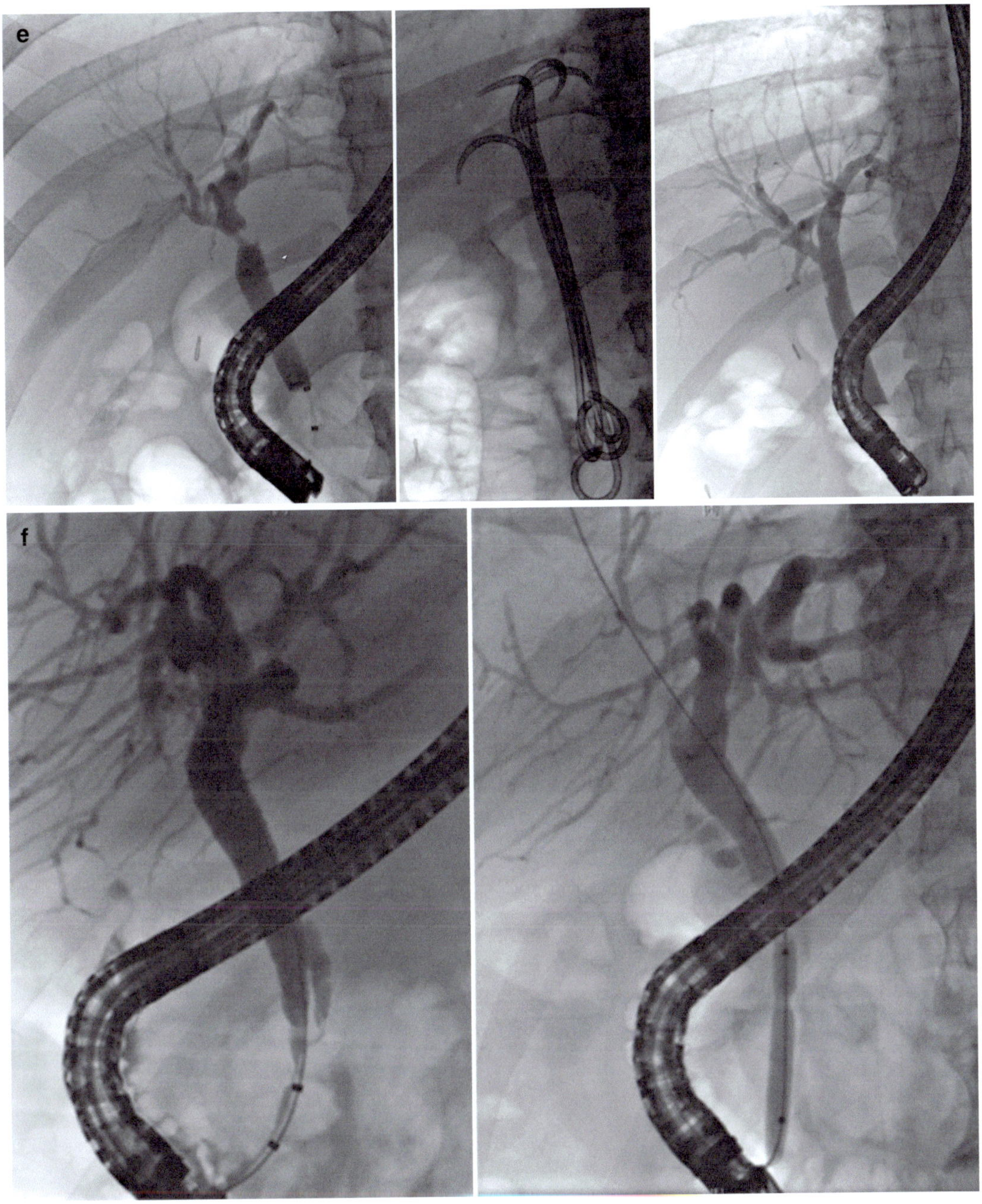

Fig. 44.3 (continued)

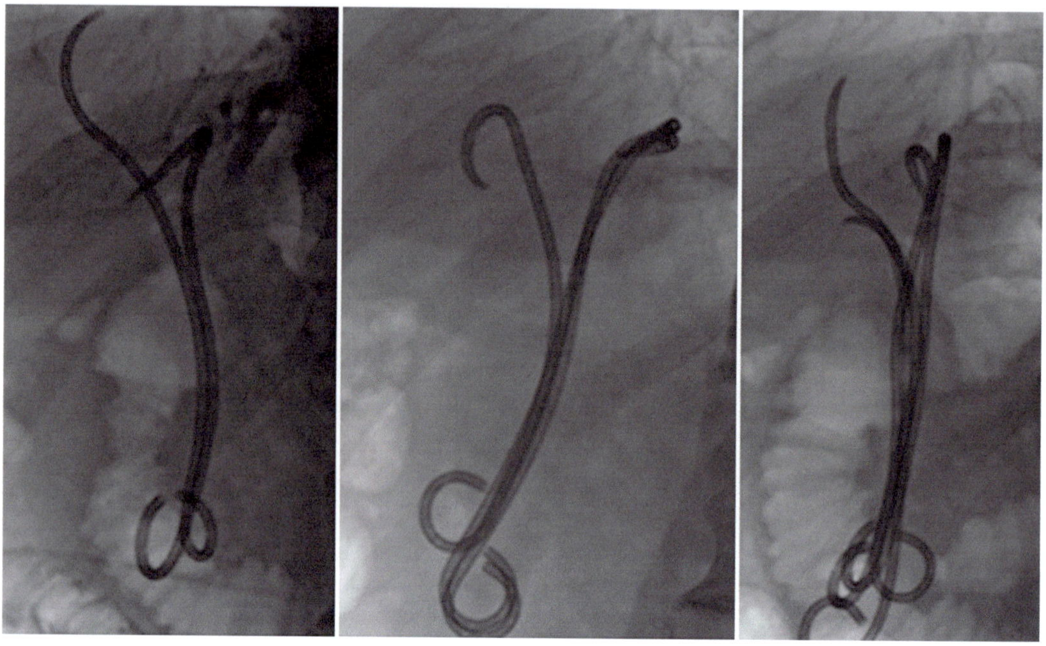

Fig. 44.3 (continued)

Table 44.1 Amsterdam Academic Medical Center classification of BDI (1996) [12]

Type	Criteria
A	Cystic duct leaks or leakage from aberrant or peripheral hepatic radicles
B	Major bile duct leaks with or without concomitant biliary strictures
C	Bile duct strictures without bile leakage
D	Complete transection of the duct with or without excision of some portion of the biliary tree

Table 44.2 Treatment approaches to different BDI types according to Strasberg [13]

Strasberg	Percutaneous	Endoscopic	Surgical	All patients
A	9	229	1	239
B	2	3	2	7
C	0	6	1	7
D	2	8	3	13
E-1	28	36	16	80
E-2	14	41	43	98
E-3	8	11	17	36
E-4	16	9	8	43
E-5	0	1	4	5
Total	79	344	105	528

44.5 Summary

In summary, a multidisciplinary team of interventional radiologists, endoscopists, and hepatobiliary surgeons is required for successfully treating BDI. If leakage is documented (sometimes requiring balloon occlusion to increase contrast hydrostatic pressure) stent therapy or sphincterotomy (or both) is recommended. Transpapillary plastic stents are usually preferred, bridging the leakage if feasible. The role of covered metal stents is promising for sealing a cystic stump leak or to treat concurrent CBD stricture and leak, but still experimental. For plastic stents, 6–8 week stenting is usually sufficient. Initial percutaneous drainage can usually be removed shortly after successful ERCP. For large defects and refractory leakage, hepato-jejunal anastomosis or other reconstructive surgery might be necessary.

References

1. Rainio M, Lindström O, Udd M, Haapamäki C, Nordin A, Kylänpää L. Endoscopic therapy of biliary injury after cholecystectomy. Dig Dis Sci. 2018;63(2):474–80. Epub 2017 Sep 25. https://doi.org/10.1007/s10620-017-4768-7.
2. Archer SB, Brown DW, Smith CD, Branum GD, Hunter JG. Bile duct injury during laparoscopic cholecystectomy: results of a national survey. Ann Surg. 2001;234(4):549–58. discussion 558-9.
3. Schmidt SC, Settmacher U, Langrehr JM, Neuhaus P. Management and outcome of patients with combined bile duct and hepatic arterial injuries after laparoscopic cholecystectomy. Surgery. 2004;135:613–8.
4. Strasberg SM, Hertl M, Soper NJ. An analysis of the problem of biliary injury during laparoscopic cholecystectomy. J Am Coll Surg. 1995;180:101–25.
5. Moreels TG. Endoscopic retrograde cholangiopancreatography in patients with altered anatomy: how to deal with the challenges ? World J Gastrointest Endosc. 2014;16:345–51.
6. Albert JG, Tal A, Bechstein WO, Trojan J, Schnitzbauer A. Three late adverse events of choledochoduodenostomy of which the endoscopist should be aware: direct retrograde cholangioscopy is helpful for diagnosis and therapy. Gastrointest Endosc. 2015;81(2):463–4. pii: S0016-5107(14)01822-7. https://doi.org/10.1016/j.gie.2014.05.324.
7. Albert JG, Finkelmeier F, Friedrich-Rust M, Kronenberger B, Trojan J, Zeuzem S, Sarrazin C. Identifying indications for percutaneous (PTC) vs. endoscopic ultrasound (EUS)-guided "rendezvous" procedure in biliary obstruction and incomplete endoscopic retrograde cholangiography (ERC). Z Gastroenterol. 2014;52(10):1157–63. Epub 2014 Oct 14. https://doi.org/10.1055/s-0034-1366629.
8. Bismuth H, Majno PE. Biliary strictures: classification based on the principles of surgical treatment. World J Surg. 2001;25:1241–4.
9. Way LW, Stewart L, Gantert W, Liu K, Lee CM, Whang K, Hunter JG. Causes and prevention of laparoscopic bile duct injuries: analysis of 252 cases from a human factors and cognitive psychology perspective. Ann Surg. 2003;237:460–9.
10. Neuhaus P, Schmidt SC, Hintze RE, Adler A, Veltzke W, Raakow R, Langrehr JM, Bechstein WO. Classification and treatment of bile duct injuries after laparoscopic cholecystectomy. Chirurg. 2000;71:166–73.
11. Bektas H, Schrem H, Winny M, Klempnauer J. Surgical treatment and outcome of iatrogenic bile duct lesions after cholecystectomy and the impact of different clinical classification systems. Br J Surg. 2007;94:1119–27.
12. Bergman JJ, van den Brink GR, Rauws EA, de Wit L, Obertop H, Huibregtse K, et al. Treatment of bile duct lesions after laparoscopic cholecystectomy. Gut. 1996;38:141–7.
13. Pitt HA, Sherman S, Johnson MS, Hollenbeck AN, Lee J, Daum MR, Lillemoe KD, Lehman GA. Improved outcomes of bile duct injuries in the 21st century. Ann Surg. 2013;258(3):490–9. https://doi.org/10.1097/SLA.0b013e3182a1b25b.

Primary Sclerosing Cholangitis

45

Christian Schäfer and Jörg G. Albert

Abbreviations

AIH	Autoimmune hepatitis
EASL	European Association for the Study of the Liver
EOC	Eosinophilic cholangitis
ERCP	Endoscopic retrograde cholangiopancreatography
ESGE	European Society of Gastrointestinal Endoscopy
IAC	IgG4-associated cholangitis
IBD	Inflammatory bowel disease
LFT	Liver function test
MRCP	Magnetic resonance cholangiopancreatography
PSC	Primary sclerosing cholangitis
UDCA	Ursodeoxycholic acid

45.1 Introduction

Primary sclerosing cholangitis (PSC) is a chronic inflammatory disease of the larger and medium-sized bile ducts with a prevalence of 6–16 cases per 100,000 in Europe and North America [1].

C. Schäfer (✉) · J. G. Albert
Abteilung für Gastroenterologie, Hepatologie und Endokrinologie, Robert-Bosch-Krankenhaus, Stuttgart, Germany
e-mail: Christian.Schaefer@rbk.de; Joerg.Albert@rbk.de

During its chronic course, this condition leads to fibrosis and strictures of the biliary tree, resulting in cholestasis, progressive cirrhosis, and hepatic failure. Median survival without liver transplantation after diagnosis ranges from 6 to 12 years [2]. In comparison to patients with cholestatic disease, asymptomatic patients have a more favorable prognosis [3].

Concomitant inflammatory bowel disease (IBD) may be found in 60–80% of all PSC patients, most often ulcerative colitis and—less frequently—Crohn's disease. Conversely, ulcerative colitis confers a risk for PSC of approximately 5 % [4, 5].

45.2 Symptoms and Diagnosis

Patients may be asymptomatic at the time of primary diagnosis, which is often made in the context of inflammatory bowel disease and abnormal liver function tests. Approximately 50% of the patients have clinical manifestations, e.g., pruritus, jaundice, and enlarged liver or spleen. Laboratory parameters show a cholestatic pattern (elevated alkaline phosphatase and bilirubin). In progressive liver disease, additional changes may occur. However, no specific laboratory parameter exists that reliably allows the diagnosis of PSC.

Thus, the primary diagnosis of PSC is based on cholangiography (ERCP or MRCP). Magnetic resonance cholangiopancreatography (MRCP) is

M. Mutignani et al. (eds.), *Endotherapy in Biliopancreatic Diseases: ERCP Meets EUS*,
https://doi.org/10.1007/978-3-030-42569-2_45

non-invasive and, therefore, the preferred method with a sensitivity of 86% and a specificity of 94% compared to ERCP or PTC [6]. ERCP might provide a higher sensitivity for detecting "early PSC" or minor ductal alterations; however therapeutic decisions are rarely influenced by these findings, and the periprocedural risks of ERCP (e.g., cholangitis or pancreatitis) are usually not justified.

In PSC, bile duct morphology is characterized by focal or extended strictures alternating with normally shaped or slightly dilated segments (Fig. 45.1). Thus, its shape reminds of a withered or gnarled tree. In most cases, both intra- and extrahepatic bile ducts are involved; isolated intrahepatic disease is observed in only 11%, and sole extrahepatic disease in 2% of all PSC patients [7]. Gallbladder abnormalities are found in a substantial portion of patients; a larger mass may be suggestive of gallbladder carcinoma requiring cholecystectomy.

Minor bile duct changes are often missed by ultrasound and CT scan, especially in early disease. CT and ultrasound, however, may show thickening of the bile duct wall or the presence of masses in some cases. In patients with suspected PSC, endoscopic ultrasound may be valuable in detecting typical changes of extrahepatic PSC, such as wall thickening (≥1.5 mm), irregular wall structure, significant changes of the caliber of the common bile duct, and perihilar lymphadenopathy [8]. In addition, EUS offers the possibility of FNA of suspicious lymph nodes or intrahepatic masses.

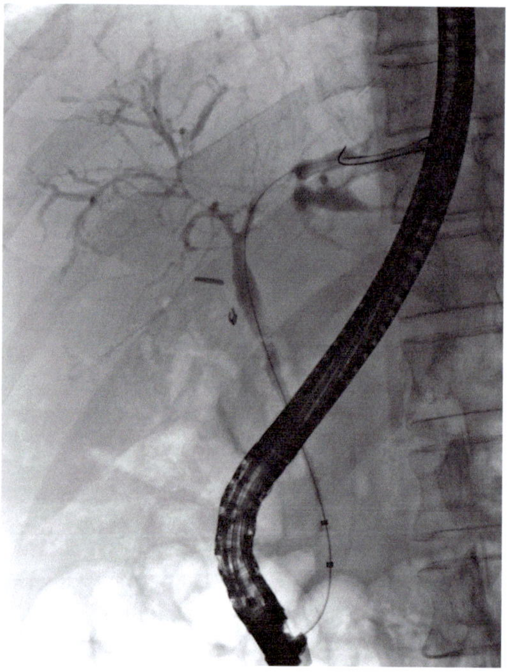

Fig. 45.1 Typical ERCP image of intra- and extrahepatic PSC: dominant stricture of the left intrahepatic duct with the guidewire in place. Diffuse sclerotic narrowing of the right intrahepatic and extrahepatic bile ducts

45.3 Variants of PSC and Differential Diagnosis

"Small duct PSC" occurs in approx. 10% of all PSC patients and is characterized by histologic changes of intrahepatic bile ducts that are confined to branches of higher degree. The diagnosis of small duct PSC might be missed by imaging modalities. Thus, histopathological examinations are required for establishing the diagnosis. Liver histology is also essential to diagnose the overlap syndrome in which both PSC and autoimmune hepatitis (AIH) are present in the same patient. PSC-AIH overlap occurs predominantly in patients of younger age.

Another bile duct disease, IgG4-associated cholangitis (IAC), might perfectly mimic PSC and usually presents with bile duct alterations similar to PSC. However, IAC is frequently associated with type 1 autoimmune pancreatitis and other IgG4-related diseases (e.g., Riedel's thyroiditis, dacryoadenitis and sialadenitis, IgG4-related aortitis, or periaortitis, tubulointerstitial nephritis, membranous glomerulonephritis). These patients show rapidly progressive liver disease (cirrhosis), but also a good response to corticosteroid treatment [9]. Diagnosis of IAC is based on HISORt criteria for IgG4-related sclerosing cholangitis, and the evaluation of a histopathological specimen is crucial to establish the diagnosis. At histopathology, IgG4-positive plasma cell infiltrates, storiform fibrosis, and obliterative phlebitis are typical for IAC. Tissue eosinophilia may also be present. For more detailed features, see Table 45.1. Raised serum

Table 45.1 Clinical and imaging differences of PSC, IAC, and eosinophilic cholangitis (EoC) [11]

	PSC	IAC	EoC
Gender, m:f	1.5:1	7:1	1:1
Age (years)	<40	>50	<40
Clinical presentation	Elevated cholestatic enzymes (AP)	Obstructive cholestasis	Cholestasis (+pain)
Serum IgG4 elevated	<20%	>70%	No
Pancreas involved	<5%	50–90%	No (?)
Multi-visceral disease	No	Yes	?
Association with IBD	80%	<10%	<10% (?)
Bile duct alterations	Generalized – Intra- and extrahepatic – Narrowing of bile ducts like a string of pearls – Picture of "defoliated tree"	DHC – Long smooth strictures – Multiple strictures – Relatively minor prestenotic dilation – Low CBD stricture	Generalized
Treatment success from steroids	Very rarely	Yes	Yes

IgG4 levels in type 1 AIP occur in approximately 60–80% of cases. However, in both type 1 autoimmune pancreatitis and IAC, serum IgG4 levels can be normal despite evidence of active disease. Presently, it remains controversial whether eosinophilic cholangitis (Fig. 45.2) represents an independent disease [10].

A broad variety of *secondary cholangiopathies* should be considered as differential diagnoses of PSC, including infectious, vascular, toxic, inflammatory, and congenital etiologies (Table 45.2).

In many of these entities, the morphologic features may not differ from PSC. Features of the patient's history, clinical course, and comorbidities may help to identify the underlying etiology.

45.4 Medical Therapy

Ursodeoxycholic acid (UDCA), used at a dose of 15 mg/kg/day, may improve liver function tests [12]. However, there is no benefit in terms of mortality or transplantation-free survival. At a higher dose (>28 mg/kg/day), UDCA was associated with an unfavorable outcome compared to placebo-treated patients [13].

The treatment of cirrhotic complications is similar to that in cirrhosis of any other etiology and shall not be considered in this review.

45.5 Role of ERCP

Endoscopic retrograde cholangiopancreatography (ERCP) may be applied in PSC for two reasons: treating symptomatic strictures and/or verifying malignancy. ERCP has a high diagnostic accuracy and allows the acquisition of biopsy material and intraductal therapy. The risk of suppurative cholangitis or ERCP-associated pancreatitis must always be weighed against the benefit of ERCP. Therefore, non-invasive clarification (e.g., MRCP together with biochemical tests) should always precede the use of ERCP.

The Amsterdam classification highlights the cholangiographic changes in PSC (Table 45.3). It was validated and shown to correlate with patient prognosis [14]. However, none of the ductographic criteria is specific for PSC, and the findings must always be interpreted in the clinical context.

Antibiotic prophylaxis is recommended for all patients with PSC undergoing ERCP (ESGE guideline; [15]).

In patients with progressive cholestasis who may not only suffer from jaundice but also from agonizing pruritus, ERCP may be warranted (Fig. 45.3). As shown by Björnsson et al. [16], a substantial percentage of these patients (45%) have a so-called "dominant stricture" defined by a diameter of ≤1.5 mm of the common bile duct,

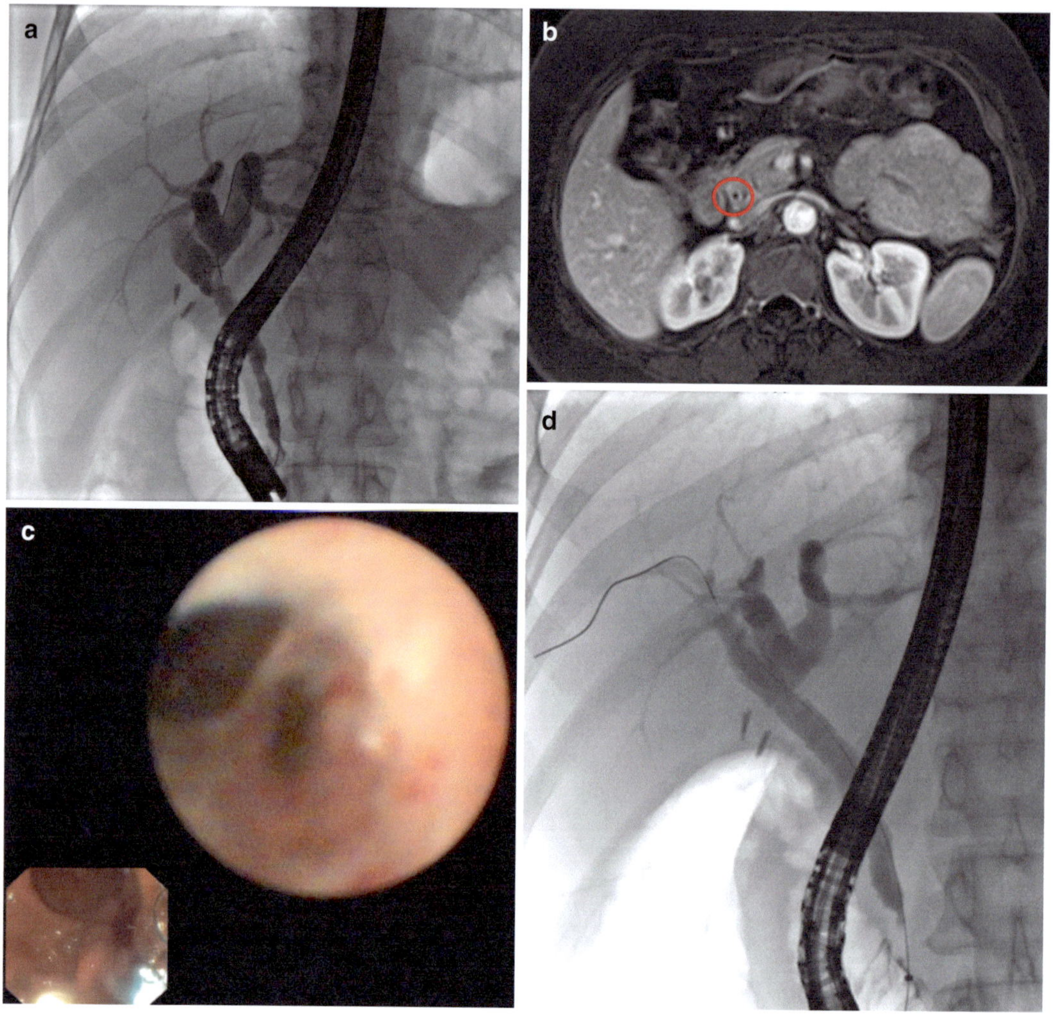

Fig 45.2 (a) 41-year old female patient with recurrent right upper quadrant pain for several years. Liver function tests showed a cholestatic pattern. ERCP indicates irregular narrowing all of the complete CBD and the hepatic hilum, with clips dating from a previous cholecystectomy. (b) At MRI, the common bile duct (CBD) shows thickening of the wall with increased uptake of contrast. (c) At cholangioscopy, diffuse sclerosing lesions of the CBD were visualized, while the intrahepatic bile ducts appeared normal. Intraductal biopsies revealed a dense infiltration of eosinophilic lymphocytes without any features of IgG4-associated cholangitis. (d) A diagnosis of eosinophilic cholangitis (EOC) was established. After 4 weeks of systemic corticosteroids, the CBD narrowing completely resolved

or ≤1.0 mm of the hepatic ducts. The question is, whether patients with such a dominant stricture may benefit from endoscopic intervention, i.e., balloon dilation and/or placement of plastic stents. This has not been evaluated by controlled trials so far. Several retrospective case series suggest that endoscopic interventions may relieve symptoms, reduce cholestasis, and contribute to a prolonged survival (Table 45.4).

The life time risk of developing cholangiocarcinoma is 10–15% [25]. Malignancy of the biliary system should be suspected, once a patient rapidly develops cholestasis, weight loss, or abdominal pain. According to a report from the large Heidelberg series [18], mainly PSC patients with concomitant inflammatory bowel disease have a significant risk of cholangiocarcinoma, and gall bladder carcinoma (as well as colorectal

Table 45.2 Classification of secondary sclerosing cholangitis and conditions that may mimic primary sclerosing cholangitis on cholangiography

Infectious	Chronic (bacterial) cholangitis
	Parasitic cholangitis
	Cholangiopathy in acquired immunodeficiencies (e.g., HIV)
Mechanical/toxic	Impacted gallstones mimicking biliary strictures
Neoplastic	Malignant conditions (cholangiocarcioma, metastases)
Ischemic	Vascular trauma
	Ischemic-type biliary lesion (ITBL) following hepatobiliary surgery or liver transplantation (e.g., hepatic artery thrombosis)
	Intra-arterial chemotherapy (e.g., transarterial chemoembolization of hepatocellular carcinoma)
	Sclerosing cholangitis in critically ill patients with biliary casts
Vascular	Portal biliopathy
Systemic inflammatory diseases	Histiocytosis
	Hypereosinophilic syndrome
	Mast cell syndrome
	Graft-versus-host disease
Congenital	Caroli's disease

Table 45.3 Amsterdam classification of cholangiographic changes in primary sclerosing cholangitis (PSC) [14]

Type	Intrahepatic	Extrahepatic
0	No visible abnormalities	No visible abnormalities
I	Multiple caliber changes; minimal dilatation	Slight irregularities of duct contour; no stricture
II	Multiple strictures; saccular dilatations, decreased arborization	Segmental strictures
III	Only central branches filled despite adequate filling pressure; severe pruning	Strictures of almost entire length of duct
IV	–	Extremely irregular margins; diverticulum-like outpouchings

cancer). In the absence of inflammatory bowel disease, no increased cancer risk was observed, even in the presence of a dominant stricture.

Despite this latter finding, any effort should be made to detect or rule out cancer as soon as possible, whenever a dominant stricture occurs. As a screening parameter, the measurement of the tumor marker CA19-9 in serum (at a cutoff at 20 U/mL) is not sensitive and non-specific and may not be recommended. A higher sensitivity level may be reached by combining CA19-9 measurements with cross-sectional imaging, i.e., ultrasound, CT, or MRI (Table 45.5). For the confirmation of the cancer diagnosis, however, methods with a higher specificity are needed. This may be achieved by transpapillary cytology brushings or forceps biopsies of suspicious strictures obtained during ERCP or by biopsies obtained during cholangioscopy. However, the sensitivity of bile duct brushings might be as low as 50% [26]. The same is true for intraductal biopsies [27]. However, newer molecular techniques may be more sensitive in visualizing cytogenetic aberrations in brush preparations, such as fluorescence in situ hybridization (FISH). In the two cited studies, combining this technique with conventional brush cytology or histology from forceps biopsies raised the specificity and sensitivity to levels above 80% [27, 28]. Whether FISH analysis proves to be broadly applicable and useful needs to be awaited.

45.6 Role of Cholangioscopy, EUS, and Intraductal Ultrasound

If the CBD diameter is large enough, cholangioscopy can be performed (e.g., using the SpyGlass System, mother-baby scopes, or in the nearest future a single-instrument cholangioscope). Apart from obtaining cytology or histology specimens, cholangioscopy may be useful in differentiating suspicious lesions from bile stones or other bile duct pathologies [29] and in performing targeted biopsies with direct visualization of the bile duct surface. However, there is no hard evidence that taking intraductal biopsies under direct visualization by cholangioscopy might improve sensitivity [30].

ESGE/EASL do not suggest routine use of endoscopic techniques other than ERCP (i.e., endoscopic ultrasound including intraductal ultrasound (IDUS), cholangioscopy, confocal endomicroscopy) [15].

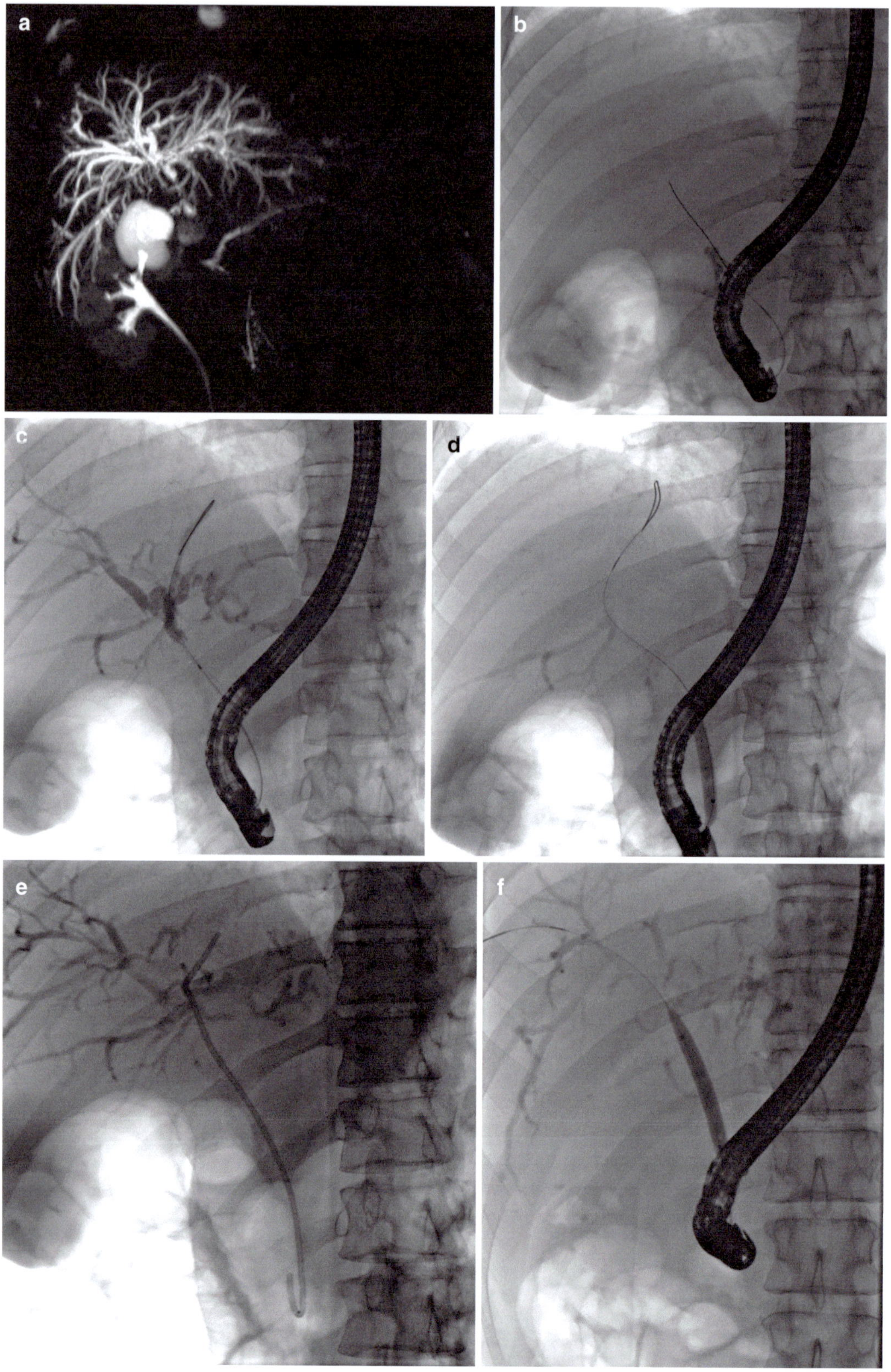
a
b
c
d
e
f

Fig. 45.3 Endoscopic treatment approach to PSC. (**a**) Non-invasive imaging: MRCP shows dilation of the intrahepatic bile ducts with a suspected stricture of the hilar region. (**b**) The guidewire "leads" at ERCP, i.e., no application of contrast into the intrahepatic bile ducts that have not been reached by the tip of the wire in order to prevent infections. (**c**) With the guidewire having passed the CBD stricture, a small amount of contrast is injected and shows diffuse stricturing of the extrahepatic bile ducts. The intrahepatic bile ducts appear normal. (**d**) Hydrostatic balloon dilation of the CBD is performed. (**e**) A plastic endoprosthesis (7 Fr) was inserted to obtain long-term drainage of the biliary system. Insertion of plastic endoprostheses has to be critically appraised in PSC because of the risk of cholangitis. However, in this case of a dominant stenosis of the CBD and absence of major intrahepatic disease, drainage by a plastic stent was performed. Plastic endoprostheses should be left no longer than four weeks. (**f**) Four weeks later, hydrostatic balloon dilation of the CBD is repeated. (**g**) Again, a plastic endoprosthesis has been placed (10 Fr), but again only for a short duration (4 weeks). (**h**) Another four weeks later, the result seems very promising. The CBD narrowing has almost completely resolved. (**i**) The gGT value rapidly decreased with the treatment

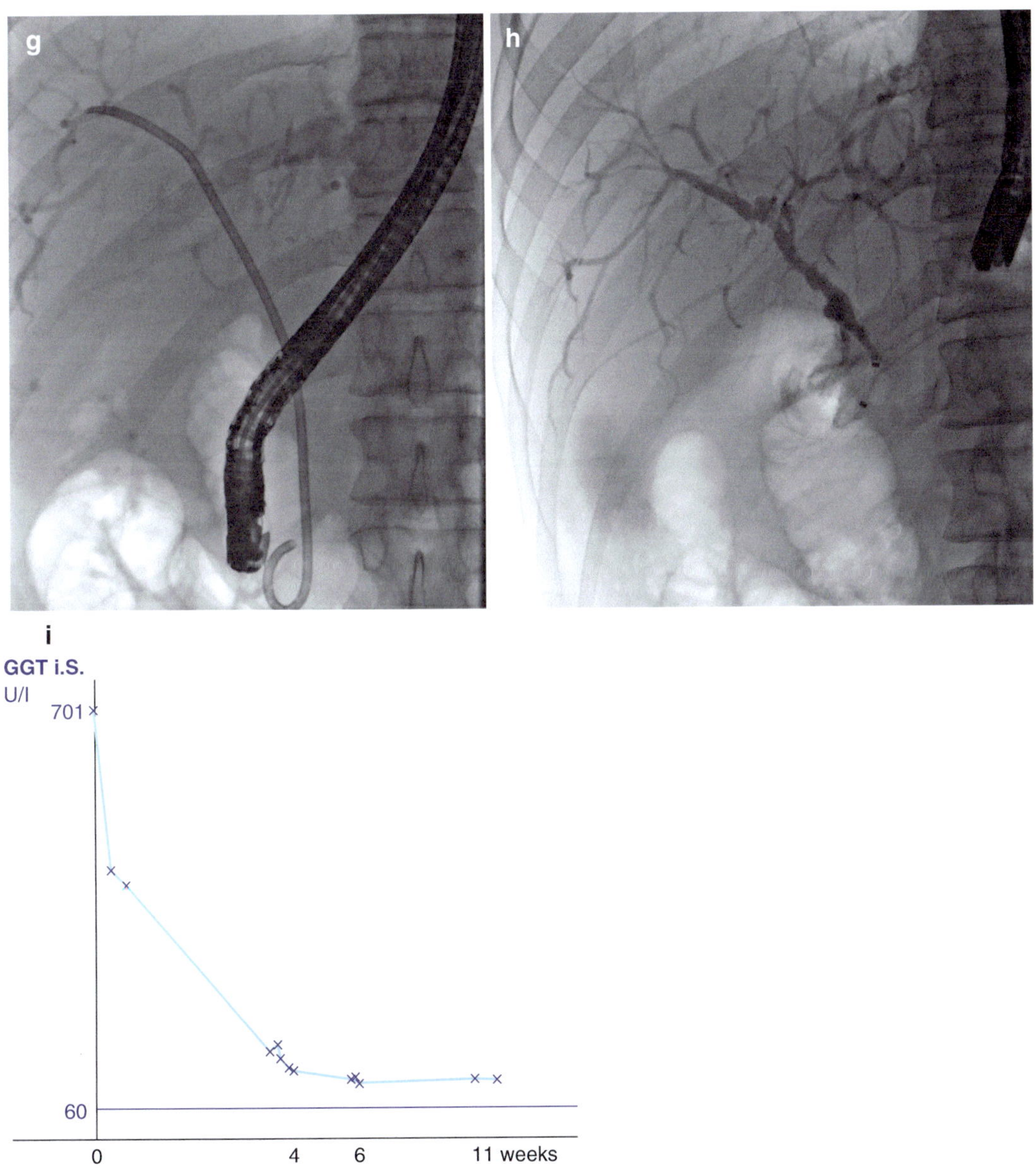

Fig. 45.3 (continued)

Table 45.4 Patient series with dominant structures

Study	Patients with dominant strictures/ total number	Intervention	Effect	Side effects
Gotthardt et al. [17] Rudolph [18]	*N* = 97/171	500 dilations 5 stents	– Improvement of pruritus and LFTs – Survival free of LTX at 5 years: 81% (at 10 years 52%)	Pancreatitis 2.2% Cholangitis 1.4% Bile duct perforation 0.2% *N* = 6 CC
May et al. [19]	*N* = 14	Dilation + stent (during ERCP or transhepatically)	– Less cholangitis, pruritus, drop in bilirubin	Postprocedural cholangitis 5/14
Chapman et al. [20]	*N* = 80/128	474 ERCPs Stent 46% Dilation 20% Dilation + stent 17%, failed: 17%	– Survival 13.7 years (patients with dominant stricture) vs. 23 years (patients without dominant stricture)	2 bile duct perforations 2 pancreatitis 1 PTD-related fistula Mild cholangitis/ pancreatitis *N* = 21 (26%) CC
Wagner et al. [21]	*N* = 12	ERCP: Dilation, nasobiliary catheter	8: effective 3: LTX 1: ineffective	None
Lee et al. [7]	*N* = 53/85	ERCP: 50 dilations, 38 stenting, 8 NB tube, 17 stone extractions	41 of 35: improvement of symptoms, LFTs, or cholangiograms	Pancreatitis *N* = 15
Ponsioen et al. [22]	*N* = 32	Stenting for 1–23 days	Symptom-free and decrease of LFTs (1 year): 80%	7 transient complications (45 ERCPs)
Baluyut et al. [23]	*N* = 63	Balloon dilation	Survival better than predicted 5-year survival	
Kaya et al. [24]	*N* = 71/1009	34 dilation 37 dilation + stent (in approx. 50% percutaneous approach)	Both groups similar in the reduction of cholastasis	More complications in stent group than in dilation group

All studies were retrospective studies. *CC* cholangiocarcinoma, *LTX* liver transplantation

Table 45.5 Role of the combination of diagnostic modalities for establishing the diagnosis of cholangiocarcinoma in PSC [28]

	Sensitivity	Specificity	PPV	NPV
CA 19-9 Cutoff 20 U/mL	78%	67%	23	96
CA 19-9 + US	91	62	23	98
CA 19-9 + CT	100	38	22	100
CA 19-9 + MRI	96	37	24	98
Subsequent cholangiograhy	91	69	42	96
Brush cytology	50	97	86	83
Aneusomy (FISH)	86	83	80	88

45.7 Surgery and Liver Transplantation

The only option that has a proven survival benefit in PSC is liver transplantation. About 25% of patients might need LTx for PSC during their lifetime [31]. LTx for PSC has similar survival rates compared to other indications, but re-transplantation rate is higher than in other indications so that 10–15% of patients need a second liver transplantation [32].

Other surgical procedures, such as bilio-enteric drainage operations, should be avoided because of significant morbidity and mortality, e.g., due to ascending cholangitis.

45.8 Conclusion

Despite improved understanding of the pathogenesis, primary sclerosing cholangitis remains a severe disease with an unfavorable prognosis. Medical therapies have no influence on the survival. ERCP plays a role as an adjunct to establish the diagnosis of malignancy in newly developed strictures and as a treatment option for symptom relief. In patients with a dominant biliary stenosis, ERCP-guided balloon dilation may reduce jaundice and agonizing pruritus. Brush cytology or biopsies obtained by cholangioscopy or ERCP may aid in the early diagnosis of cholangiocarcinoma. Patients with progressive hepatic failure need to be evaluated for liver transplantation.

References

1. Eaton JE, Talwalkar JA, Lazaridis KN, Gores GJ, Lindor KD. Pathogenesis of primary sclerosing cholangitis and advances in diagnosis and management. Gastroenterology. 2013;145:521–36.
2. Lebovics E, Palmer M, Woo J, Schaffner F. Outcome of primary sclerosing cholangitis. Analysis of long term observation of 38 patients. Arch Intern Med. 1987;147:729–31.
3. Broomé U, Olsson R, Lööf L, Bodemar G, Hultcrantz R, Danielsson A, Prytz H, Sandberg-Gertzén H, Wallerstedt S, Lindberg G. Natural history and prognostic factors in 305 Swedish patients with primary sclerosing cholangitis. Gut. 1996;38:610–5.
4. Chapman R, Fevery J, Kalloo A, Nagorney DM, Boberg KM, Shneider B, Gores GJ. Diagnosis and management of primary sclerosing cholangitis. Hepatology. 2010;51:660–78.
5. Olsson R, Danielsson A, Jarnerot G, Lindstrom E, Loof L, Rolny P, Ryden BO, Tysk C, Wallerstedt S. Prevalence of primary sclerosing cholangitis in patients with ulcerative colitis. Gastroenterology. 1991;100:1319–23.
6. Dave M, Elmunzer BJ, Dwamena BA, Higgins PD. Primary sclerosing cholangitis: meta-analysis of diagnostic performance of MR cholangiopancreatography. Radiology. 2010;256:387–96.
7. Lee JG, Schutz SM, England RE, Leung JW, Cotton PB. Endoscopic therapy of sclerosing cholangitis. Hepatology. 1995;21:661–7.
8. Lutz HH, Wasmuth HE, Streetz K, Tacke F, Koch A, Luedde T, Trautwein C, Tischendorf JJ. Endoscopic ultrasound as an early diagnostic tool for primary sclerosing cholangitis: a prospective pilot study. Endoscopy. 2012;44:934–9.
9. Björnsson E, Chari S, Silveira M, Gossard A, Takahashi N, Smyrk T, Lindor K. Primary sclerosing cholangitis associated with elevated immunoglobulin G4: clinical characteristics and response to therapy. Am J Ther. 2011;18:198–205.
10. Walter D, Peveling-Oberhag J, Schulze F, Bon D, Zeuzem S, Friedrich-Rust M, Albert JG. Intraductal biopsies in indeterminate biliary stricture: evaluation of histopathological criteria in fluoroscopy- vs. cholangioscopy guided technique. Dig Liver Dis. 2016;48:765–70.
11. Joshi D, Webster GJ. Biliary and hepatic involvement in IgG4-related disease. Aliment Pharmacol Ther. 2014;40:1251–61.
12. Triantos CK, Koukias NM, Nikolopoulou VN, Burroughs AK. Meta-analysis: ursodeoxycholic acid for primary sclerosing cholangitis. Aliment Pharmacol Ther. 2011;34:901–10.
13. Lindor KD, Kowdley KV, Luketic VA, Harrison ME, McCashland T, Befeler AS, Harnois D, Jorgensen R, Petz J, Keach J, Mooney J, Sargeant C, Braaten J, Bernard T, King D, Miceli E, Schmoll J, Hoskin T, Thapa P, Enders F. High-dose ursodeoxycholic acid for the treatment of primary sclerosing cholangitis. Hepatology. 2009;50:808–14.
14. Ponsioen CY, Reitsma JB, Boberg KM, et al. Validation of a cholangiographic prognostic model in primary sclerosing cholangitis. Endoscopy. 2010;42:742–7.
15. Aabakken L, Karlsen TH, Albert J, Arvanitakis M, Chazouilleres O, Dumonceau JM, Färkkilä M, Fickert P, Hirschfield GM, Laghi A, Marzioni M, Fernandez M, Pereira SP, Pohl J, Poley JW, Ponsioen CY, Schramm C, Swahn F, Tringali A, Hassan C. Role of endoscopy in primary sclerosing cholangitis: European Society of Gastrointestinal Endoscopy (ESGE) and European Association for the Study of the Liver (EASL) Clinical Guideline. Endoscopy. 2017;49:588–608.
16. Björnsson E, Lindqvist-Ottosson J, Asztely M, Olsson R. Dominant strictures in patients with primary sclerosing cholangitis. Am J Gastroenterol. 2004;99:502–18.
17. Gotthardt DN, Rudolph G, Klöters-Plachky P, Kulaksiz H, Stiehl A. Endoscopic dilation of dominant stenoses in primary sclerosing cholangitis: outcome after long-term treatment. Gastrointest Endosc. 2010;71:527–34.
18. Rudolph G, Gotthardt D, Kloeters-Plachky P, Rost D, Kulaksiz H, Stiehl A. In PSC with dominant bile duct stenosis, IBD is associated with an increase of carcinomas and reduced survival. J Hepatol. 2010;53:313–7.
19. May GR, Bender CE, LaRusso NF, Wiesner RH. Nonoperative dilatation of dominant strictures in

primary sclerosing cholangitis. AJR Am J Roentgenol. 1985;145:1061–4.
20. Chapman MH, Webster GJ, Bannoo S, Johnson GJ, Wittmann J, Pereira SP. Cholangiocarcinoma and dominant strictures in patients with primary sclerosing cholangitis: a 25-year single-centre experience. Eur J Gastroenterol Hepatol. 2012;24:1051–8.
21. Wagner S, Gebel M, Meier P, Trautwein C, Bleck J, Nashan B, Manns MP. Endoscopic management of biliary tract strictures in primary sclerosing cholangitis. Endoscopy. 1996;28:546–51.
22. Ponsioen CY, Lam K, van Milligen de Wit AW, Huibregtse K, Tytgat GN. Four years experience with short term stenting in primary sclerosing cholangitis. Am J Gastroenterol. 1999;94:2403–7.
23. Baluyut AR, Sherman S, Lehman GA, Hoen H, Chalasani N. Impact of endoscopic therapy on the survival of patients with primary sclerosing cholangitis. Gastrointest Endosc. 2001;53(3):308–12.
24. Kaya M, Petersen BT, Angulo P, Baron TH, Andrews JC, Gostout CJ, Lindor KD. Balloon dilation compared to stenting of dominant strictures in primary sclerosing cholangitis. Am J Gastroenterol. 2001;96:1059–66.
25. Lee YM, Kaplan MM. Primary sclerosing cholangitis. N Engl J Med. 1995;332:924–33.
26. Trikudanathan G, Navaneethan U, Njei B, Vargo JJ, Parsi MA. Diagnostic yield of bile duct brushings for cholangiocarcinoma in primary sclerosing cholangitis: a systematic review and meta-analysis. Gastrointest Endosc. 2014;79:783–9.
27. Nanda A, Brown JM, Berger SH, Lewis MM, Barr Fritcher EG, Gores GJ, Keilin SA, Woods KE, Cai Q, Willingham FF. Triple modality testing by endoscopic retrograde cholangiopancreatography for the diagnosis of cholangiocarcinoma. Therap Adv Gastroenterol. 2015;8:56–65.
28. Charatcharoenwitthaya P, Enders FB, Halling KC, Lindor KD. Utility of serum tumor markers, imaging, and biliary cytology for detecting cholangiocarcinoma in primary sclerosing cholangitis. Hepatology. 2008;48(4):1106–17.
29. Ramchandani M, Reddy DN, Gupta R, Lakhtakia S, Tandan M, Darisetty S, Sekaran A, Rao GV. Role of single-operator peroral cholangioscopy in the diagnosis of indeterminate biliary lesions: a single-center, prospective study. Gastrointest Endosc. 2011;74:511–9.
30. Walter D, Hartmann S, Herrmann E, Peveling-Oberhag J, Bechstein W, Zeuzem S, Hansmann ML, Friedrich-Rust M, Albert JG. Eosinophilic cholangitis is a potentially underdiagnosed etiology in indeterminate biliary stricture. World J Gastroenterol. 2017;23:1044–50.
31. Weismüller T, Trivedi PJ, Bergquist A, Imam M, et al. Patient age, sex, and inflammatory bowel disease phenotype associate with course of primary sclerosing cholangitis. Gastroenterology. 2017;152:1975–84.
32. Maheshwari A, Yoo HY, Thuluvath PJ. Long-term outcome of liver transplantation in patients with PSC: a comparative analysis with PBC. Am J Gastroenterol. 2004;99:538–42.

46 Acute Cholecystitis

Andrea Anderloni, Alessandro Fugazza,
Ferdinando D'Amico, and Alessandro Repici

46.1 Introduction

Acute cholecystitis (AC) is a disease frequently encountered in daily clinical practice and represents an inflammation of the gallbladder caused by obstruction of the cystic duct. The obstruction is generally related to the presence of gallstones and develops in individuals with a history of symptomatic gallstones, but there are some cases of acute cholecystitis without gallstones (acalculous acute cholecystitis, ACC).

46.2 Diagnosis

According to the Tokyo guidelines 2018, the diagnosis of AC is based on the combination of clinical, laboratory, and imaging findings [1]. Clinical signs include pain/tenderness in the right upper abdominal quadrant, fever, and positive Murphy's sign (accentuation of the pain and interruption of the inspiratory act during the subcostal palpation of the gallbladder in deep inspiration). Elevated C-reactive protein and increase of white blood cells are the most characteristic laboratory test alterations whereas thickening of the gallbladder wall and the presence of fluid collections around the gallbladder are considered the two classic imaging findings.

Ultrasonography (US) is the first-choice imaging method for the morphological diagnosis of AC (Fig. 46.1) since it is a non-invasive method widely available, simple to use, and cost-effective. Contrast-enhanced CT and MRI can be used if abdominal US does not allow a definitive diagnosis or to exclude the presence of complications.

Patients with AC may present different disease stages ranging from a mild, self-limited illness to

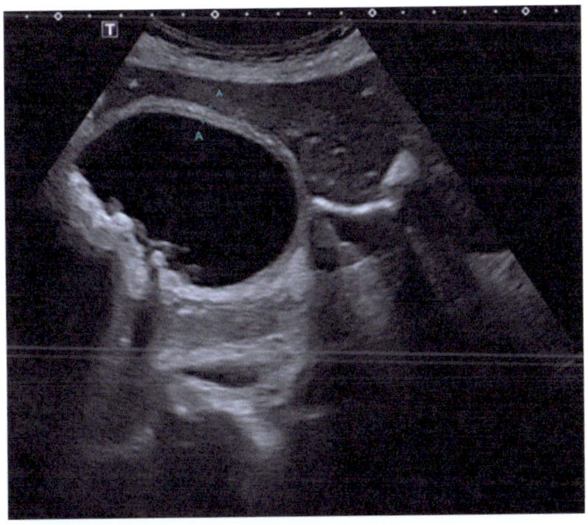

Fig. 46.1 Ultrasound image of acute cholecystitis: characteristic findings are wall thickening with hypoechoic layer, and presence of sludge and gallstones

A. Anderloni (✉) · A. Fugazza · F. D'Amico
A. Repici
Digestive Endoscopy Unit, Division
of Gastroenterology, Humanitas Research Hospital,
Rozzano, MI, Italy
e-mail: andrea.anderloni@humanitas.it

M. Mutignani et al. (eds.), *Endotherapy in Biliopancreatic Diseases: ERCP Meets EUS*,
https://doi.org/10.1007/978-3-030-42569-2_46

a fulminant and potentially life-threatening disease. Severity assessment criteria have been created, and AC is now classified into the following 3 categories: "mild (Grade I)," "moderate (Grade II)," and "severe (Grade III)" [1].

AC is defined severe if related to the presence of cardiovascular, neurological, respiratory, renal, hepatic, or hematological damage. Severe AC is a condition that affects vital prognosis, even if its mortality rate is only around 1% [2]. Patients with severe AC have a greater length of hospital stay, a greater conversion to open surgery, and higher medical costs [3, 4].

46.3 Treatment

Laparoscopic cholecystectomy is the gold standard for treatment of AC; nevertheless, therapeutic strategy should be established according to the severity of disease and general conditions of the patient.

Patients with mild and moderate AC should ideally be subjected to surgery as soon as possible. If they cannot be immediately operated, conservative treatment should be performed at first and delayed surgery considered once treatment is seen to take effect. In the case of patients with severe AC, medical therapy to support organ damage should be first applied and subsequently they should be evaluated for possible surgery. Initial medical treatment includes intravenous fluid infusion, electrolyte correction, and treatment with antimicrobials and analgesics [5].

As an alternative option to surgery, in patients considered unfit for surgery, conservative treatment and biliary drainage should be performed to control the gallbladder inflammation [5].

Therapeutic non-surgical drainage approaches are percutaneous cholecystostomy, including percutaneous transhepatic gallbladder drainage (PTGBD) and aspiration (PTGBA), transpapillary drainage of the gallbladder, and EUS-guided transmural gallbladder stent placement [6, 7].

46.4 Percutaneous Cholecystostomy

Percutaneous cholecystostomy (PC) is a widely used and established technique to perform drainage of the gallbladder. Percutaneous cholecystostomy include percutaneous transhepatic gallbladder drainage (PTGBD) and aspiration (PTGBA) without catheter placement as a simple decompression method (Figs. 46.2 and 46.3). This approach has been shown to be efficacious in approximately 90% of patients unfit for surgery and allows obtaining bile samples for microbiological and cultural analysis and to control the source of infection [8, 9]. Ultrasound is the main method for image-guided PC as it is a relatively simple technique. After ultrasound-guided puncture of the gallbladder, a guidewire is inserted into the gallbladder followed by a stent under fluoroscopic guidance. However, PC cannot be performed in patients with thrombocytopenia, coagulation disorders, and massive ascites or patients taking anticoagulants or antiplatelet drugs. Adverse events may occur in up to a quarter of patients undergoing PC, including biliary peritonitis, bleeding, pneumothorax, dislodgement, and premature tube removal. Moreover, percutaneous cholecystostomy involves the positioning of external tubes that are uncomfortable and have a negative impact on quality of life of patients [10].

46.5 Endoscopic Transpapillary Gallbladder Drainage (ETGBD)

ETGBD includes endoscopic nasogallbladder drainage (ENGBD) and gallbladder stenting (EGBS), under endoscopic retrograde cholangiopancreatography (ERCP). Drainage of the gallbladder is performed through the cystic duct with a nasobiliary tube or stent across the papilla (Fig. 46.4). ENGBD involves the successful cannulation of the main bile duct. Subsequently a

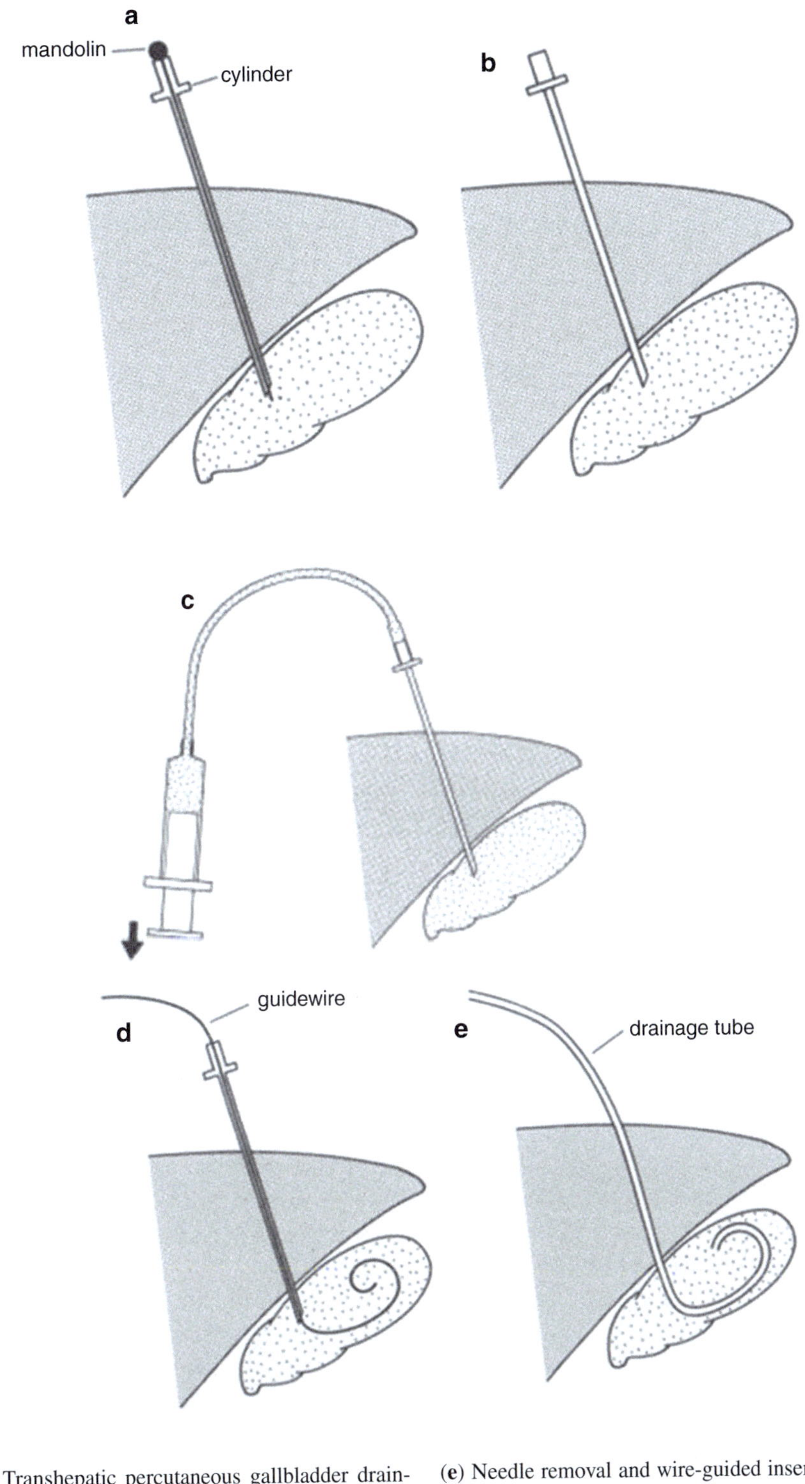

Fig. 46.2 Transhepatic percutaneous gallbladder drainage (PTGBD): (**a**) A needle with mandolin is inserted into the gallbladder through the liver. (**b**) Removal of the internal mandolin. (**c**) Aspiration of bile to verify correct positioning and perform microbiological examination of the bile. (**d**) Insertion of the guidewire inside the gallbladder. (**e**) Needle removal and wire-guided insertion of a single pigtail drainage catheter. Subsequent removal of the guidewire and fixation of the catheter to the patient's skin. (**f**) Percutaneous transhepatic gallbladder aspiration (PTGBA) [7]

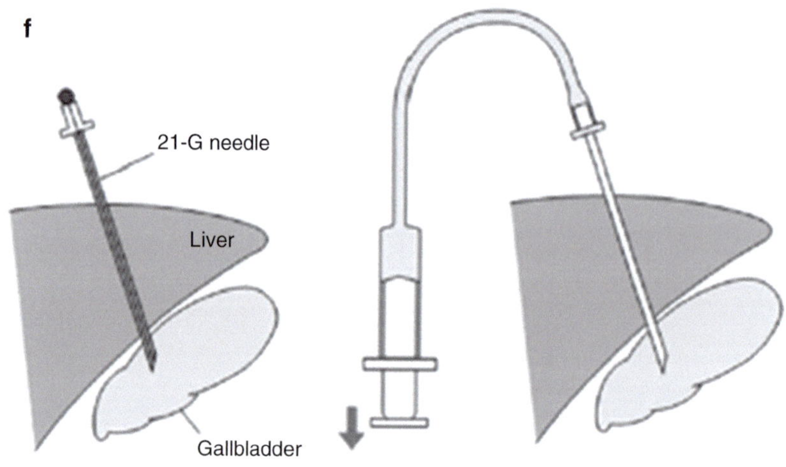

Fig. 46.2 (continued)

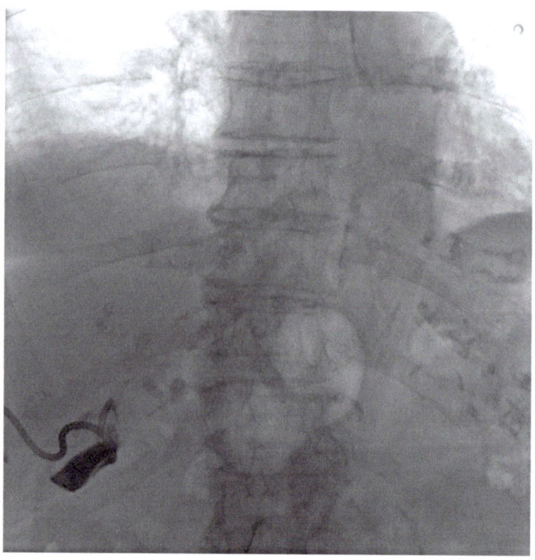

Fig. 46.3 PTGBD: Fluoroscopic image of the correct positioning of the pigtail catheter inside the gallbladder

0.025- or 0.035-in. guidewire is advanced into the cystic duct and then into the gallbladder, allowing insertion of a nasogallbladder tube into the gallbladder. EGBS is performed in the same way as ENGBD, but a double pigtail plastic stent is inserted into the gallbladder.

ETGBD appears to be suitable for patients with severe liver disease, ascites, coagulopathy, or thrombocytopenia, who cannot undergo percutaneous drainage. However, disadvantages of the transpapillary endoscopic approach are represented by anatomically inaccessible location, which does not allow selectively cannulating the cystic duct, risk of causing post-ERCP pancreatitis, and risk that plastic stents can clog, causing an exacerbation of the disease [11].

A meta-analysis that compared the two transpapillary endoscopic approach found no statistically significant difference in technical success, clinical success or adverse event rate between ENGBD and EGBS. Tokyo guidelines 2018 suggest that both ENGBD and EGBS can be considered for the gallbladder drainage and the choice of using one technique rather than another depends on the endoscopist's decision [12].

46.6 EUS-Guided Gallbladder Drainage (EUS-GBD)

Feasibility, efficacy, and safety of EUS-GBD have been recently confirmed in a systematic review and pooled analysis with overall technical success of 95.8% and a clinical success, defined as resolution of acute cholecystitis of 93.4% [13].

Different endoscopic techniques, approaches, and stents can be used to perform EUS-GBD. The gallbladder is localized by EUS from the duodenal bulb or the stomach and lack of interposing vessels are excluded using doppler flow. Both distal gastric antrum and the duodenal bulb represent good access to gallbladder. The puncture site

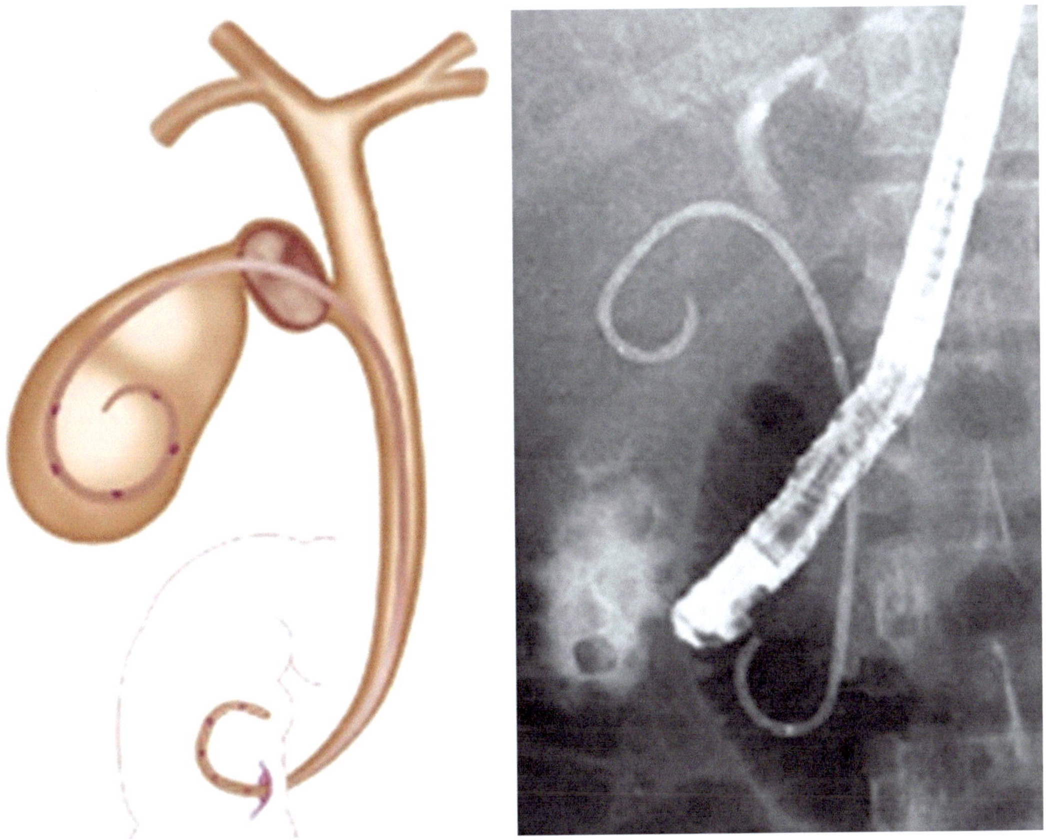

Fig. 46.4 Endoscopic transpapillary gallbladder drainage (ENGBD). Scheme of the transpapillary positioning of double pigtail biliary plastic stent into the gallbladder (left); fluoroscopic image of correct positioning (right) [7]

is usually the one in which the distance between the gastrointestinal tract and the gallbladder is lower (less than 1 cm) (Fig. 46.5).

In the past, plastic stents and self-expanding metal stent (SEMS) have been used for EUS-GBD. Since these stents were not specifically designed for EUS-GBD, adverse events such as bile leakage, stent occlusion, and migration have been described. New stents specifically designed for echoendoscopic procedures, lumen apposing metal stent (LAMS), have been recently developed to overcome these limitations [14]. LAMS are made up of braided nitinol, and they are fully covered with silicone to prevent tissue ingrowth, with wide flanges on both ends that provide anchoring and permit to avoid stent migration. More recently, the stent has been incorporated into a delivery system with an electrocautery mounted on the distal tip (Hot Axios; Boston Scientific Corp.), which allows performing the procedure in only one step, without the need for any additional exchange of accessories (Fig. 46.6).

A recent multicentric retrospective study on high-risk surgical patients with AC who underwent EUS-GBD using EC-LAMS reported technical and clinical success of 98.7% and 95.9% of cases [15]. Single-step approach reduces the time of the procedure, prevents bile leakage, and decreases radiation exposure, because unlike the multistep drainage requiring fluoroscopic control, the procedure is entirely performed under ultrasound guidance [16]. The most frequent adverse events are bleeding, uncontrolled release and migration of the stent, and recurrence of cholecystitis, related to the obstruction of LAMS. Placement of double pigtail plastic stent or SEMS trough the LAMS can be useful to avoid food impaction and ingrowth, preventing recurrences [17].

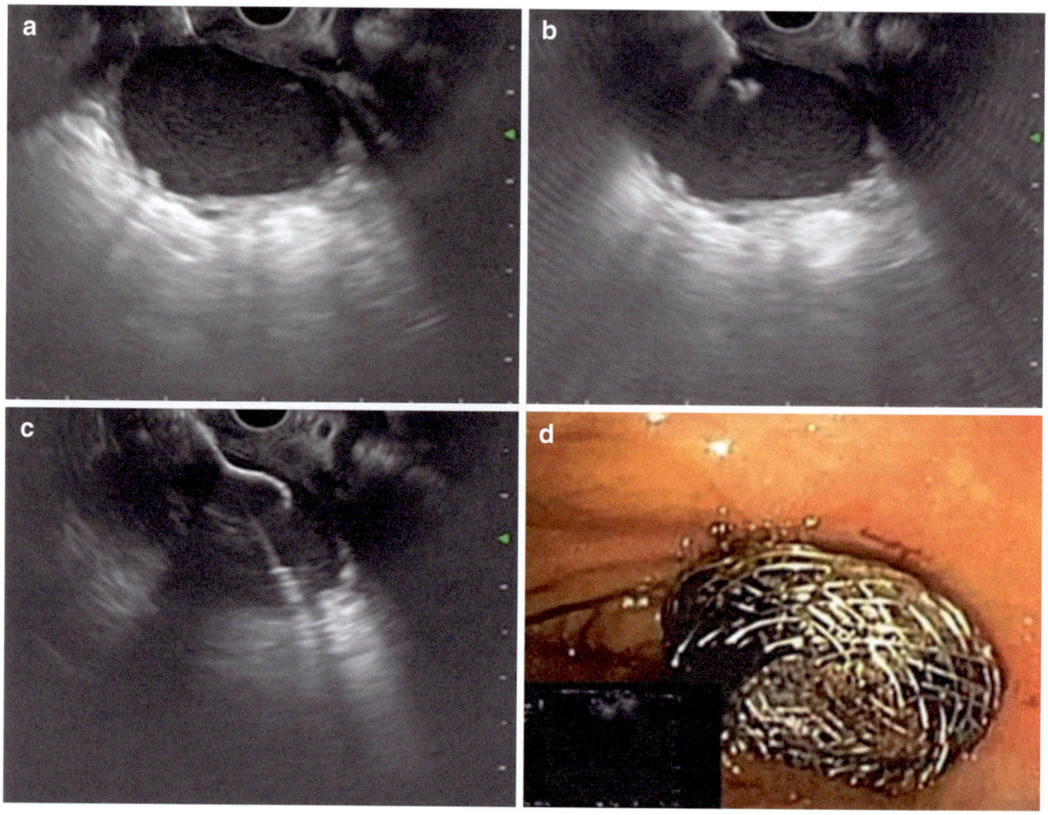

Fig. 46.5 Endoscopic ultrasound gallbladder drainage: (**a**) EUS vision of thick-walled gallbladder with sludge and biliary microcalcules. (**b**) Advancement of the LAMS inside the gallbladder by electrocautery under EUS vision. (**c**) Opening of the distal flange of the stent under EUS guidance. (**d**) Final endoscopic vision of the correct positioning of the stent

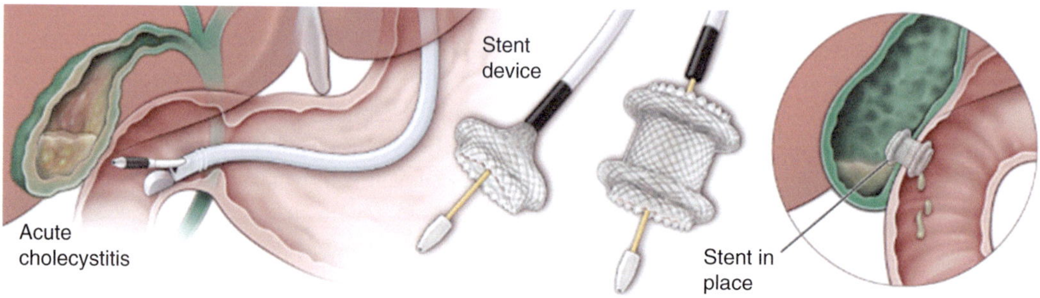

Fig. 46.6 The Hot-Axios system consists of an electrocautery device and the lumen apposing metal stent (LAMS) pre-assembled on the release system [15]

46.7 Comparison Between Non-surgical Drainage Techniques

A recent meta-analysis by O. Ahmed et al. compared the clinical outcomes of high-risk patients undergoing EUS-GBD versus percutaneous cholecystostomy for the non-surgical management of acute cholecystitis [18]. A total of five studies, including 495 patients, were selected for analysis. There were no statistically significant differences between the two groups in terms of

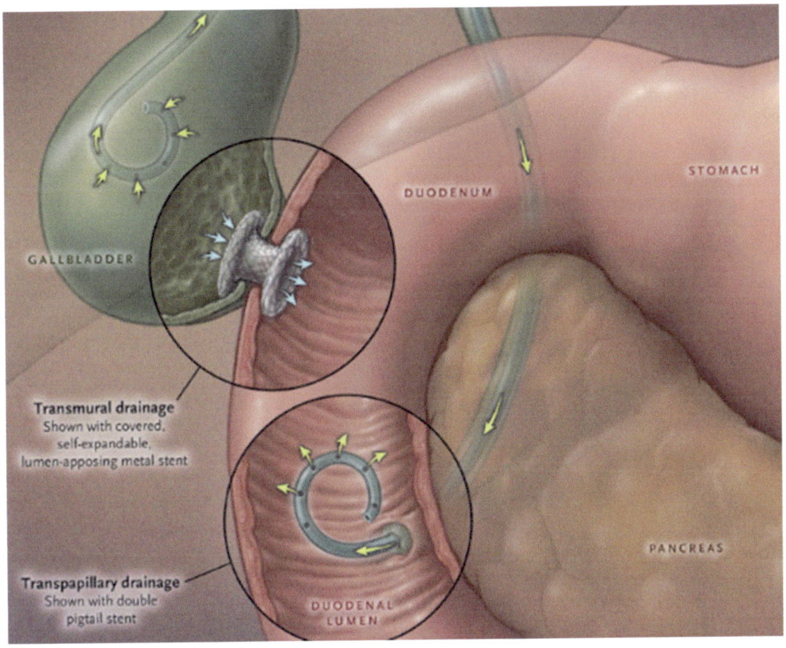

Fig. 46.7 Schematic comparison between EUS-guided gallbladder drainage by lumen apposing metal stent (LAMS) and endoscopic transpapillary gallbladder drainage (ENGBD) using a double pigtail plastic biliary stent [6]

technical and clinical success, but the pain score and re-intervention rate were significantly lower in EUS-GBD group. Moreover a multicenter, international, retrospective experience comparing percutaneous and EUS-guided gallbladder drainage showed no difference in the rate of adverse events, although the percentage of re-intervention and the length of hospital stay were smaller in patients undergoing EUS-GBD, translating into overall cost savings [19].

A retrospective comparative study between EUS-guided gallbladder drainage and endoscopic transpapillary cholecystostomy, including 172 patients, showed higher technical and clinical success rates in the EUS-guided group than in the endoscopic transpapillary group (99.3% and 99.3% vs. 86.6% and 86%, respectively, $P < 0.01$). The adverse event rate was significantly higher in the ETGBD group compared to the other (19.3% vs. 7.1%, $P = 0.02$) (Fig. 46.7) [20].

In conclusion, EUS-GBD is emerging as an attractive alternative to percutaneous drainage for the treatment of patients with AC unfit for surgery. Further prospective randomized studies are awaited to verify these results in terms of long-term outcomes and cost-effectiveness.

References

1. Yokoe M, Hata J, Takada T, Strasberg SM, Asbun HJ, Wakabayashi G, et al. Tokyo guidelines 2018: diagnostic criteria and severity grading of acute cholecystitis (with videos). J Hepatobiliary Pancreat Sci. 2018;25(1):41–54. https://doi.org/10.1002/jhbp.515.
2. Yokoe M, Takada T, Hwang TL, Endo I, Akazawa K, Miura F, et al. Descriptive review of acute cholecystitis: Japan-Taiwan collaborative epidemiological study. J Hepatobiliary Pancreat Sci. 2017;24:319–28.
3. Paul Wright G, Stilwell K, Johnson J, Hefty MT, Chung MH. Predicting length of stay and conversion to open cholecystectomy for acute cholecystitis using the 2013 Tokyo guidelines in a US population. J Hepatobiliary Pancreat Sci. 2015;22:795–801.
4. Amirthalingam V, Low JK, Woon W, Shelat V. Tokyo guidelines 2013 may be too restrictive and patients with moderate and severe acute cholecystitis can be managed by early cholecystectomy too. Surg Endosc. 2017;31:2892–900.
5. Okamoto K, Suzuki K, Takada T, Strasberg SM, Asbun HJ, Endo I, et al. Tokyo guidelines 2018: flowchart for the management of acute cholecystitis. J Hepatobiliary Pancreat Sci. 2018;25(1):55–72. https://doi.org/10.1002/jhbp.516.
6. Baron TH, Grimm IS, Swanstrom LL. Interventional approaches to gallbladder disease. N Engl J Med. 2015;373:357–65. https://doi.org/10.1056/NEJMra1411372.
7. Tsuyuguchi T, Itoi T, Takada T, Strasberg SM, Pitt HA, Kim MH, Supe AN, Mayumi T, Yoshida M, Miura F, Gomi H, Kimura Y, Higuchi R, Okamoto

K, Yamashita Y, Gabata T, Hata J, Kusachi S, Tokyo Guideline Revision Committee. TG13 indications and techniques for gallbladder drainage in acute cholecystitis (with videos). J Hepatobiliary Pancreat Sci. 2013;20(1):81–8. https://doi.org/10.1007/s00534-012-0570-2.
8. Venara A, Carretier V, Lebigot J, Lermite E. Technique and indications of percutaneous cholecystostomy in the management of cholecystitis in 2014. J Visc Surg. 2014;151:435–9.
9. Little MW, Briggs JH, Tapping CR, Bratby MJ, Anthony S, Phillips-Hughes J, Uberoi R. Percutaneous cholecystostomy: the radiologist's role in treating acute cholecystitis. Clin Radiol. 2013;68(7):654–60.
10. Jang JW, Lee SS, Song TJ, Hyun YS, Park DH, Seo DW, Lee SK, Kim MH, Yun SC. Endoscopic ultrasound-guided transmural and percutaneous transhepatic gallbladder drainage are comparable for acute cholecystitis. Gastroenterology. 2012;142:805–11.
11. Itoi T, Coelho-Prabhu N, Baron TH. Endoscopic gallbladder drainage for the management of acute cholecystitis. Gastrointest Endosc. 2010;71:1038–45.
12. Mori Y, Itoi T, Baron TH, Takada T, Strasberg SM, Pitt HA, et al. Tokyo Guidelines 2018: management strategies for gallbladder drainage in patients with acute cholecystitis (with videos). J Hepatobiliary Pancreat Sci. 2018;25:87–95. https://doi.org/10.1002/jhbp.504.
13. Anderloni A, Buda A, Vieceli F, Khashab MA, Hassan C, Repici A. Endoscopic ultrasound-guided transmural stenting for gallbladder drainage in high-risk patients with acute cholecystitis: a systematic review and pooled analysis. Surg Endosc. 2016;30:5200–8. https://doi.org/10.1007/s00464-016-4894-x.
14. Penas-Herrero I, de la Serna-Higuera C, Perez MM. Endoscopic ultrasound-guided gallbladder drainage for the management of acute cholecystitis (with video). J Hepatobiliary Pancreat Sci. 2015;22:35–43.
15. Dollhopf M, Larghi A, Will U, Rimbaş M, Anderloni A, Sanchez-Yague A, Teoh AYB, Kunda R. EUS-guided gallbladder drainage in patients with acute cholecystitis and high surgical risk using an electrocautery-enhanced lumen-apposing metal stent device. Gastrointest Endosc. 2017;86(4):636–43. Epub 2017 Mar 1. https://doi.org/10.1016/j.gie.2017.02.027.
16. Súbtil JC, Betes M, Muñoz-Navas M. Gallbladder drainage guided by endoscopic ultrasound. World J Gastrointest Endosc. 2010;2:203–9.
17. Takagi W, Ogura T, Sano T, Onda S, Okuda A, Masuda D, Imoto A, Takeuchi T, Fukunishi S, Higuchi K. EUS-guided cholecystoduodenostomy for acute cholecystitis with an anti-stent migration and anti-food impaction system; a pilot study. Therap Adv Gastroenterol. 2016;9(1):19–25. https://doi.org/10.1177/1756283X15609285.
18. Ahmed O, Rogers AC, Bolger JC, Mastrosimone A, Lee MJ, Keeling AN, Cheriyan D, Robb WB. Meta-analysis of outcomes of endoscopic ultrasound-guided gallbladder drainage versus percutaneous cholecystostomy for the management of acute cholecystitis. Surg Endosc. 2018;32(4):1627–35. Epub 2018 Feb 5. https://doi.org/10.1007/s00464-018-6041-3.
19. Tyberg A, Saumoy M, Sequeiros EV, Giovannini M, Artifon E, Teoh A, Nieto J, Desai AP, Kumta NA, Gaidhane M, Sharaiha RZ, Kahaleh M. EUS-guided versus percutaneous gallbladder drainage: Isn't it time to convert? J Clin Gastroenterol. 2018;52(1):79–84. https://doi.org/10.1097/MCG.0000000000000786.
20. Oh D, Song TJ, Cho DH, Park DH, Seo DW, Lee SK, Kim MH, Lee SS. EUS-guided cholecystostomy versus endoscopic transpapillary cholecystostomy for acute cholecystitis in high-risk surgical patients. Gastrointest Endosc. 2019;89(2):289–98. pii: S0016–5107(18)33011–6. [Epub ahead of print]. https://doi.org/10.1016/j.gie.2018.08.052.

47 Acute Pancreatitis

Andrea Tal and Jörg G. Albert

Abbreviations

ABP	Acute biliary pancreatitis
ANC	Acute necrotic collections
CT	Computed tomography
ERCP	Endoscopic retrograde cholangiopancreatography
LAM	Lumen-apposing metal stents
MRCP	Magnetic resonance cholangiopancreatography
SIRS	Systemic inflammatory response syndrome
WON	Walled-off necrosis

47.1 Introduction

Acute pancreatitis is one of the common gastroenterological conditions leading to hospitalization [1]. The worldwide burden of acute pancreatitis is rising, although incidence and aetiology varies across countries and region [2]. It can evolve to a potentially life-threatening situation with necrosis, sepsis and multiorgan failure in up to 35% of the patients facing a severe course. Different factors can lead to this local and subsequently systemic inflammatory process. Among these, alcohol, gallstones and biliary sludge play a worldwide key role accounting for up to 70–80% of all cases [1, 3, 4]. Less frequent causes of acute pancreatitis include medication, endoscopic retrograde cholangiopancreatography (ERCP), hypercalcaemia, hypertriglyceridemia, malignancies, autoimmune pancreatitis, surgery and trauma [1, 5]. Obesity as a pathophysiological co-factor of biliary pancreatitis is advancing worldwide so that the burden of gallstones will further increase [6]. Several randomised controlled trials in the past decades evaluated treatment options for acute pancreatitis, establishing endoscopy as one of the main pillars for biliary aetiology [7–9] and complications in necrotising pancreatitis [10–12].

47.2 Symptoms and Diagnosis

Patients who suffer from acute pancreatitis typically present with abdominal pain. The pain can vary in location, duration and intensity; it is often radiating to the back. Abdominal distension, jaundice and acholic faeces can be present as well as elevated temperature, nausea and diarrhoea or constipation. Rarely, periumbilical or flank hematoma can be found in severe pancre-

A. Tal (✉)
Gastroenterologic practice, IPG Hanau,
Hanau, Germany

J. G. Albert
Abteilung für Gastroenterologie, Hepatologie und Endokrinologie, Robert-Bosch-Krankenhaus,
Auerbachstraße, Stuttgart, Germany
e-mail: joerg.albert@rbk.de

M. Mutignani et al. (eds.), *Endotherapy in Biliopancreatic Diseases: ERCP Meets EUS*,
https://doi.org/10.1007/978-3-030-42569-2_47

atitis (Cullen and Grey Turner sign). In biliary pancreatitis, the pain is more often located in the right upper quadrant and epigastrium. Some patients, especially older ones, may present with jaundice and only minimal pain, though.

The diagnosis of acute pancreatitis can be established if two out of three features are present: abdominal pain consistent with acute pancreatitis, serum lipase (or amylase) activity three times greater than the upper limit of normal and characteristic findings of acute pancreatitis on contrast-enhanced computed tomography, MRI, or percutaneous ultrasound [13]. When symptoms and medical history make an acute pancreatitis probable but serum lipase is not increased (yet), imaging is needed to eliminate uncertainty (ultrasound or CT scan). In contrast to that, the yield of CT scans in several studies was low and had no implications with regard to clinical management though [14]. An early CT scan might even prolong hospital stay and protract the time to a second CT, which is needed to diagnose necrosis with possible infection.

According to the revised Atlanta classification, acute pancreatitis can be categorised as mild, moderate and severe (Fig. 47.1) [13]. This is dependent on the presence of local and systemic complications as well as transient and persistent organ failure. Local complications involve acute peripancreatic fluid collection, pancreatic pseudocyst, acute necrotic collection and walled-off necrosis whether sterile or infected [4]. Systemic complications include organ failure of one or more organs or worsening of pre-existing medical conditions (respiratory, cardiovascular, hepatic or renal).

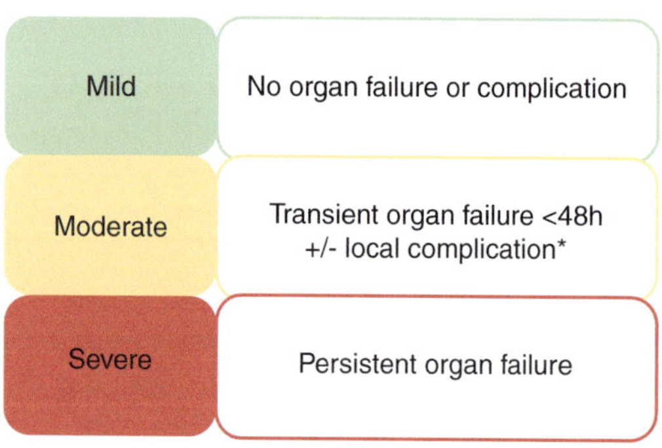

Fig. 47.1 The revised Atlanta classification for the severity of pancreatitis; * Local complications involve acute peripancreatic fluid collection, pancreatic pseudocyst, acute necrotic collection, and walled-off necrosis whether sterile or infected. Systemic complications include organ failure of one or more organs or worsening of pre-existing medical conditions (respiratory, cardiovascular, hepatic, or renal)

47.3 Scoring Systems for Severity Prediction

Various (complex) scoring systems to predict the severity and/or clinical outcome of acute pancreatitis have been proposed over the last decades. The need to identify patients with acute pancreatitis who urgently need therapy and allocation to intensive care unit demands fast, simple and overall applicable methods [15]. The Ranson score has been used for more than three decades. Since then, at least 8 additional clinical scoring systems have been developed (e.g. APACHE II, SIRS, BISAP, JSS). These scores perform with moderate accuracy in predicting persistent organ failure and seem comparable with simple tools like blood urea nitrogen, creatinine and haematocrit measurements at admission [15, 16]. With all these scores and laboratory findings, approximately 50% of the patients will be predicted a moderate to severe pancreatitis. But only a half or less of them will experience such progress [1]. In contrast to that, the patient predicted a mild pancreatitis will do so with good accuracy. Due to its simplicity and comparable accuracy, international guidelines suggest using signs of 48 h persistent systemic inflammatory response syndrome (SIRS) as a predictor for severe pancreatitis [17].

47.4 Fluid Resuscitation

Systemic and local inflammatory processes can lead to loss of fluids in the third space, causing hypovolemia, hypotension and subsequent organ failure. Great efforts in terms of randomised controlled trials have been made to evaluate the best way fluid resuscitation should be accomplished

[17]. Hydroxyethyl starch and saline might increase mortality [18, 19] whereas balanced crystalloid fluids such as Ringer's lactate are recommended by the International Association of Pancreatology (IAP) [17].

Some decades ago, fluid resuscitation for acute pancreatitis was performed in a more liberal and aggressive way until randomised control trials demonstrated potential risks. Rapid uncontrolled or too little fluid resuscitation can lead to worsening course of the disease and increased rates of infection, compartment syndrome and the need of mechanical ventilation; mortality is increased [1]. Due to the complexity of the trials, resuscitation goals and outcomes, ambigous recommendations can be found. Where the IAP suggests an early goal-directed therapy with regard to hemodynamic, clinical and laboratory parameters (e.g. heart rate, mean arterial pressure, urinary output, blood urea nitrogen, creatinine, haematocrit), other gastroenterological societies don't see any proven benefit and are therefore unwilling to give recommendations [5]. Until now, a common fluid resuscitation protocol is the administration of balanced crystalloid solution at a rate of 200–500 mL per hour, or 5–10 mL per kilogram of body weight per hour. This usually amounts in 2500–4000 mL in the first 24 h [4].

47.5 Nutrition

Historically, it was thought that an acute inflamed pancreas should be given "rest" so that a longer period without food intake was suggested. Since then, a lot has been learned through randomised trials and this dogma has changed since then. Nutrition is considered an important factor that may impact clinical outcomes in critically ill patients. Several randomised trials addressed this topic in patients experiencing acute pancreatitis [20, 21]. Enteral nutrition seems to be beneficial administered in either way (oral intake, via nasogastral or nasoduodenal tube) compared to parenteral nutrition [22]. The latter may even increase sepsis rates, infection of necrosis and mortality. However, one must be aware of aspiration risks in gastroparesis and retention stomach as these may request for a gastroduodenal tube. Based on actual data, tube feeding in predicted severe pancreatitis can be limited to those patients who have insufficient oral caloric intake after 3–5 days. An earlier (<24 h) enteral nutrition seems to have no additional benefits so far [21, 23–26]. Patients with predicted mild pancreatitis should be given a soft or solid diet as it is associated with shorter hospital stays than is a clear-liquid diet [27]. A big meta-analysis including 20 RCTs concluded that there is no specific type of enteral nutrition or immuno-nutrition that improves the outcome in acute pancreatitis [28], but when Patients are able to eat on their own, they should be offered a normal to light-fat diet. If an additional parenteral supplement is beneficial in patients with acute pancreatitis who don't achieve their energy goals remains unanswered but seems to apply for critically ill patients [29].

47.6 Role of ERCP in Biliary Pancreatitis

Temporary or permanent bile duct stone impaction within the sphincter of oddi or the common channel may cause an alteration in intrapancreatic duct pressure and subsequent activation of pancreatic digestive enzymes triggering biliary pancreatitis [30]. This is mostly caused by common bile duct stones. Whether an early ERCP with stone extraction and sphincterotomy is beneficial or not has been under investigation for almost 25 years now [7].

In patients with suspected acute biliary pancreatitis but without obstructive jaundice, early ERCP and sphincterotomy were associated with more severe adverse events and more frequent respiratory failure [8]. In case that the presence of stones remains unclear in patients with acute biliary pancreatitis, EUS is a good tool to select the patients who are bound for therapeutic ERCP [31, 32]. The diagnostic value of EUS seems to be somewhat higher than MRCP for choledocholithiasis, but MRCP may be an effective, noninvasive modality to detect CBD stones in ABP and can also help in identifying patients who require ERCP [33].

When no signs of cholangitis are present, early endoscopic intervention seems not to improve the outcome in patients with acute gallstone pancreatitis and biliopancreatic obstruction [34].

All these findings result in disapproving of early ERCP in predicted mild biliary pancreatitis in all current guidelines, reviews and meta-analysis [1, 4, 5, 9, 17].

However, consensus is lacking regarding the role of early ERCP in predicted severe ABP. Where some meta-analyses conclude that an early ERCP in severe ABP can reduce mortality and morbidity [35–37], more recent ones see no benefit [38, 39]. There is no evidence that early routine ERCP significantly affects mortality or local/systemic complications, regardless of the predicted severity of biliary pancreatitis, up to date even though a big randomised trial is ongoing [40]. This controversy may reflect the necessity for better prediction markers and scores as there are still a high number of false positive results in predicting severe course of pancreatitis. Even though the incongruent data, routine early ERCP in predicted severe ABP is recommended by most guidelines for acute pancreatitis.

There is consensus in all guidelines and meta-analyses that an endoscopic intervention, whether ERCP or endosonography, is clearly indicated in patients with cholangitis and/or signs of cholestasis. The diagnosis of cholangitis is therefore a cornerstone for clinical decision in ABP but remains challenging. Signs of cholangitis included the Charcot's triad (right upper quadrant abdominal pain, jaundice, and fever), leucocytosis and the presence of Reynold's pentad (Charcot's triad plus mental confusion and septic shock). The unquestionable clinical definition of cholangitis may be ambiguous and comparability of clinical trials, and their indication for the treatment of ABP is difficult—especially as a severe pancreatitis can mimic SIRS itself [30].

All the knowledge of ERCP indication in biliary pancreatitis has not changed the outcome of patients with ABP yet. It may be due to the fact that an intervention could potentially cause further pancreatic injury or does not always eliminate the pancreatic duct obstruction [41].

47.7 Antibiotic Therapy

In patients with cholangitis, antibiotics for empiric therapy have to be adapted to the local resistance patterns of each hospital, the severity of the cholangitis and patients' medical history (e.g. colonisation with multi-resistant bacteria, immunosuppression). Bile fluid contains a polymicrobial flora (E. coli spp., klebsiella spp., pseudomonas spp., staphylococcus spp. e.g.) so that broad spectrum antibiotics are needed for initial therapy in patients with cholangitis [2, 42].

Necrotising pancreatitis develops in 15–20% of all pancreatitis patients. Of these, 30% develop infected necrosis with high mortality rates driven by sepsis and multiorgan failure [1, 4]. Several trials tried to overcome this complication by prophylactic antibiotic therapy but failed to do so [43–48]. Nevertheless, the use of prophylactic antibiotics significantly reduced the incidence of extrapancreatic infections (lungs, urinary tract, and bloodstream) in one trial. In a Cochrane meta-analysis, a reduction in pancreatic infection in the subgroup of patients who received imipenem was seen. This may be due to the fact that carbapenem antibiotics can achieve a high pancreatic tissue concentration compared to many other substances [49]. Currently, antibiotics are only recommended for cholangitis, proven or suspected infected necrosis by all existing guidelines. If infected necrosis is suspected or proven, it is important to start a calculated antibiotic therapy. Different studies, mostly of low quality and retrospective, tried to address this issue. The best way for switching to a targeted therapy seems to be microbiological workup of specimen obtained by biopsies, necrosectomy or blood culture. The most frequently found microbes in peripancreatic fluids and necrosis are enterococci, enterobacteriaceae and fungi [50, 51].

As superinfection is thought to be triggered by bacterial translocation from the bowel, few studies investigated the role of probiotics in acute pancreatitis, showing increased rates of mesenteric ischemia and mortality. Probiotics are contraindicated in acute (severe and mild) pancreatitis [1, 4, 5, 17].

47.8 Cholecystectomy and Prevention of Relapse

Cholecystectomy can prevent recurrent biliary pancreatitis. Relapse risk for ABP when surgery is delayed ranges around 30% [52, 53]. One study could show that cholecystectomy during Index Admission lowers 30-day readmission rates [54]. Therefore, several guidelines recommend cholecystectomy during the initial admission rather than after discharge in patients with mild acute biliary pancreatitis. It seems that patients who underwent early cholecystectomy after severe pancreatitis with existing peripancreatic fluid collections or pseudocysts have an increased incidence of infected collections. In those patients, cholecystectomy should be delayed beyond 6 weeks, at which time pseudocyst drainage can safely be combined with cholecystectomy [55]. Cholecystectomy is advised for every fit patient who experienced ABP and endoscopic sphincterotomy as gallstone-related gallbladder disease has to be handled [5]. For patients who are not fit for surgery, endoscopic biliary sphincterotomy will reduce the risk of recurrent biliary pancreatitis but may not reduce the risk of subsequent acute cholecystitis and biliary colic [4].

After a first episode of acute pancreatitis, around 10% will develop chronic pancreatitis and 36% of patients after recurrent pancreatitis. The risks of recurrence and transition to chronic pancreatitis is much higher among smokers, alcoholics and men [56]. Therefore, it is crucial to encourage the patients to be abstinent. Pancreatic dysfunction (exocrine and endocrine) develops in 20–30% of patients. Factors for the transition to recurrent attacks and chronic pancreatitis include the severity of the initial attack, the degree of pancreatic necrosis and the cause of acute pancreatitis [57, 58].

47.9 Necrosectomy and Peripancreatic Fluid Collections

According to the Revised Atlanta classification [58], pancreatitis can be divided into interstitial oedematous and necrotising pancreatitis. The time of appearance and the persistence of fluid collections play an important role in therapeutic management. Interstitial oedematous pancreatitis can cause acute fluid collections at the early phase (<4 weeks) and may result in pancreatic pseudocyst formation (>4 weeks). Correspondently, necrotising pancreatitis can develop acute necrotic collections (ANC) (<4 weeks) and develop into walled-off necrosis (WON) (>4 weeks).

The treatment paradigms for walled-off necrosis (WON) have undergone extensive transitions over the past decades: from open surgical debridement to endoscopic minimally invasive treatment [10, 59]. Based on high-quality trials, interdisciplinary step-up algorithms have been proposed lately and represent the actual standard of care [11, 60] (Fig. 47.2). There is consensus all over the world that an endoscopic approach should be delayed at least 4–6 weeks after the presentation of the first fluid collection so that both necrosis and pseudocyst are allowed to develop a stable “wall”. If an endoscopic approach is better than a minimally invasive surgical, one cannot be unequivocally answered by the present knowledge, although the endoscopic step-up approach seems to have less rates of pancreatic fistulas and shorter length of hospital stay [11]. This might steer the standard of care practice towards endoscopy.

As a first step, an infected necrosis has to be drained either endoscopically or by percutaneous drainage. The latter can be established under ultrasound or CT guidance. The endoscopic approach should be performed via EUS-guided puncture of WON followed by balloon dilation of the access site under guide-wire guidance or by use of a cystotome [60]. Either plastic stents or lumen-apposing metal stents (LAM) can be used to keep the access, but long-term data on LAM are still sparse. Up to now, no recommendation for a specific stent type has been implemented in guidelines, but it seems that LAM are safe and effective [61–63]. Whether LAM can reduce the need for endoscopic necrosectomy remains to be answered. As a next step, nasocystic catheters can be placed for irrigation and might help to resolve necrosis. A concurrent endoscopic transmural drainage with percutaneous drainage should be

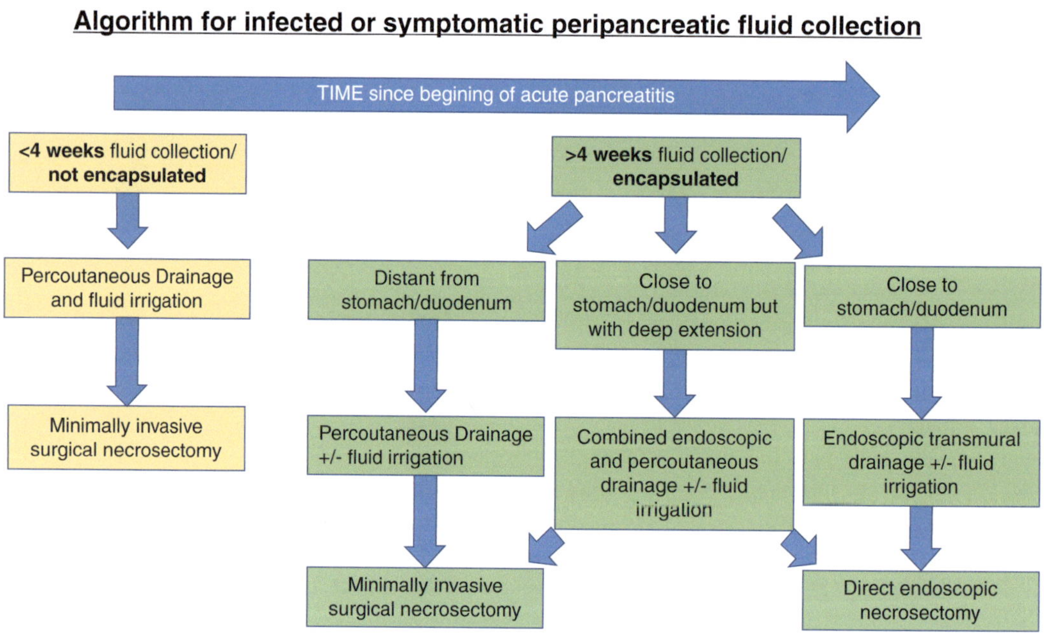

Fig. 47.2 Practical algorithm for the management of peripancreatic fluids dependent on the time since first appearance

considered in patients with walled-off necrosis extending to the pelvic para-colic gutters (combined approach).

If the first step of the therapy (drainage+/− nasocystic catheter) does not lead to clinical improvement or even shows deterioration, a CT scan should be performed. If WON is not sufficiently drained, additional drainage is needed. Otherwise, the next step is direct endoscopic necrosectomy or minimally invasive surgical debridement. Endoscopic necrosectomy is performed by a combination of suction, irrigation and mechanical removal of debris. This can be done with normal gastroscopes but always by using CO_2 insufflation as there is a significant risk for air embolism otherwise [60]. The instruments optimally used for necrosectomy (e.g. snares, Dormia basket) remain at the discretion of the endoscopist. Endoscopic necrosectomy is not free of risks. In a meta-analysis, this treatment option showed bleeding, perforation and pancreatic fistulas as the most frequent adverse events [64].

The main indication for endoscopic intervention in necrotising pancreatitis is infection of necrosis, either clinically or radiologically suspected/proven. Other possible indications are: ongoing organ failure for several weeks, ongoing gastric outlet obstruction, intestinal or biliary obstruction due to mass effect of walled-off necrosis. Moreover, disconnected pancreatic duct syndrome with ongoing symptoms would be an indication for intervention [17].

47.10 Conclusion

Acute pancreatitis is a rising clinical problem all over the world. Several scientists and clinicians have been trying to identify the optimal treatment for acute pancreatitis. Based on these advances, the management of acute (biliary) pancreatitis has changed in the past years, although many questions remain. Up to now, no effective therapeutic strategy has been developed to stop the inflammatory cascade which leads to multi-organ failure and consecutive death in patients suffering from acute pancreatitis. Further studies, many more years and brilliant scientists will be needed to find a solution for all those remaining questions. Until then, our main effort should be the implementation and dissemination of evidence-based approaches without being reluctant to overcome old paradigms.

Key Points

- Biliary obstruction is the most frequent reason for pancreatitis and amongst the most frequent gastroenterological emergencies worldwide.
- Biliary obstruction should be excluded/proven within hours of admission.
- ERCP is the best option for patient with cholangitis, ongoing biliary obstruction, and severe predicted biliary pancreatitis.
- The observance of current guidelines and evidence-based recommendations is mandatory for improving the outcome of the patient.
- Prophylactic antibiotic therapy and early CT scans are not recommended.
- Minimally invasive, endoscopic-based, and percutaneous step-up approaches are nowadays standard of care for the treatment of complications of necrotising pancreatitis.

References

1. van Dijk SM, Hallensleben NDL, van Santvoort HC, Fockens P, van Goor H, Bruno MJ, et al. Acute pancreatitis: recent advances through randomised trials. Gut. 2017;66(11):2024–32.
2. Alves JR, Silva Rdo C, SCP G, Freitas TT, Souza DL, Amico EC. Microbiological analysis of bile in patients with benign and malignant biliopancreatic diseases and its consequences. Arq Gastroenterol. 2016;53(3):156–62. http://www.scielo.br/scielo.php?script=sci_arttext&pid=S0004-28032016000300156&lng=en&tlng=en.
3. Roberts SE, Morrison-Rees S, John A, Williams JG, Brown TH, Samuel DG. The incidence and aetiology of acute pancreatitis across Europe. Pancreatology. 2017;17(2):155–65. http://www.ncbi.nlm.nih.gov/pubmed/28159463.
4. Forsmark CE, Swaroop Vege S, Wilcox CM. Acute pancreatitis. N Engl J Med. 2016;375(20):1972–81. https://doi.org/10.1056/NEJMra1505202.
5. Crockett SD, Wani S, Gardner TB, Falck-Ytter Y, Barkun AN, Crockett S, et al. American Gastroenterological Association Institute guideline on initial management of acute pancreatitis. Gastroenterology. 2018;154(4):1096–101.
6. Seidell JC, Halberstadt J. The global burden of obesity and the challenges of prevention. Ann Nutr Metab. 2015;66(Suppl 2):7–12. http://www.ncbi.nlm.nih.gov/pubmed/26045323.
7. Fan ST, Lai EC, Mok FP, Lo CM, Zheng SS, Wong J. Early treatment of acute biliary pancreatitis by endoscopic papillotomy. N Engl J Med. 1993;328(4):228–32.
8. Fölsch UR, Nitsche R, Lüdtke R, Hilgers RA, Creutzfeldt W. Early ERCP and papillotomy compared with conservative treatment for acute biliary pancreatitis. The German study group on acute biliary pancreatitis. N Engl J Med. 1997;336(4):237–42.
9. van Geenen E-JM, van Santvoort HC, Besselink MGH, van der Peet DL, van Erpecum KJ, Fockens P, et al. Lack of consensus on the role of endoscopic retrograde cholangiography in acute biliary pancreatitis in published meta-analyses and guidelines. Pancreas. 2013;42(5):774–80. http://content.wkhealth.com/linkback/openurl?sid=WKPTLP:landingpage&an=00006676-201307000-00004.
10. Seifert H, Wehrmann T, Schmitt T, Zeuzem S, Caspary WF. Retroperitoneal endoscopic debridement for infected peripancreatic necrosis. Lancet (London, England). 2000;356(9230):653–5. http://www.ncbi.nlm.nih.gov/pubmed/10968442.
11. van Brunschot S, van Grinsven J, van Santvoort HC, Bakker OJ, Besselink MG, Boermeester MA, et al. Endoscopic or surgical step-up approach for infected necrotising pancreatitis: a multicentre randomised trial. Lancet (London, England). 2018;391(10115):51–8. http://www.ncbi.nlm.nih.gov/pubmed/29108721.
12. Trikudanathan G, Attam R, Arain MA, Mallery S, Freeman ML. Endoscopic interventions for necrotizing pancreatitis. Am J Gastroenterol. 2014;109(7):969–81; quiz 982. http://www.ncbi.nlm.nih.gov/pubmed/24957157.
13. Banks PA, Bollen TL, Dervenis C, Gooszen HG, Johnson CD, Sarr MG, et al. Classification of acute pancreatitis--2012: revision of the Atlanta classification and definitions by international consensus. Gut. 2013;62(1):102–11.
14. Spanier BWM, Nio Y, van der Hulst RWM, Tuynman HARE, Dijkgraaf MGW, Bruno MJ. Practice and yield of early CT scan in acute pancreatitis: a Dutch observational multicenter study. Pancreatology. 2010;10(2–3):222–8.
15. Mounzer R, Langmead CJ, Wu BU, Evans AC, Bishehsari F, Muddana V, et al. Comparison of existing clinical scoring systems to predict persistent organ failure in patients with acute pancreatitis. Gastroenterology. 2012;142(7):1476–82; quiz e15–6.
16. Koutroumpakis E, Wu BU, Bakker OJ, Dudekula A, Singh VK, Besselink MG, et al. Admission hematocrit and rise in blood urea nitrogen at 24 h outperform other laboratory markers in predicting persistent organ failure and pancreatic necrosis in acute pancreatitis: a post hoc analysis of three large prospective databases. Am J Gastroenterol. 2015;110(12):1707–16.
17. Working Group IAP/APA Acute Pancreatitis Guidelines. IAP/APA evidence-based guidelines for the management of acute pancreatitis. Pancreatology. 2013;13(4):e1–15. http://linkinghub.elsevier.com/retrieve/pii/S1424390313005255.

18. Annane D. Effects of fluid resuscitation with colloids vs crystalloids on mortality in critically ill patients presenting with hypovolemic shock. JAMA. 2013;310(17):1809. http://jama.jamanetwork.com/article.aspx?doi=10.1001/jama.2013.280502.
19. Perel P, Roberts I, Ker K. Colloids versus crystalloids for fluid resuscitation in critically ill patients. Cochrane Database Syst Rev. 2013;(2):CD000567. https://doi.org/10.1002/14651858.CD000567.pub6.
20. Al-Omran M, Albalawi ZH, Tashkandi MF, Al-Ansary LA. Enteral versus parenteral nutrition for acute pancreatitis. Cochrane Database Syst Rev. 2010;(1):CD002837. http://www.ncbi.nlm.nih.gov/pubmed/20091534.
21. Bakker OJ, van Brunschot S, Farre A, Johnson CD, Kalfarentzos F, Louie BE, et al. Timing of enteral nutrition in acute pancreatitis: meta-analysis of individuals using a single-arm of randomised trials. Pancreatology. 2014;14(5):340–6.
22. Chang Y, Fu H, Xiao Y, Liu J. Nasogastric or nasojejunal feeding in predicted severe acute pancreatitis: a meta-analysis. Crit Care. 2013;17(3):R118. http://www.ncbi.nlm.nih.gov/pubmed/23786708.
23. Wereszczynska-Siemiatkowska U, Swidnicka-Siergiejko A, Siemiatkowski A, Dabrowski A. Early enteral nutrition is superior to delayed enteral nutrition for the prevention of infected necrosis and mortality in acute pancreatitis. Pancreas. 2013;42(4):640–6. http://www.ncbi.nlm.nih.gov/pubmed/23508012
24. Sun J-K. Effects of early enteral nutrition on immune function of severe acute pancreatitis patients. World J Gastroenterol. 2013;19(6):917. http://www.wjgnet.com/1007-9327/full/v19/i6/917.htm.
25. Bakker OJ, van Brunschot S, van Santvoort HC, Besselink MG, Bollen TL, Boermeester MA, et al. Early versus on-demand nasoenteric tube feeding in acute pancreatitis. N Engl J Med. 2014;371(21):1983–93.
26. Stimac D, Poropat G, Hauser G, Licul V, Franjic N, Valkovic Zujic P, et al. Early nasojejunal tube feeding versus nil-by-mouth in acute pancreatitis: a randomized clinical trial. Pancreatology. 2016;16(4):523–8. https://linkinghub.elsevier.com/retrieve/pii/S1424390316300175.
27. Teich N, Aghdassi A, Fischer J, Walz B, Caca K, Wallochny T, et al. Optimal timing of oral refeeding in mild acute pancreatitis. Pancreas. 2010;39(7):1088–92. http://www.ncbi.nlm.nih.gov/pubmed/20357692.
28. Petrov MS, Loveday BPT, Pylypchuk RD, McIlroy K, Phillips ARJ, Windsor JA. Systematic review and meta-analysis of enteral nutrition formulations in acute pancreatitis. Br J Surg. 2009;96(11):1243–52. http://www.ncbi.nlm.nih.gov/pubmed/19847860.
29. Heidegger CP, Berger MM, Graf S, Zingg W, Darmon P, Costanza MC, et al. Optimisation of energy provision with supplemental parenteral nutrition in critically ill patients: a randomised controlled clinical trial. Lancet. 2013;381(9864):385–93. http://linkinghub.elsevier.com/retrieve/pii/S0140673612613518.
30. Vege SS, DiMagno MJ, Forsmark CE, Martel M, Barkun AN. Initial medical treatment of acute pancreatitis: American Gastroenterological Association Institute technical review. Gastroenterol Int. 2018;154(4):1103–39. http://www.ncbi.nlm.nih.gov/pubmed/29421596.
31. Liu CL, Fan ST, Lo CM, Tso WK, Wong Y, Poon RTP, et al. Comparison of early endoscopic ultrasonography and endoscopic retrograde cholangiopancreatography in the management of acute biliary pancreatitis: a prospective randomized study. Clin Gastroenterol Hepatol. 2005;3(12):1238–44.
32. Kim DB, Paik C-N, Song DS, Kim HA, Kim Y-J, Lee JM, et al. The role of endoscopic ultrasonography and magnetic resonance cholangiopancreatography in patients with acute pancreatitis after negative computed tomography findings of the etiology. Pancreas. 2018;47(9):1165–71. http://www.ncbi.nlm.nih.gov/pubmed/30142119.
33. Lee S-L, Kim H-K, Choi H-H, Jeon B-S, Kim T-H, Choi J-M, et al. Diagnostic value of magnetic resonance cholangiopancreatography to detect bile duct stones in acute biliary pancreatitis. Pancreatology. 2018;18(1):22–8. http://www.ncbi.nlm.nih.gov/pubmed/29246689.
34. Oría A, Cimmino D, Ocampo C, Silva W, Kohan G, Zandalazini H, et al. Early endoscopic intervention versus early conservative management in patients with acute gallstone pancreatitis and biliopancreatic obstruction: a randomized clinical trial. Ann Surg. 2007;245(1):10–7.
35. Heinrich S, Schäfer M, Rousson V, Clavien P-A. Evidence-based treatment of acute pancreatitis: a look at established paradigms. Ann Surg. 2006;243(2):154–68. http://www.ncbi.nlm.nih.gov/pubmed/16432347.
36. Ayub K, Imada R, Slavin J. Endoscopic retrograde cholangiopancreatography in gallstone-associated acute pancreatitis. Cochrane Database Syst Rev. 2004;(4):CD003630. http://www.ncbi.nlm.nih.gov/pubmed/15495060.
37. Moretti A, Papi C, Aratari A, Festa V, Tanga M, Koch M, et al. Is early endoscopic retrograde cholangiopancreatography useful in the management of acute biliary pancreatitis? A meta-analysis of randomized controlled trials. Dig Liver Dis. 2008;40(5):379–85. http://www.ncbi.nlm.nih.gov/pubmed/18243826.
38. Petrov MS, Uchugina AF, Kukosh MV. Does endoscopic retrograde cholangiopancreatography reduce the risk of local pancreatic complications in acute pancreatitis? A systematic review and metaanalysis. Surg Endosc. 2008;22(11):2338–43. http://www.ncbi.nlm.nih.gov/pubmed/18528624.
39. Uy MC, Daez MLO, Sy PP, Banez VP, Espinosa WZ, Talingdan-Te MC. Early ERCP in acute gallstone pancreatitis without cholangitis: a meta-analysis. JOP. 2009;10(3):299–305. http://www.ncbi.nlm.nih.gov/pubmed/19454823.

40. Schepers NJ, Bakker OJ, Besselink MGH, Bollen TL, Dijkgraaf MGW, van Eijck CHJ, et al. Early biliary decompression versus conservative treatment in acute biliary pancreatitis (APEC trial): study protocol for a randomized controlled trial. Trials. 2016;17(1):5. http://trialsjournal.biomedcentral.com/articles/10.1186/s13063-015-1132-0.
41. Dubravcsik Z, Madácsy L, Gyökeres T, Vincze Á, Szepes Z, Hegyi P, et al. Preventive pancreatic stents in the management of acute biliary pancreatitis (PREPAST trial): pre-study protocol for a multicenter, prospective, randomized, interventional, controlled trial. Pancreatology. 2015;15(2):115–23. https://linkinghub.elsevier.com/retrieve/pii/S1424390315000344.
42. Kipp F. Analysis of bile colonization and intestinal flora may improve management in liver transplant recipients undergoing ERCP. Ann Transpl. 2015;20:249–55. http://www.annalsoftransplantation.com/abstract/index/idArt/893549.
43. García-Barrasa A, Borobia FG, Pallares R, Jorba R, Poves I, Busquets J, et al. A double-blind, placebo-controlled trial of ciprofloxacin prophylaxis in patients with acute necrotizing pancreatitis. J Gastrointest Surg. 2009;13(4):768–74. http://www.ncbi.nlm.nih.gov/pubmed/19082671.
44. Wittau M, Mayer B, Scheele J, Henne-Bruns D, Dellinger EP, Isenmann R. Systematic review and meta-analysis of antibiotic prophylaxis in severe acute pancreatitis. Scand J Gastroenterol. 2011;46(3):261–70.
45. Lim CLL, Lee W, Liew YX, Tang SSL, Chlebicki MP, Kwa AL-H. Role of antibiotic prophylaxis in necrotizing pancreatitis: a meta-analysis. J Gastrointest Surg. 2015;19(3):480–91. http://www.ncbi.nlm.nih.gov/pubmed/25608671.
46. Ukai T, Shikata S, Inoue M, Noguchi Y, Igarashi H, Isaji S, et al. Early prophylactic antibiotics administration for acute necrotizing pancreatitis: a meta-analysis of randomized controlled trials. J Hepatobiliary Pancreat Sci. 2015;22(4):316–21. http://www.ncbi.nlm.nih.gov/pubmed/25678060.
47. Dellinger EP, Tellado JM, Soto NE, Ashley SW, Barie PS, Dugernier T, et al. Early antibiotic treatment for severe acute necrotizing pancreatitis: a randomized, double-blind, placebo-controlled study. Ann Surg. 2007;245(5):674–83. http://www.ncbi.nlm.nih.gov/pubmed/17457158.
48. Isenmann R, Rünzi M, Kron M, Kahl S, Kraus D, Jung N, et al. Prophylactic antibiotic treatment in patients with predicted severe acute pancreatitis: a placebo-controlled, double-blind trial. Gastroenterol Int. 2004;126(4):997–1004. http://www.ncbi.nlm.nih.gov/pubmed/15057739.
49. Büchler M, Malfertheiner P, Friess H, Isenmann R, Vanek E, Grimm H, et al. Human pancreatic tissue concentration of bactericidal antibiotics. Gastroenterol Int. 1992;103(6):1902–8. http://www.ncbi.nlm.nih.gov/pubmed/1451983.
50. Negm AA, Poos H, Kruck E, Vonberg RP, Domagk D, Madisch A, et al. Microbiologic analysis of peri-pancreatic fluid collected during EUS in patients with pancreatitis: impact on antibiotic therapy. Gastrointest Endosc. 2013;78(2):303–11. https://doi.org/10.1016/j.gie.2013.03.001.
51. Schmidt PN, Roug S, Hansen EF, Knudsen JD, Novovic S. Spectrum of microorganisms in infected walled-off pancreatic necrosis—impact on organ failure and mortality. Pancreatology. 2014;14(6):444–9. http://www.ncbi.nlm.nih.gov/pubmed/25266641.
52. Gurusamy KS, Nagendran M, Davidson BR. Early eversus delayed laparoscopic cholecystectomy for acute gallstone pancreatitis. Cochrane Database Syst Rev. 2013;(9):CD010326. http://www.ncbi.nlm.nih.gov/pubmed/23996398.
53. van Baal MC, Besselink MG, Bakker OJ, van Santvoort HC, Schaapherder AF, Nieuwenhuijs VB, et al. Timing of cholecystectomy after mild biliary pancreatitis: a systematic review. Ann Surg. 2012;255(5):860–6. http://www.ncbi.nlm.nih.gov/pubmed/22470079.
54. Krishna SG, Kruger AJ, Patel N, Hinton A, Yadav D, Conwell DL. Cholecystectomy during index admission for acute biliary pancreatitis lowers 30-day readmission rates. Pancreas. 2018;47(8):996–1002. http://www.ncbi.nlm.nih.gov/pubmed/30028444.
55. Nealon WH, Bawduniak J, Walser EM. Appropriate timing of cholecystectomy in patients who present with moderate to severe gallstone-associated acute pancreatitis with peripancreatic fluid collections. Ann Surg. 2004;239(6):741–9; discussion 749–51. http://www.ncbi.nlm.nih.gov/pubmed/15166953.
56. Sankaran SJ, Xiao AY, Wu LM, Windsor JA, Forsmark CE, Petrov MS. Frequency of progression from acute to chronic pancreatitis and risk factors: a meta-analysis. Gastroenterol Int. 2015;149(6):1490–1500.e1. http://www.ncbi.nlm.nih.gov/pubmed/26299411.
57. Bertilsson S, Swärd P, Kalaitzakis E. Factors that affect disease progression after first attack of acute pancreatitis. Clin Gastroenterol Hepatol. 2015;13(9):1662–9.e3. http://www.ncbi.nlm.nih.gov/pubmed/25911118.
58. Gupta R, Wig JD, Bhasin DK, Singh P, Suri S, Kang M, et al. Severe acute pancreatitis: the life after. J Gastrointest Surg. 2009;13(7):1328–36. http://www.ncbi.nlm.nih.gov/pubmed/19415400.
59. van Brunschot S, Hollemans RA, Bakker OJ, Besselink MG, Baron TH, Beger HG, et al. Minimally invasive and endoscopic versus open necrosectomy for necrotising pancreatitis: a pooled analysis of individual data for 1980 patients. Gut. 2018;67(4):697–706. https://doi.org/10.1136/gutjnl-2016-313341.
60. Arvanitakis M, Dumonceau J-M, Albert J, Badaoui A, Bali M, Barthet M, et al. Endoscopic management of acute necrotizing pancreatitis: European Society of Gastrointestinal Endoscopy (ESGE) evidence-based multidisciplinary guidelines. Endoscopy.

2018;50(5):524–46. http://www.thieme-connect.de/DOI/DOI?10.1055/a-0588-5365.
61. Saunders R, Ramesh J, Cicconi S, Evans J, Yip VS, Raraty M, et al. A systematic review and meta-analysis of metal versus plastic stents for drainage of pancreatic fluid collections: metal stents are advantageous. Surg Endosc. 2018;33(5):1412–25. http://link.springer.com/10.1007/s00464-018-6416-5.
62. Puga M, Consiglieri C, Busquets J, Pallarès N, Secanella L, Peláez N, et al. Safety of lumen-apposing stent with or without coaxial plastic stent for endoscopic ultrasound-guided drainage of pancreatic fluid collections: a retrospective study. Endoscopy. 2018;50(10):1022–6. http://www.thieme-connect.de/DOI/DOI?10.1055/a-0582-9127.
63. Han D, Inamdar S, Lee CW, Miller LS, Trindade AJ, Sejpal DV. Lumen apposing metal stents (LAMSs) for drainage of pancreatic and gallbladder collections. J Clin Gastroenterol. 2018;52(9):835–44. Available from: http://insights.ovid.com/crossref?an=00004836-900000000-97985.
64. van Brunschot S, Fockens P, Bakker OJ, Besselink MG, Voermans RP, Poley J-W, et al. Endoscopic transluminal necrosectomy in necrotising pancreatitis: a systematic review. Surg Endosc. 2014;28(5):1425–38. http://www.ncbi.nlm.nih.gov/pubmed/24399524.

48 Chronic Pancreatitis

Myriam Delhaye

48.1 Introduction

Abdominal pain is the dominant symptom of chronic pancreatitis (CP), reported by 80–90% of patients [1], either as episodic pain (or Type A pain pattern) or as continuous pain (or Type B pain pattern) [2].

Endoscopic therapy (ET) in CP aims to provide pain relief by using the decompression of the pancreatic duct, based on the rationale that pain is related to ductal hypertension caused by an outflow obstruction of the main pancreatic duct (MPD). Indeed, according to a multicenter study of more than 1000 patients who had been selected for ET of painful CP, MPD obstruction was caused by pancreatic stones alone, ductal strictures alone, and a combination of stones and strictures in 18%, 47%, and 32% of cases, respectively [3].

Therefore ET is indicated for selected patients with both:

- Persistent (continuous or recurrent) pain related to CP after failed conservative management.
- Outflow obstruction of the MPD (i.e., MPD dilatation ≥5 mm) secondary to ductal stricture(s) and/or stone(s) amenable to ET [4], corresponding to the most severe grade of the Cambridge's classification of pancreatitis [5].

ERCP can achieve MPD drainage by pancreatic sphincterotomy of the major and/or minor papilla (Fig. 48.1), by temporary stent(s) placement or by pancreatic stone(s) extraction, usually after fragmentation with extracorporeal shock waves lithotripsy (ESWL). The effectiveness of ET is usually the result of these combined procedures.

The development of endoscopic ultrasonography (EUS) has expanded the possibilities in MPD drainage, for patients in whom conventional ERCP is not feasible or fails.

Biliary obstruction complicates the course of CP in 3–23% of patients [6] due to peribiliary inflammation and fibrosis and less frequently due to biliary compression by a pseudocyst. Endoscopy is the preferred initial management for CP-related common bile duct (CBD) strictures. The primary goal is to resolve bile duct obstruction, achieve long-term duct patency, and maintain liver function.

Overall, the goals of treatment in CP patients are pain management, management and prevention of complications of pancreatitis, and improvement or prevention of pancreatic insufficiencies.

M. Delhaye (✉)
Department of Gastroenterology, Hepatopancreatology and Digestive Oncology, Erasme Hospital, Brussels, Belgium
e-mail: Myriam.Delhaye@erasme.ulb.ac.be

M. Mutignani et al. (eds.), *Endotherapy in Biliopancreatic Diseases: ERCP Meets EUS*,
https://doi.org/10.1007/978-3-030-42569-2_48

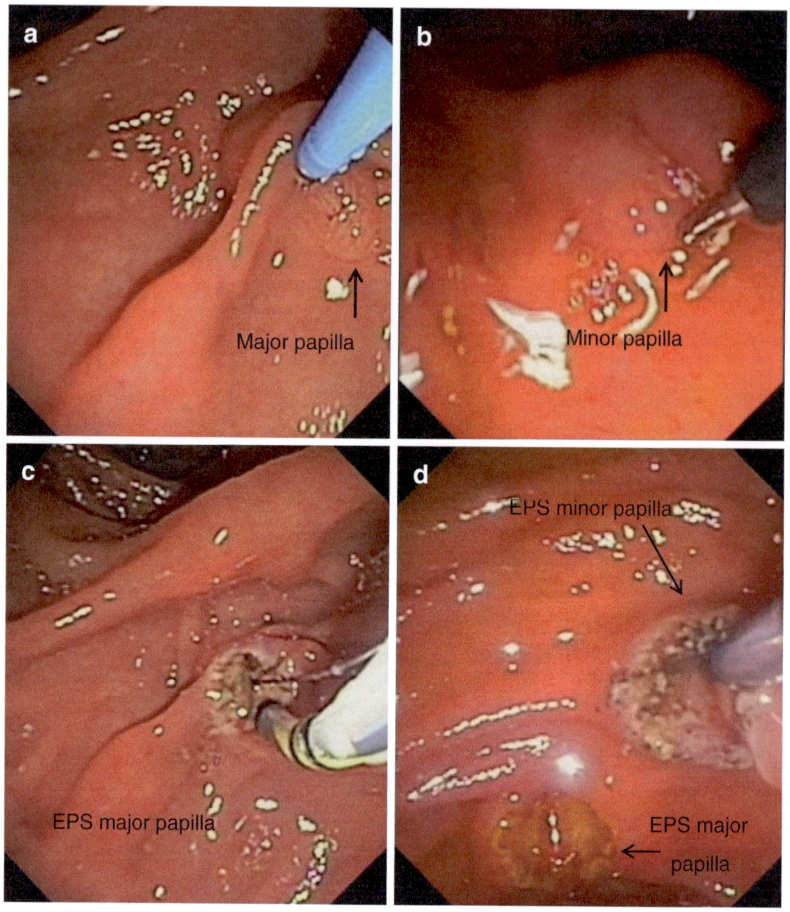

Fig. 48.1 Cannulation and endoscopic pancreatic sphincterotomy. (**a**) Major papilla approached with a ball tip catheter. (**b**) Minor papilla approached with a minor papilla cannula. (**c**) Endoscopic pancreatic sphincterotomy (EPS) at the major papilla. (**d**) Endoscopic pancreatic sphincterotomy (EPS) at the minor papilla and already performed at the major papilla

48.2 Main Pancreatic Duct Drainage

Pain in CP has a highly variable clinical presentation, differing in chronicity and severity [7]. Moreover, the multifactorial nature of pain is recognized in CP patients, including ongoing inflammation, alterations in pancreatic nerves, and central sensitization secondary to chronic nociceptive input, all of which being not affected by MPD drainage [4].

Some studies define clinical response as subjective improvement in abdominal pain, others use complete or partial pain relief, and still others combine pain relief with other more objective outcomes such as reduction in analgesic use or decreased rate of hospitalization for pain.

Pain relief can be assessed by one-dimensional scales, usually numeric (often from 0 to 10) verbal or visual analogue scale (VAS) that quantify only the intensity of pain [4].

Multidimensional scales, such as the Izbicki pain scores [8], are based on frequency of pain, intensity (as indicated by VAS), need for analgesics, and disease-related inability to work during the 12 months prior to the time point of pain assessment and are commonly used to assess pain relief in CP patients.

Other clinical benefits from ET include increase in body weight, improvement of pancreatic exocrine/endocrine functions, and improvement in quality of life.

48.2.1 Main Pancreatic Duct Drainage by ERCP

48.2.1.1 Clinical Results

Stricture-Predominant Disease

Benign dominant strictures of the MPD are generally due to inflammation or fibrosis and are usually located in the pancreatic head.

Dilatation alone is not a standard treatment option for MPD strictures, and various modalities of pancreatic duct stenting have been attempted following strictures' dilatation (Fig. 48.2) to obtain a sustained response. About two-thirds of patients with advanced CP require pancreatic stenting to achieve appropriate ductal decompression.

Single Plastic Stenting

Immediate pain relief after single MPD plastic stenting was recorded in 82% [9] to 94% [10] of patients and can be expected when drainage of the MPD is adequate [11, 12]. In the absence of early symptomatic improvement, the stent should be removed because ductal hypertension is not likely to be the cause of pancreatic pain and other causes of pain should be considered.

For long-term evaluation, the European Society of Gastrointestinal Endoscopy (ESGE) suggests using the absence of pain (relapse) at 1-year post-stent removal as a reasonable and workable definition of pain relief [13]. Long-term pain relief was experienced by about two-thirds of patients, as shown in many retrospective non-randomized studies (Table 48.1).

In a metaanalysis, with a subgroup analysis of CP patients with MPD stricture, including 9 studies and 536 patients, the pooled estimate of the proportion of patients with long-term pain relief was 67.5% (95% CI: 51.5–80.2%) [29].

However, in a prospective randomized controlled trial (RCT) comparing ET and surgical MPD drainage in painful CP patients, the rate of complete or partial pain relief assessed by the Izbicki pain scores measured during the first 2 years after ET (n = 19 patients), and also after a mean follow-up period of 7 years (n = 16 patients), was only 32% at 2 years [30] and 38% at 7 years of follow-up [31].

These very low clinical success rates could be explained partly by the low technical success rate of ET (53%) in the Cahen's study [30], the high proportion of patients with chronic pain (Type B pain pattern in 63% of patients), and maybe the

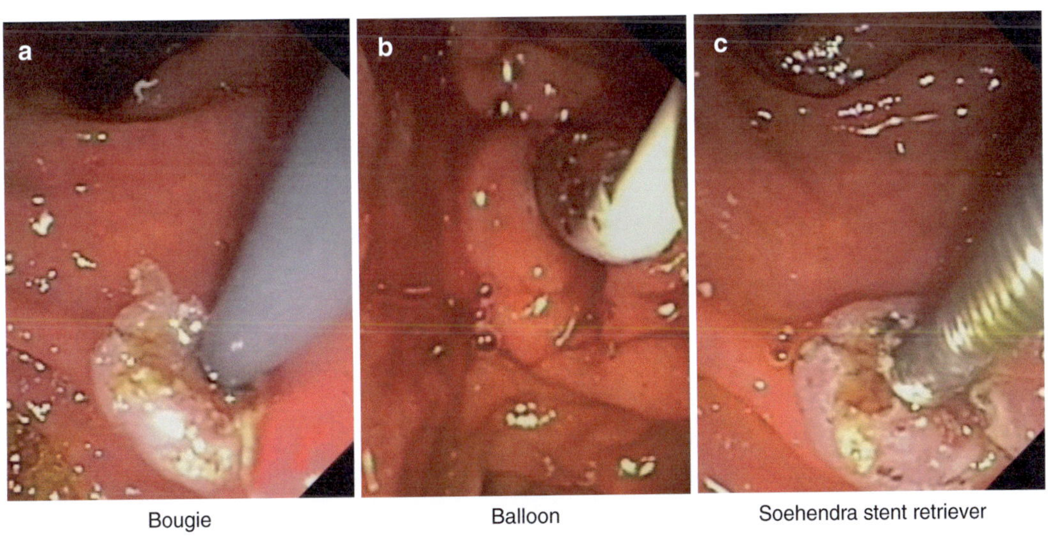

Fig. 48.2 Main pancreatic duct stricture dilatation. Dilatation of main pancreatic duct stricture is usually done before stenting and can be performed using a bougie (**a**), a wire-guided balloon (4–6 mm) (**b**), or a Soehendra stent retriever (**c**)

Table 48.1 MPD drainage for stricture-predominant disease

Author, year	Study design, *n* patients	Pain type A/B	Duration of disease before ET (y)	% ESWL/% stenting	Technical success	Sustained clinical success	Stenting duration, m	Need for restenting	Need for surgery	FU duration, m
SPS										
Binmoeller, 1995 [11]	R, 93	NA	5.6	37%/100%	100%	65%	15.7	27%	26%	59
Smits, 1995 [9]	R, 51	NA	2.4	6%/96%	96%	71% (22/31)	6.3 ($n = 31$)	NA	12%	34
Rösch, 2002 [3]	R, 1018	73%/27%	NA	26%/57%	88%	85% (681/801)	NA	NA	23%	59
Dite, 2003 [14]	P; 64 Partly RCT 36 randomized	NA	NA	0%/52%	97%	65% ($n = 64$) 61% ($n = 36$)	16	NA	NA	60
Vitale, 2004 [15]	R, 89	NA	NA	0%/100%	NA	83% (62/75)	5.3	NA	12%	43 ($n = 75$)
Eleftheriadis, 2005 [16]	R, 100	NA	3 years	51%/100%	100%	62%	23	38%	4%	69
Farnbacher, 2006 [17]	R, 98	68%/32%	NA	61%/100%	100%	78%	10	18%	23%	46 ($n = 57$)
Clarke, 2012 [18]	R, 71	58%/42%	NA	8%/75%	85%	51% (28/55)	NA	NA	31% (17/55)	58 ($n = 63$)
He, 2014 [19]	P, 89	48%/52%	NA	0%/87%	NA	87% (72/83)	11	NA	4%	24 ($n = 83$)
MPS										
Costamagna, 2006 [20]	P, 19	NA	NA	32%/100%	NA	84%	7	16%	NA	38
Bove, 2017 [21]	NA, 48	NA	NA	NA/100%	NA	77%	6	17%	NA	114
FC SEMS										
Park, 2008 [22]	P, 13	NA	NA	0%/100%	100%	100%	2	NA	NA	5
Sauer, 2008 [23]	P, 6	NA	NA	67%/100%	100%	67%	3	NA	NA	NA
Moon, 2010 [24]	P, 32	NA	NA	59%/100%	100%	84%	3	9%	3%	5
Giacino, 2012 [25]	R, 10	NA	NA	NA/100%	100%	90%	5.7	NA	0%	20
Matsubara, 2016 [26]	P, 10	NA	NA	NA/100%	100%	38% (3/8)	3.5	20%	10%	35 ($n = 8$)
Oh, 2018 [27]	R, 18	NA	NA	50%/100%	100%	72%	7.5	22%	6%	47 ($n = 15$)
Tringali, 2018 [28]	P, 15	NA	NA	27%/100%	NA	53%	7.1	NA	NA	38 ($n = 9$)

ET endoscopic therapy, *ESWL* extracorporeal shock waves lithotripsy, *FU* follow-up, *y* years, *m* months, *R* retrospective, *P* prospective, *RCT* randomized controlled trial, *NA* not available short duration of MPD stenting (6.2 months). Indeed, in 7 series totalizing 521 patients [9, 11, 14–17, 19], the average stenting duration was 13 months (range 5.3–23 months) (Table 48.1).

Resolution of the MPD stricture was reported in 5 studies (145 patients) [10, 12, 30, 32, 33], in 9% of patients [10] to 50% of patients [30].

However symptomatic improvement may persist after pancreatic stent removal despite persistence of the stricture [12], suggesting that stricture resolution is not a prerequisite for symptomatic improvement.

Comparable clinical results were observed when pancreatic duct stents were exchanged only if patients developed relapsing pain (on-demand stent exchange strategy) or at fixed, predetermined interval, irrespective of symptoms [13]. Indeed, stent clogging occurs very early and frequently [34] but does not correlate with symptoms [35, 36].

Factors associated with stent occlusion within 90 days were identified by Farnbacher MJ et al. [36] and included stent diameter >8.5 Fr (RR 4.93), stent length >8 cm (RR 2.31), female gender (RR 2.80) and oral enzyme supplementation (considered as a surrogate marker for severe pancreatic exocrine insufficiency) (RR 2.90).

On the other hand, with respect to stent diameter, it was shown in a retrospective study of 163 patients [37] that CP patients with stents ≤8.5 Fr were 3.2 times more likely to be hospitalized for abdominal pain than those who had received 10 Fr stents. So the ESGE recommends treating dominant MPD stricture by inserting a single 10 Fr plastic stent with stent exchange planned within 1 year even in asymptomatic patients to prevent complications related to long-standing stent occlusion [13].

Relapsing pain after "definitive" single plastic stent removal occurred in about 25% (6–56%) of patients [11, 31–33, 38, 39], mostly during the first 2 years following stent removal [16]. Re-stenting after definitive single stent removal was indicated in 26% (10–38%) of patients [11, 16, 17, 30, 32, 39].

Surgical procedures were performed in about 20% of patients after pancreatic stenting (Table 48.1), in patients who had not responded to ET, to cure complications or for patients who despite clinical improvement after stenting required too frequent stent replacements during the follow-up [40].

The impact of ET on the body weight was reported in 4 series [11, 14, 15, 17], showing increase or no change in body weight for about 74% of patients after MPD stenting.

Regarding pancreatic exocrine function, a single prospective non-randomized comparative study in 42 CP patients reported preservation of exocrine function in the stenting group after a single plastic stenting duration of 15.2 months ($n = 20$ patients), and significant worsening of the pancreatic exocrine function in the non-stenting group ($n = 22$) while no differences were observed for overt diabetes during a mean follow-up of 5.2 years [39].

However, 3 other studies have not reported such favorable impact of pancreatic duct stenting on pancreatic exocrine function with de novo development after pancreatic exocrine insufficiency in about 30% of patients at the end of follow-up [16, 30, 31].

Similar progressive deterioration of the pancreatic endocrine function was noted in CP patients after single plastic stenting of the MPD with 18–44% of de novo diabetes at 5 years follow-up after stenting [3, 11, 14, 16, 31].

No significant improvement was observed in physical and mental scores of the quality of life (QoL) scores in the RCT at 2 years following single plastic stenting [30].

Multiple Plastic Stenting

Single plastic stent could not be definitively removed in approximately one-third of patients because of symptomatic persistent or recurrent strictures [11, 16, 17]. In such refractory cases, insertion of multiple plastic stents (MPS), side-by-side, in the MPD provides more rigorous dilatation of the MPD stricture and allows pancreatic juice flow alongside the stents even if there is stent clogging (Fig. 48.3). Consequently, a shorter duration of stenting to achieve stricture resolution, a decrease in the number of stents exchanges, and a more durable result after stent removal could be expected.

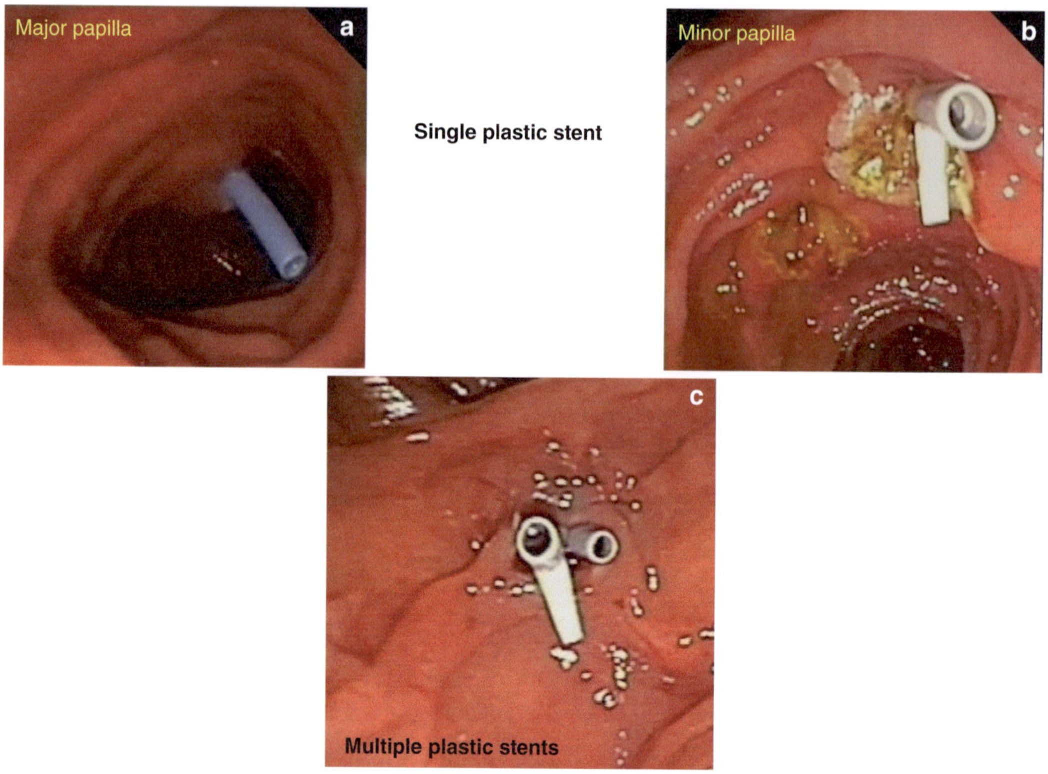

Fig. 48.3 Pancreatic duct stenting. Single plastic 10 Fr stent protruding from the major papilla (**a**) and 8.5 Fr stent from the minor papilla (**b**). Two side-by-side plastic 8.5 Fr stents placed through the major papilla (**c**)

Temporary placement of MPS (median of 3 simultaneous stents 8.5–11.5 Fr) for 6–12 months (mean 7 months) in refractory cases provided persistent pain resolution in 84% of cases (16/19) during long-term follow-up after stents removal (mean 38 months) [20] (Table 48.1).

Resolution of the stricture was observed in 95% of cases (18/19); relapsing pain after "definitive" stents removal occurred in 11% of cases with a need for re-stenting in 16% (3/19) [20].

Only one further observational study was published in abstract form, regarding the temporary insertion for 6 months of multiple side-by-side plastic stents in 48 patients [21]. In this study, stricture resolution was obtained in 89.5% of cases and pain relief, at 9.5 years of follow-up, in 77.1% of patients [21]. Symptomatic MPD stricture recurrence occurred in 23% of cases (11/48) after a mean time of 26.4 months from MPS removal.

Self-Expandable Metal Stenting

For refractory MPD strictures, the temporary insertion of self-expandable metal stent (SEMS) could be an option, the main advantage of SEMS compared to plastic stents being a larger diameter.

Uncovered and partially covered SEMS have provided disappointing results [41] because of the high dysfunction rate and the inability to remove the stent because of tissue hyperplasia through the wire mesh.

According to a systematic review of 4 prospective series (total 61 patients), temporary placement of a fully covered SEMS (FC-SEMS) had provided pain improvement in 85% of the patients during a short follow-up time after stent removal [22–25, 42].

Less encouraging results were recently reported in 3 small series (<20 patients) during follow-up periods ranging from 35 months to

47 months, with an average sustained clinical success of 59% (24/41) [26–28] (Table 48.1).

Stricture improvement was noted in 96% of cases [22, 24–26, 28]. The duration of stenting with FC-SEMS ranged from 2 months to 7.5 months (Table 48.1), but the optimal duration of stenting has yet to be determined, 3 months being safe for stent removal but maybe insufficient for stricture resolution and 6 months being maybe too long for easy SEMS removal.

Symptomatic recurrent MPD stricture after FC-SEMS removal occurred in 20% of cases [24, 26, 27] and require either repeat stenting (15%) or surgery (4%) (Table 48.1).

In a pilot study, a biodegradable non-covered self-expandable stent has provided clinical success at 1-year follow-up in 10 (53%) of 19 patients who had no stricture resolution at least 6 months after previous plastic stent insertion (median, 10 months) [43]. In this study, stricture resolution was obtained in 58% of cases (11/19) while repeat stenting and surgery were needed in 4 (21%) and 5 patients (26%), respectively [43].

Stone(s)-Predominant Disease

Intraductal stones are found in 32–90% of patients presenting with CP [44], are solitary in 10–62% of patients, are most frequently located in the pancreatic head, and are associated with stricture(s) in approximately 50% of the patients [45] (Table 48.2).

ERCP alone using pancreatic sphincterotomy and a basket or a balloon allows stone extraction (Fig. 48.4) in a minority of patients: 9% of 1041 patients in 2 retrospective studies [47, 51] and 14% of 1834 patients in a survey of 125 hospitals [55].

Failed stone extraction is associated with stones >10 mm, a diffused location, stone impaction, and location upstream from a stricture [51, 56]. So, primary endoscopic attempt at pancreatic stone extraction is reserved to selected patients based on reasonable expected success of endoscopic extraction after endoscopic pancreatic sphincterotomy, namely small (<5 mm), non-calcified stones located in the cephalic portion of the MPD, with no associated ductal stricture. However, in 70–90% of cases, pancreatic stones cannot be extracted without pre-ERCP fragmentation [47, 57].

ESWL was proven useful for treating obstructive stone-associated painful CP in several meta-analyses [58, 59].

In the first metaanalysis [58] including 588 patients from 17 studies, ESWL effectively relieves MPD obstruction and alleviates pain in CP most often in combination with ET. The mean effect size was 0.62 ± 0.17. The more recent metaanalysis including 27 studies (with 6 prospective ones) and 3189 patients [59] reported that pancreatic ESWL allowed a complete/partial MPD clearance in 70%/22% of the patients, respectively. The pooled proportion of patients with absence of pain at follow-up was 53% (95% CI: 51–55) and mild-to-moderate pain at follow-up was 33% (95% CI: 31–36). Narcotic use was decreased in 80% (95% CI: 77–82) of the pooled proportion of patients.

Pancreatic ESWL was shown as safe and effective also in a pediatric population of patients with pancreatic stones, with similar outcome as that in a matched adult population of patients [54].

Pain relapses occurred in approximately one-third of patients, more frequently in patients with stones and strictures than in those with stones alone [3]. They were usually related to stone migration or recurrence [52], progressive stricturing of the MPD, or pancreatic stent obstruction or dislodgement [47, 49, 60].

All these situations could be further managed successfully by ERCP ± ESWL with a similar response rate as that for initial therapy [47]. The timing of pain relapse for stone-predominant disease was reported most often within the 3 first years of follow-up [48, 49, 51].

In one retrospective study of 128 patients [61], pain relapse occurred at an early date (at 38.6 ± 5.3 months) in patients with incomplete stone removal, compared with 83.7 ± 5.5 months in the complete removal group ($p < 0.001$).

Surgery was required in 4.4% (95% CI: 4–5) of the pooled proportion of patients for various reasons, mainly for inadequate pain control with ERCP ± ESWL [59]. The need for surgery in stone-predominant disease ranged from 1.4% to 21%, with a mean of 6.3% in 10 series including

Table 48.2 MPD drainage for stone-predominant disease

Author, year	Study design, *n* patients	Pain type A/B	Duration of disease before ET (y)	% stenting/% ESWL	Technical success	Complete ductal stone clearance	Sustained clinical success	Need for surgery	FU duration, m
Adamek, 1999 [46]	R, 80	NA	NA	NA/100%	54%	NA	76%	10%	40
Farnbacher, 2002 [47]	R, 125	72%/28%	5.9	56%/91%	85%	51%	48% (40/84)	12%	29 ($n = 84$)
Delhaye, 2004 [40]	R, 56	55%/45%	5 y	48%/100%	86%	NA	66%	21%	173
Inui, 2005 [48]	R 237 ESWL + ET 318 ESWL alone	NA	NA	0%/100%	73%	73%	76% (382/504)	4% (22/504)	44.3 ($n = 504$)
Tadenuma, 2005 [49]	R, 117	NA	NA	12%/100%	NA	56%	70% (49/70)	1.4% (1/70)	77.5 ($n = 70$)
Seven, 2012 [50]	R, 120	NA	2.9	95%/100%	NA	NA	85%	16% (9/55)	52
Suzuki, 2013 [51]	R, 540	NA	NA	NA/85%	NA	74%	84%	1.9%	42
Tandan, 2013 [52]	R, 636	NA	NA	56%/100%	100%	78%	87%	9%	24–60
Korpela, 2016 [53]	R, 83	NA	NA	NA/100%	83%	83%	69%	6%	42
Wang, 2017 [54]	P	A/B/RAP		NA/100%	NA				
	72 children	70%/8% 22%	5.3			86%	78% (52/67)	6% (4/67)	36
	72 matched adults	58%/9% 34%	7.8			94%	80% (55/69)	1.4% (1/69)	34

ET endoscopic therapy, *ESWL* extracorporeal shock waves lithotripsy, *FU* follow-up, *y* years, *m* months, *R* retrospective, *P* prospective, *NA* not available, *RAP* recurrent acute pancreatitis

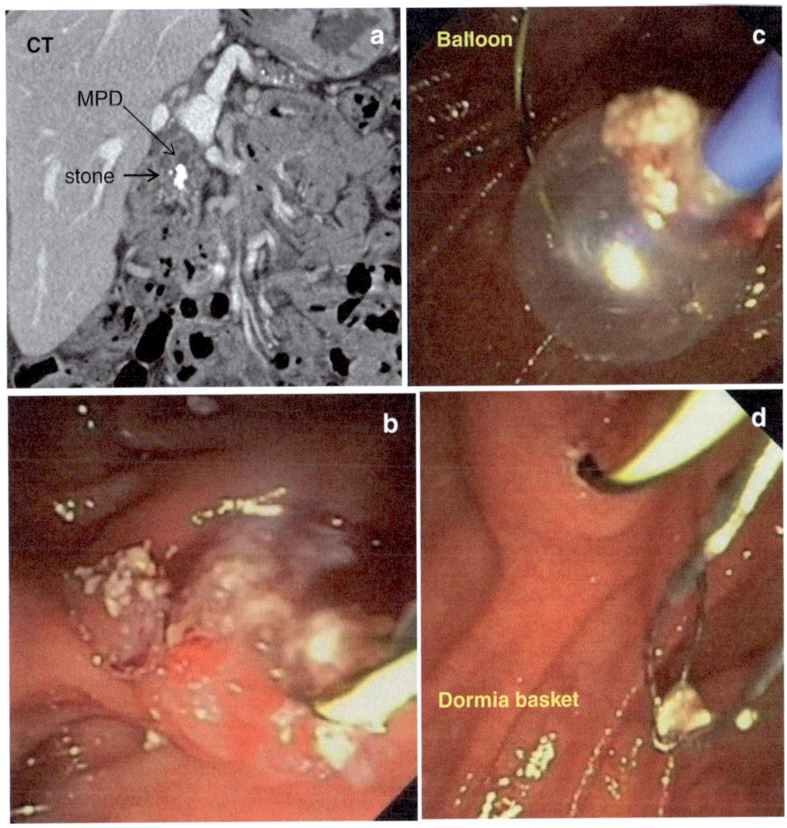

Fig. 48.4 Stone-predominant disease. (**a**) A coronal CT picture showing a big obstructive calcified stone (arrow) in the head of pancreas with upstream main pancreatic duct (MPD) dilatation (arrow). (**b**) Stone fragments seen in the duodenal lumen after extracorporeal shock waves lithotripsy. Stones fragments were removed by using balloon catheter (**c**) and/or Dormia basket (**d**)

2218 patients (Table 48.2), which is significantly lower than in 8 series with stricture-predominant disease (20.5% of 1591 patients) (Table 48.1) ($p < 0.0001$) [45].

Regarding the changes in body weight occurring after ERCP ± ESWL, the patient's weight was constant or increased in 81% (95% CI: 79–84) of the pooled proportion of patients and weight decrease was noted in only 8% (95% CI: 6–10) [59].

In most long-term studies, the pancreatic exocrine/endocrine functions deteriorated during follow-up after ERCP ± ESWL [40, 46, 49, 50, 52].

However, compared with the natural history of the progression of exocrine insufficiency in CP patients treated conservatively [2], pancreatic exocrine insufficiency after endoscopic ductal drainage in alcohol-induced CP seemed to occur up to 10 years later and to be dependent on early relief of ductal obstruction [40].

Exocrine as well as endocrine pancreatic functions deteriorated more significantly in the incomplete removal group and in the continuing drinking group as shown in a retrospective study of 70 patients followed at long-term [49].

In another long-term study, it was also noted that endocrine function seems mainly dependent on alcohol consumption habits, the risk of developing de novo diabetes mellitus being significantly associated with alcohol-related CP [40].

Finally, in the metaanalysis, the proportion of patients requiring a decreased quantity of antidiabetic medications after ERCP ± ESWL management was only 5.2% (95% CI: 4–7) [59].

The improvement in QoL is a combination of relief of pain, improvement in food intake, a decreased use of analgesics, and a decrease in the rate of hospitalization [52]. Most studies used non-validated subjective, numeric [1–10] scale assessing overall QoL [50, 52]. Taking into account these limitations, QoL improved in 88.8% (95% CI: 77–82) of the pooled proportion of patients in the metaanalysis [59].

48.2.1.2 Factors Predictive of Clinical Results

Factors predicting favorable clinical outcome after endoscopic pancreatic duct drainage have been identified.

Immediate pain relief was independently associated with MPD stone clearance [57, 62], with successful decompression of the MPD (i.e., a decrease in MPD diameter) [12, 60, 63] and with a low frequency of pain attacks before ET (i.e., Type A pain pattern) [57, 60, 62, 63].

Pre-therapeutic factors predicting long-term pain relief (≥2 years) and/or absence of pain relapse following ET of CP include:

- The location of obstructive calcifications in the head of pancreas [64].
- A short disease duration prior to treatment [11, 18, 19, 40, 57, 65].
- A low frequency of pain attacks or Type A pain pattern or non-severe pain with low rate of patients taking narcotics daily, before ET [17–19, 57, 66].
- Absence of MPD stricture at initial ET [12, 49, 57].
- Presence of steatorrhea [65].

Factors identified after initial completion of MPD drainage by ERCP and *associated with long-term pain relief* (≥2 years) and/or absence of pain relapse following treatment include:

- Complete MPD stone clearance [49, 61, 67].
- MPD stricture resolution after stenting [12, 49, 57].
- Low alcohol intake (<20 g/day) or discontinuation of alcohol [17, 49, 68].
- Non-smoking or discontinuation of tobacco [40, 50, 68].
- Short duration of ET, low number of ERCP procedures [17, 40].

Interestingly, pain duration ≤3 years, no preoperative use of opioids, and≤5 endoscopic procedures prior to surgery were also factors, all independently associated with higher rates of pain relief after surgery with ORs 1.8, 2.1, and 2.5, respectively [69].

As complete MPD stone clearance is associated with favorable clinical outcome, *factors associated with complete MPD stone clearance* have also been recorded:

- The presence of a single stone vs. multiple stones [46, 49, 57, 61, 63, 65].
- The absence of MPD stricture [49, 61].
- A lower density of stones (<820 HU [61], <1000.45 HU [70]).
- Stone(s) located in the pancreatic head [65].
- Performance of ESWL prior to endoscopic attempt at stone extraction [57].

Predictive factors for the need of re-stenting within 1 year of stent removal or *continuing ET* include:

- The presence of pancreas divisum [16].
- The presence of pain immediately prior to pancreatic stenting [17].
- Alcohol continuing consumption [17].

Factors associated with the development of de novo *steatorrhea* include:

- Alcohol-induced cause of CP [40].
- Long duration of symptomatic ductal obstruction (as suggested by a long duration of ET and a high number of hospitalizations for pain after initial ET) [40].

Alcohol-induced cause of CP was also associated with the *development of* de novo *diabetes* [40].

From these results, the best candidates for successful treatment of painful CP with first-line ET should be patients in the early stage of the disease with episodic, non-severe pain, with no need for opioid use, with distal obstruction of the MPD (low-density single stone in the head of the pancreas) and no MPD stricture, in whom complete MPD stone clearance and adequate ductal drainage should be achieved with a low number of ERCP procedures. Recommendations about alcohol and tobacco discontinuations should be obviously provided.

48.2.2 Main Pancreatic Duct Drainage by EUS

EUS-guided drainage of the MPD is indicated for symptomatic MPD obstruction as a second-line procedure after failed conventional transpapillary MPD drainage, in patients with painful CP who are not suitable for surgery (i.e., patients who have already had pancreatic surgery).

Failure of transpapillary MPD drainage could occur in inaccessible papilla (post-surgical altered anatomy), in disconnected pancreatic duct (i.e., secondary to MPD rupture), in tight ductal stricture (Fig. 48.5), in pancreas divisum (i.e., failure of minor papilla cannulation), in cystic dystrophy of the duodenal wall (failure to recognize papilla) [71–74].

EUS-guided MPD drainage is technically challenging. In a review of 222 reported patients (including a mix of indications), technical success was noted in 77% (170/222), with complications reported in 42/222 patients (19%) (involving mainly post-procedural abdominal pain, pancreatitis, and bleeding) [75].

A minimum MPD dilatation of 6 mm is required to achieve EUS-guided puncture of the MPD. Four to eight weeks after the first procedure, patients were scheduled for the replacement of the initial small-caliber stent by either a larger stent or more often 2 stents implanted side-by-side. Stent could be placed in the direction of the head of the pancreas (anterograde stent placement, transpapillary, or transluminal, when the stent does not cross the site of ductal obstruction, the papilla, or the anastomosis) or in the direction of the tail of the pancreas (retrograde stent placement). Sometimes a rendez vous procedure, with an EUS-guided MPD puncture and insertion of a guidewire through the papilla, was followed by ERCP and conventional transpapillary drainage of the MPD [76].

Compared to EUS-guided biliary drainage, a lower success rate for EUS-guided pancreatic duct drainage was reported probably due to the small diameter of the MPD compared to the bile duct, the hard pancreatic parenchyma in CP patients, and the relatively short length for guidewire insertion [72].

Complete or major pain relief has been reported in 69–88% of patients in the largest series of patients (36–94 patients, totalizing 239 patients) with painful obstructive CP after successful EUS-guided drainage of the MPD [73, 77–79] (Table 48.3).

In a retrospective, single-center study including 45 patients (8 CP patients), a prior ERCP performed during the same procedure as EUS-guided MPD drainage was the only statistically significant risk factor for failed stent placement [76]. In the same study, many patients (19/23 = 83%) will have a durable clinical benefit after a stenting duration of 4 months. During a follow-up period of 32 months, recurrence of symptoms occurred in 4 patients after a median of 14 months [76].

A malignant etiology, as the cause of the complete MPD obstruction, should always be excluded as it was diagnosed in 5 patients (14%) within 1 year after the procedure in one series of 36 patients [73].

48.3 Common Bile Duct Drainage

CP-associated biliary strictures occur in the distal common bile duct (CBD) with proximal bile duct dilatation and delayed run-off of contrast. Symptomatic biliary stricture can lead to a variety of adverse outcomes, including chronic cholestasis, jaundice, recurrent cholangitis, and rarely secondary biliary cirrhosis. The objectives of biliary drainage in CP patients is long-term stricture resolution with clinical success being defined as an improvement in biochemical markers of liver function, a radiographic resolution of biliary dilatation, absence of cholangitis during follow-up, and no need for further therapy after removal of the stent(s) [81, 82].

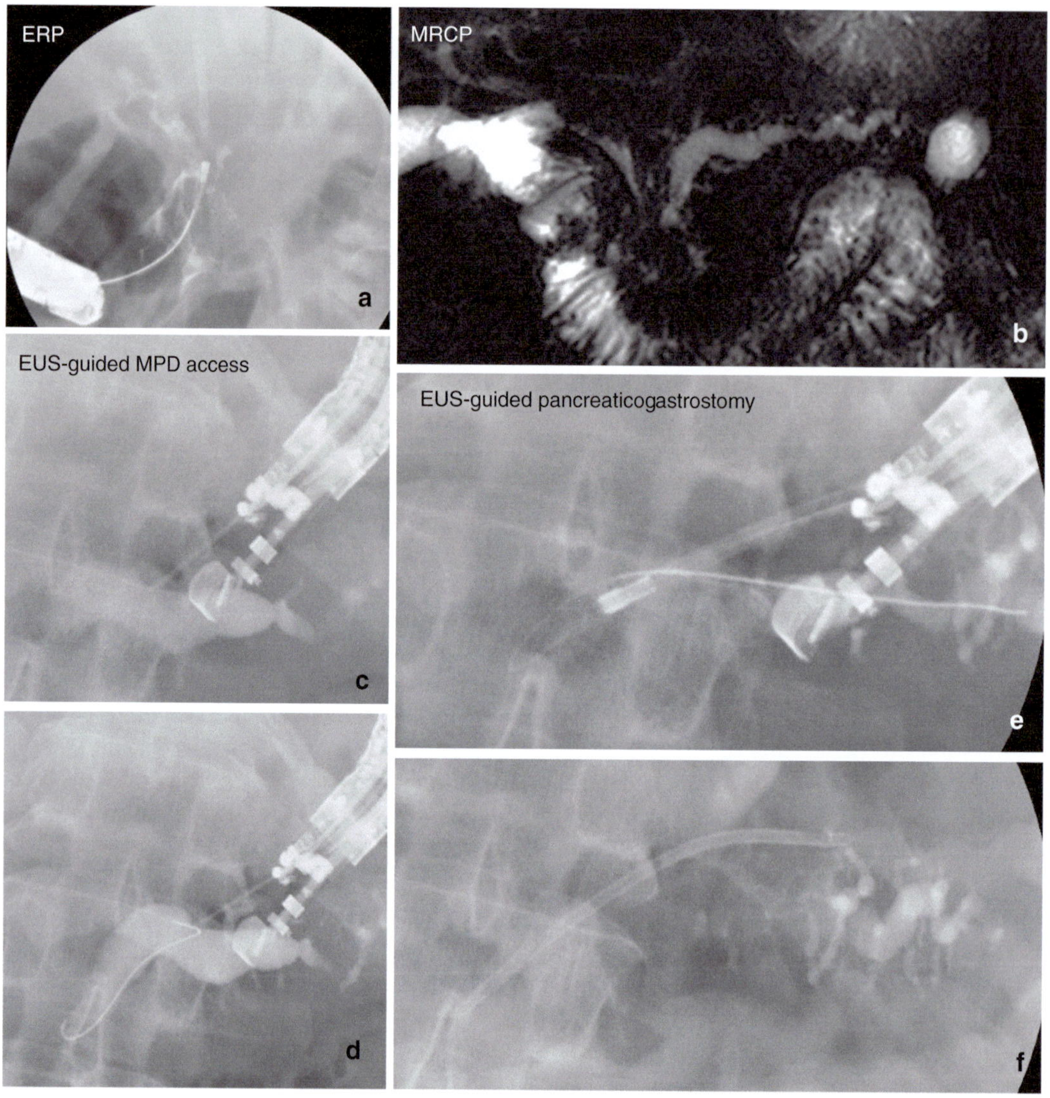

Fig. 48.5 EUS-guided pancreaticogastrostomy. (**a**) Downstream complete obstruction of the main pancreatic duct (MPD) due to a tight stricture during endoscopic retrograde pancreatography (ERP). (**b**) In the same patient, the MPD was dilated (9 mm) above a long prepapillary stricture (25 mm) as shown by magnetic resonance cholangiopancreatography (MRCP). A 3 cm pseudocyst was seen in the tail of the pancreas. There was no suspicion of malignancy in the head of pancreas. (**c**) Opacification of the dilated MPD after EUS-guided puncture with a needle catheter and contrast injection. (**d**) A guidewire was advanced into the MPD. (**e**) A 8.5 Fr cystotome with diathermic metal tip was passed over the guidewire to enlarge the tract between the stomach and the MPD. (**f**) A 7 Fr, 7 cm-long pancreaticogastric plastic stent was placed in the MPD

Table 48.3 MPD drainage under EUS guidance (> 20 patients)

Author, year	Study design, *n* patients	Duration of disease before ET (y)	Technical success	Clinical success	Need for surgery	FU duration, m
Tessier, 2007 [73]	R, 36 (2 centers) 20 CP	NA	EPG $n = 29$ EPD $n = 7$ 92%	69%	8%	14.5
Will, 2015 [77]	R, 94 35 CP	NA	57% (47/83) RV technique $n = 21$ Antegrade technique $n = 26$	82% (68/83)	13%	15
Oh, 2016 [80]	R, 25 10 CP	NA	FC-SEMS EPG $n = 23$ EPD $n = 1$ EPJ $n = 1$ 100%	92% (23/25) (early pain improvement) Stent in place	NA	NA
Chen, 2017 [78]	R, 40 (7 centers) RAP or CP $n = 17$	NA	92.5%	87.5%	NA	NA
Tyberg, 2017 [79]	R, 80 (4 centers) 29 CP	NA	EPG $n = 75$ EPD $n = 5$ 89%	81%	1.3%	24 ($n = 70$)

MPD main pancreatic duct, *EUS* endoscopic ultrasonography, *CP* chronic pancreatitis, *ET* endoscopic therapy, *y* years, *FU* follow-up, *m* months, *R* retrospective, *RAP* recurrent acute pancreatitis, *EPG* endoscopic pancreaticogastrostomy, *EPD* endoscopic pancreaticoduodenostomy, *RV* rendez vous, *FC-SEMS* fully covered self-expandable metal stent, *EPJ* endoscopic pancreaticojejunostomy, *NA* not available

48.3.1 Common Bile Duct Drainage by ERCP

There has been a gradual evolution in the endoscopic management of distal biliary strictures secondary to CP. ERCP with stent(s) placement is the first-line treatment modality for the management of CP-related CBD stricture. Biliary drainage may be performed with single or multiple side-by-side plastic stents or SEMS.

48.3.1.1 Clinical Results

Single Plastic Stenting

Most early series used biliary sphincterotomy and single (usually 10 Fr) plastic stents for varying time periods (Table 48.4).

Endoscopic biliary drainage was technically successful in 100% of patients and provided short-term clinical resolution of symptoms in all cases [83–87].

Most often single plastic stents were exchanged at 3–4 month intervals for up to 12 months to avoid complications of clogging and resulting cholangitis.

Long-term sustained clinical benefit after single plastic stent removal was, however, reported in only about 30% of 350 patients (ranging from 11% to 80%) 8–49 months after stent removal (Table 48.4).

The only prospective study was from Kahl's group [89] who treated 61 patients for 12 months with a single 10 Fr stent changed every 3 months. During a median follow-up of 40 months post-stenting, long-term success was achieved in 26% of patients (Table 48.4).

The discordant better clinical success rate in the study by Vitale et al. [87] could be related to the lower rate of calcifications present in the head of the pancreas in this study (16%) compared to a rate of 60–70% in other series, suggesting a less severe disease.

Table 48.4 Stents for CBD strictures in patients with CP

Author, year	Study design, *n* patients	Duration of disease before biliary stenting, y	Calcifications in the head	Length of the stenosis	Stenting duration, m	Long-term success	Stent dysfunction of any cause	Need for surgery	FU duration, m
Single plastic stent									
Devière, 1990 [83]	R, 25	3.3	NA	NA	NA	12%	72%	28%	14 ($n = 19$)
Barthet, 1994 [84]	R, 19	7	84%	26 mm	10	11%	NA	21%	18
Smits, 1996 [85]	R, 58	1.1	71%	NA	10	28%	64%	28%	49
Farnbacher, 2000 [86]	R, 31	NA	16%	19.8 mm	10	32%	52%	6%	28
Vitale, 2000 [87]	R, 25	1.1	16%	15 mm	13.3	80%	20%	8%	32
Eickhoff, 2001 [88]	R, 39	3.4	5%	17.6 mm	9	31%	44%	28%	58
Kahl, 2003 [89]	P, 61	6	64%	NA	12	26%	34%	49%	40
Catalano, 2004 [90]	R, 34	NA	44%	NA	21	24%	41%	41%	50
Cahen, 2005 [91]	R, 58	1.9	NA	NA	9	38%	48%	29%	45
Multiple plastic stents									
Draganov, 2002 [92]	R, 9	NA	67%	NA	14	44%	NA	11%	48
Catalano, 2004 [90]	P, 12	NA	50%	NA	14	92%	8%	8%	47
Pozsar, 2004 [93]	R, 29	4.4	NA	NA	21	62%	28%	10%	12
Regimbeau, 2012 [94]	R, 33	6.5	100%	NA	21 MPS 12 SEMS	76%	21%	52%	44
Haapamäki, 2015 [95]	P, RCT, 30	NA	77%	25 mm	6	88% (22/25)	23%	0%	37

Okyama, 2017 [96]	P, 10	8.8	100%	24 mm	12	60%	20%	NA	21
Self-expandable metal stent									
Cahen, 2008 [97]	P, 6	NA	NA	NA	5	50%	33%	17%	28
Behm, 2009 [98]	P, 20	NA	75%	NA	5	80%	5%	0%	22
Mahajan, 2009 [99]	P, 19	NA	NA	NA	3	58%	11%	NA	4
Perri, 2012 [100]	P, 17	NA	65%	NA	6	53% (8/15)	65%	18%	24
Devière, 2014 [101]	P, 127	2.3	NA	NA	11	80%	22%	NA	20
Haapamäki, 2015 [95]	P, RCT, 28	NA	82%	30 mm	6	91% (20/22)	29%	4%	41
Saxena, 2015 [102]	R, 30	NA	NA	NA	3–6	90%	NA	NA	18

FU follow-up, *m* months, *MPS* multiple plastic stents, *SEMS* self-expandable metal stent, *R* retrospective, *P* prospective, *RCT* randomized controlled trial, *NA* not available

Multiple Plastic Stenting

Temporary (12 months) placement of multiple side-by-side plastic biliary stents allowed obtaining gradual and sustained CBD stricture resolution with clinical success reported in 44–92% of cases (Table 48.4), which was higher compared with the placement of a single plastic stent.

Catalano et al. [90] treated 46 patients with CP-related biliary strictures, including a first group of 34 patients who received a single 10 Fr plastic stent changed at 3–6 months interval over a mean of 21 months and a second group of 12 patients who were prospectively enrolled to receive 4–5 stents over 14 months. The overall clinical success rate in patients receiving a single plastic stent was 24% after a mean follow-up of 4.2 years compared with 92% for those treated with multiple plastic stents followed for a mean of 3.8 years ($p < 0.01$) [90].

From the available evidence, it appears that the sequential placement of multiple plastic stents is an effective treatment for the majority of patients with CBD strictures secondary to CP [103]. Stents should be left in place for at least 12 months and then removed.

However, using this approach, multiple endoscopic procedures are required for scheduled stent upsizing and exchanges to prevent adverse events related to stent occlusion [82].

Recurrent stricture at 2 years of follow-up has been documented in 10% of patients (3/30) in the RCT comparing multiple plastic stenting and SEMS stenting in biliary strictures related to CP [95].

Self-Expandable Metal Stenting

The main advantages of SEMS compared to plastic stents are [103, 104]:

- A larger diameter: one 10 mm SEMS has a width equivalent to that of approximately 7 plastic stents sized 10 Fr with as a consequence, a prolonged stent patency with a low rate of stent occlusions.
- A fewer endoscopic sessions: only 2 ERCP sessions are required compared to 4–5 sessions for a 1-year stenting duration with plastic stents exchanged every 3 months.
- A technically easy placement and removal.

The use of both uncovered and partially covered SEMS for biliary strictures due to CP has been disappointing because of stent-associated endoluminal epithelial hyperplasia involving the uncovered portions of the SEMS, resulting in late stent occlusion with difficulty of removal [81, 103, 105].

So, fully covered SEMS (FC-SEMS) are currently preferred for benign biliary strictures to prevent tissue ingrowth or stent embedment and for easy removal [103].

A systematic review including 13 studies on plastic stenting ($n = 570$ patients but only 90 CP) and 12 studies on FC-SEMS ($n = 376$ patients but only 128 CP) showed that FC-SEMS achieved a higher success rate (77%) than plastic stent(s) (33%) at 12 months follow-up in resolving benign biliary strictures [104].

The median number of ERCP interventions with FC-SEMS was significantly lower than that with plastic stent(s) (1.5 vs. 3.9, $p = 0.002$), and the median duration of stenting was shorter in the FC-SEMS (4.5 months) than in the plastic stent(s) group (11 months) ($p = 0.001$) [104].

However, a randomized controlled trial in 60 patients with CP-related CBD strictures (30 patients received multiple plastic stents (up to 6 plastic stents 10 Fr) and 28 patients a single 10 mm FC-SEMS, during 6 months) found that multiple plastic stenting and FC-SEMS provided similar success rates, 2 years after stent removal (88% in the multiple plastic stents group and 91% in the FC-SEMS group, $p = 0.405$) (Fig. 48.6) [95].

In a metaanalysis of 22 studies including 1298 patients (470 CP), the weighted pooled rate of CP-related biliary stricture resolution with FC-SEMS was 75% (95% CI: 61–85) [82].

Considering only the 4 RCT (213 patients) comparing multiple plastic stenting and FC-SEMS in benign biliary strictures of various origins, similar results for stricture resolution, stricture recurrence and adverse events were reported following temporary insertion of either multiple plastic stents or a FC-SEMS, while fewer ERCPs were required with FC-SEMS [82].

In a large multicenter prospective study including 127 patients with biliary stricture

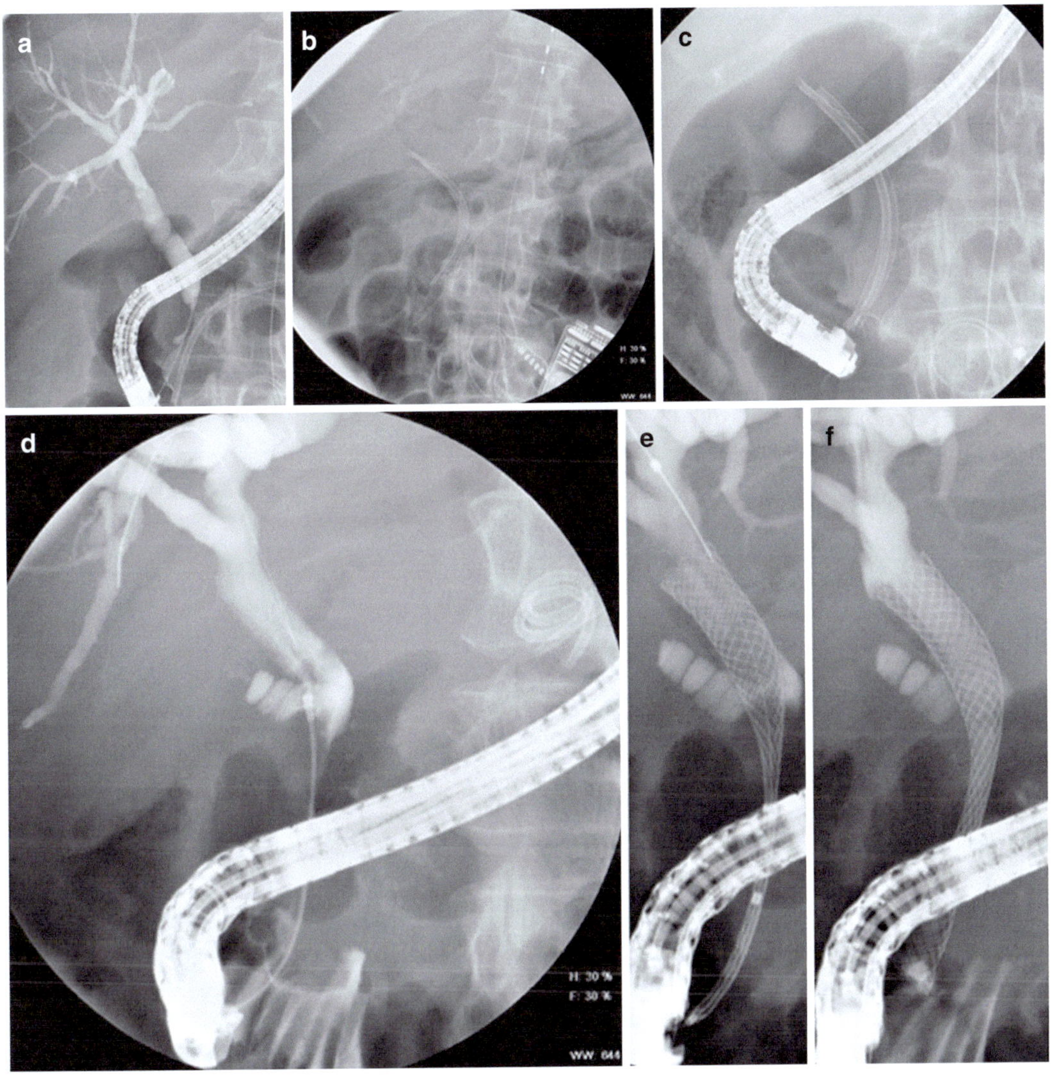

Fig. 48.6 Common bile duct stenting. (**a**) Distal stricture of the common bile duct (CBD) in a patient with chronic pancreatitis. A single plastic 10 Fr, 7 cm-long stent was previously placed in the main pancreatic duct. (**b**) Two biliary plastic stents (10 Fr + 7 Fr) could be successfully placed followed, 3 months later, by placement of 3 new plastic stents (8.5 Fr, 7 cm-long) (**c**). (**d**) Another patient with a CBD stricture-related to chronic pancreatitis and prior cholecystectomy. (**e**, **f**) A fully covered 10 mm, 6 cm-long self-expandable metal stent (Wallflex) was deployed, allowing bile ducts drainage into the duodenum

related to CP, treated with FC-SEMS during a period of 11 months, the restenting of a previously resolved stricture was needed in only 10.5% of cases at 20 months follow-up [105]. The weighted pooled rate for stricture recurrence after FC-SEMS insertion for benign biliary stricture was 16% (95% CI: 11–22) in the metaanalysis [82].

Stent migration is the most frequent adverse events related to FC-SEMS and occurred in 9% of the cases in a metaanalysis of 37 studies (1677 patients with benign biliary strictures) [106].

From the available evidence, FC-SEMS appear to have an excellent efficacy in CP-related biliary stricture. They are as effective as multiple plastic stents but require fewer ERCP to achieve clinical success.

48.3.1.2 Factors Associated with Clinical Success

CP-associated biliary strictures tend to be refractory because of periductal fibrotic tissue and calcifications.

Pancreatic Calcifications in the Head of Pancreas

In a prospective study including 61 patients treated with a single 10 Fr plastic stent, changed every 3 months for a total stenting duration of 12 months, Kahl et al. [89] found pancreatic head calcification was associated with a worse long-term stricture outcome (successful treatment in 8% (3/39) of patients with calcification of the pancreatic head vs. 59% (13/22) of patients without calcification of the pancreatic head, RR 17.3 (4.1–74), $p < 0.001$).

Similar observation was recorded in another study [90] (7% (1/15) vs. 37% (7/19) of patients with and without pancreatic head calcifications, respectively) among patients treated with a single plastic stent.

In contrast, this factor may be less relevant if simultaneous multiple plastic stents are used (success in 5/6 with calcific pancreatitis vs. 6/6 with non-calcific pancreatitis) [90] or if FC-SEMS are used (stricture resolution at the 6-month scheduled removal in 7/11 patients with pancreatic head calcifications vs. 5/6 patients without pancreatic head calcifications, $p = 0.39$) [100].

Concomitant Acute Pancreatitis

Biliary stenting resulted in complete resolution of the CBD stenosis in 11/12 patients (92%) with concomitant acute pancreatitis as opposed to only 11/46 patients (24%) in the group without concomitant acute pancreatitis (OR 33 (2.9–333), $p = 0.005$ in multivariate analysis) [91]. This suggests that CBD stenosis due to compression by an edematous pancreas instead of a fibrotic pancreatic parenchyma could resolve spontaneously when the inflammation subsides.

Stricture Length

In one small study (10 patients), the stricture length was significantly associated with complete stricture improvement (stricture length of 20.5 ± 3.0 mm in the complete group ($n = 6$) vs. 29.0 ± 5.1 mm in the incomplete group ($n = 4$), $p = 0.011$) [96]. Successful results after multiple plastic stenting, during a mean period of 1 year, were recorded only in patients with a stricture length of <24 mm [96].

Finally, despite the feeling that CP patients likely needed longer duration of stenting to allow for adequate stricture remodeling [84, 102], no consistent association was identified between the stricture resolution rate and the duration of biliary SEMS therapy in the metaanalysis [82].

48.3.2 Common Bile Duct Drainage by EUS

ERCP is the preferred procedure for biliary drainage in both benign and malignant obstructions. However, about 3–5% of cases cannot be managed by ERCP because of surgically altered anatomy, variant anatomy, duodenal obstruction, gastric outlet obstruction, periampullary diverticulum, or ampullary pathology.

Conventionally, such patients undergo percutaneous transhepatic biliary drainage. EUS-guided biliary drainage has emerged as an alternative procedure after failed ERCP.

Two approaches have been described, the extra-hepatic approach, where the CBD is accessed through the duodenum or through the gastric antrum with transluminal stent placement (choledochoduodenostomy) or transpapillary stent placement (via the rendez vous technique), and the intra-hepatic approach, where the left intra-hepatic bile ducts were accessed from the gastric wall with transluminal stent placement (hepaticogastrostomy) or transpapillary stent placement (via the rendez vous technique or via the antegrade technique in case of inaccessible papilla) [107].

EUS-guided biliary drainage has mostly been used in malignant conditions. For example, in the metaanalysis by Khan MA et al., [107] including 20 studies and 1186 patients, only 163 patients (14%) had benign biliary strictures from various etiologies. In addition to the heterogeneity among studies, there was no separate analysis for efficacy and safety in malignant vs. benign diseases.

In another systematic review [108], including 42 studies and 1192 patients, data for benign diseases could be extracted from 7 studies ($n = 71$ patients) and reported a technical success rate of 95.8% and a functional success rate of 82.3%.

Overall, no difference statistically significant was identified between transduodenal and transgastric approaches regarding technical and functional success rate.

The average complication rate was 18.9% in a review of 14 studies with more than 50 patients, including 1244 patients [72].

Bile leakage and bleeding were found to be the most common post-procedure adverse events in both the extra-hepatic and intra-hepatic approaches [108] while choledochoduodenostomy appeared significantly safer as compared to hepaticogastrostomy (pooled OR 0.40 (0.18–0.87), $p = 0.022$) [107].

A higher technical success rate was associated with the distal location of the bile duct stricture ($p = 0.0001$), and a higher clinical success rate was associated with the transpapillary method of drainage ($p = 0.0037$) [107].

Functional success rate for malignant conditions was higher than that for benign diseases although both of them had similar technical success rate [108].

So biliary obstruction after failed ERCP that is caused by malignant diseases may be better suited for EUS-guided biliary drainage than benign diseases.

48.4 Conclusions

In painful chronic obstructive pancreatitis, MPD drainage through ERCP ± ESWL or under EUS guidance could provide adequate pain relief, in the long-term, for about two-thirds of patients. However, the quality of evidence of reported results remains low because most published series were retrospectively performed, in single centers, without control group, and the few RCTs were very small sized.

Factors predictive of clinical success have been identified, and it is suggested to treat appropriate candidates early in the disease course, i.e., within the first 2–3 years after symptom onset, with a limited number of endoscopic interventions. It should be acknowledged that ET remains a potential option for patients with co-morbidities occurring in CP such as portal hypertension.

If no persistent pain relief was obtained after a limited trial of endoscopic treatments ± ESWL, that means that other factors than increased pancreatic ductal pressure could be involved in the pain syndrome and for these patients no further attempts at MPD drainage should be proposed.

Treatment of CBD stricture related to CP with a single plastic stent or uncovered SEMS has long been abandoned because of poor long-term results. Both multiple plastic stents and FC-SEMS are effective in the management of benign biliary stricture caused by CP.

References

1. Frulloni L, Falconi M, Gabbrielli A, et al. Italian consensus guidelines for chronic pancreatitis. Dig Liver Dis. 2010;42S:S381–406.
2. Ammann RW, Muellhaupt B. The natural history of pain in alcoholic chronic pancreatitis. Gastroenterology. 1999;116:1132–40.
3. Rösch T, Daniel S, Scholz M, et al. Endoscopic treatment of chronic pancreatitis: a multicenter study of 1000 patients with long-term follow-up. Endoscopy. 2002;34:765–71.
4. Drewes AM, Bouwense SAW, Campbell CM, et al. Guidelines for the understanding and management of pain in chronic pancreatitis. Pancreatology. 2017;17:720–31.
5. Sarner M, Cotton PB. Classification of pancreatitis. Gut. 1984;25:756–9.
6. Abdallah AA, Krige JEJ, Bornman PC. Biliary tract obstruction in chronic pancreatitis. HPB (Oxford). 2007;9:421–8.
7. Mullady DK, Yadav D, Amann ST, et al. Type of pain, pain-associated complications, quality of life, disability and resource utilisation in chronic pancreatitis: a prospective cohort study. Gut. 2011;60:77–84.

8. Bloechle C, Izbicki JR, Knoefel WT, Kuechler T, Broelsch CE. Quality of life in chronic pancreatitis—results after duodenum-preserving resection of the head of the pancreas. Pancreas. 1995;11:77–85.
9. Smits ME, Badiga SM, Rauws EA, Tytgat GN, Huibregtse K. Long-term results of pancreatic stents in chronic pancreatitis. Gastrointest Endosc. 1995;42:461–7.
10. Cremer M, Devière J, Delhaye M, Baize M, Vandermeeren A. Stenting in severe chronic pancreatitis: results of medium-term follow-up in seventy-six patients. Endoscopy. 1991;23:171–6.
11. Binmoeller KF, Jue P, Seifert H, Nam WC, Izbicki J, Soehendra N. Endoscopic pancreatic stent drainage in chronic pancreatitis and a dominant stricture: long-term results. Endoscopy. 1995;27:638–44.
12. Ponchon T, Bory RM, Hedelius F, et al. Endoscopic stenting for pain relief in chronic pancreatitis: results of a standardized protocol. Gastrointest Endosc. 1995;42:452–6.
13. Dumonceau JM, Delhaye M, Tringali A, et al. Endoscopic treatment of chronic pancreatitis: European Society of Gastrointestinal Endoscopy (ESGE) clinical guideline. Endoscopy. 2012;44:784–800.
14. Díte P, Ruzicka M, Zboril V, Novotný I. A prospective, randomized trial comparing endoscopic and surgical therapy for chronic pancreatitis. Endoscopy. 2003;35:553–8.
15. Vitale GC, Cothron K, Vitale EA, et al. Role of pancreatic duct stenting in the treatment of chronic pancreatitis. Surg Endosc. 2004;18:1431–4.
16. Eleftheriadis N, Dinu F, Delhaye M, et al. Long-term outcome after pancreatic stenting in severe chronic pancreatitis. Endoscopy. 2005;37:223–30.
17. Farnbacher MJ, Mühldorfer S, Wehler M, Fischer B, Hahn EG, Schneider HT. Interventional endoscopic therapy in chronic pancreatitis including temporary stenting: a definitive treatment? Scand J Gastroenterol. 2006;41:111–7.
18. Clarke B, Slivka A, Tomizawa Y, et al. Endoscopic therapy is effective for patients with chronic pancreatitis. Clin Gastroenterol Hepatol. 2012;10:795–802.
19. He Y-X, Xu H-W, Sun X-T, et al. Endoscopic management of early-stage chronic pancreatitis based on M-ANNHEIM classification system: a prospective study. Pancreas. 2014;43:829–33.
20. Costamagna G, Bulajic M, Tringali A, et al. Multiple stenting of refractory pancreatic duct strictures in severe chronic pancreatitis: long-term results. Endoscopy. 2006;38:254–9.
21. Bove V, Tringali A, Valerii G, et al. Endoscopic dilation of pancreatic duct strictures in chronic pancreatitis with multiple plastic stents: results in 48 patients. Gastrointest Endosc. 2017;85:AB236.
22. Park DH, Kim MH, Moon SH, Lee SS, Seo DW, Lee SK. Feasibility and safety of placement of a newly designed, fully covered self-expandable metal stent for refractory benign pancreatic ductal strictures: a pilot study (with video). Gastrointest Endosc. 2008;68:1182–9.
23. Sauer B, Talreja J, Ellen K, Ku J, Shami VM, Kahaleh M. Temporary placement of a fully covered self-expandable metal stent in the pancreatic duct for management of symptomatic refractory chronic pancreatitis: preliminary data (with videos). Gastrointest Endosc. 2008;68:1173–8.
24. Moon SH, Kim MH, Park DH, et al. Modified fully covered self-expandable metal stents with antimigration features for benign pancreatic-duct strictures in advanced chronic pancreatitis, with a focus on the safety profile and reducing migration. Gastrointest Endosc. 2010;72:86–91.
25. Giacino C, Grandval P, Laugier R. Fully covered self-expanding metal stents for refractory pancreatic duct strictures in chronic pancreatitis. Endoscopy. 2012;44:874–7.
26. Matsubara S, Sasahira N, Isayama H, et al. Prospective pilot study of fully covered self-expandable metal stents for refractory benign pancreatic duct strictures: long-term outcomes. Endosc Int Open. 2016;4:E1215–22.
27. Oh D, Lee JH, Song TJ, et al. Long-term outcomes of 6-mm diameter fully covered self-expandable metal stents in benign refractory pancreatic ductal stricture. Dig Endosc. 2018;30:508–15.
28. Tringali A, Vadalà di Prampero SF, Landi R, et al. Fully covered self-expandable metal stents to dilate persistent pancreatic strictures in chronic pancreatitis: long-term follow-up from a prospective study. Gastrointest Endosc. 2018;88:939–46.
29. Jafri M, Javed S, Sachdev A, et al. Efficacy of endotherapy in the treatment of pain associated with chronic pancreatitis: a systematic review and meta-analysis. JOP. 2017;18:125–32.
30. Cahen DL, Gouma DJ, Nio Y, et al. Endoscopic versus surgical drainage of the pancreatic duct in chronic pancreatitis. N Engl J Med. 2007;356:676–84.
31. Cahen DL, Gouma DJ, Laramée P, et al. Long-term outcomes of endoscopic vs surgical drainage of the pancreatic duct in patients with chronic pancreatitis. Gastroenterology. 2011;141:1690–5.
32. Topazian M, Aslanian H, Andersen D. Outcome following endoscopic stenting of pancreatic duct strictures in chronic pancreatitis. J Clin Gastroenterol. 2005;39:908–11.
33. Ishihara T, Yamaguchi T, Seza K, Tadenuma H, Saisho H. Efficacy of s-type stents for the treatment of the main pancreatic duct stricture in patients with chronic pancreatitis. Scand J Gastroenterol. 2006;41:744–50.
34. Ikenberry SO, Sherman S, Hawes RH, Smith M, Lehman GA. The occlusion rate of pancreatic stents. Gastrointest Endosc. 1994;40:611–3.
35. Morgan DE, Smith JK, Hawkins K, Wilcox CM. Endoscopic stent therapy in advanced chronic pancreatitis: relationships between ductal changes, clinical response, and stent patency. Am J Gastroenterol. 2003;98:821–6.

36. Farnbacher MJ, Radespiel-Tröger M, König MD, Wehler M, Hahn EG, Schneider HT. Pancreatic endoprostheses in chronic pancreatitis: criteria to predict stent occlusion. Gastrointest Endosc. 2006;63:60–6.
37. Sauer BG, Gurka MJ, Ellen K, Shami VM, Kahaleh M. Effect of pancreatic duct stent diameter on hospitalization in chronic pancreatitis: does size matter? Pancreas. 2009;38:728–31.
38. Sasahira N, Tada M, Isayama H, et al. Outcomes after clearance of pancreatic stones with or without pancreatic stenting. J Gastroenterol. 2007;42:63–9.
39. Seza K, Yamaguchi T, Ishihara T, et al. A long-term controlled trial of endoscopic pancreatic stenting for treatment of main pancreatic duct stricture in chronic pancreatitis. Hepatogastroenterology. 2011;58:2128–31.
40. Delhaye M, Arvanitakis M, Verset G, Cremer M, Devière J. Long-term clinical outcome after endoscopic pancreatic ductal drainage for patients with painful chronic pancreatitis. Clin Gastroenterol Hepatol. 2004;2:1096–106.
41. Eisendrath P, Devière J. Expandable metal stents for benign pancreatic duct obstruction. Gastrointest Endosc Clin N Am. 1999;9:547–54.
42. Shen Y, Liu M, Chen M, Li Y, Lu Y, Zou X. Covered metal stent or multiple plastic stents for refractory pancreatic ductal strictures in chronic pancreatitis: a systematic review. Pancreatology. 2014;14:87–90.
43. Cahen DL, Van der Merwe SW, Laleman W, Poley J-W, Bruno MJ. A biodegradable non-covered self-expandable stent to treat pancreatic duct strictures in chronic pancreatitis: a proof of principle. Gastrointest Endosc. 2018;87:486–91.
44. Issa Y, van Santvoort HC, van Goor H, Cahen DL, Bruno MJ, Boermeester MA. Surgical and endoscopic treatment of pain in chronic pancreatitis: a multidisciplinary update. Dig Surg. 2013;30:35–50.
45. Dumonceau JM, Delhaye M, Tringali A, et al. Endoscopic treatment of chronic pancreatitis: European Society of Gastrointestinal Endoscopy (ESGE) Clinical Guideline—Updated August 2018. Endoscopy. 2019;51(2):179–93.
46. Adamek HE, Jakobs R, Buttmann A, Adamek MU, Schneider AR, Riemann JF. Long term follow up of patients with chronic pancreatitis and pancreatic stones treated with extracorporeal shock wave lithotripsy. Gut. 1999;45:402–5.
47. Farnbacher MJ, Schoen C, Rabenstein T, Benninger J, Hahn EG, Schneider HT. Pancreatic duct stones in chronic pancreatitis: criteria for treatment intensity and success. Gastrointest Endosc. 2002;56:501–6.
48. Inui K, Tazuma S, Yamaguchi T, et al. Treatment of pancreatic stones with extracorporeal shock wave lithotripsy: results of a multicenter survey. Pancreas. 2005;30:26–30.
49. Tadenuma H, Ishihara T, Yamaguchi T, et al. Long-term results of extracorporeal shockwave lithotripsy and endoscopic therapy for pancreatic stones. Clin Gastroenterol Hepatol. 2005;3:1128–35.
50. Seven G, Schreiner MA, Ross AS, et al. Long-term outcomes associated with pancreatic extracorporeal shock wave lithotripsy for chronic calcific pancreatitis. Gastrointest Endosc. 2012;75:997–1004.
51. Suzuki Y, Sugiyama M, Inui K, et al. Management for pancreatolithiasis: a Japanese multicenter study. Pancreas. 2013;42:584–8.
52. Tandan M, Reddy DN, Talukdar R, et al. Long-term clinical outcomes of extracorporeal shockwave lithotripsy in painful chronic calcific pancreatitis. Gastrointest Endosc. 2013;78:726–33.
53. Korpela T, Udd M, Tenca A, et al. Long-term results of combined ESWL and ERCP treatment of chronic calcific pancreatitis. Scand J Gastroenterol. 2016;51:866–71.
54. Wang D, Bi YW, Ji JT, et al. Extracorporeal shock wave lithotripsy is safe and effective for pediatric patients with chronic pancreatitis. Endoscopy. 2017;49:447–55.
55. Inui K, Masamune A, Igarashi Y, et al. Management of pancreatolithiasis: a Nationwide Survey in Japan. Pancreas. 2018;47:708–14.
56. Sherman S, Lehman GA, Hawes RH, et al. Pancreatic ductal stones: frequency of successful endoscopic removal and improvement in symptoms. Gastrointest Endosc. 1991;37:511–7.
57. Dumonceau JM, Devière J, Le Moine O, et al. Endoscopic pancreatic drainage in chronic pancreatitis associated with ductal stones: long-term results. Gastrointest Endosc. 1996;43:547–55.
58. Guda NM, Partington S, Freeman ML. Extracorporeal shock wave lithotripsy in the management of chronic calcific pancreatitis: a meta-analysis. JOP. 2005;6:6–12.
59. Moole H, Jaeger A, Bechtold ML, Forcione D, Taneja D, Puli SR. Success of extracorporeal shock wave lithotripsy in chronic calcific pancreatitis management: a meta-analysis and systematic review. Pancreas. 2016;45:651–8.
60. Delhaye M, Vandermeeren A, Baize M, Cremer M. Extracorporeal shock-wave lithotripsy of pancreatic calculi. Gastroenterology. 1992;102:610–20.
61. Ohyama H, Mikata R, Ishihara T, et al. Efficacy of stone density on noncontrast computed tomography in predicting the outcome of extracorporeal shock wave lithotripsy for patients with pancreatic stones. Pancreas. 2015;44:422–8.
62. Sauerbruch T, Holl J, Sackmann M, Paumgartner G. Extracorporeal lithotripsy of pancreatic stones in patients with chronic pancreatitis and pain: a prospective follow up study. Gut. 1992;33:969–72.
63. Brand B, Kahl M, Sidhu S, et al. Prospective evaluation of morphology, function, and quality of life after extracorporeal shockwave lithotripsy and endoscopic treatment of chronic calcific pancreatitis. Am J Gastroenterol. 2000;95:3428–38.
64. Dumonceau J-M, Costamagna G, Tringali A, et al. Treatment for painful calcified chronic pancreatitis: extracorporeal shock wave lithotripsy versus

endoscopic treatment: a randomised controlled trial. Gut. 2007;56:545–52.
65. Hu L-H, Ye B, Yang Y-G, et al. Extracorporeal shock wave lithotripsy for Chinese patients with pancreatic stones: a prospective study of 214 cases. Pancreas. 2016;45:298–305.
66. Vaysse T, Boytchev I, Antoni G, et al. Efficacy and safety of extracorporeal shock wave lithotripsy for chronic pancreatitis. Scand J Gastroenterol. 2016;51:1380–5.
67. Lapp RT, Wolf JS, Faerber GJ, et al. Duct diameter and size of stones predict successful extracorporeal shock wave lithotripsy and endoscopic clearance in patients with chronic pancreatitis and pancreaticolithiasis. Pancreas. 2016;45:1208–11.
68. Tantau A, Mandrutiu A, Leucuta D-C, Ciobanu L, Tantau M. Prognostic factors of response to endoscopic treatment in painful chronic pancreatitis. World J Gastroenterol. 2017;23:6884–93.
69. Ahmed Ali U, Nieuwenhuijs VB, van Eijck CH, et al. Clinical outcome in relation to timing of surgery in chronic pancreatitis: a nomogram to predict pain relief. Arch Surg. 2012;147:925–32.
70. Liu R, Su W, Gong J, Zhang Y, Lu J. Noncontrast computed tomography factors predictive of extracorporeal shock wave lithotripsy outcomes in patients with pancreatic duct stones. Abdom Radiol (NY). 2018;43:3367–73.
71. Chapman CG, Waxman I, Siddiqui UD. Endoscopic ultrasound (EUS)-guided pancreatic duct drainage: the basics of when and how to perform EUS-guided pancreatic duct interventions. Clin Endosc. 2016;49:161–7.
72. Dhir V, Isayama H, Itoi T. Endoscopic ultrasonography-guided biliary and pancreatic duct interventions. Dig Endosc. 2017;29:472–85.
73. Tessier G, Bories E, Arvanitakis M, et al. EUS-guided pancreatogastrostomy and pancreatobulbostomy for the treatment of pain in patients with pancreatic ductal dilatation inaccessible for transpapillary endoscopic therapy. Gastrointest Endosc. 2007;65:233–41.
74. Seicean A, Vultur S. Endoscopic therapy in chronic pancreatitis: current perspectives. Clin Exp Gastroenterol. 2015;8:1–11.
75. Fujii-Lau LL, Levy MJ. Endoscopic ultrasound-guided pancreatic duct drainage. J Hepatobiliary Pancreat Sci. 2015;22:51–7.
76. Fujii LL, Topazian MD, Abu Dayyeh BK, et al. EUS-guided pancreatic duct intervention: outcomes of a single tertiary-care referral center experience. Gastrointest Endosc. 2013;78:854–64.
77. Will U, Reichel A, Fueldner F, Meyer F. Endoscopic ultrasonography-guided drainage for patients with symptomatic obstruction and enlargement of the pancreatic duct. World J Gastroenterol. 2015;21:13140–51.
78. Chen Y-I, Levy MJ, Moreels TG, et al. An international multicenter study comparing EUS-guided pancreatic duct drainage with enteroscopy-assisted endoscopic retrograde pancreatography after Whipple surgery. Gastrointest Endosc. 2017;85:170–7.
79. Tyberg A, Sharaiha RZ, Kedia P, et al. EUS-guided pancreatic drainage for pancreatic strictures after failed ERCP: a multicenter international collaborative study. Gastrointest Endosc. 2017;85:164–9.
80. Oh D, Park DH, Cho MK, et al. Feasibility and safety of a fully covered self-expandable metal stent with antimigration properties for EUS-guided pancreatic duct drainage: early and mid-term outcomes (with video). Gastrointest Endosc. 2016;83:366–73.
81. Craig PI. Role of endoscopic stenting for biliary strictures in chronic pancreatitis. Dig Endosc. 2012;24(Suppl 1):38–42.
82. Khan MA, Baron TH, Kamal F, et al. Efficacy of self-expandable metal stents in management of benign biliary strictures and comparison with multiple plastic stents: a meta-analysis. Endoscopy. 2017;49:682–94.
83. Deviere J, Devaere S, Baize M, Cremer M. Endoscopic biliary drainage in chronic pancreatitis. Gastrointest Endosc. 1990;36:96–100.
84. Barthet M, Bernard JP, Duval JL, Affriat C, Sahel J. Biliary stenting in benign biliary stenosis complicating chronic calcifying pancreatitis. Endoscopy. 1994;26:569–72.
85. Smits ME, Rauws EA, van Gulik TM, Gouma DJ, Tytgat GN, Huibregtse K. Long-term results of endoscopic stenting and surgical drainage for biliary stricture due to chronic pancreatitis. Br J Surg. 1996;83:764–8.
86. Farnbacher MJ, Rabenstein T, Ell C, Hahn EG, Schneider HT. Is endoscopic drainage of common bile duct stenoses in chronic pancreatitis up-to-date? Am J Gastroenterol. 2000;95:1466–71.
87. Vitale GC, Reed DN, Nguyen CT, Lawhon JC, Larson GM. Endoscopic treatment of distal bile duct stricture from chronic pancreatitis. Surg Endosc. 2000;14:227–31.
88. Eickhoff A, Jakobs R, Leonhardt A, Eickhoff JC, Riemann JF. Endoscopic stenting for common bile duct stenoses in chronic pancreatitis: results and impact on long-term outcome. Eur J Gastroenterol Hepatol. 2001;13:1161–7.
89. Kahl S, Zimmermann S, Genz I, et al. Risk factors for failure of endoscopic stenting of biliary strictures in chronic pancreatitis: a prospective follow-up study. Am J Gastroenterol. 2003;98:2448.
90. Catalano MF, Linder JD, George S, Alcocer E, Geenen JE. Treatment of symptomatic distal common bile duct stenosis secondary to chronic pancreatitis: comparison of single vs. multiple simultaneous stents. Gastrointest Endosc. 2004;60:945–52.
91. Cahen DL, van Berkel A-MM, Oskam D, et al. Long-term results of endoscopic drainage of common bile duct strictures in chronic pancreatitis. Eur J Gastroenterol Hepatol. 2005;17:103–8.
92. Draganov P, Hoffman B, Marsh W, Cotton P, Cunningham J. Long-term outcome in patients with

benign biliary strictures treated endoscopically with multiple stents. Gastrointest Endosc. 2002;55:680–6.
93. Pozsár J, Sahin P, László F, Forró G, Topa L. Medium-term results of endoscopic treatment of common bile duct strictures in chronic calcifying pancreatitis with increasing numbers of stents. J Clin Gastroenterol. 2004;38:118–23.
94. Regimbeau J-M, Fuks D, Bartoli E, et al. A comparative study of surgery and endoscopy for the treatment of bile duct stricture in patients with chronic pancreatitis. Surg Endosc. 2012;26:2902–8.
95. Haapamäki C, Kylänpää L, Udd M, et al. Randomized multicenter study of multiple plastic stents vs covered self-expandable metallic stent in the treatment of biliary stricture in chronic pancreatitis. Endoscopy. 2015;47:605–10.
96. Ohyama H, Mikata R, Ishihara T, et al. Efficacy of multiple biliary stenting for refractory benign biliary strictures due to chronic calcifying pancreatitis. World J Gastrointest Endosc. 2017;9:12–8.
97. Cahen DL, Rauws EA, Gouma DJ, Fockens P, Bruno MJ. Removable fully covered self-expandable metal stents in the treatment of common bile duct strictures due to chronic pancreatitis: a case series. Endoscopy. 2008;40:697–700.
98. Behm B, Brock A, Clarke BW, et al. Partially covered self-expandable metallic stents for benign biliary strictures due to chronic pancreatitis. Endoscopy. 2009;41:547–51.
99. Mahajan A, Ho H, Sauer B, et al. Temporary placement of fully covered self-expandable metal stents in benign biliary strictures: midterm evaluation (with video). Gastrointest Endosc. 2009;70:303–9.
100. Perri V, Boskoski I, Tringali A, et al. Fully covered self-expandable metal stents in biliary strictures caused by chronic pancreatitis not responding to plastic stenting: a prospective study with 2 years of follow-up. Gastrointest Endosc. 2012;75:1271–7.
101. Deviere J, Nageshwar Reddy D, Püspök A, et al. Successful management of benign biliary strictures with fully covered self-expanding metal stents. Gastroenterology. 2014;147:385–95.
102. Saxena P, Diehl DL, Kumbhari V, et al. A US multicenter study of safety and efficacy of fully covered self-expandable metallic stents in benign extrahepatic biliary strictures. Dig Dis Sci. 2015;60:3442–8.
103. Hu B, Sun B, Cai Q, et al. Asia-Pacific consensus guidelines for endoscopic management of benign biliary strictures. Gastrointest Endosc. 2017;86:44–58.
104. Siiki A, Helminen M, Sand J, Laukkarinen J. Covered self-expanding metal stents may be preferable to plastic stents in the treatment of chronic pancreatitis-related biliary strictures: a systematic review comparing 2 methods of stent therapy in benign biliary strictures. J Clin Gastroenterol. 2014;48:635–43.
105. Deviere J, Cremer M, Baize M, Love J, Sugai B, Vandermeeren A. Management of common bile duct stricture caused by chronic pancreatitis with metal mesh self expandable stents. Gut. 1994;35:122–6.
106. Zheng X, Wu J, Sun B, et al. Clinical outcome of endoscopic covered metal stenting for resolution of benign biliary stricture: systematic review and meta-analysis. Dig Endosc. 2017;29:198–210.
107. Khan MA, Akbar A, Baron TH, et al. Endoscopic ultrasound-guided biliary drainage: a systematic review and meta-analysis. Dig Dis Sci. 2016;61:684–703.
108. Wang K, Zhu J, Xing L, et al. Assessment of efficacy and safety of EUS-guided biliary drainage: a systematic review. Gastrointest Endosc. 2016;83:1218–27.

49 Pancreatic Fistulas

Stefanos M. Dokas

49.1 Initial Diagnosis: Symptoms

The clinical symptoms related with a pancreatic fistula are usually non-specific such as abdominal discomfort, bloating, nausea, and abdominal pain. These symptoms usually accompany a non-typical postoperative course. Delayed gastric emptying is another frequent sign especially when a collection is formed [1]. Fever, along with increased leukocyte count and elevated CRP, denotes the presence of infection and possibly sepsis. Elevated procalcitonin and CRP may provide early evidence of complications including the presence of pancreatic fistula in the early postoperative period [2].

Identifying amylase-rich fluid in the postoperative drain provides the first working diagnosis. Amylase activity cut-off point between normal and abnormal values was defined by the International Study Group on Pancreatic Fistula (ISGPF) [3] as three times the upper normal serum amylase activity value at or after postoperative day 3. A more precise diagnosis requires locating the site of leakage. This is crucial to management. Both invasive and non-invasive methods can be used to localize the leak.

S. M. Dokas (✉)
Endoscopy Department, St. Luke's Private Hospital, Thessaloniki, Greece
e-mail: altair@med.auth.gr

The first imaging modality used is usually computed tomography (CT). The preferred protocol is thin slice, contrast-enhanced CT. The leak is usually close to the fluid collection. The pancreatic duct can be visualized by applying post-processing techniques such as multiplanar reformation [4, 5]. The site of ductal disruption can be recognized during this process [6]. The presence of air bubbles within a peripancreatic collection is a valid indication for the presence of a pancreatic fistula [7].

Magnetic resonance is another option for localizing the site of ductal leak. MRCP with or without secretin enhancement has been shown to identify the leak in most cases [8]. Moreover, MRCP provides additional information regarding concurrent conditions such as pancreatic duct stenosis or stones and ultimately for assessing the integrity of the pancreatic duct [9]. An important advantage is the ability to visualize the pancreatic duct upstream a complete disruption.

Fistulography is a valuable imaging technique to establish the diagnosis of pancreatic fistula. It is easy to perform, readily available, and cost effective. Fistulograms are especially useful after pancreatectomy and particularly after Whipple's procedure, in order to access the integrity of the pancreatic anastomosis and reveal dehiscence or anastomotic leaks [10]. This retrograde approach has therapeutic possibilities in some cases.

M. Mutignani et al. (eds.), *Endotherapy in Biliopancreatic Diseases: ERCP Meets EUS*,
https://doi.org/10.1007/978-3-030-42569-2_49

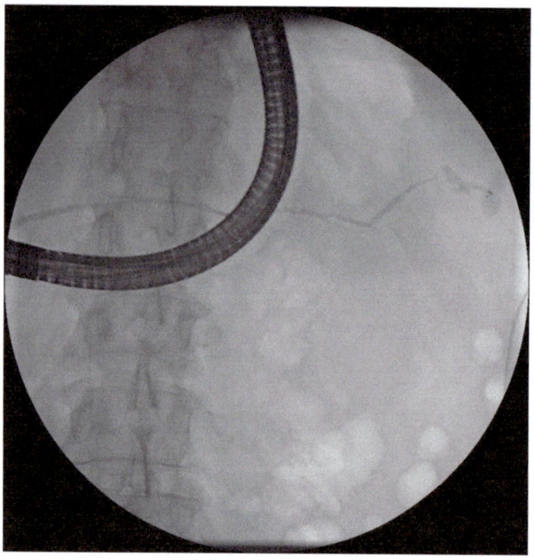

Fig. 49.1 Pancreatic leak from pancreatic tail (fluoroscopic view) (Kindly granted by M. Mutignani)

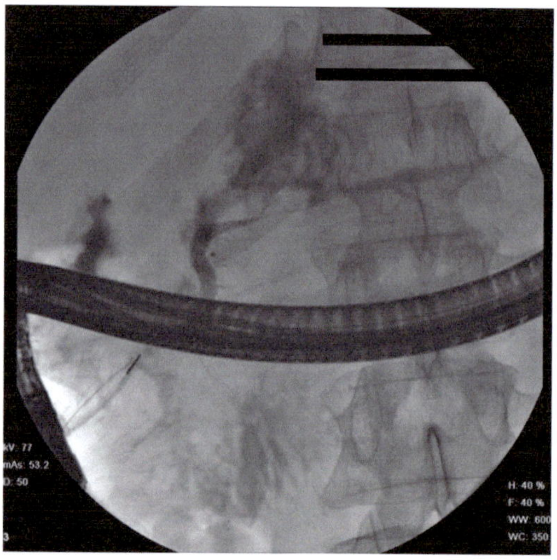

Fig. 49.2 Pancreatic leak due to traumatic transection of the main pancreatic duct (fluoroscopic view) (Kindly granted by M. Mutignani)

The gold standard in evaluating pancreatic leaks is Endoscopic Retrograde Cholangiopancreatography (ERCP). The real-time filling of the pancreatic duct with contrast medium is unique in revealing the site of the leak (Figs. 49.1, 49.2, and 49.3). The major disadvantage is that the method is invasive and carries a small but nonnegligible risk of complications. ERCP should be considered whenever endotherapy can be provided on the spot. This entails careful

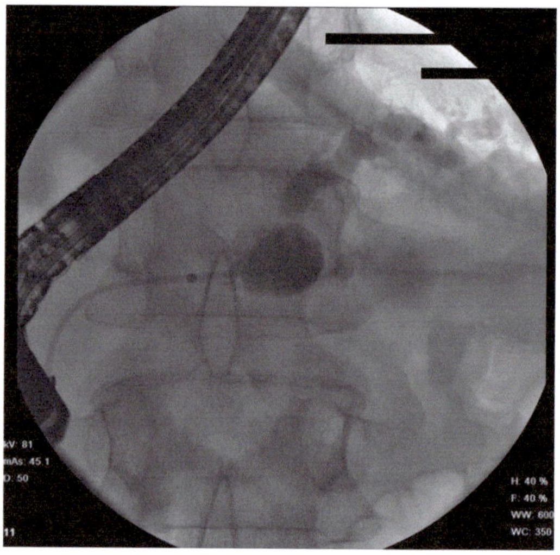

Fig. 49.3 Pancreatic leak due to surgical transection of the main pancreatic duct with closed distal portion of the main pancreatic duct (fluoroscopic view) (Kindly granted by M. Mutignani)

assessment of the clinical condition and preoperative and intraoperative imaging. Otherwise, the invasive nature of the procedure adds unnecessary risk to the treatment plan.

49.2 Management of Pancreatic Fistula

Pancreatic leaks vary in severity. The ISGPF in 2005 defined and graded the severity of postoperative pancreatic fistulas [1]. The group classified postoperative pancreatic fistulas in three grades according to severity (Table 49.1). It is clear from the parameters used that prevention of infection and sepsis is crucial in the clinical course of these patients. Obviously one of the most important actions is to minimize the risk of infection early in the course of the leak. Electrolyte and fluid balance is another keystone. In particular sodium and bicarbonate depletion may be severe and depending on the volume of the leaking fluid may further deteriorate the general condition. Patient stabilization, resuscitation, and early control of infection are therefore the first steps toward successful management. Finally nutritional support with early enteral feeding or total parenteral nutrition aids in reversing the catabolic state.

Table 49.1 Postoperative pancreatic fistula clinical severity classification

Grade	A	B	C
Clinical conditions	Well	Often well	Ill appearing/bad
Specific treatment[a]	No	Yes/no	Yes
Ultrasonography/CT (if obtained)	Negative	Negative/positive	Positive
Persistent drainage (after 3 weeks)[b]	No	Usually yes	Yes
Reoperation	No	No	Yes
Death related to fistula	No	No	Possibly yes
Signs of infections	No	Yes	Yes
Sepsis	No	No	Yes
Readmission	No	Yes/no	Yes/no

Reproduced from [3]
[a]Partial (peripheral) or total parenteral nutrition, antibiotics, enteral nutrition, somatostatin analogue, and/or minimal invasive drainage
[b]With or without a drain in situ

The first steps in managing pancreatic fistulas are therefore supportive and common in all cases, regardless of etiology. Drainage of the fluid and all associated collections is the next step. All collections should be appropriately drained in order to minimize the risk of infection. Undrained collections, if discovered, should be drained percutaneously. Broad-spectrum antibiotics are mandatory at this stage. Nutritional support should be aggressive through either enteral feeding or total parenteral nutrition (TPN). Enteral feeding maintains the intestinal mucosal barrier function; it is easy to perform and cost-effective [11], but the longstanding presence of a nasoenteric tube is not well tolerated. On the other hand, TPN minimizes the pancreatic exocrine function; it is well tolerated but may be associated with line infections and parenteral nutrition–associated liver disease in prolonged cases [12].

Somatostatin inhibits the exocrine pancreatic function, as well as biliary and enteric secretions. In theory, it could aid in the treatment of pancreatic fistulas, promoting fistula closure time. Systematic reviews on the few trials/case series published concluded in conflicting results. Somatostatin is regularly used during the perioperative period in order to reduce the incidence of pancreatic fistula [13]. Yet, after the occurrence of a pancreatic fistula, the use of somatostatin offers no major benefit on fistula closure [14]. More research is needed in order to clarify the proper use of somatostatin and its analogues.

49.3 Biliary and Pancreatic Leaks

Biliary leaks are easily managed endoscopically. The treatment of choice is endoscopic sphincterotomy with or without biliary stent or nasobiliary drainage complemented with drainage of the bilious fluid [15]. In general, the same principles are employed for a pancreatic fistula. The two conditions share many similar attributes but also crucial differences.

The main difference is in the fluid secretion pattern from the liver and the pancreas. Bile is secreted from hepatocytes [16] and modified by cholangiocytes as bile courses through the ducts. Bile production follows tonic pattern with low extrinsic interference. The rate of bile production is around 25 mL/h, or approximately 620 mL/day [17].

On the other hand, pancreatic fluid secretion is a highly regulated process with both tonic and phasic pattern of production. In the fasting state, human pancreatic exocrine secretion is cyclical and closely correlated with upper gastrointestinal motility. Ingestion of a regular meal induces postprandial enzyme secretion. When maximally stimulated, from acetylcholine and cholecystokinine, pancreatic juice production reaches a rate of 30–100 mL/min. As a consequence, this phasic burst in pancreatic juice production leads to high intraductal pressure at the same time. This is the reason why a simple pancreatic sphincterotomy is not enough to cure the leak.

49.4 General Principles of Fluid Circulation

Fluid flows following the pressure gradient from a region of high pressure to a lower pressure zone. This is a fundamental principle with application in fistula management and closure. In every case, the intraabdominal pressure is the highest, followed by the enteric intraluminal pressure and the atmospheric pressure, which is the lowest of all. Furthermore, the presence of an intaabdominal drain modifies the pressure balance around it. A drain placed very close to the leakage lowers the local pressure and diverts the fluid through the drain, thus maintaining the external fistula.

For the fistula to close, the goal is to divert the fluid from the leakage site toward the intestine. The preferable route is through the existing anatomic structures, i.e., the pancreatic duct. If this is impossible, the next best thing is to create a new route, usually through gastric or enteric wall puncture and stent placement. Bearing in mind all these barometric conditions, a review of current literature on the endoscopic management of pancreatic fistulas follows.

49.5 Endoscopic Management of Pancreatic Fistulas

The majority of uncomplicated type A fistulas will close spontaneously a few weeks after drainage. In patients with a stable course and low-volume leaks, a gradual drain removal can be performed. This begins with the removal of suction at first. Later, if the condition remains good, downsizing of the drainage catheter is done and afterward the catheter is withdrawn slightly every day while monitoring the volume of drained fluid. Grade B and C fistulas will, most certainly, require some sort of further intervention.

Endoscopic therapy for pancreatic leaks is being performed for more than 20 years. The progress made during these two decades is considerable, given the low incidence of the condition.

As mentioned above, the goal is to establish a favorable pressure gradient so as to facilitate fluid flow toward the intestine. The choice of endotherapy offered depends on the location (side branch/main pancreatic duct, head, body, and tail) and the postsurgical anatomy. In many cases, especially when leaks develop in the context of chronic pancreatitis, pancreatic duct stones or stenosis downstream may represent a key factor of fistula perpetuation. Such conditions, whenever encountered, should be accordingly dealt with, either with dilation/stenting or stone extraction to ensure free flow within the Wirsung duct. A comprehensive endoscopic classification including a treatment algorithm from a recent publication from our group is listed in Table 49.2 [18].

Small side branch leaks or "parenchymal" leaks can be treated with stenting of the main pancreatic duct (Fig. 49.4). Pancreatic head and body leaks are the easiest to treat. A pancreatic stent, after sphincterotomy, placed beyond the leakage site is the treatment of choice.

Table 49.2 Endoscopy-oriented classification of pancreatic leaks

Leak type	Subtype	Endoscopic intervention
I (Parenchymal or small side branch leaks)	Head (IH)	Bridging stent or nasopancreatic drain (NPD)
	Body (IB)	Bridging stent or NPD
	Tail (IT)	Bridging stent if duct caliber allows Cyanoacrylate/fibrin glue/other polymer injection at pancreatic tail/fistulous tract
II (Main pancreatic duct leaks)	Open proximal stump (IIO)	Bridging stent or NPD Extrapancreatic transpapillary protruding stent
	Closed proximal stump (IIC)	EUS + transmural drain of fluid collection from the distal gland into stomach/intestine EUS-guided pancreaticogastrostomy Conversion to open + bridging stent/NPD
III (Post pancreatectomy leaks)	Proximal (IIIP)	Transpapillary protruding stent to drain the collection
	Distal (IIID)	Drain the CBD and the jejunum at the level of anastomosis + EUS for transmural drain of peripancreatic collections or pancreaticogastrostomy

Reproduced from [18]

Obstruction of the duct (stricture/stone), whenever encountered, should be accordingly addressed to complement proposed endotherapy

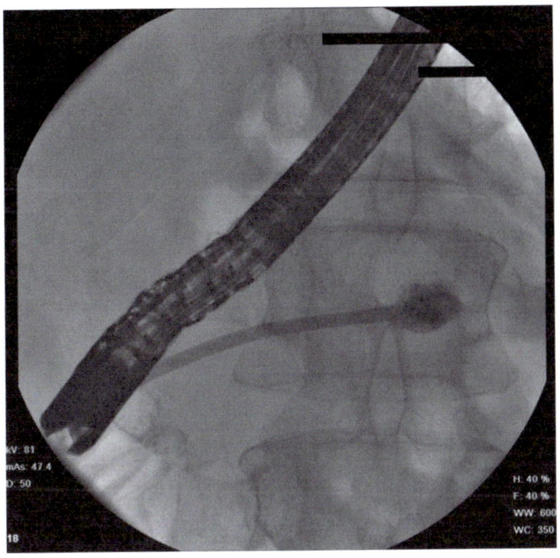

Fig. 49.4 Pancreatic leak treated by stent placement in the main pancreatic leak (fluoroscopic view) (Kindly granted by M. Mutignani)

Nasopancreatic drain is an alternative, but problematic for long-term treatment due to patient discomfort. The stenting treatment has been validated from many studies and has high success rates. The series from Kozarek et al. were among the first published on the topic [19, 20]. Others have published series with similar results [21].

Pancreatic tail leaks, on the other hand, may present with technical difficulties for the endoscopist. The narrow caliber of a normal pancreatic duct at the tail is the main difficulty. A stent may not be able to reach beyond the leakage site in the tail. Furthermore, if the leak is at the very end of the tail, there is no distal duct to stent. This may hinder endoscopic therapy, but in any case stenting of the duct up to the closest to the leak should be attempted.

To overcome this difficulty, plugging the leak with different sealing material has been proposed. Fibrin glue can be injected into the distal pancreatic duct to seal the leak. The treatment is complemented with nasopancreatic drainage and possibly with several and sequential fibrin glue injections [22]. The retrograde approach, i.e., injecting through the fistulous tract has been used to deliver fibrin glue successfully [23]. Other substances used for the same purpose are cyanoacrylates and Onyx [24–26]. Both substances act as plugs. The experience with cyanoacrylate and Onyx is limited and better be reserved only as a rescue method to avoid surgery in persisting cases and/or high-risk surgical candidates.

When the leakage originates from the main pancreatic duct, we use the term "disruption" to describe a partial transection. The term "disconnected pancreatic duct" is used to describe total transection of the Wirsung duct. Both conditions are usually accompanied by peripancreatic fluid collections and/or pseudocysts. In every case, the goal of endoscopic treatment is to bridge the duct and restore continuity and ductal patency. This can be accomplished in most cases of disruption. Fluid collections can be drained transpapillary with stenting or nasopancreatic drainage at the same time.

Kozarek et al. [19] were the first to publish their series. Both transpapillary stenting and transpapillary drainage of peripancreatic fluid were performed with success. Varadarajulu et al. [27] published their retrospective series which is the largest in the literature. They studied 92 cases in 7 years and they treated successfully 52 patients. They concluded that ductal disruption and bridging stenting were associated with a positive outcome. Similarly, Telford et al. [28] concluded that bridging stenting and prolonged stenting was associated with a positive outcome. In the study by Rana et al. [29], the authors used nasopancreatic drain instead of stents. The advantage of the nasopancreatic drain catheter is that it can be flushed and cleaned with saline in case of obstruction. Furthermore, a pancreatogram can be obtained easily without the need for ERCP.

In the scenario of disconnected pancreatic duct, quite often the proximal stump at the time of ERCP is already closed, so access to the distal duct is impossible in most cases. Endoscopic ultrasonographic (EUS)-guided transmural drain of the fluid collection maintained with double pigtail stents is probably the best and easiest approach. The technique is well known. Under EUS guidance, a puncture is made on the gastric or duodenal wall in order to enter the fluid collection. After dilation with dilating balloon, two or more double pigtail stents are inserted into the cavity. These stents are to be left indefinitely as shown by the only prospective study in the field by Arvanitakis et al. [30]. The effectiveness of this approach has been validated also from other studies [31–34]. Another option is to perform an EUS-guided distal pancreaticogastrostomy in order to divert the distal gland juice into the stomach [35, 36]. Pancreaticoduodenostomy is another similar repair [31]. A final option is to perforate the closed proximal stump with a stiff wire, or a catheter, and try to cannulate the distal duct with bridging stenting being the ultimate goal [18].

Recently, there is a trend to treat associated fluid collections with the implantation of fully covered lumen-apposing metal stents (LAMS), placed under EUS guidance. Some delivery systems have an electrocautery tip, enabling the procedure to be completed very fast, as a single-step intervention. This technique is particularly valuable in the case of walled-off necrosis where endoscopic necrosectomy may be indicated [37, 38].

Leaks after pancreatic resection is another condition encountered relatively frequently. Several risk factors (gland texture, underlying pathology, blood loss during surgery, technical issues regarding the anastomosis, etc.) have been identified that may affect the occurrence of pancreatic fistula in the postoperative period. Leaks after distal pancreatectomy are best amenable to endoscopic treatment because the access to the papilla is not hampered. The endotherapy of choice is transpapillary stenting with the stent protruding outside the gland into the collection in order to divert fluid toward the intestine, which is very effective in closing the leak [39, 40]. If a percutaneous drain is in placed at the vicinity, the tube should be withdrawn slightly to facilitate internal drainage.

Leaks after pancreaticoduodenectomy are more complex (Figs. 49.5 and 49.6). These leaks are most likely due to anastomotic dehiscence rather than true pancreatic fistulas (Fig. 49.7). The condition usually deteriorates quickly partly due to enzyme activation in the presence of enterokinase. The limited access to the anastomosis due to altered anatomy after pancreaticoduodenectomy is another major factor limiting the implementation of endotherapy. The best approach is to drain thoroughly the leaking fluid (both enteric and pancreatic) and to avoid sepsis. EUS-guided transgastric drainage and, in the presence of a dilated pancre-

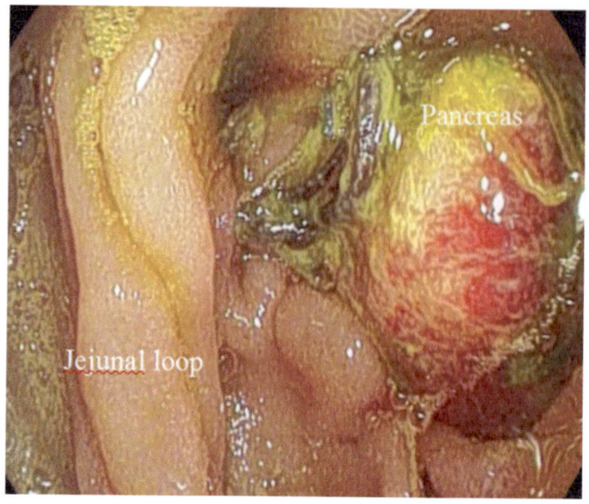

Fig. 49.5 Leak of telescopic pancreatic-jejunal anastomosis (endoscopic view) (Kindly granted by M. Mutignani)

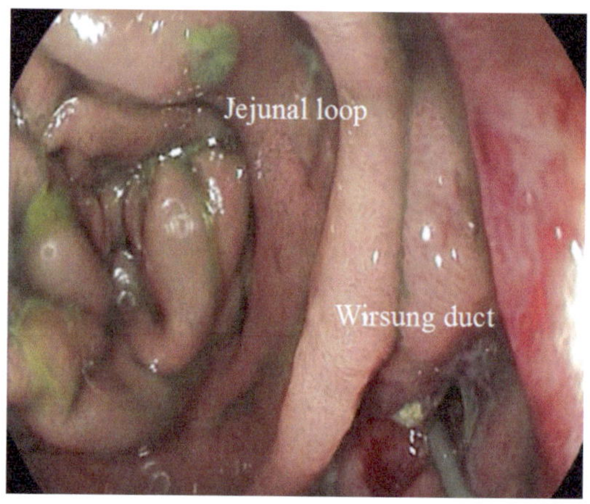

Fig. 49.6 Leak of Wirsung-to-jejunum anastomosis (endoscopic view) (Kindly granted by M. Mutignani)

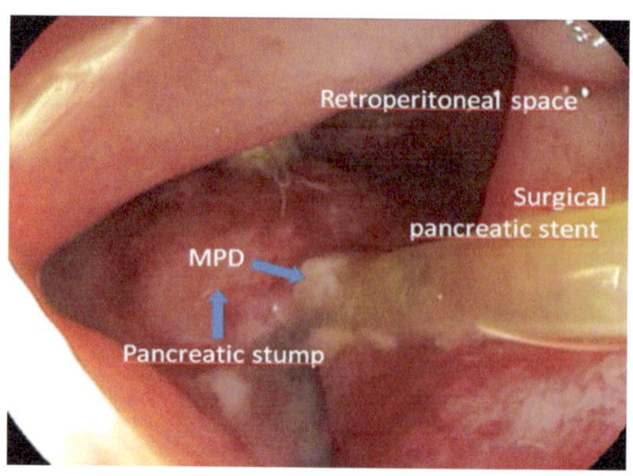

Fig. 49.7 Complete dehiscence of Wirsung-to-jejunum anastomosis (endoscopic view). *MPD:* main pancreatic duct (Kindly granted by M. Mutignani)

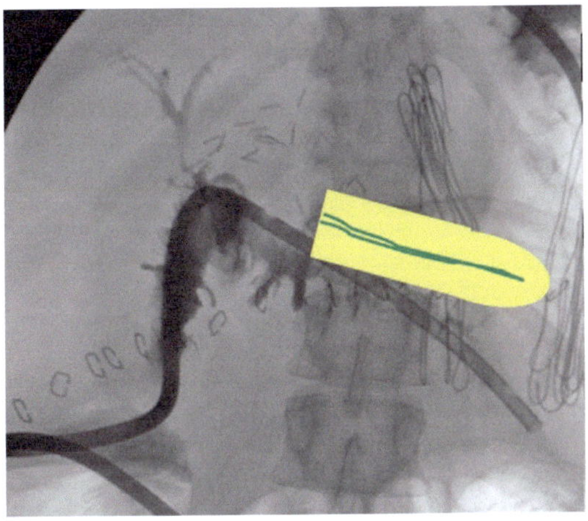

Fig. 49.8 Pancreatic fistula after duodenopancreatectomy treated by naso-retroperitoneal drain. The yellow pancreatic stump has been drawn to illustrate the complete dehiscence (Kindly granted by M. Mutignani)

atic duct, EUS transgastric pancreaticogastrostomy are valid and tested options with good results [41]. Access to the dehiscence site is easy when a pancreaticogastric anastomosis is performed. In this situation, the dehiscence is easily identified with a gastroscope and double pigtail stents can be inserted to maintain internal drainage (Fig. 49.8) as described by Bartoli et al. [42].

49.6 Endotherapy Complications

Although safe, endotherapy may be complicated with adverse events. Besides the usual complications related with sedation, post-ERCP pancreatitis is the most frequent adverse event, especially if stenting fails. But even in this case, a small stent may help downgrading the severity of post-ERCP pancreatitis by maintaining papillary flow [43]. Bleeding from the sphincterotomy or perforations occur with the usual incidence. Bacterial contamination of fluid collections is another serious complication. Administration of antibiotics prior to ERCP should be the rule in such cases. If however contamination occurs, continuation of antibiotics and percutaneous drainage are indicated.

In the long term, stents can induce pancreatic duct changes [44]. Stent caliber should be selected not to exceed the ductal width. Stent length should also be chosen wisely according to the distance between the papilla and the leak. A 5Fr stent suits most normal caliber ducts and can be inserted over a 0.035 wire, whereas a 3Fr stent is inserted over a 0.025 guide, thus requiring wire exchange. Moreover, 3Fr stents tend to migrate easily. In dilated ducts, 7Fr or even 8.5Fr stents may be inserted depending on duct diameter. In order to minimize stent-related ductal changes [44] and to reduce the risk of pancreatic sepsis [45], transpapillary stents should be removed within 7–10 days after fistula closure.

49.7 Surgical Treatment

Surgical treatment is the final solution in pancreatic leaks not responding to conservative and minimally invasive management. The main indications are the disconnected pancreatic duct syndrome, surgical debridement of pancreatic necrosis, and concurrent ductal stenosis not responding to endotherapy in the context of chronic pancreatitis. The usual approach is distal pancreatectomy, especially when splenic vein thrombosis is present [46]. When the leak is located at the head/jenu region, a fistulojejunostomy after maturing of the fistulous tract is another valid option in order to preserve the pancreas [47]. Total pancreatectomy is the last resort.

49.8 Conclusion

Patients presenting with pancreatic leaks are best managed by a multidisciplinary group of surgeons, gastroenterologists, and interventional radiologists. Endotherapy provided during ERCP is a pillar in current management. Transpapillary stenting is the most frequent intervention to treat pancreatic leaks. EUS-guided transmural drainage is a valuable and effective treatment option for disconnected pancreatic duct syndrome and pseudocysts. Surgical treatment is related with substantial morbidity and mortality and therefore should be reserved for cases refractory to endotherapy or other interventional treatments.

References

1. Malleo G, Crippa S, Butturini G, Salvia R, Partelli S, Rossini R, et al. Delayed gastric emptying after pylorus-preserving pancreaticoduodenectomy: validation of International Study Group of Pancreatic Surgery classification and analysis of risk factors. HPB (Oxford). 2010;12(9):610–8. https://doi.org/10.1111/j.1477-2574.2010.00203.x. S1365-182X(15)30343–9 [pii].
2. Giardino A, Spolverato G, Regi P, Frigerio I, Scopelliti F, Girelli R, et al. C-Reactive protein and procalcitonin as predictors of postoperative inflammatory complications after pancreatic surgery. J Gastrointest Surg. 2016;20(8):1482–92. https://doi.org/10.1007/s11605-016-3171-6. 1007/s11605-016-3171-6 [pii].
3. Bassi C, Dervenis C, Butturini G, Fingerhut A, Yeo C, Izbicki J, et al. Postoperative pancreatic fistula: an international study group (ISGPF) definition. Surgery. 2005;138(1):8–13. https://doi.org/10.1016/j.surg.2005.05.001. S0039606005002291 [pii].
4. Itoh S, Ikeda M, Ota T, Satake H, Takai K, Ishigaki T. Assessment of the pancreatic and intrapancreatic bile ducts using 0.5-mm collimation and multiplanar reformatted images in multislice CT. Eur Radiol. 2003;13(2):277–85. https://doi.org/10.1007/s00330-002-1516-x.
5. Kakihara D, Yoshimitsu K, Irie H, Tajima T, Asayama Y, Hirakawa M, et al. Usefulness of the long-axis and short-axis reformatted images of multidetector-row CT in evaluating T-factor of the surgically resected pancreaticobiliary malignancies. Eur J Radiol. 2007;63(1):96–104. https://doi.org/10.1016/j.ejrad.2007.01.022. S0720-048X(07)00046-0 [pii].
6. O'Toole D, Vullierme MP, Ponsot P, Maire F, Calmels V, Hentic O, et al. Diagnosis and management of pancreatic fistulae resulting in pancreatic ascites or pleural effusions in the era of helical CT and magnetic resonance imaging. Gastroenterol Clin Biol. 2007;31(8-9 Pt 1):686–93. MDOI-GCB-09-2007-31-8-9-C1-0399-8320-101019-200520009 [pii].
7. Raman SP, Horton KM, Cameron JL, Fishman EK. CT after pancreaticoduodenectomy: spectrum of normal findings and complications. AJR Am J Roentgenol. 2013;201(1):2–13. https://doi.org/10.2214/AJR.12.9647.
8. Gillams AR, Kurzawinski T, Lees WR. Diagnosis of duct disruption and assessment of pancreatic leak with dynamic secretin-stimulated MR cholangiopancreatography. AJR Am J Roentgenol. 2006;186(2):499–506. https://doi.org/10.2214/AJR.04.1775. 186/2/499 [pii].
9. Drake LM, Anis M, Lawrence C. Accuracy of magnetic resonance cholangiopancreatography in identifying pancreatic duct disruption. J Clin Gastroenterol. 2012;46(8):696–9. https://doi.org/10.1097/MCG.0b013e31825003b3.
10. Malleo G, Pulvirenti A, Marchegiani G, Butturini G, Salvia R, Bassi C. Diagnosis and management of postoperative pancreatic fistula. Langenbecks Arch Surg. 2014;399(7):801–10. https://doi.org/10.1007/s00423-014-1242-2.
11. Schorghuber M, Fruhwald S. Effects of enteral nutrition on gastrointestinal function in patients who are critically ill. Lancet Gastroenterol Hepatol. 2018;3(4):281–7. https://doi.org/10.1016/S2468-1253(18)30036-0. S2468-1253(18)30036-0 [pii].
12. Buchman AL, Iyer K, Fryer J. Parenteral nutrition-associated liver disease and the role for isolated intestine and intestine/liver transplantation. Hepatology. 2006;43(1):9–19. https://doi.org/10.1002/hep.20997.
13. Jin K, Zhou H, Zhang J, Wang W, Sun Y, Ruan C, et al. Systematic review and meta-analysis of somatostatin analogues in the prevention of postoperative complication after pancreaticoduodenectomy. Dig Surg. 2015;32(3):196–207. https://doi.org/10.1159/000381032. 000381032 [pii].
14. Gans SL, van Westreenen HL, Kiewiet JJ, Rauws EA, Gouma DJ, Boermeester MA. Systematic review and meta-analysis of somatostatin analogues for the treatment of pancreatic fistula. Br J Surg. 2012;99(6):754–60. https://doi.org/10.1002/bjs.8709.
15. Lakhtakia S, Reddy DN. Pancreatic leaks: endo-therapy first? J Gastroenterol Hepatol. 2009;24(7):1158–60. https://doi.org/10.1111/j.1440-1746.2009.05926.x.
16. Forker EL. Two sites of bile formation as determined by mannitol and erythritol clearance in the Guinea pig. J Clin Invest. 1967;46(7):1189–95. https://doi.org/10.1172/JCI105612.
17. Esteller A. Physiology of bile secretion. World J Gastroenterol. 2008;14(37):5641–9.
18. Mutignani M, Dokas S, Tringali A, Forti E, Pugliese F, Cintolo M, et al. Pancreatic leaks and fistulae: an endoscopy-oriented classification. Dig Dis Sci. 2017;62(10):2648–57. https://doi.org/10.1007/s10620-017-4697-5. 10.1007/s10620-017-4697-5 [pii].
19. Kozarek RA, Ball TJ, Patterson DJ, Freeny PC, Ryan JA, Traverso LW. Endoscopic transpapillary therapy for disrupted pancreatic duct and peripancreatic fluid collections. Gastroenterology. 1991;100(5 Pt 1):1362–70. S0016508591001774 [pii].
20. Kozarek RA, Ball TJ, Patterson DJ, Raltz SL, Traverso LW, Ryan JA, et al. Transpapillary stenting for pancreaticocutaneous fistulas. J Gastrointest Surg. 1997;1(4):357–61. S1091255X97800571 [pii].
21. Cicek B, Parlak E, Oguz D, Disibeyaz S, Koksal AS, Sahin B. Endoscopic treatment of pancreatic fistulas. Surg Endosc. 2006;20(11):1706–12. https://doi.org/10.1007/s00464-005-0764-7.
22. Engler S, Dorlars D, Riemann JF. Endoscopic fibrin gluing of a pancreatic duct fistula following acute pancreatitis. Dtsch Med Wochenschr. 1996;121(45):1396–400. https://doi.org/10.1055/s-2008-1043159.

23. Fischer A, Benz S, Baier P, Hopt UT. Endoscopic management of pancreatic fistulas secondary to intraabdominal operation. Surg Endosc. 2004;18(4):706–8. https://doi.org/10.1007/s00464-003-9087-8.
24. Seewald S, Brand B, Groth S, Omar S, Mendoza G, Seitz U, et al. Endoscopic sealing of pancreatic fistula by using N-butyl-2-cyanoacrylate. Gastrointest Endosc. 2004;59(4):463–70. S0016510703027081 [pii].
25. Mutignani M, Tringali A, Khodadadian E, Petruzziello L, Spada C, Spera G, et al. External pancreatic fistulas resistant to conventional endoscopic therapy: endoscopic closure with N-butyl-2-cyanoacrylate (Glubran 2). Endoscopy. 2004;36(8):738–42. https://doi.org/10.1055/s-2004-825672.
26. Zuber-Jerger I, Herold T, Kullmann F. Transpapillary sealing of a pancreatic fistula with Onyx. Gastrointest Endosc. 2006;63(7):1068–9. https://doi.org/10.1016/j.gie.2005.11.006; discussion 9. S0016-5107(05)03213-X [pii].
27. Varadarajulu S, Noone TC, Tutuian R, Hawes RH, Cotton PB. Predictors of outcome in pancreatic duct disruption managed by endoscopic transpapillary stent placement. Gastrointest Endosc. 2005;61(4):568–75. S0016510704028329 [pii].
28. Telford JJ, Farrell JJ, Saltzman JR, Shields SJ, Banks PA, Lichtenstein DR, et al. Pancreatic stent placement for duct disruption. Gastrointest Endosc. 2002;56(1):18–24. S0016510702000020 [pii].
29. Rana SS, Bhasin DK, Nanda M, Siyad I, Gupta R, Kang M, et al. Endoscopic transpapillary drainage for external fistulas developing after surgical or radiological pancreatic interventions. J Gastroenterol Hepatol. 2010;25(6):1087–92. https://doi.org/10.1111/j.1440-1746.2009.06172.x. JGH6172 [pii].
30. Arvanitakis M, Delhaye M, Bali MA, Matos C, De Maertelaer V, Le Moine O, et al. Pancreatic fluid collections: a randomized controlled trial regarding stent removal after endoscopic transmural drainage. Gastrointest Endosc. 2007;65(4):609–19. https://doi.org/10.1016/j.gie.2006.06.083. S0016-5107(06)02407-2 [pii].
31. Arvanitakis M, Delhaye M, Bali MA, Matos C, Le Moine O, Deviere J. Endoscopic treatment of external pancreatic fistulas: when draining the main pancreatic duct is not enough. Am J Gastroenterol. 2007;102(3):516–24. https://doi.org/10.1111/j.1572-0241.2006.01014.x. AJG1014 [pii].
32. Pelaez-Luna M, Vege SS, Petersen BT, Chari ST, Clain JE, Levy MJ, et al. Disconnected pancreatic duct syndrome in severe acute pancreatitis: clinical and imaging characteristics and outcomes in a cohort of 31 cases. Gastrointest Endosc. 2008;68(1):91–7. https://doi.org/10.1016/j.gie.2007.11.041. S0016-5107(07)03178-1 [pii].
33. Varadarajulu S, Bang JY, Phadnis MA, Christein JD, Wilcox CM. Endoscopic transmural drainage of peripancreatic fluid collections: outcomes and predictors of treatment success in 211 consecutive patients. J Gastrointest Surg. 2011;15(11):2080–8. https://doi.org/10.1007/s11605-011-1621-8.
34. Bang JY, Wilcox CM, Navaneethan U, Hasan MK, Peter S, Christein J, et al. Impact of disconnected pancreatic duct syndrome on the endoscopic management of pancreatic fluid collections. Ann Surg. 2016;267:561. https://doi.org/10.1097/SLA.0000000000002082.
35. Francois E, Kahaleh M, Giovannini M, Matos C, Deviere J. EUS-guided pancreaticogastrostomy. Gastrointest Endosc. 2002;56(1):128–33. S001651070200024X [pii].
36. Kahaleh M, Hernandez AJ, Tokar J, Adams RB, Shami VM, Yeaton P. EUS-guided pancreaticogastrostomy: analysis of its efficacy to drain inaccessible pancreatic ducts. Gastrointest Endosc. 2007;65(2):224–30. https://doi.org/10.1016/j.gie.2006.05.008. S0016-5107(06)01953-5 [pii].
37. Walter D, Will U, Sanchez-Yague A, Brenke D, Hampe J, Wollny H, et al. A novel lumen-apposing metal stent for endoscopic ultrasound-guided drainage of pancreatic fluid collections: a prospective cohort study. Endoscopy. 2015;47(1):63–7. https://doi.org/10.1055/s-0034-1378113.
38. Siddiqui AA, Adler DG, Nieto J, Shah JN, Binmoeller KF, Kane S, et al. EUS-guided drainage of peripancreatic fluid collections and necrosis by using a novel lumen-apposing stent: a large retrospective, multicenter U.S. experience (with videos). Gastrointest Endosc. 2016;83(4):699–707. https://doi.org/10.1016/j.gie.2015.53.020. S0016-5107(15)03036-9 [pii].
39. Grobmyer SR, Hunt DL, Forsmark CE, Draganov PV, Behrns KE, Hochwald SN. Pancreatic stent placement is associated with resolution of refractory grade C pancreatic fistula after left-sided pancreatectomy. Am Surg. 2009;75(8):654–7; discussion 7–8.
40. Reddymasu SC, Pakseresht K, Moloney B, Alsop B, Oropezia-Vail M, Olyaee M. Incidence of pancreatic fistula after distal pancreatectomy and efficacy of endoscopic therapy for its management: results from a tertiary care center. Case Rep Gastroenterol. 2013;7(2):332–9. https://doi.org/10.1159/000354136. crg-0007-0332 [pii].
41. Onodera M, Kawakami H, Kuwatani M, Kudo T, Haba S, Abe Y, et al. Endoscopic ultrasound-guided transmural drainage for pancreatic fistula or pancreatic duct dilation after pancreatic surgery. Surg Endosc. 2011;26(6):1710–7. https://doi.org/10.1007/s00464-011-2097-z.
42. Bartoli E, Rebibo L, Robert B, Fumery M, Delcenserie R, Regimbeau JM. Efficacy of the double-pigtail stent as a conservative treatment for grade B pancreatic fistula after pancreatoduodenectomy with pancreatogastric anastomosis. Surg Endosc. 2013;28(5):1528–34. https://doi.org/10.1007/s00464-013-3347-z.
43. Fazel A, Quadri A, Catalano MF, Meyerson SM, Geenen JE. Does a pancreatic duct stent prevent post-ERCP pancreatitis? A prospective randomized study. Gastrointest Endosc. 2003;57(3):291–4. https://doi.org/10.1067/mge.2003.124. S0016-5107(02)00240-7 [pii].

44. Kozarek RA. Pancreatic stents can induce ductal changes consistent with chronic pancreatitis. Gastrointest Endosc. 1990;36(2):93–5. S0016-5107(90)70958-3 [pii].
45. Kozarek R, Hovde O, Attia F, France R. Do pancreatic duct stents cause or prevent pancreatic sepsis? Gastrointest Endosc. 2003;58(4):505–9. S0016-5107(03)01891-1 [pii].
46. Murage KP, Ball CG, Zyromski NJ, Nakeeb A, Ocampo C, Sandrasegaran K, et al. Clinical framework to guide operative decision making in disconnected left pancreatic remnant (DLPR) following acute or chronic pancreatitis. Surgery. 2010;148(4):847–56. https://doi.org/10.1016/j.surg.2010.07.039; discussion 56–7. .S0039-6060(10)00407-1 [pii].
47. Behrns KE, Howard TJ. Pancreatic necrosis: when to scope, poke, or cut? Gastrointest Endosc. 2010;72(6):1326–7. https://doi.org/10.1016/j.gie.2010.03.1072; author reply 7–8. S0016-5107(10)01371-4 [pii].

Part VI

The Cytopathologist's Point of View

EUS Tissue Sampling: What Are We Talking About?

50

Luca Saragoni

50.1 Introduction

EUS-guided FNA has been in use since the early 1990s [1, 2], and its role has increased exponentially. EUS FNA permits the pathological diagnosis by means of tissue acquisition (TA) in otherwise difficult anatomic locations within abdomen, retroperitoneum, mediastinum, and perirectal space. Pancreatic neoplasms, diseases involving lymph nodes at various mediastinal and abdominal sites, gastrointestinal submucosal lesions, perirectal, adrenal, and mediastinal masses are now routinely diagnosed by EUS FNA. Despite its important diagnostic role, this technique has some limitations: the need of on-site cytopathologist, dependence sometimes on histology to achieve diagnostic material, and inability to reliably assess for molecular markers.

EUS FNA is a multistep procedure that requires proper clinical indication, correct selection of needles and adoption of evidence-based techniques for tissue sampling.

EUS FNA is most commonly performed to confirm the diagnosis of cancers clinically suspected.

Although EUS FNA has changed the landscape of diagnosis in gastrointestinal endoscopy by increasing the accuracy of tissue acquisition, it is important to recognize its pitfalls. In situations such as pancreatic masses in chronic pancreatitis (CP) and autoimmune pancreatitis (AIP), EUS FNA can yield false positivity as atypical cells in CP as well as in AIP may mimic malignancy.

Similarly, false negativity, due to technical difficulties, sampling, or interpretative errors, is also an area of concern. Moreover, diagnosing malignancy in hypocellular samples, marked desmoplastic background, and well-differentiated adenocarcinoma are challenging [3].

The basic difference between EUS FNA and EUS FNB is that the last technique allows mantaining tissue architecture. In particular, core biopsy is needed when FNA is nondiagnostic or inadequate, in special pathological fields (AIP), when special stains (immunoistochemistry) are necessary for the diagnosis (gastro intestinal stromal tumors, lymphomas) and in cases in which tissue profiling or cell cultures are needed for targeted therapies. The American Society of Gastroenterology and Endoscopy has recommended that the use of new FNB needles because highly effective for the acquisition of core specimens. They should be considered first-line for tissue sampling of nonpancreatic mass lesions, as a rescue technique after inadequate FNA samples and for lesions requiring immunoistochemistry (IHC).

L. Saragoni (✉)
Department of Pathology,
G.B. Morgagni-L. Pierantoni Hospital, Forlì, Italy
e-mail: luca.saragoni@auslromagna.it

M. Mutignani et al. (eds.), *Endotherapy in Biliopancreatic Diseases: ERCP Meets EUS*,
https://doi.org/10.1007/978-3-030-42569-2_50

50.2 Handling of Aspirated Samples

The use of stylet, as material is expelled drop by drop is the technique preferred to spread the material onto the slides after aspiration.

50.2.1 Fixation of Slides

Fixation is done either by air dry or alcohol:

1. Air-dried fixation: The slides are dried using air blower or hair dryer until their complete drying. After air fixation, slides are usually stained with Romanowsky-type staines.
2. Alcohol fixation: As soon as the slides are prepared and still wet, they are immersed in ethanol or sprayed on. These slides are stained with Papanicolau stain.

50.2.2 Rapid On-Site Diagnostic Evaluation (ROSE)

There is a theoretical advantage that on-site evaluation of slides would lead to less false-negative results as well as few passes would be required to ascertain the diagnosis. Studies have shown that ROSE increases diagnostic accuracy by up to 20%, also decreasing inadequate samples and the number of passes [4–8]. However, published meta-analyses concluded that ROSE is associated with improvement in adequacy rates (AR) at sites where AR without ROSE is less than 90% [9, 10]. Apart from these considerations, an on-site cytopathologist may have a role during the training phase and in centers with a low diagnostic accuracy [11].

50.2.3 Cell Block

In clinical situations, such as pancreatic ductal malignancy, lymphoma, neuroendocrine tumor (NET), and gastro intestinal stromal tumors (GIST), cell blocks provide additional material for histology as well as IHC and molecular profiling. Cell blocks are prepared by expelling the sample from the FNA needle into a container with a cell-preservative solution. The container with the sample is centrifugated to harvest the cells, and fibrin glue is commonly used to hold the cells and to form tissue fragments. Then, tissue is processed for histological examination.

50.3 Handling of Core Biposy Specimens

Once FNB specimen is procured, it can be processed in one of the following ways:

1. Tissue sample is transferred to 10% formalin containing solution and then processed for histopathological examination.
2. Sample is placed on a glass slide and with the help of needle is microdissected to form tissue cores.

50.4 Diagnostic Role of EUS-Guided Sampling

The increased cellularity along with preserved histologic architecture of the FNB samples makes this technique ideal for the diagnosis and eventual ancillary studies. FNB may provide benefit for nonpancreatic solid masses and lesions where FNA has been nondiagnostic [11, 12].

Solid pancreatic lesions mostly include ductal adenocarcinoma, but also lymphoma, neuroendocrine tumors, matastases, and other neoplasms together with benign conditions such as autoimmune pancreatitis and focal pancreatitis. In the last two cases (benign conditions), especially when associated with pancreatic masses, EUS-guided sampling that does not confirm cancer should be interpreted with caution. EUS-guided sampling has become the method of choice for the pathological diagnosis of solid pancreatic masses as it is very accurate [9, 13, 14], and it is an advantage staging method that allows the sampling of locoregional and distant lymph nodes, liver lesions, and small amounts of ascites undetected by other imaging techniques [15].

EUS-guided sampling could be useful also in diagnosing indeterminate biliary strictures, either as an alternative or in combination with endoluminal biliary sampling, while there is not sufficient evidence to recommend it for the diagnosis of ampullary lesions.

For pancreatic cystic lesions (PCLs), EUS-guided sampling should be used for biochemical analyses plus cytopathological examination if a precise diagnosis may change patient management, except for lesions <10 mm in diameter with no high-risk signs. Anyway, cytopathological examination of PCL aspirate was found to present low sensitivity in differentiating mucinous from nonmucinous cysts [16]. Moreover, mucin or mucin-producing cells of the gastrointestinal wall should not be misinterpreted as the mucin or epithelial cells of a mucinous cyst [17]. In mucinous cysts, the cytopathological diagnosis serves to triage patients for surgery as it is strongly correlated with the risk of malignancy [18].

For subepithelial lesions (SEL) of the gastrointestinal tract, bite-on-bite biopsy is considered the first diagnostic procedure. The term "SEL" refers to lesions located in the deep mucosa or beneath it, and they mostly correspond to benign or premalignant neoplasms and rarely to overtly malignant tumors [19]. If bite-on-bite biopsy does not yield a diagnostic specimen, EUS-guided sampling is suggested in the following clinical situations:

1. Asymptomatic hypoechoic SEL >2 cm of the stomach or gastroesophageal junction if surveillance is being considered,
2. Targeted therapy of a suspected gastrointestinal stromal tumor is being considered.
3. A carcinoma, neuroendocrine tumor, lymphoma, or intramural metastasis is suspected.

Moreover, EUS-guided sampling is always suggested as the first choice in the following clinical situations:

1. Symptoms making resection necessary.
2. Small (<2 cm) lesion located in the esophagus or stomach.
3. Pathognomonic EUS appearance of a lipoma or duplication cyst.
4. Patient is not candidated for treatment.

It is important for pathologists to remember that the mitotic count (Ki-67) determined on samples acquired under EUS guidance from gastro intestinal stromal tumors should not be used as evidence of low malignant potential of the tumor, due to the risk of underestimating the tumor proliferative activity [20, 21].

For duodenal and colorectal SELs, data are not sufficient to allow recommendations.

In patients with diffuse esophageal/gastric/rectal wall thickening, after failure of standard biopsy techniques, EUS-guided sampling is suggested with the aim to obtain a core biopsy. Diffuse GI wall thickening is predominantly observed in the stomach and, less frequently, in the esophagus and rectum. Malignant causes include linite plastica and lymphoma or diffuse metastasis. Benign causes are multiple, including eosinophilc infiltration, Zollinger-Ellison syndrome, Menetrier's disease, amyloidosis, and newly recognized entity such as IgG4-related disease [22, 23]. The possibility of a GI lymphoma should always be evaluated in patients with GI wall thickening as, in such cases, similarly to those of nodal lymphomas, samples should be preserved in conditions that will permit the application of ancillary methods.

For esophageal luminal cancers, EUS-guided sampling is suggested for the assessment of regional lymph nodes (Lns) in T1 adenocarcinomas and of lesions suspicious for metastasis such as distant Lns, left liver lobe lesions, and suspected peritoneal carcinomatosis. The true impact of EUS-guided sampling on patient management is difficult to measure because treatment decisions are influenced, not only by the presence of Lns or distant metastases but also by many other factors, including patient performance status and tumor location, histology, and infiltration depth (T-stage).

For lymph nodes restaging and for predicting complete pathological response after neoadjuvant therapy, EUS-guided sampling should only be considered in highly selected cases.

In patients with gastric cancer, the main utility of EUS-guided sampling is to avoid unnecessary surgery by demonstrating distant metastasis. Malignant involvement of distant intra-abdominal Lns or mediastinal Lns distant from the tumor is

Table 50.1 Common indications for EUS-guided sampling

1. Pancreatic mass (solid and cystic)
2. Bile duct strictures
3. Focal solid liver lesions (matastasis, hepatocellular carcinoma)
4. Diffuse esophageal or gastric wall thickening
5. Nodal staging in the setting of esophageal, gastric, rectal, or lung cancer
6. Subepithelial tumors (GIST, schwannoma, leiomyoma, NET, others)
7. Evaluation of lymphadenopathy (mediastinal, abdominal, pelvic)
8. Adrenal gland lesions (left adrenal more common)
9. Prostate mass
10. Peritoneal carcinomatosis
11. Splenic mass
12. Perivascular tumor extension, tumor thrombus, extramural tumor recurrence

indicative of metastatic disease that qualifies the patients suitable for palliation rather than resection with curative intent [24].

In rectal cancer staging, EUS-guided technique is not indicated for sampling of local Lns. Instead, it should be useful in patients with a history of rectal cancer for sampling perirectal masses if it may influence treatment decisions.

In general, the possibility of a false-positive diagnosis should be kept in mind when interpreting cytopathological samples, particularly in patients with a cancer located in GI lumens.

Common indications for EUS-guided sampling are shown in Table 50.1.

50.5 Conclusions

The currently available FNB needles have the potential to change the way the diseases of pancreas, GI tract, and deep lymph nodes are diagnosed. The increased cellularity along with the preserved histologic architecture of samples makes this technique ideal for ancillary analyses, such as immunoistochemistry and molecular biology. With such promising advantages, the use of EUS FNB is going to be widespread. A multidisciplinary team including the endosonographer and the pathologist is recommended in order to manage these techniques in the best way and to reach a diagnostic accuracy >90% as international guidelines suggest.

References

1. Vilmann P, Jacobsen GK, Henriksen FW, et al. Endoscopic ultrasonography with guided fine needle aspiration biopsy in pancreatic disease. Gastrointest Endosc. 1992;38:172–3.
2. Wiersema MJ, Hawes RH, Tao LC, et al. Endoscopic ultrasonography as an adjunct to fine needle aspiration cytology of the upper and lower gastrointestinal tract. Gastrointest Endosc. 1992;38:35–9.
3. Atul R, Surinder SR. Endoscopic ultrasound-guided tissue acquisition: techniques and challenges. J Cytol. 2019;36(1):1–7.
4. Klapman JB, Logrono R, Dye CE, et al. Clinical impact of on-site cytopathology interpretation on endoscopic ultrasound-guided fine needle aspiration. Am J Gastroenterol. 2003;98:1289–94.
5. Erickson RA, Sayage-Rabie L, Beissner RS. Factors predicting the number of EUS-guided fine-needle passes for diagnosis of pancreatic malignancies. Gastrointest Endosc. 2000;51:184–90.
6. Iglesias-Garcia J, Dominguez-Munoz JE, Abdulkader I, et al. Influence of on-site cytopathology evaluation on the diagnostic accuracy of endoscopic ultrasound-guided fine needle aspiration (EUS-FNA) of solid pancreatic masses. Am J Gastroenterol. 2011;106:1705–10.
7. Kulesza P, Eltoum IA. Endoscopic ultrasound-guided fine needle aspiration: sampling, pitfalls, and quality management. Clin Gastroenterol Hepatol. 2007;5:1248–54.
8. Wani S, Mullady D, Early DS, et al. The clinical impact of immediate on-site cytopathology evaluation during endoscopic ultrasound-guided fine needle aspiration of pancreatic masses: a prospective multicenter randomized controlled trial. Am J Gastroenterol. 2015;110:1429–39.
9. Hebert-Magee S, Bae S, Varadarajulu S, et al. The presence of a cytopathologist increases the diagnostic accuracy of endoscopic ultrasound-guided fine needle aspiration cytology for pancreatic adenocarcinoma : a meta-analysis. Cytopathology. 2013;24:159–71.
10. Schimdt RL, Witt BL, Matynia AP, et al. Rapid on-site evaluation increases endoscopic ultrasound-guided fine needle aspiration adequacy for pancreatic lesions. Dig Dis Sci. 2013;58:872–82.
11. Wani S, Muthusami VR, Komanduri S. EUS-guided tissue acquisition: an evidence-based approach (with videos). Gastrointest Endosc. 2014;80:939–59.
12. Aadam AA, Wani S, Amick A, et al. A randomized controlled cross-over trial and cost analysis comparing endoscopic ultrasound fine needle aspiration and fine needle biopsy. Endosc Int. 2016;4:E497–505.

13. Hewitt MJ, Mc Phail MJW, Possamai L, et al. EUS-guided FNA for diagnosis of solid pancreatic neoplasms: a meta-analysis. Gastrointest Endosc. 2012;75:319–31.
14. Puli SR, Bechtold ML, Buxbaum JL, et al. How good is endoscopic ultrasound-guided fine needle aspiration in diagnosing the correct etiology for a solid pancreatic mass? A meta-analysis and systematic review. Pancreas. 2013;42:20–6.
15. Suzuki R, Irisawa A, Bhutani MS, et al. An automated spring-loaded needle for endoscopic ultrasound-guided abdominal paracentesis in cancer patients. World J Gastrointest Endosc. 2014;6:55–9.
16. Thornton GD, Edelweiss M, Tong LC, et al. Endoscopic ultrasound guided fine needle aspiration for the diagnosis of pancreatic cystic neoplasms: a meta-analysis. Pancreatology. 2013;13:48–57.
17. Sigel CS, Edelweiss M, Tong LC, et al. Low interobserver agreement in cytology grading of mucinous pancreatic neoplasms. Cancer Cytopathol. 2015;123:40–50.
18. Tanaka M, Fernandcz-del Castillo C, Adsay V, et al. International consensus guidelines 2012 for the management of IPMN and MCN of the pancreas. Pancreatology. 2012;12:183–97.
19. Menon L, Buscaglia JM. Endoscopic approach to subepithelial lesions. Ther Adv Gastroenterol. 2014;7:123–30.
20. Lee M, Min BH, Lee H, et al. Feasibility and diagnostic yield of endoscopic ultrasonography-guided fine needle biopsy with a new core biopsy needle device in patients with gastric subepithelial tumors. Medicine (Baltimore). 2015;94:e1622.
21. Ricci R, Chiarello G, Attili F, et al. Endoscopic ultrasound-guided fine needle tissue acquisition biopsy sample do not allow a reliable proliferation assessment of gastrointestinal stromal tumors. Dig Liver Dis. 2015;47:291–5.
22. Reeder MM, Olmsted WW, Cooper PH. Large gastric folds, local or widespread. JAMA. 1974; 230:273–4.
23. Kawano H, Ishii A, Kimura T, et al. IgG4-related disease manifesting the gastric wall thickening. Pathol Int. 2016;66:23–8.
24. Waddell T, Verheij M, Allum W, et al. Gastric cancer: ESMO-ESSO-ESTRO clinical practice guidelines for diagnosis, treatment and follow-up. Radiother Oncol. 2014;110:189–94.

51 Molecular Biology of Biliopancreatic Lesions

Michela Visani, Giorgia Acquaviva, Annalisa Pession, Giovanni Tallini, and Dario de Biase

51.1 Molecular Biology of Biliopancreatic Lesions

The management of patients with a pancreatic lesion is still challenging. Endoscopic ultrasound–guided fine-needle aspiration (EUS-FNA) has improved pre-operative diagnosis [1–3]. Although EUS-FNA plus cytological evaluation increase clinical sensitivity, in a subset of cases the pre-operative diagnosis remains inconclusive with an atypical/suspicious cytopathologic diagnoses [4]. Molecular testing could help in solve these inconclusive cases.

Genetic alterations can be classified in (1) mutational activation of oncogenes (e.g. *KRAS*-mutation, found in >90% of pancreatic cancers), (2) inactivation of tumor suppressor genes (e.g. *TP53*, *p16/CDKN2A*, and *SMAD4*), or (3) inactivation of genome maintenance genes controlling the repair of DNA damage (e.g. *hMLH1* and *MSH2*). However, to date, there are not targetable molecules for personalized patient treatment in clinical practice, as stated by the current ESMO (European Society for Medical Oncology) guidelines [5].

M. Visani · A. Pession · D. de Biase (✉)
Department of Pharmacy and Biotechnology (Dipartimento di Farmacia e Biotecnologie)—Molecular Diagnostic Unit, Azienda USL di Bologna, University of Bologna, Bologna, Italy
e-mail: dario.debiase@unibo.it

G. Acquaviva · G. Tallini
Department of Experimental, Diagnostic and Specialty Medicine, University of Bologna-Molecular Diagnostic Unit, Azienda USL di Bologna, Bologna, Italy

51.2 Deep Sequencing of PDAC

Pancreatic adenocarcinoma (PDAC) contains an average of about 60 genetic alterations according to whole exome sequencing analyses, the majority of which are point mutation [6, 7]. These alterations may define a core of 12 cellular pathways that are genetically altered in pancreatic tumors [6]. Deep sequencing studies performed on PDAC samples revealed some genes significantly mutated, discovering known mutated genes (e.g. *KRAS, TP53, CDKN2A, SMAD4, MLL3, TGFBR2, ARID1A, SF3B1, and ROBO1) or* novel ones. The novel mutated genes may be involved in chromatin modification (*EPC1* and *ARID2*), DNA damage repair (*ATM*), or pancreatic carcinogenesis (*KDM6A* and *PREX2*) [8].

According to expression analysis, it is possible to cluster PDAC in four subtypes: (1) squamous, (2) pancreatic progenitor, (3) immunogenic, and (4) aberrantly differentiated endocrine exocrine [9].

Moreover, according to the structural alteration found in PDAC, it has been possible to identify other four subtypes of pancreatic cancer: (1) "stable" (tumors containing ≤50 structural

M. Mutignani et al. (eds.), *Endotherapy in Biliopancreatic Diseases: ERCP Meets EUS*,
https://doi.org/10.1007/978-3-030-42569-2_51

variation); (2) "locally rearranged" (tumors exhibiting a significant focal event on one or two chromosomes); (3) "scattered subtype" (tumors exhibiting a mild range of non-random chromosomal damage and <200 structural variations); (4) "unstable" (tumors exhibiting >200 structural variation events) [10].

Whole-exome sequencing of pancreatic cancer has defined some putative therapeutic targets, as *RBM10* mutations associated with longer survival, *KRAS*-Q61H mutation associated with improved survival or *BRAF* mutations defining sensitivity to vemurafenib in PDAC models [11].

51.3 Most Commonly Mutated Genes in Biliopancreatic Lesions

51.3.1 *KRAS*

KRAS is the most frequently mutated gene in pancreatic cancers (>95%) [6, 12] (Table 51.1).

KRAS protein bound to guanosine triphosphate (GTP) mediates cell survival and differentiation. Mutations in *KRAS* gene inhibit the ability to hydrolyze GTP, leaving the protein constitutively active. *KRAS* alterations are harbored by over 90% of pancreatic intraepithelial neoplasia (PanIN) [13]. Targeting of mutant *KRAS* specifically to the murine pancreas is sufficient to initiate development of PanINs and IPMNs [14–18]. In PDAC, the acquisition of a mutation in *KRAS* is an early and initiating event; however, the low frequency of progression of precursor lesions to PDAC suggests that additional genetic aberrations are needed for disease progression [16].

Mutation in *KRAS* gene were identified in carcinomas of the exocrine pancreas in 1988 for the first time [19]. *KRAS* is the most frequent gene mutated up to 90% of pancreatic adenocarcinoma (from 70 to 95%) [11] (Table 51.1).

Mutations in *KRAS* gene in PDAC have been detected not only in exon 2 but also in exon 3 [8, 11, 20]. While all mutations in *KRAS* exon 2 exhibited similar association with survival, it has been observed that cases mutated in *KRAS* exon 3 had a remarkably favorable prognosis [11].

In pancreatic specimens, multiple *KRAS* mutations could be detected in the same tumoral mass [20–22].

Several studies have suggested that cytopathology together with *KRAS* analysis improves

Table 51.1 Main genetic alteration detectable in pancreatic tumors

Features	Reported frequency of genetic alterations	Type of pancreatic lesion	Preferable Detection methods
KRAS	90–95% 45–50% 20–50%	PDAC IPMN MCN	Extractive techniques
TP53	50–75% 30–40%	PDAC PAAC	Extractive techniques, IHC
CDKN2A/p16	90–98%	PDAC	IHC
SMAD4	40–60%	PDAC	IHC
GNAS	35–50% 25–50%	IPMN MCN	Extractive techniques
CTNNB1	90–100% 5–10%	SPN PAAC	Extractive techniques, IHC
VHL	45–50%	SCA	IHC
MGMT promoter methylation	10–40%	PDAC	Extractive techniques
BRAF	1.3%	PDAC	Extractive techniques
MSI	0–1%	PDAC	Extractive techniques, IHC

PDAC Pancreatic Ductal Adenocarcinoma, *IPMN* Intraductal Papillary Mucinous Neoplasms, *SPN* Solid Pseudopapillary Neoplasm, *PAAC* Pancreatic Acinic Adenocarcinoma, *SCA* Serous Cystoadenoma, *IHC* Immunohistochemistry. The percentages quoted are estimated from the literature cited in the text the diagnosis of PDAC in EUS-FNA material [23–30].

KRAS analysis may be particularly useful mainly in case of inconclusive (e.g. acellular samples) or doubtful diagnoses (e.g. specimens with presence of cytological atypia). Even if molecular tests cannot replace a morphological diagnosis, the presence of a *KRAS* mutation in EUS-FNA material may support a re-evaluation of the original cytopathology report (especially if doubtful), an indication for a second FNA or surgery [20], and allows a significant reduction of false-negative diagnoses [31].

KRAS is the most frequently mutated gene in IPMN (45–50%) and MCN (20–50%), while it is not altered in SCA (Serous Cystoadenoma) and SPN (pancreatic solid pseudopapillary neoplasms) [32–34]. Mutations in *KRAS* are more frequently observed in gastric and pancreatobiliary-type IPMN [32].

Analysis of pancreatic cyst fluid is useful in identifying IPMNs and MCNs from non-neoplastic pancreatic cysts. This has significant implications in clinical intervention and on personalized follow-up strategies. The presence of a *KRAS* mutation is highly specific for mucinous differentiation (Table 51.1) but is inadequate in identifying MCNs [35]. In fact, *KRAS* has a very high specificity but a low (~70%) or very low sensitivity (~15%) for IPMNs and MCNs, respectively. This sensitivity increases when *KRAS* analysis is combined with *GNAS* [36, 37].

Moreover, *KRAS* mutations are found in strictures induced by pancreatic cancers and are less frequently found in those induced by bile duct cancers [38]. For biliary tract cancers, the rates of *KRAS* mutations vary widely, ranging between 0% and 100% [39].

KRAS mutations together with the loss of heterozygosity (LOH) and analysis of PCR-amplified DNA from biliary brush cytology allow discriminating reactive from malignant cells [40].

The analysis of *KRAS* and LOH helps also in the differential diagnosis of cystic mucinous pancreatic lesions (IPMN and MCN) when pre-operative cytology is non-diagnostic or carcinoembryonic antigen (CEA) cyst fluid levels are indeterminate [41].

In contrast with the majority of pancreatic cancers, cholangiocarcinomas does not show *KRAS* mutations, or the frequency of *KRAS* mutations is lower than in pancreatic ductal adenocarcinomas [40]. Thus, the presence of a *KRAS* mutation in the cytology specimens of a biliary stricture is no reason to assume that the malignancy is of pancreatic origin.

KRAS mutations in PDAC may also help in prognostic stratification of patients. In fact, coexistence of *KRAS* mutations together with *TP53* alterations and SMAD4 loss of function has been associated with worst prognosis [42, 43].

Of the several markers investigated, *KRAS* remains the one most commonly utilized for single gene testing, although its use is greatly limited by the identification of mutated *KRAS* in about 10% of chronic pancreatitis and/or low-grade pancreatobiliary epithelial cell dysplasia [44–47]. Thus, "The Papanicolaou Society of Cytopathology guidelines" does not support *KRAS* testing of solid pancreatic masses and bile duct strictures as a useful single gene ancillary test.

51.3.2 *TP53*

P53 protein plays a key role in cell–cycle regulation, in the maintenance of genomic stability, and in the apoptotic process. Mutations in the *TP53* gene lead to inactivation of the normal protein function. A large majority of *TP53* inactivating alterations are single point mutations [48]. Functional loss of the protein leads to cellular survival also in the presence of DNA damage, promoting the accumulation of more genetic mutations [49].

Inactivation of the *TP53* gene is a very common event in almost all human cancers, and from 50% to 75% of pancreatic cancers demonstrate *TP53* mutations [6, 48, 50] (Table 51.1).

TP53 status evaluation can improve the sensitivity of EUS-FNA to diagnose pancreatic malignant lesions [51–53].

P53 protein overexpression was observed in FNA biopsy specimens with pancreatic cancer but not in samples with chronic pancreatitis. Combining p53 protein evaluation and histological examination, the sensitivity of diagnosis of pancreatic cancers improve, maintaining a high specificity [51, 52]. Combining p53 and Ki67 staining increases further the sensitivity of EUS-FNA in the diagnosis of PDAC [52]. Also, the combination of p53 and CA19.9 echances the sensitivity of cytology [53]. However, the combination of cytology with p53 and CA19.9 evaluation may decrease the specificity [53].

Loss of p53 protein was correlated with a worst patient prognosis, mainly if combined with *KRAS* mutation and loss of expression of SMAD4 protein [42, 43].

In IPMN, mutations in *TP53* are not a common event (~10%). The overexpression of TP53 was more commonly observed in IPMNs of the pancreatobiliary type with invasion [32]. Loss of SMAD4 and overexpression of TP53 were strongly associated with patient survival in a cohort of IPMN patients [32].

51.3.3 *SMAD4*

SMAD4/DPC4 is located on chromosome arm 18q and plays a key role in the signal transduction cascade involving TGF-β. Loss of SMAD4 protein gives rise to unregulated cellular proliferation [54]. *SMAD4* is inactivated in about 50% of pancreatic cancers by homozygous deletion and by intragenic mutations (Table 51.1) [55–58]. Loss of SMAD4 nuclear reactivity is generally observed late in pancreatic carcinogenesis. SMAD4 loss of function frequently occurs in pancreatic adenocarcinomas, but not in extrapancreatic lesions [59].

SMAD4 nuclear reactivity is preserved in reactive and inflammatory diseases of the pancreas, such as chronic pancreatitis. In PDAC, loss of SMAD4 has been associated with a worst prognosis and an increased risk of metastases [42, 43, 58, 60, 61].

The loss of SMAD4 was observed also in IPMN, and more commonly in IPMNs of the pancreatobiliary type with invasion [32].

51.3.4 *CTNNB1*

Codons from 32 to 37 of the *CTNNB1* gene encode for a region critical for the regulation of the protein β-catenin [62, 63]. When phosphorylated at residues between codons 32 and 37, β-catenin is degraded by ubiquitin ligases. Mutations within this region that blocks the phosphorylation inhibit the degradation of the β-catenin protein [64].

CTNNB1 gene mutations are molecular hallmark for pancreatic solid pseudopapillary neoplasms (SPN) [65–67]. In these types of tumors, *CTNNB1* mutations are the only molecular alteration detected [68], and, on the contrary, *CTNNB1* mutations are uncommon in PDAC [11, 67].

51.3.5 *GNAS*

The *GNAS* gene encodes the α-subunit of the stimulatory G-protein (Gαs), which mediates the regulation of adenylate cyclase activity. Mutated *GNAS* may alter the expression profiles of several other genes, as that of mucin ones (e.g. *MUC2* and *MUC5AC*). These molecular alterations may determine the characteristic IPMN phenotype [69].

GNAS activating mutations are reported prevalently in IPMN (~40–60%) (Table 51.1) [32, 33, 36, 68, 70], and in some invasive pancreatic cancers only if arising in association with an IPMN [13, 71]. At least one of *GNAS* or *KRAS* genes is mutated in the vast majority (~90%) of IPMNs [72].

In about 40% of IPMN, *GNAS* mutation coexists with *KRAS* alterations [70]. The combination of *GNAS* and *KRAS* mutation analysis provides high sensitivity and specificity for distinguishing between serous carcinomas (SCAs) and IPMNs. Most IPMNs has a *GNAS* and/or a *KRAS* whereas no SCAs have either mutation.

In addition, the presence of a *GNAS* mutation in cyst fluid can also help in distinguishing IPMNs from MCNs [73].

51.3.6 *CDKN2A*

CDKN2A/p16 maps on chromosome 9p and encodes the proteins p14^{ARF} and p16^{INK4a}. The p16 protein suppresses the progression of the cell cycle at the G1-S checkpoint by binding the cyclin-dependent kinases (CDKs), as CDK4 and CDK6 [57]. *CDKN2A/p16* was the first tumor suppressor gene that was shown to undergo promoter hypermethylation and silencing in pancreatic cancer [74]. The Rb/p16 pathway was abrogated in about all pancreatic adenocarcinoma, all through inactivation of the p16 gene [74].

Mutations in the *CDKN2A* gene are associated with an increased risk of several cancers. This gene is inactivated in more than 95% of sporadic pancreatic carcinomas (Table 51.1) by several different mechanisms, such as intragenic mutation coupled with the loss of the other allele, homozygous deletion of both alleles, or promoter hypermethylation [75–77]. Moreover, *CDKN2A* is a causative gene in familial pancreatic cancer [78], even if it has been observed that germline mutations of *CDKN2A* among patients with pancreatic cancer are uncommon (0.6%) [79]. However, patients carrying *CDKN2A* mutations are more likely to report a family history of pancreatic cancer [79].

It has been described a tendency for the tumor to be larger in patients with decreased expression of p16 protein than in those with normal expression levels. Patients with pancreatic carcinoma with p16 mutation or hypermethylation have a tumor significantly larger, and the survival period is significantly shorter if compared with patients with a pancreatic carcinoma harboring an intact p16 gene [43, 80, 81].

Other than in pancreatic adenocarcinoma, inactivating mutations of *CDKN2A/p16* are found also in IPMNs with high-grade dysplasia [82].

51.3.6.1 Other Genetic Alterations

Besides genes previously reported as important in pancreatic cancer (e.g. *KRAS, TP53, SMAD4, CDKN2A, GNAS)*, other molecular markers have been observed mutated at lower prevalence. *ARID1A* oncosuppressor protein deficiency was significantly associated with poor outcome PDAC, and mutations have been identified in *KDM6A* gene [11]. It has been observed that pancreatic tumors may harbor amplifications and copy-number gains of known oncogenes as *ERBB2, MET, FGFR1* [10]. An aberrant WNT signaling is implicated due to the frequent inactivation of several genes as *ROBO1, ROBO2, SLIT2,* and *RNF43* [10].

Contrarily to what happens in melanoma, *BRAF* gene is rarely mutated in biliopancreatic lesions (Table 51.1) [83]. Similarly, microsatellite instability (MSI) phenotype is found in only less than 1% of pancreatic adenocarcinoma (Table 51.1) [84].

Unresectable non-metastatic pancreatic carcinomas may harbor mutations in *ARID*, *GRM8*, and *TRIM33* [85].

VHL mutations are frequently (~40% of cases) reported in SCA [34] (Table 51.1).

Mutations in *BRCA* pathway genes and defects in DNA maintenance (genomic instability and the *BRCA* mutational signature) have potential implications for therapeutic selection for pancreatic cancer [10].

An additional tumor suppressor pathway altered in pancreatic cancers involves *STK11/LKB1* genes: germline mutations of *STK11/LKB1* are responsible for Peutz-Jeghers syndrome and are associated with IPMNs and invasive pancreatic cancer [86, 87]. In addition, somatic mutations of *STK11/LKB1* are observed in 5% of patients with sporadic IPMNs and pancreatic cancers [86, 87].

Cyclin E is overexpressed in a small fraction (~5%) of pancreatic adenocarcinomas [88].

O-6-methylguanine-DNA methyltransferase (*MGMT*) promoter can be found hypermethylated in PDAC [42, 89] (Table 51.1). *MGMT* promoter hypermethylation confers sensitivity to alkylating agents (e.g. temozolomide) in patients with gliomas [90]. The treatment of advanced pancreatic cancer with temozolamide has been attempted in a phase II study in 1998 [91], but no clinical response was seen in the 15 patients subjected to treatment. However, it is worth noting that treatment was performed without selecting patients according to MGMT promoter methylation status.

Malignant cystic lesions are identifiable, also evaluating the pancreatic cyst fluid: in fact, an elevated amount of DNA and high-amplitude mutations are indicators of malignancy [37]. Moreover, the presence of a *KRAS* mutation in cyst fluid may help in the diagnosis of mucinous cysts [37].

51.4 Techniques

Immunohistochemistry is usually the gold standard to evaluate the protein expressed and cellular localization. Some antibodies allow recognizing the mutated protein and could be used for "mutation detection." In this case, it could be reported which type of mutation(s) the antibody is able to recognize or if the antibody is against the mutated isoform of the protein or the wild-type one.

Extractive techniques (e.g. sequencing or mutation specific assay) are usually used for the evaluating gene mutations. These techniques include Sanger sequencing, next-generation sequencing [6], real-time PCR, or digital PCR [92].

References

1. Dumonceau JM, Polkowski M, et al. Indications, results, and clinical impact of endoscopic ultrasound (EUS)-guided sampling in gastroenterology: European Society of Gastrointestinal Endoscopy (ESGE) Clinical Guideline. Endoscopy. 2011;43(10):897–912.
2. Hong SK, Loren DE, et al. Targeted cyst wall puncture and aspiration during EUS-FNA increases the diagnostic yield of premalignant and malignant pancreatic cysts. Gastrointest Endosc. 2012;75(4): 775–82.
3. Jenssen C, Hocke M, et al. EFSUMB Guidelines on Interventional Ultrasound (INVUS), Part IV—EUS-guided interventions: general aspects and EUS-guided sampling (long version). Ultraschall Med. 2016;37(2):E33–76.
4. Varadarajulu S, Fockens P, et al. Best practices in endoscopic ultrasound-guided fine-needle aspiration. Clin Gastroenterol Hepatol. 2012;10(7):697–703.
5. Ducreux M, Cuhna AS, et al. Cancer of the pancreas: ESMO Clinical Practice Guidelines for diagnosis, treatment and follow-up. Ann Oncol. 2015;26(Suppl 5):v56–68.
6. Jones S, Zhang X, et al. Core signaling pathways in human pancreatic cancers revealed by global genomic analyses. Science. 2008;321(5897):1801–6.
7. Wang L, Tsutsumi S, et al. Whole-exome sequencing of human pancreatic cancers and characterization of genomic instability caused by MLH1 haploinsufficiency and complete deficiency. Genome Res. 2012;22(2):208–19.
8. Biankin AV, Waddell N, et al. Pancreatic cancer genomes reveal aberrations in axon guidance pathway genes. Nature. 2012;491(7424):399–405.
9. Bailey P, Chang DK, et al. Genomic analyses identify molecular subtypes of pancreatic cancer. Nature. 2016;531(7592):47–52.
10. Waddell N, Pajic M, et al. Whole genomes redefine the mutational landscape of pancreatic cancer. Nature. 2015;518(7540):495–501.
11. Witkiewicz AK, McMillan EA, et al. Whole-exome sequencing of pancreatic cancer defines genetic diversity and therapeutic targets. Nat Commun. 2015;6:6744.
12. Hruban RH, van Mansfeld AD, et al. K-ras oncogene activation in adenocarcinoma of the human pancreas. A study of 82 carcinomas using a combination of mutant-enriched polymerase chain reaction analysis and allele-specific oligonucleotide hybridization. Am J Pathol. 1993;143(2):545–54.
13. Kanda M, Matthaei H, et al. Presence of somatic mutations in most early-stage pancreatic intraepithelial neoplasia. Gastroenterology. 2012;142(4):730–3.. e739
14. Guerra C, Schuhmacher AJ, et al. Chronic pancreatitis is essential for induction of pancreatic ductal adenocarcinoma by K-Ras oncogenes in adult mice. Cancer Cell. 2007;11(3):291–302.
15. Hingorani SR, Petricoin EF, et al. Preinvasive and invasive ductal pancreatic cancer and its early detection in the mouse. Cancer Cell. 2003;4(6):437–50.
16. Morris JP IV, Wang SC, et al. KRAS, Hedgehog, Wnt and the twisted developmental biology of pancreatic ductal adenocarcinoma. Nat Rev Cancer. 2010;10(10):683–95.
17. Pylayeva-Gupta Y, Grabocka E, et al. RAS oncogenes: weaving a tumorigenic web. Nat Rev Cancer. 2011;11(11):761–74.
18. Seidler B, Schmidt A, et al. A Cre-loxP-based mouse model for conditional somatic gene expression and

knockdown in vivo by using avian retroviral vectors. Proc Natl Acad Sci U S A. 2008;105(29):10137–42.
19. Almoguera C, Shibata D, et al. Most human carcinomas of the exocrine pancreas contain mutant c-K-ras genes. Cell. 1988;53(4):549–54.
20. de Biase D, Visani M, et al. Next generation sequencing improves the accuracy of KRAS mutation analysis in endoscopic ultrasound fine needle aspiration pancreatic lesions. PLoS One. 2014;9(2):e87651.
21. Gormally E, Caboux E, et al. Circulating free DNA in plasma or serum as biomarker of carcinogenesis: practical aspects and biological significance. Mutat Res. 2007;635(2-3):105–17.
22. Visani M, de Biase D, et al. Multiple KRAS mutations in pancreatic adenocarcinoma: molecular features of neoplastic clones indicate the selection of divergent populations of tumor cells. Int J Surg Pathol. 2013;21(6):546–52.
23. Bournet B, Selves J, et al. Endoscopic ultrasound-guided fine-needle aspiration biopsy coupled with a KRAS mutation assay using allelic discrimination improves the diagnosis of pancreatic cancer. J Clin Gastroenterol. 2015;49(1):50–6.
24. Bournet B, Souque A, et al. Endoscopic ultrasound-guided fine-needle aspiration biopsy coupled with KRAS mutation assay to distinguish pancreatic cancer from pseudotumoral chronic pancreatitis. Endoscopy. 2009;41(6):552–7.
25. Ginesta MM, Mora J, et al. Genetic and epigenetic markers in the evaluation of pancreatic masses. J Clin Pathol. 2013;66(3):192–7.
26. Maluf-Filho F, Kumar A, et al. Kras mutation analysis of fine needle aspirate under EUS guidance facilitates risk stratification of patients with pancreatic mass. J Clin Gastroenterol. 2007;41(10):906–10.
27. Ogura T, Yamao K, et al. Clinical impact of K-ras mutation analysis in EUS-guided FNA specimens from pancreatic masses. Gastrointest Endosc. 2012;75(4):769–74.
28. Pellise M, Castells A, et al. Clinical usefulness of KRAS mutational analysis in the diagnosis of pancreatic adenocarcinoma by means of endosonography-guided fine-needle aspiration biopsy. Aliment Pharmacol Ther. 2003;17(10):1299–307.
29. Tada M, Komatsu Y, et al. Quantitative analysis of K-ras gene mutation in pancreatic tissue obtained by endoscopic ultrasonography-guided fine needle aspiration: clinical utility for diagnosis of pancreatic tumor. Am J Gastroenterol. 2002;97(9):2263–70.
30. Takahashi K, Yamao K, et al. Differential diagnosis of pancreatic cancer and focal pancreatitis by using EUS-guided FNA. Gastrointest Endosc. 2005;61(1): 76–9.
31. Bournet B, Gayral M, et al. Role of endoscopic ultrasound in the molecular diagnosis of pancreatic cancer. World J Gastroenterol. 2014;20(31):10758–68.
32. Kuboki Y, Shimizu K, et al. Molecular biomarkers for progression of intraductal papillary mucinous neoplasm of the pancreas. Pancreas. 2015;44(2):227–35.
33. Rosenbaum MW, Jones M, et al. Next-generation sequencing adds value to the preoperative diagnosis of pancreatic cysts. Cancer. 2017;125(1):41–7.
34. Springer S, Wang Y, et al. A combination of molecular markers and clinical features improve the classification of pancreatic cysts. Gastroenterology. 2015;149(6):1501–10.
35. Nikiforova MN, Khalid A, et al. Integration of KRAS testing in the diagnosis of pancreatic cystic lesions: a clinical experience of 618 pancreatic cysts. Mod Pathol. 2013;26(11):1478–87.
36. Dal Molin M, Matthaei H, et al. Clinicopathological correlates of activating GNAS mutations in intraductal papillary mucinous neoplasm (IPMN) of the pancreas. Ann Surg Oncol. 2013;20(12):3802–8.
37. Khalid A, Zahid M, et al. Pancreatic cyst fluid DNA analysis in evaluating pancreatic cysts: a report of the PANDA study. Gastrointest Endosc. 2009;69(6):1095–102.
38. Van Laethem JL, Bourgeois V, et al. Relative contribution of Ki-ras gene analysis and brush cytology during ERCP for the diagnosis of biliary and pancreatic diseases. Gastrointest Endosc. 1998;47(6): 479–85.
39. Gress TM. Molecular diagnosis of pancreatobiliary malignancies in brush cytologies of biliary strictures. Gut. 2004;53(12):1727–9.
40. Khalid A, Pal R, et al. Use of microsatellite marker loss of heterozygosity in accurate diagnosis of pancreaticobiliary malignancy from brush cytology samples. Gut. 2004;53(12):1860–5.
41. Al-Haddad M, DeWitt J, et al. Performance characteristics of molecular (DNA) analysis for the diagnosis of mucinous pancreatic cysts. Gastrointest Endosc. 2014;79(1):79–87.
42. Masetti M, Acquaviva G, et al. Long-term survivors of pancreatic adenocarcinoma show low rates of genetic alterations in KRAS, TP53 and SMAD4. Cancer Biomark. 2018;21(2):323–34.
43. Oshima M, Okano K, et al. Immunohistochemically detected expression of 3 major genes (CDKN2A/p16, TP53, and SMAD4/DPC4) strongly predicts survival in patients with resectable pancreatic cancer. Ann Surg. 2013;258(2):336–46.
44. Layfield LJ, Ehya H, et al. Utilization of ancillary studies in the cytologic diagnosis of biliary and pancreatic lesions: the Papanicolaou Society of Cytopathology guidelines for pancreatobiliary cytology. Diagn Cytopathol. 2014;42(4):351–62.
45. Lohr M, Kloppel G, et al. Frequency of K-ras mutations in pancreatic intraductal neoplasias associated with pancreatic ductal adenocarcinoma and chronic pancreatitis: a meta-analysis. Neoplasia. 2005;7(1):17–23.
46. Lohr M, Maisonneuve P, et al. K-Ras mutations and benign pancreatic disease. Int J Pancreatol. 2000;27(2):93–103.
47. Luttges J, Reinecke-Luthge A, et al. Duct changes and K-ras mutations in the disease-free pancreas: analysis

of type, age relation and spatial distribution. Virchows Arch. 1999;435(5):461–8.
48. Forbes SA, Beare D, et al. COSMIC: exploring the world's knowledge of somatic mutations in human cancer. Nucleic Acids Res. 2015;43(Database issue):D805–11.
49. Vogelstein B, Kinzler KW. Cancer genes and the pathways they control. Nat Med. 2004;10(8):789–99.
50. Scarpa A, Capelli P, et al. Pancreatic adenocarcinomas frequently show p53 gene mutations. Am J Pathol. 1993;142(5):1534–43.
51. Itoi T, Takei K, et al. Immunohistochemical analysis of p53 and MIB-1 in tissue specimens obtained from endoscopic ultrasonography-guided fine needle aspiration biopsy for the diagnosis of solid pancreatic masses. Oncol Rep. 2005;13(2):229–34.
52. Jahng AW, Reicher S, et al. Staining for p53 and Ki-67 increases the sensitivity of EUS-FNA to detect pancreatic malignancy. World J Gastrointest Endosc. 2010;2(11):362–8.
53. Mu DQ, Wang GF, et al. p53 protein expression and CA19.9 values in differential cytological diagnosis of pancreatic cancer complicated with chronic pancreatitis and chronic pancreatitis. World J Gastroenterol. 2003;9(8):1815–8.
54. Siegel PM, Massague J. Cytostatic and apoptotic actions of TGF-beta in homeostasis and cancer. Nat Rev Cancer. 2003;3(11):807–21.
55. Hahn SA, Schutte M, et al. DPC4, a candidate tumor suppressor gene at human chromosome 18q21.1. Science. 1996;271(5247):350–3.
56. Iacobuzio-Donahue CA, Wilentz RE, et al. Dpc4 protein in mucinous cystic neoplasms of the pancreas: frequent loss of expression in invasive carcinomas suggests a role in genetic progression. Am J Surg Pathol. 2000;24(11):1544–8.
57. Maitra A, Hruban RH. Pancreatic cancer. Annu Rev Pathol. 2008;3:157–88.
58. Tascilar M, Skinner HG, et al. The SMAD4 protein and prognosis of pancreatic ductal adenocarcinoma. Clin Cancer Res. 2001;7(12):4115–21.
59. Schutte M, Hruban RH, et al. DPC4 gene in various tumor types. Cancer Res. 1996;56(11):2527–30.
60. Blackford A, Serrano OK, et al. SMAD4 gene mutations are associated with poor prognosis in pancreatic cancer. Clin Cancer Res. 2009;15(14):4674–9.
61. Singh P, Srinivasan R, et al. SMAD4 genetic alterations predict a worse prognosis in patients with pancreatic ductal adenocarcinoma. Pancreas. 2012;41(4):541–6.
62. Nelson WJ, Nusse R. Convergence of Wnt, beta-catenin, and cadherin pathways. Science. 2004;303(5663):1483–7.
63. Rubinfeld B, Robbins P, et al. Stabilization of beta-catenin by genetic defects in melanoma cell lines. Science. 1997;275(5307):1790–2.
64. Tanaka Y, Kato K, et al. Frequent beta-catenin mutation and cytoplasmic/nuclear accumulation in pancreatic solid-pseudopapillary neoplasm. Cancer Res. 2001;61(23):8401–4.
65. Abraham SC, Klimstra DS, et al. Solid-pseudopapillary tumors of the pancreas are genetically distinct from pancreatic ductal adenocarcinomas and almost always harbor beta-catenin mutations. Am J Pathol. 2002;160(4):1361–9.
66. Kubota Y, Kawakami H, et al. CTNNB1 mutational analysis of solid-pseudopapillary neoplasms of the pancreas using endoscopic ultrasound-guided fine-needle aspiration and next-generation deep sequencing. J Gastroenterol. 2015;50(2):203–10.
67. Zeng G, Germinaro M, et al. Aberrant Wnt/beta-catenin signaling in pancreatic adenocarcinoma. Neoplasia. 2006;8(4):279–89.
68. Wu J, Jiao Y, et al. Whole-exome sequencing of neoplastic cysts of the pancreas reveals recurrent mutations in components of ubiquitin-dependent pathways. Proc Natl Acad Sci U S A. 2011a;108(52):21188–93.
69. Komatsu H, Tanji E, et al. A GNAS mutation found in pancreatic intraductal papillary mucinous neoplasms induces drastic alterations of gene expression profiles with upregulation of mucin genes. PLoS One. 2014;9(2):e87875.
70. Amato E, Molin MD, et al. Targeted next-generation sequencing of cancer genes dissects the molecular profiles of intraductal papillary neoplasms of the pancreas. J Pathol. 2014;233(3):217–27.
71. Furukawa T, Kuboki Y, et al. Whole-exome sequencing uncovers frequent GNAS mutations in intraductal papillary mucinous neoplasms of the pancreas. Sci Rep. 2011;1:161.
72. Singhi AD, Nikiforova MN, et al. Preoperative GNAS and KRAS testing in the diagnosis of pancreatic mucinous cysts. Clin Cancer Res. 2014;20(16):4381–9.
73. Wu J, Matthaei H, et al. Recurrent GNAS mutations define an unexpected pathway for pancreatic cyst development. Sci Transl Med. 2011b;3(92):92ra66.
74. Schutte M, Hruban RH, et al. Abrogation of the Rb/p16 tumor-suppressive pathway in virtually all pancreatic carcinomas. Cancer Res. 1997;57(15):3126–30.
75. Bartsch D, Shevlin DW, et al. Frequent mutations of CDKN2 in primary pancreatic adenocarcinomas. Genes Chromosomes Cancer. 1995;14(3):189–95.
76. Caldas C, Hahn SA, et al. Frequent somatic mutations and homozygous deletions of the p16 (MTS1) gene in pancreatic adenocarcinoma. Nat Genet. 1994;8(1):27–32.
77. Rozenblum E, Schutte M, et al. Tumor-suppressive pathways in pancreatic carcinoma. Cancer Res. 1997;57(9):1731–4.
78. Bartsch DK, Sina-Frey M, et al. CDKN2A germline mutations in familial pancreatic cancer. Ann Surg. 2002;236(6):730–7.
79. McWilliams RR, Wieben ED, et al. Prevalence of CDKN2A mutations in pancreatic cancer patients: implications for genetic counseling. Eur J Hum Genet. 2011;19(4):472–8.
80. Gerdes B, Ramaswamy A, et al. p16INK4a is a prognostic marker in resected ductal pancreatic cancer: an

analysis of p16INK4a, p53, MDM2, an Rb. Ann Surg. 2002;235(1):51–9.

81. Ohtsubo K, Watanabe H, et al. Abnormalities of tumor suppressor gene p16 in pancreatic carcinoma: immunohistochemical and genetic findings compared with clinicopathological parameters. J Gastroenterol. 2003;38(7):663–71.
82. Abe T, Fukushima N, et al. Genome-wide allelotypes of familial pancreatic adenocarcinomas and familial and sporadic intraductal papillary mucinous neoplasms. Clin Cancer Res. 2007;13(20):6019–25.
83. Forbes SA, Beare D, et al. COSMIC: somatic cancer genetics at high-resolution. Nucleic Acids Res. 2017;45(D1):D777–83.
84. Laghi L, Beghelli S, et al. Irrelevance of microsatellite instability in the epidemiology of sporadic pancreatic ductal adenocarcinoma. PLoS One. 2012;7(9):e46002.
85. Valero V 3rd, Saunders TJ, et al. Reliable detection of somatic mutations in fine needle aspirates of pancreatic cancer with next-generation sequencing: implications for surgical management. Ann Surg. 2016;263(1):153–61.
86. Sato N, Rosty C, et al. STK11/LKB1 Peutz-Jeghers gene inactivation in intraductal papillary-mucinous neoplasms of the pancreas. Am J Pathol. 2001;159(6):2017–22.
87. Su GH, Hruban RH, et al. Germline and somatic mutations of the STK11/LKB1 Peutz-Jeghers gene in pancreatic and biliary cancers. Am J Pathol. 1999;154(6):1835–40.
88. Calhoun ES, Jones JB, et al. BRAF and FBXW7 (CDC4, FBW7, AGO, SEL10) mutations in distinct subsets of pancreatic cancer: potential therapeutic targets. Am J Pathol. 2003;163(4):1255–60.
89. Peng DF, Kanai Y, et al. DNA methylation of multiple tumor-related genes in association with overexpression of DNA methyltransferase 1 (DNMT1) during multistage carcinogenesis of the pancreas. Carcinogenesis. 2006;27(6):1160–8.
90. Hegi ME, Diserens AC, et al. MGMT gene silencing and benefit from temozolomide in glioblastoma. N Engl J Med. 2005;352(10):997–1003.
91. Moore MJ, Feld R, et al. A phase II study of temozolomide in advanced untreated pancreatic cancer. Invest New Drugs. 1998;16(1):77–9.
92. Azuara D, Ginesta MM, et al. Nanofluidic digital PCR for KRAS mutation detection and quantification in gastrointestinal cancer. Clin Chem. 2012;58(9):1332–41.

Part VII

Clinical Algorithms

52 Suspected Common Bile Duct Stones (Algorithm)

Maximilian David Schneider

Abbreviations

CBDS	Common bile duct stone
CT	Computed tomography
EHL	Electrohydraulic lithotripsy
EPBD	Endoscopic papillary balloon dilation
ERCP	Endoscopic retrograde cholangiopancreatography
EST	Endoscopic sphincterotomy
EUS	Endoscopic ultrasound
LFTs	Liver function tests
LL	Laser lithotripsy
MRCP	Magnetic resonance cholangiopancreatography
PTCD	Percutaneous transhepatic cholangial drainage
US	Ultrasound

Explanation

Common bile duct stones can be suspected in a patient presenting with biliary colic, elevated liver enzymes, jaundice, cholangitis or pancreatitis. Beside clinical features, laboratory evaluation and adequate abdominal imaging (primarily abdominal ultrasound) have to be performed to assess the likelihood for the presence of CBDS. Recent ESGE guidelines recommend direct ERCP in patients with visible stones or cholangitis only. In other cases (intermediate likelihood) EUS or MRCP before ERCP are recommended.

ERCP is the standard treatment for CBDS. Stone extraction should be performed with a basket or a balloon catheter after sphincterotomy. When stone extraction is incomplete, further treatment can be performed using endoscopic papillary balloon dilation and/or lithotripsy (mechanical, electrohydraulic, laser) during index ERCP or at a second timepoint. In more complex cases alternative procedures like PTCD, surgical CBD exploration or EUS-guided bile duct cannulation are treatment options in referral centres.

An elective cholecystectomy in nearly all patients is mandatory to avoid stone recurrence.

M. D. Schneider (✉)
Department of Gastroenterology, Hepatology and Endocrinology, Robert-Bosch-Hospital, Stuttgart, Germany
e-mail: maximilian.schneider@rbk.de

M. Mutignani et al. (eds.), *Endotherapy in Biliopancreatic Diseases: ERCP Meets EUS*,
https://doi.org/10.1007/978-3-030-42569-2_52

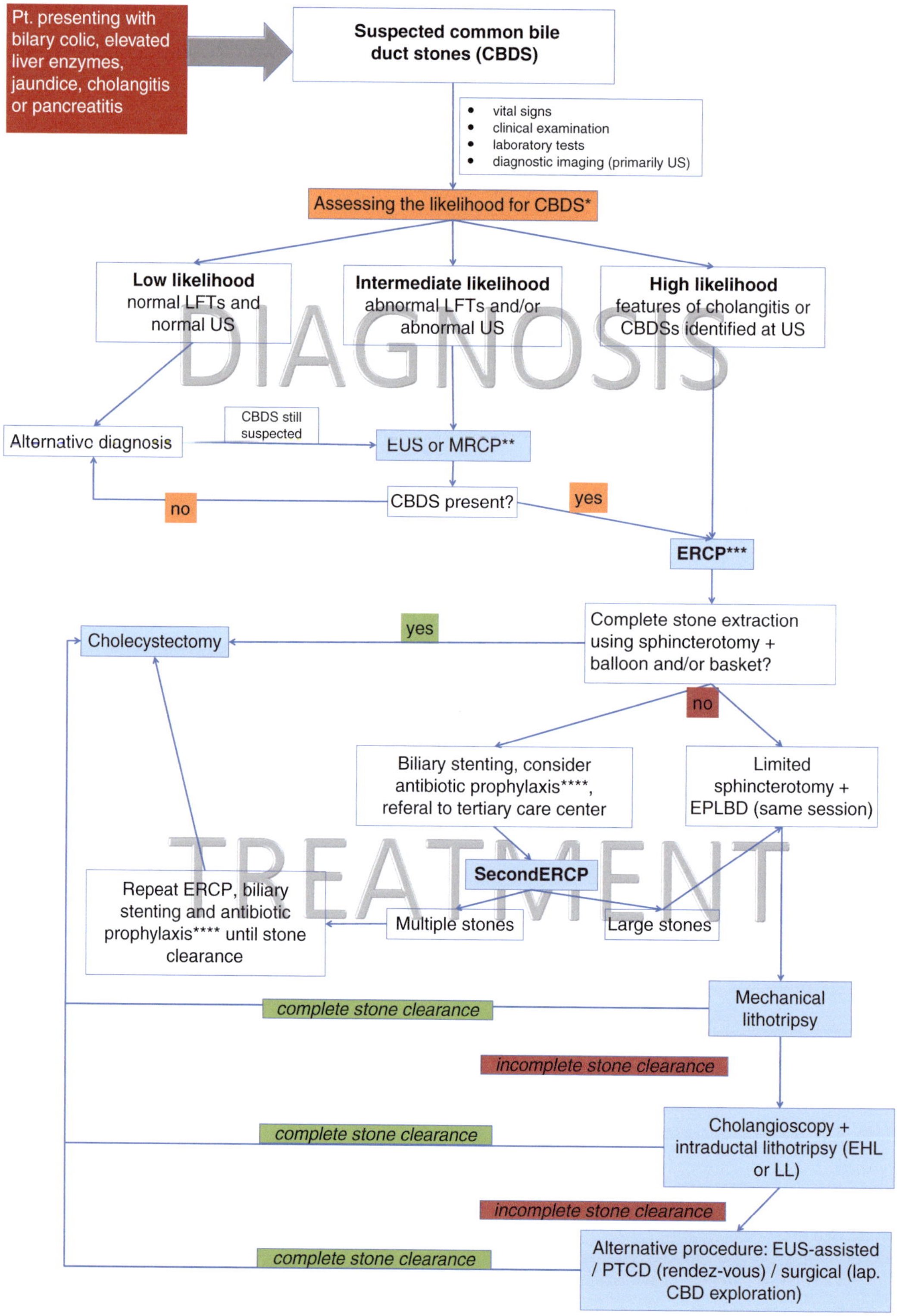
Pt. presenting with biliary colic, elevated liver enzymes, jaundice, cholangitis or pancreatitis
Suspected common bile duct stones (CBDS)
vital signs
clinical examination
laboratory tests
diagnostic imaging (primarily US)
Assessing the likelihood for CBDS*
Low likelihood normal LFTs and normal US
Intermediate likelihood abnormal LFTs and/or abnormal US
High likelihood features of cholangitis or CBDSs identified at US
DIAGNOSIS
Alternative diagnosis
CBDS still suspected
EUS or MRCP**
CBDS present?
no
yes
ERCP***
Complete stone extraction using sphincterotomy + balloon and/or basket?
yes
Cholecystectomy
no
Biliary stenting, consider antibiotic prophylaxis****, referal to tertiary care center
Limited sphincterotomy + EPLBD (same session)
TREATMENT
SecondERCP
Repeat ERCP, biliary stenting and antibiotic prophylaxis**** until stone clearance
Multiple stones
Large stones
complete stone clearance
Mechanical lithotripsy
incomplete stone clearance
complete stone clearance
Cholangioscopy + intraductal lithotripsy (EHL or LL)
incomplete stone clearance
complete stone clearance
Alternative procedure: EUS-assisted / PTCD (rendez-vous) / surgical (lap. CBD exploration)

Footnotes:

*The assessment of the likelihood for the presence of CBDS is different between European and American Guidelines. A retrospective analysis showed that the positive predictive value of ASGE high-risk criteria (bilirubin level >4 mg/dL or CBD stone on US or bilirubin level 1.8–4 mg/dL plus dilated CBD or clinical cholangitis) is 64%, therefore around one-third of patients receive unnecessary ERCP. Recent ESGE guidelines are more strict in suggesting direct ERCP and recommend using EUS or MRCP in patients without visible stones on US or cholangitis (intermediate likelihood).

**Alternatively direct cholecystectomy with intraoperative cholangiography or laparoscopic ultrasound can be performed.

***The timepoint of ERCP mainly depends on the presence of acute cholangitis (see Flowchart Acute Cholangitis) or acute pancreatitis (see Chap. 31 Acute Pancreatitis).

****Antibiotic prophylaxis is recommended, if biliary drainage is incomplete.

Bibliography

Chathadi KV, Chandrasekhara V, Acosta RD, Decker GA, Early DS, Eloubeidi MA, et al. The role of ERCP in benign diseases of the biliary tract (ASGE guideline). Gastrointest Endosc. 2015;81:795–803.

EASL. Clinical Practice Guidelines on the prevention, diagnosis and treatment of gallstones. J Hepatol. 2016;65(1):146–81.

Gutt C, et al. New S3-guidelines for diagnosis and treatment of gallstones (DGVS Guideline 2018). 2018. https://www.dgvs.de/wp-content/uploads/2018/04/Leitlinie-Gallensteine-11.04.2018.pdf.

He H, Tan C, Wu J, Dai N, Hu W, Zhang Y, et al. Accuracy of ASGE high-risk criteria in evaluation of patients with suspected common bile duct stones. Gastrointestinal Endoscopy. 2017;86(3):525–32.

Manes G, Paspatis G, Aabakken L, Anderloni A, Arvanitakis M, Ah-Soune P, et al. Endoscopic management of common bile duct stones: European Society of Gastrointestinal Endoscopy (ESGE) guideline. Endoscopy. 2019;51:472–91.

Maple JT, Ben-Menachem T, Anderson MA, Appalaneni V, Banerjee S, Cash BD, et al. The role of endoscopy in the evaluation of suspected choledocholithiasis (ASGE guideline). Gastrointest Endosc. 2010;71:1–9.

Maple JT, Ikenberry SO, Anderson MA, Appalaneni V, Decker GA, Early D, et al. The role of endoscopy in the management of choledocholithiasis (ASGE guideline). Gastrointest Endosc. 2011;74:731–44.

Williams E, Beckingham I, El Sayed G, Gurusamy K, Sturgess R, Webster G, et al. Updated guideline on the management of common bile duct stones (CBDS). Gut. 2017;66:765–82.

Acute Cholangitis (Algorithm)

53

Maximilian David Schneider

Abbreviations

AC	Acute cholangitis
Amp/Sul	Ampicillin/sulbactam
CRP	C-reactive protein
CT	Computed-tomography
DDx	Differential diagnosis
Dori	Doripenem
ERCP	Endoscopic retrograde cholangiopancreatography
Erta	Ertapenem
EST	Endoscopic sphincterotomy
Gen.	Generation
ICU	Intensive care unit
Imi	Imipenem-cilastatin
Mero	Meropenem
MRCP	Magnetic resonance cholangiopancreatography
PCT	Procalcitonin
Pip/Taz	Piperacillin/tazobactam
T	Temperature
US	Ultrasound
Vanco	Vancomycin
WBC	White blood count

Explanation

AC can be suspected in a patient with clinical or laboratory signs of infection and abdominal pain, jaundice, or a former history of cholangitis, especially when a biliary stent is implanted.

According to the Tokyo Guidelines clinical or laboratory signs of infection plus laboratory markers of cholestasis and/or biliary pathology on abdominal imaging are necessary to diagnose AC. When AC is confirmed, severity assessment of the disease is mandatory for the development of the further treatment strategy: For example, patients with evidence of organ dysfunction (e.g. sepsis) need broad spectrum antibiotics and urgent biliary drainage after clinical stabilization, whereas mildly affected patients can be treated in a more conservative manner.

M. D. Schneider (✉)
Department of Gastroenterology, Hepatology and Endocrinology, Robert-Bosch-Hospital, Stuttgart, Germany
e-mail: maximilian.schneider@rbk.de

M. Mutignani et al. (eds.), *Endotherapy in Biliopancreatic Diseases: ERCP Meets EUS*,
https://doi.org/10.1007/978-3-030-42569-2_53

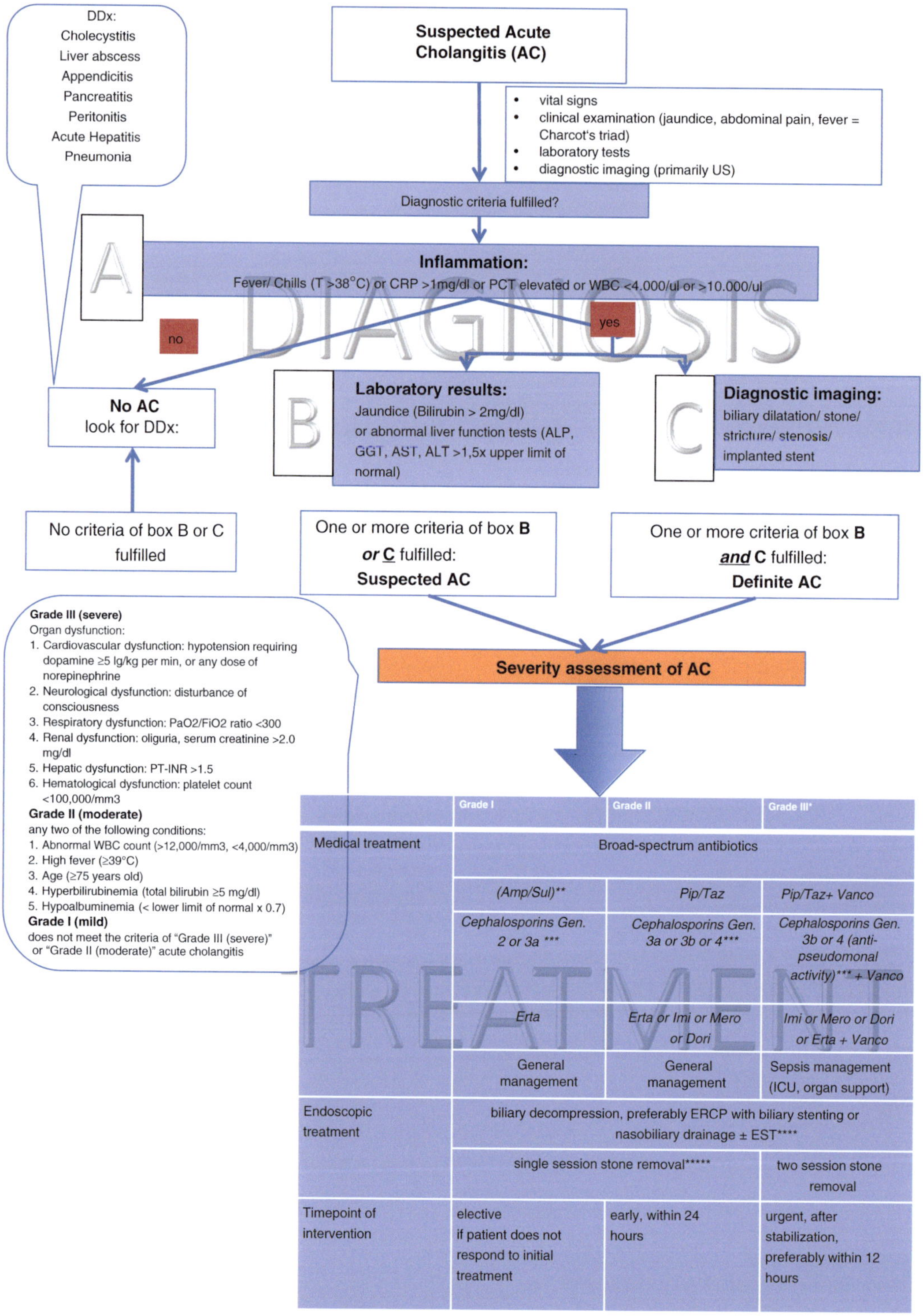

	Grade I	Grade II	Grade III*
Medical treatment	Broad-spectrum antibiotics		
	*(Amp/Sul)***	*Pip/Taz*	*Pip/Taz+ Vanco*
	*Cephalosporins Gen. 2 or 3a ****	*Cephalosporins Gen. 3a or 3b or 4****	*Cephalosporins Gen. 3b or 4 (anti-pseudomonal activity)*** + Vanco*
	Erta	*Erta or Imi or Mero or Dori*	*Imi or Mero or Dori or Erta + Vanco*
	General management	General management	Sepsis management (ICU, organ support)
Endoscopic treatment	biliary decompression, preferably ERCP with biliary stenting or nasobiliary drainage ± EST****		
	single session stone removal*****		two session stone removal
Timepoint of intervention	elective if patient does not respond to initial treatment	early, within 24 hours	urgent, after stabilization, preferably within 12 hours

Footnotes:

*Antibiotic therapy in healthcare-associated/nosocomial infections is equal to grade III infections; in case of colonization or high-rates of vancomycin-resistant enterococci (VRE) or prior vancomycin exposure, linezolid, daptomycin or tigecyclin should be used instead

**Low susceptibility rates especially for E. coli

***Addition of anti-anerobic therapy (e.g. metronidazole) is recommended in case of biliary-enteric anastomosis

****EST generally not required for biliary drainage, caution especially in case of coagulopathy (medical and sepsis-induced) and antithrombotic therapy. PTCD is an alternative option, when ERCP is not possible, surgery should be avoided

*****Consider two sessions if endoscopic papillary large balloon dilation for large or multiple stones is required

Bibliography

EASL. Clinical Practice Guidelines on the prevention, diagnosis and treatment of gallstones. J Hepatol. 2016;65(1):146–81.

Gomi H, Solomkin JS, Schlossberg D, Okamoto K, Takada T, Strasberg SM, et al. Tokyo Guidelines 2018: antimicrobial therapy for acute cholangitis and cholecystitis. J Hepatobiliary Pancreat Sci. 2018; 25:3–16.

Karvellas CJ, Abraldes JG, Zepeda-Gomez S, Moffat DC, Mirzanejad Y, Vazquez-Grande G, et al. The impact of delayed biliary decompression and anti-microbial therapy in 260 patients with cholangitis-associated septic shock. Aliment Pharmacol Ther. 2016;44: 755–66.

Kiriyama S, Kozaka K, Takada T, Strasberg SM, Pitt HA, Gabata T, et al. Tokyo Guidelines 2018: diagnostic criteria and severity grading of acute cholangitis (with videos). J Hepatobiliary Pancreat Sci. 2018; 25:17–30.

Miura F, Okamoto K, Takada T, Strasberg SM, Asbun HJ, Pitt HA, et al. Tokyo Guidelines 2018: initial management of acute biliary infection and flowchart for acute cholangitis. J Hepatobiliary Pancreat Sci. 2018;25:31–40.

Mukai S, Itoi T, Baron TH, Takada T, Strasberg SM, Pitt HA, et al. Indications and techniques of biliary drainage for acute cholangitis in updated Tokyo Guidelines 2018. J Hepatobiliary Pancreat Sci. 2017;24: 537–49.

Solomkin JS, Mazuski JE, Bradley JS, Rodvold KA, Goldstein EJ, Baron EJ, et al. Diagnosis and management of complicated intra-abdominal infection in adults and children: guidelines by the Surgical Infection Society and the Infectious Diseases Society of America. Clin Infect Dis. 2010;50: 133–64.

54 Diagnosis of Etiology in Acute Pancreatitis

Nicolò de Pretis and Luca Frulloni

Acute pancreatitis is an acute inflammatory disease of the pancreas representing a leading cause of hospital admission in Gastroenterology units [1].

Different etiological factors have been described over the last decades. A correct identification of etiology is crucial for the clinical management of acute pancreatitis and to prevent recurrent attacks.

The aim of this chapter is to review the etiology of acute pancreatitis, suggesting a clinical approach to identify the cause of the disease. Post-ERCP acute pancreatitis and acute pancreatitis secondary to pancreatic trauma are not considered in the present chapter.

Biliary pancreatitis, mainly secondary to gallstones, is the most frequent form of acute pancreatitis and accounts for up to 70% of cases [2]. The obstruction of the main pancreatic duct due to stones and/or to papillary edema might lead to pancreatic ductal hypertension, which is considered the main trigger of the inflammatory process.

In patients with biliary pancreatitis, liver tests (particularly AST and ALT) are generally elevated. In detail, the higher the serum level of ALT, the greater are specificity and positive predictive value in diagnosing biliary pancreatitis. The probability of biliary pancreatitis is up to 95% with a threefold elevation of ALT [3]. Therefore, transaminase dosage is suggested in patients with acute pancreatitis as the first step of diagnostic process. A transient elevation of liver tests is so specific that, even with negative imaging (US, MRI, or EUS), a diagnosis of biliary acute pancreatitis can be achieved. Biliary acute pancreatitis includes mainly gallstones and microlithiasis, but also, more rarely, sphincter of Oddi disfunction, anatomic abnormalities, or peri-ampullary tumors. MRI or EUS can be performed in patients with persistent elevation of transaminases to better define the cause of biliary obstruction [4]. If transaminases are normal, a biliary etiology may be safely excluded, even in the presence of sludge or stones in gallbladder at imaging at the clinical onset of the disease.

The second most common etiological factor of acute pancreatitis is alcohol, which is responsible for 20–30% of cases [5]. The underlying mechanism of pancreatic injury is still not understood. A correct medical and personal history is important to identify these patients. A threshold of alcohol consumption definitely associated to the development of acute and/or chronic pancreatitis has not been identified yet. Therefore, even considering the low prevalence of pancreatitis in heavy alcohol drinkers, a definitive diagnosis of alcohol-related acute pancreatitis should be made with caution. Some authors suggest 40 or 50 g/day of alcohol consumption as a clinically useful

N. de Pretis · L. Frulloni (✉)
Department of Medicine, Pancreas Institute, University of Verona, Verona, Italy
e-mail: luca.frulloni@univr.it

M. Mutignani et al. (eds.), *Endotherapy in Biliopancreatic Diseases: ERCP Meets EUS*, https://doi.org/10.1007/978-3-030-42569-2_54

threshold under which a pancreatitis should not be considered as alcohol related [5–7]. In patients with personal history of heavy alcohol consumption, with normal or slightly (but not transient) elevated transaminase, alcohol should be considered as possible etiology of the pancreatitis. However, in these patients, an imaging technique needs to be performed to exclude other causes of acute pancreatitis or the presence of chronic pancreatitis.

Hypertriglyceridemia has been identified as another important cause of acute pancreatitis accounting for 1–14% of cases [8]. Serum triglyceride levels >1000 mg/dL are considered necessary to induce acute pancreatitis. However, there is no clear threshold above which hypertriglyceridemia is known to trigger the inflammatory process. Serum triglyceride levels >1000 mg/dL has been suggested as a criterion to make a definitive diagnosis of hypertriglyceridemic acute pancreatitis. Diagnosis might be considered as probable if serum triglycerides levels are between 500 and 1000 mg/dL [9]. Considering that the hypertriglyceridemia may be transient, we strongly suggest dosing triglycerides at admission to avoid a misdiagnosis of hypertriglyceridemic acute pancreatitis. Moreover, hypertriglyceridemic acute pancreatitis seems to be clinically more aggressive compared to other forms [10], and a correct diagnosis might have a significant prognostic impact.

In patients with normal liver tests, low or absent alcohol intake, and triglycerides levels lower than 500 mg/dL, other rare causes of acute pancreatitis should be investigated. First, in all these patients, an imaging procedure (MRI and/or CT scan) is strongly suggested for evaluating both the pancreatic parenchyma and the ductal system. Benign, pre-malignant, and malignant tumors might be associated to acute pancreatitis. Solid and/or cystic lesions detected at imaging might be considered the etiological factor of acute pancreatitis if the more frequent causes have been excluded. Autoimmune pancreatitis may be a cause of acute pancreatitis. In these patients, imaging should suggest the diagnosis particularly in diffuse but also in focal forms. International Consensus Diagnostic Criteria need to be applied to confirm the autoimmune etiology [11]. In patients without typical imaging features of autoimmune pancreatitis, the diagnosis can be excluded and serum IgG4 should not be measured.

Anatomic abnormalities of the pancreatic ductal system, such as pancreas divisum, have been suggested as a cause of acute pancreatitis. However, the true role of pancreas divisum in the pathogenesis of acute pancreatitis is still debated. The postulated mechanism is an obstruction of the pancreatic juice outflow through the minor papilla, too small to drain adequately the large part of pancreatic secretion, leading to an increased ductal pressure able to induce acute pancreatitis. However, considering the high prevalence of pancreas divisum (up to 10%) in the general population [12], the detection of pancreas divisum as an etiological factor should be carefully managed. More investigations are required before considering the pancreatitis as related to pancreas divisum. The presence of dilation of pre-papillary main pancreatic duct (Santorinicele) can be considered the cause of pancreatitis. A secretin-enhanced US or MRI is able to better define the presence of Santorinicele and, also, to show a prolonged dilation of the main pancreatic duct that might be considered as indirect signs of outlet obstruction [13]. In these selected patients, pancreas divisum should be strongly considered as a probable cause of the pancreatitis.

If all the above-reported causes of acute pancreatitis are not diagnosed, pharmacological history should be carefully investigated. More than 100 medications have been identified as related to pancreatitis, but acute pancreatitis due to medications is rare, probably less than 5% [14]. Only few medications have been clearly related to acute pancreatitis based on a large body of evidence. The great majority of drugs are considered as potential cause of pancreatitis based on few or single case reports. Some authors proposed a classification of drugs associated to pancreatitis, based on the strength of the scientific evidence, into four categories. Drugs belonging to class 1 have at least one case report with positive rechallenging after the exclusion of the most frequent causes of pancreatitis while drugs belonging to class 4 are based on a single case report [15]. Therefore, a diagnosis of drug-related acute pancreatitis should be made with caution only after a rigorous exclusion of other etiological factors.

Etiological factor of acute pancreatitis remains unknown in around 20% of patients. In this clinical setting, the search for gene mutations may be considered. Genetic tests are suggested in young patients with the clinical onset of the disease before 20 years and in patients with positive family history for pancreatitis, independently from the presence of other causes of pancreatitis.

Many pancreatitis-associated genetic mutations have been identified over the last decades. Patients with genetic predisposition for pancreatitis might present as acute, recurrent, or chronic pancreatitis. In the clinical management, the most important mutations have been described on the following genes, PRSS1, SPINK1, and CFTR.

PRSS1 encodes a cationic trypsinogen, and its mutation is related to a premature activation of digestive enzymes in the pancreas, leading to a dominantly inherited hereditary pancreatitis [16]. SPINK1 encodes a pancreatic secretory trypsin inhibitor, and a mutation in SPINK1 may interfere with its protective action, promoting the development of pancreatitis with low penetrance [17]. Mutations in the gene of cystic fibrosis (CFTR) is related to pancreatitis not only in homozygous and compound mutations (patients suffering from cystic fibrosis), but even in patients with heterozygous mutations (patients not affected by cystic fibrosis) [18].

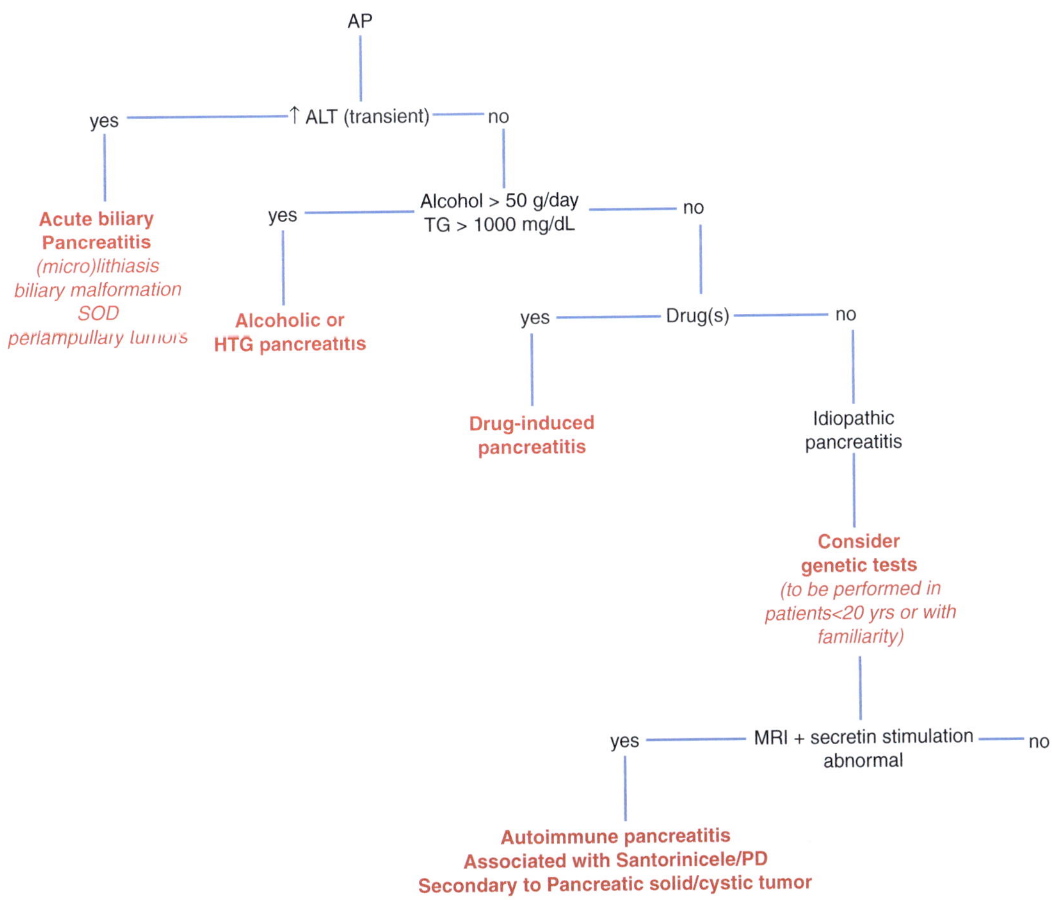

Diagnostic algorithm for diagnosis of etiology in acute pancreatitis. AP is acute pancreatitis; HTG is hyertriglyceridemia; PD is pancreas divisum. In the algorithm post-ERCP acute pancreatitis and post-traumatic pancreatitis are excluded

References

1. Peery AF, Dellon ES, Lund J, Crockett SD, McGowan CE, Bulsiewicz WJ, et al. Burden of gastrointestinal disease in the United States: 2012 update. Gastroenterology. 2012;143:1179–87.
2. Forsmarkk CE, Baillie J, AGA Institute Clinical Practice and Economics Committee, AGA Institute Governing Board. AGA Institute technical review on acute pancreatitis. Gastroenterology. 2007;132:2022–44.
3. Tenner S, Dubner H, Steinberg W. Predicting gallstone pancreatitis with laboratory parameters: a meta-analysis. Am J Gastroenterol. 1994;89:1863–6.
4. De Lèdinghen V, Lecesne R, Raymond JM, Gense V, Amouretti M, Drouillard J, et al. Diagnosis of choledicholithiasis: EUS or magnetic resonance cholangiography? A prospective controller study. Gatrointest Endosc. 1999;49:26–31.
5. Yang AL, Vadhavkar S, Singh G, Omary MB. Epidemiology of alcohol-related liver and pancreatic disease in the United States. Arch Intern Med. 2008;168:649–56.
6. Samokhvalov AV, Rehm J, Roerecke M. Alcohol consumption as a risk factor for acute and chronic pancreatitis: a systematic review and a series of meta-analyses. EBioMedicine. 2015;2:1996–2002.
7. Setiawan VW, Monroe K, Lugea A, Yadav D, Pandol S. Uniting epidemiology and experimental disease models for alcohol-related pancreatic disease. Alcohol Res. 2017;38:173–82.
8. Scherer J, Singh VP, Pitchumoni CS, Yadav D. Issues in hypertriglyceridemic pancreatitis: an update. J Clin Gastroenterol. 2014;48:195–203.
9. de Pretis N, Amodio A, Frulloni L. Hypertriglyceridemic pancreatitis: epidemiology, pathophysiology and clinical management. United European Gastroenterol J. 2018;6:649–55.
10. Carr RA, Rejowski BJ, Cote GA, Pitt HA, Zyromski NJ. Systematic review of hypetriglyceridemia-induced acute pancreatitis: a more virulent etiology? Pancreatology. 2016;16:469–76.
11. Shimosegawa T, Chari ST, Frulloni L, Kamisawa T, Kawa S, Mino-Kenudson M, et al. International consensus diagnostic criteria for autoimmune pancreatitis: guidelines of the International Association of Pancreatology. Pancreas. 2011;40:352–8.
12. Buelow R, Simon P, Thiel R, Thamm P, Messner P, Lerch MM, et al. Anatomic variants of the pancreatic duct and their clinical relevance: an MR-guided study in the general population. Eur Radiol. 2014;24:3142–9.
13. Manfredi R, Pozzi Mucelli R. Secretin-enhanced MR imaging of the pancreas. Radiology. 2016;279:29–43.
14. Tenner S. Drug induced acute pancreatitis: does it exist? World J Gastroenterol. 2014;20:16529–34.
15. Badalov N, Baradarian R, Iswara K, Li J, Steinberg W, Tenner S. Drug-induced acute pancreatitis: an evidence-based review. Clin Gastroentreol Hepatol. 2007;5:648–61.
16. Whitcomb DC. Genetic aspects of pancreatitis. Annu Rev Med. 2010;61:413–24.
17. DiMagno MJ, DiMagno EP. Chronic pancreatitis. Curr Opin Gastroentreol. 2005;21:544–54.
18. Rowntree RK, Harris A. The phenotypic consequences of CFTR mutations. Ann Hum Genet. 2003;67:471–85.

Periampullary Biliary Strictures (Algorithm)

55

Juan J. Vila

Abbreviations

CT	Computerized tomography
ERCP	Endoscopic retrograde cholangiopancreatography
EUS	Endoscopic ultrasound
FNA	Fine needle aspiration

J. J. Vila (✉)
Endoscopy Unit, Gastroenterology Department,
Complejo Hospitalario de Navarra, Pamplona, Spain

M. Mutignani et al. (eds.), *Endotherapy in Biliopancreatic Diseases: ERCP Meets EUS*,
https://doi.org/10.1007/978-3-030-42569-2_55

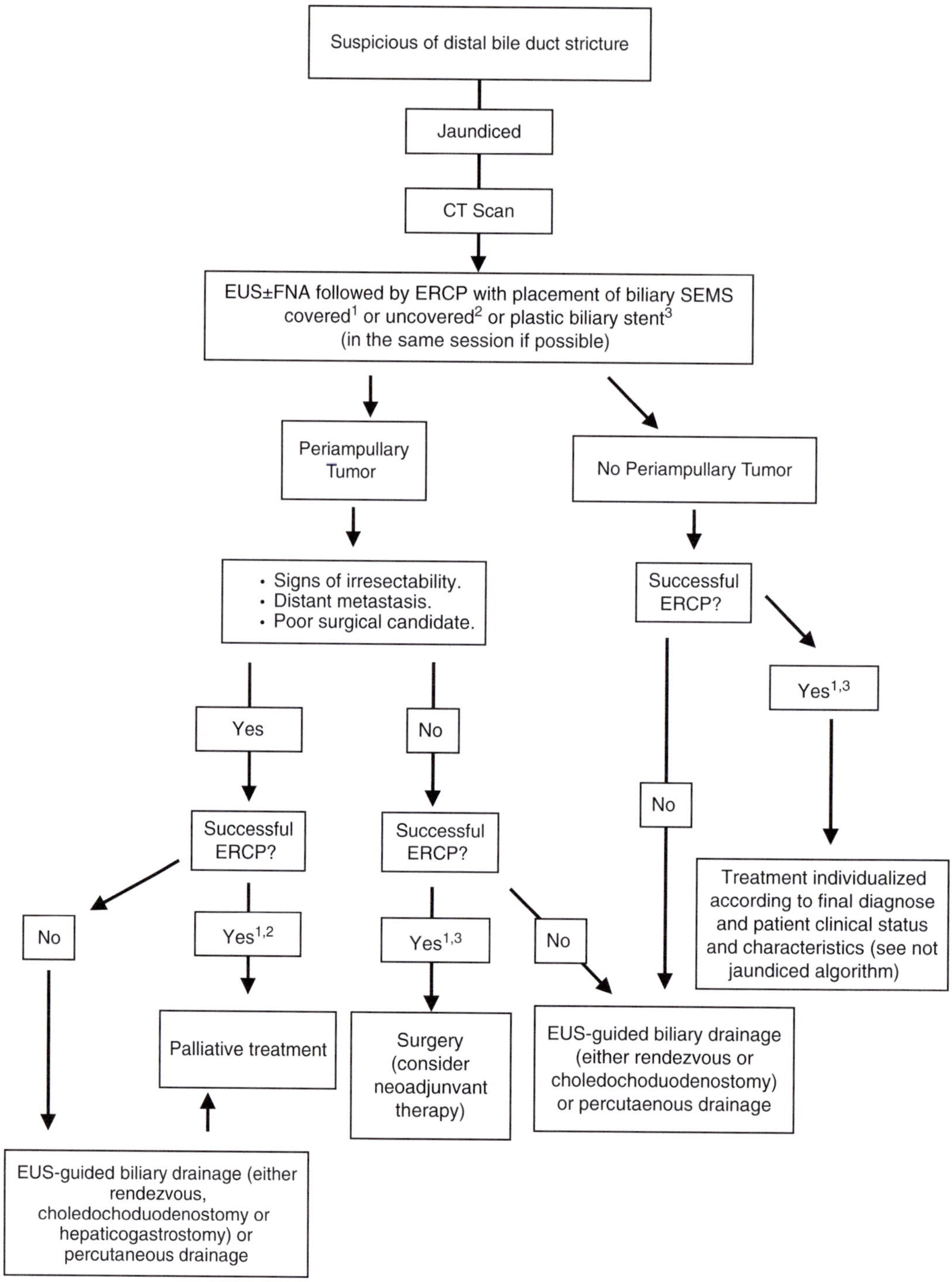
Suspicious of distal bile duct stricture
Jaundiced
CT Scan
EUS±FNA followed by ERCP with placement of biliary SEMS covered[1] or uncovered[2] or plastic biliary stent[3] (in the same session if possible)
Periampullary Tumor
No Periampullary Tumor
• Signs of irresectability.
• Distant metastasis.
• Poor surgical candidate.
Successful ERCP?
Yes[1,3]
Yes
No
Successful ERCP?
Successful ERCP?
No
No
Yes[1,2]
Yes[1,3]
No
Treatment individualized according to final diagnose and patient clinical status and characteristics (see not jaundiced algorithm)
Palliative treatment
Surgery (consider neoadjuvant therapy)
EUS-guided biliary drainage (either rendezvous or choledochoduodenostomy) or percutaenous drainage
EUS-guided biliary drainage (either rendezvous, choledochoduodenostomy or hepaticogastrostomy) or percutaneous drainage

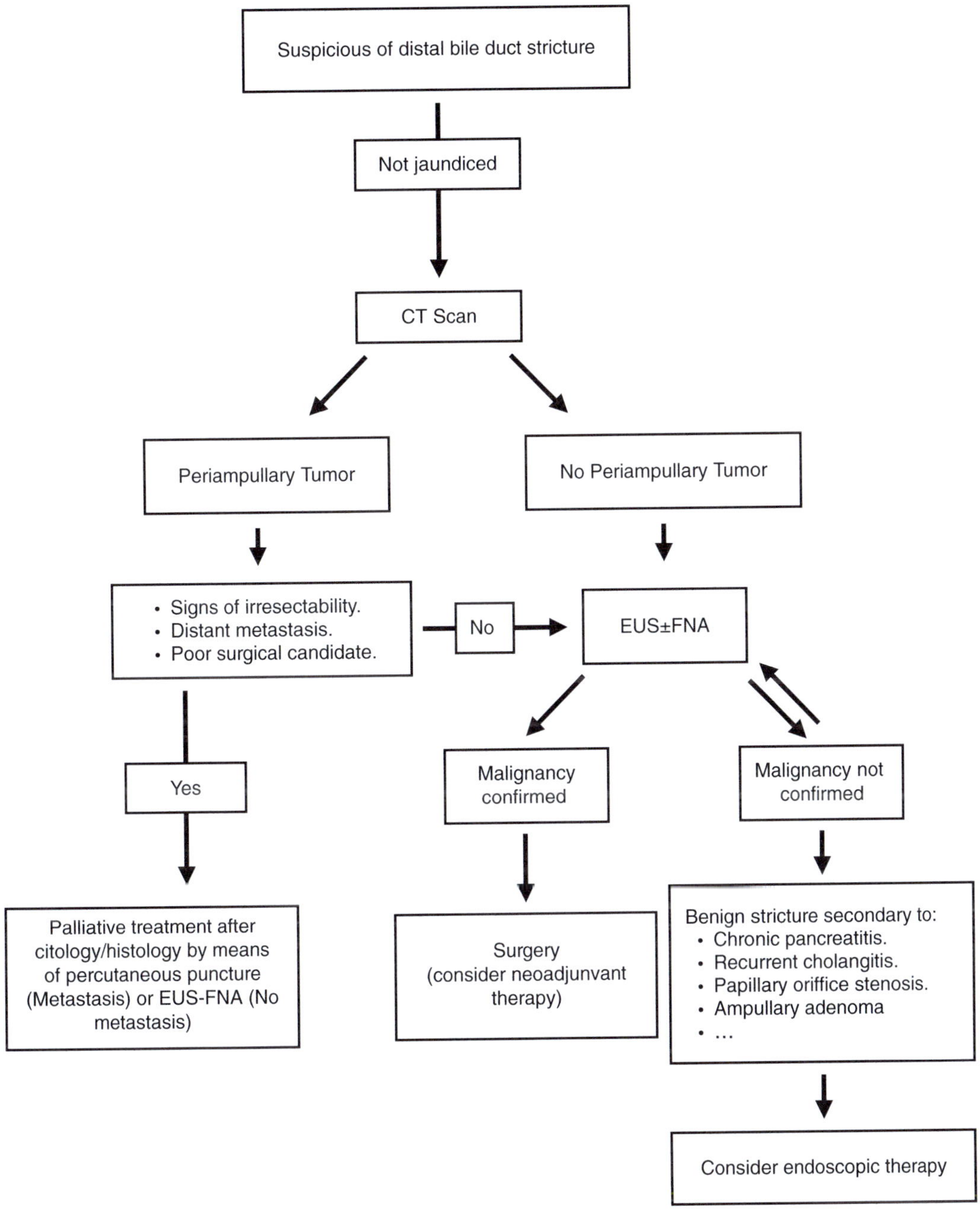
Suspicious of distal bile duct stricture
Not jaundiced
CT Scan
Periampullary Tumor
No Periampullary Tumor
• Signs of irresectability.
• Distant metastasis.
• Poor surgical candidate.
No
EUS±FNA
Yes
Malignancy confirmed
Malignancy not confirmed
Palliative treatment after citology/histology by means of percutaneous puncture (Metastasis) or EUS-FNA (No metastasis)
Surgery (consider neoadjunvant therapy)
Benign stricture secondary to:
• Chronic pancreatitis.
• Recurrent cholangitis.
• Papillary oriffice stenosis.
• Ampullary adenoma
• …
Consider endoscopic therapy

56 Hilar Strictures: Algorithm

Mario de Bellis and Elena Di Girolamo

Hilar biliary strictures (HBS) are both a diagnostic and a therapeutic challenge. Although the majority of HBS are malignant, approximately 20% of them are benign and, therefore it is mandatory to determine their etiology [1]. If a diagnosis cannot be made after a complete diagnostic work-up, HBS strictures are considered to be indeterminate [1, 2]. However, new imaging and endoscopic techniques, with ameliorated sampling methods, and broader knowledge of hepato-biliary diseases have significantly reduced the number of patients diagnosed with indeterminate HBS.

The diagnostic approach to patients with HBS strictures varies according to the presence or absence of jaundice, the location of obstruction in the intrahepatic biliary system, and evidence of a mass lesion in the liver [2]. Laboratory tests, physical examination, and acquisition of a detailed history are the initial steps of the diagnostic work-up. Elevated CA19.9 (>130 U/mL), hypoalbuminemia, leukocytosis, thrombocytosis, anorexia, weight loss, and symptoms duration have been associated with malignant HBS [3, 4]. The subsequent radiological work-up includes abdominal ultrasound, magnetic resonance imaging (MRI), and magnetic resonance cholangiopancreatography (MRCP), multidetector computed tomography (MDCT), with rapid injection of contrast media, and positron emission tomography (PET) [1, 2, 4, 5]. These imaging techniques allow us to define the level of the stricture, and the presence or absence of intrahepatic biliary dilation evaluating its severity; moreover, they are crucial for excluding the presence of intrahepatic stones and ruling out a mass lesion [1, 2, 5]. If this is identified and the subsequent staging of the patient suggests that the mass is resectable, then the patient should undergo surgery directly [1, 4, 5].

In approximately 30% of cases, a definite diagnosis is not obtained and there is a need for further investigation to rule out malignancy. Serum levels of immunoglobulin G4 should be measured in all patients with HBS, since IgG4-related diseases can mimic cholangiocarcinoma [4]. EUS+FNAB should be considered the first choice in potentially resectable patients because it avoids bile contamination. ERCP with multiple brushing is recommended in patients with indeterminate HBS, in order to obtain cytology specimens for making a diagnosis [2, 5]. FISH, Kras/p53 analysis, and flow cytometry should be used to improve the yield of brush cytology [2]. If a certain diagnosis is not made and there is still a clinical suspicion of malignancy, a repeat ERCP with cholangioscopy could obtain more tissue by means of targeted biopsies under direct cholangioscopic vision [1, 2, 4, 5]. Lastly, intraductal ultrasonography (IDUS) and confocal laser endomicroscopy

M. de Bellis (✉) · E. Di Girolamo
Division of Gastroenterology and Digestive Endoscopy, Department of Abdominal Oncology, Istituto Nazionale Tumori – IRCCS – Fondazione G. Pascale, Napoli, Italy
e-mail: m.debellis@istitutotumori.na.it

M. Mutignani et al. (eds.), *Endotherapy in Biliopancreatic Diseases: ERCP Meets EUS*,
https://doi.org/10.1007/978-3-030-42569-2_56

(CLE) could be useful to identify patients with malignant HBS [2, 5]. However, these techniques are not widely used in clinical practice.

If eventually a diagnosis of malignancy is not made, close observation and follow-up of the patients with HBS are recommended to confirm the benign etiology of HBS [1, 2, 4, 5].

The decision-making process for the diagnosis of patients with HBS can be summarized in the following algorithm (Fig. 56.1):

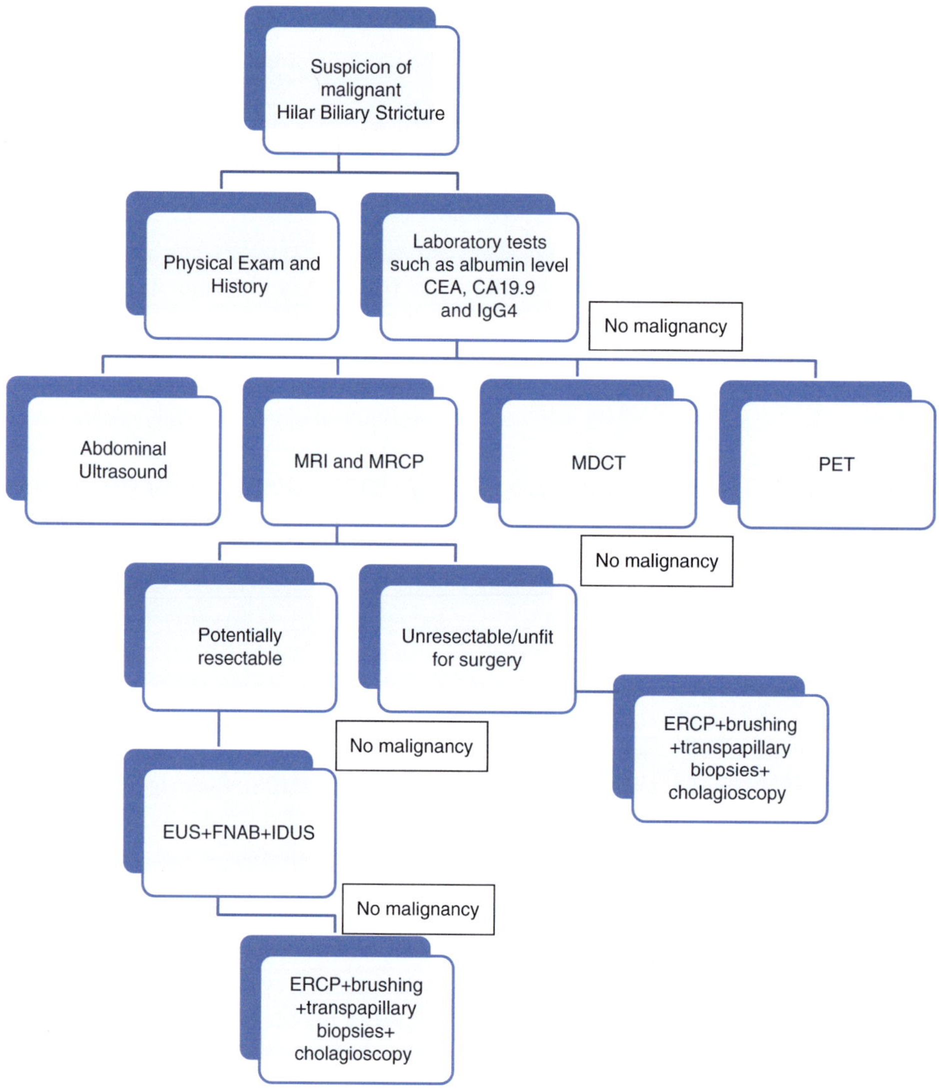

Fig. 56.1 Diagnostic work-up of patients with hilar biliary strictures

References

1. NCCN Guidelines. Version I. 2018. NCCN org. February 14, 2018.
2. Singh A, Gelrud A, Agarwal B. Biliary strictures: diagnostic considerations and approach. Gastroenterol Rep. 2015;3:22–31.
3. Thomasset SC, Saunders D, Holland A, et al. Malignant biliary strictures in patients with a normal bilirubin and/or normal liver enzymes. HPB. 2015;17:969–74.
4. Razumilava N, Gores GJ. Classification, diagnosis, and management of cholangiocarcinoma. Clin Gastroenetrol Hepatol. 2013;11:13–21.
5. Dioscoridi L, Staiano T, Carrara S, et al. Gestione multidisciplinare del colangiocarcinoma. Oncology Update. Giornale Italiano di Endoscopia Digestiva. 2016;4:19–32.

57 Diagnosis of Pancreatic Cyst: Algorithm

Stefano Francesco Crinò

Abbreviations

AP	Acute pancreatitis
BD-IPMN	Branch-duct intraductal papillary mucinous neoplasm
CE-CT	Contrast-enhanced computed tomography
CE-EUS	Contrast-enhanced endoscopic ultrasound
EUS	Endoscopic ultrasound
HGD	High-grade dysplasia
IPMN	Intraductal papillary mucinous neoplasm
MCN	Mucinous cystic neoplasm
MPD	Main pancreatic duct
MRCP	Magnetic resonance cholangiopancreatography
MRI	Magnetic resonance imaging
NET	Neuroendocrine Tumor
RP	Recurrent pancreatitis
SCA	Serous cystadenoma
SPN	Solid pseudopapillary neoplasm
TA	Tissue acquisition (fluid cytology, cyst wall fine-needle aspiration/biopsy, through-the-needle biopsy)

S. F. Crinò (✉)
Gastroenterology and Digestive Endoscopy Unit, The Pancreas Institute, University Hospital of Verona, Verona, Italy
e-mail: stefanofrancesco.crino@aovr.veneto.it

M. Mutignani et al. (eds.), *Endotherapy in Biliopancreatic Diseases: ERCP Meets EUS*, https://doi.org/10.1007/978-3-030-42569-2_57

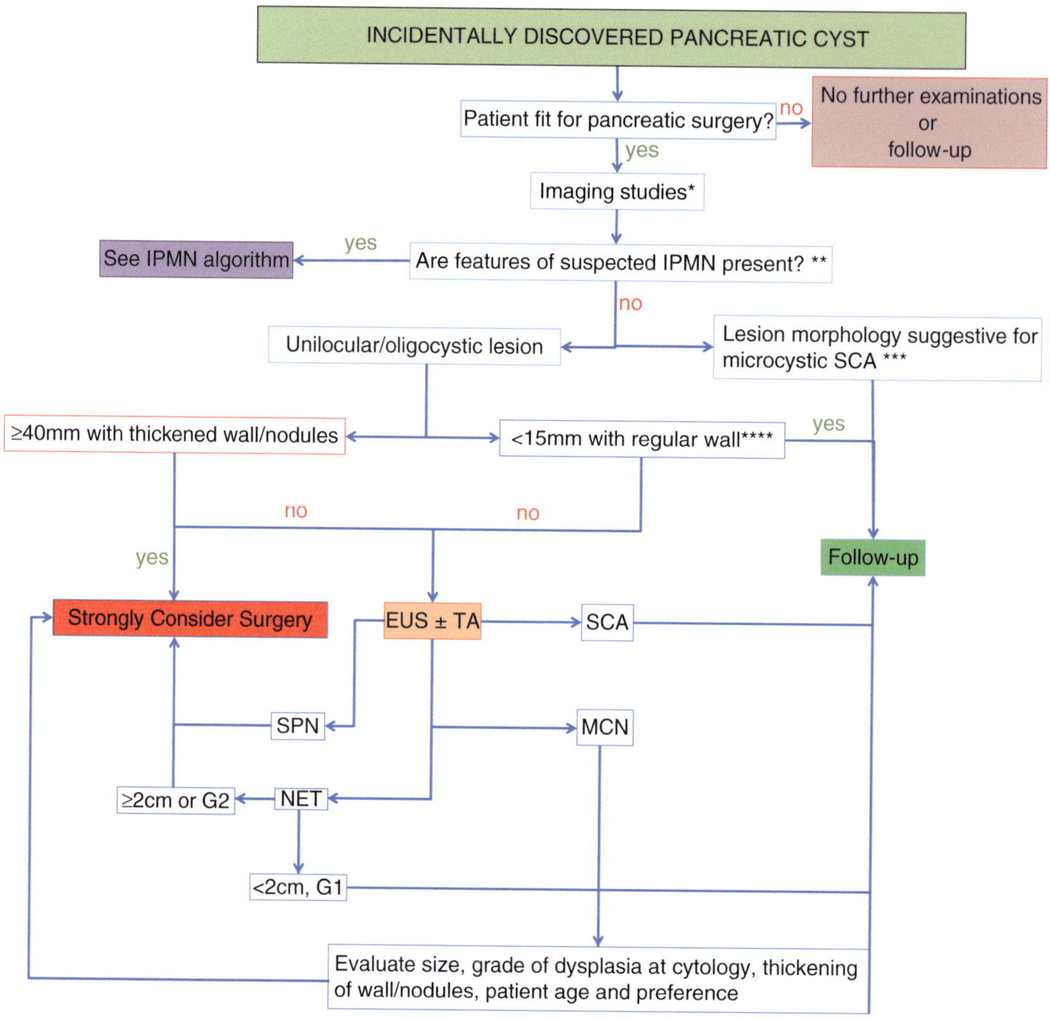

Footnotes:

∗Gadolinium-enhanced MRI with MRCP (preferred) and/or pancreatic protocol CE-CT

∗∗Communication with pancreatic ducts, multifocality, bunch of grapes morphology

∗∗∗Lobulated honeycomb shape ± central scar/calcification

∗∗∗∗Consider a first close follow-up for the risk of retention cyst in isodense pancreatic cancer

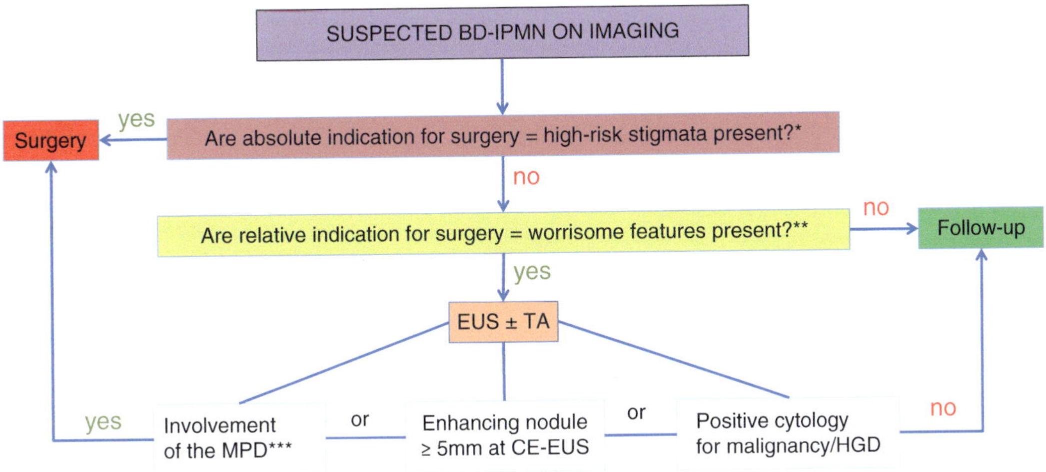

Footnotes:
∗Solid mass, enhancing mural nodule ≥5 mm, MPD ≥10 mm
∗∗Enhancing mural nodule <5 mm, MPD 5–9 mm; thickened/enhancing wall, abrupt change in caliber of MPD with distal atrophy; lymphadenopathy; new onset of diabetes mellitus; CA 19-9 ≥37 U/mL; grow rate ≥5 mm/year (or 2 years, depending on evaluated guideline); cyst size ≥30 mm (or 40 mm, depending on evaluated guideline)
∗∗∗MPD thickened wall/nodule or intraductal mucin

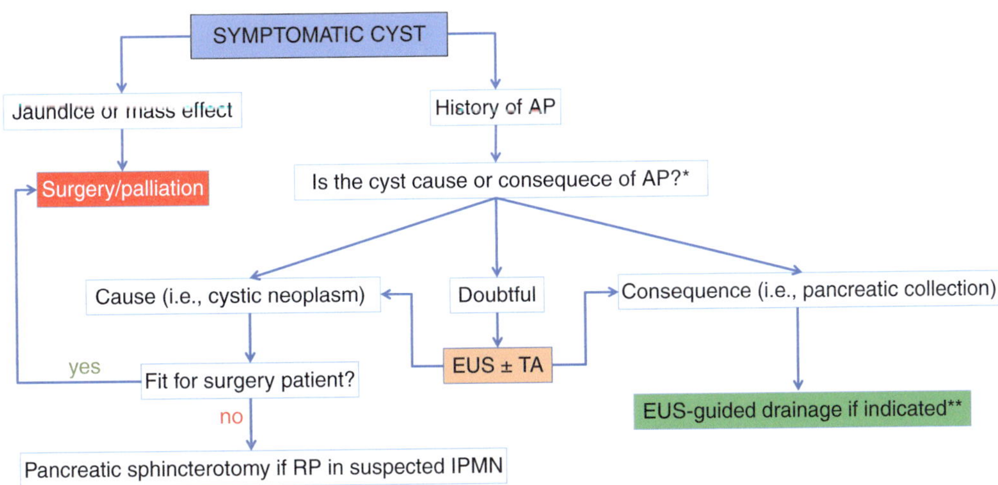

Footnotes:
∗Evaluate the relation between the presence of the cyst and the onset of pancreatitis (i.e., was the cyst already present at the time of AP?) and the cyst morphology
∗∗Symptoms (mass effect, vomiting, jaundice, abdominal pain), sign of infection, or increasing size

Bibliography

Arvanitakis M, et al. Endoscopic management of acute necrotizing pancreatitis: European Society of Gastrointestinal Endoscopy (ESGE) evidence-based multidisciplinary guidelines. Endoscopy. 2018;50(5):524–46.

Bernardoni L, et al. Preliminary experience with pancreatic sphincterotomy as treatment for intraductal papillary mucinous neoplasm-associated recurrent pancreatitis. Endosc Int Open. 2017;5(11):E1144–50.

Buscarini E, et al. Italian consensus guidelines for the diagnostic work-up and follow-up of cystic pancreatic neoplasms. Dig Liver Dis. 2014;46(6):479–93.

Sahani DV, et al. Diagnosis and management of cystic pancreatic lesions. Am J Roentgenol. 2013;2002(2):343–54.

Tanaka M, et al. Revisions of international consensus Fukuoka guidelines for the management of IPMN of the pancreas. Pancreatology. 2017;17(5):738–53.

The European Study Group on Cystic Tumours of the Pancreas. European evidence-based guidelines on pancreatic cystic neoplasms. Gut. 2018;67(5):789–804.

MIX
Papier aus verantwortungsvollen Quellen
Paper from responsible sources
FSC® C105338

If you have any concerns about our products,
you can contact us on
ProductSafety@springernature.com

In case Publisher is established outside the EU,
the EU authorized representative is:
Springer Nature Customer Service Center GmbH
Europaplatz 3, 69115 Heidelberg, Germany

Printed by Libri Plureos GmbH
in Hamburg, Germany